Clinical Pain Management

Practice and Procedures

ems can be recall

by post, please ensure t
n the Post Office; othe

6/2015

Clinical Pain Management

Practice and Procedures

2nd edition

Edited by

Harald Breivik MD DMSc FRCA
Professor, University of Oslo and Section of Anaesthesiology and Intensive Care Medicine
Rikshospitalet University Hospital
Oslo, Norway

William I Campbell MD PhD FRCA FFARCSI DPMedCARCSI
Consultant in Anaesthesia and Pain Medicine
The Ulster Hospital
Belfast, UK

Michael K Nicholas PhD
Director, ADAPT Pain Management Programme, Pain Management Research Institute
University of Sydney at Royal North Shore Hospital
Sydney, Australia

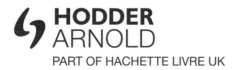

HODDER
ARNOLD
PART OF HACHETTE LIVRE UK

First published in Great Britain in 2003
This second edition published in 2008 by
Hodder Arnold, an imprint of Hodder Education,
part of Hachette Livre UK, 338 Euston Road, London NW1 3BH

http://www.hoddereducation.com

Hachette Livre UK's policy is to use papers that are natural, renewable, and recyclable products and made from
wood grown in sustainable forests. The logging and manufacturing processes are expected to conform to the
environmental regulations of the country of origin.

Whilst the advice and information in this book are believed to be true and accurate at the date of going to press,
neither the author[s] nor the publisher can accept any legal responsibility or liability for any errors or omissions
that may be made. In particular, (but without limiting the generality of the preceding disclaimer) every effort has
been made to check drug dosages; however it is still possible that errors have been missed. Furthermore, dosage
schedules are constantly being revised and new side-effects recognized. For these reasons the reader is strongly
urged to consult the drug companies' printed instructions before administering any of the drugs recommended
in this book.

British Library Cataloguing in Publication Data
A catalogue record for this book is available from the British Library

Library of Congress Cataloging-in-Publication Data
A catalog record for this book is available from the Library of Congress

ISBN 978-0-340-94009-9 (Acute Pain)
ISBN 978-0-340-94008-2 (Chronic Pain)
ISBN 978-0-340-94007-5 (Cancer Pain)
ISBN 978-0-340-94006-8 (Practice and Procedures)
ISBN 978-0-340-93992-5 (4 vol set: Acute Pain/Chronic Pain/Cancer Pain/Practice and Procedures/Web edition)

1 2 3 4 5 6 7 8 9 10

Commissioning Editor: Joanna Koster
Project Editor: Zelah Pengilley
Production Controller: Joanna Walker
Cover Design: Helen Townson

Typeset in 10 pt Minion by Macmillan India
Printed and bound in the UK by MPG Books, Bodmin, Cornwall
Text printed on FSC accredited material

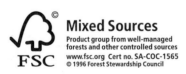

Mixed Sources
Product group from well-managed
forests and other controlled sources
www.fsc.org Cert no. SA-COC-1565
© 1996 Forest Stewardship Council

What do you think about this book? Or any other Hodder Arnold title?
Please visit our website: **www.hoddereducation.com**

Contents

Please note: The table of contents and a combined index for all four volumes in the series can be found on the Clinical Pain Management website at: www.clinicalpainmanagement.co.uk.

Contributors

Frank Andrasik PhD
Distinguished University Professor
Department of Psychology, University of West Florida
Pensacola, USA

Lars Arendt-Nielsen Prof Dr Med Sci PhD
Professor
Center for Sensory-Motor Interaction (SMI), Laboratory for
Experimental Pain Research, Aalborg University
Aalborg, Denmark

Nancy F Bandstra BSc
Doctoral Student in Clinical Psychology
Dalhousie University, Halifax, Canada

Jonathan Bannister MB ChB FRCA
Consultant in Pain Medicine and Anaesthesia
Honorary Senior Lecturer, Ninewells Hospital and Medical School
Dundee, UK

Andrew P Baranowski MD FRCA
Fellow of the Faculty of Pain Medicine of the
Royal College of Anaesthetists
Consultant in Pain Medicine
The Pain Management Centre, The National Hospital for
Neurology and Neurosurgery, University College London
Hospitals NHS Foundation Trust, London, UK

Fabrizio Benedetti MD
Professor of Physiology and Neuroscience
Department of Neuroscience and National Institute of
Neuroscience, University of Turin, Turin, Italy

David Bennett MBPhD MRCP
Wellcome Trust Clinical Scientist Fellow and Honorary Specialist
Registrar in Neurology
Wolfson Centre for Age Related Diseases, Department of
Neurology, Guy's and St Thomas' NHS Trust, London, UK

Else K Breivik Hals DDS PhD
Oral-Maxillofacial Surgeon
Section of Maxillofacial Surgery, ENT Department, Rikshospitalet
University Hospital, Oslo, Norway

Harald Breivik MD DMSc FRCA
Professor
University of Oslo, Section of Anaesthesiology and Intensive
Care Medicine, Rikshospitalet University Hospital
Oslo, Norway

William I Campbell MD PhD FRCA FFARCSI Dip Pain Med CARCSI
Consultant in Anaesthesia and Pain Medicine
The Ulster Hospital, Belfast, UK

George Chalkiadis MB BS DA (LON) FANZCA FFPMANZCA
Staff Anaesthetist and Pain Medicine Specialist, Head
Children's Pain Management Service, Royal Children's Hospital
Melbourne; and
Clinical Associate Professor
University of Melbourne, Murdoch Children's Research Institute
Department of Paediatrics, Victoria, Australia

Christine T Chambers PhD RPsych
Associate Professor of Pediatrics and Psychology
Canada Research Chair in Pain and Child Health, Dalhousie
University and IWK Health Centre, Halifax, Canada

Chetwyn CH Chan PDOT BScOT MSc PhD
Professor and Head of Department
Department of Rehabilitation Sciences, The Hong Kong
Polytechnic University, Kowloon, Hong Kong, SAR

Luana Colloca MD PhD
Research Associate
Department of Neuroscience and National Institute of
Neuroscience, University of Turin, Turin, Italy

Ron Cooper MD FFARCSI FIPP
Consultant in Anaesthesia and Pain Relief
Pain Relief Clinic, Causeway Hospital, Coleraine, UK

David Counsell MB ChB FRCA PhD
Fellow of the Faculty of Pain Medicine of the
Royal College of Anaesthetists
Consultant Anaesthetist
Department of Anaesthesia, Wrexham Maelor Hospital
Wrexham, UK

Geert Crombez PhD
Professor of Health Psychology
Department of Experimental Clinical and Health Psychology
Ghent University, Ghent, Belgium

Ben JP Crul
Professor of Pain Management
Pain Expertise Centre, Department of Anesthesiology, Radboud
University Medical Centre, Nijmegen, The Netherlands

Timothy Culbert MD
Medical Director
Integrative Medicine and Cultural Care, Children's Hospitals and
Clinics of Minnesota, Minneapolis, MN, USA

Mike Cummings MB ChB Dip Med Ac
Medical Director
British Medical Acupuncture Society, London, UK

Michele Curatolo MD PhD
Professor and Head, Division of Pain Therapy; and
Vice Chief
University Department of Anaesthesiology and Pain Therapy,
Inselspital, Bern, Switzerland

Natasha C Curran FRCA
Consultant in Pain Medicine and Anaesthesia
University College London Hospitals, London, UK

Huw TO Davies BA MA MSc PhD
Professor of Health Care Policy and Management
Social Dimensions of Health Institute, Universities of Dundee
and St Andrews, Dundee, UK

Jeroen De Jong MSc
Kinesiologist and Behavioural Therapist
Department of Rehabilitation Medicine, University Hospital
Maastricht, Maastricht, The Netherlands

Peter JD Evans MB BS FRCA DMS
Fellow of the Faculty of Pain Medicine of the
Royal College of Anaesthetists
Consultant in Pain Medicine
Pain Management Centre, Charing Cross Hospital, Imperial
College Healthcare NHS Trust, London, UK

Damien G Finniss MSc Med
Clinical Lecturer
Pain Management Research Institute, University of Sydney and
Royal North Shore Hospital, Sydney, Australia

Herta Flor PhD
Central Institute of Mental Health, Department of
Neuropsychology, Ruprecht-Karls-University of Heidelberg
Mannheim, Germany

Stefan Friedrichsdorf MD
Medical Director
Pain and Palliative Care, Children's Hospitals and Clinics of
Minnesota, Minneapolis, MN, USA

Robert J Gatchel PhD ABPP
Professor and Chair
Department of Psychology, College of Science, University of
Texas at Arlington, Arlington, TX, USA

Louis Gifford FCSP MappSc BSc
Chartered Physiotherapist
Falmouth Physiotherapy Clinic, Falmouth, UK

Ian D Goodall FRCA
Consultant
Chelsea and Westminster Healthcare NHS Foundation Trust
London, UK

Kate Grady BSc FRCA
Consultant in Pain Medicine and Anaesthesia
Department of Anaesthesia, University Hospital of South
Manchester Foundation Trust, Wythenshawe, UK

Gerbrand J Groen MD PhD
Associate Professor
Department of Anesthesiology and Pain Treatment, Utrecht
University Medical Centre, Utrecht, The Netherlands

Hilde Berner Hammer MD PhD
Consultant in Rheumatology
Department of Rheumatology, Diakonhjemmet Hospital
Oslo, Norway

Peter HTG Heuts MD PhD
Consultant in Rehabilitation Medicine
Rehabilitation Center Leijpark, Tilburg, The Netherlands

Henrik Högström MD
Senior Consultant, Pain Unit
Department of Anesthesiology, Aker University Hospital
Oslo, Norway

David Hill MD FCARCSI DIP PAIN MED RCSI
Consultant in Anaesthesia and Pain Medicine
Ulster Hospital; and
Honorary Senior Lecturer
Queen's University, Belfast, UK

Richard F Howard BSc MB ChB FRCA
Fellow of the Faculty of Pain Medicine of the
Royal College of Anaesthetists
Consultant and Clinical Director
Department of Anaesthesia, Great Ormond Street Hospital and
the Institute of Child Health, London, UK

Aage Indahl MD DMSc
Hospital for Rehabilitation, Rikshospitalet Medical Center
Stavern, Norway

Humaira Jamal PhD MRCP
Consultant in Palliative Medicine
Mount Vernon and Harefield Hospitals, Northwood, UK

Marie Johnston BSc PhD FBPsS FRSE FMedSci AcSS
Professor in Health Psychology
College of Life Sciences and Medicine, University of Aberdeen
Aberdeen, UK

Ellen Jørum MD PhD
Professor
Rikshospitalet University Hospital
Oslo, Norway

Jan Willem Kallewaard MD
Consultant Anesthetist, Specialist in Pain
Alysis Zorggroep, Arnhem, The Netherlands

Ulf E Kongsgaard MD PhD
Professor
The Norwegian Radium Hospital, Division of Anaesthesiology
and Intensive Care Medicine, Rikshospitalet University
Hospital; and Medical Faculty, University of Oslo, Oslo, Norway

Leora Kuttner PhD Reg Psych
Clinical Professor
Department of Paediatrics, University of British Columbia and
BC Children's Hospital, Vancouver, Canada

Gunnvald Kvarstein MD PhD
Medical Director
Section of Pain Management, Rikshospitalet University Hospital
Oslo, Norway

Michael Lee MBBS FRCA
MRC Clinical Research Training Fellow
Oxford Centre for Functional Magnetic Resonance Imaging of
the Brain, FMRIB Centre, UK

Steven J Linton
Professor of Clinical Psychology
Sweden Center for Health and Medical Psychology, Department
of Behavioral, Social and Legal Sciences—Psychology
Örebro University, Örebro, Sweden; and
Pain Management Research Institute, University of Sydney
Sydney, Australia

Stephan Locher MD
University Department of Anaesthesiology and Pain Therapy
Inselspital, Bern, Switzerland

Pamela E Macintyre BMedSc MBBS MHA FANZCA FFPMANZCA
Director
Acute Pain Service, Department of Anaesthesia, Pain Medicine
and Hyperbaric Medicine, Royal Adelaide Hospital and
University of Adelaide, Adelaide, Australia

William A Macrae MB ChB FRCA
Consultant in Pain Medicine
Honorary Senior Lecturer, Ninewells Hospital and Medical School
Dundee, UK

Leif Måwe MD
Section of Pain Management, Rikshospitalet University Hospital
Oslo, Norway

Malvern May MRCP FRCA
Fellow of the Faculty of Pain Medicine of the
Royal College of Anaesthetists
Consultant in Pain Medicine and Anaesthesia
Basildon and Thurrock University Hospitals, Essex, UK

Lance M McCracken PhD
Consultant Clinical Psychologist and Clinical Lead
Bath Centre for Pain Services, Royal National Hospital for
Rheumatic Diseases NHS Foundation Trust; and
Senior Visiting Fellow
Department of Psychology, University of Bath, Bath, UK

Christine Miaskowski RN PhD FAAN
Professor and Associate Dean
Department of Physiological Nursing, University of California
San Francisco, CA, USA; and
Consultant
The Centre for Shared Decision Making and Nursing Research
Rikshospitalet University Hospital, Oslo, Norway

Vanessa Morris MD FRCP
Consultant Rheumatologist
Centre for Rheumatology, University College Hospital London
and University College London, London, UK

Paul R Nandi FRCP FRCA
Consultant in Neuroanaesthesia and Pain Medicine
University College London Hospitals Pain Management Centre
The National Hospital for Neurology and Neurosurgery
London, UK

Timothy P Nash MBBS DObstRCOG FRCA
Fellow of the Faculty of Pain Medicine of the
Royal College of Anaesthetists
Honorary Senior Lecturer
Pain Research Institute, Clinical Sciences Centre, University
Hospital Aintree, University of Liverpool, UK

Toby Newton-John BA(Hons) MPsych(Clin) PhD
Clinical Psychologist and Program Director
Innervate Pain Management
Broadmeadow; and
Honorary Associate, Faculty of Medicine
University of Sydney, NSW, Australia

Michael K Nicholas PhD
Director
ADAPT Pain Management Programme, Pain Management
Research Institute, University of Sydney at Royal North Shore
Hospital, St Leonards, NSW, Australia

Rachael Powell BSc(Hons) PhD MSc
RCUK Fellow
School of Life and Health Sciences, Aston University
Birmingham, UK

Alison E Powell MA PhD
Centre for Public Policy and Management, University of
St Andrews, St Andrews, UK

Ivan N Ramos-Galvez FRCA
Consultant in Pain Medicine
Royal Berkshire NHS Foundation Trust, Berkshire, UK

Jon Raphael MSc MD FRCA
Professor
Faculty of Health, Birmingham City University, Edgbaston
Birmingham, UK

Andrew SC Rice MB BS MD FRCA
Reader in Pain Research
Department of Anaesthetics, Pain Medicine and Intensive Care
Imperial College London; and
Honorary Consultant in Pain Medicine
Chelsea and Westminster Hospital Foundation NHS Trust
London, UK

Jonathan Richardson MD FRCP FRCA FIPP
Consultant Anaesthetist
Specialist in Pain, Bradford Royal Infirmary, Pain Clinic
Bradford, UK

Steve Robson MCSP BSc(Hons)
Chartered Physiotherapist
Aspen Physiotherapy Clinic, Prudhoe, UK

Tone Rustoen RN PhD
Professor and Senior Researcher
The Centre for Shared Decision Making and Nursing Research
Rikshospitalet University Hospital and Oslo University College
Oslo, Norway

Michael Shipley MA MD FRCP
Consultant Rheumatologist
Centre for Rheumatology, University College Hospital London
and University College London, London, UK

Lesley A Smith BSc PhD
Senior Research Fellow
School of Health and Social Care, Oxford Brookes University
Oxford, UK

David Spiegel MD
Willson Professor in the School of Medicine, Associate Chair
Department of Psychiatry and Behavioral Sciences, Stanford
University, CA, USA

Audun Stubhaug MD DMSc
Professor
Oslo University, Department of Anaesthesiology and Intensive
Care Medicine, Rikshospitalet University Hospital
Oslo, Norway

Brian R Theodore MS
PhD Candidate, Department of Psychology, College of Science
University of Texas at Arlington, Arlington, TX, USA

Simon Thomson MBBS FRCA FIPP
Fellow of the Faculty of Pain Medicine of the
Royal College of Anaesthetists
Consultant in Pain Medicine and Anaesthesia
Basildon and Thurrock University Hospitals, London, UK

Irene Tracey PhD
Nuffield Professor of Anaesthetic Science, Director
Oxford Centre for Functional Magnetic Resonance Imaging of
the Brain, FMRIB Centre, Oxford University Department of
Clinical Neurology and Nuffield Department Anaesthetics, John
Radcliffe Hospital, Oxford, UK

Ivan F Trotman MBBS MD FRCP
Consultant in Palliative Medicine
Mount Vernon Hospital, Northwood, UK

Johannes Van Der Merwe BA Hons Clin Psych MA Clin Psych DTh Dip Clin Hyp
Consultant Clinical Psychologist and Unit Manager
The Real Health Institute, London, UK

Maarten Van Kleef MD PhD
Professor of Anesthesiology
Department of Anaesthesiology and Pain Management
University Hospital of Maastricht, Maastricht, The Netherlands

Jan HM Van Zundert MD PhD
Head of Multidisciplinary Pain Center
Ziekenhuis Oost-Limburg, Genk, Belgium; and University Hospital
of Maastricht, Maastricht, The Netherlands

Jeanine A Verbunt MD PhD
Rehabilitation Foundation Limburg, Hoensbroek, The Netherlands

Johan WS Vlaeyen PhD
Professor of Behavioural Medicine
Research Center for Health Psychology, Department of
Psychology, University of Leuven, Leuven, Belgium; and
Department of Clinical Psychological Science, University of
Maastricht, Maastricht, The Netherlands

Kevin E Vowles PhD
Research Fellow and Clinical Psychologist
Centre for Pain Research, School for Health, University of
Bath; and Bath Centre for Pain Services, Royal National Hospital
for Rheumatic Diseases, Bath, UK

Mads U Werner MD DMSc
Associate Professor
Cancer Pain Service, Department of Oncology, University
Hospital, Lund, Sweden

Peter R Wilson MB BS PhD
Professor of Pain Medicine, Mayo Clinic College of Medicine
Rochester, MN, USA

Amanda C de C Williams PhD CPsychol
Reader in Clinical Health Psychology
University College London; and
Consultant Clinical Psychologist
National Hospital for Neurology and Neurosurgery
London, UK

Harriët M Wittink PhD MS PT
Professor, Research Group Lifestyle and Health
University of Applied Sciences Utrecht, Utrecht, The Netherlands

Series preface

Since the successful first edition of *Clinical Pain Management* was published in 2002, the evidence base in many areas of pain medicine has changed substantially, thus creating the need for this second edition. We have retained the central ethos of the first volume in that we have continued to provide comprehensive coverage of pain medicine, with the text geared predominantly to the requirements of those training and practicing in pain medicine and related specialties. The emphasis continues to be on delivering this coverage in a format that is easily accessed and digested by the busy clinician in practice.

As before, *Clinical Pain Management* comprises four volumes. The first three cover the main disciplines of acute, chronic, and cancer pain management, and the fourth volume covers the practical aspects of clinical practice and research. The four volumes can be used independently, while together they give readers all they need to know to deliver a successful pain management service.

Of the 161 chapters in the four volumes, almost a third are brand new to this edition while the chapters that have been retained have been completely revised, in many cases under new authorship. This degree of change reflects ongoing progress in this broad field, where research and development provide a rapidly evolving evidence base. The international flavor of *Clinical Pain Management* remains an important feature, and perusal of the contributor pages will reveal that authors and editors are drawn from a total of 16 countries.

A particularly popular aspect of the first edition was the practice of including a system of simple evidence scoring in most of the chapters. This enables the reader to understand quickly the strength of evidence which supports a particular therapeutic statement or recommendation. This has been retained for the first three volumes, where appropriate. We have, however, improved the system used for scoring evidence from a three point scale used in the first edition and adopted the five point Bandolier system which is in widespread use and will be instantly familiar to many readers (www.jr2.ox.ac.uk/bandolier/band6/b6-5.html).

We have also retained the practice of asking authors to highlight the key references in each chapter. Following feedback from our readers we have added two new features for this edition: first, there are key learning points at the head of each chapter summarizing the most salient points within the chapter; and second, the series is accompanied by a companion website with downloadable figures.

This project would not have been possible without the hard work and commitment of the chapter authors and we are deeply indebted to all of them for their contributions. The volume editors have done a sterling job in diligently editing a large number of chapters, and to them we are also most grateful. Any project of this magnitude would be impossible without substantial support from the publishers – in particular we would like to acknowledge our debt to Jo Koster and Zelah Pengilley at Hodder. They have delivered the project on a tight deadline and ensured that a large number of authors and editors were kept gently, but firmly, "on track."

Andrew SC Rice, Douglas Justins, Toby Newton-John,
Richard F Howard, Christine A Miaskowski
London, Newcastle, and San Francisco

I would also like to add my personal thanks to the Series Editors who have given their time generously and made invaluable contributions through the whole editorial process from the very outset of discussions regarding a second edition in deciding upon the content of each volume and in selecting Volume Editors. More recently, they have provided an important second view in the consideration of all submitted chapters, not to mention stepping in and assisting with first edits where needed. The timely completion of the second edition would not have been possible without this invaluable input.

Andrew SC Rice
Lead Editor

Introduction to Clinical Pain Management: Practice and Procedures

Despite extensive research into the origins and mechanisms of acute and chronic pain, its management remains a challenge to all involved in health care. This is partly due to our incomplete knowledge of the subject and the plasticity of the mechanisms involved. The need to educate patients and develop therapeutic means that are effective but are well tolerated, are additional problems encountered in daily practice. Each chapter in *Practice and Procedures* can stand alone or work to complement the chapters in preceding volumes – *Acute Pain*, *Chronic Pain,* and *Cancer Pain*. Authors have been chosen as having a special interest and expertise in the practical applications they describe. They have been invited to present their work in a style that is not only comprehensive but also easy to read, with summaries of key points and evidence-based references. The editors and authors have endeavored to provide the reader with a contemporary text that utilizes our latest knowledge on the management of pain to maximize a favorable outcome.

Practice and Procedures covers various forms of pain assessment in addition to a wide range of therapies that can be provided by a diverse range of healthcare disciplines, including practical procedures and applications in the management of acute, chronic, and cancer pain. The volume concludes with valuable chapters about clinical research methods and writing medicolegal reports.

We trust that this volume will be of value to all healthcare workers, regardless of their discipline, and that it will help them to keep abreast of developments and challenges in the maturing discipline of applied pain medicine.

Harald Breivik, William I Campbell, and Michael K Nicholas
Oslo, Belfast, and Sydney

How to use this book

SPECIAL FEATURES

The four volumes of *Clinical Pain Management* incorporate the following special features to aid the readers' understanding and navigation of the text.

Key learning points

Each chapter opens with a set of key learning points which provide readers with an overview of the most salient points within the chapter.

Cross-references

Throughout the chapters in this volume you will find cross-references to chapters in other volumes in the *Clinical Pain Management* series. Each cross-reference will indicate the volume in which the chapter referred to is to be found.

Evidence scoring

In chapters where recommendations for surgical, medical, psychological, and complementary treatment and diagnostic tests are presented, the quality of evidence supporting authors' statements relating to clinical interventions, or the papers themselves, are graded following the Oxford Bandolier system by insertion of the following symbols into the text:

[I]   Strong evidence from at least one published systematic review of multiple well-designed randomized controlled trials
[II]   Strong evidence from at least one published properly designed randomized controlled trial of appropriate size and in an appropriate clinical setting
[III]   Evidence from published well-designed trials without randomization, single group pre-post, cohort, time series, or matched case-controlled studies
[IV]   Evidence from well-designed non-experimental studies from more than one center or research group
[V]   Opinions of respected authorities, based on clinical evidence, descriptive studies or reports of expert consensus committees.

Oxford Bandolier system used by kind permission of Bandolier: www.jr2.ox.ac.uk/Bandolier

Where no grade is inserted, the quality of supporting evidence, if any exists, is of low grade only (e.g. case reports, clinical experience, etc).

Other textbooks devoted to the subject of pain include a tremendous amount of anecdotal and personal recommendations, and it is often difficult to distinguish these from those with an established evidence base. This text is thus unique in allowing the reader the opportunity to do this with confidence.

Reference annotation

The reference lists are annotated with asterisks, where appropriate, to guide readers to key primary papers, major review articles (which contain extensive reference lists), and clinical guidelines. We hope that this feature will render extensive lists of references more useful to the reader and will help to encourage self-directed learning among both trainees and practicing physicians.

A NOTE ON DRUG NAMES

The authors have used the international nonproprietary name (INN) for drugs where possible. If the INN name differs from the US or UK name, authors have used the INN name followed by the US and/or UK name in brackets on first use within a chapter.

Abbreviations

5-HT	5-hydroxytryptamine	CHEOPS	Children's Hospital of Eastern Ontario Pain Scale
AC	acromioclavicular	CIDP	chronic inflammatory demyelinating polyradiculoneuropathy
ACC	anterior cingulate cortex		
ACMP	Access to Controlled Medicines Program	CK	creatine kinase
ACR	American College of Rheumatology	CLBP	chronic low back pain
ACT	acceptance and commitment therapy	CMT	Charcot–Marie–Tooth
AD	Alzheimer's disease	CNS	central nervous system
ADA	Americans with Disabilities Act	COMT	catechol-O-methyltransferase
AHCPR	Agency for Health Care Policy and Research	CONSORT	Consolidated Standard of Reporting Trials
AIDS	acquired immunodeficiency syndrome	COPM	Canadian Occupational Performance Measure
aINS	anterior insula		
ALAT	alanine aminotransferase	COX	cyclooxgenase
ALP	alkaline phosphatase	COX-2	cyclooxygenase-2
ANA	antinuclear antibody	CPG	clinical practice guidelines
ANCA	antineutrophil cytoplasmic antibody	CPNB	continuous peripheral nerve blockade
ANS	autonomic nervous system	CPS	chronic pain service
anti-CCP	anti-cyclic citrullinated protein	CPVI	Chronic Pain Values Inventory
AP	anteroposterior	CQI	continuous quality improvement
APS	American Pain Society; or acute pain service	CRP	C-reactive protein
		CRPS	complex regional pain syndrome
APTT	activated partial thromboplastin time	CSCI	continuous subcutaneous infusion
ASA	American Society of Anesthesiologists	CSF	cerebrospinal fluid
ASAT	aspartate aminotransferase	CSQ	Coping Strategies Questionnaire
ASIS	anterior superior iliac spine	CT	computed tomography
AUC	area under the curve	CUA	cost-utility analysis
BAPQ	Bath Adolescent Pain Questionnaire	DA	dopamine
BDI	Beck Depression Inventory	DAPOS	Depression, Anxiety, and Positive Outlook Scale
BNF	British National Formulary		
BOLD	blood oxygen level dependent	DASS	Depression, Anxiety and Stress Scale
BP	blood pressure	DESS	Échelle Douleur Enfant San Salvadour
BPI	Brief Pain Inventory	DLPFC	dorsolateral prefrontal cortex
		DNIC	diffuse noxious inhibitory control
CARF	Commission on Accreditation of Rehabilitation Facilities	DRG	dorsal root ganglion
		DSM	Diagnostic and Statistical Manual of Mental Disorders
CBF	cerebral blood flow		
CBT	cognitive-behavioral therapy	DTI	diffusion tensor imaging
CCBT	contextual cognitive-behavioral therapy		
CCK	cholecystokinin	ECG	electrocardiogram
CCP	content, context, and process	EDA	electrodermal activity
CEO	Chief Executive Officer	EDTA	ethylenediaminetetraacetic acid
CGH	cervicogenic headache	EEG	electroencephalography
CGRP	calcitonin gene-related peptide	ELISA	enzyme-linked immunosorbent assay

EMG	electromyogram	IPA	Impact on Participation and Autonomy
EOP	external occipital protuberance	IPG	abdominal implantable pulse generator
ERP	early receptor potential	IQ	intelligence quotient
ES	epidural space	IRB	institutional review board
ESI	epidural steroid injection	ITS	iontophoretic transdermal system
ESR	erythrocyte sedimentation rate	ITT	intention to treat
		i.v.	intravenous
FABQ	Fear-Avoidance Beliefs Questionnaire	i.v. PCA	intravenous patient-controlled opioid analgesia
FAS	Functional Activity Scale		
FBSS	failed back surgery syndrome		
FBT	fentanyl buccal tablets	JCAHO	Joint Commission on Accreditation of Healthcare Organizations
FDI	Functional Disability Inventory		
FEV	forced expiratory volume		
FLACC	Face, Legs, Arms, Cry, Consolability	LA	local anesthesia
fMRI	functional magnetic resonance imaging	LAAJ	lateral atlantoaxial joint
FPS	Faces Pain Scale	LBP	low back pain
FPS-R	Faces Pain Scale-Revised	LC	locus coeruleus
FT4	free thyroxine	LED	light-emitting diode
FVC	forced vital capacity	LFCN	lateral femoral cutaneous nerve
		LMWH	low molecular weight heparin
gammaGT	γ-glutamyl transferase	LOC	locus of control
GAN	greater auricular nerve	LOCF	last observation carried forward
GCP	Good Clinical Practice	LON	lesser occipital nerve
GI	gastrointestinal	LORT	technique of loss of resistance
GMP	good manufacturing practice	LP	lumbar puncture
GON	greater occipital nerve	LTP	long-term potentiation
HA	hyaluronic acid	M3G	morphine-3-glucuronide
HIV	human immunodeficiency virus	M6G	morphine-6-glucuronide
HIZ	high intensity zones	MAAS	Mindful Attention Awareness Scale
HLA	human leukocyte antigen	MB	medial branch
HMO	health maintenance organization	MCP	metacarpophalangeal
HPA	hypothalamic–pituitary–adrenal	MCTD	mixed connective tissue disease
HR	hazard ratio	MD	difference in means
HRV	heart rate variability	MDT	multidisciplinary teams
HSAN	hereditary sensory autonomic neuropathy	MEAC	minimum effective analgesic concentration
Hb	hemoglobin		
		MEC	minimum effective concentration
IASP	International Association for the Study of Pain	MEG	magnetoencephalography
		MHC	major histocompatibility complex
IBS	irritable bowel syndrome	mPFC	medial prefrontal cortex
ICD	International Classification of Diseases	MPI	multidimensional pain inventory
ICF	International Classification of Functioning, Disability and Health	MPO	myeloperoxidase
		MPQ	McGill Pain Questionnaire
IDET	intradiscal electrothermal therapy	MR	magnetic resonance
IDTA	intradiscal thermal annuloplasty	MRI	magnetic resonance imaging
IEC	independent ethics committee	MRS	magnetic resonance spectroscopy
IFN-γ	interferon-gamma	MST	morphine sulfate tablet
IHN	ilio-hypogastric nerve	mTh	medial thalamus
IIN	ilio-inguinal nerve		
IL-2	interleukin-2	NAA	N-acetyl aspartate
IL-6	interleukin 6	NACs	national advisory committees
i.m.	intramuscular	NCA	nurse-controlled analgesia
IMMPACT	Iniative on Methods, Measurement, and Pain Assessment	NCCPC	Non-Communicating Children's Pain Checklist
INCB	International Narcotic Control Board	NE	noradrenaline
INR	international normalized ratio	NFCS	Neonatal Facial Coding System

NGC	nucleus reticularis gigantocellularis
NH	natural history
NHMRC	National Health and Medical Research Council
NHS	National Health Service
NICE	National Institute for Health and Clinical Excellence
NIH	National Institutes of Health
NMDA	N-methyl-D-aspartic acid
NNH	number needed to harm
NNT	number needed to treat
NPY	neuropeptide Y
NRD	nucleus reticularis dorsalis
NRS	numerical rating scale
NSAID	nonsteroidal anti-inflammatory drug
OA	osteoarthritis
OBT	operant behavioral therapy
ODI	Oswestry Disability Index
OR	odds ratio
OrbF	orbitofrontal cortex
OTC	over the counter
OTFC	oral transmucosal fentanyl citrate
PACU	Post Anesthesia Care Unit
PAD	peptidylarginine deiminase
PAG	periaqueductal gray
PAR	pain relief scale
PASS	Pain Anxiety Symptoms Scale
PBCL	Procedure Behavior Check List
PBRS-R	Procedure Behavioral Rating Scale-Revised
PCA	patient-controlled analgesia
PCC	percutaneous cervical cordotomy
PCEA	patient-controlled epidural analgesia
PCINA	patient-controlled intranasal analgesia
PCQ	Pain Coping Questionnaire
PCS-C	Pain Catastrophizing Scale for Children
PCTS	patient-controlled transdermal system
PDA	personal digital assistants
PDPH	postdural puncture headache
PET	positron emission tomography
PFC	prefrontal cortices
PGIC	Patients Global Impression of Change
PGP	protein gene product
PHN	postherpetic neuralgia
PHODA	Photograph Series of Daily Activities
PID	pain intensity difference
PIPP	Premature Infant Pain Profile
PNS	peripheral nerve stimulator
POMS	Profile of Mood States
PONV	postoperative nausea and vomiting
POQ	Patient Outcome Questionnaire
POQ-VA	Pain Outcome Questionnaire-VA
PP	per protocol
PPG	photoplethysmography
PPI	present pain intensity; or proton pump inhibitor

PPP	Pediatric Pain Profile
PPPM	Parents' Postoperative Pain Measure
PPQ	Pediatric Pain Questionnaire
PR3	proteinase 3
PRF	pulsed radiofrequency
PRI	pain rating index
PSIS	posterior superior iliac spine
PTSD	posttraumatic stress disorder
QALY	quality-adjusted life years
QI	quality improvement
QRC	qualified rehabilitation counselor
QST	quantitative sensory testing
QoL	quality of life
RA	rheumatoid arthritis
rACC	rostral anterior cingulate cortex
RCT	randomized controlled trial
RD	risk difference
RF	radiofrequency; or rheumatoid factor
ROM	range of motion
RR	risk ratio
RSD	reflex sympathetic dystrophy
RVM	rostral ventromedial medulla
SAA	serum amyloid A
SCM	sterno-cleidomastoid
SCS	spinal cord stimulation
SDT	signal detection theory
SEP	somatosensory-evoked potential
SF-36	Short-Form 36
SF-MPQ	Short-Form McGill Pain Questionnaire
SLE	systemic lupus erythematosus
SLR	straight leg raise
SMD	standardized mean difference
SMK	Sluijter–Metha
SMP	sympathetically maintained pain
SNAG	sustained natural apophyseal glides
SNL	superior nuchal line
SNS	sympathetic nervous system
SOPA	Survey of Pain Attitudes
SPC	superior parietal cortex
SPID	summed pain intensity difference
SpO_2	oxygen saturation
SPTLC1	serine palmitoyl transferase long chain base subunit 1
SS	spinal stenosis
SSNRI	specific serotonin- and noradrenaline-reuptake inhibitors
SSRI	specific serotonin-reuptake inhibitors
STAI	State Trait Anxiety Inventory
TCA	tricyclic antidepressants
TENS	transcutaneous electrical nerve stimulation
THA	triamcinolone hexacetonide
TM	trapezius muscles

TMD	temporomandibular pain and dysfunction	VCUG	voiding cystourethrogram
TNFα	tumor necrosis factor-alpha	VIP	vasoactive intestinal peptide
TON	third occipital nerve	VRS	verbal rating scale
TOTPAR	total pain relief		
TSH	thyroid-stimulating hormone	WAD	whiplash-associated disorder
TSK	Tampa Scale for Kinesiophobia	WHO	World Health Organization
		WMA	World Medical Association
US	ultrasound	WMD	weighted mean difference
		WOMAC	Western Ontario and MacMaster
VA	Veterans Administration		universities
VAS	visual analog scale		

PART I

PRINCIPLES OF MEASUREMENT AND DIAGNOSIS

History-taking and examination of the patient with chronic pain

PAUL R NANDI AND TOBY NEWTON-JOHN

KEY LEARNING POINTS

- The initial medical interview should aim to establish rapport as well as obtain information.
- Case note paper with printed headings may assist in the structured recording of information.
- Behaviors are valuable physical signs in the chronic pain patient, but over-reaction does not mean that pain is psychogenic.

- The pain psychology interview should ideally gather data, as well as begin to introduce treatment concepts.
- Explaining the purpose of the assessment at the outset can allay fears or correct misunderstandings.
- The use of self-report assessment tools is a vital part of the assessment process, but not a substitute for careful clinical evaluation.

MEDICAL ASSESSMENT

Chronic pain patients are often seen as "difficult." This perception should be considered in context. Chronic pain sufferers may feel that their symptoms are trivialized or frankly disbelieved by doctors, and present to a pain specialist for the first time holding this view. By definition, these patients will have had their pain for at least three months, and in practice often considerably longer. The factors contributing to this include delays between referral from primary care to diagnostic specialists, waiting for investigations and the results of these, and in some situations a long wait for the pain clinic consultation itself.

During this period, patients often experience a variety of frustrations. They may see a number of clinicians and undergo tests which they expect to reveal the nature of their problem, but ultimately give no clear answers and they may even be given differing diagnoses by different doctors, furthering a sense of mistrust in clinicians. They may receive numerous unsuccessful treatments. Over the same period, their employment may come under threat or be lost, their recreations may be curtailed, their relationships suffer. Their clinicians may imply, or even directly state, that there is nothing wrong with them. In a recent study of patients with chronic back pain consulting specialists, it was found that patients valued explanation, information, reassurance, discussion of psychosocial issues, and management options, and (perhaps above all) being taken seriously.[1]

This chapter is not intended to provide a comprehensive guide to history-taking and examination in the chronic pain patient, several aspects of which may be found in the relevant chapters on clinical situations (see Chapter 9, Chronic pain, impairment, and disability; Chapter 10, The psychological assessment of pain in patients with chronic pain; Chapter 14, Outcome measurement in chronic pain in the *Chronic Pain* volume of this series; and Chapter 3, Selecting and applying pain measures); nor is it intended to substitute for useful current texts on general clinical history-taking and examination to which the interested reader is referred.[2, 3, 4] We will initially consider aspects of history-taking and examination generally applicable in the chronic pain patient, proposing a structure for the initial clinical interview and physical examination. We will focus on specific aspects of the clinical assessment in two important groups – nonspecific musculoskeletal pain and pain in disorders of the nervous system. Finally, we will explore the pain management psychologist's approach to the clinical interview.

Obtaining a clear medical history and performing a physical examination are traditional clinical skills with the primary purpose of establishing diagnosis with a view to a rational basis for treatment. Advances in medical technology have challenged the importance of these traditional skills,[5] but in recent years there has been a growing appreciation that the clinician's first encounter with a patient should seek more than diagnosis. It can lay the foundations of a good doctor–patient relationship and impart, as well as receive, information. This has been referred to as the three-function model[6] and might be seen as particularly appropriate in the context of chronic pain assessment; frequently, by the time a patient is referred to a pain clinic, the primary diagnosis, or diagnoses, will be clear. However, psychosocial issues are almost invariably important, and this is reflected in the coauthorship of a medical doctor and a clinical psychologist in the writing of this chapter.

Numerous questionnaires have been devised as tools to evaluate a wide range of sensory and affective elements of pain, as well as associated factors, such as physical disability and erroneous beliefs about pain causation. Some of these will be referred to later in this chapter; the subject is considered in greater depth in Chapter 10, The psychological assessment of pain in patients with chronic pain; Chapter 13, Psychological effects of chronic pain: an overview; and Chapter 14, Outcome measurement in chronic pain in the *Chronic Pain* volume in this series.

PHYSICIAN–PATIENT INTERVIEW

The patient attending a pain clinic consultation for the first time may have little idea what to expect from the service (by contrast, for example, with an appointment with a general physician). The clinician should be aware of this and it is often helpful at some point to ask the patient what his or her expectations are, concerning the assessment process as well as treatment, as this varies widely between individuals. Some expect a diagnosis (or a test that will lead to diagnosis); some just want their pain relieved. Some may have unrealistic expectations of what is achievable and it is as well for the clinician to be alerted to this early on.

Patients vary greatly in their ability to give a fluent, relevant, and thorough account of their symptoms. Some are quiet and unforthcoming, others garrulous, some distressed or angry. The clinician's interviewing style needs to be adaptable and it is important for the clinician to be concerned, engaged, and calm. Simple courtesies should not be overlooked. The clinician should greet the patient formally; unless invited to do so, calling the patient by their first name is often regarded as inappropriately familiar by some patients.[7]

When starting to take a history, allow the patient to tell their story in their own words as far as possible, rather than continually interrupting with specific or leading questions. Later in the interview, garrulous patients may need to be "brought back on track" with some direct questioning, and unforthcoming patients may need gentle leading questions, but any guiding questions should be brief, clear, and initially as open as possible rather than suggesting a desired answer. This approach (the patient-centered interviewing technique)[8, 9] allows the patient to place emphasis on those aspects of the problem that (s)he considers most important, and to feel "listened to." This helps to build a rapport between patient and clinician and to empower the patient; it may also elicit more information than is obtained by enforcing a structure on the patient's account of events.[10]

In contrast to the patient's unstructured narrative, the clinician's recording of the history needs to be logically structured. There is some evidence that the use of structured questionnaires may improve the quality of data collection and reduce the omission of important information.[11] It may be helpful to use a printed form with headings for the recording of the history (and examination).

When the patient has completed telling their story of the main complaint, it is necessary to fill in the gaps and explore relevant symptoms in more detail by applying a more traditional "doctor-centered" interviewing technique, which can be structured as outlined below.

Pain history

The following aspects of the presenting painful condition should be noted largely in the context of establishing diagnosis.

- **Location**. This should be as precise as possible. It may be helpful to ask the patient to indicate the site and extent of the pain on a body line-drawing. In some conditions, the diagnosis may be made with near-certainty on the basis of this alone, for example meralgia paresthetica. In other circumstances, identifying the exact location of the pain may call into question a preconceived pain diagnosis – for example, a patient with multiple sclerosis and unilateral leg pain attributed to demyelinating myelopathy, but whose pain is restricted to a single dermatome, is more in keeping with a lumbar root lesion.

- **Onset**. Was this sudden, rapid, or insidious? Was there any identifiable precipitant?
- **Intensity**. Most patients attending a pain clinic will have pain that is of at least moderate intensity some of the time. Variations in intensity are important and duration and frequency of severe exacerbations should be noted.
- **Temporal pattern**. Is the pain constant/fluctuating/ intermittent? Pain that is totally unremitting is often neuropathic, and if it additionally varies little, and is little influenced by anything the patient does, this may suggest a central origin.
- **Quality**. For example, is the pain sharp, aching, burning, or shooting. The patient should be encouraged to describe what he feels rather than applying a medical term that he may have heard (e.g. sciatica). Shooting, electrical, or burning sensations are characteristic of neuropathic pains, while nociceptive pains are more likely to be described as aching, dull, cramping, or throbbing. Some patients have considerable difficulty describing the quality of their pain and this is perhaps especially the case with some neuropathic pains; in this situation, the difficulty in finding appropriate words to describe the pain can itself be informative.
- **Current trend**. Is the pain evolving in its location or quality? Is it improving or deteriorating in intensity, or static?
- **Exacerbating/alleviating factors**. This refers to pain modifiers noticed by the patient, and not to treatments (which are considered separately below under Treatment history). Examples are exacerbation of back pain by spinal movement or loading, or of a painful extremity by light touch; or alleviation of back pain by lying flat or placing the painful extremity in cold water.
- **One pain or more?** Many patients have pain of more that one phenotype, and/or in more than one location, in which case all the features listed above should be obtained for each pain. This is of practical relevance; the patient with central poststroke pain may also have a painful frozen shoulder on the affected side which may be far more amenable to successful treatment than the neurogenic component of the pain.

The past pain history (if any) may conveniently be taken following the history of the presenting complaint. A previous history of pain with a similar character or location to the current symptoms may be particularly relevant if attributed to a serious cause.

Medical history

The medical history is important for several reasons in the patient with chronic pain. Enquiry should initially be made into the patient's general health. Apart from the value of this as a screening question to exclude serious morbidity, patients who consider themselves generally healthy may respond differently to a chronic pain condition than those with a history of chronic ill health.[12]

Serious comorbidity may complicate or even contra-indicate some pain treatment options. Particular hazards of systemic drug treatments may be posed by seriously impaired liver or kidney function. Some invasive treatments carry greater risk in patients with an increased bleeding tendency, either from a hemorrhagic disorder (e.g. thrombocytopenia, hemophilia) or anticoagulant treatment. Neuraxial nerve blocks, and some sympathetic blocks producing large regional vasodilatation, may be dangerous in patients with impaired cardiac reserve. Potent opioids should be used with caution in patients with severe chronic respiratory disease.

Many patients with diseases related or unrelated to their painful condition will be taking drugs long term which may potentially give rise to adverse interactions with pain medication.

Nonpain contingent causes of disability, e.g. some neurological diseases, may limit attainable objectives of physical rehabilitation.

Treatment history

This can conveniently be divided into pharmacological treatments and other forms of treatment.

PHARMACOLOGICAL

All drug treatments for pain, present and past, should be documented. For each drug, information about the dosage given and duration of treatment should be sought, as well as the effect on the pain, side effects, and (in the case of past treatments) the reason why the drug was discontinued. Often patients with chronic pain will be taking drugs likely to produce dependence, especially opioids. The specific issue of substance abuse in the chronic pain patient is addressed in Chapter 46, Pain management and substance misuse in the *Chronic Pain* volume in this series.

Topical treatments should specifically be inquired about, as they may be overlooked by the patient; likewise, the patient should specifically be asked about complementary and alternative treatments, such as homeopathic medicines, vitamin and mineral supplements, and also herbal remedies which the patient may erroneously assume to be irrelevant. Many herbal medicines have pronounced pharmacological effects and interact with other drugs; St John's Wort, in particular, is involved in numerous drug interactions among which are the reduction in plasma levels of amitriptyline and carbamazepine. Some herbal medicines can also cause serious side effects in their own right, including allergic reactions, interference with coagulation, and hepatotoxicity.

Drugs used for reasons other than pain treatment should be recorded. Some are of particular relevance to the pain clinician, for example anticoagulant therapy in patients scheduled for injection treatment. The risk of adverse drug interactions should always be considered. It is impossible to remember them all; the British National Formulary (BNF) currently lists in the order of 2500 interactions, and the clinician should have ready access to a comprehensive and regularly updated reference source such as this. Some interactions are the result of enzyme induction or inhibition; for example, corticosteroids inhibit the metabolism of tricyclic antidepressants, and carbamazepine is an enzyme inducer that reduces the effect of coumarin anticoagulants and oral contraceptives.

The patient should be asked about allergies to drugs; the nature of any reported adverse reaction should be sought (many patients report allergy when in fact they have experienced a nonimmune-mediated adverse reaction, for example diarrhea following antibiotic therapy).

NONPHARMACOLOGICAL

This should include all physical therapies, with some description of the types of treatment given including forms of noninvasive stimulation, such as transcutaneous electrical nerve stimulation (TENS). The question, "Have you ever been to a pain clinic before?" may provide a useful starting point for discussing these treatments. Specific enquiry should be made as to whether the patient has seen a physiotherapist with particular experience in chronic pain management. Injection treatments should be documented, with details of exactly what was done if this is known to the patient.

Surgical procedures will probably be volunteered by the patient but should be asked about nevertheless, and nonpharmacological complementary and alternative treatments, such as acupuncture, should also be noted. In every case, the patient should be asked whether the treatment had any beneficial effect on the pain, and whether there were any ill effects.

The patient should also be asked whether they have seen a psychologist regarding their pain. This inquiry sometimes provokes a hostile response for which the clinician should be prepared; some tact is often required in the timing of this line of questioning, and it may be prudent to wait until later in the interview in case the patient raises the issue first.

Psychosocial history

This is invariably important in patients with chronic pain of any severity and the proportion of time allocated to it in the history-taking should reflect this. An appropriate starting point is the patient's personal circumstances (Who is at home? Are you working? What is your job?). The clinician should ask specifically about the effect of the pain on activity and behavior – occupational, domestic, social, recreational, and sexual – as appropriate. (S)he should ask about effect and emotions (anxiety, depression, anger, frustration). These issues are addressed in more depth below under Psychological pain interview, but should at least be touched upon during the initial interview.

PHYSICAL EXAMINATION

During the interview

The physical examination should start as soon as the patient enters the consulting room, and continue throughout the interview. Behaviors can be considered as valuable physical signs in the context of the chronic pain sufferer. Is the patient calm or agitated? Animated or "flat"? Does (s)he appear cheerful or sad? (If tearful at any point, note should be made of what appears to trigger this in the interview). Does the patient's behavior seem appropriate? Does the patient appear comfortable in the interview chair, or restless? Is the patient well presented or unkempt? Does the patient present a lucid account of events or seem distracted, confused, drowsy, or intoxicated?

What terms does the patient use to describe symptoms? Are they largely descriptive without undue emotive dramatization (e.g. "It's like having a bad toothache in your back") or catastrophic (e.g. "It's like a million wasps stinging me") or attributional/medicalized (e.g. "It's because the surgeon operated in the wrong place"/"I've got sciatica because the L4/5 disk is prolapsing and compressing the nerve root")?

It is often informative to observe the patient's behavior while preparing to be examined (rising from the interview chair, walking to and getting onto the examination couch, etc.). Note whether there is elaborated behavior of disability or distress.

Formal physical examination

The majority of chronic pain problems presenting to pain clinics have their origin in the musculoskeletal system and the nervous system, and due emphasis is accordingly given to the examination of these two systems. The scope of the examination deemed necessary is determined partly by the nature of the presenting problem, and partly by the source of referral. A patient with typical postherpetic neuralgia who is otherwise entirely well probably does not need complete systematic examination. A patient referred from a medical generalist in primary care should probably undergo a comprehensive examination at first attendance;

a more focused examination is appropriate if the patient has been assessed by a specialist in the field of the patient's disorder.

CHRONIC PAIN IN DISORDERS OF THE MUSCULOSKELETAL SYSTEM: ADDITIONAL NOTES

This group of conditions includes diseases such as rheumatoid arthritis and ankylosing spondylitis, which have clear diagnostic criteria, a relatively well-understood pathology and well-established treatments, some of which are fairly disease-specific (e.g. gold injections for rheumatoid disease). These diseases are usually readily recognized by medical generalists, reflecting their high profile in teaching at medical school, and if referral to a specialist is deemed necessary, this will usually be a rheumatologist in the first instance. In contrast, conditions such as nonspecific back pain and myofascial pain, which are undoubtedly more common, receive little attention in undergraduate medical teaching and general medical practitioners may be less confident in the assessment and treatment of these cases than they are with the primary inflammatory arthropathies.

The following key questions/features apply to chronic back/spinal pain, as follows.

Key questions in the history

- Elicit risk factors for serious spinal pathology (red flags) (see Chapter 37, Chronic back pain in the *Chronic Pain* volume in this series).
- Is the pain midline or to one side?
- Was there an initiating event?
- What factors influence the pain?
- Does the pain radiate into one or both lower limbs?
- Are there deficits of sensation/power of the lower limbs?
- What activities does the pain restrict/prevent?

Key features of the examination

The patient needs to be examined adequately undressed and in good lighting. Remember to ask the patients' permission to touch them before doing so, and tell them what you intend to do before you do it.

Look for:

- stigmata of specific rheumatological disease, e.g. osteoarthritis;
- abnormalities of posture/gait, and fixed deformity (inspect from the back to detect scoliosis, from the side to detect abnormality of the cervical and lumbar lordoses and thoracic kyphosis);
- general level of fitness (muscular development, obesity);
- scars of previous surgery;
- abnormalities of skin and subcutaneous soft tissue – e.g. erythema *ab igne* from prolonged application of local heat, loss of lumbar paraspinal muscle bulk from disuse.

- range of movement (flexion, extension, lateral bending, rotation). Test with patient's hips and feet in alignment.
- antalgic movements and distress behavior.

Feel for:

- local tenderness/swelling/heat;
- myofascial tender points.

Test additionally for:

- straight leg raise. Dorsiflexion of the foot characteristically increases the pain of radicular compression, as does flexing the hip with the knee bent and then extending the knee (Lasegue's test). Reduced straight leg raise is generally regarded as having high sensitivity for lumbar disk herniation but poor specificity,[13, 14] although a recent publication suggests that both sensitivity and specificity are lower than previously believed, and that these maneuvers add little to the information gained from the history.[15]
- sacroiliac joint stressing tests for buttock pain;

It is suggested that discogenic pain is significantly correlated with pain centralization on repetitive movement testing, lumbar facet joint pain with absence of provocation when rising from sitting, and sacroiliac pain with specific mechanical stressing.[16] However, high degrees of disability and distress may be associated with reduced specificity of provocative tests of spinal pain and complicate their interpretation (see below under Over-reaction and related issues).[17]

CHRONIC PAIN IN DISORDERS OF THE NERVOUS SYSTEM: ADDITIONAL NOTES

Chronic pain associated with disorders of the nervous system may be nocigenic (usually musculoskeletal) or neuropathic. The reader is referred to Chapter 24, Pain in neurological disease in the *Chronic Pain* volume in this series, for a fuller discussion of this. In addition to the general aspects of history-taking and examination, the clinical assessment of this group of patients should aim to establish:

- the primary neurological diagnosis;
- whether there is a single pain phenotype or more than one;
- for each pain phenotype, whether the pain is nocigenic or neuropathic;
- for each neuropathic pain phenotype, whether the lesion(s) is peripheral or central.

In some cases, the primary diagnosis will be clearly established by the time the patient presents to the pain clinic. In other cases it may be suspected but unproven, or frankly obscure. However, in every case the clinician should seek to establish the likely cause of the pain, not only in terms of primary diagnosis, but in terms of broad pathophysiological mechanisms of pain generation. Some neurological conditions, such as trigeminal neuralgia, produce a highly stereotyped pain syndrome. Others, such as multiple sclerosis, may give rise to a broad range of phenotypically diverse clinical pains with a variety of putative pain-generating mechanisms.

In the patient with an established neurological disease, it is likely that he will have been seen by a neurologist and undergone a thorough general neurological examination. However, the examination may not have been closely focused on abnormalities of sensation, which are important in neuropathic pain.

Key questions in the history

- Is the pain in an area of sensory deficit?
- Are there elements of burning or shooting/electrical sensations?
- Is there accompanying paresthesia or dysesthesia? This includes Lhermitte's phenomenon, a widely spreading paresthesia provoked by neck flexion and characteristic of multiple sclerosis (see Chapter 24, Pain in neurological disease in the *Chronic Pain* volume in this series).
- Are there associated abnormalities, past or present, of altered color, temperature, or sweating, edema or dystrophic changes?
- Is there allodynia (pain evoked by stimulation that is normally innocuous, like light touch)?
- Is there hyperalgesia (supranormally intense perception of stimulation that is normally painful, like pinprick)?
- Is there hyperpathia (increased somatosensory detection threshold, with development of pain of increasing intensity with repetitive or sustained stimulation – this is pathognomonic of neuropathic pain)?
- Is there an associated movement disorder?

Key features of physical examination

Look for:

- abnormalities of posture or gait;
- abnormal involuntary movement;
- focal wasting;
- local changes of color or swelling.

Feel for:

- locally altered temperature/sweating;

Test (motor) for:

- tone;
- power;
- reflexes.

Test (sensory) for:

- light touch – deficit/allodynia;
- warm/cool – deficit/allodynia;
- pinprick – deficit/hyperalgesia;
- proprioception/vibration;
- movement- or pressure-evoked sensation (if appropriate to presentation) – e.g. Tinel's test (paresthesia in the hand/fingers provoked by percussion over the median nerve at the wrist in carpal tunnel syndrome).

Full quantitative sensory testing utilizes specialized techniques and is not part of routine physical examination. However, some basic equipment for semi-quantitative sensory testing (von Frey filaments, constant temperature rollers for non-noxious warm and cold) can be considered routine clinical tools in this group of patients and are valuable assets in assessing both sensory deficits and hypersensitivity phenomena.

OVER-REACTION AND RELATED ISSUES

Much emphasis has been placed on some aspects of behavior in chronic pain patients which are commonly cited as evidence of either a psychogenic basis of the pain, conscious symptom exaggeration, or even frank malingering. As a general rule, these conclusions are not justified. However, they may usefully draw attention to the probability of prominent psychosocial issues.

Examples of the types of presentation and behavior liable to make this sort of impression on the attending clinician are:

- "accoutrements of disability" without an obvious objective need – crutches, dark glasses, wheelchair, etc;
- florid displays of distress during the history-taking and (especially) examination – wincing, groaning, and slow, antalgic movement;
- "nonorganic signs," such as those cited by Waddell and colleagues.[18] These are grouped into the following categories:
  - tenderness – e.g. widespread superficial tenderness to light palpation over the lumbar spine;
  - simulation, e.g. "rotating" the spine with the shoulders and pelvis remaining in the same plane;
  - distraction, e.g. wide disparity between sitting and supine straight leg raise;
  - regional disturbance, e.g. "give way" weakness or nondermatomal sensory loss.
  - over-reaction, e.g. slow movement, grimacing, and sighing.

It should be emphasized that Waddell's signs are indicators of distress, not evidence of malingering or absence of a genuine cause for the pain.

PSYCHOLOGICAL PAIN INTERVIEW

As with the taking of the medical history, there are multiple objectives involved in the psychological pain interview. Obviously one is attempting to obtain clear, factual information relating to the patient's pain history – what was done, when, by whom, and to what outcome. However, it is more than that. As was noted above, patients have a need to "tell their story" and allowing them to do that tends to lead to better outcomes.[19] The psychological pain interview should also gain an understanding of how the patient understands his or her pain – to find out how they think about the problem which has brought them to your office. This may involve the verbalization of thoughts and understandings which have hitherto been only implicit, never been made public before, even to the speaker. Finally, unlike the medical assessment, the psychological pain interview is also often the first step in a process of engagement in a treatment model which is unfamiliar at best. The challenge is to achieve all of these objectives in the time limitation that all clinicians observe – no easy task.

How one goes about the psychological pain interview also depends to some extent upon the basis on which it is conducted. It might be the second or third in a series of assessments that the patient has been through in the one visit, having been seen by the pain specialist and perhaps a physiotherapist or nurse, prior to a team case conference. It might be an assessment that has followed from a referral from the pain specialist who has been treating the patient from within the same service, in the same building, with ready access to shared notes and "corridor case discussions." Or the assessment might be a stand-alone affair, the result of a referral from one practitioner to another working in physically and organizationally disparate services. Generally speaking, the more remote one is from the interdisciplinary team assessment format, the more reliant one is upon information obtained from the psychological assessment in order to generate a treatment formulation.

The interview is also shaped to some extent by the amount of information obtained from psychometric assessment as part of the assessment process. The more extensive the questionnaire battery, the more latitude there is in the interview to explore areas in greater detail. See Chapter 9, Chronic pain, impairment, and disability; Chapter 10, The psychological assessment of pain in patients with chronic pain; Chapter 14, Outcome measurement in chronic pain in the *Chronic Pain* volume in this series; and Chapter 3, Selecting and applying pain measures for a full discussion of self-report assessment instruments in chronic pain. Inclusion of the partner is an invaluable aid to the assessment process, as this offers the opportunity of obtaining a different perspective on the patient's coping ability, a second interpretation of the impact of pain on family life, and a chance to observe directly some of the behavioral interactions known to maintain pain-related disability.[20]

Content

There is often cause for concern when clinicians are carrying out sequential interdisciplinary assessments that patients are being asked the same questions by each team member. While there is obviously the potential for redundancy and a loss of rapport with the patient ("I already told the last guy all of this!"), judicious use of common questioning can be valuable. Occasionally a second prompt helps a patient to recall information that they had forgotten or neglected to give the first time. It may also be that with greater trust or rapport with one clinician, the patient feels more comfortable to divulge information. Inconsistent responses to the same kinds of questions can also alert the clinical team to a patient who is not giving honest answers to unambiguous questions. Finally, most patients with chronic pain will expect to be asked questions about pain modulators, treatments undertaken, and so on. Covering this familiar territory early on can help to build rapport, particularly with patients who may be skeptical if not overtly hostile about the role of a clinical psychologist in the pain treatment team.

There is no definitive set of questions that should comprise the psychological interview. However, the following topic areas represent a broad set of categories for exploration in conjunction with the medical history. The clinical psychologist may also need to begin the interview with a brief explanation of the nature of pain psychology. It can be worthwhile to state openly that the purpose of the assessment is not to expose the underlying psychological causes of pain, but to explore how the persistent pain problem has impacted upon various life areas (as it so often does), so that optimum treatment plans can be developed. It can also be useful at the outset to invite the patient to change position during the interview (stand, lean against the wall, pace the room), rather than continue sitting in discomfort. Not only does this invitation help to build rapport, it is a tacit acceptance of the reality of the patient's pain.

PAIN HISTORY

Information about the onset of the pain, diurnal variations, modulators of pain, and in particular what the patient does (and does not do) in response to pain flare-ups, are important and expected components of the assessment. In particular, the pain psychologist should be looking for behavioral contingencies that may be influencing disability, such as positive or negative reinforcement for pain behavior.[21]

Past treatment, current treatments, and expectations of future treatment should be assessed. Use of pain medications, their perceived benefits and any identified side effects should be noted. Alcohol and other drug use (especially marijuana) are important to assess, as this information may not be freely offered, but may impact upon treatment significantly.

UNDERSTANDING OF PAIN MECHANISMS

Both the patient and the partner should be asked questions such as "Why do you think that this pain has persisted X months/years after it originally started?" Concerns about undetected but sinister disease processes are particularly important.

Beliefs about the risk of further damage through normal movement and gentle exercise should also be elicited, as any physical therapy that is proposed will need to be accommodated in this.

DAILY ROUTINE

Time to bed, time out of bed, the elements of a typical day and evening, and how the current routine compares to premorbid activity levels are important. For the non-working patient who describes his or her day as "just pottering about at home," several key follow-up questions include: How many household chores are still your responsibility? Other than to attend medical appointments, how often do you leave the house? How much time during the typical day do you spend lying down?

WORK

A brief vocational history provides useful information not only about the impact of pain on psychosocial functioning, but also about the patient's expectations and beliefs. Determining the educational level obtained, the type of work being done at the time of injury, whether work was sustained or discontinued because of pain, attempts to return to work and their outcome, and future expectations for work are important assessment questions.[22] In particular, for patients in receipt of financial support for not working, a careful exploration of the incentives for returning to work should be made.

IMPACT OF PAIN ON FAMILY LIFE

Following on from the above, specific inquiry should be made as to how roles within the family have changed since the onset of the pain and how the family has adjusted to those changes.[23] What does the spouse do more of now, as well as less of now, because of pain? How has communication changed within the relationship? What about intimacy – not just sexual activity, but physical and emotional closeness? Clearly, the responses given to these questions must be interpreted in the context of the premorbid relationship quality.

PSYCHOLOGICAL DISORDERS

By leaving direct questioning about depression, anxiety, and other psychological disorders until relatively late in the interview, the clinician has had a chance to build enough trust and rapport with the patient to obtain unguarded responses. Screening for current mood disorders, as well as obtaining a history of mental health, is important for treatment planning. It is often useful to find out about previous exposure to psychological or psychiatric treatment, as negative personal experiences of such treatment can create significant barriers to engaging in any future intervention. Further discussion of the issues concerning the assessment of psychopathology in the context of chronic pain is given in Chapter 13, Psychological effects of chronic pain: an overview in the *Chronic Pain* volume in this series, as well as Chapter 3, Selecting and applying pain measures.

SOCIAL HISTORY

A brief childhood and family history can shed light on developmental issues which may be relevant for future treatment – for example, a family history of depression, childhood abuse or neglect, attention deficit disorder, or other early psychobehavioral disorders, even family responses to illness during childhood, may all be fruitful areas for evaluation.

INTERPERSONAL SKILLS

The pain psychology assessment is not concerned solely with analyzing information given by the patient, but with how that information is given. Displays of pain behavior should of course be noted, but the careful clinician will try to observe when those behaviors occur to determine whether patterns can be detected. They may happen during discussion of more emotionally challenging topics, or after a prolonged period of immobility, or at the beginning of the interview, but not towards the end. Attention should also be paid to the patient's communication skills as these might shed light on any relationship difficulties discussed, or need to be taken into account when considering a group-based treatment program.

As a final point, by definition, taking a history is an exercise in retrospection – what happened, when, and why. However, the first contact with a pain psychologist is often the starting point to a new treatment direction. The assessment often marks the ending of medical efforts to find sustainable pain relief, and the beginning of a self-management model of pain – which might be an entirely foreign concept to the patient. For this reason, the emphasis in the assessment should err on the future rather than retelling the past. The clinician really wants to know what the patient thinks about where to go next, rather than where he or she has been before.

CONCLUSIONS

Skilled history-taking and physical examination are important in the assessment of the chronic pain patient;

however, there are some differences of emphasis between the main objectives of history-taking and examination in these patients compared with most primary medical specialties. Patient-, as well as doctor-centered interviewing is desirable for optimum gathering of information and for establishing a productive clinician–patient relationship.

REFERENCES

1. Laerum E, Indahl A, Skouen JS. What is 'the good back consultation'? A combined qualitative and quantitative study of chronic low back pain patients' interaction with and perception of consultations with specialists. *Journal of Rehabilitation Medicine*. 2006; **38**: 255–62.

∗ 2. Bickley LS. *Bates' guide to physical examination and history taking*, 9th edn. Philadelphia: Lippincott Williams & Wilkins, 2007.

3. Douglas G, Nicol F, Robertson C (eds). *Macleod's clinical examination*, 11th edn. Edinburgh: Elsevier Churchill Livingstone, 2005.

4. Tierney LM, Henderson MC (eds). *The patient history evidence-based approach*. New York: Lange Medical Books/McGraw-Hill, 2005.

5. Ende J, Fosnocht KM. Clinical examination: still a tool for our times? *Transactions of the American Clinical and Climatological Association*. 2002; **113**: 137–50.

6. Bird J, Cohen-Cole SA. The three-function model of the medical interview. *Advances in Psychosomatic Medicine*. 1990; **20**: 65–88.

7. Conant EB. Addressing patients by their first names. *New England Journal of Medicine*. 1998; **308**: 1107.

8. Engel GL. The need for a new medical model: a challenge for biomedicine. *Science*. 1977; **196**: 129–36.

9. Smith RC, Lyles JS, Mettler J *et al*. The effectiveness of intensive training for residents in interviewing. A randomized, controlled study. *Annals of Internal Medicine*. 1998; **128**: 118–26.

10. Beckman HB, Frankel RM. The effect of physician behaviour on the collection of data. *Annals of Internal Medicine*. 1984; **101**: 692–6.

11. Ramsey PG, Curtis JR, Paauw DS *et al*. History taking and preventative medicine skills among primary care physicians: An assessment using standardized patients. *American Journal of Medicine*. 1998; **104**: 152–8.

12. Linton SJ, Althoff B, Melin L *et al*. Psychological factors related to health, back pain and dysfunction. *Journal of Occupational Rehabilitation*. 1994; **5**: 1–10.

13. Ballantyne JC. *The Massachusetts General Hospital handbook of pain management*, 3rd edn. Philadelphia: Lippincott Williams & Wilkins, 2006: 42.

14. Supik LF, Broom MJ. Sciatic tension signs and lumbar disc herniation. *Spine*. 1994; **19**: 1066–9.

15. Vroomen PC, de Krom MC, Wilmink JT *et al*. Diagnostic value of history and physical examination in patients suspected of lumbosacral nerve root compression. *Journal of Neurology, Neurosurgery and Psychiatry*. 2002; **72**: 630–4.

16. Young S, April C, Laslett M. Correlations of clinical examination characteristics with three sources of chronic low back pain. *Spine Journal*. 2003; **3**: 460–5.

17. Laslett M, Oberg B, April CN, McDonald B. Centralization as a predictor of provocation discography results in chronic low back pain, and the influence of disability and distress on diagnostic power. *Spine Journal*. 2005; **5**: 370–80.

18. Waddell G, McCulloch JA, Kummel E, Venner RM. Non-organic signs in low back pain. *Spine*. 1980; **5**: 117–25.

19. Charon R. Suffering, storytelling and community: an approach to pain treatment from Columbia's program in Narrative Medicine. In: Flor H, Kalso E, Dostrovsky J (eds). *Proceedings of the 11th World Congress on Pain*. Seattle: IASP Press, 2006: 19–27.

∗ 20. Newton-John TRO. Solicitousness and chronic pain: a critical review. *Pain Reviews*. 2002; **9**: 7–27.

∗ 21. Sanders SH. Operant conditioning with chronic pain: back to basics. In: Gatchel R, Turk DC (eds). *Psychological approaches to pain management: a practitioners handbook*. New York: Guilford Press, 1996: 112–30.

22. Linton SJ, Gross D, Schultz IZ *et al*. Prognosis and the identification of workers risking disability: research issues and directions for future research. *Journal of Occupational Rehabilitation*. 2005; **15**: 459–74.

23. Schwartz L, Ehde DM. Couples and chronic pain. In: Schmaling K, Sher TG (eds). *The psychology of couples and illness: theory, research and practice*. Washington, DC: American Psychological Association, 2000: 191–216.

2

Practical methods for pain intensity measurements

WILLIAM I CAMPBELL AND KEVIN E VOWLES

KEY LEARNING POINTS

- Pain is a complex and multifaceted experience that is affected by sensory, emotional, physiological, and environmental factors, as well as past experiences. Only the person experiencing the pain can accurately indicate its intensity.
- Appropriate pain assessment relies on an appreciation of its complex nature and only measures with proven reliability and validity should be used.
- Simple assessment tools can be easy and quick to use, while more complex assessment tools may be more sensitive and provide more information about the pain experience.
- Visual analog scales, verbal rating scales, and numerical rating scales are reliable and valid measures of pain

intensity, although each has limitations. Current consensus statements recommend that an 11-point numerical rating scale be used to rate average pain.
- Questionnaire measures may take into account the various dimensions of pain, but can be complex for the patient to use and the clinician to score.
- Regardless of the pain assessment tool used, it is important to be aware of the degree of change on that scale that is clinically meaningful, or analysis of the results will be of little value. While individual patients will differ in what they define as clinically meaningful, it appears that a pain reduction of 30–50 percent is sufficient for the majority of pain sufferers.

INTRODUCTION

The measurement of pain intensity is essential in health care. The experience of pain is exceedingly common, with one recent study indicating that 83 percent of patients presenting to emergency departments report the experience of significant pain,[1] and arguments have been made that this aspect of patient care has been neglected.[2] Accurate and appropriate pain assessment offers many

potential advantages. First, if pain is not assessed, it is not likely that it will be appropriately treated. Second, the specific characteristics of pain, such as its intensity, quality, and impact, may be useful in determining the type of treatment offered. Third, in many settings, pain intensity is an important indicator of treatment efficacy, in conjunction with measures of functioning. Fourth, qualitative and temporal features of pain may have a diagnostic value. Finally, pain and suffering are often inexorably linked – appropriate treatment of pain may significantly reduce the suffering of the individual in pain. There is no doubt that this is an important area to consider in most, if not all, healthcare settings.

Although the importance of pain measurement in health care is obvious, it must be carried out with care. Pain is an extremely complex experience. It is a private internal event which cannot be directly observed by others. It is widely accepted that the rating of pain should be carried out by the pain sufferer whenever possible, since observers cannot accurately assess the feelings of another person and inaccurate judgments are therefore likely. It appears that healthcare providers, in particular, tend to underestimate the severity of pain in comparison to ratings made by sufferers of both acute and chronic pain.[3, 4] Furthermore, although historical views of pain intensity have tended to view it purely as nociception, an overwhelming amount of evidence suggests that the pain experience is an amalgamation of nociception, emotion, cognition, environment, and prior learning.[5, 6] Therefore, any assessment of pain must take this complexity into account if the assessment itself is to be of value.

Accurate and appropriate pain measurement is also made more difficult by the fact that pain is a construct, like depression, anxiety, and intelligence.[7, 8] Constructs are best understood as descriptive terms that categorize related groups of observations. The constructs themselves cannot be directly assessed, but the related observations can be, particularly when they co-occur or are related to one another in a fairly predicable fashion. The various components that comprise pain can be considered to be its intensity, quality, and impact on emotional, social, and physical functioning.[6] Intensity may be defined as how much a pain "hurts" or how severe it is in relation to certain defined anchor points. Quality ratings tend to be more concerned with other aspects of the pain experience, such as affective or sensory qualities. Finally, impact on functioning can be assessed by determining how pain interferes with normal "everyday" activities or how it relates to symptoms of psychological distress.

The purpose of this chapter is to provide a comprehensive review of pain measurement. We will focus on psychometrically sound assessment methods and will include a discussion of pain measurement in those who may not be able to appropriately utilize the standard approaches. Our hope is that this chapter will be of direct assistance in the clinic by providing a concise and up-to-date reference. The interested reader is also encouraged to consult Chapter 3, Selecting and applying pain measures for a conceptual discussion of assessment.

FACTORS AFFECTING THE PERCEPTION OF PAIN

It is a common belief that the intensity of pain is closely, if not directly, related to the extent of injury. This belief is grossly untrue since pain and suffering are more closely associated with the meaning of pain and psychosocial factors, including learning history. For example, Beecher's[9, 10] classic observations clearly illustrate that pain intensity and severity of injury can vary independent of one another, findings which have been replicated many times in that similar acute or chronic pain experiences are often associated with a wide variety of pain intensity ratings.

While injury severity or degree of tissue damage is not consistently related to pain ratings, there are a number of other factors that have consistent relations. This topic is covered in detail in Chapter 9, Chronic pain, impairment, and disability; Chapter 10, The psychological assessment of pain in patients with chronic pain; and Chapter 13, Psychological effects of chronic pain: an overview, in the *Chronic Pain* volume of this series. It seems prudent, however, to at least discuss this issue briefly in the present chapter as well, given the close relations of these factors to pain intensity.

All things considered, demographic factors, such as age, education, and marital status, have fairly weak relations with pain intensity ratings across studies. There are, however, two notable exceptions. First, men tend to have higher pain tolerance and rate similar types of pain as less intense in comparison to women.[11] There may be several reasons for this discrepancy, including differences in learning histories, as well as psychological, social, and biological factors.[11, 12] Second, there is a moderate amount of evidence that white people tend to rate pain experiences as less intense and less distressing in comparison to other ethnicities, particularly black and Hispanic individuals.[13, 14, 15, 16] Perhaps most concerning, several studies have found evidence of disparities among the ethnicities in access to pain treatment (see Cintron and Morrison[17] for a review).

Across studies, settings, and populations, psychosocial factors are the strongest predictors of pain. The most studied emotional experiences include depression and anxiety (including anxiety specific to pain), although anger has been the subject of study as well.[18, 19] In general, as these emotional experiences worsen, pain ratings are higher (see Chapter 10, The psychological assessment of pain in patients with chronic pain; Chapter 13, Psychological effects of chronic pain: an overview; and Chapter 36, Neck pain and whiplash, in the *Chronic Pain* volume of this series for a more detailed treatment of this subject).

Other factors which may influence the perception, and therefore the assessment, of pain are climatic conditions and time of day when the measurement is carried out. Patients suffering from chronic pain often have exacerbations of their symptoms as the weather changes. Many of these observations have been reflected in folklore – e.g. "aches and pains, coming rains."[20] The most frequently reported meteorological factors which alter pain complaint are temperature and humidity. These weather conditions alter pain perception mostly in disorders involving joints, muscles, and postoperative scars.[21] Most patients are aware of a fluctuation in pain intensity according to the time of day.[22] Those patients who do not convey regular trends of pain intensity throughout the day also report significantly higher ratings of emotional stress. Ideally, patients should rate their pain at the same time of day. There is no control over climatic conditions but the observer should be aware that it may affect pain scores.

THE MEMORY OF PAIN

The ability to remember pain is needed to create an upper anchor point for most pain intensity scales. The ability to recall pain intensity for up to one week is fairly accurate, with correlations generally in the range of 0.90.[22, 23, 24] After several weeks, recall continues to be strongly related to its original value, although it can vary according to a number of factors, including "status" of assessor (i.e. ratings made to research assistants were 86 percent higher than those made to treating physician two weeks after a procedure[25]), consistency of pain episodes (i.e. recall of episodic pain is less accurate than more consistent pain[26]), variability in pain intensity (i.e. recall of more variable pain is less accurate[27]), and whether or not current pain complaints are present.[28] Furthermore, within individual variability appears greater than if recall data are collapsed across individuals,[29] thus caution should be used when asking individuals to make ratings about pain episodes that are more temporally distant. Based on the results of these and other studies, it seems prudent to restrict time frames for recalled pain to a period of several weeks, perhaps as long as a month, in order to increase reliability and validity of measurements.

In addition to the issues inherent in recalled pain intensity, memory for the specific qualities of the pain and the patient's mood at the time of pain is less accurate than for intensity when assessed after several weeks.[30] A high affect, such as anxiety at the time of initial registration of pain, is thought to interfere with recall and results in an exaggerated memory of pain intensity.[31] Further episodes of acute pain may also interfere with accurate recall. In the chronic pain situation, the current level of pain and mood influences the accuracy of remembered pain, for example patients with lower levels of pain at the moment of recall tend to underestimate their past pain levels and vice versa.[32] There is strong evidence for a post-pain modulation phenomenon, in which cognitive processes influence both pain recall and future pain report.[33] Attempts to assess pain by longer-term recall is therefore not recommended since it may be inaccurate both in intensity and quality – contemporary pain scores are much more appropriate and less prone to error.

SCALES USED TO RATE PAIN INTENSITY

The most frequently assessed dimension of pain is its intensity. Although the concept is readily understood by patients, intensity is best considered as a complex measure of nocioception, pain quality, and pain history, as well as aspects of emotional functioning and current environment, as each of these factors seems to have an influence. Any single rating of pain is best considered within this multidimensional framework. Although pain ratings are most frequently carried out verbally or in writing, emerging evidence supports the use of electronic and computerized assessment methods as well.[34, 35, 36, 37]

Typically used single ratings of pain include the numerical rating scale (NRS), verbal rating scale (VRS), visual analog scale (VAS), and faces rating scale, each of which is outlined in the following. These relatively simple, often single item measures are easy to administer, brief to complete, and have all been used effectively in clinical and research settings. Therefore, it is likely that any of them will work in most settings, allowing test selection to be made based on the information that is being sought and specific characteristics of the population being sampled. Regardless of the type of scale used, however, it is important to consider the descriptive terms that are used as the anchor points, particularly for the maximal anchor. A series of studies have suggested that descriptors used as anchor points can have an effect on pain ratings[38, 39, 40] and it is recommended that anchor points be consistent between patients, with descriptors such as "no pain" or "pain at its least" be used at the lower end of the scale and "pain as bad as you can imagine" or "worst pain possible" at the higher end.[6] In particular, one study found that "worst pain imaginable" as the maximal anchor produced the most normally distributed sample of scores.[41] Furthermore, the ratings obtained by individual measures do not appear interchangeable with one another,[42] which makes comparisons among them difficult and best avoided.

Numerical rating scales

The NRS is one of the most convenient ways of determining pain intensity and has proven reliability and validity.[7, 43] NRSs have demonstrated positive and significant correlations with other measures of pain intensity.[7, 44] The recent statement from the Initiative on Methods, Measurement, and Pain Assessment (IMMPACT)[43] recommended the use of an 11-point (i.e. 0–10) NRS as a key outcome measure for clinical trials and this recommendation also seems sensible for use in clinical applications. This committee also recommended that the time frame for the pain rating should be over the past 24 hours or past seven days, whichever is most appropriate. It is potentially useful to obtain ratings of current, average pain (over past 24 hours/seven days/etc.), highest, and lowest pain as well. A recent study by

Nicholas and collagues[45] provided normative data on a large sample of pain sufferers ($n = 4250$). Within this sample, mean average pain intensity over the past week was 6.4 (SD = 2.1) with means of 6.2 (SD = 2.0) for men and 6.5 (SD = 2.1) for women.

Although it is possible to use additional numbers on an NRS (e.g. 101 point scale), it is not clear that they offer greater utility. At least one study has shown that most patients use a 101-point NRS as though pain intensity changed in steps of 10 units, i.e. they treated the scale as though there were 11 points.[44] This phenomenon is particularly likely to occur if the patient gives a verbal indication of pain intensity rather than marking the scale themselves. It seems that little information is lost by using an 11-point NRS over a 101-point scale. A similar finding seems apparent in scales that are composed of fewer numbers (i.e. seven or fewer), as sensitivity can be reduced to the extent that it is difficult to detect the mean change in an actively treated group compared to a placebo group.[7, 33] It is important to note that the specific numbers used in these scales may not refer strictly to rank order but they may also possess ratio properties, i.e. a change from 6 to 3 indicates a reduction in pain which equates to a 50 percent reduction in pain intensity.[7, 46]

Verbal rating scales

A VRS contains lists of adjectives reflecting various levels or categories of pain intensity from no pain through to the most intense pain possible. There should be a sufficient number of adjectives to permit the patient to express a graded range of pain intensities. Patients are asked to read over the list of words and choose the one best describing their pain intensity. Like the NRSs, the VRS is simple and fast to use and may use four or more words (e.g. none, mild, moderate, severe).[47, 48, 49] It suffers from similar problems as the NRS. The magnitude of change between any two points on the scale cannot be assumed to be the same, i.e. the extent of the difference between mild and moderate pain cannot be interpreted as the same as that between moderate and severe pain. In addition, each patient will interpret the difference between any two specific adjectives differently. Since the gradations of pain intensity vary between adjectives, the VRS does not possess any ratio properties.[50]

The recent IMMPACT statement[6] recommended that a VRS composed of four descriptors (i.e. none, mild, moderate, severe) is likely sufficient for most settings. In addition, given that similar VRSs have been used in a variety of clinical studies, use of this measure can allow cross-study comparisons.

Visual analog scales

A VAS consists of a line labeled at either end with the extremes of the feeling to be measured. The patient is asked to make a mark or otherwise indicate which point along the scale best represents their pain intensity. If there is any difficulty in understanding the concept this may be overcome by describing the scale in terms of a thermometer indicating pain intensity, which gradually changes from no pain to worst pain possible. In general, line length is 100 mm. Pain intensity is scored numerically as the distance in millimeters from zero. This type of scale has the advantages of being fast, sensitive to small changes and the data can be analyzed relatively easily. The VAS was originally employed in 1923 for educational purposes but was not widely used for pain assessment until the 1960s.[51, 52] It is considered an excellent communication bridge between patient and observer and avoids some of the problems which arise through the use of categorical scales, since the scale is continuous. Perhaps the primary drawback of the VAS is that it usually demonstrates more missing or incomplete data in comparison to NRS measures.[7] Furthermore, difficulty completing VAS measures is associated with analgesic intake and older age.[7, 53, 54]

The VAS may be vertical or horizontal with the lowest ratings located on the bottom and left sides, respectively (see **Figure 2.1**). The use of graduations, numbers, or words along the line is inappropriate, since it causes clustering of results around these points, interfering with what would otherwise be an even distribution.[55] It could be argued that the use of any marks or words along a VAS renders it a categorical scale. It is essential that the same type and orientation of scale is used throughout any series of measurements, otherwise the variation in measurement method may no longer render the results suitable for meaningful scrutiny. Care must be taken when reproducing these scales since photocopying can result in changes in the size of the scale.[48] Although the overall change in scale size may appear insignificant, it can lead to erroneous measures, especially if some of the pain scores are small.

The VAS has been used very widely over the last few decades in research associated with all types of pain. It has been shown to be reliable, valid, and internally consistent. This consistency does not alter as a function of pain intensity or time. The VAS is considered to have ratio properties inferring that the changes throughout the scale are accepted by the patient in a continuous manner, i.e. it may be assumed that a drop in pain intensity from 50 to 25 mm is a 50 percent reduction in pain.[50]

Pain measurement by pictures and toys

Pictorial pain rating scales frequently use diagrams of facial expression ranging from an appearance of being content to extreme distress[56] (see **Figure 2.2**). The Faces Pain Scale-Revised (FPS-R) utilizes a six-face scale.[57] Its validity is supported by a strong positive correlation with the VAS and also conforms closely to linear interval scales. The pictures are ranked and assigned a score. Patients are

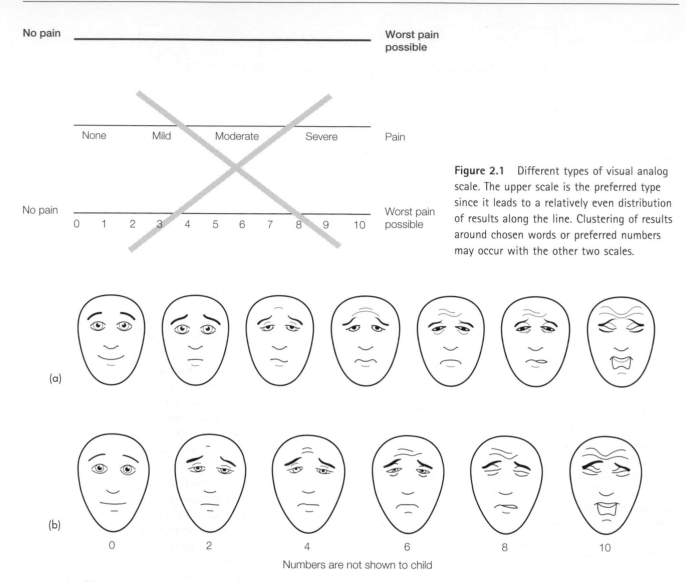

Figure 2.1 Different types of visual analog scale. The upper scale is the preferred type since it leads to a relatively even distribution of results along the line. Clustering of results around chosen words or preferred numbers may occur with the other two scales.

Numbers are not shown to child

Figure 2.2 (a) The Faces Pain Scale. (b) The Faces Pain Scale – revised. The faces are ranked from no pain on the extreme left (pain score 0), through to severe pain on the extreme right (pain score 6). Part (a) redrawn from Bieri D, Reeve RA, Champion GD, et al. The Faces Pain Scale for the self-assessment of the severity of pain experienced by children: development, initial validation, and preliminary investigation for ratio scale properties. *Pain.* 1990; **41**: 139-50, and part (b) redrawn from Hicks CL, von Baeyer CL, Spafford PA, et al. The Faces Pain Scale-Revised: toward a common metric in pediatric pain measurement. *Pain.* 2001; **93**: 173-83, with permission from IASP.

asked to indicate which picture best indicates their pain experience, the number associated with the chosen picture being the pain score. The main advantage of this type of scale over others is that the patient does not need to be literate but in other respects it has limitations similar to the NRSs or VRSs.

Toys and other pictorial methods have been successfully used to assess pain intensity in children. Most of these devices are modifications of the VAS (see **Figure 2.3**). Some observers prefer to use a neutral facial expression rather than one of contentment to convey the absence of pain. They therefore have the advantages of a continuously variable scale combined with the ease of communication with nonliterate patients. In its simplest form, neither the visual analog toy nor the faces scale

differentiates between pain intensity and the reaction to pain. One device, however, incorporates a colored analog scale to assess intensity and a facial affective scale to assess the aversive component of pain.[58] Test–retest data suggest that there is good rank ordering of the faces in association with pain in children.

PAIN ASSESSMENT BY QUESTIONNAIRE

The McGill Pain Questionnaire

Perhaps one of the most widely used composite measures of the qualitative and quantative experience of pain is the

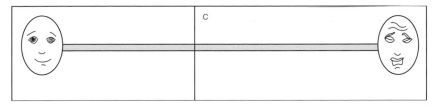

Figure 2.3 The visual analog toy. The toy depicts two facial expressions to illustrate the extremes of pain experienced. A cursor or sliding indicator (c) is positioned by the patient between the two facial expressions to indicate current pain intensity, and the distance to the cursor is used to estimate the pain score. Some devices have a graduated scale on the reverse side of the toy, so that the score under the back of the cursor may be read off directly.

McGill Pain Questionnaire (MPQ)[59] (see **Figure 2.4**). The MPQ consists of 78 words describing pain in sensory, affective, and evaluative terms. The sensory part of the questionnaire uses words describing the quality of the pain (e.g. throbbing, burning, or aching). These words have been arranged in groups each with similar sensory qualities and ranked according to their intensity. Affective words such as tiring, sickening, and frightful, together with evaluative words like annoying and troublesome are also arranged in groups and ranked. A miscellaneous group of sensory adjectives are also included. A six-point VRS for pain intensity is also included. A numerical score for the sensory, affective, and evaluative components of pain can now be obtained by adding the scores for the ranked words chosen in each subclass.

The MPQ has demonstrated itself to be reliable, valid, and temporally consistent across a multitude of studies and is available in at least 19 different languages (see Melzack and Katz[47] for a review). In general, the questionnaire is to be completed in a pen-and-paper format. It can be administered verbally, although at least one study has found that this method is associated with higher pain ratings.[60] Completion time is brief, estimated to be 5–15 minutes.[47]

A more concise form of the MPQ was introduced in 1987, the short-form McGill pain questionnaire (SF-MPQ). The measure consists of 15 descriptors (11 sensory and four affective), each of which is rated on an intensity scale from 0 ("none") to 3 ("severe") (**Figure 2.5**).[61] Three pain scores are derived from the sum of the ranked values obtained from the chosen descriptors – sensory, affective, and total. A VAS and a present pain intensity scale are also included within the SF-MPQ. These permit sensitivity of pain intensity measurement to be combined with qualitative information within a questionnaire, which is quicker to administer than the original MPQ.

Composite measures that include a pain subscale

There are a number of assessment inventories available that assess many aspects of the pain experience in addition to pain intensity. These measures provide a viable means of obtaining a breadth of information in a time-efficient manner, when the use of more lengthy assessment batteries is not practical. The measures reviewed each have evidence of acceptable reliability and validity.

Brief pain inventory

The Brief Pain Inventory (BPI) was originally developed to assess cancer pain but its use can be extended to evaluate chronic nonmalignant pain.[62, 63] Much like the MPQ, the BPI has proven utility across a broad range of clinical settings, including chronic musculoskeletal,[64, 65] neuropathic,[66, 67] and procedural pain,[68, 69] as well as human immunodeficiency virus (HIV)/acquired immunodeficiency syndrome (AIDS).[70, 71] The BPI includes three items measuring pain severity and quality, as well as seven additional items assessing the interference pain has on functioning (e.g. mood, function, sleep, interpersonal relationships). Recent consensus statements have recommended the BPI for use in clinical trials.[72, 73] Finally, two subscale scores can be computed: pain intensity and interference from pain, although there is some evidence for a three-factor structure (pain intensity, impact of pain on mood, impact of pain on activity), particularly in cancer pain.[64, 74, 75]

West Haven–Yale Multidimensional Pain Inventory

In addition to pain intensity, the Multidimensional Pain Inventory (MPI)[76] assesses affect/distress, functioning in typical activities, and spouse/partner responses to pain, as reported by the respondent. Subscale scores are expressed as *t*-scores (mean: 50, SD: 10) that are based on comparisons with the original normative sample of Kerns and colleagues.[76] The MPI has been widely used and is appropriate for a range of pain conditions.[77, 78] Furthermore, a series of cluster analyses that took place after the measure's initial validation derived a classification scheme, allowing respondents to be categorized, for example as "adaptive" or "dysfunctional" copers, or as "interpersonally distressed," and these categories are related to a number of measures of patient functioning.[79, 80, 81] A particular strength of the MPI is its use of standardized scores and the range of domains assessed.

McGill Pain Questionnaire

Patient's Name ______________________ Date ______________ Time ________ am/pm

DATE PAIN COMMENCED ______________________

PR1: S __________ (1–10) **A** __________ (11–15) **E** __________ (16) **M** __________ (17–20) **PRI(T)** __________ (1–20) **PPI** __________

DATE FIRST TREATMENT ______________________ **DATE TREATMENT COMPLETED** ______________________

1 FLICKERING, QUIVERING, PULSING, THROBBING, BEATING, POUNDING	11 TIRING, EXHAUSTING
2 JUMPING, FLASHING, SHOOTING	12 SICKENING, SUFFOCATING
3 PRICKING, BORING, DRILLING, STABBING, LANCINATING	13 FEARFUL, FRIGHTFUL, TERRIFYING
4 SHARP, CUTTING, LACERATING	14 PUNISHING, GRUELLING, CRUEL, VICIOUS, KILLING
5 PINCHING, PRESSING, GNAWING, CRAMPING, CRUSHING	15 WRETCHED, BLINDING
6 TUGGING, PULLING, WRENCHING	16 ANNOYING, TROUBLESOME, MISERABLE, INTENSE, UNBEARABLE
7 HOT, BURNING, SCALDING, SEARING	17 SPREADING, RADIATING, PENETRATING, PIERCING
8 TINGLING, ITCHY, SMARTING, STINGING	18 TIGHT, NUMB, DRAWING, SQUEEZING, TEARING
9 DULL, SORE, HURTING, ACHING, HEAVY	19 COOL, COLD, FREEZING
10 TENDER, TAUT, RASPING, SPLITTING	20 NAGGING, NAUSEATING, AGONIZING, DREADFUL, TORTURING
	PPI: 0 NO PAIN, 1 MILD, 2 DISCOMFORTING, 3 DISTRESSING, 4 HORRIBLE, 5 EXCRUCIATING

BRIEF	RHYTHMIC	CONTINUOUS
MOMENTARY	PERIODIC	STEADY
TRANSIENT	INTERMITTENT	CONSTANT

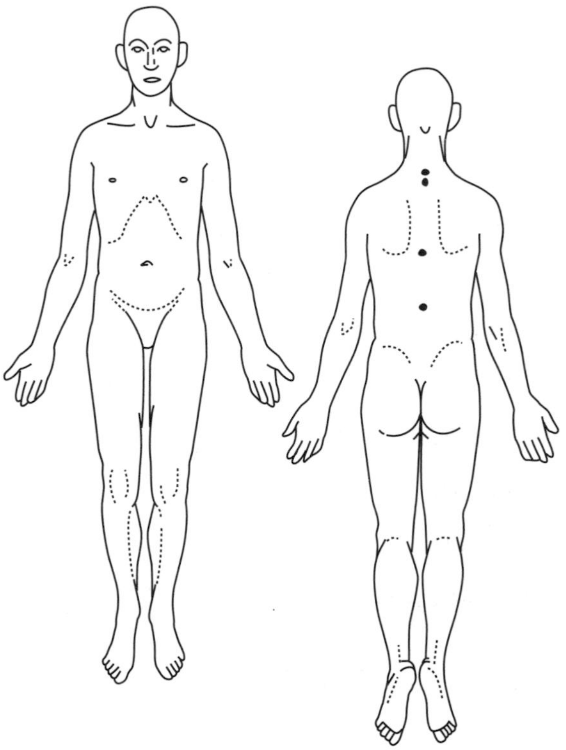

E = EXTERNAL I = INTERNAL

COMMENTS:

Figure 2.4 The McGill Pain Questionnaire. The descriptors are grouped into four categories: sensory (sections 1–10, flickering–splitting), affective (sections 11–15, tiring–blinding), evaluative (section 16, annoying–unbearable), and miscellaneous (sections 17–20, spreading–torturing). Scoring is carried out for each category by summating the rank value of each chosen word. The rank value is based on its position within each set of words, for example throbbing in section 1 would be given a score of 4. Scoring all sections 1–20 provides the pain rating index (PRI), whereas scoring sections 1–10 and 11–15 separately permits an estimate of the sensory and affective components of pain independently. Present pain intensity is determined from the six-point rating scale. Reprinted from Melzack R. The McGill Pain Questionnaire: major properties and scoring methods. *Pain*. 1975; **1**: 277–99, with permission.

SHORT-FORM McGILL PAIN QUESTIONNAIRE
RONALD MELZACK

PATIENT'S NAME: _____   DATE: _____

	NONE	MILD	MODERATE	SEVERE
THROBBING	0) _____	1) _____	2) _____	3) _____
SHOOTING	0) _____	1) _____	2) _____	3) _____
STABBING	0) _____	1) _____	2) _____	3) _____
SHARP	0) _____	1) _____	2) _____	3) _____
CRAMPING	0) _____	1) _____	2) _____	3) _____
GNAWING	0) _____	1) _____	2) _____	3) _____
HOT–BURNING	0) _____	1) _____	2) _____	3) _____
ACHING	0) _____	1) _____	2) _____	3) _____
HEAVY	0) _____	1) _____	2) _____	3) _____
TENDER	0) _____	1) _____	2) _____	3) _____
SPLITTING	0) _____	1) _____	2) _____	3) _____
TIRING–EXHAUSTING	0) _____	1) _____	2) _____	3) _____
SICKENING	0) _____	1) _____	2) _____	3) _____
FEARFUL	0) _____	1) _____	2) _____	3) _____
PUNISHING–CRUEL	0) _____	1) _____	2) _____	3) _____

NO
PAIN _____ WORST
POSSIBLE
PAIN

PPI

0	NO PAIN	_____
1	MILD	_____
2	DISCOMFORTING	_____
3	DISTRESSING	_____
4	HORRIBLE	_____
5	EXCRUCIATING	_____

(PPI is Present Pain Intensity)

Figure 2.5 The short-form McGill Pain Questionnaire. The descriptors are divided into two groups: sensory (throbbing-splitting) and affective (tiring–exhausting – punishing–cruel). Scoring is carried out by summating the checked values beside the appropriate descriptor, according to the intensity of each. The provision of a visual analog scale and a present pain intensity scale permits a more direct estimation of pain intensity. Reprinted from the Short-Form McGill Pain Questionnaire. *Pain.* 1987; **30**: 191-79, with permission.

Medical outcomes study Short–Form

The Short-Form 36 (SF-36)[82] is an international standard when it comes to the quantification of functioning. It includes a bodily pain subscale, composed of two items assessing pain severity and interference. In addition, the measure includes subscales assessing physical functioning, general health, vitality, social functioning, and mental health. It was developed to be a generic measure, thus it is not pain specific. The measure has been used in multiple healthcare settings and has proven utility.[83, 84, 85, 86]

Pain Outcome Questionnaire-VA

More recently, the Veterans Administration (VA) hospitals in the United States have developed a measure for assessing outcomes following chronic pain treatment. The Pain Outcome Questionnaire-VA (POQ-VA)[87] has been the result of this effort. Pain quality is one of the primary domains assessed, as are emotional and physical functioning. While the measure is relatively new and has been primarily used within VA hospitals,[87, 88] a slightly modified version has also been tested in other settings.[89]

ASSESSMENT OF PAIN AT THE EXTREMES OF AGE

The vast majority of information on pain assessment comes from middle-aged samples. Of course, the findings of these studies do not necessarily extend to those who are significantly younger or older. Empirical work in the past two decades has increasingly focused on this area and, although these literatures remain in need of development, it is now possible to approach assessment of pain at the extremes of age in a manner informed by empirical findings.

Children

The assessment of children's pain is a major challenge for a number of reasons. Effective communication of pain often involves the ability to verbally communicate. Pain responding is affected by previous encounters with painful stimuli, thus, individuals with shorter histories of pain experience may respond differently. Finally, parents or caregivers are often present when pain is being assessed and their presence can have an affect on the assessment process. The area of pediatric pain is fairly well established and a full review of this area is beyond the scope of the present chapter. There are at least two recent reviews on the subject, which will be of use to those with a particular interest in this area.[90, 91]

Pain intensity measures in younger individuals may be carried out by using behavioral, physiological, or psychological means.[92] In pre-verbal or early verbal children, behavioral and physiological indicators have been the most widely studied and a number of psychometrically sound instruments exist. A recent systematic on behalf of the Pediatric IMMPACT consortium[91] evaluated 20 observational pain scales and provided recommendations for use in various pain assessment contexts. For procedural pain, the Face, Legs, Arms, Cry, Consolability (FLACC) scale[93] or Children's Hospital of Eastern Ontario Pain Scale for ages one to seven[94] were recommended. For postoperative pain, the FLACC and the Parents' Postoperative Pain Measure[95] were recommended for use at hospital and home, respectively. For critical care, the COMFORT scale[96] was recommended. For chronic pain, the authors were not able to provide recommendations as they noted that behavioral signs of chronic pain often change over time.

When children are more verbally proficient, estimated to occur around the age of five,[97] self-report is the preferred method of assessment.[98, 99] Pictorial scales are the most commonly used measure (e.g. FPS-R,[57] the Oucher scale[100]), although the single item measures commonly used in adults (e.g. NRS, VAS) appear adequate as well.[101] As is the case with adults, pain in children is understood to be a complex construct and measuring pain intensity alone may be inadequate and may benefit from the inclusion of measures of the impact of pain on functioning (see Eccleston et al.[102] and Jordan et al.[103] for a review of relevant measures).

Older adults

The measurement of pain in older adults is also complex. This complexity is compounded by the frequency with which pain is experienced in this population, with some estimates indicating that 25–50 percent of community dwelling older adults suffer from significant pain which interferes with functioning.[104] Furthermore, as part of the aging process, degenerative changes occur at the receptor organs, such as Pacini's and Meissner's corpuscles.[105, 106] Peripheral nerves undergo segmental demyelination and the degeneration which occurs within the central nervous system leads to neurotransmitter changes with altered sensory processing.[107, 108] The ability to tolerate deep pain is consistent through childhood and adolescence but declines by the age of 60 years. Tolerance to cutaneous pain becomes elevated with aging.[109, 110] These changes do not seem to confer many advantages, given the common experience of pain in older populations. Any of the pain rating scales mentioned above may be used in the elderly but difficulties in understanding the abstract concept of VASs seem to be particularly prevalent in this age group,[7, 53, 54] and this may result in errors or the inability to obtain a pain measure from some patients. In this situation it may therefore be more appropriate to assess pain intensity with a VRS or an NRS. The FPS-R is also a viable alternative and is worth considering.[111, 112] At least one measure of pain has been developed that is specifically for use with older adults, the Geriatric Pain Measure,[113] a 24-item measure of pain intensity and interference. A 12-item short form has also recently been developed, which appears to have retained much of the reliability and validity of the longer version.[114]

CHRONIC NONMALIGNANT PAIN

Chronic pain assessment is a complex issue. Unlike acute pain where intensity may be altered mainly by affect alone, behavior and mood can become a greater issue than the pain itself. The scales mentioned earlier can be used to measure pain intensity in chronic pain conditions, but it is important that they are interpreted with the understanding that the results are understood to be affected by mood, beliefs, current environmental circumstances, and history. If outcome of treatment is to be assessed in these patients, the measurement of pain intensity alone will therefore be inadequate. A wide variety of specialized questionnaires have been developed for patients who suffer from chronic pain and these incorporate scales to determine the patients' pain beliefs, expectations, coping skills together with analgesic use, as well as affective and intensity measures. There are book-length treatments of the subject of measurement selection in chronic pain,[115] as well as shorter articles and chapters.[116, 117] If pain intensity alone is to be evaluated, it is preferable to perform multiple measurements over time. As stated earlier, memory for pain is not as accurate as contemporary ratings, so the use of a "pain diary" utilizing categorical or analog scales at set times during the day is a more satisfactory way of recording pain during the day rather than estimating a daily average.

CANCER PAIN

The measurement of pain in patients with cancer can be more difficult than in those with benign disease. Multiple item measures of pain intensity (e.g. MPQ) are reliable, but it is believed that there is insufficient evidence concerning their validity in this type of pain.[118] The BPI may be a more appropriate tool,[62] and indeed NRSs for pain and function can be very valuable.[119] Mood disturbance and beliefs about the meaning of the pain in relation to the illness are known to be significant predictors of perceived pain intensity. Concerns about social and spiritual matters add to the complexity. In addition to the psychological distress of the cancer patient affecting pain measurement, several differing pain problems may coexist – for example acute nociceptive pain due to bone or visceral carcinoma, in conjunction with neuropathic pain from nerve root involvement. One must also bear in mind the pain induced by investigative and therapeutic processes which may add to any suffering. Detailed evaluation of pain intensity in these situations is pivotal to effective therapeutic decision-making.[120] Regular pain intensity measurements of each symptomatic site will then be necessary when titrating towards optimum analgesia, in keeping with individual patients needs. A full assessment of the patient with cancer would not be complete without an evaluation of all the factors which alter pain perception as well as its intensity, but this is beyond the scope of this chapter. Pain intensity measures are generally carried out by one of the scales mentioned above. The MPQ can be used during the initial assessment since it permits evaluation of various qualities of pain. The use of a pain diary is useful in this situation and may even help some patients to cope with their pain. The use of any pain rating scale in these circumstances should be perceived to be clinically relevant by the patient, family, and staff. Scoring by a trained observer using a 4–5 point categorical VRS may in fact be the most appropriate.

In patients suffering from persistent pain:

- any of the scales mentioned previously may be used;
- the assessment of psychological and behavioral factors often proves to be much more valuable than evaluating pain intensity alone;
- simple forms of pain assessment are the most appropriate if the patient is seriously ill or dying.

SERIAL MEASURES OF PAIN

The measurement of pain should be carried out at the time during which it is perceived, whenever possible. A single measurement is therefore like a "snapshot" of the pain intensity and as such may not reflect the pain experienced over a period of hours or days. A series of measurements carried out at regular time intervals can build up a better picture of the overall problem. The arithmetic sum of the scores over a set time can therefore provide an "area under the pain curve" against time value, e.g. for four VAS ratings of say 75, 55, 45, and 25 at three-hourly intervals, the sum of the VAS (SUMVAS) would be 200 over a nine-hour period. Another method is to determine the pain intensity difference (PID), at set times, from the original pain score and calculate the sum of these over a set time period, as shown in **Table 2.1**. A correction factor is applied to each PID, depending on the time difference between the current rating and the previous one – this gives a corrected "time-weighted" PID and the sum of these over the set time period provides the SPID. If pain relief is now assessed in a similar fashion the total pain relief (TOTPAR) can be calculated, as shown in **Table 2.2**.[121]

HANDLING AND INTERPRETING MEASUREMENT RESULTS

Data from pain intensity measures using ranked scales such as the VRS or the NRS may not be normally distributed and nonparametric tests, such as the Mann–Whitney U-test, are appropriate. The wide range of words available through the MPQ are normally assessed by nonparametric means although Melzack originally suggested that the t-test could be used to assess differences in mean pain scores.[59] Ratio scale data such as that derived

Table 2.1 The handling of serial measurements of pain over a period of time.

Time (hours)	Current pain score (A)	Initial pain score (B)	Pain intensity difference (B–A)	Correction factor	Corrected PID
0.5	2	3	1	0.5	0.5
1	1	3	2	0.5	1
2	1	3	2	1	2
3	2	3	1	1	1
4	3	3	0	1	0
Sum of pain intensity differences (SPID)					4.5
Maximum possible SPID[a]					12
Percentage of maximum possible pain intensity difference rating					37.5%

[a]Initial pain rating × number of hours over which ratings were recorded.

Table 2.2 If pain relief is now assessed in a similar fashion the total pain relief (TOTPAR) can be calculated.[121]

Time (hours)	Current pain Relief	Correction factor	Corrected score
0.5	2	0.5	1
1	3	0.5	1.5
2	3	1	3
3	2	1	2
4	1	1	1
TOTPAR			8.5
Maximum TOTPAR[a]			12
Percentage of maximum TOTPAR			70.83%

[a]Maximum relief score × time in hours.

from the VAS, although continuously variable, should also be tested by nonparametric means, such as the Wilcoxon ranked-sums test or Kruskal–Wallis one-way analysis of variance. Some statisticians suggest that arcsin or logistic transformation of the raw data leads to increased sensitivity at the extreme ends of the scale with a more normal distribution of results, thus making appropriate the use of the more powerful parametric tests such as the *t*-test, analysis of variance, or regression analysis.[122] Although parametric tests permit a much more flexible and powerful analysis to be carried out than the nonparametric methods, their power is reduced when data come from a non-normal distribution. Tests for normal distribution of data may be easily performed using standard statistical programs such as SPSS.

Establishing sample sizes for research purposes can be a difficult problem and it is often necessary to revert to methods using expressions assuming a normal distribution. The number of patients or subjects needed for a study will depend on the magnitude of change one wishes to detect and the variance of the observations. This information can be derived from previously published work or a pilot study. Sample size to achieve 90 percent

power at the 95 percent level of statistical significance can be estimated using the following formula:

$$n > 21 \times (S/d)^2 \text{ for independent samples}$$

(where S is the standard deviation of the observed data; d is the difference in the outcome measure to be detected, between individuals; n is the number of subjects per group).[122] When observations are made on paired data the same power and level of significance are achieved as above using the formula:

$$n > 10.5 \times (SD/d)^2 \text{ for paired samples}$$

(where SD is the standard deviation of the differences within subjects; d is the difference in the outcome measure to be detected, within each individual; n is the number of individuals, which will create pairs of observations). A power of 80 percent is calculated by replacing 21 with 15.8 and 10.5 with 7.9 in these formulae.

Determining the magnitude of a meaningful change is of prime importance in both the clinical and research situations. It is not only important in determining sample size but in evaluating the efficacy of treatment. Various ways of determining the change in magnitude which is considered meaningful have been proposed. These correspond to an approximate reduction in pain of 20 percent using an NRS in moderate postoperative pain.[123] An NRS may not be considered sensitive enough to detect supple changes, with a single category improvement on a pain relief scale exceeding the minimal clinical significance on a ten-point NRS.[124] Using a VAS in the acute moderate pain situation, a 27–29 percent change appears to equate with a meaningful change.[125] It is interesting to note that healthy adults rate pain intensity cut points for mild, moderate, and severe pain much as patients who are in pain, using VAS or NRS respectively.[125, 126] For chronic pain, several studies have suggested that a reduction of 30 percent appears clinically meaningful for many patients,[6, 127, 128, 129] although some have also used the more stringent cut-point of a 50 percent reduction. Furthermore, pain reduction is only one of a myriad of potentially meaningful outcomes for people with chronic pain and reductions in pain have been shown to have fairly weak relations with patient satisfaction with treatment.[130] Contemporary recommendations have identified a number of important outcome domains identified by pain sufferers which often include an assessment of whether treatment has aided in the improvement of functioning and quality of life, which may be useful additional measures of clinical effect.[6, 130, 131]

CONCLUDING REMARKS

There are a variety of methods by which pain intensity can be assessed, each having limitations and advantages. Self-report scales have established psychometric properties and are the metric of choice whenever possible, particularly as ratings of observers tend to differ from patients. Ratings of observers, however, may be useful in providing adjunctive information, particularly when the observer is a caregiver of the one in pain or has an established history of close contact (e.g. parents). The specific scale to be used depends to a large extent on the setting and purposes for which it is used. A single-item VAS may be the most appropriate for rapid assessment of the effects of titrating analgesia in acute or hospital settings, whereas a more comprehensive measure might be most appropriate for initial assessment and treatment selection. Regardless of the measure that is used, it seems prudent to keep in mind the complex and multi-dimensional nature of pain, which will affect even the simplest of single-item pain measures.

Pain intensity measures are also a useful metric by which to evaluate treatment effectiveness, particular those in which pain reduction is a primary goal. When assessing response within a single patient (across time or different treatment), raw pain scores can be used, however, when collapsing data across multiple patients, it is advisable to convert scores to a ratio (e.g. a percentage change) from the original baseline score in each individual, given that many scales have ratio, not continuous, properties.

The vast majority of measures available were normed on adults samples, thus care must be exercised when using these measures with children and older individuals. There are now a fair number of specific measures for use in these populations and it is advised that these specific measures be used whenever feasible.

Finally, the experience of pain is exceedingly common and is often correctly referred to as a ubiquitous human experience. The ability to accurately assess and interpret pain ratings is a foundational skill for many who are involved in health care. It is our hope that the preceding paragraphs will be of use to those involved in this area and will facilitate the effective treatment of those experiencing, and all to often suffering from, significant pain.

REFERENCES

1. Todd KH, Ducharme J, Choiniere M et al. Pain in the emergency department: results of the pain and emergency medicine initiative (PEMI) multicenter study. Journal of Pain. 2007; 8: 460–6.
2. Tcherny-Lessenot S, Karwowski-Soulie F, Lamarche-Vadel A et al. Management and relief of pain in an emergency department from the adult patients' perspective. Journal of Pain and Symptom Management. 2003; 25: 539–46.
3. Prkachin KM, Solomon PE, Ross J. Underestimation of pain by health-care providers: towards a model of the process of inferring pain in others. Canadian Journal of Nursing Research. 2007; 39: 88–106.
4. Kappesser J, Williams AC, Prkachin KM. Testing two accounts of pain underestimation. Pain. 2006; 124: 109–16.
* 5. Melzack R, Wall PD. The challenge of pain, 2nd edn. London: Penguin, 1988.
* 6. Dworkin RH, Turk DC, Farrar JT et al. Core outcome measures for chronic pain clinical trials: IMMPACT recommendations. Pain. 2005; 113: 9–19.
* 7. Jensen MP, Karoly P. Self-report scales and procedures for assessing pain in adults. In: Turk DC, Melzack D (eds). Handbook of pain assessment, 2nd edn. New York: Guilford Press, 2001: 15–34.
* 8. Melzack R, Torgerson WS. On the language of pain. Anesthesiology. 1971; 34: 50–9.
* 9. Beecher HK. Relationship of significance of wound to pain experienced. Journal of the American Medical Association. 1956; 161: 1609–13.
10. Beecher HK. Pain in men wounded in battle. Annals of Surgery. 1946; 123: 96–105.
* 11. Riley 3rd JL, Robinson ME, Wise EA et al. Sex differences in the perception of noxious experimental stimuli: a meta-analysis. Pain. 1998; 74: 181–7.
12. Greenspan JD, Craft RM, LeResche L et al. Studying sex and gender differences in pain and analgesia: a consensus report. Pain. 2007; 132: S26–45.
13. Rahim-Williams FB, Riley 3rd JL, Herrera D et al. Ethnic identity predicts experimental pain sensitivity in African Americans and Hispanics. Pain. 2007; 129: 177–84.
14. Campbell CM, Edwards RR, Fillingim RB. Ethnic differences in responses to multiple experimental pain stimuli. Pain. 2005; 113: 20–6.
15. Edwards RR, Doleys DM, Fillingim RB, Lowery D. Ethnic differences in pain tolerance: clinical implications in a chronic pain population. Psychosomatic Medicine. 2001; 63: 316–23.
16. Riley 3rd JL, Wade JB, Myers CD et al. Racial/ethnic differences in the experience of chronic pain. Pain. 2002; 100: 291–8.
* 17. Cintron A, Morrison RS. Pain and ethnicity in the United States: A systematic review. Journal of Palliative Medicine. 2006; 9: 1454–73.
18. Rhudy JL, Meagher MW. Noise stress and human pain thresholds: divergent effects in men and women. Journal of Pain. 2001; 2: 57–64.

* 19. Klossika I, Flor H, Kamping S et al. Emotional modulation of pain: a clinical perspective. Pain. 2006; 124: 264–8.

20. Toth J. Old weather sayings are rational – and here's their rationale. Science Digestest. 1979; 50: 70–3.

21. Shutty Jr MS, Cundiff G, DeGood DE. Pain complaint and the weather: weather sensitivity and symptom complaints in chronic pain patients. Pain. 1992; 49: 199–204.

22. Folkard S, Glynn CJ, Lloyd JW. Diurnal variation and individual differences in the perception of intractable pain. Journal of Psychosomatic Research. 1976; 20: 289–301.

23. Jamison RN, Raymond SA, Slawsby EA et al. Pain assessment in patients with low back pain: comparison of weekly recall and momentary electronic data. Journal of Pain. 2006; 7: 192–9.

24. Hunter M, Philips C, Rachman S. Memory for pain. Pain. 1979; 6: 35–46.

* 25. Williams DA, Park KM, Ambrose KR, Clauw DJ. Assessor status influences pain recall. Journal of Pain. 2007; 8: 343–8.

26. Kikuchi H, Yoshiuchi K, Miyasaka N et al. Reliability of recalled self-report on headache intensity: investigation using ecological momentary assessment technique. Cephalalgia. 2006; 26: 1335–43.

27. Stone AA, Schwartz JE, Broderick JE, Shiffman SS. Variability of momentary pain predicts recall of weekly pain: a consequence of the peak (or salience) memory heuristic. Personality and Social Psychology Bulletin. 2005; 31: 1340–6.

28. Brauer C, Thomsen JF, Loft IP, Mikkelsen S. Can we rely on retrospective pain assessments?. American Journal of Epidemiology. 2003; 157: 552–7.

29. Stone AA, Broderick JE, Shiffman SS, Schwartz JE. Understanding recall of weekly pain from a momentary assessment perspective: absolute agreement, between- and within-person consistency, and judged change in weekly pain. Pain. 2004; 107: 61–9.

30. Ekblom A, Hansson P. Pain intensity measurements in patients with acute pain receiving afferent stimulation. Journal of Neurology, Neurosurgery, and Psychiatry. 1988; 51: 481–6.

31. Kent G. Memory of dental pain. Pain. 1985; 21: 187–94.

* 32. Feine JS, Lavigne GJ, Dao TT et al. Memories of chronic pain and perceptions of relief. Pain. 1998; 77: 137–41.

* 33. Gedney JJ, Logan H. Pain related recall predicts future pain report. Pain. 2006; 121: 69–76.

34. Jamison RN, Gracely RH, Raymond SA et al. Comparative study of electronic vs. paper VAS ratings: a randomized, crossover trial using healthy volunteers. Pain. 2002; 99: 341–7.

35. Burton C, Weller D, Sharpe M. Are electronic diaries useful for symptoms research? A systematic review. Journal of Psychosomatic Research. 2007; 62: 553–61.

36. Cook AJ, Roberts DA, Henderson MD et al. Electronic pain questionnaires: a randomized, crossover comparison with paper questionnaires for chronic pain assessment. Pain. 2004; 110: 310–17.

37. Jamison RN, Fanciullo GJ, Baird JC. Computerized dynamic assessment of pain: comparison of chronic pain patients and healthy controls. Pain Medicine. 2004; 5: 168–77.

* 38. Dannecker EA, George SZ, Robinson ME. Influence and stability of pain scale anchors for an investigation of cold pressor pain tolerance. Journal of Pain. 2007; 8: 476–82.

39. Robinson ME, George SZ, Dannecker EA et al. Sex differences in pain anchors revisited: further investigation of "most intense" and common pain events. European Journal of Pain. 2004; 8: 299–305.

40. Williams ACdC. Simple pain rating scales hide complex idiosyncratic meanings. Pain. 2000; 85: 457–63.

41. Seymour RA, Simpson JM, Charlton JE, Phillips ME. An evaluation of length and end-phrase of visual analogue scales in dental pain. Pain. 1985; 21: 177–85.

42. Lund I, Lundeberg T, Sandberg L et al. Lack of interchangeability between visual analogue and verbal rating pain scales: a cross sectional description of pain etiology groups. BMC Medical Research Methodology. 2005; 5: 31.

* 43. Dworkin RH, Turk DC, Wyrwich KW et al. Interpreting the clinical importance of treatment outcomes in chronic pain clinical trials: IMMPACT recommendations. Journal of Pain. 2008; 9: 105–21.

44. Jensen MP, Turner JA, Romano JM. What is the maximum number of levels needed in pain intensity measurement?. Pain. 1994; 58: 387–92.

* 45. Nicholas MK, Asghari A, Blyth FM. What do the numbers mean? Normative data in chronic pain measures. Pain. 2008; 134: 158–73.

46. Price DD, Bush FM, Long S, Harkins SW. A comparison of pain measurement characteristics of mechanical visual analogue and simple numerical rating scales. Pain. 1994; 56: 217–26.

47. Melzack R, Katz J. The McGill Pain Questionnaire: Appraisal and current status. In: Turk DC (ed.). Handbook of pain assessment, 2nd edn. New York: Guilford Press, 2001: 35–52.

* 48. Jensen MP, Karoly P, Braver S. The measurement of clinical pain intensity: a comparison of six methods. Pain. 1986; 27: 117–26.

49. Frank AJ, Moll JM, Hort JF. A comparison of three ways of measuring pain. Rheumatology and Rehabilitation. 1982; 21: 211–17.

* 50. Price DD, Harkins SW. Psychophysical approaches to measurement of the dimensions and stages of pain. In: Turk DC, Melzack D (eds). Handbook of pain assessment, 2nd edn. New York: Guilford Press, 2001: 53–75.

51. Freyd M. The graphic rating scale. Journal of Educational Psychology. 1923; 43: 83–102.

* 52. Aitken RC. Measurement of feelings using visual analogue scales. Proceedings of the Royal Society of Medicine. 1969; 62: 989–93.

53. Herr KA, Spratt K, Mobily PR, Richardson G. Pain intensity assessment in older adults: use of experimental pain to compare psychometric properties and usability of selected

pain scales with younger adults. *Clinical Journal of Pain.* 2004; **20**: 207–19.

54. Williamson A, Hoggart B. Pain: a review of three commonly used pain rating scales. *Journal of Clinical Nursing.* 2005; **14**: 798–804.

55. Huskisson EC. Measurement of pain. *Journal of Rheumatology.* 1982; **9**: 768–9.

∗ 56. Bieri D, Reeve RA, Champion GD *et al.* The Faces Pain Scale for the self-assessment of the severity of pain experienced by children: development, initial validation, and preliminary investigation for ratio scale properties. *Pain.* 1990; **41**: 139–50.

∗ 57. Hicks CL, von Baeyer CL, Spafford PA *et al.* The Faces Pain Scale-Revised: toward a common metric in pediatric pain measurement. *Pain.* 2001; **93**: 173–83.

58. McGrath PA, Seifert CE, Speechley KN *et al.* A new analogue scale for assessing children's pain: an initial validation study. *Pain.* 1996; **64**: 435–43.

∗ 59. Melzack R. The McGill Pain Questionnaire: major properties and scoring methods. *Pain.* 1975; **1**: 277–99.

60. Klepac RK, Dowling J, Rokke P *et al.* Interview vs paper-and-pencil administration of the McGill Pain Questionnaire. *Pain.* 1981; **11**: 241–6.

∗ 61. Melzack R. The short-form McGill Pain Questionnaire. *Pain.* 1987; **30**: 191–7.

∗ 62. Cleeland CS, Ryan KM. Pain assessment: global use of the Brief Pain Inventory. *Annals of the Academy of Medicine, Singapore.* 1994; **23**: 129–38.

∗ 63. Tan G, Jensen MP, Thornby JI, Shanti BF. Validation of the Brief Pain Inventory for chronic nonmalignant pain. *Journal of Pain.* 2004; **5**: 133–7.

64. Mendoza T, Mayne T, Rublee D, Cleeland C. Reliability and validity of a modified Brief Pain Inventory short form in patients with osteoarthritis. *European Journal of Pain.* 2006; **10**: 353–61.

65. Gammaitoni AR, Galer BS, Lacouture P *et al.* Effectiveness and safety of new oxycodone/acetaminophen formulations with reduced acetaminophen for the treatment of low back pain. *Pain Medicine.* 2003; **4**: 21–30.

66. Jensen MP, Ehde DM, Hoffman AJ *et al.* Cognitions, coping and social environment predict adjustment to phantom limb pain. *Pain.* 2002; **95**: 133–42.

67. Semenchuk MR, Sherman S, Davis B. Double-blind, randomized trial of bupropion SR for the treatment of neuropathic pain. *Neurology.* 2001; **57**: 1583–8.

68. Mendoza TR, Chen C, Brugger A *et al.* The utility and validity of the modified brief pain inventory in a multiple-dose postoperative analgesic trial. *Clinical Journal of Pain.* 2004; **20**: 357–62.

69. Su L, Tucker R, Frey SE *et al.* Measuring injection-site pain associated with vaccine administration in adults: a randomised, double-blind, placebo-controlled clinical trial. *Journal of Epidemiology and Biostatistics.* 2000; **5**: 359–65.

70. Evans S, Fishman B, Spielman L, Haley A. Randomized trial of cognitive behavior therapy versus supportive psychotherapy for HIV-related peripheral neuropathic pain. *Psychosomatics.* 2003; **44**: 44–50.

71. Smith MY, Egert J, Winkel G, Jacobson J. The impact of PTSD on pain experience in persons with HIV/AIDS. *Pain.* 2002; **98**: 9–17.

∗ 72. Turk DC, Dworkin RH, Allen RR *et al.* Core outcome domains for chronic pain clinical trials: IMMPACT recommendations. *Pain.* 2003; **106**: 337–45.

73. Caraceni A, Cherny N, Fainsinger R *et al.* Pain measurement tools and methods in clinical research in palliative care: recommendations of an Expert Working Group of the European Association of Palliative Care. *Journal of Pain and Symptom Management.* 2002; **23**: 239–55.

74. Saxena A, Mendoza T, Cleeland CS. The assessment of cancer pain in north India: the validation of the Hindi Brief Pain Inventory – BPI-H. *Journal of Pain and Symptom Management.* 1999; **17**: 27–41.

75. Cleeland CS, Nakamura Y, Mendoza TR *et al.* Dimensions of the impact of cancer pain in a four country sample: new information from multidimensional scaling. *Pain.* 1996; **67**: 267–73.

76. Kerns RD, Turk DC, Rudy TE. The West Haven-Yale Multidimensional Pain Inventory (WHYMPI). *Pain.* 1985; **23**: 345–56.

77. Jacob MC, Kerns RD. Assessment of the psychosocial context of the experience of chronic pain. In: Turk DC, Melzack D (eds). *Handbook of pain assessment,* 2nd edn. New York: Elsevier, 2001: 362–84.

∗ 78. Hopwood CJ, Creech SK, Clark TS *et al.* The convergence and predictive validity of the multidimensional pain inventory and the personality assessment inventory among individuals with chronic pain. *Rehabilitation Psychology.* 2007; **52**: 443–50.

79. Turk DC, Rudy TE. The robustness of an empirically derived taxonomy of chronic pain patients. *Pain.* 1990; **43**: 27–35.

80. Soderlund A, Denison E. Classification of patients with whiplash associated disorders (WAD): Reliable and valid subgroups based on the Multidimensional Pain Inventory (MPI-S). *European Journal of Pain.* 2006; **10**: 113–19.

81. Greco CM, Rudy TE, Manzi S. Adaptation to chronic pain in systemic lupus erythematosus: Applicability of the multidimensional pain inventory. *Pain Medicine.* 2003; **4**: 39–50.

82. Ware JE, Sherbourne CD. The MOS 36-item short-form health survey (SF-36). 1. Conceptual-framework and item selection. *Medical Care.* 1992; **30**: 473–83.

83. Bullinger M, Alonso J, Apolone G *et al.* Translating health status questionnaires and evaluating their quality: the IQOLA Project approach. International Quality of Life Assessment. *Journal of Clinical Epidemiology.* 1998; **51**: 913–23.

84. Gandek B, Ware Jr JE, Aaronson NK *et al.* Tests of data quality, scaling assumptions, and reliability of the SF-36 in eleven countries: results from the IQOLA Project. International Quality of Life Assessment. *Journal of Clinical Epidemiology.* 1998; **51**: 1149–58.

85. Wagner AK, Gandek B, Aaronson NK *et al*. Cross-cultural comparisons of the content of SF-36 translations across 10 countries: results from the IQOLA Project. International Quality of Life Assessment. *Journal of Clinical Epidemiology.* 1998; **51**: 925–32.

86. Keller SD, Ware Jr JE, Gandek B *et al*. Testing the equivalence of translations of widely used response choice labels: results from the IQOLA Project. International Quality of Life Assessment. *Journal of Clinical Epidemiology.* 1998; **51**: 933–44.

87. Clark ME, Gironda RJ, Young RW. Development and validation of the Pain Outcomes Questionnaire-VA. *Journal of Rehabilitation Research and Development.* 2003; **40**: 381–95.

88. Clark ME, Bair MJ, Buckenmaier 3rd CC *et al*. Pain and combat injuries in soldiers returning from Operations Enduring Freedom and Iraqi Freedom: implications for research and practice. *Journal of Rehabilitation Research and Development.* 2007; **44**: 179–94.

89. Schatman M, Campbell A. Innovations in outcomes assessment in pain management. *Pain Practice.* 2004; **14**: 6–8.

∗ 90. Cohen LL, Lemanek K, Blount RL *et al*. Evidence-based assessment of pediatric pain. *Journal of Pediatric Psychology.* 2007.

∗ 91. von Baeyer CL, Spagrud LJ. Systematic review of observational (behavioral) measures of pain for children and adolescents aged 3 to 18 years. *Pain.* 2007; **127**: 140–50.

∗ 92. McGrath PA. An assessment of children's pain: a review of behavioral, physiological and direct scaling techniques. *Pain.* 1987; **31**: 147–76.

93. Merkel SI, Voepel-Lewis T, Shayevitz JR, Malviya S. The FLACC: a behavioral scale for scoring postoperative pain in young children. *Pediatric Nursing.* 1997; **23**: 293–7.

94. McGrath PJ, Johnson G, Goodman JT *et al*. CHEOPS: A behavioral scale for rating postoperative pain in children. In: Fields HL, Dubner R, Cervero F (eds). *Advances in pain research and therapy.* New York: Raven Press, 1985: 395–402.

∗ 95. Chambers CT, Reid GJ, McGrath PJ, Finley GA. Development and preliminary validation of a postoperative pain measure for parents. *Pain.* 1996; **68**: 307–13.

96. Ambuel B, Hamlett KW, Marx CM, Blumer JL. Assessing distress in pediatric intensive care environments: the COMFORT scale. *Journal of Pediatric Psychology.* 1992; **17**: 95–109.

97. von Baeyer CL. Children's self-reports of pain intensity: scale selection, limitations and interpretation. *Pain Research and Management.* 2006; **11**: 157–62.

∗ 98. Finley GA, McGrath PJ. Introduction: The roles of measurement in pain management and research. In: Finley GA, McGrath PJ (eds). *Measurement of pain in infants and children, progress in pain research and management.* Seattle, WA: International Association for the Study of Pain, 1998: 1–4.

99. Blount RL, Piira T, Cohen LL, Cheng PS. Pediatric procedural pain. *Behav Behavior Nodification.* 2006; **30**: 24–49.

100. Beyer JE, Denyes MJ, Villarruel AM. The creation, validation, and continuing development of the Oucher: A measure of pain intensity in children. *Journal of Pediatric Nursing.* 1992; **7**: 335–46.

101. Von Baeyer CL. Children's self-reports of pain intensity: scale selection, limitations and interpretation. *Pain Research and Management.* 2006; **11**: 157–62.

102. Eccleston C, Jordan AL, Crombez G. The impact of chronic pain on adolescents: a review of previously used measures. *Journal of Pediatric Psychology.* 2006; **31**: 684–97.

103. Jordan A, Eccleston C, Crombez G. Parental functioning in the context of adolescent chronic pain: A review of previously used measures. *Journal of Pediatric Psychology.* 2008; **33**: 640–59.

104. Barsky AJ. Forgetting, fabricating, and telescoping: the instability of the medical history. *Archives of Internal Medicine.* 2002; **162**: 981–4.

105. Pare M, Albrecht PJ, Noto CJ *et al*. Differential hypertrophy and atrophy among all types of cutaneous innervation in the glabrous skin of the monkey hand during aging and naturally occurring type 2 diabetes. *Journal of Comparative Neurology.* 2007; **501**: 543–67.

106. Gibson SJ, Helme RD. Age differences in pain perception and report: a review of physiological, psychological, laboratory and clinical studies. *Pain Reviews.* 1995; **2**: 111–37.

107. Jacobs JM, Love S. Qualitative and quantitative morphology of human sural nerve at different ages. *Brain.* 1985; **108**: 897–924.

108. Gescheider GA, Beiles EJ, Checkosky CM *et al*. The effects of aging on information-processing channels in the sense of touch: II. Temporal summation in the P channel. *Somatosensory and Motor Research.* 1994; **11**: 359–65.

109. Farrell M, Gibson S. Age interacts with stimulus frequency in the temporal summation of pain. *Pain Medicine.* 2007; **8**: 514–20.

110. Woodrow KM, Friedman GD, Siegelaub AB *et al*. Pain tolerance: differences according to age, sex and race. *Psychosomatic Medicine.* 1972; **34**: 548–56.

111. Miro J, Huguet A, Nieto R *et al*. Evaluation of reliability, validity, and preference for a pain intensity scale for use with the elderly. *Journal of Pain.* 2005; **6**: 727–35.

112. Kim EJ, Buschmann MT. Reliability and validity of the Faces Pain Scale with older adults. *International Journal of Nursing Studies.* 2006; **43**: 447–56.

113. Ferrell BA, Stein WM, Beck JC. The Geriatric Pain Measure: validity, reliability and factor analysis. *Journal of the American Geriatrics Society.* 2000; **48**: 1669–73.

114. Blozik E, Stuck AE, Niemann S *et al*. Geriatric Pain Measure short form: development and initial evaluation. *Journal of the American Geriatrics Society.* 2007; **55**: 2045–50.

∗115. Turk DC, Melzack R. *Handbook of pain assessment,* 2nd edn. New York: Elsevier, 2001.

116. Williams AC. Outcome assessment in chronic non-cancer pain treatment. *Acta Anaesthesiologica Scandinavica.* 2001; **45**: 1076–9.

*117. Vowles KE, Gross RT, McCracken LM. Evaluating outcomes in the interdisciplinary treatment of chronic pain: A guide for practicing clinicians. In: Schatman M, Campbell A (eds). *Chronic pain management: guidelines for multidisciplinary program development.* New York: Informa, 2007: 203–20.

*118. Jensen MP. The validity and reliability of pain measures in adults with cancer. *Journal of Pain.* 2003; **4**: 2–21.

119. Serlin RC, Mendoza TR, Nakamura Y *et al.* When is cancer pain mild, moderate or severe? Grading pain severity by its interference with function. *Pain.* 1995; **61**: 277–84.

120. Cherry NI, Portenoy RK. Cancer pain: Pinciples of assessment and syndromes. In: Wall PD, Melzack R (eds). *Textbook of pain.* New York: Churchill Livingstone, 1994: 787–823.

121. Max MB, Laska EM. Single-dose analgesic comparisons. In: Max MB, Portenory RK (eds). *The design of analgesic clinical trials. Advances in pain research and therapy.* New York: Raven Press, 1991: 55–95.

*122. Armitage P. *Statistical methods in medical research.* Oxford: Blackwell Scientific Publications, 1977.

*123. Cepeda MS, Africano JM, Polo R *et al.* What decline in pain intensity is meaningful to patients with acute pain?. *Pain.* 2003; **105**: 151–7.

124. Bernstein SL, Bijur PE, Gallagher EJ. Relationship between intensity and relief in patients with acute severe pain. *American Journal of Emergency Medicine.* 2006; **24**: 162–6.

125. Campbell WI, Patterson CC. Quantifying meaningful changes in pain. *Anaesthesia.* 1998; **53**: 121–5.

126. Palos GR, Mendoza TR, Mobley GM *et al.* Asking the community about cutpoints used to describe mild, moderate, and severe pain. *Journal of Pain.* 2006; **7**: 49–56.

127. Ostelo RW, Deyo RA, Stratford P *et al.* Interpreting change scores for pain and functional status in low back pain: towards international consensus regarding minimal important change. *Spine.* 2008; **33**: 90–4.

128. Farrar JT, Portenoy RK, Berlin JA *et al.* Defining the clinically important difference in pain outcome measures. *Pain.* 2000; **88**: 287–94.

*129. Farrar JT, Young Jr JP, LaMoreaux L *et al.* Clinical importance of changes in chronic pain intensity measured on an 11-point numerical pain rating scale. *Pain.* 2001; **94**: 149–58.

*130. McCracken LM, Evon D, Karapas ET. Satisfaction with treatment for chronic pain in a specialty service: preliminary prospective results. *European Journal of Pain.* 2002; **6**: 387–93.

*131. Turk DC, Dworkin RH, Revicki D *et al.* Identifying important outcome domains for chronic pain clinical trials: An IMMPACT survey of people with pain. *Pain.* in press.

3

Selecting and applying pain measures

JOHANNES VAN DER MERWE AND AMANDA C DE C WILLIAMS

KEY LEARNING POINTS

- Clarity on the aims of treatment is essential before selecting outcome measures.
- The range of available measures associated with pain treatment is bewildering, since the effects of pain are so far reaching.
- The choice of measures is a compromise between content, psychometric qualities, and demands on the responder.
- Content can be guided by defining domains of outcome; commonly in pain management these approximate to:
  - pain;
  - physical functioning;
  - emotional and cognitive functioning;
    - social and occupational function;
    - participant ratings of impact of treatment;
    - other symptoms and adverse events.
- Psychometric qualities of measures must be understood for valid interpretation.
- The psychometric properties of a measure, reliability, validity, and sensitivity to change, are not unconditional qualities of the measure but describe its performance in particular conditions of population, time, and extent of change.
- There will inevitably be important psychological variance in outcome which is not captured by standard measures selected.

INTRODUCTION

The range of possible measures associated with pain treatment can be bewildering, since the effects of pain are so far reaching. While the aims of assessment (such as diagnosis) or treatment should determine the choice of measures, and they certainly provide the basis, there is still huge choice among pain-specific or general measurement instruments, long-established or more recently developed, broad scope or narrow focus. Eventually the choice is often made pragmatically, guided by recommendations from fellow clinicians, and by practical considerations such as length. In this process, important considerations may be lost, and this chapter aims to help

to address those to enable the reader to make a more confident choice of what best suits the evaluation in hand.

The first major area is that of domains of outcome: measures should be straightforward to interpret with reference to the aims and methods of treatment. Many evaluations of acute and of chronic pain problems rely heavily or solely on pain as an outcome, even where it is acknowledged that changing pain is not the main or sole target of treatment. Some broad measures (such as quality of life) appear to promise almost a panacea to measurement problems, but a total score can be no more than the sum of its constituent item scores, interpreted according to data on its use in the real world, with all the limitations of those data. An appreciation of the conceptual basis of any measurement domain, and of unresolved conceptual problems which are inevitably represented in measures which arise from them, engenders a critical and strong interpretation of study results.

The second major area is that of the psychometric qualities of measures, appreciation of which provides an aid to their interpretation. Distinguishing true from error variance is like detecting the signal against a background of noise, so that choosing a less noisy instrument, and recognizing that in a different location (population) it may pick up different noise, provides more confident identification of the signal, such as variance due to treatment. The section on psychometric qualities of measures (see Quality of measures and interpretation of their output), which is not exhaustive but covers the most common areas of concern, also incorporates a short section on definition of clinically significant change.

A comprehensive guide to measures requires not a chapter but a book; two are repeatedly recommended (Turk and Melzack[1] and McDowell and Newell[2]), as are the output of the Initiative on Methods, Measurement, and Pain Assessment in Clinical Trials (IMMPACT) project, and other chapters in these volumes (see Chapter 8, Assessment, measurement, and history in the *Acute Pain* volume; Chapter 10, The psychological assessment of pain in patients with chronic pain in the *Chronic Pain* volume; Chapter 14, Outcome measurement in chronic pain in the *Chronic Pain* volume; and Chapter 2, Practical methods for pain intensity measurements).[3] During the IMMPACT initiative, 27 specialists from academia, governmental agencies, and the pharmaceutical industry participated in a consensus meeting and identified core outcome domains that should be considered in clinical trials of treatments for chronic pain. There was a consensus that chronic pain clinical trials should assess outcomes representing six core domains: (1) pain, (2) physical functioning, (3) emotional functioning, (4) participant ratings of improvement and satisfaction with treatment, (5) symptoms and adverse events, and (6) participant disposition.[3] The project is important, not least for its attempt to propose common metrics across a wide range of treatment modalities.

There is no short answer with adequate scientific credibility to the question of what is the "success rate" in a single study of a treatment for pain. Attempts at evaluation require time and effort from patients, clinicians, and researchers, and the guidelines in this chapter aim to make their investment as productive as possible by judicious choice, analysis, and interpretation of measures.

CONTENT OF MEASURES AND CONSIDERATIONS FOR THEIR SELECTION

The outcomes to be assessed are effectively determined by the aims of treatment, and may also be required by methods of treatment. However, the statement of treatment aims is often rather narrow (e.g. pain relief), leaving implicit the associated gains which are often listed as part of the rationale for trying to improve pain treatment: mood, function, activity, overall quality of life, greater independence in health care. For this reason, it can be helpful to use a short checklist of outcome domains, to ensure that relevant outcomes are covered. Most clinicians and patients embark on treatment with multiple aims, usually, but not necessarily, reductions in pain experience and healthcare use, and improvements in activity levels, mood and well-being, and physical state. Despite mutual influence among these areas, it is not the case that improvement in one domain implies proportional improvements in all others. So, outcome measurement requires attention to as many of these domains as are targets of treatment. Measurement of associated variables, which are not targeted by treatment but are relevant to understanding outcome data, is worth a brief reminder, since it is surprisingly often overlooked. For instance, in trials of a new drug in a family with marked adverse effects on a minority of users, data on previous use and reactions among those in the trial sample is important.

Method of measurement

An important consideration is that of sampling method used in the measures available. If the target of assessment is what a person feels (symptom, mood, experience), then it can only be sampled by self-report. If the target of assessment is what a person does, then either self-report or direct measurement are options. Self-report is the common choice, as substantial practical obstacles may be presented by prolonged observation, or difficulties in obtaining independent sources of relevant information (such as work or health records). This is not a problem where the selected self-report measure is well validated, as described below, but in some current instruments the "gold standard" used for validation was simply a longer-established self-report measure, not infrequently developed using both concepts and psychometric methods which have been superseded as our understanding improves – perhaps a "fool's gold" standard. Behavioral measures are generally underused in the health field, surprisingly in pain treatment where several of the major targets of pain treatment are behavioral: increased activity in general, return to work or other improvement in work activities, greater independence in health care resulting in less use of health and disability-related resources. However, self-report and observation measure separate but related aspects of the behavior of interest; they cannot be expected to be perfectly correlated.[4, 5]

Domains of outcome

One of the most frequently asked questions concerning outcome of pain treatment, particularly in chronic pain, is whether there is not a single, simple measure of treatment success. If there were, it would be of enormous benefit to patients, pain treatment staff, and those who fund treatment. But can pain treatment ever have a single relevant outcome? Even the briefest assessment of experimentally produced pain in healthy subjects must address the multiple dimensions of pain. So when subjects are clinical patients, with some degree of interference by pain in their lives, a single outcome is inconceivable.

There are many possible ways of grouping possible outcomes: here, the broad domains of biomedical variables, psychosocial variables, and behavior and function are used as headings; further distinctions are made between domains derived in a meta-analysis of cognitive-behavioral therapy (CBT) for chronic pain in adults, also applicable to children.[6]

BIOMEDICAL DOMAINS

Biomedical assessment tends to be most specific to the symptom or problem, except for pain itself, and is covered in Chapter 11, Assessment of the patient with neuropathic pain and Chapter 12, Diagnostic procedures in chronic pain, both in the *Chronic Pain* volume of this series. The critical reader may wish to investigate further some of the statements about reliability and validity and the population/s within which those parameters were established. Interrogation of interrater (and even intrarater) reliability for reading x-rays and quantifying clinical examination findings has revealed widespread shortcomings.[7, 8] Some measures of disease processes, of performance in clinical tests, or in general use (e.g. aerobic capacity), may show good reliability but may lack the validation and comparison data that is required to render them interpretable in pain populations, that is, they may be poor proxies for everyday function and mobility.[7] Such measures may be of interest in their own right, or they may be used to investigate what variance they explain in the overall function of the patient. In some cases, they belie the use of an outdated model which attempts to predict pain from extent of physical pathology.

Pain experience incorporates multiple dimensions of pain, variously described. The simplest classification is three-fold: as sensory or discriminative, affective (emotional) and cognitive, and behavioral (interference), and spans several domains of measurement. Although not easily separable, there is good evidence for attempting to do so in experimental and clinical settings.[9] While intensity may not change at all, the meaning of the pain to the individual can change, and with it, behavior, emotions, and others' responses (see Chapter 15, Contextual cognitive-behavioral therapy). A single or global pain rating represents pain dimensions in unknown quantities, and probably in combinations which vary between patients and across assessment contexts, obscuring their meaning. More detailed consideration of the advantages and disadvantages of particular pain measurement techniques and instruments can be found in Chapter 2, Practical methods for pain intensity measurements.

Pain relief is at last being studied to ascertain better its meaning to patients who use it. By far the most common pain relief outcome criterion is 50 percent, which has considerable face validity, provides a ratio scale for analysis, and has been refined to provide a cumulative measure.[10] However, the 50 percent criterion does not arise from studies either of patients' stated goals or of changes in target behaviors in relation to pain relief, and there are indications that in relation to behavioral change it may be higher than necessary. For instance, a study which compared cancer patients' ratings of breakthrough pain and pain relief after an analgesic with their request for further analgesic found that nearer 30 percent pain relief sufficed.[11] While they interpret this conservatively, since other variables affect patients' willingness to ask for analgesia, it suggests the need to examine pain relief criteria further, and demonstrates a more patient-based and clinically useful approach to measuring analgesic effectiveness than is often used.

Other symptoms which are inherently unpleasant and impact on quality of life, such as fatigue, nausea, and numbness, may also be important to assess, particularly in chronic illness such as cancer or where they may occur as adverse effects of treatment. They can be measured by the same methods as pain.

PSYCHOSOCIAL DOMAINS

Psychosocial variables include separate although often related areas – affect, cognitive content and process, and coping – which cannot be represented by a single measure. What the measures share is that the latent constructs to which they refer are hypothetical, dependent on their definitions and therefore on their theoretical origins, and representing a late conscious phase of complex non-conscious processes. Because most have heuristic value, they take on a meaning beyond the limits of their definitions and origins which confounds their interpretation (see Chapter 2, Practical methods for pain intensity measurements). Particular examples of the over-interpretation of constructs represented by measures whose total can be no more than the sum of their items, answered without reference to context or consequences, are those of pain behavior and of coping (see below under Behavior and activity). Assigning numbers to extent of agreement with a statement or degrees of intensity of an emotion does not mean that the construct is linear and distinct from related constructs. Some of the issues of importance to patients' welfare may be better addressed by sensitive open-ended questioning, responses to which can at best be categorized.

Affect or emotion measured in pain studies includes constructs such as depression, anxiety, anger, or, more broadly, distress or negative and positive affect. The possible list of overlapping terms for emotions is a long one, and those terms tend to draw heavily on psychiatric and personality psychology models, where more normal psychology, particularly cognitive psychology, probably offers more appropriate ones. Anxiety may be more helpfully construed in terms of worry and specific fears; depression in terms of a distress related to impact of pain on the patient's life, negative view of the self, and functional and physical disturbance.[12, 13, 14] Positive emotion (well-being, happiness) is often overlooked, although it may provide better measurement of mood improvement than depression and anxiety measures. Patients may describe their emotions in terms such as frustration for which there is no psychological model or measure. For this reason, simple numerical or visual analog ratings scales for emotions can be appropriate and are represented in some quality of life measures.[2]

Like pain, emotions have no unequivocal referents for validation: all have – and share – correlates in overt behavior, physiology, cortical and subcortical activity. Comparison with psychiatric diagnosis, with which the measures share a theoretical framework, is common but problematic. Anxiety and depression show systematic differences from their parent constructs in psychiatry. Generalized anxiety has proved much less relevant in experimental and clinical pain than pain-related fear, and several fear measures have recently been developed.[13, 15] In depression or depressed mood, drawing on a psychiatric model produced measures with somatic items which, unlike in psychiatric populations, are often preferentially endorsed by patients in pain. The only measures of cognitive content (such as self-blame, guilt, sense of punishment) and affective content (such as feeling sad, loss of interest, feeling hopeless) without somatic items, are the Depression, Anxiety and Stress Scale (DASS) and the Depression, Anxiety, and Positive Outlook scale (DAPOS).[16, 17] Otherwise, interpretation of measures should include a check on somatic item endorsement. If the purpose is diagnosis of depressive disorder, as, for instance, in trials of antidepressants, then psychiatric interview is superior to self-report measures.

Cognitive measures are used to sample patients' thinking about pain, but without an agreed model of the mind, there is no satisfactory classification. They can be grouped approximately into those of content, process, and coping strategies (in measures which may also sample behavioral strategies). Cognitive content covers beliefs, such as those concerning control, self-efficacy, and attribution, and some beliefs may also appear as the cognitive statements in coping lists and as the cognitive content of emotion measures. Cognitive processes, particularly biases in appraisal and interpretation such as catastrophizing, are central to cognitive theory of emotion, and there is some overlap with emotion measures; for instance, the Beck Depression Inventory (BDI) contains self-referential appraisals.[18] Cognitive strategies, such as distraction, are also processes but over which the patient is assumed to

have greater voluntary control; however, measures may cover both (e.g. the Coping Strategies Questionnaire (CSQ)).[19] As with emotion, effective measurement tends toward the pain-specific, exemplified by the move from general locus of control, which poorly predicted patients' thinking and behavior in relation to pain, to pain-specific appraisal (using cognitive measures of beliefs about pain discussed above), and self-efficacy.[20] Careful consideration of the purpose of evaluation is needed to select measures, and for general treatment studies, a way to select among the many measures on offer is to examine their validation data. Those which involve prediction of behavior, such as adherence to treatment, or prediction of change in variables which were not too closely related, can be interpreted more confidently than those which provide only concurrent validation against a similar instrument (for these details see Refs 2, 21, 22).

Coping as a construct requires radical overhaul. It has considerable face validity, and is part of lay discourse, usually implying a positive means of managing. However, negative strategies, behavioral or cognitive, may have more important effects on the individual's life. The labels positive and negative are in themselves problematic, in that the efficacy of a coping strategy depends on its appropriateness to the problem and to the context, and on the short- and long-term outcome (not necessarily the same) for the individual patient, information which is difficult to collect. In its place, checklists use generalizations to classify strategies, relying on characteristics which may lack empirical support, of which active/passive is the most common. Any strategy – seeking social support, attempting distraction, using analgesics – can be effective in one set of circumstances, irrelevant in another, and disastrous in a third, thus such classifications are not reliably agreed by researchers. Selection among existing coping checklists, and particularly any use of interpretative rather than descriptive subtotals, should be made with these points in mind.

The concept of acceptance in pain is still in development; concepts are already elaborated in the pain field and measures are available.[23, 24, 25]

BEHAVIOR AND ACTIVITY

This broad area of assessment can be subdivided into specific and summary measures of behavior and physical function, by observer or by self-report; broader measures of function, disability, and quality of life which include some psychosocial content and which take as focus the interference with a variety of roles and activities by functional deficits rather than the deficits themselves; and behaviors which are not necessarily the target of change for the patient, but reflect societal goals and those of the referrers and funders, such as reduction of use of health and welfare resources. The move towards replacing the coping construct by more specific cognitive and behavioral constructs is welcome.

Physical performance is an easily accessible measure in any treatment program that includes exercise classes. However, interpretation is more problematic, as performance varies with psychological as well as physical state.[26] The different standard tests and various measures only overlap partially, or not at all, in what they test, and validation is rarely adequately addressed, making interpretation difficult.[27, 28] Thorough examination of what influences these measures will result in clearer recommendations.

Pain behavior presents particular problems as a hypothetical construct defined differently by different measuring instruments, and almost without exception, like measures of coping, making assumptions of in/appropriateness and in/effectiveness. The functions of pain behavior, including decreasing disability as well as increasing it, deliberate communication and attempts not to communicate, and pain relief, require further exploration before measures of pain behavior provide the information desired. Some observational measures can provide high reliability, and used in contexts such as medical consultation and domestic activity with the spouse have extended understanding, but the measures themselves cannot incorporate context or consequences and therefore serve poorly to describe treatment outcome. Pain behaviors can be understood best in relation to their communicative function.[29]

Within a behavioral formulation of chronic pain, behaviors, such as limping or guarding, were theoretically and empirically associated with greater disability and therefore an appropriate target of treatment. Within a cognitive behavioral framework, and with appreciation that the association is not as straightforward as assumed, pain behavior is less appropriate as a treatment outcome measure. For instance, while walking with a stick or cane may be associated with greater disability than walking unaided, it may enable the user to be more mobile and active than he or she would otherwise be, and thus protect against greater disability as well as contributing to better quality of life. Measurement of specific behaviors may relate to processes of change: limping in relation to mobility, groaning in relation to communication, and if those are targets of treatment, observational pain behavior scales offer means of measurement. Specific behaviors or functions are covered by the comments on observed physical performance in the biomedical domain: good reliability is often attainable, but validation is less satisfactorily tackled for many, requiring demonstration of a relationship with relevant everyday physical performance.

A specific component of pain behavior, for which detailed measurement usually requires videotaping and training of observers, is that of facial expression of pain. For nonverbal subjects unable to use pictorial scales, behavioral measures of pain are the only option.[30, 31] However, it is important to remember that report of one's own pain and another's observation of pain-related behavior are only weakly related.[5, 32] Pain behavior may be reported by others than the patient, particularly for children, where general behavioral scales may be used at home or in school as accessory measures of a child's distress or disturbance (see Chapter 44, Chronic pain in children, in the *Chronic Pain* volume in this series). There has been an upsurge of interest in measurement of pain in elderly cognitively impaired adults, with several scales in early stages of testing but none yet well enough documented to merit unconditional endorsement.[33]

Items concerning social support, including the quality of intimate relationships, are rare in pain studies other than as coping resources or pain behaviors. However, in many areas of health, close confiding relationships promote good physical and mental health and health maintenance, and arguably should be better represented as outcomes of treatments which aim towards more normal life through pain relief or pain management.

QUALITY OF LIFE AND OTHER COMPOUND MEASURES

An important but unresolved dilemma in quality of life measurement is how to recognize respondents' subjectivity with an objective measure.[34] Quality of life and other compound measures were intended in part to address the desire for a single comprehensive measure, since overall improvement in quality of life summarizes the aims of many treatments for pain. All of the many in use in the pain field rely on self-report, and combine different behaviors and functions ascribed different weightings to obtain one or more totals. Attention to content can help selection, and **Table 3.1** gives the number of items, response options, and an impression of the content of some of the most popular along a rough dimension from physical to psychosocial. A review by Wittink *et al.*[35] of three instruments in common use in pain studies, the Short-Form-36 (SF-36), Multidimensional Pain Inventory (MPI), and Oswestry Disability Index (ODI), shows both differences and overlap in coverage. The wider the range of activities covered by items in the measure, the more relevant are influences other than pain and physical impairment, such as beliefs and mood, lifestyle preferences, availability of resources, and cultural norms. The more comprehensive disability questionnaires effectively rank order the various degrees of compromise of mobility, and suggest goals which are observable within the clinic setting. The narrower the range of activities included, the higher the risk of excluding some of importance to reasonable numbers of pain respondents. Consideration of content affects both selection and interpretation of the measure.

In part, the complexity of quality of life measures reflects their multiple purposes, described by Higginson and Carr:[36] to prioritize problems, facilitate communication, screen for potential problems, identify preferences, monitor changes or response to treatment, and

Table 3.1 Content of widely used measures of function and disability in pain.

Measure	Summary	Content [number of items] — More physical ←→ More psychosocial
Short form 36 of Medical Outcomes Study SF-36[20]	9 separate domains rescaled 0–100; age-sex norms available	Physical functioning [10]; Role physical [4]; Bodily pain [2]; Vitality [4]; Social functioning [2]; General health [5]; Mental health [5]; Role emotional [3]
Sickness Impact Profile SIP[21]	Single total (%) or physical and psychosocial separately	Ambulation [12]; Body care and movement [23]; Mobility [10]; Eating [9]; Work [9]; Home management [10]; Sleep and rest [7]; Recreation and pastimes [8]; Communication [9]; Emotional behavior [9]; Alertness behavior [10]; Social interaction [20]
Roland and Morris short SIP[22]	Single total 0–24	Physical function [18]; Activity [3]; Sleep and rest [7]; Irritability [1]; Appetite [1], Sleep
Nottingham Health Profile NHP[23]	Total of domains or "profile"	Pain [8]; Physical abilities [8]; Sleep [5]; Energy levels [3]; Emotional reactions [9]; Social isolation [5]

(Continued over)

Table 3.1 Content of widely used measures of function and disability in pain (continued).

Measure	Summary	Content [number of items] More physical ←——→ More psychosocial
Multidimensional Pain Inventory (MPI/WHYMPI)[24]	Domain totals as mean 0–6, or patient type	Pain and pain interference including control and mood [20] · Activity [18] · Spouse response [14]
Pain Disability Index (PDI)[25]	Single total 0–70	Self-care [1] · Life-support activity [1] · Family/home responsibilities [1] · Recreation [1] · Social activity [1] · Occupation [1] · Sexual activity [1]
Brief Pain Inventory (BPI)[26]		Pain [4] · Walking ability [1] · General activity [1] · Normal work [1] · Sleep [1] · Mood [1] · Relationships [1]
Oswestry Low Back Pain Disability Questionnaire[27]	Single total as % of possible maximum	Pain intensity · Lifting [6] · Walking [6] · Sitting [6] · Standing [6] · Sleep [1] · Personal care [6] · Sleeping [6] · Sex life [6] · Travelling [6] · Enjoyment [1] · Social life [6]

Numbers in square brackets represent the number of questions on each content area.

train new staff. Other properties of measures which may guide choice concern the population on which it was developed (e.g. chronicity of the pain, specificity of the type of pain or pain site, inclusion or not of intermittent pain such as headache, the proportion working, the sex ratio, age range, and similar characteristics); and the number of response levels available, from two (yes/no) to a 10-point or 101-point (visual analog scale (VAS)) rating of difficulty or frequency, given the extent of change expected.

Satisfaction ratings belong among psychosocial measures rather than those of activity and function, but are the simplest form of a single outcome measure, and are extensively used in audit of treatments. They constitute a very transparent measure and are rarely adequately tested for bias arising from the context of testing, and are therefore unsuitable as the major or only outcome assessment; they may bear a weak to nonexistent relationship with other outcomes.[37]

Interference with social roles, such as domestic work and employment, family involvement, and community activity, is included in many compound measures, and it is important not to assume that severe physical disability necessarily restricts family or social life or even work. However, work quality and hours may be significantly reduced by pain even when the person with pain continues in employment.[38] Independent sources of information are available for some aspects: employment or welfare records may provide number of workdays lost, welfare benefits claimed, or state-provided help with domestic and family duties. Of course, extent of state provision varies between and within countries, and people differ in what they attempt to manage independently, making comparisons difficult.

THIRD PARTY-DEFINED OUTCOMES

Some questionnaires have been adapted for significant others and others designed *de novo*. Overall, the assessment of significant others of chronic pain patients with a reasonable degree of confidence is possible on a number of different dimensions including behavioral responses, mood and perceptions of marital adjustment and pain-related cognitions and beliefs.[39] Once more, these can be expected to give somewhat different accounts: when proxies complete questionnaires in privacy they may consistently under-report the burden of morbidity compared to subjects.[40]

Third party-defined outcomes also describe those identified not by patients or those close to them but by treatment staff, treatment funders, and national policies. Particularly those concerned with cost may override patient-defined outcomes such as extent of improvement. There are many stakeholders in the treatment of an individual patient: family members, employers, work colleagues, as well as funders, insurance companies, and

policymakers, may subscribe to diverse and even conflicting anticipated outcomes.[41] For instance, patients may reduce work hours or demands when the effort to maintain employment adversely affects their lives outside work, and while this change may improve their quality of life and that of their families, reduction in work is usually seen to represent a deterioration in patients' function and is unlikely to be the goal of treatment providers. Another example is that of welfare provision, which may improve the quality of life for patients and their families, but represents a target of treatment to reduce costs to society. Other goals, while associated with health improvement, may be substantially determined by variables beyond the control of patient or health carers: it is not uncommon for patients to reach a level of function which is compatible with work, but for employers to find them poor prospects, or for the patients' skills not to match requirements in the local job market. Setting goals of treatment, such as return to work, need to take this into account.

Healthcare resources are a particularly important outcome which may be identified by the patient and/or by others. They can be described using a range of events from daily drug use to surgery, or visits to primary carer to specialist level hospital treatments. Concern over veracity and accuracy of patients' accounts of drugs consumed and treatments undertaken can lead to an overcritical approach to an area where multiple sources of information may be examined for convergence (availability of health records permitting), and a best estimate made. Another source of reluctance to quantify post-treatment recourse to pain-related drugs and other health care may be differences within the treatment team, as there are within the pain community, about the aim of treatment: is it abstinence from all analgesics, or from all drugs prescribed for pain or mood, or restriction to nonopioids? And is all further pain-related treatment undesirable, or might a patient build on treatment gains by individual physiotherapy or psychological therapy? Specifying agreed goals of treatment is essential not only for selection of measures, but also for consistent interpretation of results. Similar considerations may apply as to third party-identified outcomes: it may be that intervention with health carers rather than patients is required to achieve an outcome such as less repeated unnecessary treatment, or adequate postoperative analgesia, or to curb excessive opioid prescription.

Nonoutcome variables: treatment process

While considering measurement, it is worth asking whether treatment methods or processes require assessment. In general, treatment is given with confidence that it is what it claims to be: that relaxation is relaxing, that the epidural analgesic is delivered epidurally, that the drug tested in a four-week trial is taken as directed for four weeks, that the no treatment control group is having no treatment. Not only does monitoring of treatment components contribute to confidence in findings of the trial, but can in some cases allow substudies, for instance of dose–response relationships, of subgroup responses, or of differences among care providers. Self-report is the most common way of assessing adherence, but reliability and validity are variable and often not addressed.[42] There is a tendency for the patient to overestimate adherence by self-report, and this will often contribute to the underestimation of treatment effects. However, self-report accesses beliefs and expectations which are not always picked up by other methods. Accuracy can be affected by time period, memory, desire to please, the wording and skills of the interviewer, patient culture, understanding etc. Clear and direct questions often lead to better accuracy.[43]

QUALITY OF MEASURES AND INTERPRETATION OF THEIR OUTPUT

The psychometric properties of a measure, reliability, validity, and sensitivity to change, are not unconditional qualities of the measure, but describe its performance in particular conditions of population, time, and extent of change. This makes it relevant to consider their likeness to those of the study for which outcome measures are sought. Psychometric qualities of tests are established over time. Newer tests may have better established psychometric qualities; older instruments, although they have acquired a track record, may have been tested to standards which are now superseded. Long clinical use is no guarantee of reliability, as is evident from the data on many clinical tests. Details of wording, question order, wording and format can have surprisingly large and systematic effects on responses: for example, different answers may be given to open-ended questions than from checklist or closed questions, or assumptions about intended reference period for frequency judgments.[43]

Reliability

Reliability describes the extent to which the instrument will give a consistent result, minimally affected by error, across content, time, and observers if not the subject. Reliability is calculated by ratio of true variance to that of true variance plus error variance. The error variance, in turn, is made up of systematic error plus random error, thus minimizing both systematic and random error improves reliability. Some random error is inevitable, but some arises from poor wording or problematic response categories. For instance, you might ask your patients "Can you climb stairs?", providing the responses "yes" or "no." A patient who can only climb them with great difficulty, or using a handrail, might on one occasion

decide that this qualified as yes, and on another decide that it did not meet the questioner's expectations and answer no. The more specific the question and/or response categories, the more consistent the responses. Such concerns are beyond the needs of someone selecting among existing tests, but are covered in texts such as McDowell and Newell.[2]

Low reliability effectively wastes the efforts of measurement, and erodes confidence in data obtained and in its interpretation. A scale with poor internal consistency can mislead. If it is measuring more than one construct, the total becomes a complex amalgam of the constructs, and change or difference between two totals could represent all sorts of processes which cannot be distinguished from one another. A scale or measure with poor test–retest reliability is responding to influences other than changes in the construct of interest, and since those influences are likely to vary across assessment occasions in ways which are not observed or taken into account, their variance is misattributed to variance in the construct. This might equally obscure real change and give an illusion of change where there is none: there would be no means to identify either. A measure or observation with poor interrater reliability is likewise subject to substantial influences unrelated to the construct of interest, and usually attributable to particular characteristics or beliefs of the raters. Again, this is as likely to miss real differences as to report them mistakenly. So how good is good enough? Reliability coefficients run from 0, where all variance is error variance, to 1.0, where there is no error variance.

Internal consistency is a measure of closeness of all items to the underlying construct, and is usually expressed as Cronbach's alpha. It is improved by dropping items which have a low correlation (that is, share little variance) with the total score and with other items. The disadvantages of high consistency is that some of the most interesting content may be lost, items which represented diversity within the original development population, and this limits applicability and generalizability. It also explains why some widely used tests with good reliability are rather repetitive, a fact which does not escape patients. An alpha of 0.85 may be considered acceptable.[44]

Test–retest reliability, or repeatability, effectively stability over time, is often calculated by simple correlation but better by intraclass correlation or kappa. The ideal, assuming stability of the underlying construct, is identical scores across time in the absence of identifiable sources of change, as measured by intraclass correlation, rather than identical rank order of scores across the population, as measured by simple parametric or nonparametric correlation. Of course, people do vary across time for an infinite number of reasons, and the highest test–retest reliability coefficients tend to occur where time between tests is short, not infrequently 24 or 48 hours. However, change in clinical treatments often involves time spans of weeks, months or years, and there is often no untreated control group which provides repeated assessment data over this time. However, extrapolating from a good 24-hour test–retest reliability to good reliability over 24 days or 12 months is wishful thinking. A good test–retest correlation is 0.9 or more; 0.8 to 0.9 is often considered acceptable; for kappa it is 0.6 or more.[2]

Interrater reliability used to be measured by bivariate correlation, parametric or nonparametric, or by percentage agreement between raters of all possible ratings. Consensus now requires intraclass correlation or kappa, which gives a more conservative estimate by calculating actual agreement (not relative order) and discounting for chance agreement by reference to the base rate of the event of interest. Good intraclass correlation indicates high variance in ratings due to subjects and low variance due to raters; a high kappa indicates high level of agreement between raters. Use of video allows multiple raters to observe the same subject, and can be used for calibration of raters on the same material. Iterative training with discussion of differences and, where possible, rectification of their causes can be used to attain satisfactory levels of reliability. It cannot be assumed without such procedures that raters are making the judgments intended. For both ICC and kappa, 0 represents no agreement and 1 perfect agreement; Dworkin and Sherman[44] suggest that an ICC below 0.8 or kappa below 0.6 is unacceptable.

Validity

Validity identifies the extent to which a test measures what it is intended to measure, which may be a real quality or a hypothetical construct, and does not measure instead, or as well, some unknown construct/s. A measure can be reliable but lack a clear relationship with a construct. For instance, there are several measures of "somatization," and tests of "fibromyalgia," but far from universal agreement on what they tell us, even on the existence of either phenomenon. Validity is estimated by comparison of the output of the measure with its object – the real quality or construct, or as close as possible an approximation. A noninvasive and low risk new diagnostic test, for instance, can be compared with biopsy or other findings from invasive or high risk procedures or from longer-term outcome, and to the extent that the data coincide, both for positive and negative results, that diagnostic test can be said to be valid in that population. Its validity in a population with a very different base rate of the event/s of interest (disease, item content) would have to be reestablished. For instance, a self-report inventory of function developed largely on students may be heavily weighted towards certain types of social activity which are characteristic of young independent adult life. This could cause decreasing validity the older the population to which it is applied, and a fit and active 70 year old might find little to endorse and thereby be scored as functioning poorly.

Many tests lack such a concrete "gold standard" for establishing validity. This may be because the construct poses practical difficulties for measurement, but more often it is hard to define and operationalize. Many of the constructs in everyday use – fitness, health, distress, motivation, social support – are so well understood that it is hard to recognize that there is no agreed definition or measurement. Tests are compiled from a wide pool of definitions, observations, and expert opinions on the construct, then content is narrowed until a reliable measure is achieved. The choice of referent can be difficult and controversial, as is well exemplified by "intelligence." As is also the case with intelligence, what is measured by the test (IQ) comes to be taken for the construct itself, leading to culturally inappropriate use of the tool, and attempts to locate the construct in the cortex.

Construct validity is best established by using one or more behavioral referents, but they can be difficult to identify and/or to measure. However, measures vary considerably in the extent to which they address this problem, or have acquired validation over time by being shown to predict behavior, and those which have such data allow more confident interpretation than those without. Details of validation are usually published with the test, and are available in texts on measures.[2, 21]

Concurrent validity is an aspect of validity which is generally the easiest to establish. The referent is an existing measure purportedly of the same construct, and if scores on the new measure correlate well with scores of the same subjects on the existing measure, and this "gold standard" is itself well validated, convergent validity is established. The gold standard, constructed, tested, and published according to norms which have been substantially improved over the intervening decades, may not be adequate or entirely appropriate, but through passage of time and scarcity of alternative measures has acquired criterion status.

Divergent validity is a variant of convergent validity, obtained by demonstrating relatively poor correlation with measures of unlike constructs, or those for which the new instrument might inadvertently be a proxy measure. Careful choice is needed in order that this does not become a superficial exercise. For example, it is important that a measure of coping (depending on how it is defined) is not too highly related to measures of mood, range of activities, or social desirability of self-presentation; it might, however, share more variance with measures of problem-solving and confidence.

Cutpoints are a special case of validity and are often used with little respect for their specificity to the population in which they were derived. The subject is beyond the scope of this chapter and is easily found in texts on test validity; for the choice of test, the only information required is the base rate of the problem in the original population and the population under study.[2, 44] If the populations are substantially different, the structure of the measuring instrument in the new population needs to be checked. Even where the populations are similar, some caution needs to be exercised, in that depending on the consistency of items within the measurement instrument, all patients with the same score are not identical. The number of possible combinations of items for an instrument with N items is 2^N. Thus, for instance, a five-item questionnaire has 32 possible item combinations: dichotomizing responses using a cutpoint of 3 would give 16 possible combinations of items in each category.

Sensitivity to change

Sensitivity to change, or responsiveness, is related to validation and subject to some of the same problems. It is estimated by comparing scores on the instrument before and after change with a referent which is known to indicate change, and so is a function of the measurement instrument within population parameters. Overlooking this and using it on sufficiently different populations results in floor and ceiling effects before or after treatment which can prevent calculation of change. It is increasingly tested in new measuring instruments; sometimes establishing sensitivity to differences between a healthy and a pain group is substituted. This can be an issue if the treatment is not expected to bring about large changes, and/or if the population is not expected to achieve the healthy norm, as in many chronic pain and cancer populations. Details of testing sensitivity to change are beyond the range of this chapter, but can be found in texts on measurement.[2, 44]

Estimating change or difference

Use of an unsuitable or unsatisfactory measure, or poor choice of statistical test, can obscure positive or null outcomes. Reporting an effect where none exists, type I error, is analogous to the specificity of a test, and reporting no effect where it exists, type II error, analogous to sensitivity of a test.[45] In clinical treatment studies, numbers are often small and so power of tests is low, and variance is often high (in a heterogeneous clinical population), raising the likelihood of type II error. Although surprisingly common even in respectable journals, the solution is not to perform multiple tests and set a low criterion for statistical significance (increasing the likelihood of type I error) and then to select the "significant" results according to researchers' expectations. By contrast, in a large and relatively homogeneous group, a mean change in a 100 mm pain VAS of 5 mm will achieve statistical significance, but is likely to be considerably less than patients hoped and clinicians intended. The substitution of statistical significance for clinical significance is unfortunate and misses the opportunity to describe the changes anticipated from treatment, of major interest to readers.

Clinical significance of change can be variously defined and calculated. The first focuses on return to a healthy or healthier state; the second to the meaningfulness of the change achieved; the third to the broader improvements brought about by specific treatment. The interested reader is referred to Kendall,[46] Kazdin,[45] Evans et al.,[47] and Jacobson et al.[48]

1. A criterion is set, by reference to healthy norms (empirically established, as in a few self-report instruments such as the SF-36 and in many diagnostic tests, or no more than the local mean such as of workdays lost through sickness), to a proportional change agreed or argued to be meaningful (such as the use of 50 percent pain relief, or a doubling of distance walked in a specified time), or to nonoccurrence of an event characteristic of the ill population (such as no further investigations or treatments for pain, or no waking from sleep due to pain). The proportion of the treated population meeting this criterion (given that none did so before treatment) is reported.

2. Reliable change is calculated by reference to the standard deviation: assuming normally distributed and not extensively overlapping healthy and dysfunctional scores, a post-treatment score which falls within two standard deviations of the healthy mean, or which falls outside two standard deviations to the healthy side of the dysfunctional mean, or which falls the healthy side of the intersection of the distributions, can be considered to indicate significant change.[48] Again, the proportion of the treated population meeting this criterion is reported.

3. Meaningfulness of clinical change in a specific problem, such as pain, can also be defined by the extent to which it is associated with overall change in quality of life or function.

These methods of defining clinical change can be combined, but their results do not necessarily coincide. For all three, it can be a problem that the aim of treatment in chronic and cancer pain is usually not total cure but improvement of the specific symptom or the overall quality of life. Healthy norms, where available, may therefore not be appropriate or attainable. Particularly where there is steady deterioration and the aim of treatment is to slow or halt it, quality of life may be the most suitable measure of whether treatment is worthwhile. Even in acute pain, as mentioned by Campbell (Chapter 2, Practical methods for pain intensity measurements), absence of pain may not be a realistic end point and the decision must be made on what's meaningful change. Patients are too rarely asked this question and researchers too rarely consider it.

There are certainly well-established options for analyzing the results of uncontrolled treatment studies, and where regular recordings are made, as in diary studies, multilevel statistical procedures can clarify relationships between variables and influences over time.[47, 49] Options include effect size calculations, effectively mean change calculated in units of standard deviation, and therefore comparable across measures and even across domains.[50, 51]

Weiss *et al.*[52] emphasize the tension between researchers and clinicians as an obstacle in the quest for clinical significance and the implementation of evidence-based treatments. They view direct interaction with patients as the foundation for assessing clinical significance; researchers may lack practical experience while clinicians may doubt research relevance. However, measuring goal attainment may serve for clinical purposes but cannot adequately be standardized across patients, and even over the course of treatment a patient may reasonably change goals entirely, change priorities, and change what marks achievement or brings satisfaction. Issues of treatment evaluation are also discussed in Morley and Williams.[51]

Inspecting raw data plots can be helpful in deciding on tests. Variability in response is of clinical interest, and planned tests are better than *post hoc* snooping of data. **Figures 3.1** and **3.2** show data for 200 patients on a questionnaire scored 0–60, where 0 represents a very poor state and 60 a very good one. The overall population has a pretreatment mean of 22 (S.D. 11) and a post-treatment mean of 27 (S.D. 16), a gain of mean 5 points. This change is statistically significant ($t = 8.2$, $p < 0.0001$), and it would be easy to stop at this point and conclude that treatment was successful in bringing about significant change, problematically equating clinical change (equal to half a standard deviation) with statistical significance.

However, both the pre-post scatterplot of data in **Figure 3.1**, in which differences appear larger the higher the pretreatment score, and the histograms in **Figure 3.2** which suggest a roughly bimodal response, invite further investigation. A median split (at 20) of the pretreatment scores shows the lower half scoring a mean of 13 (S.D. 5) pretreatment and 14 (S.D. 7) post-treatment, no real change at all; the upper half score a mean of 30 (S.D. 7) pretreatment and 38 (S.D. 12) post-treatment, a change of over one standard deviation, and arguably of clinical as well as statistical significance. The implications for treatment are that the lower scorers pretreatment need something more to enable them to change, information which does not emerge from the overall analysis.

SUMMARY AND EXAMPLE

Increasing pressure for clinical services to audit their performance demands the use of measures. How should those responsible choose among the possibilities?

- Aims of treatment are defined in general terms, such as "reducing pain, improving function," mainly by

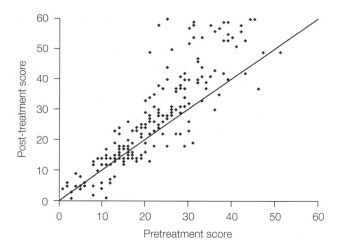

Figure 3.1 Scatterplot of pre and post-treatment scores, showing line of no change.

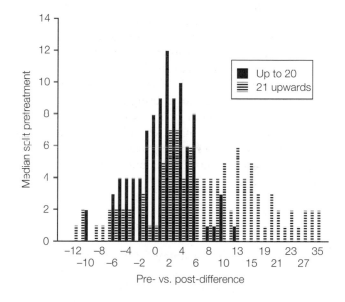

Figure 3.2 Histogram of pre and post-treatment scores.

treatment staff using experience of the service and knowledge of the literature, but patient groups, treatment facility mission statements, or local or national charters, may all contribute. These aims are then operationalized in achievable terms such as "at least 50 percent pain relief by discharge," and "significant reduction in disability in nonworkers, and reduction to local sickness absence norm in workers" for x percent of treated patients. Particularly where patients may present relatively intractable problems, minimum expectations may be appropriate: an example might be "All patients will gain an explanation of their pain and feel that they are believed and understood by staff," operationalized in terms of patients' ratings of such statements.

- Treatment aims determine which domains require measurement, and the headings in this chapter can be used as a checklist. A pain clinic which serves mainly early referrals from primary care may focus more on rapid pain abolition or substantial reduction, and use measures of affect and cognition to screen for patients with or at risk of developing psychological problems, and a brief measure of function to check that pain relief is accompanied by recovery of previous activity levels. A pain clinic with a large proportion of chronic pain patients, referred from other specialists, is likely to have more modest pain reduction goals and to use more extensive measures of affect, cognition, and function or disability, since major aims will be reduction of problems in these areas, that is, improvement in quality of life. Pain ratings would be recorded at every visit (perhaps with use of diary measures by the patient in the interim); pain relief at specific points in treatment evaluation. Psychosocial and functional measures would be taken at longer intervals, or only at initial assessment and discharge. Both clinics might sample satisfaction with a range of aspects of the service at discharge.
- In choosing these measures, concerns of test–retest reliability and validation in settings as near as possible to everyday life will be paramount. In addition, the existence of healthy population norms, or norms of comparable treated and untreated pain patients, help to set criteria for clinical significance of change.
- Processes of treatment also require specific measures so that outcomes can be investigated adequately. Patient adherence to recommended treatment, whether pharmacotherapy, exercise, relaxation, or thought monitoring, should be sampled. Therapist adherence to treatment guidelines may also be sampled, since therapists' skills can affect treatment efficacy. Data such as numbers of visits, numbers of treatments, dropout before discharge, length of time to discharge, and re-referral after discharge, are relevant for service audit.
- Most measures in use in the pain field rely on self-report, so that attention to minimizing demand characteristics is important: by computerized measures where possible, or by administration in a standard fashion by staff not involved in the patient's treatment. If possible, third party reports should be added, for instance, from employment sources or primary care physician; or a family member can confirm that a patient now walks a set local distance without a stop, or without a stick.
- The package of measures, piloted on an unselected sample of patients, may prove too long or repetitive, compromising reliability. Increasing use of computerized questionnaires and scanning of paper versions leaves the patient, rather than data entry personnel, bearing the burden of overlong assessments. However, patients' altruism should not be underestimated, and for many, the assurance that the clinic uses their responses better to understand the needs of future patients and to improve services is enough to obtain full cooperation.

REFERENCES

1. Turk DC, Melzack R (eds). *Handbook of pain assessment.* New York: Guilford Press, 1992.
2. McDowell I, Newell C. *Measuring health: a guide to rating scales and questionnaires,* 2nd edn. New York: Oxford University Press, 1996.
3. Turk DC, Dworkin RH, Allen RR *et al.* Core outcome domains for chronic pain clinical trials: IMMPACT recommendations. *Pain.* 2003; **106**: 337–45.
* 4. Wittink H, Rogers W, Sukiennik A, Carr DB. Physical functioning: self-report and performance measures are related but distinct. *Spine.* 2003; **28**: 2407–413.
5. Labus JS, Keefe FJ, Jensen MP. Self-reports of pain intensity and direct observations of pain behavior: when are they correlated? *Pain.* 2003; **102**: 109–24.
6. Morley SJ, Eccleston C, Williams ACdeC. Systematic review and meta-analysis of randomised controlled trials of cognitive behaviour therapy and behaviour therapy for chronic pain in adults, excluding headache. *Pain.* 1999; **80**: 1–13.
7. Waddell G, Turk DC. Clinical assessment of low back pain. In: Turk DC, Melzack R (eds). *Handbook of pain assessment,* 2nd edn. New York: Guilford Press, 2001: 431–53.
8. Rudy TE, Turk DC, Brody MC. Quantification of biomedical findings in chronic pain: problems and solutions. In: Turk DC, Melzack R (eds). *Handbook of pain assessment.* New York: Guilford Press, 1992: 447–72.
9. Price DD. *Psychological mechanisms of pain and analgesia.* Seattle: IASP Press, 1999.
10. Moore A, Moore O, McQuay H, Gavaghan D. Deriving dichotomous outcome measures from continuous data in randomised controlled trials of analgesics: use of pain intensity and visual analogue scales. *Pain.* 1997; **69**: 311–15.
11. Farrar JT, Portenoy RK, Berlin JA *et al.* Defining the clinically important difference in pain outcome measures. *Pain.* 2000; **88**: 287–94.
12. Aldrich S, Eccleston C, Crombez G. Worry about chronic pain: vigilance to threat and misdirected problem solving. *Behaviour Research and Therapy.* 2000; **38**: 457–70.
13. Vlaeyen JWS, Linton SJ. Fear-avoidance and its consequences in chronic musculoskeletal pain: a state of the art. *Pain.* 2000; **85**: 317–32.
14. Pincus T, Morley SJ. Cognitive processing bias in chronic pain: a review and integration. *Psychological Bulletin.* 2001; **127**: 599–617.

15. Williams ACdeC. Measures of function and psychology. In: Melzack R, Wall PD (eds). *Textbook of pain*, 4th edn. Edinburgh: Churchill Livingstone, 1999: 427–44.

16. Lovibond SH, Lovibond PF. *Manual for the depression, anxiety, stress scales*, 2nd edn. Sydney: Psychology Foundation, 1995.

17. Pincus T, Williams ACdeC, Vogel S, Field A. The development and testing of the depression, anxiety, and positive outlook scale (DAPOS). *Pain*. 2004; **109**: 181–8.

18. Beck AT, Ward CH, Mendelson M *et al*. An inventory for measuring depression. *Archives of General Psychiatry*. 1961; **4**: 561–71.

19. Rosenstiel AK, Keefe FJ. The use of coping strategies in chronic low back pain patients: relationship to patient characteristics and current adjustment. *Pain*. 1983; **17**: 33–44.

20. Nicholas MK. The pain self-efficacy questionnaire: taking pain into account. *European Journal of Pain*. 2007; **11**: 153–63.

21. Turk DC, Melzack R (eds). *Handbook of pain assessment*, 2nd edn. New York: Guilford Press, 2001.

22. Turk DC, Okifuji A. Matching treatment to assessment of patients with chronic pain. In: Turk DC, Melzack R (eds). *Handbook of pain assessment*, 2nd edn. New York: Guilford Press, 2001: 400–14.

23. McCracken LM, Eccleston C. A comparison of the relative utility of coping and acceptance-based measures in a sample of chronic pain sufferers. *European Journal of Pain*. 2006; **10**: 23–30.

24. Hofmann SG, Asmundson GJG. Acceptance and mindfulness-based therapy: new wave or old hat? *Clinical Psychology Review*. 2008; **28**: 1–16.

25. McCracken LM, Vowles KE, Eccleston C. Acceptance of chronic pain: component analysis and a revised assessment method. *Pain*. 2004; **107**: 159–66.

26. Simmonds MJ, Olson SL, Jones S *et al*. Psychometric characteristics and clinical usefulness of physical performance tests in patients with low back pain. *Spine*. 1998; **23**: 1412–21.

27. Filho IT, Simmonds MJ, Protas EJ, Jones S. Back pain, physical function, and estimates of aerobic capacity. What are the relationships among methods and measures? *American Journal of Physical Medicine and Rehabilitation*. 2002; **81**: 913–20.

28. Grotle M, Brox JI, Vøllestad NK. Functional status and disability questionnaires: what do they assess? A systematic review of back-specific outcome questionnaires. *Spine*. 2004; **30**: 130–40.

29. Williams AC de C, Craig KD. Editorial – A science of pain expression? *Pain*. 2006; **125**: 202–03.

30. Craig KD, Prkachin KM, Grunau RVE. The facial expression of pain. In: Turk DC, Melzack R (eds). *Handbook of pain assessment*, 2nd edn. New York: Guilford Press, 2001: 153–69.

31. Hadjistavropoulos T, von Baeyer C, Craig KD. Pain assessment in persons with limited ability to communicate. In: Turk DC, Melzack R (eds). *Handbook of pain assessment*, 2nd edn. New York: Guilford Press, 2001: 134–49.

∗ 32. Hadjistavropoulos T, Craig KD. A theoretical framework for understanding self-report and observational measures of pain: a communications model. *Behaviour Research and Therapy*. 2002; **40**: 551–70.

33. Zwakhalen SMG, Hamers JPH, Abu-Saad HH, Berger MPF. Pain in elderly people with severe dementia: A systematic review of behavioural pain assessment tools. *Biomedicine Central BMC Geriatrics*. 2006; **6**: 3.

34. Stenner PHD, Cooper D, Skevington SM. Putting the Q into quality of life; the identification of subjective constructions of health-related quality of life using Q methodology. *Social Science and Medicine*. 2003; **57**: 2161–72.

35. Wittink H, Turk DC, Carr DB *et al*. Comparison of the redundancy, reliability, and responsiveness to change among SF-36, Oswestry Disability Index, and Multidimensional Pain Inventory. *Clinical Journal of Pain*. 2004; **20**: 133–42.

36. Higginson IJ, Carr AJ. Measuring quality of life using quality of life measures in the clinical setting. *British Medical Journal*. 2001; **322**: 1297–300.

37. Lunnen KM, Ogles BM. A multiperspective, multivariable evaluation of reliable change. *Journal of Consulting and Clinical Psychology*. 1998; **66**: 400–10.

38. Blyth M, March LM, Nicholas MK, Cousins MJ. Chronic pain, work performance and litigation. *Pain*. 2003; **103**: 41–7.

39. Sharp TJ, Nicholas MK. Assessing the significant others of chronic pain patients: the psychometric properties of significant other questionnaires. *Pain*. 2000; **88**: 135–44.

40. Grootendorst PV, Feeny DH, Furlong W. Does it matter whom and how you ask? Inter- and intra-rater agreement in the Ontario Health Survey. *Journal of Clinical Epidemiology*. 1997; **50**: 127–35.

41. Young AE, Wasiak R, Roessler RT *et al*. Return to work outcomes following work disability: stakeholder motivations, interests and concerns. *Journal of Occupational Rehabilitation*. 2005; **15**: 543–56.

42. Rand CS. "I took the medicine like you told me, doctor": self-report of adherence with medical regimens. In: Stone AA, Turkkan JS, Bachrach CA *et al*. (eds). *The science of self-report: implications for research and practice*. Mahwah, NJ: Lawrence Erlbaum Associates, 1999: 257–76.

∗ 43. Schwarz N. Self-reports: how the questions shape the answer. *American Psychologist*. 1999; **54**: 93–105.

∗ 44. Dworkin SF, Sherman JJ. Relying on objective and subjective measures of chronic pain: guidelines for use and interpretation. In: Turk DC, Melzack R (eds). *Handbook of pain assessment*, 2nd edn. New York: Guilford Press, 2001: 619–38.

45. Kazdin AE. The meanings and measurement of clinical significance. *Journal of Consulting and Clinical Psychology*. 1999; **67**: 332–9.

46. Kendall PC. Clinical significance. *Journal of Consulting and Clinical Psychology.* 1999; **67**: 283–4.

* 47. Evans C, Margison F, Barkham M. The contribution of reliable and clinically Significant change methods to evidence-based mental health. *Evidence Based Mental Health.* 1998; **1**: 70–2.

48. Jacobson NS, Roberts LJ, Berns SB, McGlinchey JB. Methods for defining and determining the clinical significance of treatment effects: description, application, and alternatives. *Journal of Consulting and Clinical Psychology.* 1999; **67**: 300–307.

49. Affleck G, Zautra A, Tennen H, Armeli S. Multilevel daily process designs for consulting and clinical psychology: a preface for the perplexed. *Journal of Consulting and Clinical Psychology.* 1999; **67**: 746–54.

50. Cohen J. *Statistical power analysis for the behavioral sciences.* New Jersey: Lawrence Erlbaum Associates, 1988.

51. Morley S, Williams ACdeC. Conducting and evaluating treatment outcome studies. In: Turk DC, Gatchel R (eds). *Psychological approaches to pain management: a practitioners handbook*, 2nd edn. New York: Guilford Press, 2002: 52–68.

52. Weiss D, Edwards W, Weiss JW. The clinical significance decision. Cited November 3, 2006. Available from: http://instructional1.calstatela.edu/dweiss/PSY504/clinsig.htm.

4

Sensory testing and clinical neurophysiology

ELLEN JØRUM AND LARS ARENDT-NIELSEN

KEY LEARNING POINTS

- Results of sensory testing and neurophysiological evaluation must be correlated with the symptoms and the clinical findings of the patient.
- Of all quantitative sensory testing procedures, determination of thermal thresholds assessing small fiber function/dysfunction is most appropriate in the evaluation of pain patients.
- Von Frey nylon filaments may be used in the assessment of mechanical detection and pain thresholds as well as in mapping of areas of secondary hyperalgesia to punctate stimuli.

- Although electromyography/neurography does not assess the function of small nerve fibers, it is recommended to be included in the evaluation of patients with painful neuropathies and nerve damages to obtain an overall view of the nerve fibers affected.
- Sensory-evoked potentials following CO_2 laser stimulation relate to pain and nociceptive impulses projected in the spinothalamic tract. The method has been used in the evaluation of pain patients, although mainly as a research tool

INTRODUCTION

The diagnosis of neuropathic (and nociceptive pain) is in most cases based on a thorough interview and a clinical examination of the patient. In many cases, however, there is a need for further classification of a painful syndrome, and the question arises as to which testing procedures are adequate. This chapter describes the different clinical neurophysiological and sensory testing methods available and their role in the evaluation of painful syndromes. The conventional clinical neurophysiological methods such as neurography (nerve conduction studies) and somatosensory-evoked potentials using peripheral electrical stimulation are of little value since they assess the function of the fast-conducting $A\beta$-fiber and dorsal column system, which does not mediate the sensation of pain.

Somatosensory potentials following CO_2 laser stimulation relate to pain and nociceptive impulses projected in the spinothalamic tract, but the large interindividual variation in the amplitude of the laser-evoked potentials suggests that they may not be suitable for routine examinations in clinical practice.

In most cases neuropathic pain is characterized by sensory abnormalities that are caused by lesions of sensory nerve fibers or sensory pathways within the central nervous system (CNS). Further diagnostic and descriptive characterization of a painful syndrome may be obtained by performing quantitative sensory testing (QST), which allows a quantitative evaluation of sensory thresholds to tactile, vibratory, pressure, and temperature stimuli. Because neuropathic pain is often characterized by dysfunctions of the sensory qualities that are mediated by thin Aδ- and C-fibers, thermotesting (quantitative evaluation of thermal thresholds), which allows testing of heat, cold, and heat and cold pain, is of special importance. Testing for allodynia/hyperalgesia to tactile and thermal stimulation as well as testing for abnormal temporal summation or "windup-like" pain is of great value in the evaluation of neuropathic pain, and may be helpful in assessing underlying pathophysiological mechanisms.

NEUROPHYSIOLOGICAL MECHANISMS

It is beyond the scope of this chapter to describe in detail the complicated pathophysiological mechanisms involved in acute and, particularly, chronic pain. The mechanisms of nociception and inflammatory and neuropathic pain are discussed in detail in Chapter 1b, Mechanisms of inflammatory hyperalgesia and Chapter 1a, Applied physiology of nociception in the *Acute Pain* volume of this series and Chapter 1, Applied physiology: neuropathic pain in the *Chronic Pain* volume of this series. To a large extent, most mechanisms are still unknown. However, it may be helpful to have some understanding of the known basic mechanisms. The sensation of acute pain is the result of activation of normal (not sensitized) nociceptors classified as Aδ- or C-nociceptors, according to the peripheral nerve fiber transmitting the neural impulses. Several classes of C-nociceptors in humans have been identified by the technique of microneurography.[1] Of special importance for pathophysiological mechanisms may be the discovery of mechano-insensitive or silent nociceptors, i.e. nociceptors that are not activated by normal noxious stimuli but become active in a state of injury, particularly following inflammation.[2]

If a peripheral injury occurs, the C-nociceptors may become sensitized as a result of the effect of a large number of inflammatory substances released at the site of the injury. Sensitization of C-nociceptors may produce sensory changes that are restricted to this site. The sensory changes that are produced are, first and foremost, a lowering of the heat pain threshold or allodynia to heat (allodynia is defined as pain produced by a nonpainful stimulus) and, second, hyperalgesia to heat (hyperalgesia is defined as an increased response to a stimulus that is normally painful). It is important to note that sensory changes due to nociceptor sensitization will be detectable within the site of injury alone, and not in the surrounding tissue.

In the event of acute pain, the incoming stimuli to the spinal cord are processed normally, and the nociceptive impulses are passed over to second-order neurons and transmitted in central projection pathways. If sustained peripheral injury (or an injury to a peripheral nerve) occurs, an increased barrage of nociceptive impulses reaches the dorsal horn of the spinal cord and central sensitization may occur. This general term includes a complicated series of events in neurons in the dorsal horn. Windup, a cumulative increase of action potentials caused by nociceptive stimulation, is considered to be a possible first initial step that is mediated by the activation of *N*-methyl-D-aspartate (NMDA) receptors.[3] A state of central hyperexcitability is produced, which is characterized in animal experiments by allodynia to light mechanical stimulation and an increase in the size of the peripheral receptive fields of the central neurons.[4] It may not yet be possible to explain all of the clinical symptoms, findings, and sensory abnormalities in patients with chronic pain using the theory of central sensitization, but the demonstration of central hyperexcitability has had a tremendous impact on the understanding of some of the phenomena observed in patients with chronic pain. For instance, allodynia to mechanical stimulation, which is frequently encountered in neuropathic pain patients, and the increase (over time) in the extent of the areas of pain have been accredited to central hyperexcitability. Whether the occurrence of spontaneous and paroxysmal pain may be explained entirely or partly by the same mechanisms remains an unresolved question. In general, a substantial amount of research is still needed to understand fully the different aspects of clinical pain.

Traditionally, clinical pain syndromes have been treated according to the etiology of the pain (e.g. postherpetic neuralgia, painful diabetic neuropathy). Because of the current knowledge of the possible common neurophysiological mechanisms involved in different pain entities, it has recently been suggested that, instead of focusing on the different etiologies, it might be possible to assess and treat pain according to the underlying neurophysiological mechanisms involved, i.e. mechanism-based classification of pain.[5]

This opens up new perspectives for the future management of pain, and represents a huge challenge for developing test procedures that will enable us to distinguish between different mechanisms in a clinical setting.

SOMATOSENSORY EVALUATION OF PAIN

A patient's subjective estimate of the magnitude of pain intensity may be determined by means of a visual analog scale (VAS). However, for better classification and documentation of a painful syndrome, supplementary investigations are often required. The aim of this chapter is to give an overview of the available supplementary tests. The purposes of employing such tests will fall mainly into the categories of diagnostic or objective documentation of a pain condition. Ideally, the results of testing could be used as a basis for treatment algorithms. Until now, sensory testing and some clinical neurophysiological tests have been mainly used in clinical research, for classifying the different abnormalities found in painful syndromes, and in clinical pharmacological trials. However, sensory testing is increasingly employed in the clinical evaluation of pain syndromes. Procedures, as well as equipment in use, vary between different laboratories. To give simple recommendations and general practical guidelines for the use of such testing in a purely clinical setting is, therefore, difficult. The aim of this chapter is to give some guidelines as to when and how to perform clinical neurophysiological or sensory testing.

It will be strongly emphasized throughout the chapter that all supplementary testing must be correlated to the clinical symptoms and findings of the patient and that it is not appropriate to make a diagnosis of a painful syndrome based on the results from sensory testing or clinical neurophysiological testing alone. The chapter will focus on the methods that are currently in use, but will also present methods that are currently more experimental and are still not regarded as conventional tools in the diagnosis of pain.

PAIN CONDITIONS

Pain conditions may be categorized in many ways – one approach is to describe the pain as nociceptive or neuropathic, depending on its cause. This is a general classification disregarding the etiology of the pain. Pain can also be categorized as acute or chronic, according to whether its duration is less than or more than three months respectively. Most patients referred for supplementary sensory or clinical neurophysiological testing will suffer from chronic pain. The neuropathic pain condition is primarily known to produce sensory abnormalities and, thus, deserves special attention. For the clinician, it is important to note that nociceptive pain may also produce sensory changes.[6]

Visceral pain referred to the skin may show sensory abnormalities that are detectable by sensory testing.[7] The same is true for referred muscle pain.[8] For the reader, it is important to be aware of the existence of such findings, in the sense that the usefulness of sensory assessment is not restricted to neuropathic pain conditions. The finding of sensory abnormalities in different pain types may reflect the involvement of some common neurophysiological mechanisms.

NOCICEPTIVE PAIN

Nociceptive pain derives from the activation of nociceptors alone. The nociceptors may be normal or sensitized. When cutaneous nociceptors are normal, no sensory abnormalities have been described. When nociceptors become sensitized as a result of injuries to peripheral tissues and the subsequent release of inflammatory agents, sensory changes will result.

As mentioned above, sensitization of nociceptors will result in allodynia/hyperalgesia to heat and possibly some types of mechanical stimuli within the site of injury[9, 10] – changes that are detectable with sensory testing.

In contrast to cutaneous pain, muscle pain is described as aching and cramping, is difficult to localize, and has characteristic referred pain patterns. Unfortunately, knowledge of the basic aspects of muscle pain in humans is still very poor as most of the information originates from experiments using anesthetized animals. Furthermore, the data on the neurophysiology of pain have mainly been obtained from studies of cutaneous nociception. This lack of knowledge about the neural mechanisms involved in muscle pain has led to much debate and speculation about the mechanisms related to the etiology, pathogenesis, diagnosis, and treatment.

Experimental approaches to the study of muscle pain in humans are a way of increasing knowledge. This is important as the socioeconomic impact of musculoskeletal pain disorders is substantial, and new insight into the pathophysiological mechanisms can help to prevent chronicity.

Experimental methods can be used in the laboratory for basic studies (e.g. central hyperexcitability or screening of treatment procedures) and also in the clinic to characterize patients with musculoskeletal disorders (e.g. fibromyalgia).

The primary advantages of experimental approaches to assess pain sensitivity under normal and pathological conditions are:

- the stimulus can be controlled, i.e. the pain intensity and quality do not vary over time;
- pain reactions to controlled stimuli can be assessed quantitatively;
- pain reactions can be compared quantitatively between controls and patients.

One disadvantage of experimental pain research is that the stimulus paradigm (intensity, duration, and modality) might not mimic clinical pain conditions completely.

Several experimental models have been used to induce and assess muscle pain in humans. Intramuscular (i.m.)

injection of algogenic substances (bradykinin, serotonin, capsaicin, hypertonic saline), i.m. electrical stimulation, ischemia, or eccentric exercise are some examples.

Injection of hypertonic saline has been used extensively in the past because the quality of the induced pain is similar to clinical muscle pain that is localized and referred. Injections of chemical substances are, however, not suitable if the muscle pain needs to be turned on and off more rapidly. A model has been developed based on continuous intramuscular electrical stimulation in which the local and referred pain vanish immediately when the stimulation is terminated.[11]

Infusion of a variety of algogenic substances has been tested, and a combination of, for example, serotonin and bradykinin is particularly effective in causing muscular hyperalgesia to muscle pressure stimulation. It seems that the severity of the referred pain is related to the intensity and duration of the ongoing muscle pain and most likely also to the degree of central hyperexcitability.[12] In patients with chronic pain syndromes such as fibromyalgia or whiplash, the pain responses to experimental muscle pain are substantially exaggerated compared with controls.[13] Experimental models are valuable for assessing the basic aspects of muscle pain in volunteers and in patients with musculoskeletal disorders.

NEUROPATHIC PAIN

Neuropathic pain results from a lesion or a dysfunction of the nervous system (peripheral or central). One may distinguish between nociceptive neuropathic pain, which is caused by the activation of nociceptors connected to nervous tissue (e.g. cervical or lumbar radiculopathy), and the deafferentation type of neuropathic pain, which often involves mechanisms of central sensitization. It is this latter form of neuropathic pain that will be described here. A painful condition may develop immediately after injury or after a long delay, such as days, weeks, or even months. The results of sensory and, eventually, clinical neurophysiological testing need to be correlated with the patient's symptoms and clinical findings. Typically, the patient may complain of several types of pain, but there is a large interindividual variability (**Table 4.1**). Most

patients will complain of constant pain, the quality of which may vary; commonly used descriptors include "burning," "aching," and "sore." The constant pain may vary spontaneously in intensity, but will typically be intensified by physical activity and exposure to cold. Many patients will suffer from paroxysmal pain, lasting for seconds up to minutes, within the painful area and with radiation from this area. The frequency of paroxysms may vary, from several times a day until a few times every week. The quality of the paroxysmal pain may be described as "shooting," "intense," or "sharp." Typically, the patient also complains of evoked pain, which is mostly caused by lightly touching the skin or by exposure to wind. A painful condition may develop from the time of onset, often resulting in an increase in the area of pain or an intensification of the constant pain. In most cases, neuropathic pain is accompanied by sensory abnormalities[14, 15] that are related to lesions in the sensory nerve fibers or sensory pathways within the CNS.[16] Sensory disturbances may develop from both causes, as shown in **Table 4.2**.

Sensory disturbances may sometimes be detected by routine neurological sensory examination (light touch with a cotton swab or pinprick with a needle). However, hypoesthesia is often masked by allodynia to light mechanical stimulation. Nevertheless, reduced sensibility to light touch may be reported by some patients. Hyperalgesia to pinprick is often reported as a different, more painful, sensation, often with radiation and an unpleasant aftersensation.

Table 4.2 Sensory abnormalities in neuropathic pain.

Type	Example	
Quantitative	Hypoesthesia	Hypoalgesia
	Hyperesthesia	Hyperalgesia
Qualitative	Allodynia	
	Paresthesia	
	Dysesthesia	
Spatial	Dyslocalization	
	Radiation	
Temporal	Abnormal latency	
	Abnormal aftersensation	
	Abnormal summation	

Table 4.1 Characteristics of neuropathic pain.

Type of pain	Description	Duration, frequency, and intensity
Spontaneous pain	Burning, aching, squeezing, cutting, piercing, pricking, sore (and other descriptions)	Constant, but with possible variation in intensity
Spontaneous paroxsymal pain	Shooting, sharp, stinging, throbbing, radiating	Duration, seconds to minutes; frequency, from none to several per day
Evoked pain	Pain or unpleasant sensation by stimulation of painful area (usually light touch)	

The diagnosis of neuropathic pain may in most cases be confirmed by careful interviewing of the patient and a routine neurological examination. Further diagnostic and descriptive characterization is obtained by performing QST, which allows, as indicated by the name, a quantitative evaluation of the different sensory qualities.

SENSORY QUALITIES

The sensation of touch, pressure, and vibration are all mechanosensitive modalities that are transmitted in large-diameter myelinated AⓇ afferent neurons, spinal dorsal columns, and medial lemniscal pathways, which are accessible to testing through conventional neurophysiological techniques such as neurography and electrically induced sensory-evoked potentials.

For testing modalities such as fast pain (Aδ-fibers), dull, burning, aching pain (C-fibers), heat and heat pain (C-fibers), and cold (Aδ-fibers) and cold pain (Aδ- and C-fibers), neurography and somatosensory-evoked potentials (SEP) are of little value.

Many disorders, for example diabetic neuropathy, affect the small-diameter fibers before the large-diameter fibers, and a clinical diagnosis concerning nerve impairment can only be obtained when the large-diameter fibers start to show measurable signs of dysfunction. At that time, the thin fibers may be severely affected, with the possibility of developing severe neuropathic chronic pain. Methods to assess early impairment of the thin-fiber function are needed.

BASIS FOR SENSORY TESTING

Routine neurological sensibility testing is inadequate for a quantitative, modality-specific assessment of sensory disturbance. Sensory testing has developed in recent years as a valuable supplement to the quantitative determination of modality-specific disturbances. In general, sensory testing in humans involves a large variety of disciplines (auditory, visual, somatic, kinesthetic, etc.). In particular, sensory testing involves the standardized activation of the specific sensory pathways system and the measurement of evoked responses. The ultimate goal of advanced human sensory testing is to obtain a better understanding of mechanisms involved in sensory transduction, transmission, and perception under normal and pathophysiological conditions. Sensory testing can be applied in the laboratory for basic studies or in the clinic to characterize patients with dysfunctions affecting pain pathways. At present, there are different stimulation techniques available in the laboratory, including electrical, thermal, and mechanical techniques; however, commercially available equipment needed to apply these techniques is scarce.

To differentiate between the dysfunctions that are related to various disorders of the sensory system, it is necessary to establish a series of sensory tests with different stimulus modalities activating different pathways. The design of adequate regimes to test sensory fibers involves two separate topics:

1. standardized activation;
2. measurement and quantification of the evoked reactions.

QUANTITATIVE SENSORY TESTING

QST is used to measure the intensity of stimuli needed to produce specific sensory perceptions. Tests have been developed for the determination of sensory thresholds for tactile, vibratory, pressure, and temperature stimulation.

Various laboratories have used different approaches and paradigms.

All quantitative sensory tests are psychophysical tests that require patients to be awake and alert, to fully understand the instructions given, and to be fully capable of cooperating during testing.

ESTIMATION OF TACTILE SENSIBILITY BY VON FREY NYLON FILAMENTS

For quantitative testing of tactile sensibility, von Frey nylon filaments are easy to use. They consist of a series of filaments of varying thickness, calibrated according to the force required to make them bend. The hairs primarily stimulate the rapidly adapting cutaneous receptors when hairs with low bending pressures are applied to the skin. One method of assessing tactile sensation is to apply the hairs in an ascending and descending order of magnitude and to record both the appearance and disappearance threshold. In neuropathic pain, tactile sensibility, as measured by von Frey hairs, may be reduced in the affected skin areas.[17] This is a typical finding that may be observed in a routine neurological examination, in which testing for tactile sensibility with a cotton swab may only give a sensation of hyperesthesia (in fact, allodynia to light mechanical stimulation) that masks an eventual reduction in tactile sensibility. Another way of assessing the tactile threshold is to determine the value of the bending force of the filament which is detected in 50 percent of applications. One should be aware that the nominal bending force of von Frey hairs varies with temperature and humidity, and it may be necessary to calibrate the bending force against a balance for each experimental session.[18]

The von Frey hairs increasingly excite skin nociceptors with increasing bending force, and may be used to determine tactile pain detection thresholds.

The nylon filaments have been used for the determination of allodynia/hyperalgesia to punctate stimuli in human experimental models.[19] The von Frey hairs may also be employed for mapping areas of secondary hyperalgesia to punctate stimuli (owing to central sensitization) in experimental models of pain[19] or in a clinical context.[20] It has been shown that secondary hyperalgesia to punctate stimuli is mediated by conduction in Aδ-nociceptive fibers,[21] in contrast to the Aβ-fiber-mediated secondary hyperalgesia to light brush.

Summary of von Frey hair testing

- **Indication**: for quantitative testing of tactile sensibility.
- **How it is executed**: apply the hairs in an ascending and descending order of magnitude and record both the appearance and disappearance thresholds, or determine the value of the bending force of the filament which is detected in 50 percent of applications:
  - with increasing bending force, the von Frey hairs will excite skin nociceptors and may be used to determine tactile pain detection thresholds;
  - may be used to map the area of hyperalgesia to punctate stimuli.
- **Contraindications**: none.
- **Typical findings and interpretations**: reduced tactile sensibility as well as hyperalgesia to punctate stimuli.

DETERMINATION OF VIBRATORY THRESHOLDS BY VIBRAMETER

The vibrameter (equipment for quantitative evaluation of vibratory thresholds) may be used for the evaluation of both vibratory and vibratory pain thresholds. The vibrameter determines the stimulus level needed to produce the sensation of vibration and is easily and quickly performed. The vibratory perception threshold can be determined on any point of the human body.

The determination of vibratory thresholds is primarily of value in the quantitative evaluation of vibratory sensory deficit. Hyperalgesia to vibration has been described in the evaluation of pain patients.[22] In an investigation of patients with neuralgia, it was found that the vibration frequency could be raised to 130 Hz without causing pain, in both normal volunteers and patients' uninjured areas (hands). In all patients with neuralgia, allodynia to vibration in the affected part was demonstrated.

Summary of vibrameter testing

- **Indication**: quantitative evaluation of vibratory perception and vibratory pain thresholds.
- **How it is executed**: the vibrameter may be applied on any point of the human body.

- **Contraindications**: none.
- **Typical findings**: increased vibratory threshold (reduced sensibility) and allodynia/hyperalgesia to vibration.

DETERMINATION OF PRESSURE THRESHOLDS BY ALGOMETER

The algometer is used for quantitative determination of thresholds to pressure or pinching. The measurement of pressure pain thresholds has been used in a large variety of test situations. In clinical practice, the pressure algometer is usually applied over a bony surface (for instance the tibia) or over muscles. The essence of pressure algometry is that increasing pressure is applied to the part of the body that is being investigated and the outcome is the patients' or volunteers' reaction to the pressure. The outcome measures in pressure algometry are the pain detection threshold and/or the pain tolerance threshold. Pressure rate and pressure area have been shown to be important factors for reliable results. To date, pressure algometry has, for instance, been used to assess the effects of drugs, different treatment modalities, pain thresholds in children, experimental pain in muscles, pain thresholds in populations studies, head and neck pain,[23] masseter muscle soreness, myofascial trigger points, and pain in patients with fibromyalgia.[24] The method seems to be well suited for the determination of pressure hyperalgesia in musculoskeletal disorders.

Summary of algometer testing

- **Indication**: quantitative determination of the threshold to pressure or pinching.
- **How it is executed**: the algometer is applied over bony surface or muscle (for pressure threshold) or is used for pinching a fold of the skin.
- **Contraindications**: none.
- **Typical findings**: reduced sensibility or allodynia/hyperalgesia to pressure or pinching.

THERMOTEST

Painful syndromes (mainly neuropathic pain) are often characterized by dysfunctions in the sensory qualities that are mediated by thin nerve fibers, which are not easily investigated by conventional electrophysiological testing such as neurography. Thermotest (quantitative evaluation of thermal thresholds) allows the testing of qualities such as heat, cold, and heat and cold pain sensations (**Figure 4.1**). It is important to note that, whereas neurography tests dysfunction of peripheral nerve fibers, the thermotest describes the status of temperature somatosensory afferents all the way from the cutaneous receptors to the

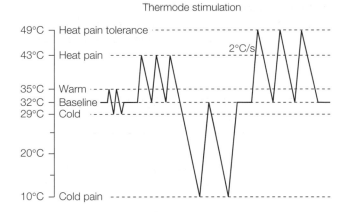

Figure 4.1 Normal thermal thresholds measured by thermotest from a baseline of 32°C.

brain, but it is not possible to determine the level of any lesion. There are different thermotest devices commercially available that have varying technical parameters. Testing for thermal sensory abnormalities is employed not only in the evaluation of pain patients but also in patients with thermal sensory abnormalities in general, such as thin-fiber neuropathies. Some devices are primarily designed to evaluate the sensory deficits of heat, cold, and heat pain. Prominent findings in neuropathic pain conditions are heat and cold hyperalgesia. Testing only for heat and cold functions in patients with neuropathic pain will give inconclusive results because heat and cold hyperalgesia may occur in the presence of normal heat and cold thresholds. When evaluating neuropathic pain patients, all four thermal qualities should be tested – heat, cold, heat pain, and cold pain.[25] As well as determining the threshold values, it is important to ask the patient about the quality of the sensation. Paradoxical sensations are frequently reported, most often that cold pain is perceived as heat. Heat and cold pain are often described as having a sudden onset, with radiation and after-sensations, which is valuable information in the evaluation of hyperalgesia. It is important to note that the interindividual variability in sensory abnormalities is large and may develop in both directions, as shown in **Figure 4.2**.

There are two different methods of thermal sensory testing that are generally available: the two-alternative forced choice method and the method of limits. The two-alternative forced choice method implies that a stimulus at a given level of intensity is presented to the patient during only one of a pair of stimulus events and the patient has to indicate which of the stimuli is perceived. Success or failure at this level results in subsequent stimuli being delivered at lesser or greater stimulus intensities respectively.[26] The forced choice method reduces the response bias and therefore seems better suited for a psychophysical examination, but the method is time-consuming. The method has mainly been employed in the evaluation of neurological patients with sensory deficits in general and not in pain patients in particular. For the evaluation of pain patients, the method of limits, in which the intensity of stimulation is continuously increased from 0 (or from skin temperature) to the point of detection threshold, is probably the most appropriate. This is mainly because of ethical considerations as a suprathreshold stimulus may evoke severe pain, which is often sustained. For the same reason, it is desirable to use as few stimuli as possible to determine a pain threshold. The pain tolerance threshold may also be determined; however, for some patients, the detection threshold itself will represent the level of tolerance. For cold and heat detection thresholds, it is usual to use a total of 5–10 repeated tests, whereas for cold and heat pain three repeated measurements are often used.

There are many parameters that may influence the results of the testing. The baseline skin temperature is an important factor that may influence the ability to discriminate between a rise or fall in temperature. In many laboratories, the contact probe is applied at a standard temperature of 32°C, thereby reducing the interindividual variability in perception thresholds. Alternatively, the temperature of the contact probe may be set at a lower or a higher temperature. By employing a higher baseline temperature, heat thresholds would be assessed at the baseline temperature itself or at a very short interval from baseline. A lower baseline temperature would create a bias in favor of a cold threshold at a short interval from baseline. It is not recommended that

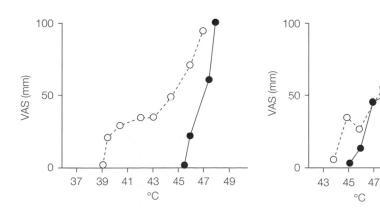

Figure 4.2 Patterns of abnormal sensory disturbances to heat stimulation of patient with neuropathic pain. Open circles, nonaffected side; filled circles, affected side.

the patient's skin should be warmed before testing. Another possibility is to adjust the temperature of the contact probe to be the same as the patient's skin temperature. One should be aware that, because of autonomic dysfunction in patients with complex regional pain syndromes, the skin temperature may be 1–3°C lower in the affected part. It may be difficult to compare sensory thresholds in affected and normal skin areas in these patients if the baseline temperature of the contact probe is set at different levels within the same individual. The baseline temperature should therefore be kept constant for each individual. It is difficult to give strict recommendations regarding the choice between using a fixed baseline of 32°C or a baseline temperature adjusted to the skin temperature. However, using a fixed temperature of 32°C allows easier comparison of sensory thresholds between individuals.

The rate of stimulus rise may also influence the sensory threshold. The most commonly employed rate of temperature change is 1°C/second. Quicker rates may induce reaction time artifacts, whereas slower changes create stimuli that are too long.

Due to the influence of spatial summation of sensory modalities, the size of the contact probe may also influence the sensory thresholds, in the sense that recruitment of more receptors will lower the threshold. For practical reasons, it means that thresholds are not comparable when probes of different sizes have been employed. Surface areas may vary from 9 to 12.5 cm^2, and smaller contact probes are used to test the face or fingertip.

A major question is to decide which skin areas should be tested. For the individual evaluation of pain patients, it is recommended that the patient should serve as their own control by testing normal contralateral "mirror" areas; of course, this is not possible in bilateral disease states such as diabetic or human immunodeficiency virus (HIV)-related neuropathy. Since thermal sensibility normally varies between regions of the body (e.g. higher sensitivity in the thenar eminence than in proximal parts of the extremities or the truncus), testing of a contralateral asymptomatic skin area is often performed. However, one should be aware that because of central plasticity (central sensitization), sensory thresholds in contralateral regions may be abnormal. Therefore, in many cases, it may be recommended that sensory thresholds are tested in a third skin area as a supplementary control. Testing all four modalities in three different skin regions may be time-consuming, but in many cases it is worthwhile.

In order to prevent injuries to the skin, the maximum temperature limit is recommended to be 50°C and the minimum to be 5°C.

Once again, it is emphasized that the results of thermotesting should be correlated with the patient's symptoms and clinical findings, and that a diagnosis or an evaluation of a painful syndrome based on thermotest alone is of little value.

Summary of thermotesting

- **Indications**: to test perception thresholds of heat and cold; to determine heat and cold pain thresholds; to detect possible qualitative abnormalities in thermal perception; to examine for possible allodynia/hyperalgesia to heat or cold.
- **How it is executed**: thermotesting may be performed in many ways. We recommend:
  - using the method of limits;
  - testing all four thermal qualities;
  - keeping a constant baseline temperature for each individual;
  - that the maximum temperature limit is 50°C and the minimum is 5°C.
- **Contraindications**: none (when used appropriately).
- **Typical findings**: there are large variations in the results obtained. In patients with neuropathic pain, findings may be reduced sensibility to heat and cold as well as allodynia/hyperalgesia to thermal stimuli, especially cold.

TESTING FOR ABNORMAL TEMPORAL SUMMATION

Temporal summation of neural impulses in nociceptive nerve fibers is a physiologically important mechanism by which the sensation of pain can be intensified.[27] From clinical practice, it is well known that repetitive stimulation of a painful skin area in a patient suffering from neuropathic pain may produce an intense and long-lasting pain. This is referred to as an abnormal temporal summation (often called "windup like pain,"[17] even though no direct correlation to the windup phenomenon in the neurons of the dorsal horn that has been observed in animal studies can be confirmed). The abnormal temporal summation seen in patients may be assessed very roughly by repetitive stimulation (usually with a frequency of 2–3 Hz) of the skin by a von Frey hair, for up to 20–30 seconds. If the phenomenon of abnormal temporal summation is present, the patient will report the sudden onset of an intense pain within the stimulated area, often occurring within a few seconds, that is associated with the presence of aftersensation and radiation. Abnormal temporal summation may be regarded as a sign of central hyperexcitability. By measuring latency, duration of aftersensation, and area of radiation, it is possible to quantify the phenomenon. For scientific purposes, more elegant techniques are available, either by von Frey application by standardized pressure and frequencies or by the use of electrical skin stimulation.

CONVENTIONAL NEUROPHYSIOLOGICAL TECHNIQUES

The practical details of conventional neurophysiological techniques, such as neurography or the measurement of evoked potentials, will not be given since these tests should be performed by trained clinical neurophysiologists. However, the indications for ordering such investigations will be discussed.

Neurography

Neurography is a generic term for the measurement of parameters such as conduction velocity, distal delay, motor and sensory amplitudes, and latency of late volleys such as the H- and F-wave. Nerve conduction studies play an important role in precisely delineating the extent and distribution of a peripheral nerve lesion and give some indication of nerve-root pathology (by evaluation of late reflexes). Neurography does not evaluate the function of thin nerve fibers such as Aδ-fibers that mediate cold/sharp pain nor that of C-fibers mediating the sensation of heat, heat pain, and some forms of tactile pain. The indication for neurography would be to evaluate whether there is a peripheral nerve lesion in the context of a general or polyneuropathy that is also affecting large myelinated nerve fibers. (The diagnosis of polyneuropathy cannot be excluded on basis of a normal neurography since a pure thin-fiber polyneuropathy may only be demonstrated by means of thermotesting.)

Sensory-evoked potentials

In routine neurophysiological practice, sensory-evoked potentials are measured following peripheral electrical stimulation. Unfortunately, some clinical papers assume that the evoked potentials to painful electrical stimulation represent aspects of nociceptive transmission. Based on reported evidence, it is obvious that the electrically evoked potentials that project to the dorsal columns are associated with sensory qualities such as light touch, vibration, and pressure. On the other hand, sensory-evoked potentials following CO_2 laser stimulation relate to pain and nociceptive impulses projected in the spinothalamic tract.

The potentials evoked by nonpainful and painful electrical stimulation are surprisingly similar. None of the components of the evoked potentials elicited by painful electrical stimuli can be considered as pain specific in the sense that they appear only following stimuli above the pain threshold.[28, 29] The shape or amplitude of the vertex potential does not change when the intensity of the electrical stimulus exceeds the pain threshold.[29, 30] This has led to the suggestion that vertex potentials evoked by nociceptive electrical stimuli are not reliable correlates for changes within the nociceptive system.[31]

The large interindividual variation in the amplitude of the laser-evoked potentials suggests that they may not be suitable for routine examinations in clinical practice. A large set of normative data based on laser-evoked potentials from normal, healthy, age- and sex-adjusted controls is essential. A statistical criterion of three standard deviations might be used to categorize sensory abnormality associated with laser-evoked potentials. In studies in which the patient and control groups serve as their own controls, for example by comparing the differences in amplitude for potentials evoked from two areas or by follow-up after surgery, measurement of laser-evoked potentials is suitable for monitoring purposes. Laser-evoked potentials can also provide useful information that is not accessible by conventional electrophysiological techniques. Laser-evoked potentials have been shown to be of value in assessing impairment of pain and temperature sensation in patients with peripheral neuropathies.[32]

A correlation between pain/temperature impairment and changes in the laser-evoked potential measurement has been found in patients with syringomyelia,[33] patients with multiple sclerosis,[34] and in neurological patients with various dissociated sensory deficits.[35] Sensory testing and clinical neurophysiology studies have indicated that patients with central pain syndromes occasionally have impairment of pain and temperature sensation. Central pain syndromes could be caused by disinhibition of spinothalamic excitability or by the reduction of spinothalamic function as a result of other central changes or disease in the brain. Casey et al.[36] found that central pain patients (cerebral or brainstem infarctions) with normal tactile sensation had significantly lower laser evoked potentials on the affected side than on the nonaffected side. This study supports a deficit in spinothalamic tract function, but does not suggest excessive central responses to the activation of cutaneous nociceptive pathways. The laser-evoked potential may also be pathologically exaggerated.

Fibromyalgia patients show a dramatically exaggerated reaction to muscle stimulation.[37] Evoked potentials to cutaneous laser stimulation have indicated larger amplitudes in these patients than in controls.[38] The major alteration in laser-evoked potentials is found only in the late components (N170–P390). These effects suggest the presence of exogenous factors such as reduced cortical and subcortical inhibition or central hypervigilance to the nociception, probably involving the limbic midcingulate generator. However, it has been shown that hypnotically induced hyperalgesia can also increase the laser-evoked vertex potentials.[39]

OTHER NEUROPHYSIOLOGICAL TECHNIQUES

Microneurography

Microneurography is an invasive technique that was developed by Swedish neurophysiologists Hagbarth and Vallbo to make single-fiber recordings from nerve fibers in subjects who are awake. Erik Torebjörk was the first to record from single afferent C-fibers in humans in 1974.[40] Since then, he has described the human nociceptive system, both mapping the different classes of C-nociceptors[1] and describing the pathophysiology of C-nociceptors in peripheral injury.[2, 9] Few reports have been published on this technique in patients, but recently some studies have been performed showing sensitization of mechano-insensitive fibers and spontaneous activity[41] as well as catecholamine-induced activation of nociceptors.[42]

Microneurography is technically a very difficult and time-consuming process, often requiring repeated investigations in one subject; therefore, it is only suitable for research purposes. Since the technique is also invasive, it should only be employed by those trained in its use and following discussion of the risks of nerve injury with the patient.

FUTURE PERSPECTIVE IN ADVANCED SENSORY TESTING

It has been proposed[5] that pain assessment and management should be mechanism-based. For this to be feasible, it is necessary to have quantitative techniques available that are capable of accurately determining which mechanisms are operative in the individual patient. This has not yet been achieved, and further concerted efforts are required to develop clinically useful techniques.

It is very important that sensory tests should be combined with the information obtained from the clinical history and examination of the patient to produce a comprehensive picture of the abnormalities in that patient, and possibly an indication of the mechanisms involved in the generation of that patient's pain.[43] A battery of sensory tests should consist of those that selectively activate the different afferent pathways – Aβ-, Aδ-, and C-fibers – and hence their respective spinocortical pathways. Clinical symptoms related to, for example, neuropathic pain can manifest themselves in many ways, and the results of sensory testing can be just as diverse. However, quantitative measures for follow-up are mandatory. As substantial plasticity can take place in the CNS, it is therefore important to include tests that quantitatively evaluate this aspect, e.g. tactile hyperalgesia or allodynia to touch.

In many cases, no abnormalities to a single stimulus may be measured, but when the stimulus is repeated, pain is elicited. The facilitation of central summation is an example of mechanism-based assessment. In complex regional pain syndromes (reflex dystrophy or causalgia) and neuropathic pain syndromes, repetitive tactile stimuli summate and evoke pain as a result of facilitation of the central integrative mechanisms, most likely in second-order dorsal horn neurons.

Without a controlled electronic device, it can be difficult to apply repetitive tactile von Frey hair stimulation at a fixed frequency. In a number of experimental studies, a 2-Hz train of repetitive stimuli seems to be adequate to generate "windup-like" pain and aftersensations in patients with neuropathic pain. Laboratory models exist in which the frequency and stimulus duration can be adjusted electronically, and different stimulation probes can be attached.

The currently available thermode stimulators have very slow rates of temperature change (e.g. 2°C/second), therefore they are not applicable for repetitive thermal stimulation. Recently, a thermal stimulator based on heat-foil technology has been developed for repetitive thermal stimulation (**Figure 4.3**). This device can provide a pulse rise time of up to 40°C/second and hence deliver pulses

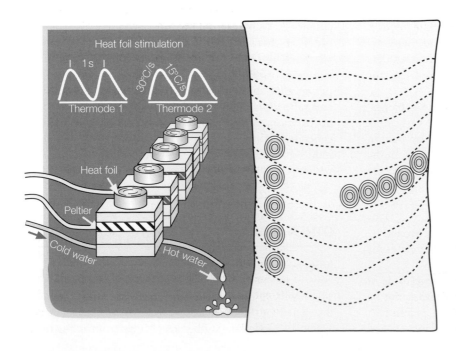

Figure 4.3 Thermal stimulation based on heat-foil technology. The example shows how temporal summation (response to repeated stimulation) can be assessed within and between dermatomes.

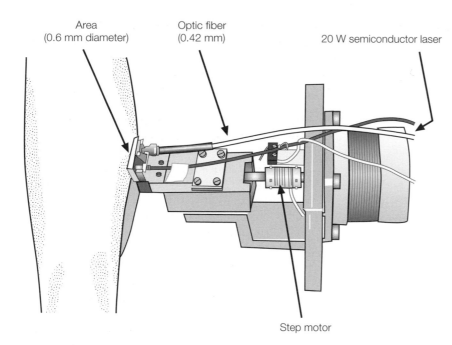

Area (0.6 mm diameter) Optic fiber (0.42 mm) 20 W semiconductor laser

Step motor

Figure 4.4 Heat pulses can be delivered to the skin by a semiconductor laser without touching the skin. The laser selectively activates the thin nerve fibers. The dark fiber is another optical fiber used by a low-intensity laser for determining the distance to the skin. As the heat beams diverge, a step motor will constantly adjust the distance to the skin so that the diameter of the stimulated skin is constant. The heat pulse can also be used to generate brain-evoked potentials.

at, for example, 2 Hz. Another problem can arise in patients with severe allodynia to touch when the heat thresholds to thermode or heat-foil stimulation have to be measured. Applying the thermode to the skin evokes pain and hampers the determination of the heat threshold.

In experimental pain research, high-energy laser has been used as a selective thin-fiber activator. The currently available lasers are very expensive and are complicated to operate; hence, they are not suitable for clinical routine and bedside testing. In recent years, the developments within the field of semiconductor lasers (e.g. 20 W, 970 nm) are promising, and such lasers may be available in the near future (**Figure 4.4**).

Due to accessibility, cutaneous stimulation has predominantly been used in sensory testing. Most often, the abnormalities are not restricted to the skin but may also manifest in deeper structures. At a minimum, the general sensitivity of muscles should be assessed by pressure algometry or electrical stimulation.

In conclusion, quantitative sensory testing has a role to play in clinical neurophysiology, neurology, and pain management. The challenge for the future is to develop techniques to:

1. assess not only the pain pathways as such but also, in more detail, the various mechanisms involved;
2. investigate pain originating not only from skin but also from deeper structures.

REFERENCES

∗ 1. Schmidt R, Schmelz M, Forster C *et al.* Novel classes of responsive and unresponsive C nociceptors in human skin. *Neuroscience.* 1995; **15**: 333–41.

∗ 2. Schmelz M, Schmidt R, Ringkamp M *et al.* Sensitization of insensitive branches of C nociceptors in human skin. *Journal of Physiology.* 1994; **480**: 389–94.

3. Davies SN, Lodge D. Evidence for involvement of N-methyl-d-aspartate receptors in "wind-up" of class 2 neurones in the dorsal horn of the rat. *Brain Research.* 1987; **424**: 402–6.

4. Woolf CJ, King AE. Dynamic alterations in the cutaneous mechanosensitive receptive fields of dorsal horn neurons in the rat spinal cord. *Journal of Neuroscience.* 1990; **10**: 2717–26.

∗ 5. Woolf C, Bennett GJ, Doherty M *et al.* Towards a mechanism-based classification of pain. *Pain.* 1998; **77**: 227–9.

6. Hansson P, Lindblom U. Quantitative evaluation of sensory disturbances accompanying focal or referred nociceptive pain. In: Vecchiet L, Albe-Fessard D, Lindblom U (eds). *New trends in referred pain and hyperalgesia.* Amsterdam: Elsevier Science Publishers, 1993: 251–8.

7. Vecchiet L, Giamberardino MA, Dragani L, Albe-Fessard D. Pain from renal/ureteral calculosis: evaluation of sensory thresholds in the lumbar area. *Pain.* 1989; **36**: 289–95.

8. Graven-Nielsen T, Arendt-Nielsen L, Svensson P, Jensen TS. Stimulus–response functions in areas with experimentally induced referred muscle pain – a psychophysical study. *Brain Research.* 1997; **744**: 121–8.

∗ 9. LaMotte RH, Thalhammer JG, Torebjörk HE, Robinson CJ. Peripheral neural mechanisms of cutaneous hyperalgesia following mild injury by heat. *Journal of Neuroscience.* 1982; **2**: 765–81.

∗ 10. Kilo S, Schmelz M, Koltzenburg M, Handwerker HO. Different patterns of hyperalgesia induced by experimental inflammation in human skin. *Brain.* 1994; **117**: 385–96.

11. Laursen R, Graven-Nielsen T, Jensen TS, Arendt-Nielsen L. The effect of compression and regional anaesthetic block on referred pain intensity in humans. *Pain*. 1999; **80**: 257–63.

12. Babenko V, Graven-Nielsen T, Svensson P *et al.* Experimental human muscle pain and muscular hyperalgesia induced by combinations of serotonin and bradykinin. *Pain*. 1999; **8**: 21–8.

13. Sörensen J, Graven-Nielsen T, Henriksson KG *et al.* Hyperexcitability in fibromyalgia. *Journal of Rheumatology*. 1998; **25**: 152–5.

* 14. Lindblom U, Verrillo RT. Sensory functions in chronic neuralgia. *Journal of Neurology, Neurosurgery, and Psychiatry*. 1979; **42**: 422–35.

* 15. Lindblom U. Assessment of abnormal evoked pain in neurological pain patients and its relation to spontaneous pain: a descriptive and conceptual model with some analytical results. In: Fields HL, Dubner R, Cervero F (eds). *Advances in pain research and therapy*. New York: Raven Press, 1985: 409–23.

* 16. Boivie J, Leijon G, Johansson I. Central post-stroke pain – a study of the mechanisms through analyses of the sensory abnormalities. *Pain*. 1989; **37**: 173–85.

17. Eide PK, Jørum E, Stubhaug A *et al.* Relief of post-herpetic neuralgia with the N-methyl-d-aspartic acid receptor antagonist ketamine: a double-blind, cross-over comparison with morphine and placebo. *Pain*. 1994; **58**: 347–54.

18. Andrews K. The effect of changes in temperature and humidity on the accuracy of von Frey hairs. *Journal of Neuroscience Methods*. 1993; **50**: 91–3.

19. Warncke T, Stubhaug A, Jørum E. Ketamine, an NMDA receptor antagonist, suppresses spatial and temporal properties of burn-induced secondary hyperalgesia in man: a double-blind, cross-over comparison with morphine and placebo. *Pain*. 1997; **72**: 99–106.

20. Stubhaug A, Breivik H, Eide PK *et al.* Mapping of punctate hyperalgesia around a surgical incision demonstrates that ketamine is a powerful suppressor of central sensitisation to pain following surgery. *Acta Anaesthesiologica Scandinavica*. 1997; **41**: 1124–32.

21. Ziegler EA, Magerl W, Meyer RA, Treede RD. Secondary hyperalgesia to punctate mechanical stimuli. Central sensitization to A-fibre nociceptor input. *Brain*. 1999; **122**: 2245–57.

22. Engkvist O, Wahren LK, Wallin G *et al.* Effects of regional intravenous guanethidine block in posttraumatic cold intolerance in hand amputees. *Journal of Hand Surgery*. 1985; **10**: 145–50.

23. Bovim G. Cervicogenic headache, migraine and tension-type headache. Pressure–pain threshold measurements. *Pain*. 1992; **51**: 169–73.

24. Kosek E, Ekholm J, Hansson P. Modulation of pressure pain sensibility in fibromyalgia patients is located deep to the skin but not restricted to muscle tissue. *Pain*. 1995; **63**: 335–9.

* 25. Verdugo R, Ochoa JL. Quantitative somatosensory thermotest. A key method for functional evaluation of small calibre afferent channels. *Brain*. 1992; **115**: 1–21.

26. Dyck PJ, Karnes JL, O'Brien PC, Zimmerman IR. Detection thresholds of cutaneous sensation in humans. In: Dyck PJ, Thomas PK, Griffin J *et al.* (eds). *Peripheral neuropathy*, 3rd edn. Philadelphia, PA: WB Saunders, 1993: 706–28.

27. Lundberg LER, Jørum E, Holm E, Torebjörk HE. Intraneural electrical stimulation of cutaneous nociceptive fibres in humans: effects of different pulse patterns on magnitude of pain. *Acta Physiologica Scandinavica*. 1992; **51**: 207–19.

28. Debecker J, Desmedt JE. Les potentiels évoqués cérébraux et les potentiels de nerf sensible chez l'Homme. *Acta Neurologica et Psychiatrica Belgica*. 1965; **64**: 1212–48.

29. De Broucker T, Willer JC. Etude comparative du réflexe nociceptif et des composantes tardives du potentiel évoqué somésthésique lors de stimulations du nerf sural chez l'homme normal. *Revue d'électroencéphalographie et de neurophysiologie clinique*. 1985; **15**: 149–53.

30. Brennum J, Jensen TS. Relationship between vertex potentials and magnitude of pre-pain and pain sensations evoked by electrical skin stimuli. *Electroencephalography and Clinical Neurophysiology*. 1992; **82**: 387–90.

31. Leandri M, Campbell JA, Lahuerta J. The effect of attention on tooth-pulp evoked potentials. In: Fields HL, Dubner R, Cervero F (eds). *Advances in pain research and therapy*. New York: Raven Press, 1985: 331–6.

* 32. Kakigi R, Shibasaki H, Tanaka K *et al.* CO_2 laser-induced pain-related somatosensory evoked potentials in peripheral neuropathies: correlation between electrophysiological and histopathological findings. *Muscle and Nerve*. 1991; **14**: 441–50.

* 33. Kakigi R, Shibasaki H, Kuroda Y *et al.* Pain-related somatosensory evoked potentials in syringomyelia. *Brain*. 1991; **114**: 1871–89.

34. Kakigi R, Kuroda Y, Neshige R *et al.* Physiological study of the spinothalamic tract conduction in multiple sclerosis. *Journal of the Neurological Sciences*. 1992; **107**: 205–9.

* 35. Bromm B, Treede RD. Laser-evoked cerebral potentials in the assessment of cutaneous pain sensitivity in normal subjects and patients. *Revue Neurologique*. 1991; **147**: 625–43.

* 36. Casey KL, Beydoun A, Boivie J *et al.* Laser-evoked cerebral potentials and sensory function in patients with central pain. *Pain*. 1996; **64**: 485–91.

37. Sørensen J, Graven-Nielsen T, Henriksson KG *et al.* Hyperexcitability in fibromyalgia. *Journal of Rheumatology*. 1998; **25**: 152–5.

38. Gibson SJ, Littlejohn GO, Gorman MM *et al.* Altered heat pain threshold and cerebral event-related potentials following painful CO_2 laser stimulation in subjects with fibromyalgia syndrome. *Pain*. 1994; **58**: 185–93.

39. Arendt-Nielsen L. First pain related evoked potentials to argon laser stimuli – recording and quantification. *Journal of Neurology, Neurosurgery, and Psychiatry*. 1990; **53**: 398–404.

40. Torebjörk HE. Afferent C units responding to mechanical, thermal and chemical stimuli in human non-glabrous skin. *Acta Physiologica Scandinavica.* 1974; **92**: 374–90.

41. Ørstavik K, Weidner C, Schmidt R *et al.* Pathological C-fibres in patients with a chronic painful condition. *Brain.* 2003; **126**: 567–78.

42. Jørum E, Ørstavik K, Schmidt R *et al.* Catecholamine-induced excitation of nociceptors in sympathetically maintained pain. *Pain.* 2007; **127**: 296–301.

43. Arendt-Nielsen L. Induction and assessment of experimental pain from human skin, muscle and viscera. In: Jensen TS, Turner JA, Wiesenfeld-Hallin Z (eds). *Proceedings of the 8th World Congress on Pain.* Seattle, WA: IASP Press, 1997: 393–425.

5

Pharmacological diagnostic tests

ANDREW P BARANOWSKI AND NATASHA C CURRAN

KEY LEARNING POINTS

- Lidocaine may be useful in patients with neuropathic pain, but may not predict if oral analogs will show any benefit.
- Phentolamine helps to identify patients who may respond to sympathetic blockade.

- Ketamine can be useful in neuropathic pain and potentially help in opioid tolerance.
- Opioids are proven to reduce neuropathic pain, but long-term efficacy and tolerance, and addiction remain issues.

INTRODUCTION

A pharmacological diagnostic test is usually a drug challenge in which a drug is administered intravenously over a relatively short period of time and titrated against a patient's pain. Different drugs are thought to act upon different pathophysiological mechanisms. Subjecting a patient to a range of drugs may help in understanding which mechanisms are important in an individual patient. Different drug groups may provide clues about treatments to which a patient may respond.

Pharmacological challenges may also be combined with quantitative sensory testing (QST – see Chapter 4, Sensory testing and clinical neurophysiology) to enable alterations in sensory phenomena to be monitored. This combined approach has the potential of providing us with more information about the underlying pathophysiology than a drug challenge alone.[1] The combined approach may inform us about sensory changes that are occurring with the drug challenge independent of a reduction in pain. If a reduction in a sensory abnormality is detected

by QST independent of a reduction in pain perception, it still has to be proven whether that drug group should be continued and a further agent should be added. The list of agents and their effects on different sensory abnormalities is growing.[2, 3, 4, 5] Small doses of several different drugs may increase the chance of reducing pain with fewer side effects. Also, several different drugs may be required to reduce all the sensory phenomena and hence the pain.

In this chapter, only intravenous drug challenges will be considered. Drug challenges may also be oral or spinal (epidural/intrathecal). In clinical practice, all drugs should be titrated against effect and side effects. The practical information regarding the administration of intravenous drug challenges has changed little since the last edition of this book, but the chapter has been updated to reflect the growing scientific and clinical evidence.

Advantages of intravenous drug challenges

- The effect of a potential treatment may be rapidly ascertained.

- A number of potential treatments may be screened over a relatively short period of time.
- "Clean" drugs with single modes of action may be used to provide information about specific pathophysiological mechanisms.
- Combining intravenous drug challenges with QST may yield information about the pathophysiological mechanisms and hence possible treatments.
- Side effects will be observed in a controlled environment and serious side effects can be appropriately managed.
- Blinding and double-blinding is possible and improves the value of the information gained.

Disadvantages of intravenous drug challenges

- Side effects may be more common as the drug is titrated up to a relatively high dose within a relatively short time. For instance, when establishing opioid sensitivity, oral medication may be titrated up over weeks with fewer side effects than if the same plasma level were achieved during the short time-frame of an intravenous drug challenge. This problem with side effects may result in:
  - the benefit of a drug being missed;
  - the patient refusing a potentially helpful treatment because of concerns over side effects.
- Even within a particular drug group, different drugs may have different effects. As a consequence, using a single agent from a drug group may result in the potential benefits of another agent within that group being missed.
- A positive result to an intravenous drug challenge does not always imply that the oral equivalent will be effective.
- A drug may have benefit not easily demonstrated in an acute outpatient setting where the sole end point is a pain score.
- Intravenous drug challenges are time consuming.
- Protocols vary from site to site and, as a result, the outcomes may be difficult to interpret.

INTRAVENOUS LIDOCAINE

Background

Nerve injury is associated with a reduction of some sodium channels and the development of novel sodium channels (downregulation of $Na_v1.8$ and $Na_v1.9$ sodium channels is associated with slow tetrodotoxin-resistant currents; up-regulation of $Na_v1.3$ sodium channels is associated with fast tetrodotoxin-sensitive currents). There is also a change in the distribution of these channels (with an increase in cell body, dendrites, and tips of injured axons). The consequences of these changes are that injured cutaneous afferents become prone to generating more prolonged and higher frequency discharges. The refractory period is reduced. These changes in the characteristics of sodium channels are thought to underlie the mechanisms of mechanosensitivity, thermosensitivity, and chemosensitivity.[6] Recent data show that local anesthetics may also have pain-relieving actions via targets other than sodium channels, including neuronal G protein-coupled receptors and binding sites on immune cells.[7]

Low doses of the sodium channel blocker lidocaine (lignocaine) have been demonstrated in animal models of neuropathic pain to reduce spontaneous neuronal firing in a selective manner that does not block normal axonal firing.[8, 9] Human studies have demonstrated that low plasma doses of lidocaine reduce neuropathic pain and sensory phenomena, such as allodynia, without an effect on nociceptive pain.[10] Nociceptive pain may be reduced with intravenous lidocaine, but only with high doses.[10][III]

A positive lidocaine challenge may be followed by repeated infusions of lidocaine. Some of our patients have significant benefit from infusions for up to three months. A role for the oral analog mexiletine may also be defined.[11] Oral mexiletine has been shown to be effective in peripheral neuropathic pain.[12][III] However, in clinical experience, a positive response to infusion of lidocaine does not necessarily predict responsiveness to oral analogs. In cancer patients, subcutaneous infusions of lidocaine may be used.[13]

Indications

An intravenous lidocaine trial is indicated in patients suspected of having neuropathic pain and when there is a suggestion of central sensitization, such as some of the visceral pains with referred muscle hyperalgesia and cutaneous hypersensitivity.[14, 15, 16] In addition, some of the diffuse muscle pains, such as fibromyalgia, may benefit from repeated intravenous infusions.[17, 18][V] Lidocaine infusion has also been used to treat chronic daily headache with substantial medication overuse.[19][V] Visual analog scale (VAS) scores should be greater than 5 on the day, and the pain scores should not fluctuate significantly over short periods of time.

Contraindications

- **Absolute contraindications**: failure to obtain patient consent and allergy to lidocaine.
- **Relative contraindications**: these depend on the dose and duration of infusion. Care should be taken with those patients who have a history of cardiac disease (particularly dysrhythmias) or epilepsy. In such patients, the low-dose four-hourly regimens could be considered (see below).

Doses and paradigms

Within the pain management center of the National Hospital for Neurology and Neurosurgery, London, UK, there are three different protocols.

THE BOLUS REGIMEN

The bolus regimen consists of 1 mg/kg lidocaine slow bolus (three minutes); repeated after 15 minutes, up to three times (a maximum of 4 mg/kg over 60 minutes).

- The bolus regimen can be used as a screening tool. The problem is that side effects are common (see below under Side effects and their management). Also, the results may be debatable as the high plasma levels achieved may block different pathways to the low-dose regimen and may have a central cognitive effect associated with sedation.
- We feel that in healthy patients the above regimen is safe because higher bolus doses of lidocaine have been given by other groups without complications:
  - Marchettini et al.[4] – 1.5 mg/kg as a single bolus over 60 seconds;
  - Boas et al.[10] – 3 mg/kg over three minutes. However, it must be noted that when Tucker and Boas[20] infused 3 mg/kg over three minutes, toxic plasma levels in the range of 15 µg/mL were reached.

If higher doses are used as repeated boluses, extreme care must be exercised as toxic peak levels may be reached because of accumulation. Moreover, the strong subjective central nervous system (CNS) effects may greatly exaggerate any specific analgesic effect through an unspecific placebo response. This phenomenon has been well documented (in another context) by Romundstad et al.[21]

SHORT INFUSION REGIMEN

The short infusion regimen consists of 3 mg/kg lidocaine over one hour using an infusion pump.

- Higher doses have been given by other groups:
  - Rowbotham et al.[22] – 5 mg/kg over one hour, maximum 450 mg, all patients achieved plasma levels >1 µg/mL, the maximum being 4.8 µg/mL (see below for relevance).
  - McQuay and Moore[23] stated "The best documented effective dose of intravenous lidocaine was 5 mg/kg, which was well tolerated when infused over 30 minutes."
  - In our paper,[14] we reported on an infusion of 5 mg/kg over two hours; at one hour, plasma levels as high as 10 µg/mL were seen (see below). Caution must therefore be exercised with higher doses.

FOUR-HOUR INFUSION

The four-hour infusion administers 2 mg/kg over four hours by infusion pump.

- We also reported an infusion of 1 mg/kg over two hours. All patients achieved plasma levels >1 µg/ml after ~15 minutes, with a maximum of 2 µg/mL (± standard error of the mean (s.e.m.) 0.6) at two hours.[14]
- This is a relatively safe technique and should be considered the method of choice in those patients for whom there is concern about epilepsy or cardiac disease.
- We have extended the duration of infusion from two to four hours as we feel that the longer the infusion, the better the result.[14, 24]

An "extended" six-hour infusion, 5 mg/kg over six hours by infusion pump, has also been described. This higher dose has been given over an extended period in a small study with benefit on percentage pain intensity difference over lower doses and placebo, but larger sample sizes are required to confirm these results.[25]

To summarize:

- Plasma levels of 1–2 µg/mL appear to be adequate for a reduction in neuropathic pain.
- All patients should be "nil by mouth" for the procedure. With the four-hour infusion method, we normally feed patients after one hour of the infusion, as we feel that toxicity is unlikely and our main reason for starving relates to the rare incidence of lidocaine allergy. Diabetic patients are often not starved for the four-hour 2 mg/kg infusion.
- Informed, written consent must be obtained.
- It is the four-hour 2 mg/kg infusion that we routinely use on the ward for inpatients. With appropriate arrangements, the doctor setting up the infusion is only with the patient for the first 30 minutes and the ward staff monitor thereafter.
- Full monitoring (electrocardiograph (EKG), blood pressure (BP), and oxygen saturation (SpO_2)) is instigated. In the bolus regimen, BP is measured every five minutes for the duration of the test and 30 minutes after the last bolus. For the infusion techniques, BP is measured every five minutes for 30 minutes, then every 15 minutes for the duration of the infusion. EKG and oxygen saturation monitoring is continuous.
- Lidocaine is diluted with saline to a volume that is easy for the pump to infuse, e.g. 60 mL.
- Pain scores (VAS, short-form McGill Pain Questionnaire (MPQ) or some alternative) should be measured every 15 minutes.
- If QST is employed, it is used before and just after the infusion.

- Following a positive response to intravenous lidocaine, some patients obtain significant benefit associated with repeated infusions of lidocaine. We currently run a nurse-led clinic where some patients return every three months for their intravenous lidocaine infusion.
- The correlation of benefit to the patient between oral mexiletine and intravenous lidocaine is not clear.[26] However, following a positive low-dose lidocaine, placebo-controlled, double-blind test infusion, it is traditional for a patient to try oral mexiletine if the test is positive. The author would normally start with mexiletine 50 mg and titrate up to mexiletine 10 mg/kg/day (see Chapter 19, Antiepileptic and antiarrhythmic agents in the *Chronic pain* volume in this series and Chapter 12, Antiepileptics, antidepressants, and local anesthetic drugs, for other regimens). The failure of intravenous lidocaine to predict responsiveness to oral mexiletine may represent a lack of central effect by mexiletine.

Side effects and their management

- Allergic reactions are rare[27] and are managed as for any allergic response.
- Most side effects are dose related.[20, 28] This makes the procedure very safe, if performed with caution. Heart failure and increasing age may result in an accumulation of lidocaine, resulting in an increased risk of toxicity.
  - For neuropathic pain, therapeutic plasma levels appear to be 1–2 μg/mL.[14, 24, 26]
  - Light-headedness, feeling drunk, and sedation occur at around 4–5 μg/mL. Other minor, subjective, CNS symptoms may occur, such as circumoral numbness, dizziness, and tinnitus.
  - Serious neurotoxicity is felt to occur at levels of 10–15 μg/mL, and minor CNS symptoms should warn of the risk of the more serious convulsions.
  - Cardiac side effects due to the lidocaine, such as heart block, asystole, and negative inotropic effects, have been reported. These are usually associated with large doses of lidocaine administered over a short period of time, with children and the elderly, and with patients with severe cardiac disease. Convulsions and hypoxia may contribute to these cardiac events. Early treatment of convulsions and hypoxia may prevent cardiac complications.

Practical tips

Lidocaine should be diluted in saline to a volume that makes calculation of the infusion rate easy, e.g. 60 mL. Ensure that the lidocaine and saline are carefully and adequately mixed. All infusions should be labelled and used immediately.

Efficacy

Evidence shows that intravenous lidocaine is most effective for neuropathic pain of peripheral origin.[23, 25] It can also be tried for all conditions suspected of having components of neuropathic pain or where central sensitization may be present. Intravenous lidocaine may reduce muscular pain, such as that associated with fibromyalgia.[18] [V] A recent Cochrane review of systemically administered local anesthetic agents for neuropathic pain selected 32 controlled clinical studies using lidocaine (16 trials) and mexiletine (12 trials).[29] It concluded that lidocaine and oral analogs were safe drugs in controlled clinical trials for neuropathic pain, were better than placebo (weighted mean difference (WMD) $= -11$; 95 percent CI, -15 to -7; $p < 0.00001$), and were as effective as or equal to morphine, gabapentin, amitriptyline, and amantadine. [III] The authors suggest that future trials should enrol specific diseases and test novel lidocaine analogs, for example AN-132, with better toxicity profiles with more emphasis on outcomes measuring patient satisfaction to assess if statistically significant pain relief is clinically meaningful.

To summarize:

- repeated doses of intravenous lidocaine may be helpful for pain management;
- intravenous lidocaine is known to be safe if used judiciously and with care;
- intravenous lidocaine may indicate that an oral analog of lidocaine (e.g. mexiletine) could be helpful in managing a patient's pain. However, only a few patients respond to oral mexiletine.

INTRAVENOUS PHENTOLAMINE

Background

Animal models of neuropathic pain[30, 31] and the capsaicin model in humans[32] have indicated that the sympathetic nervous system may be involved in the development and maintenance of pain. Intravenous phentolamine has been shown to produce pain relief in some patients with chronic pain.[33, 34, 35, 36] [II] [III] In early studies, approximately 50 percent of patients with reflex sympathetic dystrophy (RSD) were thought to have sympathetically maintained pain (SMP), as determined by an intravenous phentolamine test, first described by Arner.[34] RSD was later renamed complex regional pain syndrome (CRPS) type I, because far from all patients with CRPS have sympathetically maintained pain. Pain conditions other than the CRPS may also exhibit sympathetic maintenance.

It has recently been demonstrated in a patient whose pain is relieved by symapthetic blockade, that C-fibers could be activated following strong endogenous sympathetic bursts, and for about three minutes following the injection of norepinephrine into their innervation territory.[37] The authors conclude that sensitized mechano-insensitive nociceptors can be activated by endogenously released catecholamines. This gives us the most direct evidence of sympathetically maintained pain.

Interestingly, the reduction in pain associated with intravenous phentolamine may persist even after phentolamine has theoretically been eliminated from the body.[35] Also, the onset of pain relief may be hours or even days after the infusion has ended. There is a complex relationship between the results of an active infusion and a placebo infusion. Some authors have disputed the results of intravenous phentolamine infusion trials, suggesting that the results are due to the placebo response,[38, 39, 40, 41] and the evidence base has changed little in the past five years.[42] There are other ways of investigating whether or not a pain is sympathetically maintained than intravenous phentolamine. However, these other tests have their own problems. For instance, local anesthetic sympathetic trunk blocks (including stellate ganglion blockade) may block somatic afferent input. They may also be associated with significant systemic levels of the local anesthetic being achieved. Both of these may result in false-positive tests. A regional intravenous guanethidine block (with tourniquet cuff applied to the proximal part of a limb) cannot be used to investigate whether a pain is sympathetically maintained. Such blocks are often associated with the tourniquet cuff producing a pressure blockade of the Aβ afferent neurons, which would reduce the phenomenon of allodynia. Also, over a period of time, Aδ- and C-fiber acute nociceptive afferents would also be blocked by the pressure of the cuff. Finally, the procedure often involves the use of local anesthetic that inhibits the effect of guanethidine on noradrenaline release and reuptake, and lidocaine would modify the pain pathways both peripherally and centrally.

Indications

Complex regional pain syndromes types I and II are the principal indications. The test may be used to investigate many other pains, including central neuropathic pain, visceral pain, and myofascial pains. VAS scores should be greater than 5 out of 10 on the day, and the pain scores should not fluctuate significantly over short periods of time.

Contraindications

These include conditions where hypotension may be detrimental, e.g. ischemic heart disease and cerebral vascular disease. Asthma/bronchospasm may be considered a relative contraindication as intravenous propranolol may also be required. Patients who cannot lie supine should also be excluded. Care should be exercised with patients that have peripheral vascular disease.

Doses and paradigms

At our pain management center, we use a modified version of the Baltimore protocol:[43]

- phentolamine 0.5 mg/kg over 20 minutes for frail patients;
- phentolamine 1 mg/kg over 10 minutes for fit patients.

To summarize:

- all patients should be "nil by mouth" for at least six hours before the procedure and provide informed, written consent;
- full monitoring is instigated (EKG, BP, SpO_2), with BP every five minutes. EKG and saturation monitoring are continuous. Monitoring should be continued until observations have returned to baseline with no postural hypotension and for at least 0.5 hours after the last of the phentolamine has been infused;
- the patient lies flat during the infusion phase;
- an intravenous solution of sodium lactate intravenous compound (Hartman solution) or saline is instigated (4–8 mL/kg). The intravenous line should be long enough so that, with a three-way tap, intravenous injections may be given to a patient without the patient knowing the exact timing of injection of the individual agents;
- pain scores (VAS, short-form MPQ, or some alternative) should be measured every five minutes during the test and for 30 minutes after the last dose of phentolamine;
- after 15 minutes of the Hartman/saline infusion and measuring baseline pain scores, 1–2 mg of propranolol is given as a slow intravenous injection;
- ten minutes after the intravenous propranolol, phentolamine is infused according to the above dose regimen;
- significant hypotension is unusual if the patient is fit and recumbent. However, if a fall in blood pressure does occur, it is usually treated with intravenous infusions as appropriate. Care on mobilizing the patient must be exercised, in view of the risk of postural hypotension;
- QST may be combined with the phentolamine test. Cold allodynia is said to be associated with SMP,[44] and in our laboratory we have seen cold allodynia resolved with the phentolamine test.

Side effects and their management

- Propranolol may result in bradycardia and possibly cardiac failure. Peripheral vascular disease may also be exacerbated. Bronchospasm is a real risk in asthmatics.

- Phentolamine will cause significant hypotension, which can be prevented by the patient adopting a reclined posture and receiving intravenous solutions. Without propranolol, the patient will develop tachycardia.[45]

Pharmaceutical considerations

Phentolamine (Rogitine, Regitine) 10 mg/mL is administered in 1 mL ampoules. Dilute to a manageable volume with saline 0.9 percent.

Practical tips

Both propranolol and the saline infusion prior to phentolamine serve as a placebo as well as preventing the side effects (hypotension and tachycardia). The injections should be given blind to the patient, hence the need for an intravenous drip extension with a three-way tap. A positive phentolamine test occurs when there is a significant fall in pain (30–50 percent) associated with the phentolamine and not the placebo infusion or propranolol. In the event of headaches, not using the propranolol is a consideration as propranolol may in its own right reduce the severity of certain headaches.

Efficacy

Whilst there is more acceptance that pain is sympathetically maintained in some patients, efficacy of phentolamine has not yet been adequately tested.[42] Despite this, the authors feel that the test is useful and that it helps to identify a group of patients who may respond to other types of sympathetic blockade. We will continue to use the test in our pain management center until further evidence is available. For studies on the effect of sympatholytic therapies, it is essential that the patient has sympathetically maintained pain or components of a complex pain that are sympathetically maintained. The phentolamine test is one way of selecting appropriate patients for such studies.

To summarize:

- in certain pain conditions, the pain may be maintained by the sympathetic nervous system. Blocking the sympathetic system may reduce the perceived pain;
- transient blockade of the sympathetic system by means of an intravenous phentolamine test is a specific method of investigating whether a pain is sympathetically maintained.

INTRAVENOUS KETAMINE

Background

There is accumulating evidence for the importance of the *N*-methyl-D-aspartate (NMDA) receptor channel in the development and maintenance of chronic persistent pain. It is particularly important in central sensitization and opioid tolerance.[46, 47] However, NMDA receptors may also mediate peripheral sensitization and visceral pain.[47] Ketamine has been used as a general anesthetic and as an intravenous analgesic in burns and accident and emergency units for many years. It is thought to act primarily at the NMDA receptor, although it may also have actions at sodium channels and μ-opioid receptors.[48] Ketamine has been shown in animal models of neuropathic pain to reduce central sensitization and wind up (see Chapter 16, Opioids and chronic noncancer pain in the *Chronic Pain* volume of this series; Chapter 12, Clinical pharmacology of opioids: basic pharmacology in the *Cancer Pain* volume of this series; and Chapter 10, Treatment protocols for opioids in nonmalignant pain). It has been found to be useful in a number of chronic pain states, including peripheral neuropathies with allodynia, stump and phantom pain, central pain, and cancer-related pain with and without a neurological component.[49, 50, 51, 52, 53][III] Ketamine may be useful in opioid-resistant pain in which the ketamine may restore the opioid dose–response curve toward normal.[50, 54]

Oral ketamine has a bioavailability of about 17 percent (see below under Doses and paradigms). An intravenous infusion test dose is a quick way of establishing whether treatment with oral ketamine is a possibility. Certain chronic pain patients, especially those with cancer pain, may be sent home on an infusion of ketamine, which may be either subcutaneous or intravenous. Ketamine is a drug which is associated with abuse potential, and great care must be exercised if a patient is to be managed at home on parenteral ketamine.

Topical preparations of ketamine exist, the theory of their benefit lying in ketamine's peripheral action at both opiod, sodium, and potassium channels.[55] However, the studies on its use are small, and the mechanism of action may still be via systemic absorption.[56]

Indications

- Neuropathic pain states and patients with pain that is resistant to opioids.
- Cancer pain patients: particularly in the terminal stages and patients with head and neck cancer (airway maintenance).

Contraindications

These include hypertension, cardiac disease, and psychotic states. Swallowing problems may be a relative contraindication in view of increased salivation.

Doses and paradigms

- All patients should be nil by mouth for at least six hours before the procedure and provide informed, written consent.
- Full monitoring is instigated (EKG, BP, SpO_2), with BP checked every five minutes. EKG and saturation monitoring are continuous. Monitoring should be continued until observations have returned to baseline; normally, this would be for one hour after the end of the infusion.
- Intravenous access is established, and a syringe driver is set up to deliver ketamine 0.15 mg/kg over 20 minutes. Normally, ketamine is diluted to 20 mL with saline; we use a 60-mL syringe and infuse at a rate of 60 mL/hour.
- Pain scores (VAS, short-form MPQ, or some alternative) should be measured every five minutes during the test, and for 30 minutes after the last dose of ketamine.
- QST may be combined with the ketamine test.
- The test is terminated if:
  - the pain is abolished completely or the VAS score is less than 20/100;
  - the patient experiences dysphoria or extreme drowsiness;
  - BP becomes greater than 30 percent of baseline.
- The patient may be discharged one hour after the end of the infusion providing observations have returned to normal/baseline and there are no residual central nervous system effects.
- If the patient has a significant reduction in pain and minimal side effects, oral ketamine may be substituted. The calculation for the dose is difficult. In general, the final oral dose of ketamine is calculated by taking into account the dose infused to provide analgesia and the variable bioavailability of oral ketamine, which is between 10 and 20 percent of the intravenous dose. However, the usual starting dose of oral ketamine is a maximum of about 100 mg/day,[57] the final dose being arrived at by careful titration. Some patients may not even tolerate 100 mg/day.

Side effects and their management

Tachycardia and hypertension may result in the test being abandoned. Hallucinations and psychotic states may also be a problem. These side effects are usually curtailed by stopping the infusion, but may continue for many hours.[58] Hypersalivation may also occur.

Pharmaceutical considerations

Ketamine (Ketalar) infusions may be diluted with 5 percent glucose or normal saline. Note, ketamine is a general anesthetic agent, so overdose will result in an anesthetized patient!

Practical tips

A small dose of atropine or glycopyrronium bromide (glycopyrrolate) may reduce the salivation. Psychotic states may be prevented by reduced lighting and a quiet enviroment; they may respond to midazolam.

Efficacy

The response to an intravenous ketamine infusion has been found to predict the subsequent response to an oral dextromethorphan treatment regimen in fibromyalgia patients, so the intravenous ketamine test might reduce unnecessary treatment trials.[59]

An evidence-based review found level II evidence of pain relief in fibromyalgia and ischemic pain, but for nonspecific neuropathic pain, level II and level IV studies reported divergent results with questionable long-term effects.[60] For phantom limb pain and postherpetic neuralgia (PHN), level II studies provided objective evidence of reduced hyperpathia, and pain relief was usually substantial either after parenteral or oral ketamine. This conflicts with later work which suggests that intravenous ketamine is not associated with efficacy in PHN, although this may reflect lack of data rather than lack of effect.[61] Acute or chronic episodes of severe neuropathic pain represented the most frequent use of ketamine as a "third-line analgesic," often by intravenous or subcutaneous infusion.[60][IV] Ketamine shows some promise in the treatment of CRPS, but the evidence so far is weak.[62, 63] In cancer pain, two small trials have shown that intravenous ketamine improves the effectiveness of morphine, but data are insufficient to assess the effectiveness of ketamine in this setting.[64][III]

To summarize:

- ketamine is a general anesthetic. However, in lower doses it has good analgesic properties;
- ketamine is an NMDA antagonist and appears to reduce secondary hyperalgesia by a mechanism independent of opioid effects;
- an intravenous drug trial of ketamine may be used to determine whether oral ketamine may be of benefit to a patient;
- oral bioavailability is variable and care must be taken when calculating an oral dose of ketamine from an intravenous dose. Start oral ketamine judiciously;
- evidence for efficacy of ketamine for treatment of chronic pain is moderate to weak.

INTRAVENOUS OPIOIDS

Background

Opioids are well recognized as having an important role in the management of acute pain. In nonacute pain, the role of opioids is more debatable. If opioids are to be used in nonacute pain conditions, it is important that the efficacy be proven. Prescribing opioids to a patient with an opioid-insensitive pain may not only produce unnecessary side effects, but also predispose the patient to opioid addictive behavior and, because of this, guidelines exist for prescribing opioids in chronic pain.[65, 66]

Neuropathic pains may be sensitive to opioids, although this may be a relative phenomenon in which large doses of opioids may produce an analgesic response, but side effects are limiting.[67] A recent systematic review concluded that intermediate-term studies demonstrate significant efficacy of opioids over placebo in the treatment of neuropathic pain, but that long-term efficacy has yet to be established.[68][III] Certain opioids may be more beneficial in neuropathic pains than others. For instance, methadone is thought to have NMDA receptor antagonist properties.[69] Such activity may be advantageous in the management of neuropathic pains. It must also be remembered that whereas the neuropathic component of a patient's pain may be relatively unresponsive to an opioid, the nociceptive component, frequently also present, will be responsive. Pethidine has local anesthetic properties and may therefore have certain advantages in the management of pain where aberrant sodium channel activity is an issue. However, due to its short half-life (which often leads to addictive behavior), the risk of norpethidine accumulation and subsequent convulsions, plus lack of any real evidence that it is superior to morphine for visceral pain, the authors of this chapter cannot recommend it. In fact, we actively discourage its use. Oxycodone, however, may be a useful alternative to morphine in the treatment of visceral pain syndromes.[70]

Intravenous opioid drug challenges are notoriously difficult to perform. Side effects may interfere with the test if the opioid is administered too quickly and the potential benefits from the opioid may be missed. Also, there is some debate about which opioid should be used. Should a placebo also be given and should the opioid be reversed with naloxone or such similar agent? There is an argument that, even if the intravenous opioid test is positive, an oral opioid test must be carried out before the patient is started on prolonged oral opioid treatments.

Indication

Intravenous opioids are indicated for use in nonacute pains that are not responsive to other treatments.

Contraindication

- Opioid sensitivity and allergy; drug addiction.
- Relative contraindications include a past history of drug addiction and patients with severe respiratory disease.

Doses and paradigms

- Morphine: the patient may need to be an inpatient. The Oxford group[67, 71] have used a patient-controlled analgesia system with nurse/observer measurement of analgesia, mood, and adverse effects.
- Remifentanil: this is a new approach, which may offer a more rapid procedure.[72]
- Alfentanil: in patients without previous exposure to strong opioids, we normally inject 100-µg aliquots every minute up to a maximum of 1000 µg (ten times 100-µg aliquots). Each incremental dose is given in the absence of effect or side effects. Higher doses may be required in patients either taking opioids or with a history of previous exposure to opioids. Higher doses may also be given in the absence of effect or side effects.
  - Intravenous access is obtained and oxygen supplementation is applied, as is full monitoring, including measurement of the patient's oxygen saturation. Falls in oxygen saturation may occur late, and monitoring of depth and frequency of respiratory effort as well as levels of consciousness is mandatory. VAS scores should be measured before each increment. It may be necessary to have different VAS measurements for different components of the patient's pain.
  - Reversal with naloxone should be contemplated in patients not routinely on maintenance opioids. We would normally inject naloxone 100 µg intravenously every minute to a total of 400 µg in the absence of a positive response (i.e. return of VAS to baseline).

Side effects and their management

The principal side effect is respiratory depression. Only personnel trained in the recognition and treatment of respiratory depression should perform the procedure. Full monitoring, resuscitation equipment, and naloxone must be available.

Practical tips

As a placebo, low-dose intravenous benzodiazepine could be considered. The effects of the benzodiazepine could be reversed with flumazenil (Anexate) as a part of the test.

Efficacy

Opioids are effective for both neuropathic and musculoskeletal chronic pain, but patients have not been studied in the long term with regard to tolerance and addiction.[73]

To summarize:

- opioids may have an important role in the management of chronic pain. Some form of opioid challenge (oral or intravenous) should be instigated prior to starting regular oral opioids;
- only an appropriately trained person, with full monitoring and resuscitation equipment available to them, should undertake the opioid challenge;
- different opioids may have different effects and side effects;
- there are now numerous guidelines published for the long-term use of opioids in patients with persistent pain.

REFERENCES

∗ 1. Woolf CJ, Bennett GJ, Doherty M et al. Towards a mechanism-based classification of pain? (editorial). Pain. 1998; **77**: 227–9.

2. Gottrup H, Hansen PO, Arendt-Nielsen L, Jensen TS. Differential effects of systemically administered ketamine and lidocaine on dynamic and static hyperalgesia induced by intradermal capsaicin in humans. British Journal of Anaesthesia. 2000; **84**: 155–62.

3. Park KM, Max MB, Robinovitz E et al. Effects of intravenous ketamine, alfentanil, or placebo on pain, pinprick hyperalgesia, and allodynia produced by intradermal capsaicin in human subjects. Pain. 1995; **63**: 163–72.

4. Marchettini P, Lacerenza M, Marangoni C et al. Lidocaine test in neuralgia. Pain. 1992; **48**: 377–82.

5. Attal N, Nicholson B, Serra J (eds). New directions in neuropathic pain: focusing treatment on symptoms and mechanisms. Worcester: Royal Society of Medicine Press, 2000.

6. Cummins T, Dib-Hajj S, Black J et al. Sodium channels as molecular targets in pain. In: Devor M, Rowbotham M, Wiesenfeld-Hallin Z (eds). Proceedings of the 9th World Congress on Pain, vol. 8. Seattle, WA: IASP, 2000: 77–91.

7. Amir R, Argoff CE, Bennett G et al. The role of sodium channels in chronic inflammatory and neuropathic pain. Journal of Pain. 2006; **7** (Suppl. 1): S1–S29.

8. Chabal C, Russell LC, Burchiel KJ. The effect of intravenous lidocaine, tocainide, and mexiletine on spontaneously active fibers originating in rat sciatic neuromas. Pain. 1989; **38**: 333–8.

9. Woolf CJ, Wiesenfeld-Hallin Z. The systemic administration of local anaesthetics produces a selective depression of C-afferent fibre evoked activity in the spinal cord. Pain. 1985; **23**: 361–74.

∗ 10. Boas RA, Covino BG, Shahnarian A. Analgesic responses to i.v. lignocaine. British Journal of Anaesthesia. 1982; **54**: 501–05.

11. Galer BS, Harle J, Rowbotham MC. Response to intravenous lidocaine infusion predicts subsequent

response to oral mexiletine: a prospective study. Journal of Pain and Symptom Management. 1996; **12**: 161–7.

12. Dejgard A, Petersen P, Kastrup J. Mexiletine for treatment of chronic painful diabetic neuropathy. Lancet. 1988; **1**: 9–11.

13. Brose WG, Cousins MJ. Subcutaneous lidocaine for treatment of neuropathic cancer pain. Pain. 1991; **45**: 145–8.

14. Baranowski AP, De Courcey J, Bonello E. A trial of intravenous lidocaine on the pain and allodynia of postherpetic neuralgia. Journal of Pain and Symptom Management. 1999; **17**: 429–33.

15. Ferrante FM, Paggioli J, Cherukuri S, Arthur GR. The analgesic response to intravenous lidocaine in the treatment of neuropathic pain. Anesthesia and Analgesia. 1996; **82**: 91–7.

16. Nagaro T, Shimizu C, Inoue H et al. The efficacy of intravenous lidocaine on various types of neuropathic pain. Masui Japanese Journal of Anesthesiology. 1995; **44**: 862–7 (in Japanese).

∗ 17. Bennett MI, Tai YM, Galer BS et al. Intravenous lignocaine in the management of primary fibromyalgia syndrome. Response to intravenous lidocaine infusion predicts subsequent response to oral mexiletine: a prospective study. International Journal of Clinical Pharmacology Research. 1995; **15**: 115–19.

18. Raphael JH, Southall JL, Treharne GJ, Kitas GD. Efficacy and adverse effects of intravenous lignocaine therapy in fibromyalgia syndrome. BMC Musculoskeletal Disorders. 2002; **3**: 21.

19. Williams DR, Stark RJ. Intravenous (lidocaine) infusion for the treatment of chronic daily headache with substantial medication overuse. Cephalalgia. 2003; **23**: 963–71.

20. Tucker GT, Boas RA. Pharmacokinetic aspects of intravenous regional anesthesia. Anesthesiology. 1971; **34**: 538–49.

21. Romundstad L, Breivik H, Niemi G et al. Methylprednisolone intravenously 1 day after surgery has sustained analgesic and opioid-sparing effects. Acta Anaesthesiologica Scandinavica. 2004; **48**: 1223–31.

∗ 22. Rowbotham MC, Reisner-Keller LA, Fields HL. Both intravenous lidocaine and morphine reduce the pain of postherpetic neuralgia. Neurology. 1991; **41**: 1024–8.

∗ 23. McQuay HJ, Moore RA. Systemic local anaesthetic-type drugs in chronic pain. In: McQuay HJ, Moore RA (eds). An evidence-based resource for pain relief. Oxford: Oxford University Press, 1999: 242–8.

24. Ferrante FM, Paggioli J, Cherukuri S, Arthur GR. The analgesic response to intravenous lidocaine in the treatment of neuropathic pain. Anesthesia and Analgesia. 1996; **82**: 91–7.

∗ 25. Tremont-Lukats IW, Challapalli V, McNicol ED et al. Systemic administration of local anesthetics to relieve neuropathic pain: a systematic review and meta-analysis. Anesthesia and Analgesia. 2005; **101**: 1738–49.

26. Galer BS, Harle J, Rowbotham MC. Response to intravenous lidocaine infusion predicts subsequent

response to oral mexiletine: a prospective study. *Journal of Pain and Symptom Management.* 1996; **12**: 161–7.

27. Wallace MS, Dyck JB, Rossi SS *et al.* Computer-controlled lidocaine infusion for the evaluation of neuropathic pain after peripheral nerve injury. The analgesic response to intravenous lidocaine in the treatment of neuropathic pain. Anaphylactic shock following intravenous administration of lignocaine. *Pain.* 1996; **66**: 69–77.

28. Tucker GT, Mather LE. Clinical pharmacokinetics of local anaesthetics. *Clinical Pharmacokinetics.* 1979; **4**: 241–78.

∗ 29. Challapalli V, Tremont-Lukats IW, McNicol ED *et al.* Systemic administration of local anesthetic agents to relieve neuropathic pain. *Cochrane Database of Systematic Reviews.* 2005; **CD003345**.

∗ 30. Baron R. Peripheral neuropathic pain: from mechanisms to symptoms. *Clinical Journal of Pain.* 2000; **16** (Suppl. 2): S12–20.

31. Ramer MS, Thompson SW, McMahon SB. Causes and consequences of sympathetic basket formation in dorsal root ganglia. *Pain.* 1999; **6** (Suppl.): S111–20.

∗ 32. Kinnman E, Nygards EB, Hansson P. Peripheral alpha-adrenoreceptors are involved in the development of capsaicin induced ongoing and stimulus evoked pain in humans. *Pain.* 1997; **69**: 79–85.

∗ 33. Dellemijn PL, Fields HL, Allen RR *et al.* The interpretation of pain relief and sensory changes following sympathetic blockade. *Brain.* 1994; **117**: 1475–87.

34. Arner S. Intravenous phentolamine test: diagnostic and prognostic use in reflex sympathetic dystrophy. *Pain.* 1991; **46**: 17–22.

35. Galer BS. Peak pain relief is delayed and duration of relief is extended following intravenous phentolamine infusion. Preliminary report. *Regional Anesthesia.* 1995; **20**: 444–7.

36. Raja SN, Treede RD, Davis KD, Campbell JN. Systemic alpha-adrenergic blockade with phentolamine: a diagnostic test for sympathetically maintained pain. *Anesthesiology.* 1991; **74**: 691–8.

37. Jorum E, Orstavik K, Schmidt R *et al.* Catecholamine-induced excitation of nociceptors in sympathetically maintained pain. *Pain.* 2007; **127**: 296–301.

38. Dotson RM. Causalgia – reflex sympathetic dystrophy – sympathetically maintained pain: myth and reality. *Muscle and Nerve.* 1993; **16**: 1049–55.

∗ 39. Fine PG, Roberts WJ, Gillette RG, Child TR. Slowly developing placebo responses confound tests of intravenous phentolamine to determine mechanisms underlying idiopathic chronic low back pain. *Pain.* 1994; **56**: 235–42.

40. Verdugo RJ, Ochoa JL. "Sympathetically maintained pain." I. Phentolamine block questions the concept. *Neurology.* 1994; **44**: 1003–10.

41. Verdugo RJ, Campero M, Ochoa JL. Phentolamine sympathetic block in painful polyneuropathies. II. Further questioning of the concept of "sympathetically maintained pain". *Neurology.* 1994; **44**: 1010–14.

∗ 42. Rowbotham MC. Pharmacologic management of complex regional pain syndrome. *Clinical Journal of Pain.* 2006; **22**: 425–9.

∗ 43. Raja SN, Turnquist JL, Meleka S, Campbell JN. Monitoring adequacy of alpha-adrenoceptor blockade following systemic phentolamine administration. *Pain.* 1996; **64**: 197–204.

44. Choi Y, Yoon YW, Na HS *et al.* Behavioral signs of ongoing pain and cold allodynia in a rat model of neuropathic pain. Effects of short-acting NMDA receptor antagonist MRZ 2/576 on morphine tolerance development in mice. *Pain.* 1994; **59**: 369–76.

45. Shir Y, Cameron LB, Raja SN, Bourke DL. The safety of intravenous phentolamine administration in patients with neuropathic pain. *Anesthesia and Analgesia.* 1993; **76**: 1008–11.

46. Price DD, Mayer DJ, Mao J, Caruso FS. NMDA-receptor antagonists and opioid receptor interactions as related to analgesia and tolerance. *Journal of Pain and Symptom Management.* 2000; **19** (Suppl. 1): S7–11.

∗ 47. Petrenko AB, Yamakura T, Baba H, Shimoji K. The role of *N*-methyl-D-aspartate (NMDA) receptors in pain: a review. *Anesthesia and Analgesia.* 2003; **97**: 1108–16.

48. Hirota K, Lambert DG. Ketamine: its mechanism(s) of action and unusual clinical uses. *British Journal of Anaesthesia.* 1996; **77**: 441–4.

49. Backonja M, Arndt G, Gombar KA *et al.* Response of chronic neuropathic pain syndromes to ketamine: a preliminary study [published erratum appears in *Pain* 1994; 58: 433]. *Pain.* 1994; **56**: 51–7.

∗ 50. Eide PK, Jorum E, Stubhaug A *et al.* Relief of post-herpetic neuralgia with the *N*-methyl-D-aspartic acid receptor antagonist ketamine: a double-blind, cross-over comparison with morphine and placebo. *Pain.* 1994; **58**: 347–54.

51. Eide PK, Stubhaug A, Stenehjem AE. Central dysesthesia pain after traumatic spinal cord injury is dependent on *N*-methyl-D-aspartate receptor activation. *Neurosurgery.* 1995; **37**: 1080–7.

∗ 52. Graven-Nielsen T, Aspegren KS, Henriksson KG *et al.* Ketamine reduces muscle pain, temporal summation, and referred pain in fibromyalgia patients. *Pain.* 2000; **85**: 483–91.

53. Sorensen J, Bengtsson A, Backman E *et al.* Pain analysis in patients with fibromyalgia. Effects of intravenous morphine, lidocaine, and ketamine. *Scandinavian Journal of Rheumatology.* 1995; **24**: 360–5.

∗ 54. Dickenson AH. Neurophysiology of opioid poorly responsive pain. *Cancer Surveys.* 1994; **21**: 5–16.

55. Gammaitoni A, Gallagher RM, Welz-Bosna M. Topical ketamine gel: possible role in treating neuropathic pain. *Pain Medicine.* 2000; **1**: 97–100.

56. Poyhia R, Vainio A. Topically administered ketamine reduces capsaicin-evoked mechanical hyperalgesia. *Clinical Journal of Pain.* 2006; **22**: 32–6.

57. Enarson MC, Hays H, Woodroffe MA. Clinical experience with oral ketamine. *Journal of Pain and Symptom Management.* 1999; **17**: 384–6.

58. Max MB, Byas-Smith MG, Gracely RH, Bennett GJ. Intravenous infusion of the NMDA antagonist, ketamine,

in chronic posttraumatic pain with allodynia: a double-blind comparison to alfentanil and placebo. *Clinical Neuropharmacology.* 1995; **18**: 360–8.

59. Cohen SP, Verdolin MH, Chang AS *et al.* The intravenous ketamine test predicts subsequent response to an oral dextromethorphan treatment regimen in fibromyalgia patients. *Journal of Pain.* 2006; **7**: 391–8.

∗ 60. Hocking G, Cousins MJ. Ketamine in chronic pain management: an evidence-based review. *Anesthesia and Analgesia.* 2003; **97**: 1730–9.

61. Hempenstall K, Nurmikko TJ, Johnson RW *et al.* Analgesic therapy in postherpetic neuralgia: a quantitative systematic review. *PLoS Medicine.* 2005; **2**: e164.

62. Correll GE, Maleki J, Gracely EJ *et al.* Subanesthetic ketamine infusion therapy: a retrospective analysis of a novel therapeutic approach to complex regional pain syndrome. *Pain Medicine.* 2004; **5**: 263–75.

63. Goldberg ME, Domsky R, Scaringe D *et al.* Multi-day low dose ketamine infusion for the treatment of complex regional pain syndrome. *Pain Physician.* 2005; **8**: 175–9.

∗ 64. Bell RF, Eccleston C, Kalso E. Ketamine as adjuvant to opioids for cancer pain. A qualitative systematic review. *Journal of Pain and Symptom Management.* 2003; **26**: 867–75.

65. Kalso E, Allan L, Dellemijn PLI *et al.* Recommendations for using opioids in chronic non-cancer pain. *European Journal of Pain.* 2003; **7**: 381–6.

66. The Pain Society. Recommendations for the appropriate use of opioids for persistent non-cancer pain. A consensus statement prepared on behalf of the Pain Society, the Royal College of Anaesthetists, the Royal College of General Practitioners and the Royal College of Psychiatrists. March 2004.

∗ 67. Jadad AR, Carroll D, Glynn CJ *et al.* Morphine responsiveness of chronic pain: double-blind randomised crossover study with patient-controlled analgesia. *Lancet.* 1992; **339**: 1367–71.

∗ 68. Eisenberg E, McNicol ED, Carr DB. Efficacy and safety of opioid agonists in the treatment of neuropathic pain of nonmalignant origin: systematic review and meta-analysis of randomized controlled trials. *Journal of the American Medical Association.* 2005; **293**: 3043–52.

69. Ebert B, Thorkildsen C, Andersen S *et al.* Opioid analgesics as noncompetitive *N*-methyl-D-aspartate (NMDA) antagonists. *Biochemical Pharmacology.* 1998; **56**: 553–9.

70. S taahl C, Christrup LL, Andersen SD *et al.* A comparative study of oxycodone and morphine in a multi-modal, tissue-differentiated experimental pain model. *Pain.* 2006; **123**: 28–36.

71. McQuay HJ, Jadad AR, Carroll D *et al.* Opioid sensitivity of chronic pain: a patient-controlled analgesia method. *Anaesthesia.* 1992; **47**: 757–67.

72. Gustorff B. Intravenous opioid testing in patients with chronic non-cancer pain. *European Journal of Pain.* 2005; **9**: 123–5.

∗ 73. Kalso E, Edwards JE, Moore RA, McQuay HJ. Opioids in chronic non-cancer pain: systematic review of efficacy and safety. *Pain.* 2004; **112**: 372–80.

6

The role of biochemistry and serology in pain diagnosis

HILDE BERNER HAMMER

KEY LEARNING POINTS

- Clinical examination and history of the disease is of major importance in guiding the choice of laboratory tests.
- Laboratory tests are seldom diagnostic.
- A laboratory test should only be required in an attempt to refine the diagnosis further.
- Laboratory tests may be used to assess the degree of disease activity.

INTRODUCTION

This chapter discusses the various laboratory examinations used in the elucidation of different causes of pain of more than a few days' duration. A thorough clinical examination including a history of the disease is of major importance and will guide the choice of laboratory tests. Thus, the number of tests of relevance will primarily be dependent upon the differential diagnosis.

The following basic laboratory tests will often be important in clinical examinations to assess organ function:

- hemoglobin (Hb), erythrocytes, leukocytes, platelets (bone marrow);
- alanine aminotransferase (ALAT), aspartate aminotransferase (ASAT), alkaline phosphatase (ALP), γ-glutamyl transferase (gammaGT), albumin (liver function);
- creatinine and urine examination (kidney function).

In addition, the following laboratory assessments may be useful, depending on the history and clinical examination of the pain patient.

Serum protein electrophoresis

Serum protein electrophoresis is primarily used to identify patients with multiple myeloma and other serum protein disorders. The proteins are separated based on their physical properties. A homogeneous spike-like peak in a focal region of the gamma-globulin zone indicates a monoclonal gammopathy, which is associated with a clonal process that is malignant or potentially malignant, including multiple myeloma and Waldenström's macroglobulinemia.[1] In contrast, polyclonal gammopathies may be caused by any reactive or inflammatory process.[1]

Creatine kinase

Creatine kinase (CK) is an enzyme catalyzing the reaction from creatine phosphate to creatine, and the enzyme is mainly found in skeletal muscles, heart, and brain, where there are different amounts of the isoenzymes. CK levels are usually normal in the electrolyte and endocrine myopathies (notable exceptions are thyroid and potassium disorder myopathies).[2, 3, 4] However, the CK level may be highly elevated (10–100 times normal) in the inflammatory myopathies and can be moderately to highly elevated in the muscular dystrophies.[3, 5] Other conditions that can be associated with elevated CK levels include sarcoidosis, infections, alcoholism, and adverse reactions to medications. Metabolic (storage) myopathies tend to be associated with only mild to moderate elevations in CK levels.[3, 6]

Other tests

Electrolytes (calcium, phosphate, magnesium), as well as glucose, may be useful in assessments of muscle weakness of uncertain origin.[7]

In patients with pain, it will often be necessary to examine for nutritional or hormonal causes.

NUTRITIONAL DEFICIENCIES

Vitamin B_{12}

As many as 15–20 percent of people over the age of 65 years are estimated to be deficient in B_{12}.[8, 9] Pernicious anemia is a marker of B_{12} deficiency, but it is inadequate on its own since B_{12} deficiency exists in the absence of anemia. The nonhematological manifestation of B_{12} deficiency results in nerve dysfunction, including neuropathy.[10] It is likely that the peripheral neuropathy is linked to the diffuse myalgia that is sometimes seen in B_{12} deficiency and this improves with B_{12} replacement.[10, 11] However, there are few studies on the link between nutritional deficiencies and pain syndromes.

Iron

Iron deficiency in muscle occurs when muscle ferritin is depleted. Iron is essential for the generation of energy through the cytochrome oxidase enzyme system, and deficiency causes fatigue, poor endurance, and can cause muscle pain.[12] Iron loss as determined by low ferritin levels does not correlate directly with anemia, since the first stage of iron loss is associated with depletion of freely accessible iron stores in muscle, liver, and bone marrow.[10] Chronic tiredness and unusual fatigue with exercise may be symptoms of iron deficiency. High ferritin levels are seen in hemochromatosis, where deposits may cause arthralgia and arthritis.[13]

Vitamin D

Vitamin D deficiency may be associated with musculoskeletal pain, loss of type II muscle fibers, and proximal muscle atrophy,[14, 15] and the deficiency is detected by measuring 25-OH vitamin D. A high percentage of subjects with chronic musculoskeletal pain may be found to be deficient in vitamin D.[16]

HORMONE ANALYSES

Thyroid function tests (thyroid-stimulating hormone (TSH), free thyroxine (FT4)) should routinely be performed in patients who present primarily with complaints of widespread pain and fatigue to rule out overt hypothyroidism as the cause of these symptoms.[17] Measurement of serum TSH is the best initial laboratory test of thyroid function and should be followed by measurement of free thyroxine if the TSH value is low (and of thyroid peroxidase antibody if the TSH value is high).[18] Some patients may have low T3 syndrome, with a T4 to T3 conversion disorder (possibly secondary to a long-term stress disorder), and they may need substitution of both hormones.[19]

ACUTE PHASE REACTION

As part of an examination, it will often be of interest to examine for inflammation or infection, which may be assessed indirectly by use of acute phase proteins. The acute phase reaction is a major pathophysiologic phenomenon that accompanies inflammation and/or infections. Despite its name, this reaction may be chronic if the inflammation or infection is longstanding. In all instances where inflammatory cytokines are released, increased levels of the acute phase proteins are seen, which will be the case in inflammatory diseases, infections, trauma, and various neoplasms.[20, 21, 22, 23] Acute phase protein synthesis by hepatocytes is induced largely by the cytokines that participate in the local inflammatory process and are secreted primarily by activated monocytes, macrophages, and endothelial cells. Interleukin 6 (IL-6) is the major inducer of acute-phase changes, while IL-1 and tumor necrosis factor-alpha (TNFα) play more limited roles.[20, 22] Acute phase protein levels do not always change coordinately, which suggests independently regulated mechanisms for the regulation of synthesis. They increase by at least 25 percent during inflammatory states. There are several acute phase reactants that may be used in the clinics, where those increasing in concentrations are called positive reactants (e.g. C-reactive protein (CRP), serum amyloid A (SAA), fibrinogen, ceruloplasmin, alpha-1-antitrypsin, haptoglobin, ferritin, and several complement components) and those decreasing during the acute phase are called negative reactants (e.g. albumin, transferrin, and transthyretin). The degrees of increment in concentration vary between ceruloplasmin with approximately a 50 percent increase, to a 1000-fold increase for SAA.

C-reactive protein

CRP is the most widely assessed acute phase protein. One of its functions is to activate the complement cascade resulting in opsonization and phagocytosis.[24] CRP is not only important in the host's innate immune defense, but also in the protection against autoimmune diseases by its ability to help in opsonizing and phagocyting nuclear components.[24, 25, 26] Following an acute inflammatory stimuli, the concentration of CRP may rapidly rise for two to three days, to peaks that generally reflect the extent of tissue injury. When the stimulus subsides, the levels fall rapidly, with a half-life of about 18–19 hours.[24, 27] Most apparently healthy adults have serum CRP levels of less than 2 mg/L, although concentrations up to 10 mg/L are not unusual. Concentrations between 10 and 100 mg/L can be considered moderate increases, and concentrations greater than 100 mg/L are marked increases.[28, 29] As with all the acute phase proteins, CRP is not specific. However, it has in several studies been shown to be very useful in the evaluation of the degree of inflammation, infections, and necrosis, and levels up to several hundred milligrams per liter have been found in severe inflammatory or infections diseases.[30] Some patients with inflammatory joint disease have normal/low levels in spite of active disease. However, the degree of CRP elevation is usually associated with the severity of inflamed joints.[30] In some inflammatory diseases, like systemic lupus erythematosus (without serositis or arthritis), ulcerous colitis, dermatomyositis, and Sjögren's syndrome, only a modest to absent CRP response is seen, despite active inflammation.[24] CRP may be helpful in separating viral and bacterial infections, since normal or low CRP levels are regularly found in viral infections, while elevated levels are found in bacterial infections, with the levels indicating the severity of infection.[31]

Erythrocyte sedimentation rate

Over many years, the erythrocyte sedimentation rate (ESR) has been the most widely used marker of inflammation or infection. The level reflects the degree of erythrocyte aggregation and is the measured fall or setting in a vertical column (usually a 200-mm glass tube) of red blood cells within one hour at room temperature (the classical Westergren's method).[32] The degree of sedimentation is dependent on the number and shape of the erythrocytes, as well as serum proteins, that influence the tendency to aggregate erythrocytes.[33] Asymmetric, charged proteins decrease the natural tendency of erythrocytes to repel each other, leading to red blood cell aggregation and rouleaux formation. The acute phase protein fibrinogen is the most prevalent of the asymmetric acute phase proteins and has the greatest effect on ESR levels. ESR will thus indirectly reflect the acute phase reaction. The immunoglobulins, especially the pentamer IgM as well as high amounts of IgG, will also increase red blood cell aggregation and cause increased ESR. Anemia may cause increased,[34] and polycythemia decreased,[33] levels of ESR, and in addition, alterations in size and shape of erythrocytes may physically interfere with the rouleaux formation. ESR is thus an unspecific marker of inflammation, infection, malignancies, and necrosis. However, during pregnancies, there are normally increased levels of fibrinogen and ESR will thus be elevated.[35] Under the age of 50 years, the upper limits of normal ESR are 15 mm per hour for males and 20 mm per hour for females, while over the age of 50 years, the levels are 20 mm per hour and 30 mm per hour, respectively.[36]

SEROLOGIC MARKERS

Rheumatoid factor

Rheumatoid factors (RF) are antibodies directed against the Fc portion of the IgG molecule. In routine assays, the IgM-RF is measured, while all the isotypes (IgM, IgG, and IgA) may be measured by enzyme-linked immunosorbent assays (ELISA).[37] RF was first identified in sera from patients with RA, but it is not specific for this disease. The cut-off level implies that approximately 5 percent of healthy Caucasian subjects are RF-positive, and the prevalence of positive reactions increases with age.[38] In early RA, the sensitivity for RA assessed by RF measurement have been found to be between 50 and 77 percent, while the specificity is limited.[37, 39] Positive RA tests are also found in patients with other autoimmune diseases, like Sjögren's syndrome and systemic lupus erythematosus (SLE), as well as in malignancies and in chronic infections.[40] If IgM and IgA-RF are combined, there is an increased specificity for RA.[41] Patients with IgA-RF have been reported in several studies to have a more severe RA evaluated by disease activity and radiological progression.[42, 43] A high titer of RF has been associated with a more severe disease,[44] and treatment response is followed by decrease in RF levels.[45] The assessment of RF is of clinical relevance only if the patient is suspected to have arthritis, where the presence of RF will be of diagnostic and prognostic value.

Anti-cyclic citrullinated protein

The autoantibody system most specific for RA known to date is that directed to citrullinated antigens. The citrulline moiety, which is the essential part of the antigenic determinant in these antigens, is posttranslationally generated by peptidylarginine deiminases (PAD).[46, 47] Several tests are available and they have different sensitivity and specificity for RA. All have a high specificity, most often more than 90 percent, while the sensitivity ranges from about 40–90 percent.[48, 49] The antibodies are often present in the early stages of the disease and are predictive of disease outcome.[50, 51, 52, 53, 54] One may speculate that the anti-cyclic citrullinated protein (anti-CCP) antibodies may be of pathogenetic significance, where in genetically disposed individuals (especially people having special HLA-DR alleles, so-called shared epitopes), fragments of the citrullinated proteins may be presented to the immune system in the joints, resulting in an up-regulation of the immune response. In this way anti-CCP contributes to the perpetuation of joint inflammation.[46] Analysis of anti-CCP antibodies is useful for the evaluation of prognosis in individual patients with early rheumatoid arthritis.[55] The high specificity for RA makes it useful to distinguish RA patients from patients with SLE[56] and RA-like arthropathies in chronic hepatitis C virus infections[57, 58] and polymyalgia rheumatica.[59]

Antinuclear antibody

Autoantibodies, a hallmark of SLE, are typically present several years before diagnosis.[60] Several of these antibodies, which number over 100, have been associated with disease activity.[61, 62] They target nuclear and cytoplasmic antigens. These antigens are present in all nucleated cells and have a role in transcription or translation, in the cell cycle, or as structural proteins.[63] Virtually all patients with SLE have antinuclear antibodies (ANA), while most patients with ANA do not have SLE. Positive ANA are common in the sick elderly population[64] and in about one-third of healthy individuals at the lowest dilution.[65] The test is semi-quantitative at best and is poorly standardized between laboratories consequently lacking in appropriate reference preparations. An ANA titer of lower than 1:160 makes SLE very unlikely.[65] In the laboratory, pathological ANA will be characterized further for specific ANA targeting individual antigens like double-stranded (ds)DNA, SS-A/Ro, SS-B/La, Smith, and RNP. Anti-dsDNA antibodies are specific (95 percent) for SLE, though not highly sensitive (30–76 percent), making them very useful for diagnosis when positive.[65, 66, 67] However, they are occasionally also found in other autoimmune disorders. High titers in SLE are associated with active glomerulonephritis. Anti-Smith antibodies are found in only 5–30 percent of patients with SLE, but are highly specific.[65, 68] The anti-RNP antibodies are found in 40–60 percent of SLE patients, but are primarily a defining feature of mixed connective tissue disease (MCTD), and are also found in other autoimmune diseases.[69] Anti-SSA/Ro and anti-SSB/La are found in about 50 percent of SLE patients and in up to 90 percent of

patients with Sjögren's syndrome.[70] The ANA may thus be useful in diagnosing patients with history and clinical examination, indicating a connective tissue disease.

Antineutrophil cytoplasmic antibodies

Antineutrophil cytoplasmic antibodies (ANCA) are predominantly IgG auto-antibodies directed against constituents of primary granules from neutrophiles and monocytes. Although several antigenic targets have been identified, those ANCAs directed to proteinase 3 (PR3) or myeloperoxidase (MPO) are clinically relevant, whereas the importance of other ANCAs remains unknown.[71] The MPO is the major antigenic target of perinuclear ANCA, while PR3 is the major autoantigen in the cytoplasmic ANCA pattern. ANCA is primarily useful to assist in diagnosis of small-vessel vasculitis.[72] In generalized Wegener's granulomatosis, PR3 is seen in 70–80 percent and MPO in 10 percent of patients.[73] In limited Wegener's granulomatosis, ANCA are detected in only 60 percent of cases. In patients with microscopic polyangiitis, about 60 percent have MPO and 30 percent have PR3, and in Churg–Strauss patients, 30 percent have MPO and 30 percent PR3.[73] The titers may be followed for prevention of relapse.[74, 75] Even if ANCA is part of the examination of vasculitis, it may also be found in several other diseases, such as antiglomerular basement membrane diseases,[76] ulcerative colitis,[77] and Crohn's disease.[78]

Borrelia burgdorferi antibody

Lyme disease is a complex, multisystemic disease resulting from infection with spirochete *Borrelia burgdorferi*, where the initial symptoms, including erythema migrans, may develop into the late disease if not treated with antibiotics. The late disease includes symptoms involving the musculoskeletal system,[79, 80] like arthritis and myalgia, as well as neurologic features,[81] such as peripheral neuropathy, encephalitis, and myelitis. The diagnosis should be based on history and physical findings suggesting the diagnosis. *B. burgdorferi* antibodies can confirm but should never be the sole criterion for the diagnosis.[82] Recent exposure can usually be confirmed by IgM antibodies in the serum, while IgG antibodies develop later.

GENETIC MARKERS

Human leukocyte antigen–B27

The association between a group of rheumatic diseases called spondylarthropathies and human leukocyte antigen (HLA)-B27 has been known for several decades.[83, 84] The SpA includes ankylosing spondylitis, psoriatic arthritis, reactive arthritis, and arthritis secondary to inflammatory bowel disease.[85] HLA-B27 belongs to the major histocompatibility complex (MHC) class I molecules, which are multi-subunit glycoproteins on the cell surface.[86] The sensitivity and specificity of HLA-B27 for SpA in young patients with chronic inflammatory low back pain is about 90 percent.[87] The mechanisms by which HLA-B27 confers disease susceptibility to spondylarthropathies have remained elusive despite extensive studies for several years. However, findings obtained from patients with reactive arthritis suggest that HLA-B27 modulates the interplay between reactive arthritis triggering bacteria and immune cells, leading to abnormal host–microbe interaction.[86] The importance of assessing this genetic marker is primarily when history and clinical examination indicates spondylarthropathy.

GENERAL CONSIDERATIONS

Laboratory testing for rheumatic diseases allows rapid diagnosis and appropriate management, while false-positive tests can lead to inappropriate management and unnecessary concern for the patient. A thorough history and examination are arguably the best screening tests. Clinicians should be judicious in their use of laboratory testing, and should only undertake these in an attempt to further refine the diagnosis.[88]

ALGORITHM FOR LABORATORY EXAMINATION OF A PATIENT WITH PAIN

- History and clinical examination alone do not give a definitive diagnosis, and the following tests may be useful:
  - CRP and/or ESR;
  - Hb, leukocytes, platelets;
  - ASAT, ALAT, ALP;
  - creatinine and urine reagent strips;
  - TSH and FT4.
- History and clinical examination indicates symptoms caused by nutrition deficiencies:
  - vitamin B_{12};
  - folic acid;
  - iron (ferritin);
  - 25-OH vitamin D.
- History of diabetes and neuropathic pain:
  - blood glucose;
  - HbA1c.
- History and clinical examination indicates joint inflammation:
  - RF;
  - anti-CCP;
  - ANA.
- History and clinical examination indicate connective tissue disease (joint pain, changes in the skin, alopecia, intolerance to sunshine, mouth and eye

dryness, lesions in skin or mucous membranes), or vasculitis:
  - ANA (with subgroups);
  - ANCA.
- History and clinical examination indicate muscle pathology:
  - CK;
  - glucose;
  - TSH.
- If the history and clinical examination suggest malignancy, the laboratory tests available in each country will guide the specific test(s) of choice, while a screening should include:
  - blood picture;
  - CRP/ESR;
  - bone enzyme profile;
  - liver function tests;
  - electrophoresis.

Whether more of the laboratory tests mentioned here will be necessary will depend on the history and clinical examination of the patient.

CONCLUSIONS

In examining a patient with pain, it is essential to have a detailed disease history for diagnostic purposes. Only a few laboratory tests will be diagnostically significant, but they can be useful for assessing the progression of a suspected disease. Test results should be interpreted in light of the whole clinical picture, in order to guide the diagnostic and therapeutic process. Ultimately, the physician must have sufficient knowledge of the strengths and weaknesses of laboratory tests in order to interpret their findings correctly.

REFERENCES

* 1. O'Connell TX, Horita TJ, Kasravi B. Understanding and interpreting serum protein electrophoresis. *American Family Physician.* 2005; **71**: 105–12.
* 2. Alshekhlee A, Kaminski HJ, Ruff RL. Neuromuscular manifestations of endocrine disorders. *Neurologic Clinics.* 2002; **20**: 35–58.
  3. Lacomis D. Electrodiagnostic approach to the patient with suspected myopathy. *Neurologic Clinics.* 2002; **20**: 587–603.
  4. Comi G, Testa D, Cornelio F *et al.* Potassium depletion myopathy: a clinical and morphological study of six cases. *Muscle and Nerve.* 1985; **8**: 17–21.
* 5. Targoff IN. Laboratory testing in the diagnosis and management of idiopathic inflammatory myopathies. *Rheumatic Diseases Clinics of North America.* 2002; **28**: 859–90.

6. Preedy VR, Adachi J, Ueno Y et al. Alcoholic skeletal muscle myopathy: definitions, features, contribution of neuropathy, impact and diagnosis. *European Journal of Neurology*. 2001; **8**: 677–87.

7. Saguil A. Evaluation of the patient with muscle weakness. *American Family Physician*. 2005; **71**: 1327–36.

* 8. Baik HW, Russell RM. Vitamin B12 deficiency in the elderly. *Annual Review of Nutrition*. 1999; **19**: 357–77.

* 9. Andres E, Loukili NH, Noel E et al. Vitamin B12 (cobalamin) deficiency in elderly patients. *Canadian Medical Association Journal*. 2004; **171**: 251–9.

* 10. Gerwin RD. A review of myofascial pain and fibromyalgia – factors that promote their persistence. *Acupuncture in Medicine*. 2005; **23**: 121–34.

11. Sun Y, Lai MS, Lu CJ. Effectiveness of vitamin B12 on diabetic neuropathy: systematic review of clinical controlled trials. *Acta Neurologica Taiwanica*. 2005; **14**: 48–54.

12. Gasche C, Lomer MC, Cavill I, Weiss G. Iron, anaemia, and inflammatory bowel diseases. *Gut*. 2004; **53**: 1190–7.

13. Jordan JM. Arthritis in hemochromatosis or iron storage disease. *Current Opinion in Rheumatology*. 2004; **16**: 62–6.

14. Glerup H, Mikkelsen K, Poulsen L et al. Hypovitaminosis D myopathy without biochemical signs of osteoma lacic bone involvement. *Calcified Tissue International*. 2000; **66**: 419–24.

15. Mascarenhas R, Mobarhan S. Hypovitaminosis D-induced pain. *Nutrition Reviews*. 2004; **62**: 354–9.

16. Plotnikoff GA, Quigley JM. Prevalence of severe hypovitaminosis D in patients with persistent, nonspecific musculoskeletal pain. *Mayo Clinic Proceedings*. 2003; **78**: 1463–70.

* 17. Schneider MJ, Brady DM, Perle SM. Commentary: Differential diagnosis of fibromyalgia syndrome: Proposal of a model and algorithm for patients presenting with the primary symptom of chronic widespread pain. *Journal of Manipulative and Physiological Therapeutics*. 2006; **29**: 493–501.

18. AACE/AME Task Force on Thyroid Nodules. American Association of Clinical Endocrinologists and Associazione Medici Endocrinologi medical guidelines for clinical practice for the diagnosis and management of thyroid nodules. *Endocrine Practice*. 2006; **12**: 63–102.

19. De Groot LJ. Non-thyroidal illness syndrome is a manifestation of hypothalamic–pituitary dysfunction, and in view of current evidence, should be treated with appropriate replacement therapies. *Critical Care Clinics*. 2006; **22**: 57–86.

20. Gabay C. Interleukin-6 and chronic inflammation. *Arthritis Research and Therapy*. 2006; **8** (Suppl. 2): S3.

21. Johnson HL, Chiou CC, Cho CT. Applications of acute phase reactants in infectious diseases. *Journal of Microbiology, Immunology, and Infection*. 1999; **32**: 73–82.

22. Streetz KL, Wustefeld T, Klein C et al. Mediators of inflammation and acute phase response in the liver. *Cellular and Molecular Biology*. 2001; **47**: 661–73.

23. Deans C, Wigmore SJ. Systemic inflammation, cachexia and prognosis in patients with cancer. *Current Opinion in Clinical Nutrition and Metabolic Care*. 2005; **8**: 265–9.

* 24. Vermeire S, van Assche G, Rutgeerts P. C-reactive protein as a marker for inflammatory bowel disease. *Inflammatory Bowel Diseases*. 2004; **10**: 661–5.

25. Volanakis JE. Human C-reactive protein: Expression, structure, and function. *Molecular Immunology*. 2001; **38**: 189–97.

* 26. Mortensen RF. C-reactive protein, inflammation, and innate immunity. *Immunologic Research*. 2001; **24**: 163–76.

27. Vigushin DM, Pepys MB, Hawkins PN. Metabolic and scintigraphic studies of radioiodinated human C-reactive protein in health and disease. *Journal of Clinical Investigation*. 1993; **91**: 1351–7.

28. Morley JJ, Kushner I. Serum C-reactive protein levels in disease. *Annals of the New York Academy of Sciences*. 1982; **389**: 406–18.

29. Macy EM, Hayes TE, Tracy RP. Variability in the measurement of C-reactive protein in healthy subjects: implications for reference intervals and epidemiological applications. *Clinical Chemistry*. 1997; **43**: 52–8.

30. Plant MJ, Williams AL, O'Sullivan MM et al. Relationship between time-integrated C-reactive protein levels and radiologic progression in patients with rheumatoid arthritis. *Arthritis and Rheumatism*. 2000; **43**: 1473–7.

31. Mitaka C. Clinical laboratory differentiation of infectious versus non-infectious systemic inflammatory response syndrome. *Clinica Chimica Acta*. 2005; **351**: 17–29.

32. International Council for Standardization in Haematology (Expert Panel on Blood Rheology). ICSH recommendations for measurement of erythrocyte sedimentation rate. *Journal of Clinical Pathology*. 1993; **46**: 198–203.

33. Bedell SE, Bush BT. Erythrocyte sedimentation rate. From folklore to facts. *American Journal of Medicine*. 1985; **78**: 1001–09.

34. Lascari AD. The erythrocyte sedimentation rate. *Pediatric Clinics of North America*. 1972; **19**: 1113–21.

35. Branch DW. Physiologic adaptations of pregnancy. *American Journal of Reproductive Immunology*. 1992; **28**: 120–2.

* 36. Olshaker JS, Jerrard DA. The erythrocyte sedimentation rate. *Journal of Emergency Medicine*. 1997; **15**: 869–74.

* 37. Rantapää-Dahlqvist S. Diagnostic and prognostic significance of autoantibodies in early rheumatoid arthritis. *Scandinavian Journal of Rheumatology*. 2005; **34**: 83–96.

38. Husby G, Gran JT, Johannessen A. Epidemiological and genetic aspects of IgM rheumatoid factors. *Scandinavian Journal of Rheumatology. Supplement*. 1988; **75** (Suppl.): 213–18.

39. Dorner T, Hansen A. Autoantibodies in normals – the value of predicting rheumatoid arthritis. *Arthritis Research and Therapy*. 2004; **6**: 282–4.

40. Newkirk MM. Rheumatoid factors: what do they tell us? *Journal of Rheumatology*. 2002; **29**: 2034–40.

41. Jonsson T, Steinsson K, Jonsson H et al. Combined elevation of IgM and IgA rheumatoid factor has high diagnostic specificity for rheumatoid arthritis. *Rheumatology International*. 1998; **18**: 119–22.

42. Jonsson T, Valdimarsson H. Is measurement of rheumatoid factor isotypes clinically useful? *Annals of the Rheumatic Diseases*. 1993; **52**: 161–4.

43. Houssien DA, Jonsson T, Davies E, Scott DL. Rheumatoid factor isotypes, disease activity and the outcome of rheumatoid arthritis: comparative effects of different antigens. *Scandinavian Journal of Rheumatology*. 1998; **27**: 46–53.

44. van Zeben D, Hazes JM, Zwinderman AH et al. Clinical significance of rheumatoid factors in early rheumatoid arthritis: results of a follow up study. *Annals of the Rheumatic Diseases*. 1992; **51**: 1029–35.

45. Mikuls TR, O'Dell JR, Stoner JA et al. Association of rheumatoid arthritis treatment response and disease duration with declines in serum levels of IgM rheumatoid factor and anti-cyclic citrullinated peptide antibody. *Arthritis and Rheumatism*. 2004; **50**: 3776–82.

∗ 46. Zendman AJ, van Venrooij WJ, Pruijn GJ. Use and significance of anti-CCP autoantibodies in rheumatoid arthritis. *Rheumatology*. 2006; **45**: 20–5.

∗ 47. Vossenaar ER, Zendman AJ, van Venrooij WJ, Pruijn GJ. PAD, a growing family of citrullinating enzymes: genes, features and involvement in disease. *Bioassays*. 2003; **25**: 1106–18.

∗ 48. Mimori T. Clinical significance of anti-CCP antibodies in rheumatoid arthritis. *Internal Medicine*. 2005; **44**: 1122–6.

49. Avouac J, Gossec L, Dougados M. Diagnostic and predictive value of anti-cyclic citrullinated protein antibodies in rheumatoid arthritis: a systematic literature review. *Annals of the Rheumatic Diseases*. 2006; **65**: 845–51.

50. Vossenaar ER, van Venrooij WJ. Citrullinated proteins: sparks that may ignite the fire in rheumatoid arthritis. *Arthritis Research and Therapy*. 2004; **6**: 107–11.

51. Quinn MA, Gough AKS, Green MJ et al. Anti-CCP antibodies measured at disease onset help identify seronegative rheumatoid arthritis and predict radiological and functional outcome. *Rheumatology*. 2006; **45**: 478–80.

52. Meyer O, Labarre C, Dougados M et al. Anticitrullinated protein/peptide antibody assays in early rheumatoid arthritis for predicting five year radiographic damage. *Annals of the Rheumatic Diseases*. 2003; **62**: 120–6.

53. van Jaarsveld CH, ter Borg EJ, Jacobs JW et al. The prognostic value of the antiperinuclear factor, anti-citrullinated peptide antibodies and rheumatoid factor in early rheumatoid arthritis. *Clinical and Experimental Rheumatology*. 1999; **17**: 689–97.

54. Kroot EJ, de Jong BA, van Leeuwen MA et al. The prognostic value of anti-cyclic citrullinated peptide antibody in patients with recent-onset rheumatoid arthritis. *Arthritis and Rheumatism*. 2000; **43**: 1831–5.

55. Lindqvist E, Eberhardt K, Bendtzen K et al. Prognostic laboratory markers of joint damage in rheumatoid arthritis. *Annals of the Rheumatic Diseases*. 2005; **64**: 196–201.

56. Mediwake R, Isenberg DA, Schellekens GA, van Venrooij WJ. Use of anti-citrullinated peptide and anti-RA33 antibodies in distinguishing erosive arthritis in patients with systemic lupus erythematosus and rheumatoid arthritis. *Annals of the Rheumatic Diseases*. 2001; **60**: 67–8.

57. Wener MH, Hutchinson K, Morishima C, Gretch DR. Absence of antibodies to cyclic citrullinated peptide in sera of patients with hepatitis C virus infection and cryoglobulinemia. *Arthritis and Rheumatism*. 2004; **50**: 2305–8.

58. Bombardieri M, Alessandri C, Labbadia G et al. Role of anti-cyclic citrullinated peptide antibodies in discriminating patients with rheumatoid arthritis from patients with chronic hepatitis C infection-associated polyarticular involvement. *Arthritis Research and Therapy*. 2004; **6**: R137–41.

∗ 59. Lopez-Hoyos M, Ruiz de Alegria C, Blanco R et al. Clinical utility of anti-CCP antibodies in the differential diagnosis of elderly-onset rheumatoid arthritis and polymyalgia rheumatica. *Rheumatology*. 2004; **43**: 655–7.

60. Arbuckle MR, McClain MT, Rubertone MV et al. Development of autoantibodies before the clinical onset of systemic lupus erythematosus. *New England Journal of Medicine*. 2003; **349**: 1526–33.

61. Marchini B, Dolcher MP, Sabbatini A et al. Immune response to different sequences of the EBNA I molecule in Epstein-Barr virus-related disorders and in autoimmune diseases. *Journal of Autoimmunity*. 1994; **7**: 179–91.

∗ 62. Sherer Y, Gorstein A, Fritzler MJ, Shoenfeld Y. Autoantibody explosion in systemic lupus erythematosus: more than 100 different antibodies found in SLE patients. *Seminars in Arthritis and Rheumatism*. 2004; **34**: 501–37.

∗ 63. Sheldon J. Laboratory testing in autoimmune rheumatic diseases. *Best Practice and Research. Clinical Rheumatology*. 2004; **18**: 249–69.

64. Ruffatti A, Calligaro A, Del Ross T et al. Anti-double-stranded DNA antibodies in the healthy elderly: prevalence and characteristics. *Journal of Clinical Immunology*. 1990; **10**: 300–03.

65. Kurien BT, Scofield RH. Autoantibody determination in the diagnosis of systemic lupus erythematosus. *Scandinavian Journal of Immunology*. 2006; **64**: 227–35.

66. Hahn BH. Antibodies to DNA. *New England Journal of Medicine*. 1998; **338**: 1359–68.

67. Vitali C, Bencivelli W, Isenberg DA et al. Disease activity in systemic lupus erythematosus: report of the Consensus Study Group of the European Workshop for Rheumatology Research. I. A descriptive analysis of 704 European lupus patients. European Consensus Study Group for Disease Activity in SLE. *Clinical and Experimental Rheumatology*. 1992; **10**: 527–39.

68. Hoch SO, Eisenberg RA, Sharp GC. Diverse antibody recognition patterns of the multiple Sm-D antigen polypeptides. *Clinical Immunology*. 1999; **92**: 203–8.

69. Sawalha AH, Harley JB. Antinuclear autoantibodies in systemic lupus erythematosus. *Current Opinion in Rheumatology*. 2004; **16**: 534–40.

70. Harley JB, Scofield RH, Reichlin M. Anti-Ro in Sjögren's syndrome and systemic lupus erythematosus. *Rheumatic Diseases Clinics of North America*. 1992; **18**: 337–58.

* 71. Bosch X, Guilabert A, Font J. Antineutrophil cytoplasmic antibodies. *Lancet*. 2006; **368**: 404–18.

72. Falk RJ, Jennette JC. Thoughts about the classification of small vessel vasculitis. *Journal of Nephrology*. 2004; **17** (Suppl. 8): S3–9.

73. Wiik A. Rational use of ANCA in the diagnosis of vasculitis. *Rheumatology*. 2002; **41**: 481–3.

74. Han WK, Choi HK, Roth RM et al. Serial ANCA titers: useful tool for prevention of relapses in ANCA-associated vasculitis. *Kidney International*. 2003; **63**: 1079–85.

75. Tervaert JW, Huitema MG, Hene RJ et al. Prevention of relapses in Wegener's granulomatosis by treatment based on antineutrophil cytoplasmic antibody titre. *Lancet*. 1990; **336**: 709–11.

76. Levy JB, Hammad T, Coulthart A et al. Clinical features and outcome of patients with both ANCA and anti-GBM antibodies. *Kidney International*. 2004; **66**: 1535–40.

77. Saxon A, Shanahan F, Landers C et al. A distinct subset of antineutrophil cytoplasmic antibodies is associated with inflammatory bowel disease. *Journal of Allergy and Clinical Immunology*. 1990; **86**: 202–10.

* 78. Savige J, Dimech W, Fritzler M et al. Addendum to the International Consensus Statement on testing and reporting of antineutrophil cytoplasmic antibodies. Quality control guidelines, comments, and recommendations for testing in other autoimmune diseases. *American Journal of Clinical Pathology*. 2003; **120**: 312–18.

79. Sigal LH. Musculoskeletal manifestations of Lyme arthritis. *Rheumatic Diseases Clinics of North America*. 1998; **24**: 323–51.

80. Steere AC, Schoen RT, Taylor E. The clinical evolution of Lyme arthritis. *Annals of Internal Medicine*. 1987; **107**: 725–31.

81. Logigian EL, Kaplan RF, Steere AC. Chronic neurologic manifestations of Lyme disease. *New England Journal of Medicine*. 1990; **323**: 1438–44.

* 82. Sigal LH. Pitfalls in the diagnosis and management of Lyme disease. *Arthritis and Rheumatism*. 1998; **41**: 195–204.

83. Brewerton DA, Hart FD, Nicholls A et al. Ankylosing spondylitis and HL-A 27. *Lancet*. 1973; **1**: 904–07.

84. Aho K, Ahvonen P, Lassus A et al. HL-A 27 in reactive arthritis. A study of Yersinia arthritis and Reiter's disease. *Arthritis and Rheumatism*. 1974; **17**: 521–6.

85. De Keyser F, Baeten D, Van den Bosch F et al. Gut inflammation and spondyloarthropathies. *Current Rheumatology Reports*. 2002; **4**: 525–32.

* 86. Vähämiko S, Penttinen MA, Granfors K. Aetiology and pathogenesis of reactive arthritis: role of non-antigen-presenting effects of HLA-B27. *Arthritis Research and Therapy*. 2005; **7**: 136–41.

* 87. Sieper J, Rudwaleit M. Early referral recommendations for ankylosing spondylitis (including pre-radiographic and radiographic forms) in primary care. *Annals of the Rheumatic Diseases*. 2005; **64**: 659–63.

88. Colglazier CL, Sutej PG. Laboratory testing in the rheumatic diseases: a practical review. *Southern Medical Journal*. 2005; **98**: 185–91.

7

Diagnostic algorithms for painful peripheral neuropathy

DAVID BENNETT

KEY LEARNING POINTS

- Careful classification is very helpful in understanding the underlying etiology of a peripheral neuropathy.
- Neuropathies can be classified in terms of the speed of onset (acute versus chronic), anatomical distribution, fiber type involvement (i.e. sensory, motor, and/or autonomic) and underlying pathology (axonal versus demyelinating).
- Careful clinical history, examination, and neurophysiology are essential first steps to achieve this classification.

- Small-fiber neuropathies represent a particular diagnostic challenge as neurophysiology is often normal. Assessment of epidermal innervation by skin biopsy can be particularly helpful in this situation.
- Nerve biopsy is associated with a significant morbidity and should be reserved for selected cases (i.e. investigation of a potentially treatable neuropathy).

INTRODUCTION TO NEUROPATHY

The emphasis of this chapter will be on a pragmatic diagnostic approach to painful neuropathy. Diagnosis can be viewed as having three stages; confirmation that there is indeed evidence of injury to the peripheral nervous system; classification of the neuropathy; and finally investigation of any underlying cause. As with all clinical medicine, the key to this process is clinical history and examination followed by appropriate laboratory investigations.

Neuropathies represent one of the most common neurological disorders with a prevalence of 2.4 percent in the general population rising up to 8 percent with age.[1] Nerve injury may lead to the dysfunction of motor, sensory, or autonomic fibers in various combinations. Patients can therefore present in a number of ways, including negative symptoms such as sensory loss, weakness, and autonomic dysfunction, as well as positive symptoms such as paresthesia and pain. Virtually any type of neuropathy can give rise to neuropathic pain, for instance leprosy, which was thought of as a painless neuropathy, is actually associated with a high prevalence of neuropathic pain.[2] There is no doubt that certain types of neuropathy have a particular propensity for causing pain and these are listed in **Table 7.1**.

Table 7.1 Neuropathies commonly associated with pain.

Mononeuropathy and multiple mononeuropathies	Symmetrical polyneuropathy
Entrapment, e.g. carpal tunnel syndrome	Genetic causes – Fabry's disease, amyloidosis, CMT 2B (RAB7 mutation), CMT 4F (periaxin mutation), HSAN1 (SPTCL1 mutation)
Trauma, e.g. postamputation	
Connective tissue disease/vasculitis, e.g. systemic lupus erythematosis, rheumatoid arthritis, Churg–Strauss disease, Wegener's granulomatosis, polyarteritis nodosa, nonsystemic vasculitic neuropathy	Metabolic causes – alcohol, diabetes, amyloid, beri beri
	Toxins/drugs – thallium, acrylamide, antiretrovirals, vincristine, cisplatin, thalidomide
Diabetes – mononeuropathy/proximal diabetic neuropathy	Paraneoplastic
Herpes zoster – postherpetic neuralgia	**Infective/postinfective – neuroborreliosis, HIV, hepatitis B/C, Guillain–Barré syndrome**
Malignant infiltration	Other:
Plexus neuritis	Erythromelalgia
	Idiopathic small-fiber neuropathy
	Paraprotein related, e.g. neuropathy associated with anti-MAG antibodies

Situations in which the neuropathy can present acutely in bold.
CMT, Charcot–Marie–Tooth disease; HIV, human immunodeficiency virus; HSAN, hereditary sensory and autonomic neuropathy; MAG, myelin-associated glycoprotein.

THE CLASSIFICATION OF NEUROPATHY

A classification of neuropathy is useful in providing a mental framework on which to work when undertaking the clinical history and examination.

Anatomical classification

This is based on the distribution of the nerve fibers involved in the neuropathy. Anatomically, a neuropathy may be described as a:

- **mononeuropathy** – involving a single nerve;
- **mononeuritis multiplex** – involving multiple single nerves;
- **symmetrical polyneuropathy** – involving multiple nerve fibers symmetrically, usually in a length-dependent process (polyneuropathies can also be asymmetric and can also predominantly affect proximal nerve fibers);
- the disease process may affect other regions of the peripheral nervous system including **lumbar or brachial plexopathies** – involving a nerve plexus;
- **radiculopathy** – involving nerve roots.

One disease process can give rise to multiple types of neuropathy. A good example of this is diabetes mellitus, one of the most common causes of neuropathy worldwide, which can present with a neuropathy of all the above types. The anatomical presentation does, however, give some clues to etiology. Mononeuropathies are often caused by entrapment, for example, of the median nerve in the carpal tunnel or of the ulnar nerve at the elbow. A presentation with mononeuritis multiplex may indicate an underlying infective or inflammatory process, such as vasculitis, although this mode of presentation would be very unusual for a toxic neuropathy. Symmetrical polyneuropathies are often caused by chronic metabolic disturbances, such as diabetes, renal, or hepatic impairment.

Fiber type involved

It is also helpful to define what types of peripheral nerve fiber are involved in a neuropathy, either sensory, motor, and/or autonomic fibers, in various combinations. A general schema for relating the clinical symptoms and signs of neuropathy to fiber type is shown in **Table 7.2**. This is helpful as particular disease processes may have a predilection for certain sizes of nerve fiber, as follows:

- **large fiber** – isoniazid neuropathy, some paraneoplastic neuropathies;
- **mixed** – diabetes mellitus, alcohol;
- **small fiber** – amyloidosis, Fabry's disease, hereditary sensory and autonomic neuropathy, diabetes mellitus/impaired glucose tolerance, or idiopathic small fiber neuropathy.

Pathology

Most classifications of neuropathy are broadly subdivided into axonal or demyelinating forms depending on whether the primary pathology affects the axon or myelin

Table 7.2 The symptoms and signs seen following injury to different types of nerve fiber in peripheral neuropathy.

Peripheral nerve fiber involved	Symptoms	Signs
Motor axons (large myelinated)	Weakness	Muscle weakness
		Muscle wasting
		Fasciculation
Sensory axons		Contractures
Large myelinated (Aβ-fibers)	Numbness	Reduced light touch, proprioception and vibration sense
	Paresthesia	Gait ataxia/Romberg's sign
	Incoordination	
Small (unmyelinated C and thinly myelinated Aδ-fibers)	Pain	Reduced pinprick and thermosensation
		Dysesthesia
		Ulceration
Autonomic axons (principally small unmyelinated C-fibers)	Urinary dysfunction	Horner's syndrome
	Impotence	Postural hypotension
	Gastrointestinal motility disorders	
	Hypohidrosis	

sheath. Such categorization will require investigations such as neurophysiology, cerebrospinal fluid (CSF) examination, and possibly nerve biopsy (see below under Nerve biopsy). The distinction as to whether the primary process is axonal or demyelinating can be difficult, as the relationship between axons and myelinating Schwann cells is so close that injury to one cell type ultimately leads to dysfunction in the other. As a general rule, axonal neuropathies are more likely to be painful.

- **Predominantly axonal neuropathies** – diabetes mellitus, alcohol, HIV, most toxic neuropathies, Charcot–Marie–Tooth (CMT) disease type 2.
- **Predominantly demyelinating neuropathies** – acute inflammatory demyelinating polyradiculoneuropathy variant of Guillan–Barré syndrome, chronic inflammatory demyelinating polyradiculoneuropathy (CIDP), paraprotein-related neuropathy, CMT type 1.

Time course of presentation

The distinction of acute from chronic neuropathies is somewhat arbitrary. The time points shown in **Table 7.3** were originally developed for the classification of inflammatory demyelinating neuropathies (and could be seen as too short when applied to axonal neuropathies).

The time course again gives clues to underlying etiology. For example, an acute neuropathy is most likely to be due to an inflammatory, postinfective, or vascular cause than to have a metabolic cause. Excluding entrapment neuropathies, acute painful neuropathies are unusual but important as they may have a treatable cause (such neuropathies are highlighted in bold in **Table 7.1**).

Table 7.3 Time course of presentation.

	Onset of symptoms to clinical nadir
Acute neuropathy	1 month
Subacute neuropathy	1–2 months
Chronic neuropathy	>2 months

TAKING A CLINICAL HISTORY FROM A PATIENT WITH NEUROPATHY

Presenting complaint

Explore and delineate the symptoms described above and shown in **Table 7.2**. It is also important to consider the time course and nature of presentation (progressive versus stuttering).

Past medical history

Past medical history will include coexistent conditions and their treatment. Diabetes, hypothyroidism, malignancy, renal and liver failure may make an important contribution to neuropathy.

Drugs and toxins

Alcohol use, as well as drug and toxin exposure, should be documented. Occupational toxin exposure is actually very rare; however, drug toxicity is relatively more common and thought needs to be given to the timing and dosing in relation to symptoms.

Family history

This is very important in the assessment of peripheral neuropathy. There are a number of painful neuropathies which have a genetic basis, such as CMT types 2B and 4F, hereditary sensory autonomic neuropathy (HSAN, type 1), Fabry's disease, erythromelalgia,[3] and paroxysmal extreme pain disorder.[4]

Social history

Nutritional deficiencies remain an important cause of neuropathy, so a thorough dietary history is important. Ethnic origin and travel may give clues to unusual infectious causes of neuropathy, such as leprosy.

Systems review

It is important to take account of any systemic symptoms, such as weight loss, fever, arthralgia, skin rashes, or sicca syndrome.

EXAMINING A PATIENT WITH NEUROPATHY

Neurological examination will be aimed at trying to define the neuroanatomical site of any lesion and the types of peripheral nerve fiber involved. Observation should be made of muscle bulk (in length-dependent neuropathies wasting is usually first seen in the extensor digitorum brevis muscle in the feet and the first dorsal interosseus in the hands). Fasciculation indicates muscle denervation. Pes cavus is a sign of a long-standing neuropathy which is often but not exclusively hereditary. Look/feel for any evidence of thickened nerves (the superficial radial, ulnar, and posterior auricular are particularly amenable to palpation). These are seen in some inflammatory and demyelinating neuropathies, as well as in leprosy.

Examine the cranial nerves. Fundoscopy may reveal a systemic process, such as diabetes. Ophthalmoplegia may be observed in acute neuropathies such as Guillan–Barré and Miller Fisher syndrome, but it is rare in chronic neuropathies. Facial nerve involvement is also rare, but is particularly associated with Sjögrens syndrome, neuroborreliosis, and sarcoidosis.

Document the motor power in the limbs. In the UK, use the Medical Research Council motor scale. In most neuropathies weakness is predominantly distal (e.g. of ankle dorsiflexion) and most marked in the legs. Proximal weakness (e.g. of hip flexion) is particularly associated with inflammatory demyelinating neuropathies. Deep tendon reflexes should be tested and are often absent in the context of neuropathy.

It is usual to end the neurological examination with sensory assessment. Pain should be classified as spontaneous or stimulus evoked. Tactile sensation can be mapped with cotton wool, pinprick using a Neurotip[TM], thermal sensation by warm and cold objects and vibration sense by a 128-Hz tuning fork. Document the intensity, quality, and spatiotemporal aspects of evoked sensations;[5] diagrams can be helpful in doing this. Lastly, perform a full general examination, looking in particular for any underlying systemic process, such as a purpuric rash in vasculitis or parotid enlargement in Sjögren's syndrome.

LABORATORY INVESTIGATIONS

Quantitative sensory testing

Quantitative sensory testing (QST) refers to the analysis of perception in response to defined external stimuli. Mechanical sensitivity for tactile stimuli is measured with von Frey hairs, pinprick sensation with weighted needles, and vibration sensation with an electronic vibrameter. A probe operating on the Peltier principle is used to assess thermal perception. There are actually no adequately powered class I studies demonstrating the effectiveness of QST in any context.[6] There are a number of class II and III studies which demonstrated that it is probably or possibly useful in identifying small- or large-fiber sensory abnormalities in patients with diabetic neuropathy, small-fiber neuropathies, uremic neuropathies, and demyelinating neuropathy.[6, 7] QST does not only demonstrate sensory loss but can also be used to quantify some of the abnormal perceptions, such as mechanical and thermal allodynia and hyperalgesia seen in painful neuropathies. It should be noted that QST abnormalities can be due to lesions in the central or peripheral nervous system and indeed may also be secondary to nonneuropathic pain syndromes. There is relatively large intraindividual variation and such testing cannot distinguish between true sensory neuropathy and simulated sensory loss.[8] QST therefore does have its limitations and in clinical practice it is most useful in the diagnosis of small-fiber neuropathies not amenable to assessment by standard neurophysiology (see below under Neurophysiology). The current recommendation from the American Academy of Neurology is that QST should not be used as the sole criteria for structural pathology and should be combined with clinical examination and other appropriate investigations.[6]

Blood tests

It is impossible to give an exhaustive list of blood tests used to investigate a painful neuropathy as this should be very much governed by the clinical features. Below is some guidance.

- **Blood tests checked in the majority of neuropathies.** Full blood count, erythrocyte sedimentation rate, renal profile, liver function tests, thyroid function tests, fasting plasma glucose, and a glucose tolerance test (impaired glucose tolerance is a previously under-recognized cause of painful sensory neuropathy[9]), plasma protein electrophoresis (with immunofixation), vitamin B_{12}, and folate.
- **Blood tests to consider in neuropathies which are acute, asymmetric, or where there are systemic features.** Autoimmune screen (antinuclear antibodies, extractable nuclear antigen, double-stranded DNA binding, rheumatoid factor, antineutrophil cytoplasmic antibody, antineuronal antibodies), hepatitis serology, C-reactive protein, Lyme serology, HIV testing, serum angiotensin converting enzyme.
- **Genetic tests for hereditary neuropathies which are commonly painful.** Hereditary sensory and autonomic neuropathy type-1 causes sensory loss, lancinating pain, ulceration, and autonomic involvement; it occurs due to mutations in serine palmitoyl transferase long chain base subunit 1 (SPTLC1) and is inherited in an autosomal dominant fashion. CMT 2B causes sensory loss, ulceration, lancinating pain, autonomic and motor involvement and is due to mutations in small GTPase late endosomal protein RAB7. Again, disease inheritance is autosomal dominant. CMT 4F is an autosomal recessive condition which leads to a demyelinating neuropathy with severe sensorimotor involvement. It is caused by mutations in periaxin.

Neurophysiology

Neurophysiology is an essential part of the investigation of neuropathy (for review see Ref. 10). Nerve conduction studies in combination with electromyogram (EMG) provide useful information in helping to differentiate between axonal and demyelinating neuropathies. Demyelinating neuropathies result in slowing of conduction velocity, temporal dispersion, and/or conduction block. In contrast, axonal neuropathies show reduced compound action potentials with relatively preserved conduction velocity. Neurophysiology can also be useful in localization of pathology and assessing whether a neuropathy is symmetric or asymmetric. One major disadvantage when investigating painful neuropathies is that standard techniques demonstrate conduction in large myelinated (nonnociceptive) afferents, but not C-fibers. Standard neurophysiology can therefore provide evidence for nerve injury, as well as give clues to its localization and underlying pathology. A normal examination, however, does not exclude injury to small diameter afferents which are often the culprits in neuropathic pain. Laser-evoked potentials can be used to test function in Aδ- and C-fibers,[11] but these are only available on a research basis

and do not differentiate between peripheral and central lesions.

Other measures of unmyelinated fiber function

There are a number of tests which rely on the effector function of unmyelinated fibers. An example is using laser Doppler to measure the size of the neurogenic flare in response to a chemical stimulus which activates C-fibers and this response is reduced in small-fiber neuropathy (for examples see Refs 12, 13[II]). A problem is that many other factors can alter this response. A number of tests can be used to measure sudomotor function (as a measure of dysfunction in postganglionic sympathetic neurons), including sweat testing, sympathetic skin response, and sudomotor axon reflex testing.[14] In one recent study, 98 percent of patients with clinically defined small-fiber neuropathy were found to have abnormal sudomotor function as assessed by thermoregulatory sweat test and sudomotor axon reflex testing.[15] Another group has also found a close correlation between abnormalities in sudomotor function and epidermal innervation density in painful sensory neuropathy.[16]

Nerve biopsy

As a general principle, nerve biopsy should be reserved for situations where it may be helpful in the diagnosis of a potentially treatable cause of neuropathy. Examples of such indications when investigating painful neuropathy would include vasculitis,[17, 18] sarcoidosis,[19] and amyloid neuropathy[20] (see **Figure 7.1**). As well as revealing the underlying cause of the neuropathy, it is also helpful in classification into axonal versus demyelinating forms. In the context of small-fiber neuropathies, the number of unmyelinated fibers within the nerve can be quantified;[21] however, this requires electron microscopy, is time consuming, and may not fully reflect the degree of unmyelinated fiber degeneration.[22, 23][II] The reason for a conservative approach in the use of nerve biopsy is that it is associated with a significant morbidity. Following nerve biopsy, up to 20 percent of patients report pain at the biopsy site six months following the procedure.[24] Other side effects include sensory loss and infection. The decision as to which nerve to biopsy is usually made on the basis of finding a sensory nerve which is both clinically affected and in which neurophysiology confirms a reduced or absent sensory action potential. In practice, this usually means taking the sural or superficial peroneal nerve. It is important to understand that only certain nerves are suitable for biopsy, and pathology may be proximal to the biopsy site. In certain situations, such as vasculitic neuropathy, diagnostic yield is increased by taking combined nerve and muscle biopsies.[17, 25] In selected patients, this procedure remains very helpful.

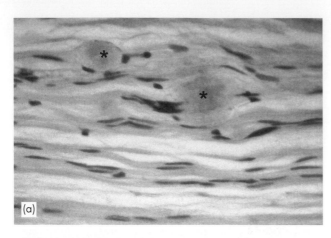

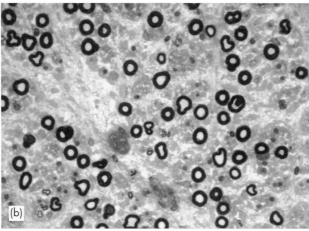

Figure 7.1 Nerve biopsy taken from a patient with familial amyloid neuropathy. (a) Congo red staining revealing two amyloid deposits (asterisks); (b) resin section showing the early effects of amyloid neuropathy with a reduction in small myelinated (and unmyelinated) fibers. Images provided by Dr M Groves, National Hospital for Neurology and Neurosurgery, London, UK.

One study has looked prospectively at the usefulness of nerve biopsy and found that in 60 percent of patients this investigation changed or was helpful in guiding the management of patients.[24]

Skin biopsy

Over the last decade, skin biopsy has been developed as a tool for the investigation of neuropathy.[26] It is especially helpful in the diagnosis of small-fiber neuropathies which are often painful and where other investigations, such as neurophysiology, are often normal.[27, 28][II] A punch skin biopsy is taken usually at the level of the lateral malleolus and thigh (two sites are chosen in order to look for a distal–proximal gradient in the neuropathy). Immunostaining is performed for a pan-neuronal marker protein gene product 9.5 and the number of epidermal nerve fibers (representing C-fibers) quantified (see **Figure 7.2**).

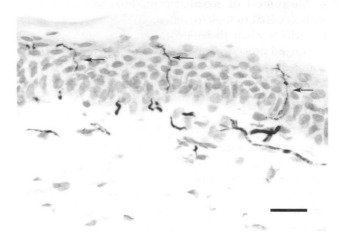

Figure 7.2 Protein gene product (PGP) 9.5 immunoreactive intra-epidermal fibers (arrows) in human distal calf skin biopsy. Scale bar = 50 μm. Image provided by Prof. P. Anand, Imperial College, London.

For sensory neuropathy, this procedure has been shown to have a positive predictive value of 75 percent and negative predictive value of 90 percent[29] and can be helpful in monitoring progression of neuropathy. Qualitative changes on nerve fiber morphology can also be shown on biopsy; for instance, epidermal fibers may demonstrate abnormal axonal swellings.[30] The use of this procedure is no longer restricted to the investigation of small-fiber neuropathies, but it can also be used to study demyelinating neuropathies.[31] In some instances it can give helpful information on the etiology of the neuropathy; for example, demonstrating the deposition of anti-MAG antibodies.[32] In the long term, this procedure may increasingly replace nerve biopsy; however, it is not available in all centers.

Imaging

In certain situations, magnetic resonance imaging may be helpful in the investigation of a painful neuropathy, especially in mononeuropathies or plexopathies when there is a possibility of nerve entrapment or an infiltrative process within the nerve.[33] Not only can this reveal the site of nerve entrapment/injury, but may also demonstrate signal change and atrophy in the relevant denervated muscle groups. Whole body fluorodeoxyglucose positron emission tomography (PET) scanning is used when investigating paraneoplastic neuropathy to reveal an occult neoplasm.[34]

Lumbar puncture

In standard practice, lumbar puncture is rarely used in the investigation of peripheral neuropathy. It may be helpful in the context of acquired demyelinating neuropathies, such as CIDP, to look for a raised CSF protein. It can also be helpful when there is concern that there may be a meningeal process, such as neuroborreliosis or malignant meningitis.

SUMMARY

Virtually any kind of neuropathy can result in the development of neuropathic pain; however, some disease processes have a particular propensity for doing this, including alcohol-related, amyloid, diabetic, and vasculitic neuropathy. It is extremely helpful to classify neuropathies in terms of the speed of onset (i.e. acute versus chronic), the anatomical distribution of involvement, the fiber type(s) affected, and whether the pathology is axonal versus demyelinating. Much of this information can be gained from appropriate clinical history and examination. Neurophysiology is an essential investigation usually allowing the differentiation between axonal and demyelinating neuropathies and determining whether the neuropathy is symmetrical or asymmetrical. Conventional neurophysiology, however, gives only limited information on small-fiber function which may require more detailed investigation, such as measurement of the flare response, the sympathetic skin response, or skin biopsy to assess epidermal innervation density. As a general principle, nerve biopsy should be reserved for situations where it may be helpful in the diagnosis of a potentially treatable cause of neuropathy, such as vasculitic neuropathy.

REFERENCES

1. Martyn CN, Hughes RA. Epidemiology of peripheral neuropathy. *Journal of Neurology, Neurosurgery, and Psychiatry.* 1997; **62**: 310–18.
2. Stump PR, Baccarelli R, Marciano LH *et al.* Neuropathic pain in leprosy patients. *International Journal of Leprosy and Other Mycobacterial Diseases.* 2004; **72**: 134–8.
3. Yang Y, Wang Y, Li S *et al.* Mutations in SCN9A, encoding a sodium channel alpha subunit, in patients with primary erythermalgia. *Journal of Medical Genetics.* 2004; **41**: 171–4.
4. Fertleman CR, Ferrie CD. What's in a name – familial rectal pain syndrome becomes paroxysmal extreme pain disorder. *Journal of Neurology, Neurosurgery, and Psychiatry.* 2006; **77**: 1294–5.
* 5. Cruccu G, Anand P, Attal N *et al.* EFNS guidelines on neuropathic pain assessment. *European Journal of Neurology.* 2004; **11**: 153–62.
* 6. Shy ME, Frohman EM, So YT *et al.* Quantitative sensory testing: report of the Therapeutics and Technology Assessment Subcommittee of the American Academy of Neurology. *Neurology.* 2003; **60**: 898–904.

7. Quantitative sensory testing: a consensus report from the Peripheral Neuropathy Association. *Neurology.* 1993; **43**: 1050–2.
8. Freeman R, Chase KP, Risk MR. Quantitative sensory testing cannot differentiate simulated sensory loss from sensory neuropathy. *Neurology.* 2003; **60**: 465–70.
9. Singleton JR, Smith AG, Bromberg MB. Increased prevalence of impaired glucose tolerance in patients with painful sensory neuropathy. *Diabetes Care.* 2001; **24**: 1448–53.
* 10. Krarup C. An update on electrophysiological studies in neuropathy. *Current Opinion in Neurology.* 2003; **16**: 603–12.
11. Treede RD, Lorenz J, Baumgartner U. Clinical usefulness of laser-evoked potentials. *Neurophysiologie Clinique.* 2003; **33**: 303–14.
12. Moller AT, Feldt-Rasmussen U, Rasmussen AK *et al.* Small-fibre neuropathy in female Fabry patients: reduced allodynia and skin blood flow after topical capsaicin. *Journal of the Peripheral Nervous System.* 2006; **11**: 119–25.
13. Walmsley D, Wiles PG. Early loss of neurogenic inflammation in the human diabetic foot. *Clinical Science.* 1991; **80**: 605–10.
14. Low PA. Testing the autonomic nervous system. *Seminars in Neurology.* 2003; **23**: 407–21.
15. Low VA, Sandroni P, Fealey RD, Low PA. Detection of small-fiber neuropathy by sudomotor testing. *Muscle and Nerve.* 2006; **34**: 57–61.
16. Novak V, Freimer ML, Kissel JT *et al.* Autonomic impairment in painful neuropathy. *Neurology.* 2001; **56**: 861–8.
17. Said G, Lacroix-Ciaudo C, Fujimura H *et al.* The peripheral neuropathy of necrotizing arteritis: a clinicopathological study. *Annals of Neurology.* 1988; **23**: 461–5.
18. Collins MP, Mendell JR, Periquet MI *et al.* Superficial peroneal nerve/peroneus brevis muscle biopsy in vasculitic neuropathy. *Neurology.* 2000; **55**: 636–43.
19. Said G, Lacroix C, Plante-Bordeneuve V *et al.* Nerve granulomas and vasculitis in sarcoid peripheral neuropathy: a clinicopathological study of 11 patients. *Brain.* 2002; **125**: 264–75.
20. Vital C, Vital A, Bouillot-Eimer S *et al.* Amyloid neuropathy: a retrospective study of 35 peripheral nerve biopsies. *Journal of the Peripheral Nervous System.* 2004; **9**: 232–41.
21. Llewelyn JG, Gilbey SG, Thomas PK *et al.* Sural nerve morphometry in diabetic autonomic and painful sensory neuropathy. A clinicopathological study. *Brain.* 1991; **114**: 867–92.
22. Periquet MI, Novak V, Collins MP *et al.* Painful sensory neuropathy: prospective evaluation using skin biopsy. *Neurology.* 1999; **53**: 1641–7.
23. Herrmann DN, Griffin JW, Hauer P *et al.* Epidermal nerve fiber density and sural nerve morphometry in peripheral neuropathies. *Neurology.* 1999; **53**: 1634–40.

∗ 24. Gabriel CM, Howard R, Kinsella N *et al*. Prospective study of the usefulness of sural nerve biopsy. *Journal of Neurology, Neurosurgery, and Psychiatry*. 2000; **69**: 442–6.

25. Vital C, Vital A, Canron MH *et al*. Combined nerve and muscle biopsy in the diagnosis of vasculitic neuropathy. A 16-year retrospective study of 202 cases. *Journal of the Peripheral Nervous System*. 2006; **11**: 20–9.

∗ 26. Lauria G, Cornblath DR, Johansson O *et al*. EFNS guidelines on the use of skin biopsy in the diagnosis of peripheral neuropathy. *European Journal of Neurology*. 2005; **12**: 747–58.

27. McCarthy BG, Hsieh ST, Stocks A *et al*. Cutaneous innervation in sensory neuropathies: evaluation by skin biopsy. *Neurology*. 1995; **45**: 1848–55.

28. Holland NR, Stocks A, Hauer P *et al*. Intraepidermal nerve fiber density in patients with painful sensory neuropathy. *Neurology*. 1997; **48**: 708–11.

29. McArthur JC, Stocks EA, Hauer P *et al*. Epidermal nerve fiber density: normative reference range and diagnostic efficiency. *Archives of Neurology*. 1998; **55**: 1513–20.

30. Lauria G, Morbin M, Lombardi R *et al*. Axonal swellings predict the degeneration of epidermal nerve fibers in painful neuropathies. *Neurology*. 2003; **61**: 631–6.

31. Li J, Bai Y, Ghandour K *et al*. Skin biopsies in myelin-related neuropathies: bringing molecular pathology to the bedside. *Brain*. 2005; **128**: 1168–77.

32. Lombardi R, Erne B, Lauria G *et al*. IgM deposits on skin nerves in anti-myelin-associated glycoprotein neuropathy. *Annals of Neurology*. 2005; **57**: 180–7.

∗ 33. Koltzenburg M, Bendszus M. Imaging of peripheral nerve lesions. *Current Opinion in Neurology*. 2004; **17**: 621–6.

34. Rees JH, Hain SF, Johnson MR *et al*. The role of [18F]fluoro-2-deoxyglucose-PET scanning in the diagnosis of paraneoplastic neurological disorders. *Brain*. 2001; **124**: 2223–31.

8

Novel imaging techniques

MICHAEL LEE AND IRENE TRACEY

KEY LEARNING POINTS

- Functional neuroimaging refers to the measurement and localization of neural activity that results from a sensory, motor, or cognitive task.
- Neuroimaging techniques differ in terms of what they measure, their invasiveness, and the spatial or temporal information they provide.
- Imaging techniques have revealed that the structure, neurochemistry, and receptor distributions in the brains of chronic pain patients differ from those of healthy individuals.

- The brain network that underlies the heightened sensitivity to pain that patients report has been shown to differ from that which is engaged during our experience of everyday or nociceptive pain.
- The chronic pain state may now be regarded as a disease in its own right, with pathophysiology that is increasingly revealed by neuroimaging.
- Neuroimaging is being rapidly developed as diagnostic and treatment monitoring tools in the pain clinic and as analgesic bioassays in research and industry.

INTRODUCTION

It is well recognized that the needs of chronic pain patients are largely unmet, creating an enormous physical, emotional, and financial burden to sufferers, carers, and society.

Although a myriad of pharmacological, physical, psychological, and interventional therapies are available, few are specific for any particular chronic pain condition. Furthermore, efficacy for these therapies as measured in clinical trials is limited and their translation from the trial population and scenario to the individual patient in the clinic is not easily achieved. What we desperately need are innovative methods that aid

diagnosis and provide data to inform decisions regarding choice and targeting of treatments, alongside conventional clinical measures in individual patients. Neuroimaging techniques that noninvasively provide functional or structural information regarding the central nervous system (CNS) can fulfill this need and have already shown that the brains of patients suffering chronic pain are significantly more affected than previously anticipated.

This chapter will focus on how magnetic resonance imaging (MRI) and positron emission tomography (PET) work as imaging techniques. Their application and contribution to the field of pain research will also be illustrated.

FUNCTIONAL IMAGING

Functional neuroimaging refers to the measurement and localization of neural activity that result from the performance of a task whether sensory, motor, or cognitive. **Figures 8.1** and **8.2** illustrate the main imaging modalities in use today and what physiological correlate of brain activity they measure. There is a cost or balance between the spatial and temporal information achievable and invasiveness if high resolution is desired in both domains. Common methods include PET, functional magnetic resonance imaging (fMRI), multichannel electroencephalography (EEG), and magnetoencephalography (MEG). PET- and fMRI-based techniques record localized changes related to cerebral blood flow (CBF) that is coupled to neural activity. As these hemodynamic changes lag behind neural activity, a limit on the order of seconds is placed on the temporal resolution of these methods. In contrast, MEG and EEG record rapid electrical fluctuations that occur during neural activity and provide excellent temporal resolution on the order of milliseconds. However, spatial resolution is poor and limited to the superficial cortex. Nonetheless, when combined with the use of laser as a radiant heat source for the stimulation of cutaneous nociceptors in humans, MEG and EEG can provide information on the integrity of the nociceptive pathway.

STRUCTURAL IMAGING – FROM SYSTEM TO MOLECULE

MRI and PET have been employed to provide information on the anatomical structure and the neurochemical composition of the CNS providing, together with functional information, a systems view of pain processing within the CNS.

More recently, advances in our ability to label receptor, neurotransmitters, or even intracellular substrates allow PET and MRI-based techniques to image their function and distribution within the CNS. These labels provide a visual report from the scene of cellular events. Molecular imaging has thus been defined as the measurement and imaging of biological processes *in vivo* at the molecular and cellular level, combining knowledge of genetics and proteomics in the creation of molecular probes that are detectable by imaging technologies.

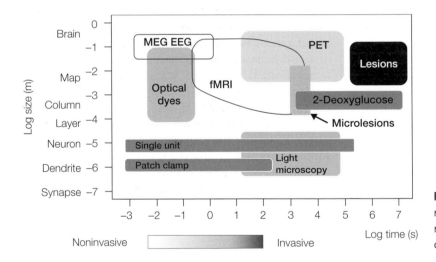

Figure 8.1 A schematic displaying the relationship between the spatial and temporal resolution in terms of their invasiveness for the current imaging tools commonly used.

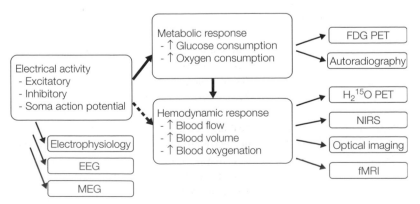

Figure 8.2 A schematic displaying the neurophysiological correlates of neural activity and what techniques detect that particular signal. EEG, electroencephalography; FDG-PET, flurodeoxyglucose positron emission tomography; fMRI; functional magnetic resonance imaging; H$_2$^{15}O-PET, water-based positron emission tomography; MEG, magnetoencephalography; NIRS, near infrared spectroscopy.

fMRI AND PET AS CBF–BASED IMAGING TECHNIQUES

The common form of fMRI used is blood oxygen level dependent (BOLD). The signal from BOLD imaging depends on the relative concentrations of oxy- and deoxyhemoglobin in the local vasculature. The disproportionate increase in cerebral blood flow that accompanies neural activity results in the relative decrease in the concentration of deoxygenated hemoglobin. Deoxygenated hemoglobin is a paramagnetic molecule. It distorts the local magnetic field and causes a loss of signal. Thus the decrease of deoxygenated hemoglobin leads to higher signal intensities that contrast against surrounding tissue (**Figure 8.3**). During image analysis, the BOLD signal that is expected to result from the stimulus is modelled mathematically. The model is compared to the signal that is measured during the experiment itself. Statistical maps are constructed and superimposed on a structural brain image to indicate where the measured signal best fits the model (**Figure 8.4**).

PET employs radioactive tracers to measure CBF. Commonly, ^{15}O, a radioactive isotope, is chemically incorporated into water and intravenously injected. [^{15}O]Water is extracted from plasma into brain tissue on passing through the brain. This extraction or uptake is highly correlated with regional cerebral blood flow. The radioisotope then undergoes positron emission decay and emits a positron, the antimatter counterpart of an electron. After travelling for a few millimeters, the positron encounters and annihilates with an electron, and produces a pair of annihilation (gamma) photons moving in opposite directions. These are detected when they reach a scintillator material in the scanner, creating a burst of light (photons) which is detected by photomultiplier tubes (**Figure 8.5**). The technique depends on simultaneous (coincidental) detection of the pair of photons; photons which do not arrive in pairs (within a few nanoseconds) are ignored. Using statistics collected from tens of thousands of coincidence events, a map of radioactivity as a function of location may be constructed and plotted.

Table 8.1 compares the PET and fMRI in terms of the information they provide and their relative advantages and disadvantages.

Over the last decade, PET and fMRI studies have revealed the large distributed brain network that is accessed during processing of noxious input. Several cortical and subcortical brain regions are commonly activated by noxious stimulation, including anterior cingulate cortex (ACC), insula cortex, frontal and prefrontal cortices (PFC), primary and secondary somatosensory cortices (S1 and S2, respectively), thalamus, basal ganglia, cerebellum, amygdala, hippocampus, and regions within the parietal and temporal cortices. This network is thought to reflect the complexity of pain as an experience and is often called the pain matrix. The matrix can be simplistically thought of as having lateral components (sensory–discriminatory, involving areas such as primary and secondary somatosensory cortices, thalamus, and posterior parts of insula) and medial components (affective–cognitive–evaluative, involving areas like the anterior parts of insula, ACC, and PFC).[1] However, because different brain regions play a more or less active role depending upon the precise interplay of the factors involved in influencing pain perception (e.g. cognition, mood, injury, etc.), the pain matrix is not a defined entity. A recent meta-analysis of human data from different imaging studies provides clarity regarding the most common regions found active during an acute pain experience as measured by PET and fMRI (**Figure 8.6**).[2] These areas include primary and secondary somatosensory, insular, anterior cingulate, and prefrontal cortices, as well as the thalamus. This is not to say that these areas are the fundamental core network of human nociceptive processing (and if ablated would cure all pain), although

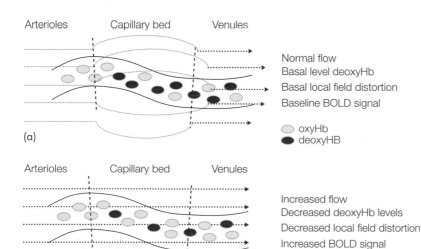

(a)

(b)

Normal flow
Basal level deoxyHb
Basal local field distortion
Baseline BOLD signal

○ oxyHb
● deoxyHB

Increased flow
Decreased deoxyHb levels
Decreased local field distortion
Increased BOLD signal

Figure 8.3 During neural activation, arteriolar blood inflow increases leading to a decrease in deoxyhemoglobin (deoxyHb)–oxyhemoglobin ratio. As deoxyHb is a paramagnetic molecule, its decrease leads to a reduction in local magnetic field distortion; the result is an increase in functional magnetic resonance imaging (fMRI) or blood oxygen level dependent (BOLD) signal in the area of neural activity. (a) basal state; (b) activated state.

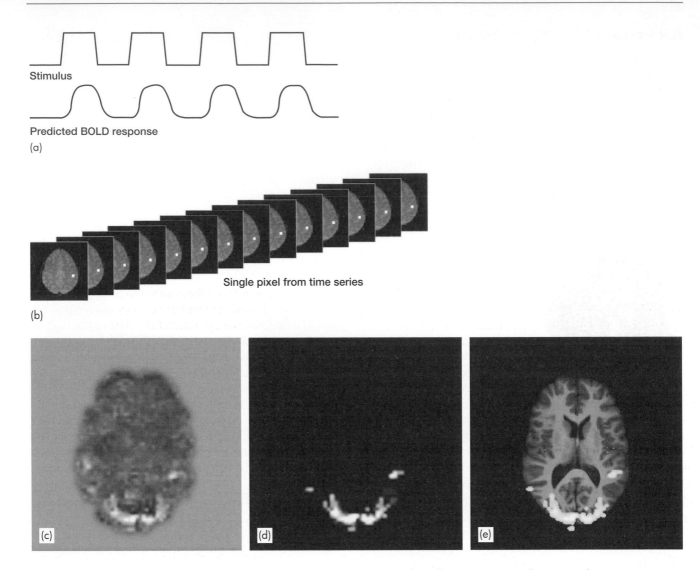

Figure 8.4 (a) Representation of the predicted blood oxygen level dependent (BOLD) response pattern (bottom line) to the repeated stimulus (top line). (b) A single pixel that activates to that repeated stimulus. (c) The statistical map obtained. (d) This map is then thresholded at an appropriate p-score and then (e) overlaid on a high quality magnetic resonance scan of the same subject's brain.

studies investigating acute pharmacologically induced analgesia do show predominant effects in this core network suggesting their overall importance in influencing pain perception.[3] Other regions, such as basal ganglia, cerebellum, amygdala, hippocampus, and areas within the parietal and temporal cortices, can also be active dependent upon the particular set of circumstances for that individual. A cerebral signature for pain is perhaps how we should define the network that is necessarily unique for each individual.[4] This is particularly relevant given the very recent awareness of how great a role our genes play in the perception of pain related to a noxious stimulus or due to injury. For example, individuals homozygous for the met158 allele of the catechol-O-methyltransferase (COMT) polymorphism (val158met) showed diminished regional mu-opioid system responses to pain (measured using PET) and higher sensory and affective ratings for experimentally induced pain compared with heterozygote.[5] The link between our genes and pain perception

during acute and chronic pain experiences is now one of the most exciting areas of pain research at present and is being led primarily by animal studies, but with fast translation to human studies.[6] Functional imaging is poised to provide phenotypic information that is based on objective mechanistic data in conjunction with reported pain symptomatology and thus provide the intermediary between genetics and behavior.

Anterior insular and prefrontal cortex

It is now clear that the CNS processing that underlies the heightened sensitivity to pain that patients report differs from the processing that occurs during the experience of everyday or nociceptive pain.[7]

Compared to healthy controls, patients have enhanced activity in response to identical noxious stimulation in several areas that form part of the above-mentioned brain

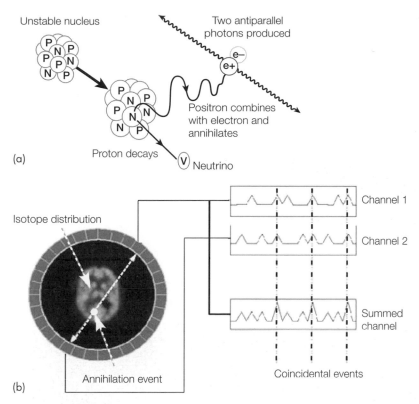

Figure 8.5 (a) The unstable radionuclide decays emit a positron which collides with a nearby electron and annihilates. Two photons are produced and travel in opposite directions (antiparallel). (b) These photons are detected by photomultiplier tubes (channel one and two). Only coincidental events are regarded (summed channels).

Table 8.1 Comparison of functional magnetic resonance imaging (fMRI) and positron emission tomography (PET) as cerebral blood flow (CBF)-based imaging techniques.

Modality	BOLD fMRI	^{15}O-water PET
Working principle	Detects changes in the magnetic field due to variations in the oxyHb/deoxyHb ratio	Detects the radioactive isotopes that is tagged on to molecule of interest
Availability	Most tertiary medical centers	Isotopes are short-lived and must be generated by a nearby cyclotron
Invasiveness	Completely noninvasive	Employs radio-isotopes. Requires intravenous access as minimum
Spatial resolution	1–2 mm	5 mm at best
Temporal resolution	Hundreds of milliseconds	Minutes
Experimental design	Flexible. Limited mainly by noise and magnetic environment	Limited by tracer half-life and radiation dose
Derived data	Unable to quantify the physiological baseline absolutely	Able to quantify the physiology baseline absolutely

BOLD, blood oxygen level dependent; CBF, cerebral blood flow; fMRI, functional magnetic resonance imaging; PET, positron emission tomography.

network. Over the last decade, two key areas have emerged that consistently show increased activation, irrespective of underlying pathology or modality of stimulation employed – the rostral anterior insula and prefrontal cortex.

A recent meta-analysis by Schweinhardt and colleagues[8] revealed that clinically relevant pain is represented more rostrally in the anterior insula than pain that is experimentally generated in healthy volunteers. Anterior insular activity is found not only during subjective feelings of pain, but is associated with anxiety, depression, irritable bowel syndrome, chronic fatigue, fibromyalgia, somatization, and fear. Its activity in chronic pain patients is consistent with current theories regarding altered interoception or body awareness.[9]

A specific role for the lateral PFC as a pain control center has been put forward in a study of experimentally induced allodynia in healthy subjects.[10] Here, increased lateral PFC activation was related to decreased pain affect, supposedly by inhibiting the functional connectivity between medial thalamus and midbrain, thereby driving the endogenous pain-inhibitory mechanisms. Such

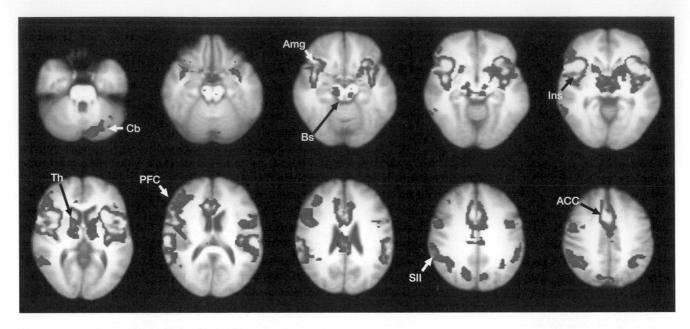

Figure 8.6 Neuroanatomy of pain processing. Brain regions that commonly activate during a painful experience are insular cortices (Ins), anterior cingulate cortex (ACC), secondary somatosensory area (SII), thalami (Th), cerebrellum (Cb). Activity in other regions, for example the brainstem (Bs), amygdala (Amg), and prefrontal cortex (PFC), depends on cognitive or emotional factors.

concepts are perhaps supported by recent studies looking at the influence of control in pain perception. Wiech and colleagues[11] performed an fMRI study in healthy controls where the level of control over their pain was manipulated, producing changes in pain ratings dependent upon both the condition and their internal locus of control. They found that the analgesic effect of perceived control relies on activation of right anterolateral PFC.[11] It is important perhaps to also note that the prefrontal cortex (specifically the dorsolateral PFC) is a site of major neurodegeneration and potential cell death in chronic pain patients.

Central sensitization and the brain stem

The descending modulatory system comprises bulbospinal circuitries that when appropriately engaged, produce facilitation (pronociception) or inhibition (antinociception). The pain-inhibiting circuitry which includes the periadqeductal gray (PAG) is best known and contributes to environmental (stress) and opiate analgesia.[12] More recent animal data have revealed that the rostroventromedial medulla (part of the brain stem reticular formation) is key to the descending pathways that facilitate pain transmission.[13]

Zambreanu and colleagues[14] were first to demonstrate involvement of the midbrain reticular formation during central sensitization in humans, using a model of secondary hyperalgesia induced by capscaicin. A subsequent pharmacological study has highlighted the influence of gold-standard agents used to treat key symptoms of neuropathic pain (gabapentin) on CNS activity related to central sensitization.[15] In this double-blind, randomized

cross-over design, a single dose of gabapentin or placebo was given to healthy controls during either a normal or centrally sensitized state. fMRI was performed during punctate stimulation of the area with and without sensitization and with either gabapentin or placebo administered. The interaction between sensitization state and drug modulation was most significant within the brain stem.

The concept that the sustained activation of facilitatory circuits or dysfunction of the descending inhibitory system underlies chronic pain has also been explored in several imaging studies. Wilder-Smith and colleagues[16] investigated whether patients with irritable bowel syndrome (IBS) had hypersensitivity and pain upon distension due to abnormalities in endogenous pain inhibitory mechanisms; they found this to be the case for patients compared with controls. Mayer and colleagues[17] examined whether visceral hypersensitivity found in patients with IBS might arise as a consequence of top-down descending influences. In a PET study, they observed greater activation of limbic and paralimbic circuits during rectal distension in patients with IBS compared with control subjects or patients with quiescent ulcerative colitis. Functional connectivity analysis suggested that the failure to activate the right lateral frontal cortex permits the inhibitory effects of limbic and paralimbic circuits on PAG activation, the consequence of which may be visceral hypersensitivity. In a more recent study, the same group examined the longitudinal change in perceptual and brain activation response to visceral stimuli in IBS patients.[18] They found, amongst other changes, that after 12 months patients had a decreased brain stem activity to both the rectal inflation, as well as during anticipation to this provocation.

While imaging studies in models of neuropathic pain and chronic pain patients continue to confirm the specific involvement of the brain stem regions in maintaining central sensitization,[19, 20, 21] the role of the spinal dorsal horn in the initiation of central sensitization, so well-described in preclinical research, remains to be confirmed in humans. Functional imaging of the spinal cord in humans is now possible and has allowed us to examine how animal data map to human neurobiology.[22] Assessing the function and thus contribution of the spinal cord, brain stem, and cortical mechanisms to the pain experience in patients is now possible; establishing functional neuroimaging as the preeminent candidate for diagnostic use in pain management.

STRUCTURAL IMAGING

Magnetic resonance volumetry

Magnetic resonance (MR) volumetry involves the use of automated analysis techniques that allow the segmentation and measurement of gray and white matter volumes of a structural brain image. Application of this technique for the sensitive assessment of cerebral atrophy in Alzheimer's disease and its progression is well established. Apkarian and colleagues[23] first reported the application of this technique to chronic pain research and found significant cerebral atrophy in chronic pain patients, even after accounting for age-related brain volume decreases. Patients with chronic back pain showed gray matter volume loss equivalent to the gray matter volume lost in 10–20 years of normal aging that was localized to the bilateral dorsolateral prefrontal cortex and right thalamus.[23] Thereafter, studies involving a range of chronic pain conditions have revealed gray matter losses in several other areas implicated in nociceptive processing.

The dramatic extent of neurodegeneration in chronic pain states evidenced by these studies has compelled the shift in approach to chronic pain from symptom to disease. There is now a pressing need to perform more advanced structural imaging measures and analyses to better quantify these effects. The challenge is in determining the possible causal factors that produce such neurodegeneration in patients. Candidate factors include the chronic pain condition itself (i.e. excitotoxic events due to barrage of nociceptive inputs), the pharmacological agents prescribed, or perhaps the physical lifestyle change subsequent to becoming a chronic pain patient. Carefully controlled longitudinal studies are now needed as this rapidly becomes an active area of research.

Diffusion tensor imaging

Diffusion of water in white matter tracts is directionally dependent (anisotrophic) on the orientation of axon bundles. Diffusion tensor imaging (DTI) is an MRI-based technique that measures the anisotropic motion of water in different regions of the brain and, after subsequent processing, calculates a principal direction of diffusion for water in each imaging voxel (**Figure 8.7**). Using DTI, Hadjipavlou and colleagues[24] defined connections between the PAG and separately for the nucleus cuneiformis (part of the brain stem reticular formation implicated in central sensitization), to the prefrontal cortex, amygdala, thalamus, hypothalamus, and rostroventral medial medulla bilaterally.[24] Such data are evidence for the existence of the anatomical circuitry that mediates the top-down influences on pain processing in humans. Characterization of anatomical connectivity by DTI in concert with neuroimaging techniques that identify areas of functional or structural alterations in chronic pain patients, will more fully inform the neurobiology that substantiates the chronic pain state.

NEUROCHEMICAL AND RECEPTOR IMAGING

Proton magnetic resonance spectroscopy

Proton magnetic resonance spectroscopy (MRS) produces signals that are reported as frequencies that may be

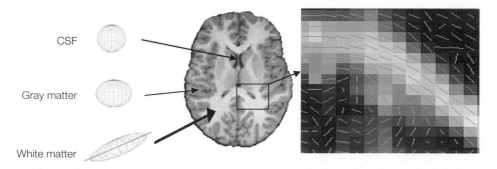

Figure 8.7 Diffusion tension imaging (DTI) is an extension of diffusion magnetic resonance imaging (MRI). If diffusion gradients are applied (i.e. magnetic field variations in the MRI magnet) in at least six directions, it is possible to calculate, for each voxel, a tensor that describes the three-dimensional shape of diffusion (a). The fiber direction is indicated by the tensor's main eigenvector. Fiber tracking algorithms can then be used to track a fiber along its whole length (b).

assigned to molecules of biological interest. An example is *N*-acetyl aspartate (NAA), an amino acid derivative located in neurons. A typical spectrum including the frequency peak due to NAA is shown (**Figure 8.8**). Grachev and colleagues[25] have demonstrated reductions in NAA concentrations (implying neuronal loss) in the dorsolateral prefrontal cortex of chronic lower back pain patients. The study adds to the current hypothesis that neurodegeneration might be occurring in the chronic pain state.

Molecular imaging and metabolic change

Receptors have a prominent role in brain function as they are the effector sites of neurotransmission at the post-synaptic membrane. Distribution, density, and activity of receptors in the brain can be visualized by radioligands labelled for PET, and the receptor binding can be quantified by appropriate tracer kinetic models. Commonly available radioligands are available for the various transmitter systems (**Table 8.2**). The quantitative imaging of opioid and dopaminergic receptors has gained importance in clinical pain research.

Early opioid ligand studies showed decreased binding in chronic pain patients that normalized after reduction of their pain symptoms.[26] Regional differences in ligand binding within key pain processing brain regions have also been reported in several neuropathic pain studies.[27, 28] A study of restless legs syndrome found that the opioid-binding potential is negatively correlated with the affective dimension of the McGill Pain Questionnaire.[29] A recent study by Maarrawi and colleagues[30] demonstrates differential brain opioid receptor availability between

Table 8.2 Common positron emission tomography (PET) ligands that are used to investigate the opiodergic and dopaminergic receptor systems.

Tracer	Abbreviation	Target
[11]C-NNC 112	–	D1 (postsynaptic dopamine receptor)
[11]C-racloprde	RAC	D2 (postsynaptic dopamine receptor)
[11]C-FLB457	–	D2 (postsynaptic dopamine receptor)
[11]C-carfentanyl	–	Opioid mu-receptor
[11]C-diprenorphine	DPN	Opioid receptor

patients with central and peripheral neuropathic pain. They found a bilateral binding decrease in both patient groups that could reflect endogenous opioid release secondary to their chronic pain, but they also found a more significant and lateralized decrease specific to the central poststroke pain patients, suggestive of opioid receptor loss or inactivation in receptor-bearing neurons. This binding decrease was more extensive than the brain anatomical lesions and not colocalized to them. These findings have important implications because if central and peripheral forms of neuropathic pain differ in the distribution of opioid system changes, this might account for a differential sensitivity to opiates. For all these studies, causation is an issue. Future studies, in particular longitudinal studies that correlate binding potential with pain intensity, are needed to help elucidate whether decreased receptor availability is caused by increased release of endogenous opioids or decreased receptor density.

There is a current resurgence of interest in how dopaminergic pathways are implicated in pain processing. Early studies in animals and patients first identified the potential relevance of this neurotransmitter system in chronic pain.[31] A recent PET study in fibromyalgia patients by Wood and colleagues[32] showed reduced pre-synaptic dopaminergic activity in several brain regions in which dopamine plays a critical role in modulating nociceptive processes. As with the endogenous opioid system, the issue of cause and effect between a functional hypodopaminergic state and pain has yet to be resolved. Reduced pain thresholds in patients with Parkinson's disease normalized after levodopa administration, and there were corresponding reductions in brain activation (insula and ACC).[33] These findings suggest that attenuation of dopaminergic activity might underlie some chronic pain states.

However, the current data from animal and patient studies on the role of dopamine mechanisms in pain, using either dopamine agonists or antagonists, is conflicting with regard to directionality (i.e. pro- or anti-nociceptive responses upon dopamine release) and location (i.e. nigrostriatal or mesolimbic pathways). A

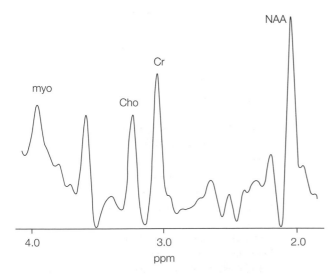

Figure 8.8 A typical ^{1}H-magnetic resonance spectroscopy (MRS) spectrum of the human brain at 3.0 T. Frequency peaks can be ascribed to a number of metabolites; creatine (Cr), *myo*-inositol (myo), choline compounds (Cho), and *N*-acetyl aspartate (NAA).

recent study by Scott and colleagues[34] has attempted to clarify this issue and showed that variations in the human pain stress experience are mediated differentially by ventral and dorsal basal ganglia dopamine activity. The role of the dopaminergic system in pain regulation remains an important issue to resolve if it is to be considered as a therapeutic target for pain.

CONCLUSION

Neuroimaging data acquisition and analytical techniques are improving rapidly. When applied to pain research, these advancements will allow us to further examine how mechanisms of chronic pain gleaned from animal studies map to human neurobiology. This is of considerable interest to all, from the laboratory-based animal researcher to chronic pain clinician. We envisage that data obtained from such techniques will not reside solely within the laboratory, but progressively move into clinical practice to aid decisions on diagnosis and treatment choices.

REFERENCES

1. Albe-Fessard D, Berkley KJ, Kruger L et al. Diencephalic mechanisms of pain sensation. *Brain Research.* 1985; **356**: 217 96.

* 2. Apkarian AV, Bushnell MC, Treede RD, Zubieta JK. Human brain mechanisms of pain perception and regulation in health and disease. *European Journal of Pain.* 2005; **9**: 463–84.

3. Wise RG, Rogers R, Painter D et al. Combining fMRI with a pharmacokinetic model to determine which brain areas activated by painful stimulation are specifically modulated by remifentanil. *Neuroimage.* 2002; **16**: 999–1014.

* 4. Tracey I, Mantyh PW. The cerebral signature for pain perception and its modulation. *Neuron.* 2007; **55**: 377–91.

5. Zubieta JK, Heitzeg MM, Smith YR et al. COMT val158met genotype affects mu-opioid neurotransmitter responses to a pain stressor. *Science.* 2003; **299**: 1240–3.

6. Tegeder I, Costigan M, Griffin RS et al. GTP cyclohydrolase and tetrahydrobiopterin regulate pain sensitivity and persistence. *Nature Medicine.* 2006; **12**: 1269–77.

* 7. Schweinhardt P, Lee M, Tracey I. Imaging pain in patients: is it meaningful? *Current Opinion in Neurology.* 2006; **19**: 392–400.

8. Schweinhardt P, Glynn C, Brooks J et al. An fMRI study of cerebral processing of brush-evoked allodynia in neuropathic pain patients. *Neuroimage.* 2006; **32**: 256–65.

* 9. Craig AD. Interoception: the sense of the physiological condition of the body. *Current Opinion in Neurobiology.* 2003; **13**: 500–05.

10. Lorenz J, Cross D, Minoshima S et al. A unique representation of heat allodynia in the human brain. *Neuron.* 2002; **35**: 383–93.

11. Wiech K, Kalisch R, Weiskopf N et al. Anterolateral prefrontal cortex mediates the analgesic effect of expected and perceived control over pain. *Journal of Neuroscience.* 2006; **26**: 11501–9.

12. Basbaum AI, Fields HL. Endogenous pain control systems: brainstem spinal pathways and endorphin circuitry. *Annual Review of Neuroscience.* 1984; **7**: 309–38.

* 13. Gebhart GF. Descending modulation of pain. *Neuroscience and Biobehavioral Reviews.* 2004; **27**: 729–37.

14. Zambreanu L, Wise RG, Brooks JCW et al. A role for the brainstem in central sensitisation in humans. Evidence from functional magnetic resonance imaging. *Pain.* 2005; **114**: 397–407.

15. Iannetti GD, Zambreanu L, Wise RG et al. Pharmacological modulation of pain-related brain activity during normal and central sensitization states in humans. *Proceedings of the National Academy of Sciences of the United States of America.* 2005; **102**: 18195–200.

16. Wilder-Smith CH, Schindler D, Lovblad K et al. Brain functional magnetic resonance imaging of rectal pain and activation of endogenous inhibitory mechanisms in irritable bowel syndrome patient subgroups and healthy controls. *Gut.* 2004; **53**: 1595–601.

17. Mayer EA, Berman S, Suyenobu B et al. Differences in brain responses to visceral pain between patients with irritable bowel syndrome and ulcerative colitis. *Pain.* 2005; **115**: 398–409.

18. Naliboff BD, Mayer EA. Brain imaging in IBS: drawing the line between cognitive and non-cognitive processes. *Gastroenterology.* 2006; **130**: 267–70.

19. Seifert F, Maihofner C. Representation of cold allodynia in the human brain – a functional MRI study. *Neuroimage.* 2007; **35**: 1168–80.

20. Mainero C, Zhang WT, Kumar A et al. Mapping the spinal and supraspinal pathways of dynamic mechanical allodynia in the human trigeminal system using cardiac-gated fMRI. *Neuroimage.* 2007; **35**: 1201–10.

21. Becerra L, Morris S, Bazes S et al. Trigeminal neuropathic pain alters responses in CNS circuits to mechanical (brush) and thermal (cold and heat) stimuli. *Journal of Neuroscience.* 2006; **26**: 10646–57.

22. Stroman PW, Tomanek B, Krause V et al. Mapping of neuronal function in the healthy and injured human spinal cord with spinal fMRI. *Neuroimage.* 2002; **17**: 1854–60.

23. Apkarian AV, Sosa Y, Sonty S et al. Chronic back pain is associated with decreased prefrontal and thalamic gray matter density. *Journal of Neuroscience.* 2004; **24**: 10410–5.

24. Hadjipavlou G, Dunckley P, Behrens TE, Tracey I. Determining anatomical connectivities between cortical and brainstem pain processing regions in humans: a diffusion tensor imaging study in healthy controls. *Pain.* 2006; **123**: 169–78.

25. Grachev ID, Fredrickson BE, Apkarian AV. Abnormal brain chemistry in chronic back pain: an in vivo proton magnetic resonance spectroscopy study. *Pain.* 2000; **89**: 7–18.

26. Jones AK, Cunningham VJ, Ha-Kawa S *et al.* Changes in central opioid receptor binding in relation to inflammation and pain in patients with rheumatoid arthritis. *British Journal of Rheumatology.* 1994; **33**: 909–16.

27. Jones AK, Watabe H, Cunningham VJ, Jones T. Cerebral decreases in opioid receptor binding in patients with central neuropathic pain measured by [11C]diprenorphine binding and PET. *European Journal of Pain.* 2004; **8**: 479–85.

28. Willoch F, Schindler F, Wester HJ *et al.* Central poststroke pain and reduced opioid receptor binding within pain processing circuitries: a [11C]diprenorphine PET study. *Pain.* 2004; **108**: 213–20.

29. von Spiczak S, Whone AL, Hammers A *et al.* The role of opioids in restless legs syndrome: an [11C]diprenorphine PET study. *Brain.* 2005; **128**: 906–17.

30. Maarrawi J, Peyron R, Mertens P *et al.* Differential brain opioid receptor availability in central and peripheral neuropathic pain. *Pain.* 2007; **127**: 183–94.

31. Hagelberg N, Jaaskelainen SK, Martikainen IK *et al.* Striatal dopamine D2 receptors in modulation of pain in humans: a review. *European Journal of Pharmacology.* 2004; **500**: 187–92.

32. Wood PB, Patterson 2nd JC, Sunderland JJ *et al.* Reduced presynaptic dopamine activity in fibromyalgia syndrome demonstrated with positron emission tomography: a pilot study. *Journal of Pain.* 2007; **8**: 51–8.

33. Brefel-Courbon C, Payoux P, Thalamas C *et al.* Effect of levodopa on pain threshold in Parkinson's disease: a clinical and positron emission tomography study. *Movement Disorders.* 2005; **20**: 1557–63.

34. Scott DJ, Heitzeg MM, Koeppe RA *et al.* Variations in the human pain stress experience mediated by ventral and dorsal basal ganglia dopamine activity. *Journal of Neuroscience.* 2006; **26**: 10789–95.

PART II

THERAPEUTIC PROTOCOLS

9

After assessment, then what? Integrating findings for successful case formulation and treatment tailoring

STEVEN J LINTON AND MICHAEL K NICHOLAS

KEY LEARNING POINTS

- The challenge of translating assessment findings into a tailored treatment plan centers on good case formulation where the mechanisms maintaining the problem are identified and treatment is tailored to the individual patient's needs.
- Assessment materials are often underutilized and used mainly to document the intensity of the problem. Case conceptualization focuses on identifying the main problems, and developing a "hypothesis" about the mechanisms supporting them for the given patient.
- Measurement techniques are important to the process since they can tell us about factors that may be unusual for the patient. However, a standard, for example normative data, is needed to judge this. Models developed in the literature are also helpful since they often capture the main mechanisms.
- Case formulation will include specific targets appropriate for treatment, a conceptualization of the mechanisms, and a specific (tailored) treatment to address these.

- However, it is vital that the patient is involved in case formulation in part to ensure that it is correct and in part to heighten engagement. Techniques such as motivational interviewing are helpful in identifying the patient's goals.
- Outcome evaluation is crucial because it provides guiding feedback as to whether the treatment is actually working. This also provides an indication of whether the case formulation is correct.
- Single-subject designs are ideal for clinical evaluations because they provide data on the individual level that can be of immediate value in judging whether treatment needs to be altered, continued, or terminated.
- Summarizing standardized assessment measures before and after treatment can be one base for judging how well a clinic is doing on the whole and may be an important part of quality control.

INTRODUCTION

Although seldom discussed, integrating assessment findings into a treatment plan is a delicate but thorny endeavor. It is delicate because seemingly small matters are important, and thorny because the process easily becomes complex. Little wonder it is often ignored. Yet, this process is the vital link between assessment and treatment: failure here risks poor treatment outcomes. Conversely, grasping the essence of the case and designing a treatment to fit these dimensions should greatly increase the potential efficacy of the treatment. The identification of the different facets of a presenting case, the formulation of a hypothesis about how the different facets may have arisen and are currently being maintained requires more than the administration of a few assessment measures. This chapter will address case formulation as a preparation for the interventions in the coming chapters.

The challenge of developing appropriate treatment

For many pain patients with chronic pain there may be no clear, treatable medical diagnosis.[1] An unfortunate consequence of the diagnostic approach is the "lumping" of patients together under a label, such as "chronic pain," when in fact they are quite heterogeneous. This has been termed the "patient uniformity myth."[2]

Furthermore, there may be no specific evidence-based treatment available. Although several reviews have concluded that cognitive-behaviorally oriented multi-dimensional programs are broadly effective,[3, 4, 5] there are numerous variations of these programs. Each program appears to have its own set of techniques and its own orientation.[4] Thus, there also seems to be a "treatment uniformity" myth that suggests that any cognitive behavioral-therapy (CBT) based pain program will be successful.

The perspective (or framework) used by clinicians to make sense of their patients' problems guides what they do. Typically, biomedical perspectives encourage further pursuit (and investigation) of possible biological mechanisms to account for the presenting problems and treatment is targeted at these mechanisms. In contrast, biopsychosocial perspectives invite an integration of biological, social, and psychological findings into a comprehensive account of the patient's presenting problems and contributing factors. A biopsychosocial framework can lead to different interventions being employed against a range of targets in different domains.

An additional challenge is selecting suitable assessment measures. The major considerations for selection of assessment measures are well canvassed in Chapter 3, Selecting and applying pain measures, so we will not repeat them here, but once we have all this information, how should we use it?

For example, we may have information on the patient's pain level, the degree to which it is interfering in their life, their level of depression as well as fear-avoidance beliefs and catastrophizing, and the nature of the responses made by the patient's family to their pain behavior. But if we are to treat this person, should we simply provide our standard pain treatment package (e.g. analgesic medication, home exercises, and relaxation training)? Alternatively,

what if we tried to integrate the information from the initial assessment to develop a formulation of the patient's presenting problems, how they interact and their contributing factors, and then instituted treatment accordingly? Thus, we would only target catastrophizing thoughts if they seemed to be contributing to the patient's problems, and we would only recommend home exercises if it seemed the patient seemed avoidant of activities. The mix of interventions could be quite different from one person to the next, even with the same diagnosis.

This "case formulation" approach is consistent with calls to match treatments to the patients' problems.[2] In a recent review, "risk" factors that have been found to maintain or enhance chronic pain were identified along with associated treatment techniques that have been found to have utility.[6] The authors found considerable potential for improving treatment efficacy by tailoring treatment to the actual risk factors found.[6]

Ideally, selection of appropriate treatments should also be based on established evidence. While randomized controlled trials are the basis for systematic reviews, they are not always possible in clinical settings.[7, 8] Furthermore, if the studies reviewed did not use patients like those presenting in a given clinic, the results may not be readily generalizable to that clinic. Thus, they may provide limited guidance on dealing with the case at hand. Accordingly, application of evidence-based treatments ought to be considered in the light of the nature of the cases in the clinic.

Other important questions concern when should a treatment be stopped (because it is not working or has worked) or when should a treatment be altered? Luckily, useful information can be acquired in the clinic that will help us determine whether our treatment is of value and indirectly whether the case formulation was correct. These aspects are considered in the next sections.

Finally, since treatment often requires the active participation of the patient, engaging the patient is another challenge. A chronic pain patient may receive instructions to do many things, and, for a lifetime. Yet the literature on adherence bears witness that dropouts, and failure to follow pain treatment regimes, is a huge problem and undoubtedly related to poor outcomes.[4, 9, 10] Thus, we have to find ways of engaging the patient in the treatment process.

CASE FORMULATION

Case formulation involves identifying problem areas and factors that seem to be maintaining the problem(s) or creating barriers for recovery. Formulation also includes integrating this information into a coherent framework, engaging the patient in this process, identifying their goals, and matching the treatment to the patient's circumstances. Finally, it involves evaluation of progress that uniquely allows for the treatment to be adjusted and tells us whether important goals are being achieved.

Let us start by scrutinizing a typical, but less than optimal, clinical procedure for a treatment plan. The patient who is suffering from a persistent spinal pain problem is assessed by an interdisciplinary team that evaluates medical, functional, disability, psychological, occupational, and socioeconomic aspects of the case. Many interviews are conducted, tests are ordered, and a set of questionnaires is completed. Cursorily, the patient is asked about her/his goals and previous treatments.

Subsequently, the team meets and hashes over the patient's condition and possible treatment options. A plan is adopted. But, we may rightly ask, on what basis? Often social aspects of the team may prevail, such as one person being dominant. Or, the selection may be based on the training of team members or "preferred interventions" rather than on the patient's specific problems and characteristics.[2] All too often, the same treatment seems to be offered despite the distinctive factors found in the assessment.

Although much information has been gathered, it may have a marginal influence on treatment decisions. So, although all clinicians would agree that patients are unique and should not be lumped into one category; and, even though there are considerable options for treatment, one patient may nevertheless be offered the same package as another. Using this approach we risk obtaining only "modest" results as treatment is designed for the "average" patient rather than for the particular patient.

A case-formulation approach offers a framework for utilizing the assessment information obtained in a way that might maximize both the patient's engagement as well as the development of the most potent treatment mix possible.

Negotiating the biopsychosocial model

Many pain clinics espouse the biopsychosocial model. This reflects current views of pain and the evidence for treatments based on this model.[11, 12, 13, 14, 15, 16] However, while providing a framework, it does not provide a specific treatment plan. The various health professionals involved in assessing a pain patient still need to negotiate a treatment plan based on their assessment. This requires conceptual, clinical, and interpersonal skills.

Using assessment materials within a biopsychosocial framework

Using a biopsychosocial framework, an adequate assessment should include the major aspects of the pain experience described above under The challenge of developing appropriate treatment. This includes the pain experience, behavioral, cognitive, emotional, and social/environmental aspects.

The role of measurement

Standardized measurement can provide reliable and valid information that is useful in developing a successful treatment plan as well as in evaluating the effect of treatment.

How to judge results

NORMS

Scores from measures of constructs such as depression, catastrophizing, and self-efficacy are not readily interpretable as we cannot know if they are typical or unusual for people in chronic pain unless we have normative data against which we can compare them.[17] Normative data represent the performance on a measure or test by a standardization sample.[18] The standardization sample should be as similar as possible to the patient we are trying to assess. Clinics that establish their own datasets may be able to readily compare new patients with that dataset. However, published norms can also be used where available and relevant.[19, 20, 21, 22, 23]

The use of normative data for comparison tells us whether the patient we are assessing is high or low on each of the assessed dimensions. For example, if someone's depression level is worse than 70 percent of those in the normative dataset it would suggest that depression is unusually high and will probably need to be addressed in a treatment plan. Conversely, if the level was at the 30th percentile of the dataset (i.e. worse than only 30 percent or better than 70 percent of similar chronic pain patients) then it would suggest that depression was not a major problem in this case and unlikely to require intervention.

This approach can help us to build a picture of a particular case and to identify potential targets for intervention. The following case example provides an illustration.

Case 1

This was a 23-year-old woman with complex regional pain syndrome (CRPS): pain is always present and located in the neck, right shoulder, arm and hand. The CRPS followed crush injury to her right hand eight months earlier (at work). An x-ray of the hand did not reveal anything significant. She presented at a pain clinic after trial of active physiotherapy (exercise), carpal tunnel release, and medication (now on gabapentin, 800 mg, four times a day; OxyContin, 10 mg, four times a day). She has returned to work three days a week, but on different duties and has a number of restrictions. At home she reports multiple limitations in her normal activities. As part of her assessment at the clinic she completed a set of questionnaires regarding her pain, mood, impact of pain on her normal activities, as well as her beliefs and responses to her pain. Her scores were compared with a normative dataset obtained from previous patients ($n = 566$) seen at the same clinic[23] with pain in the same region (**Table 9.1**).

These results indicate that, compared to other patients with pain in this region, the patient's usual pain levels, current depression, anxiety and stress levels were quite typical (and only slightly above healthy community norms).[24] In contrast, her levels of disability due to pain, fear-avoidance beliefs, self-efficacy beliefs, and catastrophizing were worse than those of 60–90 percent of the comparison group. This suggests that the patient's disability is related more to cognitive and behavioral factors rather than pain severity or mood.

Developing a conceptual model

Having identified the major presenting problems, the next step is to consider how they may interact and what factors are maintaining them. One way of providing a starting point to this process is to use a conceptual diagram like the one shown in **Figure 9.1**. The domains covered reflect the major elements in pain assessment.

The arrows will often be bidirectional (to indicate interactions) and in some cases some domains (boxes) will not apply or the effects will vary in strength (for example, many people with chronic pain do not take drugs). Equally, additional boxes may be added (e.g. lack of sleep or a comorbidity). This sort of model can help both clinician and patient to make sense of the patient's pain problems.

In case it seems the "bio" element has been omitted, the possible impact of activity changes on the body is provided for, but within the "chronic pain" box we can consider not just the pain experience but also the contributing biological mechanisms (e.g. neuropathic or nociceptive). Over time, it is likely there will be more feedback loops developed: for example, between inactivity/physical changes and pain, as well as between mood, unhelpful beliefs and pain.

This model provides a guide for what to do next. This is illustrated below in relation to case 1.

Putting the case together

The formulation of a case is like developing a hypothesis, which we can then test by intervening in specific areas and evaluating the outcome. The main steps before the intervention are as follows.

CONCEPTUALIZATION

Applying this model to case 1 would look as shown in **Figure 9.2**. Here, the key drivers for the excessive disability are high levels of unhelpful beliefs and responses (high fear-avoidance beliefs and catastrophizing); low confidence in functioning when in pain (low self-efficacy); high reliance on medication to relieve the pain (largely unsuccessful) that also causes unwanted mental side effects; and possibly relationship factors at home and at work. The evidence that the patient is more disabled at home than at work suggests that work may be a priority for her, but even though her work performance is below expectations it is having an adverse effect on her home life, where she is spending more time recovering from the effects of her work.

The pain experienced is typical of other patients with pain in this region and the level of distress (depression, anxiety) is also unremarkable for this population, so adding other medication for pain or mood would be unlikely to make much difference. However, a reduction in current medication could assist in the reduction in unwanted side effects (which are affecting work performance), but it may be at the cost of more pain, so the patient will have to weigh up this equation. This may be tested by seeing how she manages when the medication is gradually withdrawn. As high catastrophizing could adversely color her perception of pain, by helping her to modify her catastrophizing her perception of the pain could become more accepting and less alarmed.

Alternatively, if other drug options are not thought suitable, another way of limiting pain experience could be achieved through an invasive procedure. Depending on the case this might include consideration for spinal cord stimulation, radiofrequency neurotomy, or percutaneous electrical nerve stimulation, for example. However, given our formulation of this case, it is unlikely that any one of these interventions would be sufficient by itself. We would still need to help her deal with the cognitive (catastrophizing) and behavioral (avoidance) responses as well as her interactions with the social environments (home and workplace especially).

Table 9.1 Self-report measure scores for case 1 with percentile comparisons to normative dataset.

Measures	Raw scores	Percentiles (%)
Usual pain (0–10, range)	6 (2–8)	50
Disability (RMDQ) (0–24)	17	Worse than 90
Depression (DASS) (0–42)	10	45
Anxiety (DASS) (0–42)	6	50
Stress (DASS) (0–42)	14	45
Fear-avoidance beliefs (TSK) (17–68)	45	Worse than 70
Pain self-efficacy beliefs (PSEQ) (0–60)	20	Worse than 60
Catastrophizing (PRSS) (0–5)	3.9	Worse than 85

RMDQ (Roland and Morris Disability Questionnaire, modified for general pain use: Asghari and Nicholas, 2001); DASS (Depression Anxiety Stress Scales);[24] TSK (Tampa Scale for Kinesiophobia);[25] PSEQ (Pain Self-Efficacy Questionnaire);[26] PRSS (Pain Response Self-Statements).[27]

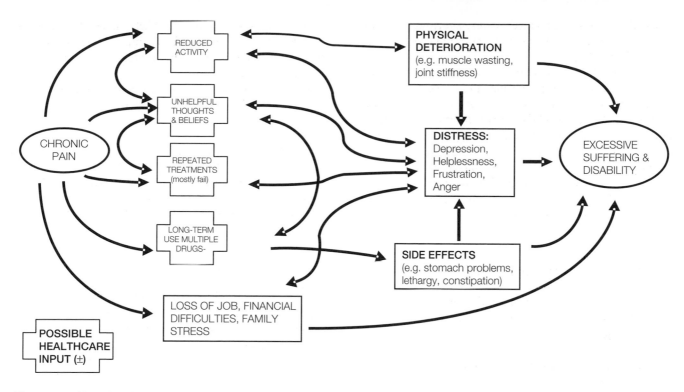

Figure 9.1 How chronic pain can become a complex problem.

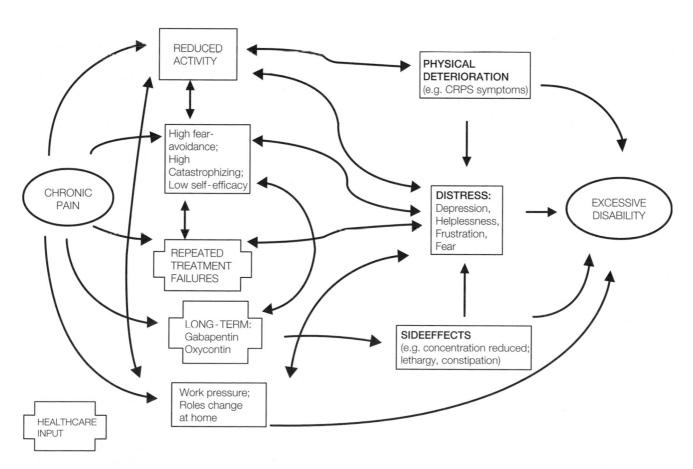

Figure 9.2 Formulation of case 1.

The difference in activity limitations between home and work suggests we should seek more information about what is happening in both places and her interactions with her family and work colleagues. This might include getting her sense of the family's and the work colleagues' views on her pain and their expectations for her condition and its management.

This approach to analyzing this patient's pain complaints illustrates how we can use clinical examinations, interviews, and self-report questionnaires to build a reasonably coherent picture of the presenting problems, their contributing factors, and to identify likely targets for intervention. This approach may be contrasted with a purely diagnostic approach (e.g. DSM-IV) which may provide a broad label for a patient, for example pain disorder, but little guidance on what to do next.[2]

TARGETS

In consultation with the patient, the treatment targets will be chosen, based on the formulation and available resources. In Case 1, the targets for intervention might include:

- increasing specific functional activities (at home and work);
- increasing work time;
- reducing side effects of medication;
- reducing pain severity.

The mechanisms for achieving these targets could include:

- gradual withdrawal of current medication;
- reduction of fear-avoidance beliefs (and behaviors);
- reduction of catastrophizing responses;
- increasing self-efficacy beliefs (for doing things despite pain);
- possibly, a trial of spinal cord stimulation (SCS).

How these mechanisms can be activated and the goals achieved will be addressed in the remaining sections. However, before any treatment can be undertaken some additional steps will be needed.

Engaging the patient

For most persisting pain conditions, effective treatment demands that the patient must play an active role. Developing a "shared understanding" where the provider and patient are on the same wavelength with regards to the problems and effective management is a key element.[10] Motivational interviewing is one method of enhancing engagement.[28, 29] Motivational interviewing involves four techniques.

1. **Developing discrepancy**. Identify the difference between the patient's current behavior and his/her important goals. The patient should be encouraged to talk openly about problems and goals and reflect upon the differences.
2. **Avoiding argumentation**. Arguing with the patient often upsets the patient and risks developing trust. Patients might also develop more reasons for why they cannot change.
3. **Rolling with resistance**. Rather than confrontation, rolling with any resistance is often more productive. The patient's standpoint can be restated to show comprehension, but then move to reframing the situation. Reflection and open questions about how one might move forward may also be helpful follow-ups.
4. **Supporting self-efficacy**. If we are viewed as the "experts" it can make it difficult to empower the patient. However, if sustainable behavior change is to be achieved, the patient must believe that he/she can actually achieve the goal. Accordingly, it is important to encourage patients to express statements of self-efficacy and to reinforce these verbally.

These elements are consistent with the communication skills of active listening and Socratic questioning. Active listening involves repeating back to the patient your understanding of what they have told you, usually in a summarized form. This allows them to confirm that you have heard them accurately. Confrontation should be avoided. Thus, it is recommended to say something like "From what you've been telling me, it sounds like …." Contrast that with the more confrontational: "You are telling me that…." The less confrontational approach can be coupled with a question to check for agreement ("is that correct?").

A Socratic style of questioning involves open questions. Rather than pose questions that begin with "Why" that can lead to defensiveness, statements that begin with words like "How," "When," "What" often work better and elicit more specific data. Examples of this interviewing style are presented in **Box 9.1**.

Such questioning enables the clinician to make a diagram of the problem such as described above under Developing a conceptual model (using the boxes for a guide). This visual representation, based directly on the patient's descriptions provides a means of confirming a "shared understanding." The assessing clinician can discuss the diagram: "so would you say that this (diagram) accurately summarizes what's been happening to you since your pain developed?" If the patient agrees, then we can move to the next step. If not, then further discussion and clarification will be needed.

ESTABLISHING WHAT THE PATIENT'S GOALS ARE

Once there is agreement on what the problems are and the major contributing factors, the goals of treatment must be

---

Box 9.1 Interview style

Obtain specific information

To develop a clear picture, it is helpful to use a Socratic style of interview. Broadly, this requires questions that begin with words like "how", "what", and "when".

For example:

- "When does your pain get worse/better?"
- "What do you usually do when the pain gets worse?"
- "What have you stopped doing because of your pain?"
- "When your pain gets worse what do you think might be happening in your body?"
- "When do you take your pain medication?"
- "How do you feel when you can't do something due to the pain?"

Checking your comprehension (and indicating you have heard)

For example:
"From what you've been saying, it sounds like the pain has had a major impact on your life – at home and at work. Is that right?"

---

negotiated. Since total pain relief is often not feasible,[30] other goals must also be considered. The main attributes of suitable goals are:

- specific (measurable);
- achievable (realistic); and
- desired by the person concerned.

These attributes can sound simple, but getting a chronic pain patient to identify their goals and commit themselves to achieving them is often quite difficult. Working through these issues can take time, but it can save time later by increasing adherence to the treatment protocol.

To promote a focus on the goals of treatment, these goals should be written down and copies kept by all parties. These can be reviewed at regular intervals to monitor progress and make necessary changes as required.

ENHANCING AND CLARIFYING MOTIVATION

McCracken and Yang[31] have proposed that it might help patients to identify goals they are prepared to work to achieve if they are encouraged to think about their values

– what gives their life meaning (for example, "to be a good parent"). Using those values as their general compass, the patient could then be asked to think about what they would need to do to achieve those values. This would lead to specific tasks or activities that can be clearly defined (e.g. sit for more than 60 minutes; carry 10 kg in each hand for 20 meters). Motivational interviewing methods can assist in this process.

ESTABLISHING WHO THE OTHER STAKEHOLDERS ARE

As well as identifying the patient's goals it will also be important to work out what has prevented their achievement (i.e. the obstacles). These may lie in the workplace, at home, or with other healthcare providers. Other people in the patient's life with an interest in the patient's progress may be called "stakeholders" because they have something to gain or lose by the patient's state. All may have equal concern for the patient's welfare, but like the patient, they also have the possibility of gains and losses depending upon the patient's progress. Compounding these different motivations, it is also possible that each stakeholder will be operating according to a different paradigm (or expectancies) in relation to the patient's pain. By identifying these other stakeholders and their roles (and likely gains/losses if there is improvement/no improvement) with the patient, the treatment planning can take these aspects into account and explore ways of dealing with them.[32] For a fuller discussion of these issues in relation to injured workers see Franche et al.[33]

Tailoring treatment to the patient

There is ample evidence that offering the same treatment to everyone with similar pain can reduce its overall efficacy.[2, 6] Ideally, an intervention should be tailored to a patient's problems and circumstances. Yet, such matching appears rare in many settings. A recent review showed that many interventions are not directed at known causal factors while some identified risk factors do not have a known treatment.[6]

SELECTING PATIENTS OR SELECTING INTERVENTIONS?

There are two basic approaches to matching patients and treatments. One attempts to select subgroups of patients who have a certain profile thought suitable for a particular intervention program. For example, if a clinic specializes in exposure programs for those with fear-avoidance features, they would select only those patients having problems due to fear-avoidance mechanisms.[34] Similarly, a clinic that focuses on stress and mood treatments would select patients with problems related to distress.[6] This approach thus starts with a treatment program and selects patients most likely to benefit.

The second approach attempts to select the treatment techniques to fit the patient's needs. This is more aligned with the case formulation approach. The findings from the assessment therefore guide the clinician in selecting which interventions might be appropriate for the particular patient. This approach might lend itself more readily to individual rather than group-based treatments, but if a clinic is sufficiently resourced the method can still be achieved by combining group and individual treatment elements. For example, it has been shown that a group-CBT program can be effectively combined with individually titrated implantable devices.[35]

Both approaches aim to increase efficiency by tailoring the match between the patient and the treatment.

TAILORING TREATMENT – FURTHER CONSIDERATIONS

Besides their different goals and factors contributing to their problems, patients will have different assets and circumstances that influence the options for tailoring. Some patients will have a long history of treatment failures and passivity that may indicate we need to start with basics, provide lots of encouraging feedback, and to progress gradually. Others will have considerable resilience, good social support, and active coping strategies allowing us to start with more advanced treatment plans that may advance quickly. Taking the patient's history and resources into account when planning treatment offers the prospect of greater success than a "one size fits all approach." By including the patient in the treatment planning they effectively share some of the responsibility for developing their treatment program and this should also enhance their acceptance of the treatment and their engagement in it.

With multiple treatments and goals, we need to consider how to proceed. Identifying a priority order for the treatments and goals can assist here. As most pain patients will have numerous problems, a good conceptualization should highlight relationships between the problems. For instance, poor communication and social skills may be linked to both problems at work, problems with friends, and problems within the family. Priority is given to those factors that are: (1) important to the patient, and (2) that may provide improvements in more than one arena. In the example, focusing on communication might then provide improvements in the areas of work, friends, and family.

Identification of barriers to change may help us design treatment plans that avoid or overcome these. Such barriers may be evident before treatment is commenced or may arise during treatment, but they can limit improvement. Often these barriers will involve other stakeholders. Several barriers for those wanting to return to work have been identified.[36, 37] For example, the patient's relationship with his/her supervisor may become a barrier if this relationship is poor (although it may enhance the process if it is good).[38, 39] Similarly, a sleeping problem may become a barrier to return to work, if the patient has difficulties getting up to go to work. Barriers are important for two reasons. First, they often disrupt an otherwise good treatment plan and may become demoralizing for the patient as well as the clinician. Second, if they are identified they may be targeted and included in the treatment plan. In this way, they may actually improve the utility of the treatment program.

In summary, while we often think about broad components of treatment programs (e.g. activity training or anxiety management), tailoring is often far more than this since it also considers how the intervention might be matched to the needs and resources of the patient. Ideally, the identification of possible barriers facilitates their targeting as part of the intervention and improves the chances of treatment success. Tailoring should be more effective than providing "a standard package" since generic approaches may well leave the patient behind, and miss important details specific to the patient at hand. These concerns may not be so important in a research study, but in the clinic they may be critical.

OUTCOME EVALUATION

Outcome evaluation enables us to determine whether the conceptualization and tailoring are correct. In turn, it also allows for adjusting the treatment plan where necessary. Fortunately, many of the initial assessment instruments may also be utilized to gauge outcome. Using them systematically provides relatively good data for judging outcome variables (e.g. disability) and process (or mechanism) variables, such as change in catastrophizing or self-efficacy.[40]

Aim of an evaluation: is treatment working?

The primary aim of clinical outcome evaluation is to judge whether treatment should be altered, continued, or terminated. This applies whether it is at the individual patient level or program level. This form of evaluation needs to be clearly differentiated from that used in treatment research studies. The perspective taken here is that outcome evaluation is an important facet of treatment for the individual patient. In contrast, the majority of published studies report average results on a group of patients. Such studies say little about the effects of your treatment on a given individual patient.

Selecting important outcomes

Selecting important outcomes may be based on the patient's goals and/or those of significance to other stakeholders. Using the goals developed with the patient provides an obvious relevance in the clinical context. Whichever measures are used, it helps if these are psychometrically sound (reliable and valid), sensitive to change, and measured often enough to monitor change during the treatment itself.

With chronic pain patients there are some common major outcome domains, some of which may be shared with various stakeholders. These are outlined in **Table 9.2**. This list is not exhaustive but it coincides with the targets outlined above:

- Is the patient feeling better (e.g. less pain, better quality of life)?
- Has function improved (e.g. daily activities)?
- Are there any physiological improvements (e.g. muscle strength)?
- Has ability to work improved?
- Is the treatment worth the economic and personal costs?

DAILY AND WEEKLY MEASUREMENTS

Generally, in treatment evaluation, some form of regular or repeated measurement is more useful than attempts to recall progress covering several months. Such data can be obtained by diary self-reports of both subjective aspects (e.g. pain intensity and satisfaction ratings), and more overt behaviors (e.g. participation in activities or hours slept). As diary reports are subjective and therefore potentially influenced by a number of factors other than treatment, it is desirable to use other measures as well. For example, activity meters may be used to measure patients' activity levels. Another option is to use standardized measurements such as questionnaires (from assessment)

on a weekly basis. Many of these are described in Chapter 3, Selecting and applying pain measures.

COMPARED TO WHAT? USING SINGLE-SUBJECT DESIGNS

An important question in evaluation is what we should compare the results to? In clinical practice it may be difficult to find a comparison group. However, normative data (see above) might be used as a benchmark to determine whether the final outcome reaches the mark. Daily or weekly data using such instruments might provide guidance during treatment as well.

Another approach is to use single-subject designs.[8] These are not to be confused with the infamous "case study." The term "case study" only reveals that a single patient is the focus of the study. They are notorious in science because they often only employ a highly selective patient, rely solely on subjective judgment (usually by the clinician), and have no control conditions. In contrast, single-subject designs should employ reliable and valid measures, repeat them over time, making systematic comparisons using the individual patient as his/her own control. This can provide for a very sensitive evaluation because it reduces the variance found in group studies where patients differ greatly.[8]

The "control" condition with a single patient is a stable baseline. **Figure 9.3** shows a simple single-subject design where pain is the outcome variable. Establish a relatively stable pretreatment level (i.e. baseline) by measuring pain ratings several times before treatment is introduced. Commence treatment once the baseline has been established. The effect of the intervention is established by viewing the data as shown in **Figure 9.3**. A benchmark

Table 9.2 Outcome domains of common interest.

Domains	Outcome examples	Interested stakeholders
Symptoms	Pain	Patient
	Sleep disturbance	Family
	Distress	Health care
		Work place
Function	Activities of daily living	Patient
	Quality of life	Family
	Ability to work	Health care
Disability	Number of days off work	Work place
	Amount of compensation payments	Insurance carrier
		Patient
Health care utilization	Medication use	Insurance carrier
	Professional care	Work place
	Complementary medical care	Patient
Patient satisfaction (with health care)	With communication	Family
	With assessment	Patient
	With treatment	Health care
	With outcome	

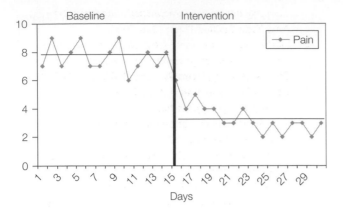

Figure 9.3 Effects of treatment on pain.

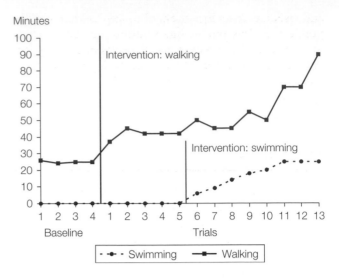

Figure 9.4 Effects of training on two activities.

can be achieved by using standardized pre- and post-treatment measures (with normative data) as well.

By using frequent measurements, with a baseline for reference, we can alter or fine-tune treatment as we proceed. We can quickly determine if a treatment is producing the expected results. In the example above, it would be counterproductive to have a patient continue with "usual graded activity" over a 16-week period if activity was not increasing – as may happen if results are not monitored and evaluated.

A variety of single-subject design are available for clinical use.[41, 42] A multiple baseline approach makes comparisons across a particular dimension (e.g. across different settings, different behaviors, or even different patients) where baselines of different lengths are utilized. The design gains strength if improvements are seen only when the treatment is applied. **Figure 9.4** shows an example employing graded activity across behaviors. Graded activity might be sequentially applied to these three types of behavior to evaluate its effects.

Final outcome evaluation

At the end of treatment, an overall evaluation may be conducted and discussed with the patient and stakeholders. Here the results of the single-subject trial may be collated with the pre- and posttreatment data in relation to the goals set.

Program evaluation

To assure service quality, a clinic may wish to continually evaluate its pain program. The use of the same standardized measures at initial assessment and treatment termination with all patients can provide a measure of overall outcome. This might be expressed in terms such as mean pain at intake was 8.5 (on a ten-point scale) and 6.2 at posttreatment which can then be compared with published outcome studies. In addition, single-subject data may be accumulated to provide success rates on an individual level. This might be expressed as 26 of 30

patients increased their daily activity levels to a specified range. As in single-subject designs, regular evaluation of progress throughout a program can also be used to fine-tune the program as it proceeds.

CONCLUSIONS

This chapter has concentrated on how to take advantage of assessment materials in formulating an accurate account of a patient's presenting problems and the factors contributing to them. The goal is to design effective treatment plans for individual patients. Rather than simply offering the same "package" to every patient, the importance of tailoring the treatment to the patients has been emphasized. By linking the assessment findings to treatment planning it is argued that treatment effectiveness should be maximized. It is also argued that assessment should not cease once treatment commences, but rather should become an integral aspect of the treatment process in the form of ongoing evaluation. This can facilitate fine-tuning treatment to achieve even better results.

It is also emphasized that in using the assessment findings clinicians should include the patient in an alliance to develop individually-relevant treatments that the patient might be motivated to pursue. Strategies such as motivational interviewing, Socratic dialogue, and valuing offer potentially good methods for promoting the patient's involvement in treatment planning and sharing responsibility for progress.

Good assessment should also identify potential barriers to change, including how other stakeholders view and deal with the patient's problems. These may need to be targeted in the treatment plan. Although often neglected, an analysis of the patient's resources can be helpful in calibrating the treatment plan. Thus, the final treatment plan will consider the patient's goals, problems, and resources in an hypothesized conceptualization of the problem. In this model, interventions may be seen as a form of hypothesis testing, which leaves open the possibility of reformulation of a case in the light of the treatment results and the development of further intervention options.

REFERENCES

1. Turk DC, Melzack R (eds). *Handbook of pain assessment*, 2nd edn. London: The Guilford Press, 2001: 760.

2. Turk DC, Okifuji A. Matching treatment to assessment of patients with chronic pain. In: Turk DC, Melzack R (eds). *Handbook of pain assessment*, 2nd edn. New York: The Guilford Press, 2001: 400–14.

3. Morley S, Eccleston C, Williams A. Systematic review and meta-analysis of randomised controlled trials of cognitive behaviour therapy and behaviour therapy for chronic pain in adults, excluding headache. *Pain*. 1999; **80**: 1–13.

4. Linton SJ. Utility of cognitive-behavioral psychological treatments. In: Nachemson A, Jonsson E (eds). *Neck and back pain: The scientific evidence of causes, diagnosis, and treatment*. Philadelphia: Lippincott Williams & Wilkins, 2000: 361–81.

5. Flor H, Fydrich T, Turk DC. Efficacy of multidisciplinary pain treatment centers: A meta-analytic review. *Pain*. 1992; **49**: 221–30.

* 6. Shaw WS, Linton SJ, Pransky G. Reducing sickness absence from work due to low back pain: How well do intervention strategies match modifiable risk factors? *Journal of Occupational Rehabilitation*. 2006; **16**: 591–605.

7. Kazdin AE. *Research design in clinical psychology*, 4th edn. London: Allyn and Bacon, 2003.

* 8. Kazdin AE (ed.). *Methodological issues and strategies in clinical research*, 2nd edn. Washington, DC: American Psychological Association, 1998: 825.

9. Turk DC, Rudy TE. Neglected topics in the treatment of chronic pain patients: Relapse, noncompliance, and adherence enhancement. *Pain*. 1991; **44**: 5–28.

10. Linton SJ. *Understanding pain for better clinical practice: A psychological perspective*. London: Elsevier, 2005: 180.

11. Waddell G. *The back pain revolution*. Edinburgh: Churchill Livingstone, 1998.

12. Waddell G. *Models of disability: Using low back pain as an example*. London: Royal society of Medicine Press Ltd, 2002: 26.

13. Turk DC. Clinical effectiveness and cost-effectiveness of treatments for patients with chronic pain. *Clinical Journal of Pain*. 2002; **18**: 355–65.

14. Turk DC, Flor H. Chronic pain: A biobehavioral perspective. In: Gatchel RJ, Turk DC (eds). *Psychosocial factors in pain: Critical perspectives*. New York: The Guilford Press, 1999: 18–34.

15. Turk DC. Biopsychosocial perspective on chronic pain. In: Gatchel RJ, Turk DC (eds). *Psychological approaches to pain management: A practitioner's handbook*, 1st edn. New York: Guilford Press, 1996: 3–32.

16. Nachemson A, Jonsson E (eds). *Neck and back pain: The scientific evidence of causes, diagnosis, and treatment*. Philadelphia: Lippincott Williams & Wilkins, 2000: 495.

17. Kendall PC, Marrs-Garcia A, Nath SR, Sheldrick RC. Normative comparisons for the evaluation of clinical significance. *Journal of Consulting and Clinical Psychology*. 1999; **67**: 285–99.

18. Anastasi A, Urbina S. *Psychological testing*, 7th edn. New York: Prentice Hall, 1997.

19. Von Korff M, Dworkin SF, Le Resche L. Graded chronic pain status: an epidemiologic evaluation. *Pain*. 1992; **40**: 279–91.

20. Kerns RD, Turk DC, Rudy TE. The West Haven-Yale Multidimensional Pain Inventory (WHYMPI). *Pain*. 1985; **23**: 345–56.

21. Wittink HM, Rogers WH, Lipman AG *et al.* Older and younger adults in pain management programs in the United States: differences and similarities. *Pain Medicine*. 2006; **7**: 151–63.

22. Chibnall JT, Tait RC. The pain disability index: factor structure and normative data. *Archives of Physical Medicine and Rehabilitation*. 1994; **75**: 1082–6.

23. Nicholas MK, Asghari A, Blyth FM. What do the numbers mean? Normative data in chronic pain measures. *Pain*. 2008; **134**: 158–73.

24. Lovibond PF, Lovibond SH. The structure of negative emotional states: comparison of the depression anxiety stress scales (DASS) with the beck depression and anxiety inventories. *Behavior Research and Therapy*. 1995; **33**: 335–43.

25. Kori SH, Miller RP, Todd DD. Kinisophobia: A new view of chronic pain behavior. *Pain Management*. 1990; Jan./Feb.: 35–43.

26. Nicholas MK. The pain self-efficacy questionnaire: Taking pain into account. *European Journal of Pain*. 2007; **11**: 153–63.

27. Flor H, Behle DJ, Birbaumer N. Assessment of pain-related cognitions in chronic pain patients. *Behavior Research and Therapy*. 1993; **31**: 63–73.

* 28. Jensen MP. Enhancing motivation to change in pain treatment. In: Turk DC, Gatchel RJ (eds). *Psychological approaches to pain management: A practitioner's handbook*, 2nd edn. New York: The Guilford Press, 2002: 71–93.

* 29. Miller WR, Rollnick S. *Motivational interviewing: Preparing people for change*. New York: Guilford Press, 1998.

30. Turk DC, Gatchel RJ (eds). *Psychological approaches to pain management: A practitioner's handbook*, Vol. 2. New York: Guilford Press, 2002: 590.

31. McCracken LM, Yang S-Y. The role of values in a contextual cognitive-behavioral approach to chronic pain. *Pain*. 2006; **123**: 137–45.

32. Nicholas MK. Reducing disability in injured workers: The importance of collaborative management. In: Linton SJ

(ed.). *New avenues for the prevention of chronic musculoskeletal pain and disability.* Amsterdam: Elsevier, 2002: 33–46.

* 33. Franche RL, Baril R, Shaw WS *et al.* Workplace-based return-to-work interventions: Optimizing the role of stakeholders in implementation and research. *Journal of Occupational Rehabilitation.* 2005; **15**: 525–42.

34. Leeuw M, Goossens MEJB, Linton SJ *et al.* The fear-avoidance model of musculoskeletal pain: State of the scientific evidence. *Journal of Behavioral Medicine.* 2007; **30**: 77–74.

35. Molloy AR, Nicholas MK, Asghari A *et al.* Does a combination of intensive cognitive-behavioural pain management and a spinal implantable device confer any advantage? A preliminary examination. *Pain Practice.* 2006; **6**: 96–103.

36. Marhold C, Linton SJ, Melin L. Identification of obstacles for chronic pain patients to return to work: evaluation of a questionnaire. *Journal of Occupational Rehabilitation.* 2002; **12**: 65–75.

37. Main CJ, Spanswick CC. *Pain management: An interdisciplinary approach.* Edinburgh: Churchill Livingstone, 2000: 438.

38. Lincoln AE, Feuerstein M, Shaw WS, Miller VI. Impact of case manager training on worksite accommodations in workers' compensation claimants with upper extremity disorders. *Journal of Occupational and Environmental Medicine.* 2002; **44**: 237–45.

39. Shaw WS, Robertson MM, Pransky G, McLellan RK. Employee perspectives on the role of supervisors to prevent workplace disability after injuries. *Journal of Occupational Rehabilitation.* 2003; **13**: 129–42.

40. Morely SJ, Keefe FJ. Getting a handle on process and change in CBT for chronic pain. *Pain.* 2007; **127**: 197–8.

41. Tripodi T. *A primer on single-subject design for clinical social workers.* Washington, DC: National Association of Social Workers Press, 1994: 153.

42. Krishef CH. *Fundamental approaches to single subject design and analysis.* Malabar, FL: Krieger Publishing, 1991: 142.

SECTION **A**

Pharmacological therapies

10

Treatment protocols for opioids in chronic nonmalignant pain

HARALD BREIVIK

KEY LEARNING POINTS

- Opioid analgesics are the most effective drugs to relieve severe, acute, and terminal pain.
- Long-term use of opioids can reduce the burden of suffering from chronic nonterminal pain, but adverse effects often reduce the beneficial effects.
- The evidence base for long-term benefits and safety is weak.
- Adverse effects of long-term opioid treatment include gastrointestinal, endocrinological, and cognitive dysfunctions, development of tolerance, hyperalgesia, and pseudoaddiction behavior.
- Problematic prescription opioid use develops in about 10 percent, and in a few, genetically predisposed people with psychosocial comorbidities, the neurobiological disease of addiction may occur, with compulsive use in spite of obvious deleterious effects of continued opioid use.

- Guidelines and recommendations for best practice of opioid use for chronic nonterminal pain are based mostly on experts' opinions.
- Steady-state regimes (stable dose of controlled/prolonged-release oral or transdermal delivery) are considered to have the best benefit/risk ratio, and they are recommended by most experts.
- Intermittent-use regimes (dose as needed) are recommended by some experts in selected patients with pain-free periods, recurrent pain, and low risk of problematic use.
- Whatever regime is chosen, long-term opioid therapy demands a major effort by physicians and patients to optimize benefits and reduce risks of serious adverse effects.

INTRODUCTION

Opioids are powerful analgesics, but they can cause a number of adverse effects. During opioid treatment of severe acute pain, respiratory depression and gastro-intestinal side effects are the most important; problematic opioid use rarely arises *de novo*. Opioid treatment of chronic pain induces gastrointestinal dysfunction in most patients, varying from slightly reduced appetite and irregular bowel movements to nausea, reflux dyspepsia, and obstinate constipation. Such adverse effects limit the usefulness of opioids for chronic pain and cause many patients to abandon opioid treatment.[1] Endocrine organs are affected with reduced production of estrogen, testosterone, and cortisol.[2] Immunological functions may be depressed.[3] More sinister is the development of compulsive opioid-seeking and other addictive behaviors that may result from long-term opioid treatment.[4, 5, 6, 7, 8] Some degree of problematic opioid use arises in about 2–10 percent of opioid-treated chronic pain patients,[7, 8, 9, 10] varying in severity from mostly nuisance problems to quite burdensome, problematic drug-related behaviors and outright addiction behavior in a few. Many of the latter have a history of nonmedical use of drug(s) or alcohol abuse before prescription opioid use.[7, 11, 12]

This backdrop sets the scene for the often difficult decisions on opioid treatment of long-lasting pain conditions when alternative treatments of lower risk have failed. The decision to start and the follow up of opioid treatment may be straightforward in elderly patients with uncomplicated nociceptive-type chronic pain. It is a more difficult decision to add an opioid to the first-line drugs for peripheral or central chronic neuropathic pain. It is a real dilemma whether to start opioid trial therapy in more complex chronic pain conditions, and whether to continue when the overall effect is somewhat positive, and there is the ever present risk of developing problematic prescription opioid use.[4, 5]

WEAK EVIDENCE BASE FOR OPIOID TREATMENT OF CHRONIC NONTERMINAL PAIN

There are only a few double-blind, placebo-controlled, randomized clinical trials (RCTs) on the benefits and side effects of opioid treatment for chronic nonterminal pain, and they are all of short duration, mostly four to eight weeks, giving no reliable evidence for long-term effects and safety.[1, 8, 13, 14, 15, 16] Pain intensity may decrease by about 30 percent,[1] some maintain satisfactory pain relief for at least three years,[10] but more than 50 percent of patients stop using opioids within one or two years because of too little pain relief or adverse effects.[1, 8]

Prolonged RCTs with large samples are probably not going to be conducted because of the problems of maintaining blinding of test-treatment and the necessity of individually titrating opioid dose to balance benefits and adverse effects.[17] Therefore, many open questions around long-term opioid treatment of chronic non-terminal pain (**Box 10.1**) will probably not be resolved by traditional RCTs. Larger, randomized, prospective, comparative studies without blinding may be the best we can hope for. The national and international agencies for medicines, responsible for the effective and safe use of drugs, do not seem to be able to take initiatives to clarify this important drug problem. They seem to be content with guidelines based mainly on expert opinion, which are a rather weak evidence-base for recommendations for a potent therapy with a rather narrow therapeutic range.[17]

The World Health Assembly recently instructed the World Health Organization (WHO) and United Nation's International Narcotic Control Board (INCB) to assure appropriate availability of opioid analgesic drugs for medical purposes worldwide and to ensure that appropriate guidelines and knowledge are present for the pharmacological treatment of acute, cancer, and chronic nonmalignant pain: the Access to Controlled Medicines Program (ACMP) was initiated and is expected to continue for at least six years.[18] Recommendations for good practice of opioid treatment for acute, cancer, and nonmalignant pain will eventually be published by the ACMP of WHO and INCB, including research agenda listing urgent research issues in this field.[18, 19, 20]

ARE SOME DRUGS OR SOME ADMINISTRATION MODES MORE PRONE TO CAUSE PROBLEMATIC PRESCRIPTION OPIOID USE?

Frequent and prolonged exposure to a potent μ-opioid receptor agonist may precipitate aberrant prescription opioid use behavior in people genetically predisposed to addiction, when circumstances are unfavorable.[4, 8] It would appear that the more rapidly the opioid drug crosses the blood–brain barrier in order to achieve a rapid onset pain relief, mood elevating, and anxiolytic effect, and the shorter the duration and the quicker the disappearance of these effects, the higher is the risk for development of problematic prescription opioid use and eventually the chronic neurobiological disease of addiction.[4, 5]

Most official guidelines therefore emphasize that long-term treatment with opioid analgesic drugs should be conducted with an opioid drug that causes a slow onset, a prolonged and slowly decaying effect on μ-opioid receptors (**Box 10.2** and **Table 10.1**).[8, 22, 23, 24, 25, 26] This makes good common sense and is generally accepted as the best practice for patients with continuously ongoing chronic pain. Opioid-treated patients appear to be less likely to develop problematic prescription opioid use when they are on a stable regime, as the steady state may be protective.[8, 27] However, this is mostly based on expert opinions and is not based on controlled trials.[28] However, the

---

Box 10.1 Some important unresolved questions about opioid therapy for chronic nonterminal pain

---

- Weak evidence-base for effectiveness and safety – how can the evidence be strengthened?
- What are reliable criteria for starting opioids for chronic nonterminal pain?
- Aims of opioid therapy: less pain, improved physical and social functions – are they realistic, or is improved mood and subjective experience of improved quality of life (QoL) appropriate goals?
- How do we determine opioid-responsiveness? Trial period? For how long? Try only one – or several opioids?
- Are some drugs more prone to cause problematic opioid usage or is it the mode of administration that determines the risk of developing problematic opioid use?
- Are some patients predisposed to become problematic patients? How do we assess risks of developing problematic opioid behavior?
- How to recognize and manage development of tolerance, physical dependence, withdrawal-exacerbation of pain, end-of-dose breakthrough pain?
- Is opioid-induced hyperalgesia a type of neurotoxicity caused by prolonged opioid therapy? Or just an accelerated development of tolerance?
- Opioid-induced gastrointestinal dysfunction, constipation, and laxative-induced distress – are they major reasons for failure of opioid therapy?
- Importance of opioid-induced endocrine dysfunction, e.g. decreased testosterone and consequences for family life and quality of life?
- Breakthrough pain: rescue fast-onset opioid dose? – or escalating the background depot opioid dose?
- Evidence for improved effectiveness of opioids with coanalgesics and opioid rotation?
- How do we recognize and manage pseudoaddiction behavior?
- How do we recognize and manage a problematic opioid-using patient who is at risk of developing the chronic neurobiological disease of addiction?
- Chronic complex pain patients who develop severe problematic opioid use: whose responsibility is this? How do we manage true addiction in pain patients and who should manage them?

Box 10.2 Some administration modes are safer than others

Administrations of opioid drugs that result in a slow-onset, prolonged, and gradually decreasing μ-opioid receptor agonist effect appear to be more easily controlled during long-term treatment than administration of a fast-onset opioid with short duration.

- Oral administration of controlled-release (depot) formulations.[4, 8]
- Transdermal administrations of opioids, e.g. buprenorphine (three- or seven-day patch) or fentanyl (three-day patch).[21]

Potent opioids with quick onset and offset and with short duration carry a higher risk of control problems.

- Parenteral injections of opioids for chronic pain are difficult to control and eventually lead to escalation of dose and difficult compliance problems. Lipophilic, potent opioids with rapid onset are likely the most risky drugs to inject.

---

success of long-term opioid treatment may be related as much to the quality of the personal relationship between physician and patient as to the characteristics of the patient, drug, or dosing regime.[4, 29]

Patients who are pain-free between recurrent painful episodes, should not be exposed to unnecessary opioid during the pain-free periods: 24 hours per day depot opioid administration may not be optimal for such patients.[8, 28]

INDICATIONS FOR LONG-TERM TREATMENT WITH A POTENT OPIOID ANALGESIC DRUG FOR CHRONIC NONTERMINAL (NONMALIGNANT) PAIN

Consideration of long-term treatment with opioid(s) as part of the management of a patient suffering from moderate to severe, debilitating chronic nonterminal pain is justified if:

- other drugs and other methods with less risk of serious side effects have failed to relieve pain and improve quality of life;
- meaningful pain relief from an opioid drug is demonstrated and is shown to be sustained with oral or transdermal administration (for intrathecal opioid administration, see Chapter 31, Intrathecal drug delivery);

- the patient's quality of life, emotional, social, and physical well-being are improved and the patient can tolerate side effects;
- the risks of adverse effects of long-term opioid therapy are acceptable;
- the patient, his family, and primary care physician understand and accept the benefits and risks of long-term opioid therapy;
- the patient and his primary care physician, and pain specialist, are prepared to make the long-term commitments and efforts needed for effective and safe opioid treatment of chronic pain.

CONTRAINDICATIONS

Opioid-unresponsive pain

Patients who do not respond with meaningful pain relief during a trial treatment period with adequate titration of an opioid should not be continued on opioid drug

Table 10.1 Oral and transdermal opioids for chronic pain.

Generic name	Analgesic starting dose in opioid naive patient
Codeine	30 mg every 4 hours
Codeine CR	100 mg every 12 hours
Dihydrocodeine	15 mg every 4 hours
Dihydrocodeine CR	60 mg every 12 hours
Tramadol	50 mg every 4 hours
Tramadol CR	100 mg every 12 hours
Tilidin+naloxone CR[a]	50+4 mg every 12 hours
Morphine	10 mg every 4 hours
Morphine CR	30 mg every 12 hours
Oxycodone	5 mg every 4 hours
Oxycodone CR	10 mg every 12 hours
Oxycodone+naloxone CR[a]	10+5 mg every 12 hours
Hydromorphone	2 mg every 4 hours
Hydromorphone CR	4 mg every 12 hours
Methadone	5 mg every 8 hours
Pethidine not for chronic pain	
Ketobemidone not for chronic pain	
Buprenorphine patch	5 μg per hour patch every 7 days
Fentanyl patch	12 μg per hour patch every 3 days

Approximate starting doses for opioid-naive adult patients above 50 kg body weight and normal general health. Doses must be reduced markedly in patients on sedative, anxiolytic, or antidepressant drugs. Sedative, cognitive, and respiratory depressant effects will be markedly enhanced by alcohol.
CR, controlled release.
[a]Naloxone-containing, controlled-release opioids markedly reduce opioid-induced gastrointestinal side effects and have no effect on analgesia due to almost complete first-pass elimination by the liver. However, in patients with liver dysfunction, first-pass elimination of naloxone is not complete, which may precipitate withdrawal syndrome.

treatment. Some pain clinicians would give the patient a second chance with one or even two different opioid agonists, hoping that the receptor population of the patient may respond better to one opioid than to another.

Neuropathic pain was formerly considered not responsive to opioid drugs.[30] However, opioid drugs are now included in guidelines for pharmacological treatment of neuropathic pain, usually as secondary drugs after the first-line drugs have failed or given insufficient relief, that is, after or in addition to antidepressants, calcium channel alpha2-delta ligands, and topical lidocaine.[21, 31, 32]

Increased risk of aberrant opioid use

The risk of developing problems from prescription opioids is increased:[4, 5, 6, 7, 8, 11, 12, 33]

- in patients with a history of previous or present drug or alcohol abuse, and
- in patients with psychiatric comorbidities.

A family history of similar problems may also imply a genetic predisposition for increased risk.

Screening instruments have been developed for evaluating the risk of problematic prescription opioid use and predicting the likelihood of successful outcome of opioid treatment.[8, 33, 34] Validation of such screening tools is ongoing.[33]

Relative contraindications?

Patients with increased risk of developing problematic opioid use, however, also need pain relief.[35] Therefore, a history of drug or alcohol abuse is not an absolute contraindication. A severely debilitating pain condition in such a patient may still warrant accepting the risk of problematic opioid seeking or possibly risking precipitating addictive behavior. Clearly, increased vigilance and monitoring of compliance with an agreed regime will be required. This will require a major effort from all parties concerned: the patient and his family, the primary healthcare professionals, the pain clinic resources, and, where available, possibly help from addiction medicine specialists.[8, 36]

PATIENT INFORMATION AND CONSENT TO OPIOID TREATMENT

Opioid treatment for chronic nonterminal ("nonmalignant") pain requires that the patient is well informed of the objectives, the expected benefits, short- and long-term adverse effects, and the risks of developing problematic use of an addictive drug. Both physician and patient awareness of goals, potential problems, and responsibilities associated with opioid treatment should be documented in writing.

- Verbal and written information, including informed consent, should be given before starting a trial for possible long-term treatment with an opioid drug.
- The patient is coresponsible for the dosing regime, compliance, adjusting dosage for breakthrough pain, and returning to baseline dosing.
- The patient must be able to understand and share responsibility for observing and reporting symptoms of development of tolerance, physical dependence, and withdrawal symptoms.
- Should problematic use develop and before the start up of opioid therapy, the patient needs to be aware of the necessity of screening urine or serum for medication level for drugs that have not been prescribed by the responsible physician.

The patient must understand that adverse effects of long-term opioid therapy may include the following.

- Confusion or changes in mental state or cognitive and thinking abilities.
- Coordination problems may make operating dangerous equipment or motor vehicles unsafe.
- Increased sleepiness, especially when combined with other drugs or alcohol.
- Constipation requiring prophylactic stool softeners and laxatives from initiating treatment.
- Respiratory depression if the dose of opioid drug is rapidly increased, especially when combined with night sedation or alcohol.
- Decreased appetite, nausea, heartburn.
- Decreased production of estrogen, testosterone, and cortisol causing infertility and decreased libido.
- Physical dependence, the physiological adaptation to the opioid drug characterized by the emergence of withdrawal symptoms when the dose is rapidly decreased. Withdrawal symptoms may be relieved by readministration of the opioid drug. Physical dependence is a predictable effect of regular, legitimate opioid use, and does not equate with addiction or drug abuse.
- Withdrawal syndrome is a constellation of signs and symptoms due to the abrupt cessation of, or reduction in, dose of a regularly administered dose of opioid. It is characterized by varying combinations and severities of the following symptoms that develop within hours to days after abrupt cessation of the opioid:
  - dysphoric, depressed mood;
  - anxiety and fear;
  - nausea, vomiting, diarrhea;
  - muscle aches and abdominal cramps;
  - lacrimation or rhinorrhea (runny nose);
  - pupillary dilation;
  - piloerection ("goose flesh");
  - sweating, fever;
  - yawning;
  - insomnia.
- Tolerance results from regular use of an opioid analgesic leading to a need for an increased dose of opioid to produce the desired effect on pain and function. Tolerance is a predictable effect of opioid use and does not imply addiction. Tolerance may develop slowly, not at all, or rapidly.
- Breakthrough pain and pseudoaddiction occur when pain for some reason increases transiently, requiring an extra opioid dose, and the patient is met with skepticism and breakthrough pain is not appropriately handled. The patient shows behavior similar to addictive behavior.
- Pseudoaddiction behavior may also occur when tolerance slowly develops and the opioid dose is not adjusted accordingly. This iatrogenic complication does not occur when there is a stable, respectful, and trusting clinician–patient relationship.
- Children born to mothers on regular opioid medication are born physically dependent on the medication and often develop a withdrawal syndrome after birth.
- Logistic problems relating to planned international travel must be anticipated and handled.
- Problematic prescription opioid use may develop in about 10 percent of patients and requires either discontinuation of opioid therapy or strict control and compliance with an agreed contract.
- Addition is a chronic neurobiological disease resulting from repeated use of opioids by persons genetically prone to develop abuse of addictive drugs, substances, and alcohol. This can occur during medical opioid treatment for chronic pain, especially in patients with psychosocial comorbidities. The prevalence is unknown.[8] Addiction is characterized by:
  - loss of control of own behavior;
  - compulsive urge to use the drug;
  - continued use despite adverse social, physical, psychological, occupational, and economic consequences.
- There should be only one prescriber (with a deputy prescriber(s) during absence for vacation, etc.) and a single dispensing pharmacy for all pain-related medication.
- There should be an agreed plan for monitoring compliance of treatment that includes the number and frequency of all prescriptions; however, only if the patient demonstrates problematic opioid use behavior is screening of urine or serum medication levels, including checks for nonprescribed medications, appropriate.
- Agreement on reasons for discontinuing opioid therapy, including loss of demonstrable beneficial effects, violation of the written agreement, and loss of control and trust.

ADDICTION AND PROBLEMATIC PRESCRIPTION OPIOID USE IN CHRONIC PAIN PATIENTS

The multifaceted problem of addiction confounds the issue of opioid treatment for chronic pain in patients with normal life expectancy. There is no agreement on how to define addiction in the context of medical treatment of chronic pain with opioid analgesic drugs.[8] The International Classification of Diseases (ICD)-10 diagnostic criteria for "drug dependence syndrome" and the Diagnostic and Statistical Manual of Mental Disorders (DSM)-IV diagnostic criteria for "substance dependence" are not applicable to chronic pain patients prescribed opioids.[4, 8, 33] The same is said of the criteria listed in the consensus document from the American pain and addiction societies: impaired control over drug use, compulsive use, continued use despite harm, and craving.[8, 37] Depending on the definition and the understanding of what comprises addiction, the prevalence in published studies varies from 0 to more than 50 percent.[33, 38, 39, 40] The true risk of developing addiction to prescription opioids is in fact not known.[8]

The term "addiction" is highly stigmatizing to pain patients and often used about patients reporting poor effect of their opioid treatment, who do not demonstrate signs and symptoms of true addiction.[39] Nevertheless, opioids are addictive drugs and a poorly controlled opioid therapy can create major problems for susceptible patients. Multiple risk factors for addiction are categorized by Ballantyne and La Forge[4, 8] in three groups as (1) psychosocial factors; (2) drug-related factors; and (3) genetic factors. When risk factors in each category occur together, a real risk of developing opioid addiction may be present in a chronic pain patient receiving opioid therapy. There seems to be agreement among experienced pain clinicians on the following statements.[5, 8]

- Pain patients are unlikely to develop addiction if they have no genetic predisposition, no psychosocial comorbidity, and are taking stable doses of opioid for the treatment of severe pain in a controlled setting.
- Pain patients are at (higher) risk of developing addiction if they have a history of personal or family substance abuse, displaying one or several psychosocial comorbidities, and if opioid treatment is not carefully organized and monitored.
- "Problematic opioid use" is a commonly used descriptive term of patients who clearly do not have optimal benefit from their opioid therapy, who need better structure and monitoring of their treatment, rather than being met with a skeptical attitude, which rapidly destroys the vitally important trustful patient–physician therapeutic relationship (**Box 10.3**).[8, 35]

> ### Box 10.3 Behaviors of pain patients who are developing problematic opioid use caused by a suboptimal opioid treatment regime
>
> - The patient is focused on opioid issues during clinic visits. This occupies a significant part of the clinic visit time, interferes with and impedes progress of other aspects of the management of the patient's pain. This behavior persists.
> - The patient develops a pattern of early refills and insists on escalating doses without any obvious change in the medical condition.
> - A pattern emerges with multiple prescription problems, e.g. demands for early refills, lost medications, lost prescriptions, stolen medications. Eventually, finding supplemental sources of opioids, obtaining opioids in emergency rooms, illegal sources, forged prescriptions.[8, 37, 39, 40]

GUIDELINES FOR TREATMENT OF CHRONIC NONTERMINAL (NONMALIGNANT) PAIN WITH OPIOIDS

National and international pain societies, expert groups, and governmental bodies have published guidelines for opioid therapy in the management of patients with chronic nonterminal/nonmalignant pain.[22, 23, 24, 25, 26] Common principles of these guidelines are outlined below, somewhat colored by the author's own experience during more than three decades of pain medicine practice.

Assessment of pain condition, opioid response, and justification for opioid therapy.

- Establish working diagnosis, differential diagnoses, analyses of the pain condition with a conclusion as to the type of pain, and possible etiological and contributory pathogenic mechanisms.
- Specific statement of the medical indication for assessment of opioid therapy:
  - reasonable attempts (but unsuccessful) at treating the pain condition with available nonopioid medications and other interventions;
  - markedly reduced quality of life.
- Potential contraindications to opioid treatment:
  - history of alcohol or substance abuse (relatively strong contraindication);
  - unstable sociopsychological background (relative contraindication).

- Blinded opioid intravenous infusion test (morphine or alfentanil; see Chapter 5, Pharmacological diagnostic tests):
  - if there is a positive beneficial response after at least one opioid on pain intensity, and preferably some effect on sensory dysfunctional symptoms (allodynia), proceed with oral trial;
  - however, the intravenous opioid test has low predictive value for the effect of orally administered opioids. It is therefore acceptable to go directly to a trial period with an oral controlled release opioid.
- Proceed with trial period of about three to six weeks with the goals of obtaining meaningful pain relief, improvements in functions and quality of life, with acceptable side effects.
- Start low with appropriate dose adjustments of:
  - one of the orally controlled release (about 12 hours) opioid drugs (e.g. dihydrocodeine, tramadol, morphine, oxycodone, hydromorphone – depending on availability and prior opioid treatment);
  - or, if compliance with oral intake is difficult, transdermal buprenorphine patch.
- Meaningful pain relief should be the goal of treatment, so that the patient's subjective overall experience is satisfactory, or about 30 percent reduction in pain intensity on a numeric rating scale.
- If these treatment goals are not obtainable with a controlled-release oral opioid or transdermal buprenorphine:
  - attempts at maintenance therapy with transdermal fentanyl may be considered;
  - the author strongly advises against parenteral opioid treatment by injection. This is too difficult to control for prolonged periods;
  - in highly selected cases, intrathecal opioid administration may be considered (Chapter 31, Intrathecal drug delivery).

THE OBJECTIVES AND TREATMENT PLAN FOR MAINTENANCE OPIOID THERAPY

Objectives of treatment

The aims of treatment should be:

- reduction in subjective pain intensity and burden of pain;
- improved ability to carry out daily activities;
- improvement in social functioning;
- improvement in subjective quality of life.

These must be measured according to principles outlined in Chapter 3, Selecting and applying pain measures and Chapter 2, Practical methods for pain intensity

measurements documented in the patient's chart, and followed over time.

Treatment plan

- The treatment plan should aim at maintaining documented effects observed during the trial period.
- It should include the type of drug, administration form, and dosage.
- There should be a frequent review of medication use, effects, and overall benefits. Initially, this should be carried out twice weekly, then weekly, and, when stable, effects, side effects, and dose required should be assessed on a monthly basis, later on possibly with longer intervals.
- Included in patients' charts at every office/clinic visit, the following should be noted:
  - efficacy of treatment on pain rating scales;
  - functional changes in ability to perform daily activities;
  - changes in ability to function at home, at work, in the community;
  - any adverse effects of opioid medication (in particular, attention should be given to opioid-induced gastrointestinal dysfunction. Offer advice on prophylaxis and treatment of constipation);
  - assessment of compliance of drug use compared with agreed plan;
  - review of the diagnosis and treatment plan.
- There should be unannounced urine or serum drug screens only when indicated.

Periodic reviews

At least every six months, there should be a review of the current status compared with previous documentation to determine whether continued opioid therapy is the best option for the patient.

TREATMENT OF ACUTE PAIN IN PATIENTS ON CHRONIC OPIOID THERAPY

When these patients have surgery, suffer trauma, or need treatment in an intensive care unit, their need for analgesic therapy is often severely underestimated. Sometimes, even misguided attempts to wean them rapidly from opioid therapy are initiated. These patients do have opioid tolerance and need a tailored titration of potent shorter-acting opioids; one should expect that the patients need doses much above "normal" acute pain doses to opioid naive patients. A restrictive approach, reducing the opioid dose rapidly in such a situation is not humane, nor is it ethical.

Consider adding clonidine to the opioid, a continuous intravenous infusion, starting with clonidine 1–2 µg/kg per hour, or 150 µg orally every six hours. Clonidine potentiates the analgesic effect of opioids and suppresses many of the autonomic and physical withdrawal symptoms.

Whenever appropriate, use a local or regional anesthetic technique, such as continuous femoral nerve or epidural block. In addition to a successful regional analgesic technique, opioid maintenance therapy is necessary to prevent tormenting the patient with a withdrawal syndrome.

TREATMENT OF BREAKTHROUGH PAIN IN PATIENTS ON CHRONIC OPIOID THERAPY

Unless the pain is episodic with pain-free intervals long enough to motivate an intermittent dosing regime, long-term opioid treatment should be based on long-acting, controlled-release opioids. When breakthrough pain occurs, experts agree that the daily dose should be adjusted, rather than treating breakthrough pain with fast-onset, short-duration opioids. Loss of control and problematic opioid use may more easily develop with the latter regime.[16]

A ceiling dose of potent opioids for chronic opioid therapy?

Whereas there does not seem to be a ceiling dose of opioids when treating acute pain in opioid-naive patients, gradually escalating doses during long-term opioid treatment for cancer and noncancer pain often do not improve pain relief, but markedly aggravate adverse effects, even causing opioid-induced hyperalgesic states. Experts do not agree on what is a reasonable ceiling dose for a trial of opioid escalation when a previously helpful opioid regime is failing.[16] No doubt careful reconsideration of overall effects are necessary when an oral dose equivalent of about morphine 200 mg per day is exceeded. However, the author has seen occasional patients have apparent successful escalation up to 200 µg per hour fentanyl patch (equivalent to about 500–700 mg per day of oral morphine?) for neuropathic pain, although endocrinological and cognitive adverse effects were apparent, eventually making detoxification necessary.

Opioid rotation when a ceiling dose or adverse effects are problematic?

Changing to another opioid must be considered as an alternative to discontinuation of opioid treatment when escalating the opioid dose has failed to improve analgesia. Sometimes this is helpful, possibly because opioids vary in their receptor interactions. When changing from one opioid to another, this can be done rapidly, making sure the new opioid is started at 50 percent less than the equivalent dose of the outgoing opioid.[16] When changing from morphine to methadone, the initial methadone dose should be even less.

AN EXAMPLE OF OPIOID TREATMENT FOR CHRONIC NOCICEPTIVE PAIN

A typical example is an elderly lady with osteoarthritis. Her sleep is severely disturbed by pain at night and she is immobilized by pain which is exacerbated by walking. She cannot tolerate major surgery and joint replacement is unavailable for socioeconomic reasons. Paracetamol (acetaminophen) is barely effective, nonsteroidal anti-inflammatory drugs (NSAIDs) and cyclooxygenase-2 (COX-2)-specific inhibitors cause unacceptable adverse gastrointestinal and renal effects. Other nonopioid analgesics, such as metamizole (dypyrone) or nefopam, are not available. Most physicians would consider it highly appropriate to prescribe an opioid analgesic to this patient.

- Treatment goals: improving quality of sleep and mobility; these are obtainable with opioids added to paracetamol with an acceptable risk of adverse effects.
- Opioid drug and dosing should be tailored to her pain profile. One of the so-called "weak opioids" may suffice, but neither codeine nor tramadol have an optimal adverse/benefit profile for this patient. Thus, a low starting dose of a controlled-release, 10–12 hours, pure µ-opioid agonist, taken once or twice daily, will be a better choice. If compliance with oral opioid is difficult in this elderly lady, the seven days buprenorphine 5 µg per hour patch, or a three days fentanyl 12 µg per hour patch may be the best option.
- Monitoring of effects and side effects: besides assuring that meaningful pain relief is maintained, it is extremely important in this patient to focus on sedative and cognitive side effects in the initial phase of treatment.

Sedation and cognitive changes are initially opioid dose-dependent. With a carefully adjusted dose, they should not be major problems unless comedications with sedatives, anxiolytics, antidepressants, or alcohol occur. All of these drugs synergistically potentiate the sedative effects of opioids, may cause confusion, or result in falls and fractures in a frail osteoporotic elderly lady.

Preventing opioid-induced gastrointestinal dysfunction is important. Appropriate emphasis should be placed on intake of nutritional fiber, stool softener, and a laxative as needed to obtain at least three bowel movements a week with normal fecal consistency. When peripherally acting opioid antagonists become available, patients like this one will benefit from coadministration of such drugs.

CHRONIC NEUROPATHIC PAIN

Patients suffering from chronic noncancer pain often have a component of neuropathic pain due to peripheral or central nervous system pathological mechanisms. Abnormal painful sensations provoked by innocuous stimuli and spontaneous pain from dysfunctional nervous tissues result in unpleasant, painful experiences.[31] A number of nonopioid drugs can modify these abnormal pain mechanisms and to some degree reduce suffering.[32] It is appropriate to prescribe an opioid for patients suffering from chronic nonnociceptive pain, when the first-line drugs and other measures fail to relieve the suffering and burden of neuropathic pain.[1, 32] The dose needed may sometimes be higher than for nociceptive pain. Otherwise the general principles described above must be adhered to.[1, 32]

CHRONIC BACK PAIN

A systematic review of 38 studies with reasonable quality concerning opioid treatment for chronic back pain was published in 2007.[38] Prevalence of opioid treatment for chronic back pain varied from 3 to 66 percent, higher in patients with reduced functional capacity. In 15 studies, opioid treatment was compared to placebo or other active treatments for up to 16 weeks. The treatment effects of opioids were marginal compared with placebo or control therapy. Problematic prescription opioid use, or what the authors considered to be "addiction," varied from 3 to 43 percent. Clearly, this commonly occurring musculoskeletal pain condition, complicated by components of neuropathic pain and psychosocial comorbidities, is a typical persistent or recurring pain condition where primary care physicians and specialists are faced with the dilemma of adding an opioid analgesic. My advice is to comply with the general principles described above under Guidelines for treatment of chronic nonterminal (nonmalignant) pain with opioids.

COMPLEX CHRONIC PAIN CONDITIONS COMPLICATED BY FAILED OPIOID THERAPY

These patients present at pain clinics with poor analgesic effect of opioid therapy, and adverse effects of long-term opioid therapy is aggravating their original pain problem.[33] They often present with behaviors indicating problematic opioid use and poor management of their opioid therapy (**Box 10.4**). They can often be helped to better effect and better control of their opioid therapy by the resources of a pain center.[41]

> ### Box 10.4 Behaviors usually indicating problematic opioid use (and suboptimal opioid regime) rather than true addiction
>
> - Aggressive complaining about the need for more drug (the patient may be right: tolerance is developing).
> - Drug hoarding during periods of reduced symptoms (makes sense).
> - The patient requests specific drug(s) (the patient may be right: all opioids are not alike; opioid receptors vary from person to person).
> - Openly acquiring similar drugs from other medical sources (a reasonable consequence?)
> - Admitting unsanctioned dose escalation on one or two occasions (patient hoping for better pain relief).[11, 12, 40]

When the patients present with behaviors that clearly indicate addictive behavior, but also with a real pain problem (**Box 10.5**), these patients will need the resources of a multidisciplinary pain center and addiction medicine specialists.[42] Rhodin and collaborators in Uppsala have demonstrated that even extremely problematic, truly addicted pain patients can be helped back to reasonable quality of life, even back to active working life, by a modified methadone treatment program.[42] Methadone is administered for pain as well as for control of addictive behavior.

CASE HISTORY ILLUSTRATING PROBLEMS FACING THE DOCTOR AND PATIENT DURING LONG-TERM OPIOID TREATMENT FOR NONMALIGNANT PAIN

A now middle-aged, former active student of political sciences and economics, now an unemployed single mother, suffered from psoriatic arthritis from the age of 12 years. Gradually, her joint pain increased, especially in the wrist joints, despite treatment with the customary regimens for arthritis. For analgesia, she took paracetamol (until low-grade hepatitis C was diagnosed, caused, most likely, by a complication from a blood transfusion after the birth of her child) and codeine or dextropropoxyphene until the age of 31 years, when she underwent surgery to her right wrist joint with a synovectomy. Her right wrist pain increased, however, and she had surgical arthrodesis six months later. Her pain did not improve and she underwent surgery four years after the first operation, when one nerve entrapped in scar tissue was released, leading to a transient improvement of the pain. By now, the patient had acquired an iatrogenic complex

---

Box 10.5 Behaviors that indicate development of true addiction in a patient on opioid for chronic pain

- Selling of prescription drugs.
- Stealing or "borrowing" drugs from others.
- Injecting oral formulations.
- Obtaining prescription drugs from nonmedical sources.
- Concurrent abuse of alcohol or illicit drugs.
- Multiple dose escalations or other noncompliance with therapy despite warnings.
- Multiple episodes of prescription "loss" and prescription forgery.
- Evidence of drug-related deterioration in the ability to function at work, in the family, or socially.
- Resistance to changes in therapy despite evidence of adverse physical and psychological effects.[11, 12]

---

regional pain syndrome in addition to her arthritis. For several years, she also had migraine and a gastrointestinal disorder with loose stools and abdominal cramps. This was aggravated by analgesic tablets, so she preferred the rectal administration of analgesics. Escalation of her opioid treatment started after the first operation, with occasional ketobemidone suppositories as rescue analgesia during periods of severe pain. From the age of 33 years, she was evaluated and treated at the pain clinic at a university hospital. She had little or no benefit from sympathetic blocks, amitriptyline, and clonazepam. She was maintained on pentazocine suppositories, which gave adequate pain relief for about three years. Gradually, the opioid was escalated to ketobemidone suppositories three to five times daily. From the age of 37 years, she was on an average dose of ketobemidone 5 mg four times daily, with two extra doses allowed every day for breakthrough pain. (Ketobemidone is equipotent with morphine.) The patient moved to a smaller town in another part of the country. In this town, it was impossible for the patient to find a doctor who was willing to continue opioid prescription. The local health authorities accused her of being addicted to opioids and only offered her withdrawal treatment. An Enforcement Court rule made it possible for her to maintain contact with her former primary care physician, who continued to prescribe opioids. This was a difficult arrangement because of the distance. She was allowed to consult him four times a year. However, this arrangement became too difficult for everybody when the patient developed breakthrough pain and aggressive pseudoaddiction behavior. It was only after two years that a doctor in the local town was willing to assume opioid prescription responsibility for the patient. However, the

patient had increasing difficulties with the child care authorities, who had received anonymous accusations of irresponsible care of her child due to opioid usage. The social circumstances in this town became impossible and she moved to the nearby community where she had grown up as a child and settled in the house in which her now ailing parents had lived until a few years previously. In this community, the district general practitioner had the knowledge and experience to take on the responsibility for managing her opioid treatment. He was able to establish a treatment regime based on a mutually trustful relationship which has been very successful for the patient. She has been able to decrease her opioid drug usage, functions socially, and is able to care well for her child. She has confidence in her primary care physician and the previous, quite dramatic, episodes of breakthrough pain with aggressive pseudoaddiction behavior disappeared.

Comments

This patient illustrates that chronic noncancer pain can be treated with potent opioids for prolonged periods. The case also illustrates well how demanding this type of treatment is for the patient and the doctors involved. Pseudoaddiction can rapidly escalate into a major problem with a vicious circle of mistrust and accusations. This develops more easily when the doctor and patient do not know each other well, and the relationship can become very difficult when the patient is unwilling to accept the treating physician's diagnosis of problematic prescription opioid use. Although the guidelines for chronic opioid treatment of noncancer pain are fairly straightforward, in practice they can be quite demanding and many doctors and pain clinicians have been taken by surprise by the many unexpected difficulties that develop. Understanding and being prepared to tackle pseudoaddiction behavior makes this task easier. Clearly, multidisciplinary pain clinic expertise and resources are needed to help primary care physicians manage such challenging patients.

CONCLUSIONS

Opioid analgesics are the most effective drugs relieving severe acute and terminal pain. Long-term use of opioids can reduce the burden of suffering from chronic non-terminal pain, but adverse effects often reduce the beneficial effects. The evidence base for long-term benefits and safety is weak. Adverse effects of long-term opioid treatment include gastrointestinal, endocrinological, and cognitive dysfunctions, development of tolerance, hyperalgesia, pseudoaddiction behavior, the chronic neurobiological disease of addiction with compulsive use in spite of obvious deleterious effects of continued opioid use. Guidelines and recommendations for best practice of opioid use for chronic nonterminal pain are based mostly on experts' opinions. Steady-state regimes (stable dose of controlled-release oral or transdermal delivery) are considered to have the best benefit/risk ratio. Intermittent-use regimes (dose as needed) are recommended by some experts in selected patients with pain-free periods, recurrent pain, and low risk of problematic use. Whatever regime is chosen, long-term opioid therapy demands a major effort by physicians and patients to optimize benefits and reduce risks of serious adverse effects.[43]

REFERENCES

* 1. Kalso E, Edwards J, Moore R, McQuay H. Opioids in chronic non-cancer pain: systematic review of efficacy and safety. *Pain.* 2004; **112**: 372–80.

2. Daniell HW. Hypogonadism in men consuming sustained-action oral opioids. *Journal of Pain.* 2002; **3**: 377–84.

3. Page GG. Immunologic effects of opioids in the presence or absence of pain. *Journal of Pain and Symptom Management.* 2005; **29**: S25–31.

* 4. Ballantyne JC. LaForge KSOpioid dependence and addiction during opioid treatment of chronic pain. *Pain.* 2007, **129**. 235–55.

5. Fields HL. Should we be reluctant to prescribe opioids for chronic non-malignant pain? *Pain.* 2007; **129**: 233–4.

6. Pletcher MJ, Kertesz SG, Sidney S *et al.* Incidence and antecedents of nonmedical prescription opioid use in four US communities. The Coronary Artery Risk Development in Young Adults (CARDIA) prospective cohort study. *Drug and Alcohol Dependence.* 2006; **85**: 171–6.

7. Edlund MJ, Steffick D, Hudson T *et al.* Risk factors for clinically recognized opioid abuse and dependence among veterans using opioids for chronic non-cancer pain. *Pain.* 2007; **129**: 355–62.

* 8. Balandyne JC. Opioid analgesia: perspectives on right use and utility. *Pain Physician.* 2007; **10**: 479–1.

9. Gramstad L, Haugtomt H, Breivik H. Use of opioids in chronic non-cancer pain – current status in Norway. In: Kalso E, Paakari P, Stenberg I (eds). *Opioids in chronic non-cancer pain. Situation and guidelines in the Nordic countries.* Helsinki: National Agency for Medicines, 1999: 49.

10. Portenoy RK, Farrar JT, Backonja MM *et al.* Long-term use of controlled release oxycodone for noncancer pain: results of a 3-year registry study. *Clinical Journal of Pain.* 2007; **23**: 287–99.

11. Savage SR. Long-term opioid therapy: assessment of consequences and risks. *Journal of Pain and Symptom Management.* 1996; **11**: 274–86.

12. Savage SR. Opioid therapy of chronic pain: assessment of consequences. *Acta Anaesthesiologica Scandinavica.* 1999; **43**: 909–17.

13. Caldwell JR, Hale ME, Boyd RE *et al.* Treatment of osteoarthritis pain with controlled release oxycodone or fixed combination oxycodone plus acetaminophen added to nonsteroidal antiinflammatory drugs: a double blind, randomized, multicenter, placebo controlled trial. *Journal of Rheumatology.* 1999; **26**: 862–9.

14. Moulin DE, Iezzi A, Amireh R *et al.* Randomised trial of oral morphine for chronic non-cancer pain. *Lancet.* 1996; **347**: 143–7.

15. McQuay H. Opioid use in chronic pain. *Acta Anaesthesiologica Scandinavica.* 1997; **41**: 175–83.

* 16. Ballantyne J, Mao J. Opioid therapy for chronic pain. *New England Journal of Medicine.* 2003; **349**: 1943–53.

17. Breivik H. Appropriate and responsible use of opioids in chronic non-cancer pain. *European Journal of Pain.* 2003; **7**: 379–80.

* 18. Scholten W, Nygren-Krug H, Zucker HA. The World Health Organization paves the way for action to free people from the shackles of pain. *Anesthesia and Analgesia.* 2007; **105**: 1–4.

19. Breivik H, Bond M. Why pain control matters in a world full of killer diseases: Pain – a silent dimension of the global top 10 diseases. *Pain: Clinical Updates.* 2004; **12**: 4.

* 20. Bond M, Breivik H, Jensen TS *et al.* Pain associated with neurological disorders. In: Aarli JA, Avanzini G, Bertolote JM *et al.* (eds). *Neurological disorders: public health challenges.* Geneva: World Health Organization, 2006: 127–39.

21. Dellemijn P, van Duijn H, Vanneste J. Prolonged treatment with transdermal fentanyl in neuropathic pain. *Journal of Pain and Symptom Management.* 1998; **16**: 220–9.

* 22. Kalso E, Allan L, Dellemijn PLI *et al.* Recommendations for using opioids in chronin non-cancer pain. In: Breivik H, Shipley M (eds). *Pain – Best practice and research compendium.* London: Elsevier, 2007: 323–8.

* 23. Federation of State Medical Boards of the United States. Model guidelines for the use of controlled substances for the treatment of pain. Last updated May 2004, cited February 2008. Available from: www.fsmb.org/pdf/2004_grpol_Controlled_Substances.pdf.

* 24. Canadian Pain Society. Use of opioid analgesics for the treatment of chronic noncancer pain – a consensus statement and guidelines from the Canadian Pain Society. *Pain Research and Management.* 1998; **3**: 197–208.

* 25. The Pain Society. Recommendations for the appropriate use of opioids in persistent non-cancer pain. Last updated March 2004, cited February 2008. Available from: www.britishpainsociety.org/pub_professional.htm#opioids.

* 26. Kalso E, Paakari P, Stenberg I (eds). *Opioids in chronic non-cancer pain. situation and guidelines in the Nordic countries.* Helsinki: National Agency for Medicines, 1999: 31–7.

27. Kreek MJ, Nielsen DA, La Forge KS. Genes associated with addiction: alcoholism, opiate, and cocaine addiction. *Neuromolecular Medicine.* 2004; **5**: 85–108.

28. Portenoy R. Appropriate use of opioids for persistent non-cancer pain. *Lancet.* 2004; **364**: 739–40.

∗ 29. Portenoy RK, Foley KM. Chronic use of opioid analgesics in non-malignant pain: report of 38 cases. *Pain.* 1986; **25**: 171–86.

30. Arnér S, Meyerson BA. Lack of analgesic effect of opioids on neuropathic and idiopathic forms of pain. *Pain.* 1988; **33**: 11–23.

31. Woolf CJ, Mannion RJ. Neuropathic pain: aetiology, symptoms, mechanisms, and management. *Lancet.* 1999; **353**: 1959–64.

∗ 32. Dworkin RH, O'Connor AB, Backonja M *et al.* Pharmacologic management of neuropathic pain: evidence-based recommendations. *Pain.* 2007; **132**: 237–51.

∗ 33. Højsted J, Sjøgren P. Addiction to opioids in chronic pain patients: a literature review. *European Journal of Pain.* 2007; **11**: 490–518.

34. Belgrade MJ, Schamber CD, Lindgren BR. The DIRE score: predicting outcomes of opioid prescribing for chronic pain. *Journal of Pain.* 2006; **7**: 671–81.

35. Rich BA. Ethics of opioid analgesia for chronic noncancer pain. *Pain: Clinical Updates.* 2007; **15**: 9.

36. Dunbar SA, Katz NP. Chronic opioid therapy for non-malignant pain in patients with a history of substance abuse: report of 20 cases. *Journal of Pain and Symptom Management.* 1996; **11**: 163–71.

∗ 37. Savage S, Covington E, Ehit H *et al. Definitions related to the use of opioids for the treatment of pain. A consensus document from the American Academy of Pain Medicine, The American Pain Society and the American Society of Addiction Medicine.* Glenview, IL: American Pain Society, 2001.

∗ 38. Martell BA, O'Connor PG, Kerns RD *et al.* Systematic review: opioid treatment for chronic back pain: prevalence, efficacy, and associations with addiction. *Annals of Internal Medicine.* 2007; **146**: 116–27.

39. Weissman DE, Haddox JD. Opioid pseudoaddiction – an iatrogenic syndrome. *Pain.* 1989; **36**: 363–6.

40. Chabal C, Erjavec M, Jacobson L *et al.* Prescription opiate abuse in chronic pain patients: clinical criteria, incidence and predictors. *Clinical Journal of Pain.* 1997; **13**: 150–5.

∗ 41. Becker N, Sjøgren P, Bech P *et al.* Treatment outcome of chronic nonmalignant pain patients managed in a Danish multidisciplinary pain centre compared to general practice: a randomized controlled trial. *Pain.* 2000; **84**: 203–11.

∗ 42. Rhodin A, Grönbladh L, Nilsson L-H, Gordh T. Methadone treatment of chronic non-malginanat pain and opioid dependence – A long-term follow-up. *European Journal of Pain.* 2006; **10**: 271–8.

43. Noble M, Tregear SJ, Treadwell JR, Schoelles K. Long-term opioid therapy for chronic noncancer pain: A systematic review and meta-analysis of efficacy and safety. *Journal of Pain and Symptom Management.* 2008; **35**: 214–28.

11

Subcutaneous drug infusion protocols for the control of cancer pain

HUMAIRA JAMAL AND IVAN F TROTMAN

KEY LEARNING POINTS

- Continuous subcutaneous infusions (CSCI) are accepted best practice for the management of cancer pain when other routes are not possible or desirable.
- The subcutaneous route can be used for the control of symptoms other than pain.
- Opioids are the main analgesics given by CSCI.
- The choice of opioids is dictated by availability, volumes, and comorbidities, such as renal and hepatic failure.

- Adverse effects are common but preventable.
- Naloxone is used to reverse opioid toxicity.
- Drug compatibilities are available on the internet and published in books.
- Local agreed syringe driver operational standards should be in place with cyclical audits and critical incident reporting to ensure good clinical governance.

INTRODUCTION

Continuous subcutaneous infusions (CSCI) are widely used for the control of pain in patients with cancer, particularly in the later stages of their illness. They have an important role in the terminal phase where drug administration by other routes is unreliable.[1, 2, 3, 4] The main indications for their use are summarized in **Box 11.1**.

Subcutaneous infusions are usually delivered by means of a mechanical syringe driver. Drug infusions by

Box 11.1 Indications for continuous subcutaneous infusion

- Unconsciousness
- Terminal care
- Vomiting
- Intestinal obstruction
- Dysphagia
- Unreliable absorption by other routes
- Pain control
- Non-compliance
- Use of specific drugs
- Patient preference

this technique have also been found useful to alleviate a number of other symptoms in patients with agitation, vomiting, and intestinal obstruction and dry secretions.[5] The use of CSCI requires a number of assumptions.

- That the physicochemical and pharmacological properties of drugs (either singly or in combination) are suitable for administration by this route.
- That the drug remains stable in solution for the duration of infusion.
- That absorption from the subcutaneous tissues is reliable and constant.

The subcutaneous route is preferred because of the following.

- **Ease of access.** Subcutaneous infusions can be administered at a wide variety of sites over the body surface. They are not dependent on finding a suitable vein and the patient does not have to be moved or turned or have their movement restricted in any way.
- **Safety.** There are fewer complications than with intramuscular or intravenous injections. Nursing staff require few special skills or experience. The infusion can be easily resited in the event of displacement without the need for specialist facilities or staff.
- **Less pain and discomfort for the patient**, particularly if repeated injections are needed. Portable devices allow the patient to remain ambulant and to be managed in the community that is rarely possible using intravenous access. Moreover, the infusion pump (syringe driver) can be concealed beneath the bed covers or in a carrying pouch causing less distraction and anxiety for the patient and family.

INDICATIONS FOR USE OF SUBCUTANEOUS INFUSIONS

The principle indications for subcutaneous infusions by syringe driver are summarized in **Box 11.1**. For the management of pain, the principle indications are:

- vomiting;
- unreliable absorption (e.g. intestinal obstruction);
- variable consciousness or dysphoria;
- uncontrolled pain;
- use of specific drugs (e.g. ketorolac, ketamine).

Commonly, syringe drivers are used to manage symptoms in patients who are dying where periods of wakefulness lessen and oral medication can no longer be taken reliably. During this time, it is generally considered important that the patient continues to receive prescribed analgesia and the only way to administer this is parenterally. The argument against the routine use of syringe drivers in this situation is that not all patients require injectable analgesia and that possibly the requirement for strong (opioid) painkillers lessens during the dying process because of multiorgan failure.

For the patient who is vomiting and in pain, a syringe driver provides a tool for dual management of symptoms with combinations of analgesic and antiemetic drugs. Continuous administration of drugs by this route diminishes the need for, and discomfort of, intermittent injections. In uncontrolled pain, the use of a syringe driver is preferred to the use of "as-required" injections for pain not only for comfort, but also to reduce the risk of tolerance and rapidly escalating opioid dose.[6]

CONTRAINDICATIONS

There are no absolute contraindications to the use of a subcutaneous infusion and it is possible to administer very large volumes by this route. Severe clotting abnormalities, particularly a depressed platelet count, predispose to the risk of hemorrhage at the injection site. Occasionally, severe skin disease makes needle placement difficult and subcutaneous needles should not be positioned into lymphedematous skin or into active tumor sites. Similarly, needles should not be inserted into skin that has been irradiated and the insertion site should be away from joints.

Phobic anxiety states may preclude the effective use of a syringe driver and patients with florid psychotic disturbance will often not tolerate their use until adequate sedation has been achieved or the cause of the mental disturbance treated.

The use of subcutaneous infusions by syringe driver requires appropriate consent from the patient.

USE OF SYRINGE DRIVERS

Syringe drivers are the most popular means to administer subcutaneous infusions.[7] They are precision instruments that are calibrated to travel a fixed distance in a given time. The volume administered to a patient will vary according to the size of syringe fitted to the driver and the dose of drug will depend upon its concentration within the syringe. There is potential for confusion in translating a prescription for a drug dose in milligrams to a driver speed in millimeters.

There are several commercially available syringe drivers and the choice of driver will often depend upon local availability and cost. Portable battery-driven units have gained widest acceptance for the management of pain in patients with cancer. In the UK, the most widely used syringe drivers are the Graseby models MS16(a) and MS26. When drugs need to be administered in a large volume of diluent, a mains-operated device may be preferred as most portable syringe-drivers will only accommodate a 35-mL syringe containing 25 mL fluid.

Portable syringe drivers enable the patient to be ambulant and can be easily transferred between hospital and community settings. The main disadvantages are that they are not fitted with malfunction alarms to warn if the device is inoperative, battery power is low, driver overspeeding, or inadvertent catheter disconnection. They do not allow significant bolus administration for breakthrough pain.

Most syringe drivers allow the rate of administration of drug to be varied. Devices which permit the patient to administer bolus doses of analgesia (patient-controlled analgesia (PCA)) have not gained wide acceptance in control of cancer pain. Potentially, the use of PCA might allow rapid titration to stable doses in opioid-naive subjects or when changing from one opioid to another when conversion factors are uncertain (e.g. morphine to fentanyl). However, the effective use of PCA requires intravenous access. Fixed rate infusions may be preferred because of the following.

- Presetting the syringe driver reduces the opportunity for error when users vary the rate during the course of an infusion.
- It enables better planning of nursing care as the syringe driver will need replenishment at a predictable time.
- It is common practice to include more than one drug in a CSCI.

STARTING A SUBCUTANEOUS INFUSION

The procedure for starting a subcutaneous infusion will be determined by local policy and procedure and influenced by the availability of drugs and equipment. The decision to administer drugs by this route will be a clinical decision made by the medical team caring for the patient in discussion with the patient and family. A careful explanation at this time is important. Patients are often frightened about the use of syringe drivers and for many it will be perceived as something that is done before death.

In all cases, setting up the infusion device (usually a portable syringe driver) should follow the manufacturer's instructions. There are some important points to observe.

Prescribing

Prescriptions should be unambiguous, legible, specify the drugs to be used, their doses, the diluent, and the duration over which they are to be infused. Standard prescription sheets may be used, although for clarity and because the dose or combination of drugs may be changed, a purpose-designed prescription sheet might be preferred. The practitioner will need to comply with national legislation and local policies for prescription of controlled drugs.

Unless there are reasons to do otherwise, it is recommended that the doses be written in milligrams per 24 hours and that the infusion pump be set to run for this time.

Priming and siting

Drugs need to be drawn up and mixed in a volume appropriate to the syringe device to be used. When preparing a subcutaneous infusion, it is important to make allowances for the additional volume needed to fill the connection catheter – in some cases this may be as much as 2 mL. This needs to be taken into account when calculating the time that the syringe will need to be replenished. Tubing should be connected using luer-locking devices.

Needles can be sited in almost any part of the body, but most convenient sites include upper chest (above the breasts), outer upper arms or thighs, the abdomen, and sometimes over the shoulders. The injection site should be covered with a transparent dressing. Once sited, ensure equipment is functioning properly and record the time the infusion starts.

Monitoring

Monitoring a subcutaneous infusion is essential. There are four main objectives:

1. to ensure the infusion delivers drugs as prescribed;
2. to monitor pain and symptom control;
3. to inspect the injection site;
4. to check for adverse events and toxicity.

Simple checklists can be used to ensure that an infusion is progressing in a satisfactory manner. These can be adapted to the clinical circumstances and frequency of observations will depend on the availability of staff and the environment in which the patient receives care. In a specialist unit, observations every four hours might be expected, while in the community setting these are inevitably less frequent. It is unnecessary and often inappropriate to perform a full profile of clinical measurements. Careful bedside observation is usually sufficient. Printed charts allow standardization of observation, act as an aide-memoir, and are useful for audit. Important items to record include:

- volume remaining in syringe (this not only provides a check that the infusion rate is as expected, but also provides an estimate of when it will need to be replenished);
- infusion device operating, connections are intact and not leaking;
- inspection of the injection site.

Simultaneously, a brief clinical assessment of the patient will include:

- level of consciousness/sedation;
- pulse and respiration;
- peripheral circulation, color, sweating;
- spontaneous movement or twitching;
- grimacing/moaning.

Monitoring pain control can be done using standard pain-assessment tools. If the patient is awake and co-operative, a simple visual analog scale (VAS), a 0–10 numeric rating scale (NRS), or a four-point verbal categorical rating scores are most commonly used. If the patient is obtunded or unconscious, pain rating has to be done by proxy, usually by the attending nurse and using visible nonverbal indicators of pain, for example, an estimate on a 0–10 NRS scale.

COMPLICATIONS

Complications with the use of subcutaneous infusions are uncommon. They can be considered under the following headings:

- equipment malfunction;
- reactions at injection site;
- drug reactions;
- prescribing errors.

Equipment malfunction

Modern infusion systems using syringe drivers are reliable and technical failure is unusual. Typical problems include:

- low power/battery failure;
- failure to recognize when syringe is fully discharged;

- disconnection of delivery tubing;
- tube blockage;
- syringe displacement in the driver;
- cracked or leaking syringe;
- driver overspeed;
- backlash – delay in infusion because the plunger on the syringe is not closely opposed to the driver mechanism at start up.

In each situation, the cause is usually obvious and remedied by appropriate action. Syringe drivers that malfunction should be inspected by an engineer and reapproved before further use. Many problems can be avoided by having local policies and procedures for use of syringe drivers.

Reactions at injection site

Minor reactions at the injection site are frequent and do not usually require intervention other than regular monitoring (Pickard, personal communication, 2004).[8] On the other hand, reactions at the injection site are the most common reason for having to resite the infusion. Reactions can vary from minor erythema to florid inflammatory lesions with abscess formation. With severe drug incompatibility, frank necrosis at the injection site may occur. The following should be considered when reactions are severe or frequent.

- Some drugs are reported to cause more frequent reactions (cyclizine, diclofenac, ketamine, and methadone).
- The risk of reactions is increased when drugs are mixed together.
- Is the correct diluent being used?
- Is there an allergic response to the drug or metal needle?
- Infection should be considered in the event of reaction.
- Host factors, such as severe clotting abnormalities, liver failure, renal failure, and immunosuppression, may increase the likelihood of reactions.

Management of reactions will depend on severity. The infusion must be resited if the reaction is severe. Simple dressings are usually all that is required, but sometimes topical or systemic steroids, antibiotics, and surgical drainage or debridement are necessary. In all severe reactions the cause should be sought and consideration given to:

- changing the drug or diluent;
- diluting the infusion;
- using single drug infusions;
- changing to a cannula made of plastic or Teflon, rather than metal;

- adding low doses of corticosteroid to the infusion (e.g. dexamethasone 1 mg);
- using an alternative route of administration;
- ensuring an aseptic technique when preparing and dispensing an infusion.

Drug reactions

Drug reactions may occur in the infusion apparatus, at the injection site, or in the body. Systemic drug reactions are no more or less common when the drug is given by subcutaneous infusion. However, there are some special circumstances, which may lead to under- or overdosing. When opioids are infused, there is a potential for narcosis in the following situations, despite there being no apparent change in the prescribed amount of drug.

- The bioavailability of a drug may be altered when two or more are mixed together. If a change is made from one combination to another, or a decision made to administer drugs singly, the opioid may become more (or less) active.
- Factors used to calculate the dose of opioid when converting from oral to subcutaneous infusion, or from one opioid to another, are only approximate with large inter- and intrasubject variation. If a subcutaneous infusion is commenced because of vomiting or intestinal obstruction, inadvertent excess may be given because the patient had not been absorbing the prescribed opioid previously given by mouth.
- At very high doses, it is unwise to apply the usual conversion factors when changing from one opioid to another as the second given opioid is likely to appear more effective. This observation has been used to advantage when opioid responsiveness is lost or adverse effects occur and has led to the concept of "opioid rotation."
- Other concomitant pain interventions may reduce the opioid requirement. Large reductions in opioid dose are sometimes needed if ketorolac or ketamine are added.
- The rate of absorption from the subcutaneous tissues may be enhanced if the patient is febrile, topical heat applied, or the ambient temperature is high. Conversely, hypotensive patients with poor peripheral circulation may receive inadequate doses of analgesia.

Management of adverse events requires identification and withdrawal of the suspected drug. Regular inspection of the infusion will detect clouding or crystallization and new solutions prepared should this happen. The clinician needs to watch for the unexpected emergence of opioid toxicity and be prepared to adjust the dose accordingly. In practice, serious opioid toxicity with subcutaneous infusions is uncommon and more likely to occur in opioid-naïve subjects or in those for whom a concomitant pain intervention is successful and the opioid dose left unchanged.

Prescribing errors

Prescribing errors can put the patient at serious risk, are a cause of great anxiety to the clinical team, can destroy confidence, and may lead to subsequent litigation. They are nearly always avoidable. Errors can occur in writing and reading a prescription, dispensing and preparing a drug, identifying the recipient, and monitoring drug administration. Although the use of subcutaneous infusion involves simple techniques, there are some important sources of error.

- The volume needed to dilute the drugs and the volume of syringe available for infusion have to be calculated.
- It may not be possible to use a full syringe because the jaws of the syringe driver will not open wide enough.
- Whether an adjustment is to be made for the capacity of the connection tubing.
- The rate of the infusion is typically measured in distance (mm) travelled along the barrel of the syringe, not the volume.
- The rate at which the driver operates may be expressed in different units of distance and time from one driver to the next.
- If the dose prescribed is altered, a completely new solution must be prepared with a new syringe.

Elimination of prescribing error is an important part of risk management for all clinicians and organizations engaged in patient care. The following are suggestions to help achieve this:

- clinicians to be fully conversant with a range of locally available drugs;
- access to specialist services;
- standardization of equipment across clinical areas;
- published protocols and guidelines for the use of subcutaneous infusions;
- documented procedures for setting up infusions and delivery systems;
- record keeping, ensuring standardization of prescription and monitoring of infusion;
- regular servicing and calibration of equipment;
- quality control and audit;
- education and training.

CHOICE OF ANALGESIC

Cancer pain is complex. It may arise directly from the tumor, from secondary deposits, or result from treatment. Pain in multiple sites is common and is often difficult to classify. Pain may have several different components (somatic, visceral, or neuropathic) and these may vary with time. It has been estimated that 60 percent or more patients will be prescribed morphine or other strong opioids during the course of their illness.[9] It must be remembered that not all patients with cancer experience pain and that opioids may be used for other indications, such as breathlessness or to relieve anxiety and distress. Cancer pain can rarely be managed by drug therapy alone and even the most skilfully crafted prescription will be ineffective if no attention is paid to the other physical, emotional, and psychological aspects of a patient's care.

The choice of analgesic and dose for use by subcutaneous infusion is influenced by several factors:

- previous analgesic requirement and opioid use;
- availability of drug;
- type of pain;
- evidence of renal or hepatic impairment.

USE OF OPIOIDS

Continuous subcutaneous infusions of opioids are routinely used to manage cancer pain. Morphine remains the strong opioid of choice worldwide for cancer pain management (**Figure 11.1**). Buprenorphine is an example of a moderately strong opioid that can be administered via the subcutaneous route. Alternative strong opioids can be used if morphine is not available or not tolerated. Adverse effects may occur in up to 20 percent of patients in a recently published survey.[10] Alternatives include diamorphine (mainly used in the UK), fentanyl, alfentanil, sufentanil, oxycodone, hydromorphone, and methadone. Analgesic actions of opioids may differ slightly and this relates to differences in affinities for the three main opioid receptor subtypes (mu, kappa, and delta) and to the production of active metabolites. Genetically determined variations in subtypes of opioid receptors cause large interindividual differences to pain-relieving effects of opioids.[11]

Morphine is well absorbed after s.c. injection and is metabolized in the liver to morphine-3-glucuronide (M3G) and morphine-6-glucuronide (M6G).[12] M6G is thought to be pharmacologically active and more potent at the mu-opioid receptor. Both M3G and M6G are renally excreted. Accumulation of M6G in renal failure is implicated as the cause of undesirable effects, such as nausea, vomiting, drowsiness, and respiratory depression.[13, 14] Other effects such as hyperalgesia, myoclonus, and agitation have been attributed to M3G in animal models.[1, 15, 16]

Alternative opioids to morphine should be considered in the following circumstances:

- the pain is opioid responsive;
- there are unacceptable side effects – nausea, vomiting, constipation, respiratory depression, drowsiness, or agitation;
- there is significant renal or liver impairment.

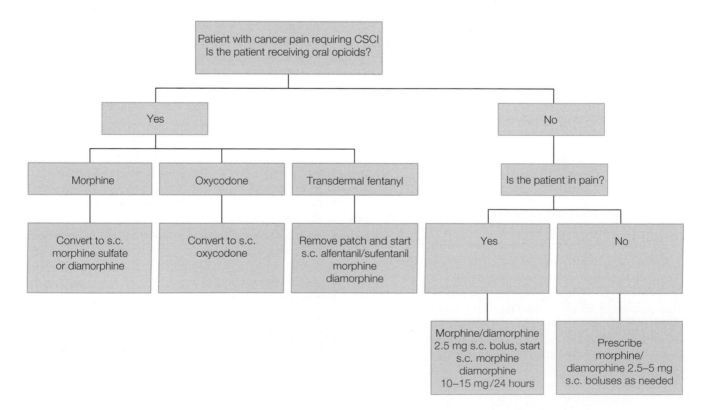

Figure 11.1 Algorithm for choice of opioid when starting continuous subcutaneous infusions (CSCI).

The most commonly used alternatives to morphine used in CSCI are listed below:

- alfentanil (particularly in the setting of renal failure);
- diamorphine (UK only);
- oxycodone (dose reduction required in severe renal failure);
- fentanyl (large volumes limit use in CSCI);
- methadone (to be initiated only with specialist supervision, relatively safe in renal and liver failure);
- hydromorphone (recommended in patients who cannot tolerate morphine, especially if diamorphine and alfentanil are not available, requires small volumes).

PRESCRIBING OPIOIDS

Often patients needing CSCI for cancer pain will be on oral morphine. Converting from the oral to the subcutaneous route, e.g. from morphine sulfate tablets (MST) to morphine, is a common clinical situation and generally this conversion is made by halving the oral dose – i.e. using a 2:1 ratio. There is variation in practice, particularly when switching between opioids, and a guide to conversion ratios is given in **Table 11.1**. It is important to remember that all conversion ratios are approximate and need to take account of interpatient variation and incomplete cross-tolerance between different opioids.

When starting a CSCI, the following points should be considered.

- Is the pain controlled on the current opioid?
- Is there a suitable parenteral preparation available?
- When changing from oral to CSCI, a rule of thumb is to use a 2:1 ratio.
- Initial dose conversion should be conservative – it is better to underestimate the dose for CSCI and make available rescue medication than potentially expose the patient to risk of becoming opioid toxic.
- Rescue doses at one-sixth of the total daily dose of opioid should be prescribed.
- Anticipatory prescribing for predictable side effects should be considered, especially laxatives for constipation and antiemetics for sickness.

OPIOID TITRATION

Regular review is required once a CSCI with opioid is commenced. If the pain is not controlled or if there is a need for frequent breakthrough doses (more than two doses per 24 hours) the total daily dose will need to be

Table 11.1 Approximate opioid equivalence for subcutaneous infusion.

Opioid	Concentration	Morphine: drug equivalence	Dose range	Evidence	Notes
Morphine sulfate	10, 15, 20, 30 mg/mL	1	No upper limit	II	Dose reduction advised in renal failure
Morphine tartrate	120 mg/mL				
Diamorphine HCl	<250 mg/mL	1:0.5	No upper limit	II	Dose reduction advised in renal failure
Fentanyl	100 µg/2 mL	1:0.01	25–50 µg/hour	III	Hepatic excretion
Alfentanil	1 mg/2 mL	1:0.25	0.5–1.0 mg/24 hours		
Sufentanil	50 µg/mL		No upper limit		Sufentanil is seven times more potent than fentanyl
Methadone HCl	10 mg/mL	1:0.25–1	No upper limit. Use only if on oral methadone initially	III	Specialist palliative care use only. No dose adjustment necessary in renal and liver failure
Hydromorphone HCl	10, 20, 50 mg/mL	1:0.2	Range 1–35 mg/hour. No maximum dose	II	Used if small volumes are required
Oxycodone	10 mg/mL, 20 mg/mL	1:0.6–1	No upper limit. Starting dose for opioid-naive patients 5–10 mg/24 hours	III	Dose reduction advised in liver and renal failure
Buprenorphine	Transdermal 35–140 µg/ hour patches	1:0.1–0.2	1600 µg/24hours		

increased. The infusion can be increased by 25–30 percent or more if necessary. Alternatively, the total amount used for breakthrough analgesia in the preceding 24 hours can be added to the CSCI driver. The aim is to have the patient pain free and mentally alert.

CHANGING OPIOIDS

Up to 30 percent of cancer patients with pain do not achieve satisfactory pain relief with morphine.[17] For these patients, changing from morphine to an alternative opioid often improves analgesia and reduces toxicity. For example, there is a clinical impression that fentanyl may give slightly less constipation while oxycodone may cause fewer hallucinations. Opioid switching is now established clinical practice. There are an increasing number of alternatives to morphine. Suggested, approximate equi-analgesic doses of opioids are shown in **Table 11.1**, but caution is advised in their interpretation.[18, 19]

OPIOID-NAIVE SUBJECTS

Occasionally, a subcutaneous infusion will be started in a patient in pain but who has not previously received opioid analgesia. The need for parenteral therapy may also indicate that the patient's clinical condition is deteriorating. Opioids should be started at very low doses, particularly in the elderly or those with renal impairment. Subsequently, an assessment of the total daily requirement can be made from the need for supplementary analgesia. It is very difficult to estimate the opioid requirements and frequent clinical review is needed both to ensure absence of toxicity and achievement of pain relief. It may be possible to advance the dose of opioid very quickly in some patients and for those in very severe pain, it is occasionally necessary to administer supplementary doses on an hourly basis.

OPIOID TOXICITY

Opioid toxicity can occur in a number of situations and can be considered in three distinct forms.

1. **Narcosis**: the classical form of opioid overdose with respiratory depression, hypotension, sedation, and small pupils. Apart from inadvertent overprescribing, it can occur in a number of special circumstances:
    a. when changing from one opioid to another;
    b. following a successful pain intervention (e.g. nerve block);
    c. following introduction of cotherapy;
    d. development of renal failure with opioids eliminated by this route (e.g. morphine).

2. **Unwanted effects**. These are predictable and may improve as tolerance develops. Sometimes they constitute an indication to stop or change the opioid. Such symptoms include:
    a. nausea and vomiting;
    b. sedation;
    c. sweating;
    d. bronchospasm;
    e. blurred vision.

3. **Adverse effects**, which arise unexpectedly and which may be profoundly disabling. In many cases, the emergence of opioid toxicity of this type requires a major revision of the treatment plan. These symptoms can be more distressing than those for which the opioid was prescribed. Adverse effects of this type are more common at very high opioid doses, where the dose has been increased very quickly and where the pain is poorly opioid responsive. They are more common in the elderly. Examples of toxic adverse effects include:
    a. cognitive dysfunction;
    b. excessive sedation;
    c. hallucinations;
    d. myoclonus;
    e. allodynia.

The management of opioid toxicity requires mature decision making and careful negotiation with the patient or, more usually, the family and carers. If a patient is dying, it is sometimes difficult to be certain that sedation or respiratory change is truly an opioid effect. Sedation, even to the point of unconsciousness, may be considered beneficial. A balance has to be achieved between reducing the opioid dose and compromising symptom control. The use of specific opioid antagonists is rarely needed, but should be considered in the event of prescribing error, narcosis after opioids are first started in naive subjects, or when vital signs are severely impaired.

Narcosis can usually be managed by temporary discontinuation of the opioid infusion and restarting it after a few hours at a lower dose rate. Unwanted effects require explanation and often a coprescription (e.g. an antiemetic). In the event of a severe adverse event a complete clinical reevaluation is mandatory. Other causes of symptoms should be sought looking specifically for hypercalcemia, renal failure, diabetes, and infection. Mental changes raise the possibility of cerebral metastases that can be excluded on clinical grounds or by scanning if appropriate. The treatment chart requires careful review, particularly to look for the number of supplementary doses of analgesic given or the use of concomitant therapy. Ultimately, the decision is whether to add treatments to counter the emergent problems, change the opioid, or explore alternative pain management techniques.

PREVENTION AND TREATMENT OF OPIOID-INDUCED BOWEL DYSFUNCTION

Opioids affect the gastrointestinal (GI) tract in a number of ways. They can stimulate the chemoreceptor trigger zone and increase vestibular sensitivity. Gastric stasis is due to direct action on the gut wall causing increased antral tone, reduced motility, and delayed gastric emptying. Gastrointestinal side effects of opioids show an inconsistent dose–response relationship. Nausea and vomiting may occur at the initiation of opioid therapy through both central and peripheral mechanisms. Patients should be warned of this and given anticipatory anti-emetic prescriptions, such as haloperidol 1.5 mg twice a day or metoclopramide 10 mg three times a day. Constipation is universal and needs prophylactic laxatives containing a combination of stimulant and softener. There is some evidence to suggest that the subcutaneous route is less likely to lead to adverse gastrointestinal side effects compared to the oral route.[20, 21]

OPIOID UNRESPONSIVENESS

Pain that fails to respond to opioids, at least to some degree, is uncommon and when present is likely to have been recognized before the decision to use a subcutaneous infusion is made. Even those pain types generally regarded as opioid unresponsive (e.g. central neuropathic pain after a stroke) are rarely completely so. However, higher doses are needed so that adverse effects limit the useful effects on such pains. Moreover, new pains frequently present themselves during the later course of an illness and regular clinical review is essential. In the event of a pain apparently not responding to the prescribed opioid:

- check that the patient is receiving the prescribed dose;
- evaluate the new pain;
- consider changing the opioid or adding another agent.

If a pain changes or a new pain emerges, a number of factors to consider are the following.

- Allodynia or cutaneous hypersensitivity may be induced by morphine and other potent opioids. Consider reducing the dose, changing the opioid or exploring other agents for neuropathic pain. Sometimes, single bolus infusions of lidocaine 100 mg intravenously may be effective.[22, 23]
- Bed-bound, semi-conscious patients may be in pain from lying in the same position for prolonged periods. Nursing measures, pressure-relieving mattresses, physiotherapy, or benzodiazepines may be helpful (the last of these for their muscle relaxant effect).
- Consider the appropriateness of adding another analgesic or using alternative pain management strategies. Weigh the patient's general condition and possible gain against the discomfort of other treatments, the lack of predictable benefit, and the risk of adverse events.
- Fear and anxiety exert powerful influences on the cognitive perception of pain. The psycho-spiritual needs of the patient must be taken into account in any pain management plan.
- Severe pain can arise from fractures, pressure sores, muscle spasms, cramps, constipation, and a distended bladder.

OPIOID PRESCRIBING IN RENAL FAILURE

The prevalence of end-stage renal failure is estimated to be 0.5 percent of the UK population and 20,000 are on dialysis.[24, 25] Drug handling in renal failure is dependent on a number of factors, including renal excretion and removal by extracorporeal techniques, such as dialysis. Active metabolites of morphine (M3G, M6G) are dependent on renal function for elimination and can accumulate in renal failure to cause undesirable effects and toxicity. The half-life of M6G is increased from three to five hours in normal renal function to about 50 hours in those with late-stage renal disease. In this situation, it is recommended that opioids that are not renally excreted e.g. alfentanil, should be used. **Table 11.2** shows suggested dose modifications for opioids in renal failure.

For those patients on dialysis, drug elimination by the procedure may precipitate a pain crisis. Appropriate anticipatory prescribing is important.

OPIOID PRESCRIBING IN LIVER FAILURE

The metabolic capacity of the liver is so great that liver disease must be extensive before effects on drug metabolism become important.[26] However, opioids that are primarily metabolized in the liver, such as fentanyl and alfentanil, may exacerbate central nervous system signs and symptoms in patients with severe hepatic dysfunction.

ADVANCED AGE

The ageing process affects all aspects of drug handling by the body.[26] In those over 65 years, there may be prolonged metabolism, a lesser inactivation over time followed by an

Table 11.2 Subcutaneous opioids in renal failure.

		Half life (hours) normal/ESRF	Dose reduction	Dialysability	Notes
First line	Alfentanil	1–4??	None	Not dialysed	
	Oxycodone	2–3/3–4	Yes	Unknown	
	Hydromorphone	2.5??	Yes	Unknown	
Third line	Morphine	1–4/unchanged	Yes	Yes	
	Diamorphine	1.7–3.5 minutes??	Yes	Yes	
Others	Methadone	13–58	No, 50% if GFR < 10 mL/minute	No	For specialist palliative care use only

ESRF, end stage renal failure; ??, half life in ESRF is unknown.

increase in duration of effects, mainly impairment of respiration. The clinical implications of this are as follows.

- Slow titration will allow for long circulation times.
- Choose a lower total dose because of increased sensitivity.
- There is a longer duration of action due to reduced clearance.
- Opioids with low plasma protein binding and no pharmacologically active metabolites should be used, e.g. fentanyl, alfentanil, methadone, and oxycodone.
- Clearance of morphine and fentanyl is decreased in the elderly who display a greater sensitivity to therapeutic doses than younger patients.

OTHER ANALGESICS

While opioids are the most common analgesic administered by CSCI, other agents have been used successfully in cancer pain management, particularly ketamine and ketorolac. It should also be remembered that other drugs added to a CSCI may make a significant contribution to pain relief even where the drug itself has no intrinsic analgesic activity. Examples include midazolam and levomepromazine.

Ketamine

Ketamine is an antagonist of the N-methyl-D-aspartate receptor and has received increasing interest as an agent for neuropathic pain syndromes.[27] It can be given by subcutaneous infusion to good effect in patients with uncontrolled pain or as a means to reduce the opioid dose in those experiencing severe adverse effects. Adverse events are common, particularly psychomimetic effects with sedation, disorientation, hallucinations, and vivid dreams. Because of the high incidence of adverse effects, ketamine should be started at the lowest dose possible and an initial test dose of 10 mg has been recommended. Subcutaneous infusions starting at a dose of 1 mg/kg/day

would seem appropriate with subsequent upward titration according to response. Adverse effects may necessitate stopping the drug, but can sometimes be managed with midazolam or haloperidol. Special precautions are needed in patients with heart disease, hypertension, and glaucoma.

PROTOCOL FOR THE USE OF KETAMINE

- The patient has poorly controlled pain despite opioid optimization and use of appropriate coanalgesia.
- Counselling and consent to treatment must be obtained.
- Commence ketamine subcutaneous infusion at 1 mg/kg/24 hours by separate syringe driver – usually either 50 or 100 mg/24 hours.
- Continue opioid, but if the patient shows signs of opioid toxicity either before or after starting ketamine, reduce opioid by 20–30 percent. Make further similar reductions if pain control is achieved.
- Give concomitant midazolam 5 mg/24 hours or haloperidol 5 mg/24 hours by subcutaneous infusion.
- Monitor pain scores and increase ketamine after 24 hours if there is no improvement.
- Use increments of 50–100 percent of previous daily dose to a maximum of 10 mg/kg/24 hours (usually < 600 mg/24 hours).
- Discontinue if there is no response or adverse effects intervene.

Nonsteroidal analgesics

Nonsteroidal anti-inflammatory agents (NSAIDs) are promoted by the World Health Organization (WHO) as coanalgesics in the analgesic stepladder. Diclofenac, naproxen, and ketorolac have been given by subcutaneous infusion with benefit. Severe, painful skin reactions prevent the use of diclofenac and naproxen.

Ketorolac has a marked morphine-sparing effect in some patients, particularly those in whom bone pain predominates. The usual initial dose of ketorolac is 60 mg/day with titration up to a maximum of 120 mg/day according to response.

NSAIDs can precipitate renal failure and cause gastrointestinal hemorrhage. It is particularly important to recognize renal failure as this may lead to the development of toxicity from other drugs eliminated by renal excretion (see above under Opioid toxicity). If NSAIDs are thought to be indicated, the usual precautions to protect against gastrointestinal side effects should be taken, particularly in the elderly. It may not be possible to provide adequate gastroprotection for patients who are unable to take drugs by mouth.

PROTOCOL FOR THE USE OF KETOROLAC

Ketorolac is a potent NSAID with strong analgesic activity.[28] It is contraindicated in patients with active peptic ulceration or evidence of active gastrointestinal bleeding. It should be used with caution in patients with renal impairment. Special precautions are also needed in the elderly and those taking warfarin or corticosteroids.

Ketorolac by CSCI may be considered in patients who have benefited from an NSAID, but are no longer able to take them by mouth or rectally, or in those with refractory pain with incomplete response to opioids, particularly if the pain is felt to be of bone origin.

In patients who benefit from ketorolac, it is often necessary to reduce the dose of background opioid and in some the benefit is such that opioid toxicity may emerge soon after the drug is introduced. It is therefore recommended that the dose of background opioid be reassessed before ketorolac is started and consideration be given to reducing this by 20 percent. The opioid dose should be adjusted as appropriate after ketorolac has been started with particular review after 6, 12, and 24 hours to check for emergence of toxicity, daily thereafter.

The usual starting dose of ketorolac is 60 mg by CSCI in 24 hours. Ketorolac must be mixed with normal saline. Other NSAIDs must be stopped.

It is sometimes preferable to give a dose of ketorolac 30 mg s.c. as soon as possible to determine possible benefit in patients who may be at risk from NSAIDs and to assess opioid-sparing potential with clinical review at four to six hours after administration. A 24-hour CSCI can subsequently be started with appropriate opioid modification.

Patients should be monitored for pain and also for the emergence of dyspeptic symptoms or bleeding. Ketorolac can be increased to 120 mg per 24 hours in increments of 30 mg.

All patients should be prescribed gastroprotection in the form of a proton pum inhibitor (PPI) and/or misoprostol. In those unable to take drugs orally, alternative routes of administration may be necessary which requires a clinical decision based on a risk/benefit appraisal.

Use of ketorolac by CSCI and for more than a few days is outside the manufacturer's product licence and its use therefore requires appropriate explanation and consent according to local policy.

DRUG COMBINATIONS

Pain often coexists with other symptoms, such as vomiting and agitation in cancer patients, and antiemetics or anxiolytic or both can be combined with an opioid.

It is common practice to use two drugs in combination from the time the infusion is first started. Some combinations of three or more drugs have been used. Factors that affect compatibility are:

- pH (most drugs given by CSCI are acidic with the exception of dexamethasone, diclofenac, ketorolac, and phenobarbital, which are alkaline);
- the type and concentrations of the drugs;
- the diluent;
- exposure to ultraviolet light;
- ambient temperature.

The stability and compatibility of many of these combinations is not known and generally an absence of precipitation is taken to imply compatibility.

However, an infusion should contain as few drugs as possible, preferably less than three. Some commonly used drug combinations are given in Table 11.3. A comprehensive and updated list can be found on internet-based databases for compatible drug combinations on the following websites: www.pallmed.net, www. palliativedrugs.com.

CLINICAL GOVERNANCE

The increasing use of CSCIs for the control of cancer pain has brought with it a need for quality assurance and risk management. This is most usefully achieved by developing locally agreed protocols and guidelines. From these, standards can be evolved. A comprehensive list can be found on the website of the Scottish Palliative Care Pharmacists' Association.[29] Setting standards enables audit to provide important information about service delivery and conformity of practice. Typical issues include:

- training requirements and currency of practice for staff;
- equipment set up;
- drug prescription;
- mixing of drugs;
- monitoring;
- reporting and managing adverse events;
- cleaning and maintaining equipment.

Table 11.3 Commonly used two-drug combinations.[7]

	Alfentanil	Clonazepam	Cyclizine	Dexamethasone	Diamorphine	Glycopyrrolate	Haloperidol	Hydromorphone	Hyoscine BBr	Hyoscine HBr	Ketamine	Ketorolac	Methadone	Levomepromazine	Metoclopramide	Midazolam	Morphine sulphate	Octreotide	Ondansetron
Alfentanil																			
Clonazepam	○																		
Cyclizine	▽	○																	
Dexamethasone	○		▽																
Diamorphine	○		▽	○															
Glycopyrrolate	○		▽	✗	○														
Haloperidol	○	○	▽	○	○														
Hydromorphone	○		✗				○												
Hyoscine BBr	○	○	●	□	○		○												
Hyoscine HBr	○	○		○	○		○												
Ketamine	○		○	○	○		○	○	○	○									
Ketorolac	○		✗	○	○		✗	○			○								
Methadone	○			○	○		○	○			○	○							
Levomepromazine	○			○	○			○	○		○	○	○						
Metoclopramide	○		●	○	○			○	○		○		○	○					
Midazolam	○		▽	○	○	○	○	○	○		○	✗	○	○	○				
Morphine sulfate	○		▽	○	○	○	○	○	○	○	○	○	○	○	○	○			
Octreotide	○		✗	○	○		○	○	○			○		○	○	○	○		
Ondansetron	○			○	○										○				
Oxycodone	○	▽	▽	▽			○		○	○	○	○		○	○	○	○	○	○

Blank square, no data; ○, compatible; ▽, compatible at usual concentrations; ●, occasionally incompatible. ✗, incompatible.

The clinical governance framework enables safe and effective practice to be monitored, sustained, evaluated, and reinforced. The process is an essential part of contemporary health care and provides a safeguard for the patient, the practitioner, and the organization.

REFERENCES

1. O'Neill WM. Subcutaneous infusions – a medical last rite. *Palliative Medicine.* 1994; **8**: 91–3.
2. David J. A survey of the use of syringe drivers in Marie Curie Centres. *European Journal of Cancer Care.* 1992; **4**: 23–8.
3. Oliver DJ. Syringe drivers in palliative care: a review. *Palliative Medicine.* 1988; **2**: 21–6.
4. Dover SB. Syringe driver in terminal care. *British Medical Journal.* 1987; **294**: 553–5.
5. Johnson I, Patterson S. Drugs used in combination in the syringe driver – a survey of hospice practice. *Palliative Medicine.* 1992; **6**: 125–30.
6. Bruera E, Brenneis C, Michaud M *et al.* Use of the subcutaneous route for the administration of narcotics in patients with cancer pain. *Cancer.* 1988; **62**: 407–11.
* 7. Dickman A, Schneider J, Varga J. *The syringe driver. Continuous subcutaneous infusions in palliative care*, 2nd edn. Oxford: Oxford University Press, 2005: 28–86.
8. Oliver D. The tonicity of solutions used in continuous infusions – the cause of skin reactions? *Hospital Pharmacy Practice.* 1991; **1**: 158–64.
9. World Health Organization. *Fighting disease, fostering development. Executive summary.* World Health Report. Geneva: World Health Organization, 1996.
10. Walsh D, Mahmoud FA, Sarhill N *et al.* Parenteral opioid rotation in advanced cancer: a prospective study. Abstracts of the MASCC/ISOO 13th International Symposium in Cancer. Copenhagen, Denmark, June 14–16, 2001 (Abstract 1429).
11. Klepstad P, Skorpen F, Borchagrevink PC, Kaasa S. Genetic variability and clinical efficacy of morphine. *Acta Anaesthesiologica Scandinavica.* 2005; **49**: 902–08.
12. McQuay HJ, Caroll D, Faura CC *et al.* Oral morphine in cancer pain: influences on morphine and metabolite concentration. *Clinical Pharmacology and Therapeutics.* 1990; **48**: 236–44.
13. Thompson PL, Bingham S, Andrews PL *et al.* Morphine 6-glucuronide: a metabolite of morphine with greater emetic potency than morphine in the ferret. *British Journal of Pharmacology.* 1992; **106**: 3–8.
14. Osborne RJ, Joel SP, Slevin ML. Morphine intoxication in renal failure: the role of morphine-6-glucuronide. *British Medical Journal (Clinical Research Ed.).* 1986; **292**: 1548–9.
15. Yaksh TL, Harty GJ. Pharmacology of the allodynia in rats evoked by high dose intrathecal morphine. *Journal of Pharmacology and Experimental Therapeutics.* 1987; **244**: 501–07.
16. Labella FS, Pinsky C, Havlicek V. Morphine derivatives with diminished opiate receptor potency show enhanced central excitatory activity. *Brain Research.* 1979; **174**: 263–71.
17. Cherny NJ, Ripamonti C, Pereira J *et al.* Strategies to manage the adverse effects of oral morphine: an evidence based report. *Journal of Clinical Oncology.* 2001; **19**: 2442–554.
18. Gordon GB, Stevenson KK, Griffie J *et al.* Opioid equi-analgesic calculations. *Journal of Palliative Medicine.* 1999; **2**: 209–18.
19. Twycross R, Wilcock A, Charlesworth S, Dickman A. *PCF2 palliative care formulary*, 2nd edn. Oxford: Radcliffe Medical Press, 2002: 159–202.
20. McDonald P, Graham P, Clayton M *et al.* Regular subcutaneous bolus morphine via an indwelling cannula for pain from advanced cancer. *Palliative Medicine.* 1991; **5**: 323–9.
21. Drexel H, Dzien A, Spiegel RW *et al.* Treatment of severe cancer pain by low dose continuous subcutaneous morphine. *Pain.* 1989; **36**: 169–76.
22. Mao J, Chen LL. Systemic lidocaine for neuropathic pain relief. *Pain.* 2000; **87**: 7–17.
23. Cassuto J, Wallin G, Hogstrom S *et al.* Inhibition of postoperative pain by continuous low dose infusion of lidocaine. *Anaesthesia and Analgesia.* 1985; **64**: 971–4.
24. Ashley C, Currie A. *The renal drug handbook*, 2nd edn. Oxford: Radcliffe Medical Press, 2004; **18**: 264; 264, 358, 396.
25. Renal Association. UK renal register, sixth annual report, December 2003. Available from: www.renalreg.com.
* 26. Doyle D, Hanks G, Nathan C, Calman K (eds). *Oxford textbook of palliative medicine*, 3rd edn. Oxford: Oxford University Press, 2004: 331.
27. Mercadente S, Lodi F, Spaio M *et al.* Long-term ketamine subcutaneous continuous infusion in neuropathic cancer pain. *Journal of Pain and Symptom Management.* 1995; **4**: 310–14.
* 28. Myers KG, Trotman IF. Use of ketorolac by continuous subcutaneous infusion for the control of cancer-related pain. *Journal of Postgraduate Medicine.* 1994; **70**: 359–62.
29. Scottish Palliative Care Pharmacists' Association. Syringe drivers in palliative care: standard. Accessed on November 26, 2006. Available from: www.palliativecarescotland.org.uk/publications/standard.pdf.

12

Antiepileptics, antidepressants, and local anesthetic drugs

HARALD BREIVIK AND ANDREW SC RICE

KEY LEARNING POINTS

- Antiepileptic, antidepressant, and local anesthetic drugs have analgesic effects in neuropathic pain conditions. About half of the patients treated report a degree of pain relief. Side effects may be burdensome and may prevent a therapeutic dose being reached.
- There are first- and second-line drugs for neuropathic pain, with opioid analgesics as last second-line drugs in selected patients.
- Antiepileptics – the following have documented efficacy in at least one randomized controlled trial (RCT), all are associated with potentially problematic side effects:
  - phenytoin;
  - carbamazepine and oxcarbazepine;
  - lamotrigine;
  - gabapentin and pregabalin;
  - valproic acid;
  - topiramate.
- Antidepressants
  - Tricyclics (TCA), especially amitriptyline, nortriptyline, and desipramine are efficacious, but may have burdensome side effects.
  - Two serotonin- and noradrenalin-reuptake inhibitors (SSNRI) – duloxetine and venlafaxine – are also effective, and have fewer side effects than TCAs.
  - The specific serotonin-reuptake inhibitors (SSRI) are generally not effective for chronic pain.
- Topical patch or gel application of lidocaine relieves allodynia and hyperalgesia locally.
- Intravenous lidocaine followed by oral mexiletine may help some patients.

INTRODUCTION

Antiepileptic, antidepressant, and local anesthetic drugs have documented antihyperalgesic and analgesic effects in pain conditions with neuropathic components. In many conditions, they are first-line drugs, with opioid analgesics as second line add-on drugs.[1, 2, 3, 4, 5, 6, 7, 8, 9, 10]

The efficacy of antidepressants, calcium channel $\alpha_2\delta1$ subunit ligands, and topical local anesthetics and opioids in neuropathic pain has been demonstrated in a number of controlled clinical trials, whereas the evidence for the effect of the other drug classes is less solid.[1] The incomplete and often modest response seen with these drugs is accepted because there are no better alternatives. In the individual patient, exploring additive analgesic effects by combining therapy with drugs of different mechanisms of action may be worthwhile. For this reason, although the generic terms "anticonvulsants" or "antiepileptic" are commonly used when referring to drugs which have efficacy in both neuropathic pain and epilepsy, this can divert the prescriber's attention from the fact that this group contains drugs of diverse mechanisms of action which should be taken into account when making therapeutic decisions, most especially when considering using a combination of therapies. However, because of the common usage of the term "antiepileptic," we will use this term, but with the above proviso.

ANTIEPILEPTICS

Carbamazepine and oxcarbazepine are effective for classic trigeminal neuralgia. The calcium channel $\alpha_2\delta 1$ subunit ligands are now well documented for several types of neuropathic pain. The other drugs in this class have equivocal evidence for effect and are therefore considered third-line drugs when first- and second-line drugs have failed or are not tolerated. Antiepileptics used in pain treatment comprise the following.[1, 3, 8, 9, 10, 11, 12]

- Nonspecific sodium channel blockers:
  - phenytoin;[8]
  - carbamazepine;[8]
  - oxcarbazepine.[3]
- Specific sodium channel blockers:
  - Lamotrigine;[3, 9]
  - topiramate (also gabaergic and antiglutaminergic effects).[1, 12]
- Calcium channel calcium channel $\alpha_2\delta 1$ subunit ligands:
  - gabapentin;[1, 3]
  - pregabalin.[1, 10]
- Gabaergic drugs:
  - valproic acid.[1, 10]

Painful conditions in which antiepileptic drugs have been shown to have an effect in some, but not all trials are:

- diabetic and other painful polyneuropathies (gabapentin, pregabalin, phenytoin, carbamazepine, lamotrigine);
- postherpetic neuralgia (gabapentin, pregabalin, valproate);
- central poststroke pain (carbamazepine, lamotrigine);
- post-spinal cord injury neuropathic pain (pregabalin);
- trigeminal neuralgia (carbamazepine, oxcarbazepine, lamotrigine).

The etiology for neuropathic pain may be less important than the phenomenology and the mechanism of pain. There is no scientific evidence for the traditional preferential use of antiepileptics in lancinating pains and antidepressants for steady burning-like pains. However, a superior outcome in the former type of pain is supported

by the effectiveness of some of the antiepileptics in trigeminal neuralgia, a condition for which there are no trials of antidepressants. Phenytoin is used infrequently because it is associated with an unfavorable side-effect profile in long-term treatment (see below under Side effects). Lamotrigine has been adequately tested in trigeminal neuralgia, in central pain, and painful polyneuropathy.

Contraindications

- Phenytoin:
  - AV block;
  - hepatic failure;
  - allergic reactions.
- Carbamazepine:
  - AV block;
  - treatment with monoamine oxidase inhibitors;
  - hepatic failure;
  - porphyria;
  - allergic reactions.
- Oxcarbazepine:
  - AV block;
  - treatment with monoamine oxidase inhibitors.
- Lamotrigine:
  - renal failure;
  - allergic skin reactions.
- Gabapentin and pregabalin:
  - none, but reduced doses in renal failure.
- Sodium valproate:
  - hepatic failure;
  - hepatic failure in relatives during treatment with sodium valproate;
  - thrombocytopenia.
- Topiramate:
  - glaucoma.

Dosing and treatment schedule

Phenytoin, carbamazepine, oxcarbazepine, topiramate, and lamotrigine are metabolized by the liver and should be used with caution in patients with liver disease. The active metabolite of oxcarbazepine (10-hydroxycarbazepine) is excreted via the kidneys. Gabapentin and pregabalin are excreted unchanged by the kidneys. Approximately 50 percent of an oral dose of sodium valproate is metabolized by the liver, and both the parent compound and the metabolites are excreted via the kidneys. Impaired renal function dictates that the dose of oxcarbazepine, gabapentin, pregabalin, and sodium valproate should be lowered. Topiramate may cause urolithiasis and extra fluid intake is recommended.

The long-term efficacy of phenytoin may be predicted by an intravenous infusion test: phenytoin 15 mg/kg body weight infused during 30 minutes. In severe acute exacerbation of trigeminal neuralgia, intravenous loading with phenytoin may also be appropriate. Oral treatment is started with 50 mg twice daily and the dose increased weekly by 50 mg until a sufficient response or until the maximal recommended serum level (80 μM) is reached. Phenytoin exhibits saturation kinetics in which minor dose increments may cause major increases in serum drug concentrations at the higher dose levels, therefore dose increments should be monitored carefully at levels over 100 mg twice daily.

When carbamazepine is used in the treatment of trigeminal neuralgia, an immediate effect is often desired. In this situation, the initial dose is 100 mg three times daily, increased by 100 mg every second day until pain relief is achieved or intolerable side effects are encountered. Later, the dose can be reduced cautiously to the lowest effective level.

In less acute cases of trigeminal neuralgia or other pain states, the treatment should be initiated very slowly, i.e. with 100 mg in the evening and dose increments of 100 mg every two to three days up to a dose of 200 mg three times daily. Further increases in the dose are guided by effects, side effects, and the upper recommended drug level (40 μM). Serum levels can be assessed every second week. In trigeminal neuralgia, it has been suggested that the effective drug level corresponds to the level recommended in the treatment of epilepsy.

If carbamazepine causes intolerable side effects, a trial of oxcarbazepine is worthwhile. In this situation, the patient can be switched directly to oxcarbazepine in a corresponding or slightly higher dose. When the treatment is started from scratch, the initial dose is 150 mg in the evening and increments of 150 mg daily are used until the dose is 450 mg twice daily. Further adjustments depend on the effect and side effects, with a top dose level defined by the upper recommended serum drug concentration (120 μM).

From clinical practice, it has emerged that the initial low dosing of lamotrigine will reduce the risk of skin rashes. In the first two weeks, 25 mg is given in the morning, and over the next two weeks the dose is 25 mg twice daily. After this phase, the dose can be increased by 50 mg every second week until an acceptable response is achieved or a maximal total daily dose of 200–300 mg twice daily. In trigeminal neuralgia, it has been suggested that the effect can be increased by using even higher doses in patients in whom standard doses produce very low serum drug concentrations. In general, however, therapeutic drug monitoring with lamotrigine is not to be recommended because there is no clear concentration–effect relationship and no defined upper recommended serum drug level.

Gabapentin should also be started slowly to minimize side effects. Over the first two days, 300 mg is given in the evening, then 300 mg twice daily for two days, and thereafter 300 mg three times daily. If there is no effect, the dose can be increased by 300–600 mg every second week according to effects and side effects, with an upper dose limit of 3600 mg daily. Several weeks can be required to reach an effective dosage, which is usually between 1800 and 3600 mg. Daily doses ≥2700 mg are often accompanied by bothersome somnolence and dizziness. In some elderly patients, gabapentin can cause or exacerbate cognitive and gait impairment.

Pregabalin is quite similar to gabapentin in effects and side effects, but onset of pain relief is more rapid and its anxiolytic effects may be of additional benefit in some patients. Pregabalin can be started with a daily dose of 150 mg (in two or three divided doses) or 75 mg at bedtime in elderly patients and in patients prone to side effects. Upward titration can reach 300 mg per day within one to two weeks and the maximum benefits occur often after two weeks of treatment at target dosages of 300–600 mg/day. The linear pharmacokinetics (90 percent oral bioavailability, excreted unchanged in urine), the more rapid onset of pain relief, and the potential for twice daily dosing of pregabalin contribute to the relative greater ease of use compared to gabapentin. In patients with reduced kidney function, doses must be reduced accordingly.[1]

Sodium valproate can be started at 500 mg/day and the dose adjusted in steps of 500 mg every week to obtain the target serum drug concentration (700 μM) according to a serum drug level measured about three weeks from the start of treatment.

Topiramate is started low (25 mg in the evening), gradually increasing the daily dose by 25 mg every two weeks, until the effect is obtained at 100–200 mg daily dose. Sufficient fluid intake to reduce risk of kidney stones must be ensured.

For all the drugs, the response is often partial and dose-related side effects may prevent a therapeutic dose being achieved.

Side effects

The antiepileptic drugs are frequently associated with side effects. The older drugs (phenytoin and carbamazepine) are more likely to do this, but the newer drugs can also cause side effects.

- Phenytoin:
  - allergic manifestations (skin);
  - sedation;
  - problems with memory and attention;
  - nystagmus, double vision, ataxia, tremor;
  - nausea, constipation;
  - peripheral neuropathy (loss of deep tendon reflexes);
  - hirsutism;
  - gingival hypertrophy.
- Carbamazepine:
  - allergic manifestations (skin, mucosa, etc.);
  - sedation;
  - ataxia, dizziness, double vision;
  - problems with accommodation;

- fluid retention, low sodium levels (clinical significance uncertain);
  - cardiac conduction disturbances (rare);
  - thrombocytopenia, agranulocytosis, aplastic anemia (rare);
  - confusion (elderly).
- Oxcarbazepine:
  - allergic manifestations (25 percent cross-reactivity with carbamazepine);
  - sedation;
  - headache;
  - ataxia, dizziness;
  - fluid retention, low sodium levels (clinical significance uncertain).
- Lamotrigine:
  - skin rash (see above under Dosing and treatment schedule);
  - insomnia;
  - headache;
  - sedation, dizziness, nausea, double vision (high doses).
- Gabapentin and pregabalin:
  - sedation;
  - ataxia, dizziness;
  - headache, nausea, vomiting;
  - erectile dysfunction.
- Valproic acid, sodium valproate:
  - increased appetite and weight gain;
  - abdominal pain, nausea, and vomiting (rare, use enteric coated tablets);
  - sedation;
  - hand tremor;
  - alopecia (rare);
  - toxic hepatitis, pancreatitis (rare, mainly children).
- Topiramate:
  - nausea, skin rash;
  - sedation, dizziness, confusion;
  - glaucoma, urolithiasis.

Treatment with sodium valproate requires special attention because of potentially serious side effects. Before treatment is started, blood tests should be carried out to determine liver function and thrombocyte count. This should be repeated after one month and thereafter every three months during the first year of treatment. In addition, the patients should be aware of the symptoms of liver disease.

For many of the antiepileptics, the speed at which doses are increased is a major determinant of the degree of side effects and the tolerability of the drugs. It is therefore recommended to "start low" and "go slowly (up)."

ANTIDEPRESSANTS

Typical antidepressants used in pain treatment (those in bold might be regarded first-line drugs because they are reputed to have a more favorable side-effect profile, although the evidence for this is not strong).

- Tricyclic antidepressants:[1, 2, 3]
  - with balanced reuptake inhibition of norepinephrine (noradrenaline) and serotonin:
    - imipramine;
    - amitriptyline; and
    - clomipramine.
  - with relatively selective reuptake inhibition of norepinephrine:
    - **desipramine**;
    - **nortriptyline**; and
    - maprotiline.
- Selective uptake inhibitors:
  - selective serotonin reuptake inhibitors (less effective or ineffective):[1, 2, 3]
    - paroxetine;
    - citalopram;
    - fluoxetine; and
    - sertraline.
- Serotonin and norepinephrine reuptake inhibitors:[1, 2, 3]
  - **venlafaxine**;[1, 4]
  - **duloxetine**.[1, 5]

The conditions in which these drugs have been shown to have an effect are:

- painful diabetic neuropathy (TCAs, SSNRIs);
- painful polyneuropathy (TCAs, SSNRIs, SSRIs);
- postherpetic neuralgia (TCAs);
- nerve injury pain (TCAs, SSNRIs);
- central poststroke pain (TCAs);
- migraine prophylaxis (TCAs);
- chronic tension type headache (TCAs).

Antidepressants have not been different from placebo in RCTs of patients with HIV neuropathy, spinal cord injury, cisplatin neuropathy, neuropathic cancer pain, phantom pain, and chronic lumbar root pain.[1]

Throughout the different neuropathic conditions, a clinically significant, but partial response with TCAs is seen in 40–60 percent of patients. The response with SSRIs is equivocal. In migraine and chronic tension-type headache, the data are equivocal.

Contraindications

The majority of problems are with TCAs:

- TCAs:
  - recent myocardial infarction (less than six months);
  - cardiac conduction disturbances, e.g. AV block;
  - uncontrolled congestive heart failure;
  - convulsive disorders;

– untreated glaucoma;
– treatment with monoamine oxidase inhibitors.
• Selective uptake inhibitor (SSRIs and SSNRIs):
– treatment with monoamine oxidase inhibitors.

SSRIs and SSNRIs should not be used in patients with convulsive disorders. Caution is also recommended when SSRIs and SSNRIs are given to patients with other contraindications to TCAs.

The serotonin syndrome characterized by hyperthermia, hyperreflexia, muscle spasms, changes in mental state, hyper- or hypotension, tachycardia, diarrhea, tremor, or problems with coordination may develop during treatment with all of these drugs. This syndrome may be seen with a single agent that potentiates serotonergic neurotransmission, but the risk of developing severe serotonin syndrome (which may be rapidly fatal) is higher when different drugs that potentiate serotonergic neurotransmission are combined and act either by the same or by different mechanisms. Caution should therefore be exercised when using tramadol in combination with antidepressant drugs.[6, 7]

Dosing and treatment schedule

TCAs, SSRIs, and SSNRIs undergo hepatic metabolism before they are excreted in the urine. Hepatic metabolism for most of these drugs depends partially on a genetic polymorphic enzyme. This is the main cause for the pronounced pharmacokinetic variability which is seen, in particular with TCAs. Together with the serum concentration–effect relationship and the known toxicity for TCAs, this is the reason for recommending monitoring of serum drug concentration when TCAs are used. Monitoring is not necessary for SSRIs, which are less toxic and have no clear concentration–effect relationships.

If there are no contraindications to TCA, amitriptyline, imipramine, or clomipramine can be started with the lowest strength tablet, 10–25 mg in the evenings of the first week, increasing the dose weekly by 25 mg in the evening until pain relief is obtained or side effects become bothersome. After five to six weeks, serum concentrations should be checked and the dose increased to yield a maximum serum concentration of:

• amitriptyline+nortriptyline of around 300 nM;
• imipramine+desipramine of around 400 nM; and
• clomipramine+desmethylclomipramine of around 400 nM.

In patients suffering severe pain, the dose adjustment can be performed more rapidly in order to achieve an adequate effect sooner or to decide whether alternative treatments should be tried because the drugs are ineffective or cause side effects. It should be noted that it is not necessary to titrate the dose for every patient treated with imipramine to serum levels of about 400 nM nor every patient treated with amitriptyline to about 300 nM because some will have a satisfactory response at lower concentrations.

The measurement of these serum drug concentrations is recommended, mainly to avoid toxicity. It is assumed that drug levels around 2000 nM are toxic, i.e. only five times higher than the therapeutic concentrations of the TCAs.

In the individual patient, it is impossible to know whether a poor response is due to inadequate dosing or whether the patient is a nonresponder. Thus, the reasons for employing therapeutic drug monitoring when TCAs are used are:

• pronounced variability in pharmacokinetics: this is primarily due to genetic variability;
• dosing according to effects and side effects is not feasible: there are nonresponders, and side effects may occur at subtherapeutic drug levels;
• low therapeutic index: for example, for imipramine and amitriptyline there is a factor of about 5–7 difference between therapeutic and toxic drug levels;
• efficacy can be increased: for imipramine, it appears that the numbers needed to treat to obtain one patient with >50 percent pain relief can be reduced from about 2 to 1.5 when dosing is guided by serum drug levels.

If the tricyclic antidepressants are ineffective, cause too severe side effects, or are contraindicated, try one of the SSNRI antidepressants with documented effects, i.e. duloxetine or venlafaxine. Less pronounced side effects make it possible to start with a relatively adequate dose level, initially at 30–60 mg duloxetine daily, increasing to a maximum dose of 120 mg. Venlafaxine should be started at 37.5 mg daily, increasing every two weeks to a maximum dose of 375 mg daily. Note that venlafaxine is mainly SSRI at lower doses, so that it is important to reach higher level dosing before the treatment attempt is cancelled due to lack of effect.[1]

The SSRIs paroxetine, citalopram, and fluoxetine have been tried as third-line drugs with limited success. Started at 10 or 20 mg daily, increasing on a weekly basis to a maximum dose of 60 mg daily.

Side effects

Treatment with TCAs is frequently associated with side effects and a substantial number of patients cannot tolerate chronic dosing with these drugs in a dose that is adequate to achieve pain relief. The SSRIs and SSNRIs are better tolerated, probably because they are devoid of postsynaptic blocking effects, but these drugs are definitely not without side effects.

- TCAs:
  - dry mouth, problems with accommodation;
  - constipation, urinary retention;
  - sweating;
  - fatigue, sedation, mental change;
  - dizziness and orthostatic hypotension;
  - cardiac conduction disturbances (AV block, intraventricular blocks);
  - confusion (elderly);
  - risk of injuries from falling.
- Selective uptake inhibitors:
  - SSRIs:
    - nausea, vomiting;
    - nervousness, anxiety, insomnia;
    - sexual dysfunction (delayed ejaculation, impotence).
  - SSNRIs:
    - headache;
    - nausea, vomiting;
    - sweating;
    - sedation, mental change;
    - hypertension.

The side effects are most pronounced soon after treatment is started and as the dose increases. Patients should therefore be encouraged to stay on the treatment for at least a few weeks. The dry mouth which occurs with TCAs may be slightly diminished by chewing gum or using artificial saliva. It is wise to recommend a mild laxative, especially for elderly patients. In particular, these patients should be warned about orthostatic phenomena, e.g. to be cautious when changing from a sitting or reclining position. The sedating properties of the TCAs can be used therapeutically by prescribing the drugs as single, evening doses because neuropathic pain is often aggravated at this time, causing sleep disturbance. However, patients should be advised against operating machinery or driving a motor vehicle until it is clear that the TCA is being administered at a stable dose which does not impair their ability to perform such tasks. Amitriptyline may be more sedating than the other TCAs with balanced reuptake inhibition as it has potent antihistaminergic and central anticholinergic properties. However, the SSRIs should be dosed in the morning to avoid insomnia.

LOCAL ANESTHETICS

Local anesthetics are used in the treatment of neuropathic pain as systemic infusion or topical application on skin areas with allodynia or hyperalgesia:[13, 14]

- lidocaine: dosing is by intravenous infusion, as oral dosing is not possible because of the high first-pass metabolism;
- mexiletine: in patients who respond with significant pain relief after lidocaine i.v., the orally active

lidocaine analog mexiletine is effective in some, but not all, lidocaine positive patients;[10, 15, 16, 17]
- topical, high concentrations of lidocaine in a patch or in a gel.[18, 19, 20]

Trials have also been performed with tocainide, procaine, and bupivacaine, but clinical utility is hampered by the high incidence of severe side effects, fast elimination, and equivocal effects.

The conditions in which the effect of these drugs are documented include:[13]

- painful diabetic polyneuropathy;
- postherpetic neuralgia;
- nerve injury pain;
- central pain.

Studies revealed benefit in conditions secondary to central nervous system lesions, as well as peripheral nerve injury pain. Systemic lidocaine is able to reduce secondary hyperalgesia and allodynia of several sensory modalities and is capable of reducing a spinally organized nociceptive reflex. Therefore, it seems most likely that systemic local anesthetics exert their effect mainly on the central nervous system. Systemic lidocaine has no impact on normal sensory thresholds.

The benefit of systemic lidocaine on spontaneous pain, pain paroxysms, dysesthesias, and allodynia may vary between studies, but its effectiveness has been seen on all modalities in clinical trials. Lidocaine infusion is used to relieve severe continuous painful conditions, and often the response is of longer duration, varying from several hours to a few weeks. A positive response to intravenous infusion of lidocaine may indicate that some effect of oral mexiletine can be expected. However, the predictive value is not strong, possibly because the tissue concentrations of mexiletine do not reach sufficient values.

Contraindications

- Systemic lidocaine:
  - any cardiac arrhythmias, especially AV blocks;
  - allergy to this drug class.
- Mexiletine:
  - any cardiac arrhythmias, especially AV blocks;
  - allergy to this drug class.

Dosing and treatment schedule

Lidocaine is infused intravenously as 5 mg/kg body weight over 30–45 minutes. Alternatively, a computer-controlled infusion paradigm can be used to obtain a serum lidocaine level of 3–4 μg/mL.[14] Doses should be reduced by 50 percent in heart failure or liver disease. Increases in blood pressure and heart rate are expected to occur during infusion.

1. Inform the patient about the procedure and side effects and confirm that driving will not take place following the procedure.
2. Establish an intravenous line with 0.9 percent saline.
3. Measure blood pressure and start electrocardiogram (ECG) monitoring.
4. Begin controlled infusion of preservative-free lidocaine in 0.9 percent saline.
5. Monitor the patient throughout the infusion and measure blood pressure every 15 minutes.
6. Continue observations as indicated for at least one hour following completion of the infusion.

Mexiletine is metabolized in the liver mainly by the iso-enzyme CYP2D6. Because of the genetic polymorphism of this enzyme, variable pharmacokinetics and drug interactions need attention.

In order to increase compliance, initiate oral mexiletine treatment with a dose of 50 mg three times daily for three days, then 100 mg three times daily for three days, and thereafter 150–300 mg three times daily (approximately 10 mg/kg body weight). Preferably dosing should be with meals.

Side effects

Acute side effects are common during intravenous lidocaine infusions at therapeutic doses:

- dizziness, sedation, confusion;
- perioral paresthesias, slurred speech, blurred vision, euphoria, lightheadedness;
- nausea.

Side effects disappear within minutes following the end of infusion.

Oral mexiletine is often accompanied by side effects:

- dizziness, lightheadedness, nausea, vomiting;
- fatigue, nervousness, tremor, unsteady gait, blurred vision;
- confusion, constipation or diarrhea, headache, paresthesias, slurred speech;
- heartburn, chest pain.

The side effects of oral mexiletine are often intolerable and it is possible that the apparent lower efficacy of this drug is because sufficiently high doses cannot be used.

SUMMARY

Antiepileptic, antidepressant, and local anesthetic drugs have analgesic effects in neuropathic pain conditions.

About half of the patients treated report a degree of pain relief. Side effects may be burdensome and may prevent a therapeutic dose being reached.

They are first- and second-line drugs for neuropathic pain, with opioid analgesics as last second-line drugs in selected patients.

REFERENCES

∗ 1. Dworkin RH, O'Connor AB, Backonja M et al. Pharmacologic management of neuropathic pain: Evidence-based recommendations. Pain. 2007; 132: 237–51.

2. McQuay HJ, Tramèr M, Nye BA et al. A systematic review of antidepressants in neuropathic pain. Pain. 1996; 68: 217–27.

∗ 3. Sindrup SH, Jensen TS. Efficacy of pharmacological treatments of neuropathic pain. An update and effect related to mechanism of drug action. Pain. 1999; 83: 389–400.

4. Sindrup SH, Bach FW, Madsen C et al. Venlafaxine versus imipramine in painful polyneuropathy: a randomized, controlled trial, Neurology. 2003; 60: 1284–9.

5. Wernicke JF, Pritchett YL, D'Souza DN et al. A randomized controlled trial of duloxetine in diabetic peripheral neuropathic pain. Neurology. 2006; 67: 1411–20.

∗ 6. Boyer EW, Shannon M. The serotonin syndrome. New England Journal of Medicine. 2005; 352: 1112–20.

7. Ripple MB, Pestaner JP, Levine BS, Smialek JE. Lethal combination of tramadol and multiple drugs affecting serotonin. American Journal of Forensic Medicine and Pathology. 2000; 21: 370–4.

8. McQuay H, Carroll D, Jadad AR et al. Anticonvulsant drugs for management of pain: a systematic review. British Medical Journal (Clinical research ed.). 1995; 311: 1047–52.

9. Luria Y, Brecker C, Daoud D et al. Lamotrigine in the treatment of painful diabetic neuropathy: a randomized, placebo-controlled study. In: Devor M, Rowbotham MC, Wiesenfeld-Hallin Z (eds). Progress in pain research and management, vol. 16. Seattle, WA: IASP Press, 2000: 857–62.

∗ 10. Finnerup NB, Otto M, Jensen TS, Sindrup SH. Algorithm for neuropathic pain treatment: an evidence based proposal, Pain. 2005; 118: 289–305.

11. Dogra S, Beydoun S, Mazzola J et al. Oxcarbazepine in painful diabetic neuropathy: a randomized, placebo-controlled study. European Journal of Pain. 2005; 9: 543–54.

12. Raskin P, Donofrio PD, Rosenthal NR et al. Topiramate vs placebo in painful diabetic neuropathy: analgesic and metabolic effects. Neurology. 2004; 63: 865–73.

∗ 13. Chaplan SR, Bach FW, Yaksh TL. Systemic use of local anesthetics in pain states. In: Yaksh TL, Lynch C, Zapol WM *et al.* (eds). *Anesthesia, biologic foundations.* Philadelphia, PA: Lippincott-Raven, 1997: 977–86.

14. Schnider TW, Gaeta R, Brose W *et al.* Derivation and cross-validation of pharmacokinetic parameters for computer-controlled infusion of lidocaine in pain therapy. *Anesthesiology.* 1996; **84**: 1043–50.

15. Attal N, Gaude V, Brasseur L *et al.* Intravenous lidocaine in central pain: a double blind, placebo controlled psychophysical study. *Neurology.* 2000; **54**: 564–74.

∗ 16. Tremont-Lukats IW, Challapalli V, McNichol ED *et al.* Systemic administration of local anesthetic agents to relieve neuropathic pain: a systematic review and meta-analysis. *Anesthesia and Analgesia.* 2005; **101**: 1738–49.

∗ 17. Kaplan KM, Mackey SC, Carroll IR. Mexiletine therapy for chronic pain: survival analysis identifies factors predicting clinical success. *Journal of Pain and Symptom Management.* 2008; **35**: 321–6.

∗ 18. Hempenstall K, Nurmikko TJ, Johnson RW *et al.* Analgesic therapy in postherpetic neuralgia: a quantitative systematic review. *Public Library of Science – Medicine.* 2005; **2**: 628–44.

19. Galer BS, Rowbotham MC, Perander J, Friedman E. Topical lidocaine patch relieves postherpetic neuralgia more effectively than a vehicle topical patch: results of an enriched enrollment study. *Pain.* 1999; **80**: 533–8.

∗ 20. Meier T, Wasner G, Faust M *et al.* Efficacy of lidocaine patch 5% in the treatment of focal peripheral neuropathic pain syndromes: a randomized, double-blind, placebo-controlled study. *Pain.* 2003; **106**: 151–8.

Psychological techniques

SECTION B

13

Self-regulation skills training for adults, including relaxation

DAVID SPIEGEL

KEY LEARNING POINTS

- Cognitive and affective dimensions of pain present important therapeutic opportunities.
- Enhancing patients' ability to control pain through self-management provides considerable pain relief even when it does not eliminate pain.
- Self-hypnosis is a powerful means of managing pain perception and the affective response to it, in both acute and chronic pain.

- Mindfulness-based stress reduction is designed to shift attention into the present, avoiding past problems and future concerns, and is helpful as an indirect analgesic intervention.
- Biofeedback can be helpful in reducing muscle tension and autonomic activity related to pain experience.
- Expectancy, including positive and negative placebo experiences, can influence pain experience through well-defined neural pathways.

INTRODUCTION

Pain is a psychophysiological phenomenon that can be either exacerbated or diminished by the emotional, cognitive, and social environment that surrounds it. Pain usually occurs within the context of the subjective distress associated with a major medical illness or physical trauma. The "pain experience" represents a combination of both tissue damage and the emotional reaction to it. There is ample evidence to suggest that psychological factors greatly influence the pain experience in either positive or negative ways. In fact, the intensity of pain is directly associated with its meaning. One critical factor that can amplify or diminish pain is the sense of helplessness that surrounds it, the perceived inability to modulate its aversive effects on consciousness. Helplessness is the key element underlying the intensity of reactions to trauma.[1, 2, 3] Pain is often intensified by the helplessness that accompanies it. Conversely, many pain patients report that they would find their pain tolerable if they could modulate it at least partially. The desire for control is a critical component of pain management.

Why, one might ask, would one contemplate utilizing a technique such as hypnosis, which is often thought to involve relinquishing control, in the treatment of a disorder that is better managed with enhanced control? Hypnosis is actually a normal state of highly focused attention, with a relative diminution in peripheral awareness.[4, 5, 6] Being hypnotized is akin to being so caught up in a good movie, play, or novel that one loses awareness of surroundings and enters the imagined world, a state termed "absorption."[7] Indeed, people who have such states spontaneously are more likely to be highly hypnotizable on formal testing.[8] Although the suspension of disbelief involved in such absorption may make hypnotized people appear more suggestible, i.e. responsive to the instructions of the person inducing hypnosis, all hypnosis is in fact self-hypnosis, a means of altering one's inner state toward an intense central focus, whether self-induced or suggested by someone else. Thus, the very state that would appear to engender loss of control can be utilized quite effectively to enhance control, especially over unwanted sensations such as pain, which can be placed at the periphery of awareness, altered, or even eliminated.

CORTICAL MODULATION OF PAIN

Pain is the ultimate psychosomatic phenomenon. It is composed of both a somatic signal that something is wrong with the body and a message or interpretation of that signal involving attentional, cognitive, affective, and social factors. The limbic system and cortex provide a means of modulating pain signals,[9, 10] by either amplifying them through excessive attention or affective dysregulation, or by minimizing them through denial, inattention, relaxation, or attention-control techniques. It is well known that many athletes and soldiers sustain serious injuries in the heat of sport or combat and are unaware of the injury until someone points out bleeding or swelling. On the other hand, some individuals with comparatively minor physical damage report being totally immobilized and demoralized by pain. A single parent with a sarcoma complained of severe unremitting pain that was interlaced with tearful concern about her failure to discuss her terminal prognosis with her adolescent son. When an appropriate meeting was arranged to plan for his future and discuss her fate with him, the pain resolved.[11]

Pain perception is influenced by one's state of consciousness. For example, chronic pain tends to be worse during evenings and weekends when people are not distracted by routine activities. It is often reduced during sleep, but may in fact interfere with sleep; more severe kinds of pain can substantially reduce sleep efficiency. Many of the more potent drugs that treat pain reduce alertness and arousal, an often unwanted side effect or one that can lead to abuse of analgesic medications.

ATTENTION TO PAIN

Like any other perceptual phenomenon, pain is modulated by attentional processes: you have to pay attention to pain for it to hurt. Novelty tends to enhance pain perception (as with an acute injury), although overwhelming and serious injury is sometimes accompanied by a surprising absence of pain perception until hours afterwards. This traumatic dissociation has been observed in victims of natural disaster, combat, and motor vehicle accidents.[12]

Somatic perception is modulated by the cortex, which enhances or diminishes awareness of incoming signals. Recent neuropsychological and brain-imaging research has demonstrated at least three attentional centers that modulate perception: a posterior parieto-occipital orienting system, a focusing system localized to the anterior cingulate gyrus, and an arousal–vigilance system in the right frontal lobe.[13, 14] These systems provide, among other things, for selective attention to incoming stimuli, allowing competing stimuli to be relegated to the periphery of awareness.

When Melzack postulated the gate control theory of pain decades ago,[15] it was observed that higher cortical input could inhibit pain signals as well. They cited Pavlov's observation that repeated shocks to dogs eventually failed to elicit pain behavior, i.e. the dogs habituated to the painful signals, and this could only be explained as cortical inhibition of pain response. Thus, in their model, there is room for descending inhibition of pain, for example via the substantia gelatinosa, as well as competitive inhibition at the spinal "gate,"[9] now thought to involve endogenous opiates. The important concept we gain from this theory is the interaction between central perception and modulation of noxious stimuli at the periphery.

MEANING OF PAIN

It has been known for half a century that the meaning structure in which pain is embedded influences the intensity of pain. In his classic study, Beecher[16] noted with surprise that soldiers who were quite badly wounded on the Anzio beachhead seemed to require very little analgesic medication. He subsequently examined a matched group of civilian surgical patients at Massachusetts General Hospital with equal or less serious surgically induced wounds. They demanded far higher levels of analgesic medication than did the combat soldiers. Beecher concluded that this disparity was based on a difference in the meaning of the pain. To combat soldiers, the pain was almost welcome as an indication that they were likely to get out of combat alive, whereas to the surgical patients it represented an interference with life and a threat to survival. This means that patients who interpret pain signals as an ominous sign of the worsening of their disease are likely to experience a greater intensity of pain. This hypothesis has been confirmed, for example, among cancer patients. Those who believe the pain represents a worsening of their disease show more pain.[17] Indeed, the meaning of the pain and associated anxiety and depression accounted for more variance in pain than did the site of metastasis.

MOOD DISORDERS AND PAIN

Anxiety and depression are often associated with a profound sense of helplessness. They are noted as frequent concomitants of pain.[18, 19, 20] This early work implied that patients with psychopathology complained more about pain. Later work suggested that there is an interaction and that perhaps chronic pain amplifies or produces depression.[21, 22] Indeed, the presence of significant pain among cancer patients is more strongly associated with major depressive symptoms than is a prior life history of depression.[23]

Depression is the most frequently reported psychiatric diagnosis among chronic pain patients. Reports of depression among chronic pain populations range from 10 to 87 percent.[24] Patients with two or more pain conditions have been found to be at elevated risk for major depression, whereas those patients with only one pain condition did not show such an elevated rate of mood disorder in a large sample of health maintenance organization (HMO) patients. The relative severity of the depression observed in chronic pain patients was illustrated by Katon and Sullivan,[25] who showed that 32 percent of a sample of 37 pain patients met criteria for major depression and 43 percent had a past episode of major depression.

Anxiety is especially common among those with acute pain. Like depression, it may be an appropriate response to serious trauma through injury or illness. Pain may serve a signal function or be part of an anxious preoccupation, as in the case of the woman with the sarcoma cited above under Cortical modulation of pain. Similarly, anxiety and pain may reinforce one another, producing a snowball effect of escalating and mutually reinforcing central and peripheral symptoms.

HYPNOSIS

Central psychological approaches to pain control can be highly effective analgesics and are underutilized.[26] It has been known since the middle of the 1800s that hypnosis is effective in controlling even severe surgical pain.[27] Hypnosis and similar techniques work through two primary mechanisms: muscle relaxation and a combination of perceptual alteration and cognitive distraction. Pain is not infrequently accompanied by reactive muscle tension. Patients frequently splint the part of their body that hurts.

Yet, because muscle tension can by itself cause pain in normal tissue and because traction on a painful part of the body can produce more pain, techniques that induce greater physical relaxation can reduce pain in the periphery. Therefore, having patients enter a state of hypnosis so that they can concentrate on an image that connotes physical relaxation, such as floating or lightness, often produces physical relaxation and reduces pain.

The second major component of hypnotic analgesia is perceptual alteration. Patients can be taught to imagine that the affected body part is numb. Temperature metaphors are often especially useful, which is not surprising given the fact that pain and temperature sensations are part of the same sensory system – the lateral spinothalamic tract. Thus, imagining that an affected body part is cooler or warmer using an image of dipping it in ice water or heating it in the sun can often help patients transform pain signals. This is especially useful for extremely hypnotizable individuals who can, for example, relive an experience of dental anesthesia and reproduce the drug-induced sensations of numbness in their cheek, which they can then transfer to the painful part of their body. They can also simply "switch off" perception of the pain with surprising effectiveness.[28, 29] Some patients prefer to imagine that the pain is a substance with dimensions that can be moved or can flow out of the body as if it were a viscous liquid. Others like to imagine that they can step outside their body to, for example, visit another room in the house. Less hypnotizable individuals often do better with distraction techniques that help them focus on competing sensations in another part of the body.

The effectiveness of the specific technique employed depends upon the degree of hypnotic ability of the subject.[30] For example, while most patients can be taught to develop a comfortable floating sensation on the affected body part, highly hypnotizable individuals may simply imagine a shot of Novocain (procain hydrochloride) in the affected area, producing a sense of tingling numbness similar to that experienced in dental work. Other patients may prefer to move the pain to another part of their body, or to dissociate the affected part from the rest of the body. As an extreme form of hypnotically induced, controlled dissociation, some highly hypnotizable patients may imagine themselves floating above their own body, creating distance between themselves and the painful sensation or experience. To some more moderately hypnotizable patients, it may be easier to focus on a change in temperature, either warmth or coolness. Low hypnotizable subjects often do better with simple distraction, focusing on sensations in another part of their body, such as the delicate sensations in their fingertips.

The images or metaphors used for pain control employ certain general principles. The first is that the hypnotically controlled image may serve to "filter the hurt out of the pain." They also learn to transform the pain experience. They acknowledge that the pain exists, but there is a distinction between the signal itself and the discomfort the signal causes. The hypnotic experience, which they create and control, helps them transform the signal into one that is less uncomfortable. So patients expand their perceptual options by having them change from an experience in which either the pain is there or it is not to an experience in which they see a third option, in which the pain is there but transformed by the presence of such competing sensations as tingling, numbness, warmth, or coolness. Finally, patients are taught not to fight the pain. Fighting pain only enhances it by focusing attention on the pain, enhancing related anxiety and depression, and increasing physical tension that can literally put traction on painful parts of the body and increase the pain signals generated peripherally (**Box 13.1**).

For patients undergoing painful procedures, such as bone marrow aspirations, the main focus is on the hypnotic imagery *per se* rather than relaxation. This works especially well with children since they are so highly hypnotizable and easily absorbed in images.[31, 32] Patients may be guided through the experience while the procedure is performed, or a given scenario can be suggested and later the patient can undergo the experience hypnotically while the procedure is under way. This enables them to restructure their experience of what is going on and dissociate themselves psychologically from pain and fear intrinsic to their immediate situation. A large-scale randomized trial compared hypnosis with nonspecific emotional support and routine care during invasive radiological procedures. All patients had access to patient-controlled intravenous analgesic medication consisting of midazolam and fentanyl. The hypnosis condition provided significantly greater analgesia and relief of anxiety, despite patient use of one-half the medication. Furthermore, with hypnosis there were fewer procedural complications such as hemodynamic instability, the procedures took on average 18 minutes less time, and the overall cost was reduced by $348 per procedure.[33] A standardized 15-minute script before surgery for breast

cancer resulted in substantial reduction in pain, medication use, procedure time, and cost.[34, 35] Modern virtual reality techniques have also been shown to enhance hypnotic analgesia.[36] Thus hypnosis is increasingly used in the medical setting in conjunction with pharmacological and other pain interventions.

SELF-HYPNOSIS

Hypnotic techniques can easily be taught to patients for self-administration.[5, 6] Pain patients can be taught to enter a state of self-hypnosis in a matter of seconds with some simple induction strategies, such as looking up while slowly closing their eyes, taking a deep breath and then letting the breath out, their eyes relax, and imagining that their body is floating and that one hand is so light it can float up in the air like a balloon. They are then instructed in the pain control exercise, such as coolness or warmth, tingling, or numbness, and taught to bring themselves out by reversing the induction procedure, again looking up, letting the eyes open, and letting the raised hand float back down. Patients can use this exercise every one to two hours initially and any time they experience an attack of pain.[37, 38] They can evaluate their effectiveness in conducting the pain control exercise by rating on a scale from 0 to 10 the intensity of their pain before and after the self-hypnosis session. As with any pain treatment technique, hypnosis is more effective when employed early in the pain cycle, before the pain has become so overwhelming that it impairs concentration. Patients should be encouraged to use this technique early and often because it is simple and effective[39] and has no side effects.[40]

Although not all patients are sufficiently hypnotizable to benefit from these techniques, two out of three adults are at least somewhat hypnotizable,[4] and it has been estimated that hypnotic capacity is correlated at a 0.5 level with effectiveness in medical pain reduction.[41] Furthermore, clinically effective hypnotic analgesia is not confined to those with high hypnotizability,[26] and many subjects who experience little analgesia still find hypnotic techniques helpful for other reasons, such as relaxation.[42]

HYPNOSIS WITH CHILDREN

Hypnosis is especially effective in comforting children who are in pain (see Chapter 40, Mind/body skills for children in pain). Several good studies have shown greater efficacy than placebo attention control.[31, 32, 43] Hypnotic techniques, including going over favorite stories, are quite effective in removing the child from the immediacy of both pain and anxiety.[43] Hypnosis seems to have advantages over distraction, especially among young children undergoing medical procedures.[43] This is likely because children as a group are more hypnotizable than adults.[44] Their

---

Box 13.1 Components of pain treatment utilizing self-hypnosis

- Explain hypnosis.
- Measure hypnotizability.
- Induce relaxation by concentrating on "floating."
- Hypnotic analgesia:
  - concentrate on a competing sensation;
  - warmth, coolness, tingling, lightness, or heaviness;
  - filter the hurt out of the pain.
- Anxiety control: screen technique.
- Exit from self-hypnotic state.
- Instructions in practicing self-hypnosis.

imaginative capacities are so intense that separate relaxation exercises are not necessary. Children naturally relax when they mobilize their imagination during the sensory alteration component of hypnotic analgesia. Self-management utilizing hypnosis and related imagination exercises is becoming a first-line treatment for such problems as headaches among children.[45] In a randomized trial involving the use of hypnosis or routine distraction techniques for children undergoing voiding cystourethrograms, hypnosis proved more effective in reducing pain and distress, facilitating catheterization, and it shortened the procedure time by an average of 17 minutes.[46]

MECHANISMS OF HYPNOTIC ANALGESIA

Recent research indicates cortical effects of hypnotic analgesia exercises, including reduced early receptor potential (ERP) amplitude in response to somatosensory stimuli[47] and increased frontal and parietal blood flow.[48] A positron emission tomography (PET) study indicated reduced activation of the anterior cingulate gyrus during hypnotic analgesia when the hypnotic instruction was that the pain would bother subjects less.[49] However, different wording during hypnosis involving a suggestion of reduced pain perception resulted in analgesia mediated by reduced activity in somatosensory cortex.[50] Thus, hypnotic alteration of nociception seems to involve cortical modulation of pain perception. A recent PET study of hypnotic alteration of color vision provides further evidence of changes in primary association cortex function.[51] When highly hypnotizable subjects were instructed to perceive a gray-tone grid as filled with color, there was a significant increase in blood flow in the lingual gyrus, the primary brain site for color processing. Conversely, when a colored image was "drained" of color hypnotically, blood flow in that region decreased. Thus, with hypnosis, "believing is seeing," and hypnotic changes in sensation are accompanied by changes in brain function that indicate an actual change in perception, not merely an altered response to perception.

A number of studies have tested the idea that endogenous opiates are involved in hypnotic analgesia. However, with one partial exception,[52] studies with both volunteers[53] and patients in chronic pain[54] have shown that hypnotic analgesia is not blocked and reversed by a substantial dose of naloxone given in a double-blind, crossover fashion. Therefore, the cortical attention deployment mechanism is currently the most plausible explanation for hypnotic reduction of pain.

OTHER FORMS OF SELF-REGULATION FOR PAIN

Nearly every self-regulation technique that is used in the treatment of pain and related anxiety and depressive symptoms, including hypnosis, combines various forms of physical relaxation with cognitive restructuring. The principle of combining imagery with physical relaxation is associated with such techniques as systematic desensitization and progressive muscle relaxation. During these treatments, patients are instructed to maintain a physical sense of relaxation, while restructuring pain-related fears. A stimulus hierarchy is then developed from least to most stressful. Patients are taught to develop their own scenarios and to augment or reduce the intensity of the stimulus within seconds, as the therapist helps them to construct and evaluate analgesic imagery. These techniques are designed to disrupt the conditioned association between pain, anxiety about disease, and somatic tension which amplifies pain and focuses more attention on it. With all such approaches, patient practice of the techniques learned is crucial to sustained effectiveness, and should encourage patients to enhance their sense of control over symptoms.[55]

Mindfulness-based stress reduction

One successful but somewhat different approach to self-regulation for pain has been mindfulness-based stress reduction. Based upon Eastern Buddhist meditative traditions, the approach involves exercises aimed at altering the management of consciousness and the experience of perception in general, rather than influencing pain in particular.[56, 57, 58, 59] In this practice, subjects are taught to spend approximately 30 minutes twice a day in a quiet state of meditation, focusing on present experience, inducing physical relaxation, and seeing anxieties as a focus on future possibilities that take away from enjoyment of the moment. The three main components of this practice are: focused attention, open presence, and compassion. Normal subjects show an increase in pain tolerance after being taught mindfulness techniques.[55] Such techniques have proven quite effective with chronic pain,[60, 61] for example among older adults with back pain,[62] and have been shown to speed healing time for patients with psoriasis.[63]

Biofeedback

A National Institutes of Health (NIH) Technology Assessment Panel reported that techniques such as hypnosis and biofeedback are effective in reducing chronic pain.[64] Although hypnosis focuses on internally generated images, biofeedback utilizes external feedback from monitors that assess heart rate, skin conductance, skin temperature, blood pressure, muscle tension, and other physiological measures. These measures are related to the functioning of the autonomic and peripheral nervous systems, and biofeedback training in modulation of perception can facilitate anxiety and pain reduction.[65, 66]

Often, pain can be attenuated by altering peripheral skin temperature in the affected area. Similarly, skill in reducing muscle tension via muscle tension biofeedback may reduce secondary intensification of pain. Thermal biofeedback is effective in reducing the sensory component of phantom limb pain[67] and muscle tension biofeedback is useful for whiplash injuries.[68] Such training is also useful for headaches, especially among children and adolescents.[69] Thus, training in reducing physiological responses to pain, such as muscle tension, sweating, and vasoconstriction, can help to interrupt the feedback cycle of somatic distress and affective preoccupation that frequently intensifies pain.

MANAGING EXPECTANCY

Expectancy has well-established effects on pain, both through placebo and nocebo (worsening) of pain. Mechanisms of such effects include classical conditioning[70, 71] which is neurologically explainable in part through coactiviation of the anterior cingulate gyrus, which engages in focal attention and conflict detection,[72, 73] and the periaqueductal gray, which process pain.[74] Negative expectancy leading to increase in pain, the nocebo effect, may be mediated by secretion of cholecystokinin.[75, 76] It is particularly important to separate the expectation of efficacy of psychological techniques from speculation about the etiology of the pain. Many patients (and doctors) assume that, if a psychological or placebo intervention reduces pain, the pain itself is "supratentorial." Nothing could be further from the truth. People can, as noted above, diminish or even ignore major injury and other forms of physical pain. The tissue injury is real, but they learn to alter their perception of it. To imply to a patient that such success means that the pain is not "real" undermines motivation and can be perceived by patients as insulting. Rather, it is best to utilize a "rehabilitation" model, teaching patients that they are learning to overcome a serious pain problem rather than proving that it was not so bad in the first place. In this way, patients can receive immediate emotional gratification from improvement, rather than feel ashamed of their ability to reduce pain.

CONCLUSION

The old dichotomy between peripheral and central pain is being replaced by a more complex and comprehensive analysis that evaluates central and peripheral components of pain and designs interventions that take advantage of therapeutic opportunities at all levels of pain perception processing. This point of view is important because it underscores the fact that successful psychosocial intervention for reducing pain may occur via understandable neurological mechanisms and does not prove that the pain is largely functional. In the same way, successful pharmacological intervention does not prove that the pain is completely peripheral in origin. Most pain syndromes are a combination of physical and neuropsychiatric distress and dysfunction and require a combination of biological and psychosocial intervention to be optimally effective. In particular, effective strategies, such as hypnosis, that provide a means for self-regulation of pain reduce the helplessness associated with pain, as well as inducing physical relaxation and literally altering pain perception, not just response to pain input. The strain in pain lies mainly in the brain.

REFERENCES

1. Koller P, Marmar CR, Kanas N. Psychodynamic group treatment of posttraumatic stress disorder in Vietnam veterans. *International Journal of Group Psychotherapy*. 1992; **42**: 225–46.
2. Spiegel D. Hypnosis in the treatment of victims of sexual abuse. *Psychiatric Clinics of North America*. 1989; **12**: 295–305.
* 3. Butler LD, Duran RE, Jasiukaitis P et al. Hypnotizability and traumatic experience: a diathesis-stress model of dissociative symptomatology. *American Journal of Psychiatry*. 1996; **153**: 42–63.
4. Spiegel H, Spiegel D. *Trance and treatment: clincial uses of hypnosis*. Washington, DC: American Psychiatric Press, 2004.
* 5. Spiegel D, Maldonado J. Hypnosis. In: Hales R, Yudsofsky S, Talbott J (eds). *American Psychiatric Press textbook of psychiatry*. Washington, DC: American Psychiatric Press, 1999.
6. Spiegel H, Greenleaf M, Spiegel D. Hypnosis. In: Sadock B, Sadock V (eds). *Comprehensive textbook of psychiatry*, 7th edn. Philadelphia, PA: Lippincott Williams & Wilkins, 2000: 2128–46.
* 7. Tellegen A, Atkinson G. Openess to absorbing and self-altering experiences ("absorption"), a trait related to hypnotic susceptibility. *Journal of Abnormal Psychology*. 1974; **83**: 268–77.
8. Tellegen A. Practicing the two disciplines for relaxation and enlightenment: comment on "Role of the feedback signal in electromyograph biofeedback: the relevance of attention" by Qualls and Sheehan. *Journal of Experimental Psychology. General*. 1981; **110**: 217–31.
9. Melzack R. From the gate to the neuromatrix. *Pain*. 1999; August (Suppl. 6): S121–6.
* 10. Golianu B, Bhandari R, Shaw R et al. Neuropsychiatric Aspects of Pain Management. In: Yudofsky S, Hales R (eds). *The American Psychiatric Publishing textbook of neuropsychiatry and behavioral neurosciences*. Washington, DC: American Psychiatric Press, 2007.
11. Kuhn CC, Bradnan WA. Pain as a substitute for the fear of death. *Psychosomatics*. 1979; **20**: 494–5.

12. Spiegel D. Dissociation and hypnosis in post-traumatic stress disorder. *Journal of Trauma and Stress.* 1988; **1**: 17–33.

13. Berger A, Posner MI. Pathologies of brain attentional networks. *Neuroscience and Biobehavioral Reviews.* 2000; **24**: 3–5.

∗ 14. Posner MI, Petersen SE. The attention system of the human brain. *Annual Review of Neuroscience.* 1990; **13**: 25–42.

∗ 15. Melzack R. Recent concepts of Pain. *Journal of Medicine.* 1982; **13**: 147–60.

∗ 16. Beecher HK. Relationship of significance of wound to pain experienced. *Journal of the American Medical Association.* 1956; **161**: 1609–13.

17. Spiegel D, Bloom JR. Pain in metastatic breast cancer. *Cancer.* 1983; **52**: 341–5.

18. Blumer D, Zorick F, Heilbronn M, Roth T. Biological markers for depression in chronic pain. *Journal of Nervous and Mental Disease.* 1982; **170**: 425–8.

19. Bond MR. Personality studies in patients with pain secondary to organic disease. *Journal of Psychosomatic Research.* 1973; **17**: 257–63.

20. Woodforde JM, Fielding JR. Pain and cancer. *Journal of Psychosomatic Research.* 1970; **14**: 365–70.

21. Peteet J, Tay V, Cohen G, MacIntyre J. Pain characteristics and treatment in an outpatient cancer population. *Cancer.* 1986; **57**: 1259–65.

22. Spiegel D, Sands S. Pain management in the cancer patient. *Journal of Psychosocial Oncology.* 1988; **6**: 205–16.

∗ 23. Spiegel D, Sands S, Koopman C. Pain and depression in patients with cancer. *Cancer.* 1994; **74**: 2570–8.

∗ 24. Dworkin SF, Von Korff M, LeResche L. Multiple pains and psychiatric disturbance. An epidemiologic investigation. *Archives of General Psychiatry.* 1990; **47**: 239–44.

25. Katon W, Sullivan MD. Depression and chronic medical illness. *Journal of Clinical Psychiatry.* 1990; **51**: 3–11; discussion 2–4.

∗ 26. Holroyd J. Hypnosis treatment of clinical pain: understanding why hypnosis is useful. *International Journal of Clinical and Experimental Hypnosis.* 1996; **44**: 33–51.

27. Esdaile J. *Hypnosis in medicine and surgery.* New York: Juian Press, 1846 (reprinted 1957).

28. Miller ME, Bowers KS. Hypnosis analgesia: dissociated experience or dissociated control? *Journal of Abnormal Psychology.* 1993; **102**: 29–38.

29. Hargadon R, Bowers KS, Woody EZ. Does counterpain imagery mediate hypnotic analgesia? *Journal of Abnormal Psychology.* 1995; **104**: 508–16.

∗ 30. Jensen M, Patterson DR. Hypnotic treatment of chronic pain. *Journal of Behavioral Medicine.* 2006; **29**: 95–124.

∗ 31. Hilgard JR, LeBaron S. Relief of anxiety and pain in children and adolescents with cancer: quantitative measures and clinical observations. *International Journal of Clinical and Experimental Hypnosis.* 1982; **30**: 417–42.

∗ 32. Zeltzer L, LeBaron S. Hypnosis and non hypnotic techniques for reduction of pain and anxiety during painful procedures in children and adolescents with cancer. *Journal of Pediatrics.* 1982; **101**: 1032–5.

∗ 33. Lang EV, Benotsch EG, Fick LJ et al. Adjunctive non-pharmacological analgesia for invasive medical procedures: a randomised trial. *Lancet.* 2000; **355**: 1486–90.

∗ 34. Montgomery GH, Bovbjerg DH, Schnur JB et al. A randomized clinical trial of a brief hypnosis intervention to control side effects in breast surgery patients. *Journal of the National Cancer Institute.* 2007; **99**: 1304–12.

35. Spiegel D. The mind prepared: hypnosis in surgery. *Journal of the National Cancer Institute.* 2007; **99**: 1280–1.

∗ 36. Patterson DR, Wiechman SA, Jensen M, Sharar SR. Hypnosis delivered through immersive virtual reality for burn pain: A clinical case series. *International Journal of Clinical and Experimental Hypnosis.* 2006; **54**: 130–42.

∗ 37. Spiegel H, Spiegel D. *Trance and treatment: clinical uses of hypnosis.* Washington, DC: American Psychiatric Press, 2004.

∗ 38. Patterson DR, Jensen MP. Hypnosis and clinical pain. *Psychological Bulletin.* 2003; **129**: 495–521.

∗ 39. Spiegel D, Bloom JR. Group therapy and hypnosis reduce metastatic breast carcinoma pain. *Psychosomatic Medicine.* 1983; **45**: 333–9.

∗ 40. Spiegel D. Oncological and pain syndromes. In: Hales R, Francis A (eds). *American Psychiatric Association annual review.* Washington, DC: American Psychiatric Association Press, 1986.

∗ 41. Hilgard ER, Hilgard ER. *Hypnosis in the relief of pain.* Los Altos, CA: Kauffman, William, 1975.

42. Jensen MP, McArthur KD, Barber J et al. Satisfaction with, and the beneficial side effects of, hypnotic analgesia. *International Journal of Clinical and Experimental Hypnosis.* 2006; **54**: 432–47.

43. Kuttner L. Favorite stories: a hypnotic pain-reduction technique for children in acute pain. *American Journal of Clinical Hypnosis.* 1988; **30**: 289–95.

44. Morgan AH, Hilgard ER. Age differences in susceptibility to hypnosis. *International Journal of Clinical and Experimental Hypnosis.* 1972; **21**: 78–85.

∗ 45. Kuttner L. Managing pain in children. Changing treatment of headaches. *Canadian Family Physician.* 1993; **39**: 563–8.

46. Butler LD, Symons BK, Henderson SL et al. Hypnosis reduces distress and duration of an invasive medical procedure for children. *Pediatrics.* 2005; **115**: e77–85.

∗ 47. Spiegel D, Bierre P, Rootenberg J. Hypnotic alteration of somatosensory perception. *American Journal of Psychiatry.* 1989; **146**: 749–54.

48. Crawford HJ, Gur RC, Skolnick B et al. Effects of hypnosis on regional cerebral blood flow during ischemic pain with and without suggested hypnotic analgesia. *International Journal of Psychophysiology.* 1993; **15**: 181–95.

∗ 49. Rainville P, Duncan GH, Price DD et al. Pain affect encoded in human anterior cingulate but not somatosensory cortex. Science. 1997; **277**: 968–71.

∗ 50. Rainville P, Carrier B, Hofbauer RK et al. Dissociation of sensory and affective dimensions of pain using hypnotic modulation. Pain. 1999; **82**: 159–71.

∗ 51. Kosslyn SM, Thompson WL, Costantini-Ferrando MF et al. Hypnotic visual illusion alters color processing in the brain. American Journal of Psychiatry. 2000; **157**: 1279–84.

52. Frid M, Singer G. Hypnotic analgesia in conditions of stress is partially reversed by naloxone. Psychopharmacology (Berl). 1979; **63**: 211–15.

53. Goldstein A, Hilgard ER. Failure of the opiate antagonist naloxone to modify hypnotic analgesia. Proceedings of the National Academy of Sciences of the United States of America. 1975; **72**: 2041–3.

54. Spiegel D, Albert LH. Naloxone fails to reverse hypnotic alleviation of chronic pain. Psychopharmacology (Berl). 1983; **81**: 140–3.

55. Kingston J, Chadwick P, Meron D, Skinner TC. A pilot randomized control trial investigating the effect of mindfulness practice on pain tolerance, psychological well-being, and physiological activity. Journal of Psychosomatic Research. 2007; **62**: 297–300.

∗ 56. Kabat-Zinn J, Massion AO, Hebert JR, Rosenbaum E. Meditation. In: Holland J (ed.). Psychooncology. New York: Oxford University Press, 1998: 767–79.

57. Kabat-Zinn J. Mindfulness meditation:health benefits of a Buddhist practice. In: Gurion GA (ed.). Mind body medicine. New York: Consumer Reports, 1993.

58. Kabat-Zinn J. An outpatient program in behavioral medicine for chronic pain patients based on the practice of mindfulness meditation:theoretic considerations and preliminary results. Revision. 1984; **7**: 71–2.

∗ 59. Kabat-Zinn J, Lipworth L, Burney R. The clinical use of mindfulness meditation for the self-regulation of chronic pain. Journal of Behavioral Medicine. 1985; **8**: 163–90.

60. Gerard S, Smith BH, Simpson JA. A randomized controlled trial of spiritual healing in restricted neck movement. Journal of Alternative and Complementary Medicine. 2003; **9**: 467–77.

61. Grossman P, Niemann L, Schmidt S, Walach H. Mindfulness-based stress reduction and health benefits. A meta-analysis. Journal of Psychosomatic Research. 2004; **57**: 35–43.

62. Morone NE, Greco CM, Weiner DK. Mindfulness meditation for the treatment of chronic low back pain in older adults: A randomized controlled pilot study. Pain. 2008; **134**: 310–19.

∗ 63. Kabat-Zinn J, Wheeler E, Light T et al. Influence of a mindfulness meditation-based stress reduction intervention on rates of skin clearing in patients with moderate to severe psoriasis undergoing phototherapy (UVB) and photochemotherapy (PUVA). Psychosomatic Medicine. 1998; **60**: 625–32.

∗ 64. NIH Technology Assessment Panel on Integration of Behavioral and Relaxation Approaches into the Treatment of Chronic Pain and Insomnia. Integration of behavioral and relaxation approaches into the treatment of chronic pain and insomnia. Journal of the American Medical Association. 1998; **276**: 313–18.

65. Spiegel D. Facilitating emotional coping during treatment. Cancer. 1990; **66**: 1422–6.

66. Titlebaum H. Relaxation. In: Zahourek RP (ed.). Relaxation and imagery: tools for therapeutic communication and intervention. Philadelphia, PA: W.B. Saunders Harcourt Brace Jovanovich, 1988: 28–52.

67. Harden RN, Houle TT, Green S et al. Biofeedback in the treatment of phantom limb pain: a time-series analysis. Applied Psychophysiology and Biofeedback. 2005; **30**: 83–93.

68. Voerman GE, Vollenbroek-Hutten MM, Hermens HJ. Changes in pain, disability, and muscle activation patterns in chronic whiplash patients after ambulant myofeedback training. Clinical Journal of Pain. 2006; **22**: 656–63.

69. Trautmann E, Lackschewitz H, Kroner-Herwig B. Psychological treatment of recurrent headache in children and adolescents – a meta-analysis. Cephalalgia. 2006; **26**: 1411–26.

70. Charron J, Rainville P, Marchand S. Direct comparison of placebo effects on clinical and experimental pain. Clinical Journal of Pain. 2006; **22**: 204–11.

71. Klinger R, Soost S, Flor H, Worm M. Classical conditioning and expectancy in placebo hypoalgesia: a randomized controlled study in patients with atopic dermatitis and persons with healthy skin. Pain. 2007; **128**: 31–9.

∗ 72. Raz A, Fan J, Posner MI. Hypnotic suggestion reduces conflict in the human brain. Proceedings of the National Academy of Sciences of the United States of America. 2005; **102**: 9978–83.

73. Raz A. Attention and hypnosis: neural substrates and genetic associations of two converging processes. International Journal of Clinical and Experimental Hypnosis. 2005; **53**: 237–58.

∗ 74. Wager TD, Scott DJ, Zubieta JK. Placebo effects on human mu-opioid activity during pain. Proceedings of the National Academy of Sciences of the United States of America. 2007; **104**: 11056–61.

∗ 75. Benedetti F, Lanotte M, Lopiano L, Colloca L. When words are painful: unraveling the mechanisms of the nocebo effect. Neuroscience. 2007; **147**: 260–71.

76. Colloca L, Benedetti F. Nocebo hyperalgesia: how anxiety is turned into pain. Current Opinion in Anaesthesiology. 2007; **20**: 435–9.

Biofeedback

FRANK ANDRASIK AND HERTA FLOR

KEY LEARNING POINTS

- Biofeedback is a self-regulation approach that is used in two basic ways in pain management.
- One approach uses feedback of muscle tension, peripheral temperature, and/or skin conductance to help facilitate overall relaxation and reduce general arousal.
- The other approach uses a comprehensive psychophysiological assessment (that includes multiple stimulus conditions and multiple response measures) to identify specific modalities to train.
- Biofeedback is rarely used in isolation; rather it is more typically combined with other cognitive and behavioral procedures to optimize effectiveness.
- Efficacy and meta-analytic reviews document its effectiveness for varied pain conditions.

INTRODUCTION

Pain is a complex, multiply determined behavior that typically requires a multifaceted, multidimensional, and multidisciplinary approach. Biofeedback is often a component of treatment and, although this chapter focuses on biofeedback as an isolated technique, it is rarely if ever applied in isolation. It is often combined with various cognitive and behavioral approaches (see Chapter 13, Self-regulation skills training for adults, including relaxation and Chapter 15, Contextual cognitive-behavioral therapy). More typically, it is one of many options that patients and therapists consider.

Biofeedback has been defined as:[1]

> ...a process in which a person learns to reliably influence physiological responses of two kinds: either responses which are not ordinarily under voluntary control or responses which ordinarily are easily regulated but for which regulation has broken down due to trauma or disease.

The process of biofeedback involves three operations. In the first step, a biological response is detected and amplified by using certain measurement devices (or transducers) and electronic amplifiers. The bioelectrical potentials detected at this stage are in a form that is difficult to utilize in biofeedback. For example, raw or unprocessed muscle tension potentials resemble the static that one usually sees between channels of a radio, and few individuals would be capable of detecting even gross changes in electrical activity when displayed in this manner. The second step involves converting the bioelectrical signals to a form that can be easily understood and easily processed by the patient. Averaging the electrical signal over a specified time period and filtering out unwanted aspects of the signals are examples of ways in which this is accomplished. The third step involves the relatively immediate feedback of a meaningful signal to the patient. This feedback is most often presented in auditory and visual modalities and in either binary (signal on/signal off at a specified threshold value; commonly used when shaping is a goal) or continuous proportional fashion (as muscle tension decreases, the tone or click rate decreases); on occasion, combinations of both are used. With all responses, care must be taken to ensure that areas of sensor placement are adequately prepped and that the measuring devices are placed on the proper locations. These factors are especially crucial in electromyography (EMG) and electroencephalography (EEG) because of the weak electrical signals that are detected. Here, electrode sites may need to be cleaned thoroughly with acetone or alcohol and lightly abraded (although advances in instrumentation are making this less necessary). With some recordings, a conductive gel or electrolyte is placed between the electrodes and the subject's skin to facilitate conductance and reduce measurement artifact (some sensors come pregelled). More detailed discussion of physiology, electrical theory, and bases of the primary responses utilized in biofeedback may be found in Peek[2] and various chapters within Andreassi,[3] Cacioppo et al.,[4] and Stern et al.[5] Various theories have been used to account for biofeedback, ranging from operant learning to cognitive and expectancy models.[6]

APPROACHES TO BIOFEEDBACK

Three different rationales or approaches have been offered for the use of biofeedback in pain management;[7, 8] here, for simplicity, they will be termed general, specific, and indirect.

General approach

The general approach employs biofeedback as an aid to general or overall relaxation training. Two assumptions underlie this use. Assumption 1 is that a reduction in general arousal leads to a concurrent reduction in central processing of peripheral sensory inputs. Assumption 2 derives from the observed relationship between anxiety and pain – anxiety is associated with decreased pain tolerance and increased reports of pain. Therefore, achievement of a more relaxed state should lead to concomitant reductions in anxiety, which in turn enhance pain tolerance and decrease pain reports. Researchers using realtime functional magnetic resonance imaging (fMRI) have shown that distraction, a component of self-regulation, activates brain structures (primarily the periaqueductal gray) associated with pain regulation.[9, 10] Activation of these brain structures has been implicated in

the anticipation of pain[11] and the anxiety associated with pain.[12] The anticipation of pain and the activation of these brain structures prior to an expected painful stimulus may account for the enhanced sensitivity to pain shown by patients with chronic pain[10] (see Andrasik and Rime[13] for a more extended discussion). Thus, one can make the case that nearly all pain patients could benefit from relaxation and tension reduction. Thus, this approach is probably the most common. It also requires the least technical proficiency.

Specific approach

The specific biofeedback approach attempts to target and modify the physiological dysfunction or response system assumed to underlie the pain condition. This approach has its origins in the pain–spasm–pain cycle first described by Bonica.[14] In implementing this approach, therapists assess psychophysiological responding, under varied stimulus conditions, in the modalities assumed to be relevant to the condition being treated. In the text to follow, comments will be restricted to peripheral measures, as these have garnered the greatest attention by researchers and clinicians. Furthermore, most of the examples presented here relate to muscle tension, as this is the response modality found most useful when working with pain patients. Readers seeking information about the much less studied central measures of pain are referred to Flor.[8]

Flor[8] has pointed out the functions, utility, and advantages of psychophysiological data collection when using the specific approach to the treatment of chronic pain. Use of this approach helps to:

- provide evidence for the role of psychological factors in maladaptive physiological functioning;
- satisfy, thus, a necessary prerequisite or justification for the use of biofeedback therapy;
- facilitate tailoring of treatments to patients;
- allow therapists and researchers to document efficacy, generalization, and transfer of treatment;
- identify potential predictors of treatment response;
- serve as a source of motivation (e.g. patients come to realize they are able to influence bodily processes by their own thoughts, emotions, and actions; their feelings of helplessness decrease; they concurrently become more open to psychological approaches in general, etc.).

Key components of the psychophysiological assessment (or "psychophysiological stress profile" as some have labelled this approach) are summarized in **Table 14.1** and are discussed more fully in Flor[8] and Arena and Schwartz,[15] among others. A brief outline of the various stages involved in carrying out a psychophysiological assessment follows.

Table 14.1 Components to a psychophysiological assessment for chronic pain.

Component	Brief description
Adaptation/habituation	Time to adjust to clinic/laboratory setting and to allow responses to stabilize
Baseline	
At rest	Serves as basis of comparison for subsequent data collection
Preexisting abilities	Assess current abilities to relax
Stress reactivity/real world	Simulate situations that occur in everyday life
Reactivity	
Somatic	Body position and posture; dynamic movement, such as standing, sitting, bending, lifting, walking, etc.; work task, such as typing on a keyboard
Psychological	Stressful imagery, such as a negative encounter with a colleague or family member
Stress recovery	Time required to return to the baseline level
Muscle scanning	Brief sequential recordings from multiple bilateral sites under varied conditions
Muscle discrimination	Estimation of muscle tension levels

ADAPTATION

The adaptation component is included for three main reasons:

1. to allow patients to become familiar with the setting and recording procedure;
2. to minimize presession effects (rushing to the appointment, temperature and humidity differences between office and outdoors);
3. to permit habituation of the orienting response and allow the response to stabilize.

Although the need for a prebaseline period is widely acknowledged, scant research has been conducted to help identify key parameters of adaptation. Most, but not all, individuals will adapt within 5–20 minutes (some individuals, though, are not fully adapted even after a standard 50/60-minute session). Practitioners are encouraged to extend this period until some stability is achieved for the key responses of interest (variability is minimized, the trend line levels off). Patients are instructed merely to sit quietly during this period.

BASELINE

Once adapted, the clinician will need to collect some type of baseline data. The baseline data serve as the basis of comparison for subsequent assessment phases and as the basis for gauging progress within and across future treatment sessions. Again, there are no definitive data to document the optimal approach (Should eyes be open or closed? Should the patient be fully reclined or sitting upright? Should conditions be neutral or designed to promote relaxation?) or the desired duration of baseline data collection. In clinical practice, the baseline period typically ranges from one to five minutes, sufficient to obtain an adequate sample.

When the goal of biofeedback is generalized relaxation, it is useful to collect a second baseline to assess preexisting abilities to regulate physiology. To accomplish this, the patient is instructed as follows: "I would now like to see what happens when you try to relax as deeply as you can. Use whatever means you believe will be helpful. Please let me know when you are as relaxed as possible." Often, it is found that the techniques currently being employed by a patient are not achieving the desired effect, which can be therapeutic in its own right.

It was once believed that elevated resting levels of muscle tension might be a unique characteristic of patients experiencing chronic pain. A review of 60 psychophysiological investigations conducted with headache, back, and temporomandibular pain and dysfunction (TMD) patients found minimal support for this notion.[16] Research on this topic, however, is compounded by questions about measurement reliability and stability.[8, 15]

REACTIVITY

The third component investigates psychophysiology in response to simulated stressors that are personally relevant or to conditions that approximate real-world events that are associated with pain onset or exacerbation. Again, there is no standard, empirically validated approach. Some examples of commonly used stimulus conditions are:

- negative imagery, wherein a patient concentrates on a personally relevant unpleasant situation (the details of which have been obtained during the intake interview);

- cold exposure (e.g. Raynaud's disease) or cold pressor test (as a general physical stressor);
- movement, such as sitting, rising, bending, stooping, or walking;
- load bearing, such as lifting or carrying an object;
- operation of a keyboard, given the ubiquitous nature of computer usage.

Although baseline differences for EMG have not been found to reliably characterize pain disorders, symptom-specific responses to stimuli have been found for certain pain conditions on a more consistent basis (for a review, see Flor[8]).

RECOVERY

Another component involves assessing recovery or return to baseline, as one of the distinguishing features of a pain or stress response is the inability to recover in a timely manner. If multiple stressful stimuli are presented to a patient, then a poststress recovery period is recommended after each stimulus presentation. This phase continues until the patient's physiology returns to a value close to that observed prior to stimulus presentation (often, responses do not fully return to their starting values).

The above components constitute the basic approach to psychophysiological assessment. The two remaining components, listed in **Table 14.1**, are less common in practice, but may be useful as well. We will return to the two remaining components in Muscle scanning and Muscle discrimination below.

Figure 14.1 provides a sample psychophysiological profile. EMG activity was recorded bilaterally from three sites (masseter, frontal, and trapezius muscles) during baseline, imagined neutral, stress, and pain situations, as well as during extended mental stress (difficult mathematical problems) and movement. Skin conductance and heart rate were monitored as well. The following information was obtained from this evaluation.

- EMG resting values were markedly elevated and asymmetrical;

- EMG values increased in response to imagery and this was particularly so for the imagined pain episodes;
- EMG values were markedly exacerbated by movement;
- Skin conductance and heart rate were found to be unresponsive.

Treatment would then be focused on reducing tension in relevant muscles and altering responding during presentations of simulated aversive situations, such as the therapist displaying verbal aggression to the patient.

MUSCLE SCANNING

Cram[17] developed an approach that permits a therapist to assess EMG activity quickly from a greater number of sites than we have disussed thus far and in a manner that does not require a large number of recording channels (only two are needed). This approach is made possible by the use of two hand-held "post" electrodes, which are used to obtain brief (around two seconds per site) sequential bilateral recordings while the patient is sitting and standing. Before his death, Cram was developing a normative database designed to help the therapist determine whether any readings are abnormally high or low and whether any asymmetries (right side versus left side differences) existed, as these were thought to be suggestive of bracing or favoring of a position or posture. The goal of biofeedback, in this application, is to return aberrant readings to a more normal state. Although this type of approach seems straightforward at first, in effect it is more complex. A number of factors can influence the readings obtained, including the angle and force by which the sensors are applied, the amount of adipose tissue present (fat acts as an insulator and dampens the signal), and the degree to which the sensors are placed in a similar location to that used for the norming sample (plus other variables that affect EMG in general). Sella[18] employs a similar approach.

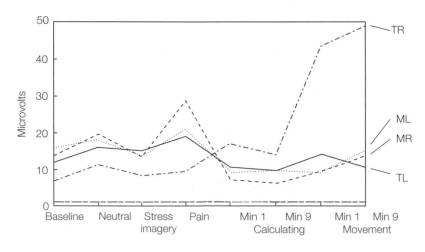

Figure 14.1 Phases of the examination, with only select measures being displayed. ML, masseter left; MR, masseter right; TL, trapezius left; TR, trapezius right. Data from Flor.[8]

MUSCLE DISCRIMINATION

Some have speculated that an inability to perceive bodily states accurately may be one of the factors serving to maintain chronic pain. Flor and colleagues found that patients with chronic pain were unable to perceive muscle tension levels accurately in both the affected and non-affected muscles and that, when exposed to tasks requiring production of muscle tension, these patients overestimated physical symptoms, rated the task as more aversive, and reported greater pain.[19, 20] These findings point to a heightened sensitivity.

Flor[8] has outlined a procedure that can be easily used to assess muscle discrimination abilities in a clinical setting.

- Present the patient with a bar of varying height that is displayed on a monitor.
- Instruct the patient to tense the targeted muscle to the level reflected in the height of the bar.
- Vary the bar height from low to high.
- Correlate the EMG readings obtained with the actual heights of the bars.
- Define as "good" discrimination abilities correlation coefficients ≥ 0.80.
- Define as "bad" or poor discrimination abilities correlation coefficients ≤ 0.50.

SUMMARY

Finally, Flor[8] has offered a number of recommendations for conducting psychophysiological assessment with pain patients. These are reproduced in **Box 14.1**.

Indirect approach

What is termed here as the "indirect" approach for employing biofeedback with pain patients is used more for clinical than for empirical reasons.[7] This model views biofeedback as a means of facilitating psychosomatic therapy. Take the case of the pain patient who steadfastly holds to a purely somatic view and refuses to accept the notion that other factors (emotional, behavioral, environmental) may be precipitating, perpetuating, or exacerbating pain and somatic symptoms. With such patients, a referral for biofeedback is likely to be less threatening (it is construed as a physical treatment for a physical problem) and to at least open the door for help. As physiological insight is acquired, such patients may begin to comprehend the broader picture, i.e. the interplay of physical and psychological factors. In fact, it is not all that uncommon for a pain patient who denies psychological factors upon entry to therapy to make a request such as the following after just a few sessions of biofeedback: "Doc, how about turning off the biofeedback equipment today. I want to talk about a few things." From this point on, session time is divided between

Box 14.1 Recommendations for psychophysiological assessment

- Use multiaxial classification of patients to identify specific somatic and psychosocial characteristics of the patients.
- If possible, use normative data from controls.
- Control for pain status (i.e. test in a pain-free and a painful state, if possible).
- Control for medication (i.e. make sure patient has not taken analgesic or psychotropic medication for several days, if possible).
- Use sites both proximal and distal to the painful site.
- Make sure that the measures selected are relevant for the specific type of pain being studied (e.g. temperature recordings for Raynaud syndrome, rather than EMG levels).
- Use ecologically valid methods of stress induction (i.e. use self-selected stressors; test stressfulness by assessing subjective stress rating, heart rate, or skin conductance levels).
- Use sufficiently long adaptation phases and baselines.
- Use a syndrome-specific and a general autonomic measure.

biofeedback and psychotherapy. Nothing further will be said about this aspect. We continue with more extended discussion of the general and specific approaches.

BIOFEEDBACK AS A GENERAL AID TO RELAXATION

Any response modality indicative of heightened arousal theoretically can serve as a target for promoting relaxation. In practice, three have served most commonly as targets for overall relaxation – muscle tension, skin conductance (perhaps better known as sweat gland activity), and peripheral temperature. These modalities, termed the workhorses of the biofeedback general practitioner,[21] are easily collected, quantified, and interpreted and are discussed below under Electromyographic-assisted relaxation, Skin conductance-assisted relaxation, and Skin temperature-assisted relaxation. Other responses can be of value as well, including heart rate, respiration, and blood volume, but these will not be addressed further (for a discussion, see Flor[8]).

Electromyographic–assisted relaxation

The rationale for employing muscle tension (and skin conductance) feedback to facilitate relaxation is straightforward. The basis of the EMG signal is the small electrochemical changes that occur when a muscle contracts. By placing a series of electrodes along the muscle fibers, the muscle action potentials associated with the ion exchange across the membrane of the muscles can be detected and processed. (When single motor units are the focus of treatment, as in the case of muscle rehabilitation, fine wire electrodes that penetrate the skin surface are used.) EMG monitoring from surface sites is accomplished by the use of two active electrodes, separated by one ground electrode, to set up two separate circuits to detect electrical activity that leaks up to the skin surface. With this arrangement, the resultant signal is the difference between the two circuits (with the amount subtracted out considered to be noise). When EMG is used for generalized relaxation, sensors are typically placed on the forehead region (one active sensor about 2.5 cm above the pupil of each eye, with the ground or reference sensor placed above the bridge of the nose). This placement, which employs large-diameter sensors, is sensitive to muscle tension from adjacent areas, possibly down to the upper rib cage.[22] Originally, it was believed that reductions in forehead muscle tension would automatically generalize to most other untrained muscles (hence, promoting a state of cultivated low arousal). This does not automatically occur,[23] so clinicians may need to train patients from several sites in the course of general relaxation treatment (or combine biofeedback with other approaches).

Surface EMG has a power spectrum ranging from about 20 to 10,000 Hz. Some of the commercially available biofeedback machines sample a very limited amount of this range. For example, some machines filter out EMG occurring below 100 Hz. This misses much of the EMG power spectrum and results in lower readings overall. Clinicians need to be aware of the bandpass of their equipment and to realize that readings obtained from one machine may not be comparable with those obtained on another machine where different settings may be employed. Some of the other factors affecting measurement quantity include sensor type and size, sensor placement on the muscle, and distance between sensors.

Skin conductance–assisted relaxation

Electrical activity of the skin, or sweating, has long been thought to be associated with arousal. In fact, in the late 1800s, Romain Virouroux included measures of skin resistance to facilitate understanding when working with cases of hysterical anesthesia.[2, 24] Electrodermal activity became popular and was thought of as a way to read the mind when used by Carl Jung in the early 1900s in word-association experiments. Two separate portions of the central nervous system are believed to be responsible for control of the electrodermal activity.[25] Sensors are typically placed on body surface areas that are most densely populated with "eccrine" sweat glands (such as the palm of the hand or the fingers), as these respond primarily to psychological stimulation and are innervated by the sympathetic branch of the autonomic nervous system.[5] Conductance measures (the reciprocal of resistance; measured in micromhos or microsiemens), as opposed to resistance measures, are preferred in clinical application because the former measures have a linear relationship to the number of sweat glands that are activated. This permits a straightforward explanation to patients (as arousal increases, so does skin conductance; focusing on decreasing skin conductance helps to lower arousal and to achieve an overall state of relaxation).

Skin temperature–assisted relaxation

It is less obvious why skin temperature has been targeted for general relaxation. This is because the first clinical application resulted from a serendipitous finding by clinical researchers at the Menninger Clinic (Topeka, KS, USA). During a standard laboratory evaluation, it was noticed that spontaneous termination of a migraine was accompanied by flushing in the hands and a rapid sizeable rise in surface hand temperature.[26] This led Sargent et al.[26] to pilot test as a treatment a procedure wherein migraineurs were given feedback to raise their hand temperatures as a way to regulate stress and headache activity. Treatment was augmented by components of autogenic training, leading to a procedure they termed "autogenic feedback." Noting that constriction of peripheral blood flow is under the control of the sympathetic branch of the nervous system, these researchers reasoned that decreases in sympathetic outflow led to increased vasodilation, blood flow, and a resultant rise in peripheral temperature (owing to the warmth of the blood). Thus, temperature feedback may be viewed as yet another way to facilitate general relaxation. With migraine headache, other approaches, assumed to be tied more directly to the underlying physiology, have also been attempted. These include blood flow in various arteries and EEG. These approaches are either quite specialized and/or have not been the focus of extensive research, so they will not be discussed further.

SELECT TREATMENT CONSIDERATIONS

Individuals seeking biofeedback treatment are often confused about the nature of their disorder, anxious and depressed, discouraged, and uncertain about their chances for improvement. Brief instructions about factors underlying their condition, pointing out those variables which potentially may be controlled by the patient, are often helpful in counteracting the patient's initial feelings of helplessness and in mobilizing his/her interest in treatment. This is followed by a description of biofeedback, what will be required during treatment (frequency and number of sessions, home practice, etc.), and any ancillary treatment that may be used. The explanation of biofeedback is best understood when accompanied by a live demonstration, which points out the steps involved in measurement and provision of feedback. Education remains an integral part of treatment, as patients continue to discover more about causes and new found ways to behave.

When used for purposes of facilitating general relaxation, initial sessions are typically held in a quiet room, lights may be dimmed, and the patient semireclined in a comfortable chair that supports the entire body. Most clinicians adopt a "coaching" model, noting that a "coach" is someone who has special skills that the patient does not yet have, but who can impart these skills by properly timed guidance. With experience, the therapist learns when the patient needs uninterrupted time to practice biofeedback and when support and assistance would be valuable. In fact, the only investigation of coaching during biofeedback found that learning was actually impeded when the therapist was overly active and intrusive.[27]

Some examples of coaching activities are provided below.

- Sharing observations for discussion. "I noticed that a couple of minutes into the session, your EMG signal shot up. It seemed you might have been clenching your teeth then. How about dropping your lower jaw and moving it just a bit forward? I wonder if anything particular might have been on your mind then?"
- Determining when breaks and encouragement might be needed. Early attempts to lower EMG or skin conductance or to raise hand temperature are often met with the opposite effect, and this situation is paradoxically worsened as patients try harder and harder. These occurrences can be of great therapeutic value as they help to demonstrate the relationship between thoughts and physiological functioning. Explaining how and why this is happening helps to counteract frustration and to get the patient back on track.
- Helping patients to articulate and consolidate learning.
- Augmenting biofeedback with instruction in complementary relaxation approaches, as appropriate.

Biofeedback involves learning a skill and this requires regular practice and eventually incorporating the learned skills into day-to-day activities. Some patients become successful simply by concentrating on the feedback stimulus and becoming aware of corresponding sensations. Others engage in various mental games or attempt to empty their minds completely and think of nothing.[28] In the early sessions, patients are encouraged to experiment with various techniques, but to remain with a given technique long enough to give it an ample trial period.

A typical treatment session involves the following components.

- Sensor attachment and time for adaptation.
- Initial progress review: discussion and review of data collection, attempts at applying skills, problems encountered, etc., while sensors are being attached and the patient is adapting.
- Resting baseline: to assess extent of change over time, as discussed previously.
- "Self-control" baseline: defined as the patient's ability to regulate the target response in the desired direction once training has begun, but in the absence of feedback;[1] this provides an index of the ability to perform the biofeedback skills outside the treatment setting and when instrumented feedback is not available.
- Actual feedback for 20–40 minutes that is continuous or interrupted by breaks.
- Final resting or self-control baseline: to assess extent of learning within the session.
- Final progress review, homework assignment, etc.

The feedback can be interspersed with stress trials or simulated work conditions to help the patient to increase his or her stress-coping skills and transfer trials where the biofeedback signal is turned off and the patient works on reaching machine-independent self-regulation.

Each session should end with a review of the strategies that were explored during the session and an appraisal of the effectiveness of each. Once the patient has shown some abilities to regulate target physiological levels in the clinic, practice outside the office is encouraged. Initially, this practice is performed in a setting maximally conducive to achieving a relaxed state or concentrating on the task at hand. Subsequently, patients are instructed to practice during everyday, but low stress, activities (when driving, shopping, standing in line, during a coffee break, etc.). The final goal is to employ learned biofeedback skills to counteract the build up of stress and physiological arousal. Skills have to be highly developed to be successful at this step.

Thus, the goals of biofeedback are for the patient to be able to discriminate when the target response is in need of control, effect the necessary change in the absence of feedback, apply the learned skills in the real world, and continue use of these skills over the long term. Therapists need, then, to be concerned with generalization and maintenance of learned skills. Lynn and Freedman[29] have identified a number of procedures for helping to make biofeedback training effects more durable. Among those which may be most easily implemented by the clinician are:

- overlearning the target response;
- incorporating booster treatments;

- fading or gradually removing feedback during treatment (which we have previously described as transfer trials);
- training under stimulating or stressful conditions (during noise and distractions, while engaged in a physical or mental task, etc.);
- employing multiple therapists (possible in group practices);
- varying the physical setting;
- providing patients with portable biofeedback for use in real-life situations;
- augmenting biofeedback with other physiological interventions and with cognitive and behavioral procedures.

A number of procedures can be used to augment biofeedback treatments for pain, especially when biofeedback is used for general relaxation.

Imagery

The first and simplest adjunctive procedure involves imagining a pleasant or relaxing scene, such as lying on a blanket at the beach while listening to the waves roll in and out or walking through a pleasant meadow on a warm, sunny day. It is best that patients avoid images that involve sexual content or vigorous physical activity (as these activities can increase rather than decrease arousal) and include as many sensory modalities (touch, sound, smell) and details as possible.[28, 30] It is recommended that patients practice employing several different relaxing images, so that they can switch to another image if the selected one is not working at a given time. With practice, images can be recalled quickly and vividly and can be used effectively to provide mental escape when situations become seemingly overwhelming.

Diaphragmatic breathing

A second procedure involves relaxed or diaphragmatic breathing. Most patients find this to be particularly useful because breathing can be readily brought under voluntary control, and it is an activity that is vital to survival. The notion of relaxed breathing is deceptively simple, so most patients need detailed instructions for correct use. Improper application can lead to blood gas imbalance and hyper- or hypoventilation. Also, patients whose initial respiration rate is high (more than 30 breaths per minute) may feel quite strange as their breathing rate approaches the relaxed range. Such patients are instructed to pay no particular attention to this and are informed that these peculiar feelings will pass with time. Gevirtz and Schwartz[31] provide an excellent discussion of the topic, which briefly reviews the physiology of breathing and provides instructions on how to teach patients to breathe slowly (to a target range of five to eight breaths per

minute), deeply (to full lung capacity), and evenly (to facilitate similar rates for exhaling and for inhaling), while concentrating on the associated physiological sensations. Having the patient subvocalize a word associated with relaxation on each exhalation can help cue subsequent relaxation.

There are various ways to promote the desired breathing pattern. Patients can practice breathing:

- while holding their arms straight overhead (which minimizes chest movement);
- while lying on a firm surface, placing a medium-weight book on the abdomen and raising and lowering the book with each respiration cycle;
- while placing one hand on the chest and the other just below the rib cage, breathing in a manner that limits movement of the hand on the chest and maximizes movement of the hand on the abdomen.

Gevirtz and Schwartz[31] discuss other approaches for promoting more relaxed breathing, including paced respiration, breath meditation, breath mindfulness, rebreathing, pursed-lip breathing, and instrument-based approaches. This very portable procedure is easily combined with other relaxation techniques.

Autogenic training

A third form of relaxation borrows from the well-developed body of literature on autogenic training – a meditation-type relaxation. Autogenic training has an extensive history and involves having patients passively concentrate on key words and phrases selected for their ability to promote desired somatic responses.[30, 32] When added to thermal biofeedback, clinicians typically utilize two of the total six components. Patients are instructed to focus on feelings/sensations of warmth and heaviness in the extremities, as this is believed to facilitate increased blood flow to the extremities, which accounts for peripheral warming and a reduction in sympathetic nervous arousal. It is recommended that patients develop their own phrasing and subvocalize these phrases numerous times (between 50 and 100) during practice in order to maximize effects.[28]

Progressive muscle relaxation training

The fourth and final technique, progressive muscle relaxation training, has the most extensive empirical basis (see below under Evidence base), but it is also the most complex. In this approach, patients engage in a systematic series of muscle-tensing and -releasing exercises, designed first to help the patient discriminate various levels of muscle tension, which makes it easier for the patient then to achieve an overall or generalized state of relaxation.

Andrasik[21] describes a typical relaxation training regimen, which is outlined in **Table 14.2**.

The following points are stressed when introducing this form of relaxation training.

- Relaxation training consists of systematic tensing and relaxing of major muscle groups.
- Tensing muscles, even for a brief period, and then releasing them results in the muscles reflexively achieving a subsequent lower level of tension.
- Experiencing a broad range of muscle tension levels enables patients to better discriminate when muscle tension is building, a goal that is consistent with Flor's work on muscle discrimination difficulties mentioned above under Muscle discrimination.
- Once discrimination abilities are improved and skills for rapidly relaxing muscles are acquired, the technique can be used to counteract tension build up as it occurs throughout the day (termed "applied relaxation").
- Achieving a deep state of relaxation is a learned skill that requires regular practice.
- The procedure will first focus on all major muscle groups, but groups will subsequently be combined over time in order to permit rapid deployment.

The procedure the authors commonly employ begins by having the patient sequentially tense and relax 14 separate muscle groupings in the 18 steps indicated in **Box 14.2**. Before formal instruction, the patient is asked to complete a few practice tension–release cycles to ensure that the tension generated is proper (neither incomplete nor overly zealous) and is confined to the target group. Muscles that are very painful or that have been strained are omitted so as not to cause further problems. Target muscle groups are tensed for five to seven seconds and then relaxed for 20–30 seconds, which constitutes a complete cycle. The patient is instructed to attend to the sensations associated with tension and relaxation during each cycle. If a patient prefers a different muscle sequence, it is acceptable to modify the sequence. However, once modified, it is important that the patient adheres to the same order. Patients may be periodically instructed to mentally scan select muscle groups that have been targeted previously in order to identify any residual tension. If detected, another tension–release cycle may be completed. Various procedures, all involving therapist suggestions, may also be used to promote a deepened sense of relaxation (such as having the therapist count out loud backwards from five to one and instructing the patient that a deeper level of relaxation will be experienced with each successive count). Relaxed breathing and imagery are added early on, in the manner described above under Select treatment considerations. Once the patient has made adequate progress at tensing and relaxing the 14 major muscle groups, the therapist begins to combine various muscle groups in order to abbreviate the procedure – first to eight total muscle groupings and then to four groupings (see **Table 14.3**).

Muscle discrimination training can be added to facilitate abilities to detect even trace amounts of tension increases. To demonstrate this aspect, a patient is asked to engage in a complete tension–release cycle involving the hand and lower arm, then to tense these muscles by only half as much. This is followed by a tension cycle involving only one-quarter as much force. Once the concept of differential tension is understood, the patient is instructed to apply differential muscle tensing to the muscles most associated with pain. This may be done while EMG activity is recorded and displayed on a monitor (see above under Muscle discrimination). Final techniques concern relaxation by recall and cue-controlled relaxation. To implement relaxation by recall, the patient is instructed first to recall the sensations associated with relaxation and then to attempt to reproduce these sensations without the aid of tension and release cycles. Actual tension–release

Table 14.2 Outline of a progressive muscle relaxation training program.

Week	Session	Introduction and treatment rationale	No. of muscle groups	Deepening exercises	Breathing exercises	Relaxing imagery	Muscle discrimination training	Relaxation by recall	Cue-controlled relaxation
1	1	X	14	X	X				
	2		14	X	X	X			
2	3		14	X	X	X	X		
	4		14	X	X	X	X		
3	5		8	X	X	X	X		
	6		8	X	X	X	X	X	
4	7		4	X	X	X	X	X	
5	8		4	X	X	X	X	X	X
6	9		4	X	X	X	X	X	X
7	None								
8	10		4	X	X	X	X	X	X

Box 14.2 Fourteen initial muscle groups and procedures for tensing in 18 steps

1. Right hand and lower arm (have client make fist, simultaneously tense lower arm)
2. Left hand and lower arm
3. Both hands and lower arms
4. Right upper arm (have client bring his/her hand to the shoulder and tense biceps)
5. Left upper arm
6. Both upper arms
7. Right lower leg and foot (have client point his/her toe while tensing the calf muscles)
8. Left lower leg and foot
9. Both lower legs and feet
10. Both thighs (have client press his/her knees and thighs tightly together)
11. Abdomen (have client draw abdominal muscles in tightly, as if bracing to receive a punch)
12. Chest (have client take a deep breath and hold it)
13. Shoulders and lower neck (have client "hunch" his/her shoulders or draw his/her shoulders up towards the ears)
14. Back of the neck (have the client press head backwards against headrest or chair)
15. Lips/mouth (have client press lips together tightly, but not so tight as to clench teeth; or have client place the tip of the tongue on the roof of the mouth behind upper front teeth)
16. Eyes (have client close the eyes tightly)
17. Lower forehead (have client frown and draw the eyebrows together)
18. Upper forehead (have client wrinkle the forehead area or raise the eyebrows)

Table 14.3 Abbreviated muscle groups.

Eight-muscle groups	Four-muscle groups
1. Both hands and lower arms	1. Arms
2. Both legs and thighs	2. Chest
3. Abdomen	3. Neck
4. Chest	4. Face (with a particular focus on the eyes and forehead)
5. Shoulders	
6. Back of neck	
7. Eyes	
8. Forehead	

cycles are used only as needed to promote the desired somatic state. Practice outside the office is necessary to maximize the effects and patients are typically instructed to practice techniques taught them once or twice per day. Audiotapes and DVDs, prepared commercially or by the therapist during an actual session with the patient, can facilitate home practice.

The reader is referred to Andrasik,[33] Arena and Blanchard,[28] Lichstein,[34] Smith,[35] and select chapters from Lehrer *et al.*[36] for further information about relaxation in general.

FINAL TREATMENT CONSIDERATIONS

There are no firm criteria for deciding when to terminate biofeedback. When biofeedback is used as a general relaxation technique, patients are typically provided with a set number of treatments, typically ranging from 8 to 12. In practice, the number of sessions is determined according to clinical response, as gauged by the degree of symptom relief and/or adequacy of control of the target physiological response. Skilled therapists come to sense when treatment has reached the point of diminishing returns or marginal utility (i.e. response reaches a plateau and further effort does not alter the situation). Some have argued for using a specific physiological training criterion as a deciding factor, e.g. ability to reduce and keep EMG levels below a certain value for a specified time, ability to raise hand temperature above a certain value within a specified time period, etc. This intuitive notion has great clinical appeal, but we are not yet at a point where it is possible to advocate for a specific approach.

Few difficulties have been reported when using biofeedback as a general relaxation procedure. A small portion of clients may experience what has been termed "relaxation-induced anxiety," noted to be a sudden increase in anxiety during deep relaxation that can range from mild to moderate intensity and that can approach the level of a minor panic attack.[37] It is important for the therapist to remain calm, reassure the patient that the episode will pass, and, when possible, have the patient sit up for a few minutes or even walk about the office when this happens. With patients who are believed to be at risk for relaxation-induced anxiety, it may be helpful to instruct them to focus more on the somatic aspects as opposed to the cognitive aspects of training[28] (see Schwartz *et al.*[38] for a discussion of other problems and solutions).

SPECIFIC BIOFEEDBACK APPROACHES

Much of the research conducted to date has focused on the value of biofeedback as a general approach to decrease stress, tension, and pain. With certain pain conditions, more specific approaches are emerging as either alternative or preferred treatments for patients with certain characteristics. A few brief examples are given for purposes of illustration.

The studies used to support claims for efficacy of EMG biofeedback for recurrent headache have monitored muscle activity almost exclusively from the forehead area, despite patients reporting other sites as being central to their pain (such as occipital, temporal, neck, and shoulders). Support exists for feedback from the upper trapezius muscles[39] and for an interesting and creative novel approach termed the "frontal–posterior neck placement."

Nevins and Schwartz[40] noted over 20 years ago that the occipitalis area is a site of headache activity for certain tension-type patients. The difficulty for clinicians has been finding an easy way to monitor EMG activity from this site (without shaving portions of the head). Nevins and Schwartz found that by placing one active electrode on the frontal area and the remaining active electrode on the posterior neck on the same side, the summated electrical activity between these sites closely approximated that which occurred in the occipital area. Hudzynski and Lawrence[41] subjected this notion to a controlled experiment, involving subjects with tension-type headache and those who were headache-free, that compared two different static sensor placements: the typical bifrontal forehead placement and a placement involving the bilateral frontal-posterior neck location. Bilateral EMG readings were also taken from the temple, masseter, sternocleidomastoid, and cervical areas utilizing muscle scanning.[17] Frontal-posterior neck readings best discriminated headache and nonheadache patients, and these readings could further distinguish headache from headache-free periods in headache patients. Hudzynski and Lawrence[42] subsequently published normative data to help clinicians gauge when EMG elevations, obtained when clients are both sitting and standing and when both narrow and wide filter settings are used, may be of clinical consequence. This approach has received limited attention, although it merits further investigation.

For TMD, in addition to frontal sites, biofeedback is provided from masseter and temporalis muscles.[43, 44, 45]

Work undertaken by Sherman[46] has helped to identify the most appropriate biofeedback treatment for patients experiencing phantom limb pain. Pain described as burning, throbbing, and tingling was associated with decreased temperature in the stump, whereas pain described as cramping was preceded by and associated with EMG changes. Targeting biofeedback accordingly leads to the greatest outcome.

Arena (cited within Arena and Blanchard[28]) describes a simplified, more straightforward approach to an individualized biofeedback treatment for chronic low back pain. Treatment begins with EMG biofeedback-assisted relaxation, initially from the frontal or forehead area, which is then followed by feedback of the trapezius muscles, all performed with the patient sitting in a comfortable chair or recliner. Once the basic strategies are acquired, positions are changed in order to facilitate generalization of training effects. The patient practices in a comfortable office chair (with arms supported), then moves to an office chair without arm support, and then to a standing position. This phase of training continues for 12–16 sessions.

If improvement is insufficient and the patient has not had a prior course of general relaxation training, then this may be pursued. If this is unwarranted or has been unsuccessful, then an abbreviated psychophysiological assessment is conducted to analyze the problem further. EMG sensors are placed bilaterally on the paraspinals (L4–L5) and the biceps femoris (back of the thigh). Recordings are made in at least two positions: sitting with back supported in a recliner and standing with arms by the side. These sites were selected because they provided greater information than other sites (such as quadriceps femoris or gastrocnemius) in previous examinations. References for these, and other EMG placement sites, may be found in Basmajian and DeLuca[47] and Lippold.[48]

The resulting data reveal one of three patterns of abnormality: (1) unusually low muscle tension levels (which Arena states most typically occurs with nerve damage and muscle atrophy); (2) unusually high muscle tension levels (which Arena states is the most common finding); and (3) left-right asymmetry, wherein one side has normal muscle activity and the other side is either abnormally high or low. Treatment centers on returning EMG values to normal levels. Arena notes that much can be learned by examining gait and posture and correcting faulty positions as well. Sella[18, 49] has also commented on these postural aspects.

The approach that Arena describes is appealing because of its simplicity. The difficulty is in determining normal versus abnormal values. Experience with a considerable number of patients is necessary for this, as Arena and colleagues do not have a developed comparison data bank, such as that prepared by Cram[17] and Sella.[18]

Finally, some researchers have turned their attention to the psychophysiological model of Travell and Simons,[50] who postulated that a large percentage of chronic muscle pain results from trigger points. Hubbard[51] has expanded upon their view using the following line of reasoning.

- Muscle tension and pain are sympathetically mediated hyperactivity of the muscle stretch receptors, or the muscle spindles.
- Muscle spindles, which are scattered throughout the muscle belly (hundreds within the trapezius muscle), are encapsulated organs that contain their own muscle fibers.
- Although traditionally viewed as a stretch sensor, the muscle spindle is now recognized to be a pain and pressure sensor and an organ that can be activated by sympathetic stimulation.
- Thus, the pain associated with trigger points arises in the spindle capsule.

Support for this model comes from studies where careful needle electrode placements have detected high levels of EMG activity in the trigger point itself, but data collected from adjacent nontender sites just 1 cm away are relatively silent.[52] Furthermore, when exposed to a stressful stimulus, EMG activity increases at the trigger point, but not at the adjacent site.[53] This work provides further evidence of the link between behavioral and emotional factors and mechanisms of muscle pain. As a result of their basic research, Gevirtz et al.[54] have developed a comprehensive treatment program that uses EMG biofeedback to facilitate muscle tension awareness in sessions and in daily life activities, to identify stressors triggering increased EMG activity, and to assist patients in finding improved ways to cope with tension-producing situations.

EVIDENCE BASE

Multiple meta-analyses have been conducted for biofeedback, other active treatments (behavioral and pharmacological), and various control conditions for recurrent headache (see Andrasik[55] for a recent review). Early meta-analyses excluded very few of the available studies; poorly designed studies were included along with expertly designed studies if sample sizes met a minimum criterion. More recent analyses have been much more selective about studies included for analysis. For example, the Agency for Health Care Policy and Research (AHCPR) meta-analysis[56] located 355 behavioral and physical treatment (acupuncture, transcutaneous electrical nerve stimulation, occlusal adjustment, cervical manipulation, and hyperbaric oxygen) articles. However, only 70 of the studies were controlled trials of behavioral treatments for migraine and only 39 of these trials met criteria for inclusion in the analysis. In a recent study on the efficacy of biofeedback in migraine headache[57] the average effect size was 0.58 with clear positive effects on frequency of migraine attacks and perceived self-efficacy. Blood volume pulse feedback yielded higher effects than peripheral temperature or EMG feedback. Effects were stable over time and treatment with home training proved more efficacious than pure clinic treatment.

In addition to meta-analytic approaches, various groups have assembled panels to conduct evidence-based reviews, wherein rigorous methodological criteria are used to evaluate every study under consideration. Evidence-based analyses have been performed by the Division 12 Task Force of the American Psychological Association[58] and the US Headache Consortium (composed of the American Academy of Family Physicians, American Academy of Neurology, American Headache Society, American College of Emergency Physicians, American College of Physicians–American Society of Internal Medicine, American Osteopathic Association, and National Headache Foundation).[59]

Consideration of the findings from the above evaluative sources leads to the following conclusions.

- Biofeedback (and other relaxation or psychologically based approaches) leads to significant reductions in headache activity, ranging from 30 to 60 percent.
- Conversely, there is a sizeable number of patients who are nonresponders or partial responders (approximately 40–70 percent). Prediction of treatment response and careful treatment planning become particularly important when attempting to improve upon this outcome.
- Improvements exceed those obtained for various control conditions.
- Nonpharmacological treatments produce benefits similar to those obtained for pharmacological treatments.
- Combining treatments can increment effectiveness, especially so for nonpharmacological combined with pharmacological. However, the net gain of adding a second treatment modality beyond a single treatment is sometimes relatively small, again stressing the importance of finding the right therapy fit for an individual patient.
- Most studies of biofeedback and related approaches have included subjects that continued their consumption of any number of pharmacological agents while undergoing nonpharmacological interventions. Only a very few studies have systematically isolated pure treatments.

The US Headache Consortium[59] concluded that behavioral treatments, such as biofeedback, may be particularly well suited for patients having one or more of the following characteristics.

- Patient prefers such an approach.
- Pharmacological treatment cannot be tolerated or is medically contraindicated.
- Response to pharmacological treatment is absent or minimal.
- Patient is pregnant, has plans to become pregnant, or is nursing.
- Patient has a long-standing history of frequent or excessive use of analgesic or acute medications that can aggravate headache.
- Patient is faced with significant stressors or has deficient stress-coping skills.

A meta-analysis has recently been completed for biofeedback-based treatments for TMD. This analysis[60] revealed a mean improvement rate of 68.6 percent for active treatment compared with 34.7 percent for various control conditions. Effect size scores for pain measures were 1.04 and 0.47 and for examination results were 1.33 and 0.26 for biofeedback and controls, respectively.

Effects noted at the end of treatment were either maintained or improved during follow-up evaluations, some of which extended over two years.

In the research literature, biofeedback treatments for chronic pain other than headache and TMD are varied in their approach and fewer in number; limited direct replications have been attempted. Reviews by various panels[61, 62] and a meta-analysis[63] provide support for biofeedback as an effective treatment for chronic pain.

REFERENCES

1. Blanchard EB, Epstein LH. *A biofeedback primer*. Reading, MA: Addison-Wesley Publishing, 1978.
* 2. Peek CJ. A primer of biofeedback instrumentation. In: Schwartz MS, Andrasik F (eds). *Biofeedback: A practitioner's guide*, 3rd edn. New York: Guilford Press, 2003: 43–87.
3. Andreassi JL. *Psychophysiology: human behavior and physiological response*, 5th edn. Mahwah, NJ: Lawrence Erlbaum Associates, 2007.
* 4. Cacioppo JT, Tassinary LG, Berntson GG (eds). *Handbook of psychophysiology*, 3rd edn. Cambridge: Cambridge University Press, 2007.
5. Stern RM, Ray WJ, Quigley KS. *Psychophysiological recording*, 2nd edn. Oxford: Oxford University Press, 2001.
6. Schwartz NM, Schwartz MS. Definitions of biofeedback and applied psychophysiology. In: Schwartz MS, Andrasik F (eds). *Biofeedback: A practitioner's guide*, 3rd edn. New York: Guilford Press, 2003: 27–39.
7. Belar CD, Kibrick SA. Biofeedback in the treatment of chronic back pain. In: Holzman AD, Turk DC (eds). *Pain management: a handbook of psychological treatment approaches*. New York: Pergamon Press, 1986: 131–50.
* 8. Flor H. Psychophysiological assessment of the patient with chronic pain. In: Turk DC, Melzack R (eds). *Handbook of pain assessment*, 2nd edn. New York: Guilford Press, 2001: 76–96.
9. Bantick SJ, Wise RG, Ploghaus A *et al.* Imaging how attention modulates pain in humans using functional MRI. *Brain*. 2002; **125**: 310–19.
10. Tracey I, Ploghaus A, Gati JS *et al.* Imaging attentional modulation of pain in the periaqueductal gray in humans. *Journal of Neuroscience*. 2002; **22**: 2748–52.
11. Fairhurst M, Wiech K, Dunckley P, Tracey I. Anticipatory brainstem activity predicts neural processing of pain in humans. *Pain*. 2007; **128**: 101–10.
12. Dunckley P, Wise RG, Fairhurst M *et al.* A comparison of visceral and somatic pain processing in the human brainstem using functional magnetic resonance imaging. *Journal of Neuroscience*. 2005; **25**: 7333–41.
* 13. Andrasik F, Rime C. Can behavioural therapy influence neuromodulation? *Neurological Sciences*. 2007; **28**: S124–9.
14. Bonica JJ. Management of myofascial pain syndromes in general practice. *The Journal of American Medical Association*. 1957; **164**: 732–8.
15. Arena JG, Schwartz MS. Psychophysiological assessment and biofeedback baselines for the front-line clinician: a primer. In: Schwartz MS, Andrasik F (eds). *Biofeedback: a practitioner's guide*, 3rd edn. New York: Guilford Press, 2003: 128–58.
16. Flor H, Turk DC. Psychophysiology of chronic pain: do chronic pain patients exhibit symptom-specific psychophysiological responses? *Psychological Bulletin*. 1989; **105**: 219–59.
17. Cram JR. EMG muscle scanning and diagnostic manual for surface recordings. In: Cram JR (ed.). *Clinical EMG for surface recordings 2*. Nevada City, CA: Clinical Resources, 1990: 1–141.
18. Sella GE. SEMG: objective methodology in muscular dysfunction investigation and rehabilitation. In: Boswell MV, Cole BE (eds). *Weiner's pain management: a practical guide for clinicians*, 7th ed. Boca Raton, FL: Taylor & Francis, 2006: 645–61.
19. Flor H, Fürst M, Birbaumer N. Deficient discrimination of EMG levels and overestimation of perceived tension in chronic pain patients. *Applied Psychophysiology and Biofeedback*. 1999; **24**: 55–66.
20. Flor H, Schugens MM, Birbaumer N. Discrimination of muscle tension in chronic pain patients and healthy controls. *Biofeedback and Self-regulation*. 1992; **17**: 165–77.
21. Andrasik F. Biofeedback. In: Mostofsky DI, Barlow DH (eds). *The management of stress and anxiety disorders in medical disorders*. Boston, MA: Allyn & Bacon, 2000: 66–83.
22. Basmajian JV. Facts versus myths in EMG biofeedback. *Biofeedback and Self-regulation*. 1976; **1**: 369–71.
23. Surwit RS, Keefe FJ. Frontalis EMG-feedback training: an electronic panacea? *Behavior Therapy*. 1978; **9**: 779–92.
24. Neumann E, Blanton R. The early history of electrodermal research. *Psychophysiology*. 1970; **6**: 453–75.
25. Boucsein W. *Electrodermal activity*. New York: Plenum, 1992.
26. Sargent JD, Green EE, Walters ED. The use of autogenic training in a pilot study of migraine and tension headaches. *Headache*. 1972; **12**: 120–4.
27. Borgeat F, Hade B, Larouche LM, Bedwani CN. Effect of therapist's active presence on EMG biofeedback training of headache patients. *Biofeedback and Self-regulation*. 1980; **5**: 275–82.
28. Arena JG, Blanchard EB. Biofeedback training for chronic pain disorders: a primer. In: Turk DC, Gatchel RJ (eds). *Psychological approaches to pain management: a practitioner's handbook*, 2nd edn. New York: Guilford Press, 2002: 159–86.
29. Lynn SJ, Freedman RR. Transfer and evaluation of biofeedback treatment. In: Goldstein AP, Kanfer F (eds). *Maximizing treatment gains: transfer enhancement in psychotherapy*. New York, NY: Academic Press, 1979: 445–84.
30. Rime C, Andrasik F. Relaxation techniques and guided imagery. In: Waldman SD (ed.). *Pain management 2*. Philadelphia, PA: Saunders/Elsevier, 2007: 1025–32.

31. Gevirtz RN, Schwartz MS. The respiratory system in applied psychophysiology. In: Schwartz MS, Andrasik F (eds). *Biofeedback: a practitioner's guide*, 3rd edn. New York: Guilford Press, 2003: 212–44.

32. Schultz JH, Luthe W. *Autogenic therapy 1*. New York: Grune & Stratton, 1969.

33. Andrasik F. Relaxation and biofeedback for chronic headaches. In: Holzman AD, Turk DC (eds). *Pain management: a handbook of psychological treatment approaches*. New York: Pergamon, 1986: 213–329.

34. Lichstein KL. *Clinical relaxation strategies*. New York: Wiley & Sons, 1988.

35. Smith JC. *Advances in ABC relaxation: applications and inventories*. New York: Springer Publishing Company, 2001.

36. Lehrer PM, Woolfolk RL, Sime WE. *Principles and practice of stress management*, 3rd edn. New York: Guilford Press, 2007.

37. Heide FJ, Borkovec TD. Relaxation-induced anxiety: paradoxical anxiety enhancement due to relaxation training. *Journal of Consulting and Clinical Psychology*. 1983; **51**: 171–82.

＊38. Schwartz MS, Schwartz NM, Monastra VJ. Problems with relaxation and biofeedback-assisted relaxation, and guidelines for management. In: Schwartz MS, Andrasik F (eds). *Biofeedback: a practitioner's guide*, 3rd edn. New York, NY: Guilford Publications, 2003: 251–64.

39. Arena JG, Bruno GM, Hannah SL, Meador KJ. A comparison of frontal electromyographic biofeedback training, trapezius electromyographic biofeedback training, and progressive muscle relaxation therapy in the treatment of tension headache. *Headache*. 1995; **35**: 411–19.

40. Nevins BG, Schwartz MS. An alternative placement for EMG electrodes in the study and treatment of tension headaches. Paper presented at the 16th Annual Meeting of the Biofeedback Society of America, New Orleans, LA, 1985.

41. Hudzynski LG, Lawrence GS. Significance of EMG surface electrode placement models and headache findings. *Headache*. 1988; **28**: 30–5.

42. Hudzynski LG, Lawrence GS. EMG surface electrode normative data for muscle contraction headache and biofeedback therapy. *Headache Quarterly*. 1990; **1**: 224–9.

43. Glass EG, Glaros AG, McGlynn FD. Myofascial pain dysfunction: treatments used by ADA members. *Journal of Craniomandibular Practice*. 1993; **11**: 25–9.

44. Glaros AG, Lausten L. Temporomandibular disorders. In: Schwartz MS, Andrasik F (eds). *Biofeedback: a practitioner's guide*, 3rd edn. New York: Guilford Press, 2003: 349–68.

45. Crider A, Glaros AG, Gevirtz RN. Efficacy of biofeedback-based treatment for temporomandibular disorders. *Applied Psychophysiology and Biofeedback*. 2005; **30**: 333–45.

46. Sherman R. *Phantom pain*. New York: Springer, 1976.

47. Basmajian JV, DeLuca CJ. *Muscles alive: their functions revealed by electromyography*. Baltimore: Williams & Wilkins, 1985.

48. Lippold DCJ. Electromyography. In: Venables PH, Martin I (eds). *Manual of psychophysiological methods*. New York: Wiley, 1967: 245–97.

49. Sella GE. Back pain: musculoskeletal pain syndrome. In: Moss D, McGrady A, Davies TC, Wickramasekera I (eds). *Handbook of mind-body medicine for primary care*. Thousand Oaks, CA: Sage Publications, 2003: 259–73.

50. Travell J, Simons D. *Myofascial pain and dysfunction: the trigger point manual*. New York: Williams & Wilkins, 1983.

51. Hubbard D. Chronic and recurrent muscle pain: pathophysiology and treatment, and review of pharmacologic studies. *Journal of Musculoskeletal Pain*. 1996; **4**: 123–43.

52. Hubbard D, Berkoff G. Myofascial trigger points show spontaneous EMG activity. *Spine*. 1993; **18**: 1803–07.

53. McNulty E, Gevirtz R, Hubbard D, Berkoff G. Needle electromyographic evaluation of trigger point response to a psychological stressor. *Psychophysiology*. 1994; **31**: 313–16.

54. Gevirtz RN, Hubbard DR, Harpin RE. Psychophysiologic treatment of chronic lower back pain. *Professional Psychology, Research and Practice*. 1996; **27**: 561–6.

55. Andrasik F. What does the evidence show? Efficacy of behavioural treatments for recurrent headaches in adults. *Neurological Sciences*. 2007; **28**: S70–7.

56. Goslin RE, Gray RN, McCrory DC *et al*. Behavioral physical treatments for migraine headache. Technical review 2.2 (prepared for the Agency for Health Care Policy and Research under contract no. 290-94-2025. Available from the National Technical Information Service; NTIS accession no. 127946), 1999.

57. Nestoriuc Y, Martin A. Efficacy of biofeedback for migraine: a meta-analysis. *Pain*. 2007; **128**: 111–27.

58. Task Force on Promotion and Dissemination of Psychological Procedures. Training in and dissemination of empirically validated psychological treatments: report and recommendations. *Clinical Psychology*. 1995; **48**: 3–23.

＊59. Campbell JK, Penzien DB, Wall EM. Evidence-based guidelines for migraine headaches: behavioral and physical treatments. Last updated September 2000, cited February 2008. Available from: http://www.aan.com/professionals/practice/pdfs/gl0089.pdf.

60. Crider AB, Glaros AG. A meta-analysis of EMG biofeedback treatment of temporomandibular disorders. *Journal of Orofacial Pain*. 1999; **13**: 29–37.

61. Keefe FJ, Hoelscher TJ. Biofeedback in the management of chronic pain syndromes. In: Hatch JP, Fisher JG, Rugh JD (eds). *Biofeedback: studies in clinical efficacy*. New York: Plenum, 1987: 211–53.

62. NIH Technology Assessment Panel on Integration of Behavioral and Relaxation Approaches into the Treatment of Chronic Pain and Insomnia. Integration of behavioral and relaxation approaches into the treatment of chronic pain and insomnia. *Journal of the American Medical Association*. 1996; **276**: 313–18.

63. Morley S, Eccleston C, Williams A. Systematic review and meta-analysis of randomized controlled trials of cognitive behaviour therapy and behaviour therapy for chronic pain in adults, excluding headache. *Pain*. 1999; **80**: 1–13.

15

Contextual cognitive-behavioral therapy

LANCE M MCCRACKEN

KEY LEARNING POINTS

- Many responses for reducing chronic pain can actually result in reduced patient functioning.
- Psychological approaches to chronic pain have evolved over the past 40 years, beginning with a focus on overt behavior and the environment, adding a relative emphasis on thoughts and beliefs, and, most recently, integrating more fully the behavioral and cognitive emphases of these earlier phases.
- In a contextual cognitive-behavioral approach, psychological events are considered in terms of their relations of influence on emotions and behavior, influence that is considered situationally dependent and determined by the patient's history.

- Core functional contextual processes of suffering and disability include experiential avoidance, cognitive fusion, values failures, and loss of contact with present moment. In turn, core therapeutic processes include acceptance, cognitive defusion, values clarification and values-based action, and mindfulness.
- A preliminary, randomized, pilot trial, a waiting phase controlled trial, and clinical significance analyses demonstrate that patients achieve significant benefits following contextual cognitive behavioral treatments for chronic pain and that these treatments operate, at least in part, according to the proposed treatment processes.

INTRODUCTION

The trouble with chronic pain is that it *is* chronic. Although the experience of chronic pain can be modifiable, this is in most cases incomplete, and can bring its own costs. It is perhaps a cruel irony that many ways to attempt to reduce pain do not improve daily living but restrict it. Effects of extended rest, avoidance, retirement, the endless search for new treatments, and side effects from medications can highlight this problem. The inevitable tradeoffs

between the rigid pursuit of pain relief and the flexible pursuit of a full life are the focus of recent treatment developments, perhaps more explicitly than they have been in the past. The question asked in these treatments is not "how can we reduce pain?" but "how can we improve participation in life by whatever means, whether pain is reduced in the process or not?"

It might be noticed that there has been a natural and healthy evolution within the cognitive and behavioral therapies for chronic pain. It is worth reviewing this process as it may point to where we will go next. Forty years ago a significant advance was made by those who called for a focus on patient behavior and social circumstances as a means for reducing the suffering and disability of those with chronic pain. This was called the operant behavioral approach.[1] In turn, roughly 25 years ago, this focus was expanded to include patients' beliefs, interpretations, attention, other cognitive processes, and pain-coping strategies. This was called the cognitive-behavioral approach or cognitive-behavioral therapy (CBT).[2] As our understanding of psychological and behavioral processes improves, and as the wider field of clinical psychology evolves, an opportunity exists for further developments of our model and methods of chronic pain management. The chapter focuses on one possible direction for these developments.

WHAT IS CONTEXTUAL COGNITIVE-BEHAVIORAL THERAPY?

Contextual cognitive behavioral therapy (CCBT) is an expansion of CBT for chronic pain.[3] It includes a broad, deep, and theoretically integrated conceptual model and adds a number of distinctive therapeutic methods to those that are currently available within CBT. Its theoretical foundation is what is called "functional contextualism."[4] While to fully describe this philosophy is beyond the scope of this chapter, what it yields in the form of CCBT can be defined briefly as a pragmatic, nonmechanistic, behaviorally focused, and cognitive approach to chronic pain. CCBT integrates the emphasis on the environment and overt behavior from the operant behavioral approach with the emphasis on the pain sufferer's cognitive and emotional experiences from CBT. The "environment" within CCBT, however is defined historically and psychologically, or functionally, and is referred to as "context." Cognitive and emotional experiences are considered in a unique way as well, not based on whether they look maladaptive, but in their relations with overt action, or the influence they exert. Thus, behavior is considered to be contextually determined via relations with events in the environment, both inside and outside the body, relations that are determined by the individual's history, their experiences, or learning. Furthermore, notions of cause and effect are not considered true or false in an ultimate sense but are merely tools for achieving practical results and are, therefore, pragmatically true to the extent they achieve desired results.

Within the CCBT framework, people suffer largely from normal processes of thinking and language, and from the ways these engender psychological inflexibility.[3, 4] In the work from our group, the focus has been on processes of suffering including experiential avoidance, cognitive fusion, values-failures, and loss of contact with present moment, or their allied therapeutic processes: acceptance, cognitive defusion, values clarification and values-based action, and mindfulness. This model of suffering and disability in chronic pain is depicted in **Figure 15.1**. The figure shows that processes of psychological inflexibility (i.e. experiential avoidance, cognitive fusion, etc.) both arise from and contribute back into the processes by which pain leads to suffering and disability. It also shows that these processes are not wholly independent, but substantially overlap in the qualities they add to behavior patterns. The purpose of this chapter is to review the framework underlying CCBT and summarize data supporting its applicability to chronic pain management.

ACCEPTANCE OF CHRONIC PAIN

We have provided a number of converging definitions of acceptance of chronic pain in the past.[5, 6] In essence it is a quality of behavior that is realistic, flexible, practical, and free from unnecessary restrictions from pain. It is the free engagement in activity with pain present and a relative absence of attempts to control or avoid pain.[6] We have most frequently measured acceptance of pain with the Chronic Pain Acceptance Questionnaire.[6, 7]

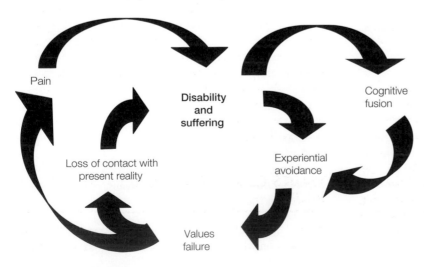

Figure 15.1 A contexual cognitive-behavioral model of chronic pain and disability.

Currently there are approximately 21 published studies of acceptance of pain including experiments,[8, 9, 10] clinical studies,[5, 6, 11, 12, 13] and treatment outcome studies.[14, 15, 16] Overall, in the clinical studies, acceptance of chronic pain has been shown to predict patient physical, social, and emotional functioning, work status, and medication use, both in retrospective and prospective analyses, and to do so independent of pain and relevant patient background variables. We have demonstrated that, as a predictor of key aspects of patient functioning, a measure of acceptance of chronic pain is significantly better than a standard measure of coping with pain[11, 17] or a measure of attention and vigilance to pain.[18]

Acceptance can be a difficult process to grasp conceptually. It can sound like a belief or way of thinking. To the patient it can sound like giving up or resignation. Ironically, it can even sound like positive thinking.[19] Technically, in our applications, it is not intended to mean any of these things. By its definition it is a process outside of the content thinking and believing. It is not a mental act but a quality of whatever action is taken in relation to pain. It is the quality of not struggling with it, of allowing space in experience for it, and being willing to have it present, whether one thinks or believes one can or not. It is not a global act of giving up but selective actions of "giving up" responding to pain as if it is a barrier to functioning or needs to change. With acceptance, contact with pain occasions awareness, watching, or flexible responding; not avoiding, bracing, wrestling, or restricted responding. Positive thinking or optimistic beliefs may achieve an ostensibly similar behavior pattern, but this is functionally a different process.

COGNITIVE DEFUSION

As humans we have an ability that other animals do not have. We can respond to events located in other places and at other times as if they are present. It is our ability to use language and thinking that makes this so. Much of the time we do not have direct contact with situations in life but only with verbally constructed versions of these situations. Our experiences are filtered and modified through our interpretations, evaluations, thoughts, and beliefs. "Cognitive fusion" is the description of this process by which our thoughts become merged with, or undistinguished from, the events they describe or the person who has them.[4]

Most cognitive-behavioral therapies in general include work with thoughts and beliefs in some way, whether that be, for example, a focus on rational or irrational beliefs,[20] or a focus on automatic thoughts and schemas.[21] Some of CBT advocates the disputing or restructuring of irrational beliefs or dysfunctional automatic thoughts. There are, however, many forms of CBT, which focus on differing levels and forms of cognition and apply differing methods for addressing these. This has led to some to criticize CBT for lacking a unifying theory of change.[22] Other studies in

patients with anxiety and depression have questioned whether changes in dysfunctional attitudes are primarily responsible for benefits of CBT[23] and whether methods directed at change in automatic thoughts or core schemas are necessary for positive treatment outcomes.[24, 25]

The model of cognition underlying CCBT is based directly on the approach of acceptance and commitment therapy (ACT).[4] Within this approach cognitive change can happen at two levels, the level of content, what thoughts look like or how frequently they occur, and the level of function or context, the impact thoughts exert on other responses. While work with both levels will have therapeutic value in different situations, a relative emphasis is placed on contextual change. A novel therapeutic process in ACT is what is called "cognitive defusion," which means a loosening of the influence of thought content on behavior and increasing contact with potential influences on behavior beyond thought content. Through cognitive defusion exercises, the chronic pain sufferer can become more aware of the process of thinking, and less entangled in the content of thinking, and can thereby act more flexibly while in contact with otherwise distressing, discouraging, or restricting thoughts. Cognitive defusion means a weakening of the role of thoughts as the sole basis for action without necessarily reformulating the content of thoughts. By bringing behavior in contact with thoughts in a different way, and altering the way they are experienced, in a broader context, cognitive defusion allows free and healthy action without the necessity of positive thoughts and beliefs, which often can be hard to achieve.

Cognitive defusion methods include the use of metaphor, paradox, humor, and experiential tasks, rather than logical confrontation, direct verbal persuasion, or empirical verification.[4] Confrontation of dysfunctional beliefs and cognitions, as is done in cognitive therapy, however, may also achieve a degree of cognitive defusion. The potential drawback of methods that direct themselves at change in content is that they can emphasize the necessity of rational thinking and reinforce the behavioral imperative of doing, or feeling emotionally, what the literal content of thought demands one do or feel. Methods directly targeting cognitive fusion will include exercises that raise awareness of (1) the experience of having a thought rather than being stuck in the content of the thought, (2) the experience of difficulties presented by trying to control thoughts, (3) the unworkability of following some thought content, and (4) the ability to act according to what the person feels is important while in contact with thoughts that "say" otherwise. This creates flexibility in the relationship between thoughts and action.

VALUES CLARIFICATION AND VALUES–BASED ACTION

"Values" are defined as chosen life directions. They can also be considered as qualities of behavior that reflect what the individual cares most about in their life. Values are made up of the answers to the question, "What do you want your life to stand for?"[4] The usefulness of values-based processes in chronic pain comes when the pain sufferer's life has become stuck in a focus on pain, and other unwanted experiences, and has lost contact with what they would hold as most important. For many chronic pain sufferers daily life can be about struggling with, trying to control, and seeking relief from, pain, and not about family, friends, intimate relations, work, health, and growth or learning, or other concerns that constitute a full and vital life. A focus of clarifying values, and enhancing values-based action, is a means for reducing this focus on pain as the primary guide for action.

Values-related processes have been discussed across a range of psychological approaches in the past, including client-centered therapy[26] and motivational interviewing.[27] However, it does not appear that they have been formally emphasized in CBT in the past as they have been in ACT. A number of recent attempts to measure values-related processes have arisen from this new emphasis with ACT and CCBT, including in general samples[28] and in chronic pain.[29]

Our first study of values included 140 consecutive patients with chronic pain seen for an assessment in a specialty pain center in the UK. For this study we developed a brief measure of values called the Chronic Pain Values Inventory (CPVI).[29] The CPVI asks patients to consider their values in domains of family, intimate relations, friends, work, health, and growth or learning, and to first rate the importance with which they hold their values and then the success they have living according to them. Results from this study demonstrated that patients' importance ratings are universally higher than their success ratings. Average success ratings positively correlated with acceptance of pain and negatively correlated with a measure of avoidance. Importantly, the average success ratings correlated significantly with measures of disability, depression, and pain-related anxiety, and, in regression analyses, predicted significant variance in patient functioning independent of acceptance of pain.[29]

Values clarification is not necessarily an easy process. In most cases it requires that patients examine circumstances that may be very painful to examine. When a patient honestly identifies what is important to them and also realizes they are not acting that way, they may experience profound loss, embarrassment, shame, or guilt. The pain of looking at values may lead patients to avoid doing it. Also, many patients find it difficult to identify what is important to them separate from what others or society specify should be important to them. It can be essential for patients to work through this. Taking a particular course of action to avoid disapproval from others is not the same behavior pattern as taking it in the service of what one about cares about most. Finally, patients may immediately close themselves off from particular directions when they label them as "impossible"

but that idea need not limit values-based action and need not lead one to reject a particular value. Directions that our minds say are impossible in one particular moment can turn out quite approachable, if possibly in small steps, when looked at more flexibly or in a different moment.

MINDFULNESS

Chronic pain sufferers often get excessively caught up with their own sensations, emotions, and thoughts and can have their behavior become disorganized, impulsive, or ineffective. They can have the natural pain, stress, and unwanted experiences in life magnified in their effects by the ways they struggle, act defensively, harden their stance toward these things, or multiply their distress by feeling and acting distressed about their distress, and so forth. These processes entail a loss of contact with the present moment and a hyperreactivity to experiences to which the individual need not react. A remedy for these processes of suffering is training in a skill set including accurate, present-focused, and accepting awareness, or what is called mindfulness.[30] To say this somewhat more technically, mindfulness is a process of contact with events in experience that alters some of the otherwise automatic functions of these events. The predominant attitudes of mindfulness include openness, curiosity, gentleness, and compassion.

Mindfulness differs from other commonly used methods, such as relaxation, for example. Relaxation is often carried out with the goal of controlling what is experienced, usually to reduce sensations or emotions of tension and stress. Mindfulness, on the other hand, is carried out to practice being aware of sensations and emotions without doing anything else about them. Guided imagery exercises are another example. These are often performed to change the content of what is being experienced and to gain the emotional and behavioral effects that come with that. Mindfulness is carried out to watch and learn from whatever content spontaneously occurs in experience while maintaining a connection with the present moment and an attitude of interested neutrality. There are many types of mindfulness exercises; some that include a focus on the body, on sensations of breathing, or on sensations during movement,[30] and some that can include the use of an imagined scene.[4]

Although mindfulness has been an interest within pain management for many years, there is still a relative lack of data regarding its usefulness. There are uncontrolled trials supporting the role of mindfulness-based methods as treatment for chronic pain[31, 32] and supportive conclusions from meta-analyses of mindfulness-based treatments for a range of conditions, including pain.[33, 34] Further study is needed.

We recently completed a study of mindfulness in patients with chronic pain.[35] In our study we administered the Mindful Attention Awareness Scale (MAAS)[36] to a sample of 105 consecutive patients with chronic pain seeking specialty treatment in the UK. The MAAS is a 15-item measure of mindfulness in which each of the items is negatively keyed (i.e. "I could be experiencing some emotion and not be conscious of it until some time later," "I find it difficult to stay focused on what's happening in the present," "I find myself preoccupied with the future or the past"). Items are rated from 1 ("almost always") to 6 ("almost never") and yield a single summary score. Correlation analyses showed that mindfulness was positively correlated with acceptance of pain and negatively correlated with measures of pain-related distress, anxiety, depression, interference with cognitive functioning, and pain medication use. Based on multiple regression analyses in which age, gender, education, duration of pain, pain intensity, and acceptance of pain, were entered first, mindfulness added a significant increment to explained variance in five of eight equations, explaining significant variance in depression, pain-related anxiety, as well as physical, psychosocial, and "other" disability. Mindfulness was a particularly good predictor of depression and "other" disability where in each case it accounted for 11 percent of the variance after the series of other potential predictors were taken into account. The variance in these equations accounted for by acceptance and mindfulness combined averaged 28 percent across the eight equations.[35]

CHRONIC PAIN IN A SOCIAL CONTEXT

A functional contextual approach to chronic pain has several implications for the role of social influences on pain and suffering. These include a potentially more sophisticated analysis of the role of significant others in chronic pain,[37] models of "self,"[38] and the role of social influence in treatment.[3]

For years, the role of social responses in chronic pain has been either framed as a process of reinforcement or punishment for overt displays of pain and disability[1] or perhaps as a buffer or stressor in the emotional experience of chronic pain.[39] Recent analyses of solicitous and punishing spouse responses suggest that the traditional operant behavioral framework is probably incomplete.[37] Social responses to pain and suffering will blend with multiple concurrent influences on behavior patterns including cognitive and emotional influences, and the effects they exert will depend on the functions they have acquired, not merely their topography. A person with pain who responds with activity avoidance may have that pattern so tightly controlled by thought and emotional content that other immediate social influences play little role (note that the role of thought content itself, however, is of a social origin). Alternatively, that pattern may be strengthened in some situations if social responses are psychologically relevant, contact the behavior, interact with it to strengthen it, and are not otherwise overwhelmed by other influences. Further still, a patient who is suffering and experiences an angry or frustrated reaction from those in their environment may feel invalidated, or like their suffering is not believed, and may act to rigidly defend the legitimacy of their problems in the future. Either of these ostensibly different patterns could lock the patient into a pattern of greater suffering and disability.[3, 37] It is not the appearance of the response as either "solicitous" or "punishing" that is critical but it is the wider context, the pain sufferer's history and the broader psychological situation, which gives those responses their meaning and function.

There are many different understandings of "self." One longstanding division is whether the self is best understood as an object or subject, "self-as know" or "self-as-knower."[40] Many authorities agree, however, that our sense of self arises in social situations and is therefore social in origin.[40, 41] We learn an awareness of who we are as this becomes important for others. In turn we expect ourselves, and are expected by others, to act consistently with this sense of our self.[4] To act unpredictably or "not like our self" is met with discouraging responses in many social situations. Two problems arise from this situation for those with chronic pain. First, unrealistic social pressure for behavioral consistency can come to bear on chronic pain sufferers whose pain leads them to experience many changes in their roles and behavior, and whose behavior changes in relation to private experiences that are not fully understood by casual observers. This can be distressing and restricting, such as when essentially arbitrary social influences press for behavior patterns that are otherwise ineffective, failing to bring desired results or bringing undesired ones. Second, through processes of thinking and speaking we can come to take too seriously a certain sense or our self, a self made up our thoughts and beliefs about who we are, but in many ways otherwise arbitrary, a self that can be referred to as "self-as-content."[4] For chronic pain sufferers, strongly held beliefs such as "I never need help from others," "I am not the sort of person to feel depressed," or "I never talk about my feelings," can be very limiting, if the person tries to defend these or deny the reality of experiences to the contrary. This is why treatment approaches for chronic pain can advocate the promotion of a different sense of self, a self that does not depend on the content of thought and belief, but recognizes a sense of self that is aware of this content, or a sense of self as the location where this content occurs, a sense of "self as context."[3, 4]

The final aspect of social context to discuss involves the context of the treatment environment. All treatment for chronic pain is inherently social, whether that is consciously considered a key therapeutic element or not. Given the nature of chronic pain there are several important social challenges to manage. First, many individuals with complex problems of chronic pain come with a history of feeling disbelieved, may be sensitive to this, and may want to avoid it. This is understandable. To suffer and to have the legitimacy of that suffering doubted can be to feel one is being called a liar, and that one will be abandoned and left with uncontrollable pain. Anyone would fight to avoid this situation, such as by trying to prove there is something wrong. Once this occurs it is a real dilemma in treatment, as it can be difficult for a person to prove they are suffering and to improve at the same time. Ways to avoid the patient feeling discounted include listening and understanding what they have lost and how they feel, being willing to feel how bad they feel, and realizing that no matter how many times you say "I believe you," it can be easily undermined. To ask a chronic pain sufferer to perform physical exercise, for example, or do something they feel is "impossible" can feel delegitimizing, as it seems to discount their pain.

A second social concern in treatment is the role of social pressure from the therapist and subtle forms of coercion. "Pressuring" patients to participate in treatment, even if done subtly, can sometimes work but it runs several risks. It may (1) provoke resistance, as most of us will resist being controlled by others, at least some of the time, (2) lead to anger at, or avoidance of, the "pressure," or (3) create behavior patterns under the control of the therapist's social approval or disapproval that are unsustainable away from the therapy environment. As discussed above, the remedy for this is to create a therapy environment that is based on the patient's willingness to participate, to give them the free choice to control what they experience when they honestly wish do to so, and to bring the patient's behavior in contact with their values as their guides for action, and in contact with concordance between what they do and what they care about, rather than social pressures of any kind.

CCBT can be a very intensive form of therapy. A primary focus of treatment includes creating occasions when patients will have painful experiences when these are a necessary part of positive change. These provide an opportunity for learning to meet these with effective action, with flexibility rather than struggling or avoidance. In order to effectively deliver treatment of this type, treatment providers will have to "be there" in treatment. The only honest way to do that is for the treatment provider to be willing to experience what they experience when patients experience what they experience. To say it another way, we are all strongly disposed to avoid pain and distress. When treatment asks the patient to be willing to face pain, treatment providers will need to demonstrate that same willingness. To not do so is to send the message that that the patient's pain is not acceptable to the treatment provider, and probably should not be to the patient. This may reinforce a long history of running away from pain on the part of the patient and may lead to functioning with significantly less freedom and vitality.

TREATMENT OUTCOME FROM CONTEXTUAL APPROACHES TO CHRONIC PAIN

Despite the relatively recent development of contextual approaches, there are a fair number of supportive studies conducted in related areas, outside of chronic pain, such as depression,[42] relapse following treatment for depression,[43] marital distress,[44] polysubstance abuse and opiate addiction,[45] psychotic symptoms,[46] and work stress.[47] There are three trials related to chronic pain;[14, 15, 16] two of these will be discussed in more detail.

All of our treatment outcome data come from the "real situation" of a Pain Management Unit set up, not to run clinical trials, but to deliver services to highly complex groups of patients who have failed other available services. In this respect our analyses of treatment outcome results are more akin to effectiveness studies than efficacy trials and, thus, seem to require no test of generality to realistic circumstances. Further, as a national tertiary care center in the National Health Service, providing services to pain sufferers who have few if any options, our patient selection criteria for services are extremely liberal.

Our first study of treatment outcome consisted of 108 chronic pain sufferers seen between March 2001 and July 2002.[15] They participated in three- or four-week, full-time, group-based, treatment courses delivered by a team of physiotherapists, occupational therapists, nurses, physicians, and clinical psychologists. Our treatments include graded physical conditioning, skills training, education, mindfulness training, and psychological methods based on the model of CCBT presented above.[3] As described above, many of the psychological methods are experiential or metaphor-based. An example of one of our treatment exercises is shown in **Box 15.1**.

Analyses in our first treatment study were based on multiple outcome measures administered at initial assessment, the start of treatment ($M = 3.9$ months later), immediately following treatment, and then at a three-month follow-up visit. In our initial report we showed that patient functioning did not significantly change during the waiting phase prior to treatment but did significantly improve in nine key domains following treatment and remained significantly improved on all measured domains at follow-up. Patients also showed significantly increased acceptance of pain during treatment and changes in acceptance were significantly correlated with changes in other key outcome variables, lending support to the notion that acceptance was an important process in the observed results.[15] **Figure 15.2** illustrates data from a sample of consecutively treated cases on our unit. It includes percentage improvements at posttreatment and follow-up and is substantially similar to the results from our earlier analyses but includes an expanded sample size, $n = 303$ rather than $n = 108$. The significant benefits patients achieved include decreased pain, anxiety, depression, physical and psychosocial disability, medication use, and physician visits, as well as

---

Box 15.1 An example of a metaphor-based, experiential, treatment exercise used in CCBT

PERSPECTIVE AND FOCUS EXERCISE

Background

When working toward life goals, maintaining focus on the circumstances that help you reach those goals is necessary. Focusing on avoidance of pain or other uncomfortable feelings can interfere with that.

Exercise

The way we view things is often a matter of focus.

1. Put a finger up in front of your face and focus on it. What do you see? How clear are other objects and people in the room? ... Now, notice what happens when you change your focus to the things several feet in front of you, or to the opposite side of the room. Now what do you see clearly and what seems to blur to a shadow? ... Which kind of focus gives you a broader picture of the world, or enables you to see more of what's around you? ... Which way would it work best if you needed to see where you are going? ... When you focus on something close up, the things in the distance blur or disappear, become unrecognizable. Likewise, it becomes more difficult to know if you are headed in the direction you want to go, or if you have arrived at your destination. If you can change what you are focusing on, the picture you have of the world might be quite different. You may have a different "perspective." The finger in front of your face is one thing you can focus on.
2. "Problems" may happen when you continue to focus only or mainly on one thing so that you can't see where you are going. After a while you may think that it is because of the FINGER itself, not because of your FOCUSING on it. Without the focusing on the finger, it is not the same matter.

Discuss

1. In concrete terms what are your "destinations" and goals?
2. Do goals have value regardless of whether pain is present or absent?
3. What happens when no pain or minimal pain is part of a goal? Does experience show that the original goal blurs or shrinks as awareness of pain increases?

Modified from: Geiser DS (1992). A comparison of acceptance-focused and control-focused psychological treatments in a chronic pain treatment center. Unpublished doctoral dissertation, University of Nevada, Reno.

---

increased walking speed, activity tolerance, and work status.

It may be noticed that most of the treatment results in **Figure 15.2** are fully maintained at follow-up but the results for some outcome measures decline and that these reduced results differ for different outcome measures. For example, there is a particular reduction in the improvements for depression. In part this may be an effect of leaving the treatment environment and facing the reality of the home situation. The more durable results for physical functioning and acceptance are, in retrospect, expected, as treatment is primarily designed to improve behavioral performance and not necessarily to reduce distressing psychological content, such as cognitive and emotional aspects of depression.

In our latest study we examined clinically significant change, but we did this in a particular subset of patients

we treat, those who are most highly disabled.[16] In this study we examined treatment outcome of 53 consecutive patients treated in a hospital-based course of treatment. These patients have extremely limited mobility and self-care and thus are unable to participate in a pain management course without a minimal amount of nursing care to assist with transfers, mobility, bathing or dressing, or other necessary activities of daily life. Our analyses demonstrated that these patients achieve significant improvement at posttreatment in pain-related distress, physical and psychosocial disability, depression, anxiety, frequency of sit-to-stand in one minute, and hours spent resting during the day due to pain. Across nine key outcome domains the highly disabled patients achieved an average effect size of $d = 0.75$, similar to the average effect size for standard treatment cases, $d = 0.77$. Reliable change analyses,[48] taking into account temporal stability of the

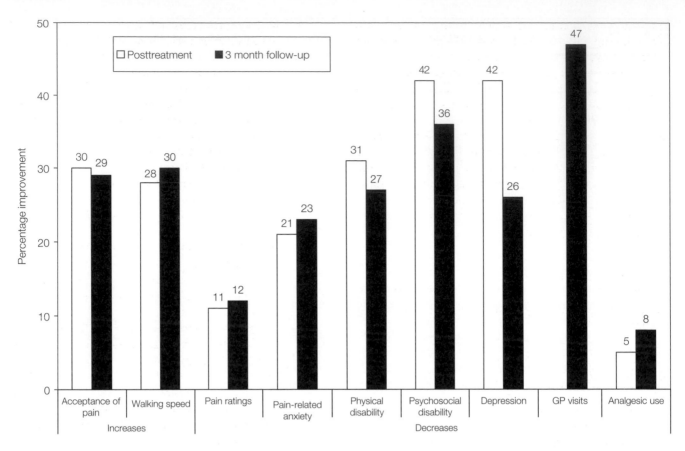

Figure 15.2 Percent improvement relative to initial baseline in key outcomes at posttreatment and three-month follow-up after a course of interdisciplinary CCBT for chronic pain ($n = 303$).

outcome measures, indicated, for example, that 47.6 percent of patients demonstrated reliable improvement in total disability and 61.9 percent demonstrated reliable improvement in depression scores. Applying criteria for "recovery" based on level of posttreatment functioning of successfully treated standard cases, 52.8 percent of the highly disabled patients met criteria for clinical recovery in a least one primary outcome domain, including physical disability, psychosocial disability, or depression.[16] This is akin to saying that for every 1.9 highly disabled patients treated from this approach one achieves recovery in at least one key domain of functioning.

SUMMARY

In many parts of the world the dominant culture says that if we do not like something, we should fix it or avoid it. This strategy works very well in some circumstances but not in others. In cases of chronic pain this can lead to significant restrictions in daily functioning and to considerable suffering. It is natural to attempt to avoid pain and it is unnatural, in some ways, to consider doing anything else.

Increasing research findings demonstrate that there is more than one way to live a free, full, and vital life once one has chronic pain. Methods available from a long tradition of behavioral and cognitive therapies are one way.[49] These methods include a wide mixture but tend to include training in coping and methods designed predominantly to control or decrease what is felt physically and emotionally, and to change the content of thought and belief.[50, 51] Another way, rather than coping with or attempting to exercise control over what is felt, thought, or believed, is to focus on contextual change.

Current contextually based therapies, such as CCBT, aim to alter the historical and situational elements that gives psychological experiences their influence over behavioral patterns and not to alter the content of psychological experiences themselves. They aim not to reduce sensations, emotions, and thoughts but to alter how they are experienced. This is not the sometimes derided "just do it" approach associated with unfair characterizations of the "old-fashioned" operant approach. Contextual change is not superficial but is an attempt to get to the core of where suffering and behavior disruption are based, primarily in processes of language and cognition. The processes in CCBT are perhaps more subtle, less logical, more metaphorical or paradoxical, less dominantly change-oriented, and more flexibly balanced between change and acceptance. Approaches such as CCBT are intensely emotional and consciously aware of social influences, as it seems it should be for patients with chronic pain who have suffered greatly, are often vulnerable, and can have complex personal histories.

We have found in our clinical service, based on the equivalent of effectiveness studies, that a treatment including processes of acceptance, cognitive defusion, mindfulness, and values is associated with significant improvements for chronic pain sufferers seen in tertiary care. These improvements include emotional, physical, and social functioning, as well as healthcare use. Together with other controlled and uncontrolled treatment studies related to pain and numerous treatment trials outside of the area of pain, these contextually based treatment methods appear promising.

ACKNOWLEDGEMENT

Thanks to Dr Miles Thompson for assistance with figure design.

REFERENCES

1. Fordyce WE. *Behavioral methods for chronic pain and illness.* St Louis: Mosby, 1976.
2. Turk DC, Meichenbaum D, Genest M. *Pain and behavioral medicine: a cognitive-behavioral perspective.* New York: Guilford Press, 1983.
* 3. McCracken LM. *Contextual cognitive-behavioral therapy for chronic pain (Progress in pain research and management)* Vol 33. Seattle: IASP Press, 2005.
* 4. Hayes SC, Strosahl K, Wilson KG. *Acceptance and commitment therapy: an experiential approach to behavior change.* New York: Guildford Press, 1999.
5. McCracken LM. Learning to live with the pain: acceptance of pain predicts adjustment in persons with chronic pain. *Pain.* 1998; **74**: 21–7.
6. McCracken LM, Vowles KE, Eccleston C. Acceptance of chronic pain: component analysis and a revised assessment method. *Pain.* 2004; **107**: 159–66.
7. Geiser DS. A Comparison of acceptance-focused and control-focused psychological treatments in a chronic pain treatment center. Unpublished Doctoral Dissertation, Reno: University of Nevada, 1992.
8. Hayes SC, Bissett RT, Korn A *et al.* The impact of acceptance versus control rationales on pain tolerance. *Psychological Record.* 1999; **49**: 33–47.
9. Gutierrez O, Luciano C, Rodriguez M, Fink BC. Comparison between an acceptance-based and a cognitive-control-based protocol for coping with pain. *Behavior Therapy.* 2004; **35**: 767–83.
10. Masedo AI, Rosa Esteve M. Effects of suppression, acceptance and spontaneous coping on pain tolerance, pain intensity and distress. *Behaviour Research and Therapy.* 2007; **45**: 199–209.
11. McCracken LM, Eccleston C. Coping or acceptance: what to do with chronic pain? *Pain.* 2003; **105**: 197–204.
12. McCracken LM, Eccleston C. A prospective study of acceptance of pain and patient functioning with chronic pain. *Pain.* 2005; **118**: 164–9.
13. Viane I, Crombez G, Eccleston C *et al.* Acceptance of pain is an independent predictor of mental well-being in patients with chronic pain: empirical evidence and reappraisal. *Pain.* 2003; **106**: 65–72.
* 14. Dahl J, Wilson KG, Nilsson A. Acceptance and Commitment Therapy and the treatment of persons at risk for long-term disability resulting from stress and pain symptoms: a preliminary randomized trial. *Behavior Therapy.* 2004; **35**: 785–801.
* 15. McCracken LM, Vowles KE, Eccleston C. Acceptance-based treatment for persons with complex, longstanding chronic pain: a preliminary analysis of treatment outcome in comparison to a waiting phase. *Behaviour Research and Therapy.* 2005; **43**: 1335–46.
* 16. McCracken LM, MacKichan F, Eccleston C. Contextual Cognitive-Behavioral Therapy for severely disabled chronic pain sufferers: effectivenss and clinically significant change. *European Journal of Pain.* 2006; **11**: 314–22.
17. McCracken LM, Eccleston C. A comparison of the relative utility of coping and acceptance-based measures in a sample of chronic pain sufferers. *European Journal of Pain.* 2006; **10**: 23–9.
18. McCracken LM. A contextual analysis of attention to chronic pain: what the patient does with their pain may be more important than their awareness or vigilance alone. *The Journal of Pain.* 2007; **8**: 230–6.
19. Nicholas MK, Asghari A. Investigating acceptance in adjustment to chronic pain: is acceptance broader than we thought? *Pain.* 2006; **124**: 269–79.
20. Ellis A. *Reason and emotion in psychotherapy.* Secaucus, NJ: Birch Lane.
21. Beck AT. *Cognitive therapy: basics and beyond.* New York: Guilford Press.
22. David D, Szentagotai A. Cognitions in cognitive-behavioral psychotherapies: toward an integrative model. *Clinical Psychology Review.* 2006; **26**: 284–98.
23. Burns DD, Spangler DL. Do changes in dysfunctional attitudes mediate changes in depression and anxiety in cognitive behavioral therapy? *Behavior Therapy.* 2001; **32**: 337–69.
24. Jacobson NS, Dobson KS, Truax PA *et al.* A component analysis of cognitive-behavioral treatment for depression. *Journal of Consulting and Clinical Psychology.* 1996; **64**: 295–304.
25. Dimidjian A, Hollon SD, Dobson KS *et al.* Randomized trial of behavioral activation, cognitive therapy, and antidepressant medication in the acute treatment of adults with major depression. *Journal of Consulting and Clinical Psychology.* 2006; **74**: 658–70.
26. Rogers CR. Toward a modern approach to values: the valuing process in the mature person. *Journal of Abnormal and Social Psychology.* 1964; **68**: 160–7.

27. Wagner CC, Sanchez FP. The role of values in motivational interviewing. In: Miller WR, Rollnick S (eds). *Motivational interviewing: preparing people for change*, 2nd edn. New York: Guilford Press, 2002: 284–98.

28. Wilson KG, Murrell AR. Values work in Acceptance and Commitment Therapy. In: Hayes SC, Follette VM, Linehan MM (eds). *Mindfulness and acceptance: expanding the cognitive-behavioral tradition*. New York: Guilford Press, 2004: 121–51.

29. McCracken LM, Yang S-Y. The role of values in a contextual cognitive-behavioral analysis of chronic pain. *Pain*. 2006; **123**: 137–45.

30. Kabat-Zinn J. *Full catastrophe living: using the wisdom of your body and mind to face stress, pain, and illness*. New York: Dell Publishing, 1990.

31. Kabat-Zinn J, Lipworth L, Burney R. The clinical use of mindfulness meditation for self-regulation of chronic pain. *Journal of Behavioral Medicine*. 1985; **8**: 163–90.

32. Kaplan KH, Goldenberg DL, Galvin-Nadeau M. The impact of a meditation-based stress reduction program on fibromyalgia. *General Hospital Psychiatry*. 1993; **15**: 284–9.

∗ 33. Baer RA. Mindfulness training as a clinical intervention: a conceptual and empirical review. *Clinical Psychology Research and Practice*. 2003; **10**: 125–43.

∗ 34. Grossman P, Niemann L, Schmidt S, Walach H. Mindfulness-based stress reduction and health benefits: a meta-analysis. *Journal of Psychosomatic Research*. 2004; **57**: 35–43.

35. McCracken LM, Gauntlett-Gilbert, Vowles K. The role of mindfulness in a contextual cognitive-behavioral analysis of chronic pain-related suffering and disability. *Pain*. 2007; **131**: 63–9.

36. Brown KW, Ryan RM. The benefits of being present: mindfulness and its role in psychological well-being. *Journal of Personality and Social Psychology*. 2003; **84**: 822–48.

37. McCracken LM. Social context and acceptance of chronic pain: the role of solicitous and punishing responses. *Pain*. 2005; **113**: 155–9.

38. Crombez G, Morley S, McCracken LM *et al.* Self, identity and acceptance in chronic pain. In: Dostrovsky JO, Carr DB, Koltzenburg M (eds). *Proceedings of the 10th World Congress on Pain*, Vol. 24. Seattle: IASP Press, 2003: 651–9.

39. Cano A, Gillis M, Heinz W *et al.* Marital functioning, chronic pain, and psychological distress. *Pain*. 2004; **107**: 99–106.

40. James W. *Principles of psychology (reprint edition)*. New York: Dover Publications, 1950.

41. Skinner BF. *Science and human behavior*. New York: The Free Press, 1953.

42. Zettle RD, Rains JC. Group cognitive and contextual therapies in treatment of depression. *Journal of Clinical Psychology*. 1989; **45**: 436–45.

43. Ma SH, Teasdale JD. Mindfulness-based cognitive therapy for depression: replication and exploration of differential relapse prevention effects. *Journal of Consulting and Clinical Psychology*. 2004; **72**: 31–40.

44. Jacobson NS, Christensen A, Prince SE *et al.* Integrative behavioral couple therapy: an acceptance-based, promising new treatment for couple discord. *Journal of Consulting and Clinical Psychology*. 2000; **68**: 351–5.

45. Hayes SC, Wilson KG, Gifford EV *et al.* A preliminary trial of twelve-step facilitation and Acceptance and Commitment Therapy with polysubstance-abusing methadone-maintained opiate addicts. *Behavior Therapy*. 2004; **35**: 667–88.

46. Bach P, Hayes SC. The use of Acceptance and Commitment Therapy to prevent the rehospitalization of psychotic patients: a randomized controlled trial. *Journal of Consulting and Clinical Psychology*. 2002; **70**: 1129–39.

47. Bond FW, Bunce D. Mediators of change in emotion-focused and problem-focused worksite stress management interventions. *Journal of Occupational Health Psychology*. 2000; **5**: 156–63.

48. Jacobson NS, Roberts LJ, Berns SB, McGlinchey JB. Methods from defining and determining the clinical significance of treatment effects: description, application, and alternatives. *Journal of Consulting and Clinical Psychology*. 1999; **67**: 300–7.

∗ 49. Morley S, Eccleston C, Williams AC. Systematic review and meta-analysis of randomized controlled trials of cognitive behaviour therapy and behaviour therapy for chronic pain in adults, excluding headache. *Pain*. 1999; **80**: 1–13.

50. De Jong JR, Vlaeyen JWS, Onghena P *et al.* Reduction of pain-related fear in complex regional pain syndrome type I: the application of graded exposure in vivo. *Pain*. 2005; **116**: 264–75.

51. Williams ACdeC, Richardson PH, Nicholas MK *et al.* Inpatient vs. outpatient pain management: results of a randomized controlled trial. *Pain*. 1996; **66**: 13–22.

16

Graded exposure *in vivo* for pain-related fear

JOHAN WS VLAEYEN, JEROEN DE JONG, PETER HTG HEUTS, AND GEERT CROMBEZ

KEY LEARNING POINTS

- Pain-related fear of pain is a normal response when pain is catastrophically misinterpreted as a sign of damage.
- Patients often consider physical activity as harmful, but may not always define their problems in terms of fear.
- In addition to clinical interview, brief questionnaires are available to identify patients with excessive pain-related fears.
- Pain-related fear is associated with hypervigilance and escape/avoidance behaviors that may have short-term

benefits in acute pain, but paradoxically worsen the problem in the long run.
- Fear reduction can be achieved with a combination of education about the harmfulness of common physical activity, the establishment of a fear hierarchy, and the actual exposure to feared activities.
- Exposure to feared activities can best be provided in the form of a behavioral experiment.
- Preliminary evidence shows that decreased pain-related fear is associated with improved daily functioning.

INTRODUCTION

In an attempt to explain how and why some individuals with musculoskeletal pain develop a chronic pain syndrome, biopsychosocial models have been developed, including the "fear-avoidance model of exaggerated pain perception,"[1] and, more recently, the cognitive–behavioral model of fear of movement/(re)injury.[2, 3] The central concept of these models is "fear of pain," or the more specific "fear that physical activity will cause (re)injury." Generally, two opposing behavioral responses to pain are postulated: "confrontation" and "avoidance." In the

absence of any serious somatic pathology, confrontation is conceptualized as an adaptive response that eventually may lead to the reduction of fear and the promotion of recovery of pain or function. In contrast, avoidance leads to the maintenance or exacerbation of fear, possibly resulting in a condition similar to a phobia. The avoidance results in the reduction of both social and physical activities, which in turn leads to a number of physical and psychological consequences augmenting the disability.[4] Prospective studies in acute low back pain patients[5] and healthy people[6] have provided support for the idea that pain-related fear may be an important precursor of pain disability.

What are the clinical consequences of these findings? In this chapter, we will first highlight the typical characteristics of pain-related fear, and the association between pain-related fear and attentional, cognitive, and behavioral processes. From a clinician's point of view, we will address cognitive–behavioral assessment methods in patients who report excessive pain-related fears. We will then describe a novel treatment approach for patients with musculoskeletal pain, which is based on the treatment methods developed for people with anxiety disorders. An adapted form of exposure *in vivo* with behavioral experiments is described which aims to provide personal evidence that the anticipated catastrophic consequences of physical performance do not occur. We critically appraise the currently available data on the effectiveness of this novel approach and address some of the complicating factors. Finally, we will provide some directions for future research and development.

CHARACTERISTICS OF PAIN-RELATED FEAR

In 1990, Kori et al.[7] introduced the term "kinesiophobia" (kinesis = movement) for the condition in which a patient has "an excessive, irrational, and debilitating fear of physical movement and activity resulting from a feeling of vulnerability to painful injury or reinjury." Recent evidence revealed that, during confrontation with feared movements, chronic low back pain patients who are fearful of movement/(re)injury typically show cognitive (catastrophic interpretations), attentional (hypervigilance), and behavioral (escape and avoidance) responses, rendering support for the idea that chronic pain and chronic fear share important characteristics.[4, 8, 9]

There is evidence that pain-related fear is associated with an exaggerated negative orientation towards pain, referred to as pain catastrophizing. Pain catastrophizing has been shown to mediate distress reactions to painful stimulation.[10] For example, Crombez et al.[11] found that pain-free volunteers with a high frequency of catastrophic thinking about pain became more fearful when threatened with the possibility of occurrence of intense pain than students with a low frequency of catastrophic thinking. In line with these findings, a strong association has been found between pain-related fear and pain catastrophizing in chronic pain patients, and it has been suggested that pain catastrophizing is likely to be a precursor of pain-related fear.[2, 12] Another study showed that when a certain sensation is interpreted as damaging, it will be perceived as more painful.[13]

PAIN–RELATED FEAR AND BEHAVIORAL PERFORMANCE

It has repeatedly been shown that pain-related fear is associated with escape/avoidance behaviors. Although in the case of chronic pain it is not possible to avoid pain completely, it is possible to avoid the perceived threat, in this case the activities that are assumed to increase pain or (re)injury. Avoidance behavior might thus be reflected in submaximal performance of activities. In a study in which chronic pain sufferers volunteered to undergo cold pressor pain, it was shown that expected danger significantly predicted avoidance of another cold pressor immersion.[14] Chronic pain patients who associate pain with damage tend to avoid activities that increase pain. Other studies that used physical performance tests reported that poor behavioral performance appeared to be more strongly associated with pain-related fear than with pain severity[15] and biomedical findings.[3]

The effects of pain-related fear on behavioral performance also appear to generalize to restrictions in daily life situations. Waddell et al.[16] demonstrated that fear-avoidance beliefs about work are strongly related to disability of daily living and work lost in the past year, and more so than pain variables such as anatomical pattern of pain, time pattern, and pain severity, and concluded that "Fear of pain and what we do about it may be more disabling than pain itself." Not only in chronic pain conditions, but also in acute back pain patients, a significant association is found between pain-related fear, poor physical performance, and self-reported disability levels.[17]

PAIN–RELATED FEAR AND ATTENTION

The cognitive theory of anxiety makes the assumption that an important function of anxiety is to facilitate the detection of potentially threatening situations. In line with this idea, it has been found that patients with phobia and anxiety disorders are hypervigilant, or overalert for threatening information:[18] they selectively attend to threatening information at the expense of other information, and have difficulties in disengaging attention from threat once it is detected. Evidence is starting to accumulate that similar attentional processes apply to pain and are relevant in pain patients.[19] Chronic back pain patients who avoid back-straining activities report not only high fear of pain and fear of (re)injury but also more attention to back sensations.[20, 21] Using structural equation modeling of self-report data, Goubert et al.[22] demonstrated that pain-related fear was a unique predictor of hypervigilance to pain and of the amount of pain experienced in low back pain patients. There is strong experimental evidence that pain-related fear induces hypervigilance for pain in healthy volunteers, but there are only a few studies that have experimentally investigated this idea in patients. Using the emotional Stroop task, several studies have demonstrated that patients with chronic pain attend selectively towards words that are thematically related to their pain and its consequences.[23] There was, however, no evidence that the attentional bias for pain words was more pronounced in patients with pain-related fear. More convincing are the results of studies that measure attention towards actual somatic stimuli or pain itself. Using a body-scanning reaction time paradigm, Peters *et al.*[24] found that in a group of fibromyalgia patients, detection latency for innocuous electrical stimuli in the arm was predicted by scores on the Pain Anxiety Symptoms Scale. In line with their findings are the results of studies using a primary task paradigm: chronic pain patients are requested to direct their attention away from pain, and to focus upon an attentionally demanding task. Degradation in task performance on the cognitive task during the experience of pain is taken as an index of attentional interference due to attention to pain and hypervigilance. A number of studies have demonstrated that degradation of task is most pronounced in chronic pain patients who reported high pain intensity,[25] high affect, somatic awareness, and high fear of (re)injury.[26] It seems then that patients who experience high fear of pain experience difficulties disengage from pain.[27]

DISCONFIRMATIONS OF HARM BELIEFS

What are the clinical implications of the above-mentioned findings? Philips[4] was one of the first to argue for the systematic application of graded exposure in order to produce disconfirmations between expectations of pain and harm, the actual pain, and the other consequences of the activity. She further suggested: "These disconfirmations can be made more obvious to the sufferer by helping to clarify the expectations he/she is working with, and by delineating the conditions or stimuli which he feels are likely to fulfill his expectations. Repeated, graded, and controlled exposures to such situations under optimal conditions are likely to produce the largest and most powerful disconfirmations."[4] Experimental support for this idea is provided by the match/mismatch model of pain,[28] which states that people initially tend to over-predict how much pain they will experience, but after some exposures these predictions tend to be corrected to match with the actual experience. A similar pattern was found by Crombez *et al.*[29] in a sample of chronic low back pain (CLBP) patients who were requested to perform four exercise bouts (two with each leg) at maximal force. During each exercise bout, the baseline pain, the expected pain, and the experienced pain were recorded. As predicted, the CLBP patients initially overpredicted pain, but after repetition of the exercise bout the overprediction was readily corrected. The expectancy did not seem to generalize to the exercise bout with the other leg as a small increase in pain expectancy reemerged. Also, expectancies were immediately corrected after another performance. In sum, it is quite plausible that, in analogy with the treatment of phobias, graded exposure to back-stressing movements may indeed be a successful

treatment approach for pain patients reporting substantial fear of movement/(re)injury.

GRADED *IN VIVO* EXPOSURE VERSUS GRADED ACTIVITY

Graded *in vivo* exposure may appear to be quite similar to the usual graded activity programs[30, 31] in that it gradually increases activity levels despite pain. However, both conceptually and practically, exposure *in vivo* is quite different from graded activity. First, graded activity is based on instrumental learning principles, and selected health behaviors are shaped through positively reinforcing predefined quota of activities. Exposure *in vivo*, originally based on extinction of pavlovian conditioning,[32] is currently viewed as a cognitive process during which fear is activated and catastrophic expectations are being challenged and disconfirmed, resulting in reductions in the threat value of the originally fearful stimuli. Second, during graded activity, special attention goes to the identification of positive reinforcers that can be provided when the individual quotas are met, whereas graded exposure pays special attention to the establishment of an individual hierarchy of the pain-related fear stimuli. Third, usual graded activity programs include individual exercises according to functional capacity and observed individual physical work demands, while graded exposure includes activities that are selected based on the fear hierarchy and the idiosyncratic aspects of the fear stimuli. For example, if the patient fears the repetitive spinal compression produced by riding a bicycle on a bumpy road, then the graded exposure should include an activity that mimics that specific activity and not just a stationary bicycle.

COGNITIVE–BEHAVIORAL ASSESSMENT

In this section we will deal with specific questionnaires, the interview, the establishment of graded hierarchies, and the behavioral tests that can be applied in order to gain sufficient information about the idiosyncratic aspects of pain-related fear responses in patients with chronic musculoskeletal pain.

Specific questionnaires

A basic question that may be asked is what the patient is afraid of or, in other words, what is the nature of the perceived threat? An answer to this question is not as simple as it seems. Patients may not view their problem as involving fear at all and may simply see difficulty in performing certain movements or activities. In addition, the specific nature of pain-related fear varies considerably, making an idiosyncratic approach almost indispensable.

Some patients fear pain. Other patients may fear not so much current pain but pain that will be experienced at a later time, for example the day after a physical exercise. Finally, patients may not fear pain itself, but the impending (re)injury that it is supposed to indicate, or they fear becoming permanently handicapped. The literature reflects this variety of fear stimuli by discussing measures for the assessment of fear of pain, fear of work and physical activity, and fear of (re)injury as a result of movement.

FEAR OF PAIN

The Pain Anxiety Symptoms Scale (PASS-20[33]) was developed to measure cognitive anxiety symptoms, fearful appraisals of pain, escape and avoidance responses, and physiologic anxiety symptoms related to pain. It is a 20-item questionnaire with internally consistent subscales. The validity of the PASS has been supported by positive correlations with measures of anxiety, cognitive errors, depression, and disability. The factor structure of the PASS-20 was found to be invariant across a fibromyalgia sample and a low back pain sample and indicated that a PASS-20 total score as well as scores on the subscales can be used.

FEAR OF WORK-RELATED ACTIVITIES

The Fear-Avoidance Beliefs Questionnaire (FABQ[16]) focuses on the patient's beliefs about how work and physical activity affect his/her low back pain. The FABQ consists of two scales: fear-avoidance beliefs of physical activity and fear-avoidance beliefs of work, the latter being consistently the stronger. The authors found that fear-avoidance beliefs about work are strongly related to disability of daily living and work lost in the past year; this was not the case for biomedical variables such as anatomical pattern of pain, time pattern, and severity of pain. On the other hand, the FABQ physical subscale is much stronger in predicting behavioral performance tests.[15]

FEAR OF MOVEMENT/(RE)INJURY

The Survey of Pain Attitudes (SOPA[34]) was developed to assess patients' attitudes towards five dimensions of the chronic pain experience: pain control, pain-related disability, medical cures for pain, solicitude of others, and medication for pain. Because of the authors' clinical observation of an association between chronic patients' hesitancy to exercise and the expressed fear of possible injury, a new scale (Harm) was added to the original instrument. As well as the Disability Scale and the Control Scale, the Harm Scale appeared to independently predict levels of dysfunction.

The Tampa Scale for Kinesiophobia (TSK[35]) is a 17-item questionnaire that is aimed at the assessment of fear of (re)injury due to movement. Each item is provided with a Likert scale, with scoring alternatives ranging from "strongly agree" to "strongly disagree." Most psychometric research has been carried out with the Dutch version of the TSK, which appears to be sufficiently reliable and valid.[2] Modest but significant correlations were found with measures of pain intensity, catastrophizing, impact of pain on daily life activities, and generalized fear. Regression analyses revealed that levels of disability were best predicted by pain-related fear, and that this was best predicted by catastrophizing. Pain intensity levels and biomedical findings were significantly less predictive of both pain-related fear and disability levels.[3] Moreover, the TSK discriminated well between avoiders and confronters during a behavioral performance task.[2, 15] Recent factor analyses revealed two subscales: these two factors were labeled *somatic focus*, which reflects the belief in underlying and serious medical problems, and *activity avoidance*, the belief that activity may result in (re)injury or increased pain. The factor structure appears invariant across pain diagnoses and Dutch, Swedish, and Canadian patients.[36]

Interview

GENERAL ISSUES

For elevated scores, the above-mentioned fear questionnaires are only indicative of the presence of pain-related fear. The assessment should be continued to further validate the hypothesis that the patient's disability is mainly determined by these fears. The semistructured interview is an additional and important tool to obtain information about the behavioral, psychophysiological, and cognitive aspects of the symptoms and to better estimate the role of pain-related fear in the maintenance of the pain problem (see **Box 16.1**). It also includes information about the antecedents (situational or internal) of the pain-related fear, and about the direct and indirect consequences. This screening might also include other areas of life stresses, as they might increase arousal levels and indirectly fuel pain-related fear. The etiologic model (**Figure 16.1**) is shown to be a useful theoretical framework that the clinician can keep in mind during the interview. Factors that often seem to be associated with the development of the fear are the characteristics of pain onset and the ambiguity around the presence or absence of positive findings on medicodiagnostics. For example, a person involved in a traffic accident may develop a fear of driving as a result of the traumatic experience. Likewise, a back pain patient may develop a fear of lifting after experiencing pain while lifting or after receiving information from a medical doctor that lifting can damage nerves in the spinal cord. Some chronic back pain patients who present with pain-related fear appear to base their conviction about vulnerability to (re)injury on the results of diagnostics tests such as radiographs and magnetic resonance imaging (MRI). The combination of (threatening) information conveyed by the medical specialist and the experience of pain and discomfort seem to strengthen that conviction. The visual confrontation with diagnostics or a medical diagnosis can be quite upsetting to some patients, as this information may be interpreted as being more threatening than intended by the specialist.

Although reports about misconceptions and misinterpretations of information can be used during the educational part of the intervention, it is more useful to identify the current level of severity and the maintaining factors of the pain problem and associated pain-related fear. The severity can often be estimated by inquiring about the extent to which the pain problem interferes with daily life, including the ability to carry on paid work, leisure activities, and normal relationships. Maintaining factors are usually negative thoughts about the danger of the physical activities, the avoidance of these activities, and hypervigilance to signals of threat. Negative thoughts can be elicited by inquiring about the client's personal theory about his pain and associated functional incapacity. Expectations about the future are also worth inquiring about: "What do you think will happen if the pain is left untreated?" For example, the back and pelvic pain complaints of a female patient started during her first pregnancy and increased after the delivery. She started worrying about the future because a relative who had received the same diagnosis finally became wheelchair bound. Her main belief was that during certain movements the tissue and nerves around the ridged symphysis pubis could be damaged or ruptured, possibly resulting in paralysis of the lower limbs. In most cases, these thoughts make people alert to bodily sensations that may signal impending danger. Situations that provoke these sensations are fearfully avoided. To gain insight into avoidance behaviors, the therapist may ask questions such as "What does the pain prevent you from doing?" and "If you no longer had this pain problem, what differences would it make to your daily life?" One can also ask directly about the situations that may worsen the pain problem. Finally, the assessment should also clarify whether other problems, such as major depression, marital conflicts, or disability claims, warrant specific attention before or after treatment. If more complicated problems are expected to arise as the pain problem diminishes, it may be better to leave the pain problem untreated.

Box 16.1 Items addressed during the interview

1. What does your pain feel like?
2. When did the pain start?
3. What were the circumstances of the pain onset?
4. If there was a sudden pain onset, what did you do, feel, and think at that moment?
5. What are you not doing because of the pain problem?
6. What do you think is causing your pain?
7. What do you think will happen in the near future if the pain remains untreated?
8. What is the influence of deep relaxation on your pain?

DETERMINING TREATMENT GOALS

There are several reasons why it is wise to spend some time on the determination of treatment goals.[37] First,

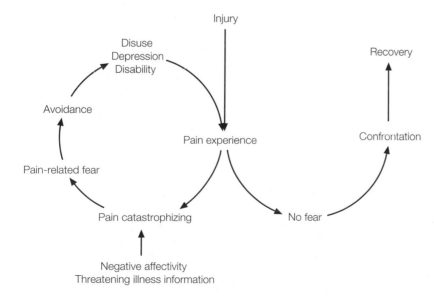

Figure 16.1 The cognitive–behavioral model of pain-related fear. Redrawn from *Pain*, **85**, Vlaeyen JW and Linton SJ, Fear-avoidance and its consequences in chronic musculoskeletal pain: a state of the art, 317–32, © Elsevier (2000).

cognitive–behavioral treatments for pain, including exposure *in vivo*, primarily aim at the restoration of functional abilities despite pain rather than at the reduction of pain. It helps to make this general goal explicit, and both patient and therapist should agree on one or more realistic and specific goals that are formulated in positive terms. Typical examples are being able to go shopping to the supermarket alone or go swimming twice a week for half an hour. In cases where the goal is to return to work, an occupational physician or vocational counselor can be consulted. Often, the exposure treatment can be synchronized with a graded resumption of work activities. Second, setting goals also helps to structure the treatment and to design the hierarchy of stimuli that will be introduced during the actual exposure *in vivo*. For example, if a patient wishes to resume his sports activities, the therapist will make sure that aspects of these will be included in the graded exposure activities. Third, setting functional goals also redirects the focus of attention from pain and physical symptoms toward daily life activities with the emphasis on the possibility of change away from the disability status. Finally, as the patient is invited to formulate his or her own goals, goal setting inadvertently reinforces the notion that active participation is an essential part of the treatment.

Graded hierarchies

Once it is identified that pain-related fear is pivotal in the maintenance of a person's pain disability, it is useful to inquire about the essential stimuli: What is the patient actually afraid of? So far, there is a lack of standardized tools for identifying these stimuli. In our experience, it is quite difficult for pain patients to verbally estimate the threat value of different situations. One of the problems is that the avoidance behaviors are not really acknowledged to be the consequences of fear but to be a direct consequence of the pain and the experienced vulnerability for (re)injury. In addition to checklists of daily activities, the presentation of visual materials such as pictures of back-stressing activities and movements might be worthwhile. They can be quite helpful in the development of graded hierarchies, reflecting the full range of situations avoided by the patient, beginning with those that provoke only mild discomfort and ending with activities or situations that are beyond the patient's present abilities. The Photograph Series of Daily Activities (PHODA[38]) is a standardized method that appears to be appropriate to design graded hierarchies. PHODA uses photographs representing various physical daily life activities, including lifting, bending, walking, bicycling, etc., that are presented to the patients, who are requested to place each photograph along a fear thermometer. (A CD-rom version of PHODA, including the pictures and a brief manual, as well as a short electronic version that can be run on a PC (PHODA-SeV[39]) is available and can be requested from phoda@hszuyd.nl.) This scale consists of a vertical line with 11 anchor points (ranging from 0 to 100) printed on a piece of cardboard that measures $60 \times 40\,cm$ (**Figure 16.2**). The fear thermometer is placed on a table in front of the patient with the following instruction: "Please look at each photograph carefully, and try to imagine yourself performing the same movement. Place the photograph on the thermometer according to the extent to which you feel that this movement is harmful to your back." In our experience, abrupt changes in movement (e.g. suddenly being hit) or activities consisting of repetitive spinal compressions (riding a bicycle on a bumpy road) are frequently mentioned stimuli in chronic back pain patients who score high for pain-related fear measures. These situations are feared because of beliefs about the causes of pain, such as ruptured or severely damaged nerves: "If I lift heavy weights, the nerves in my back might be damaged." For examples of a graded hierarchy, see **Tables 16.1** and **16.2**. Also of interest is that the same activity can be rated differently depending on the context in which the activity is performed. For example, the activity "running" receives an 80 when performed in a wood, and 50 when performed on an even terrain. It is

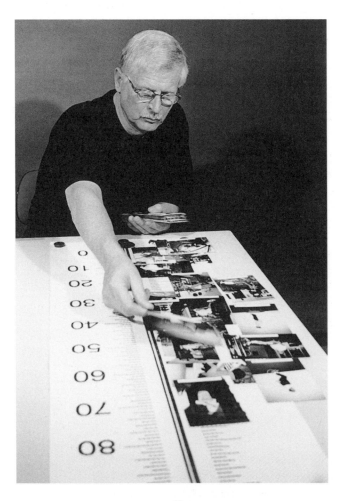

Figure 16.2 The use of PHODA[38] in establishing fear hierarchy.

Table 16.1 Graded hierarchy of pain-related fear stimuli for Ms X.

Pretreatment hierarchy	(PHODA) item	Post-treatment PHODA score
100	Throwing a trash bag	0
90	Lifting a child from squat	20
80	–	–
70	Making up the bed	0
60	Mopping the floor	10
50	Carrying a shopping bag on both arms	0
40	–	–
30	Rolling over in bed	0
20	Walking up and down stairs	0
10	Hanging out something on the clothes line	0

Table 16.2 Graded hierarchy of pain-related fear stimuli for Ms Y.

Pretreatment hierarchy	(PHODA) item	Post-treatment PHODA score
100	Carrying a small child on the shoulders	10
90	Raking leaves into a heap	20
80	Lifting a laundry basket	0
70	Riding off a curbstone with a bicycle	0
60	Lacing one's shoes while bending forward	10
50	Washing the dishes	0
40		–
30	Making up the bed	20
20	Emptying a dishwasher	0
10	Hanging something on a coat hook	0

therefore a good idea to expose patients to physical activities in a variety of contexts.

Behavioral tests

Sometimes, patients find it hard to estimate the harmfulness of an activity when it has been avoided extensively. In such cases, behavioral tests can be introduced. They consist of performing an activity that has been avoided previously while performance indices (such as time, distance, or number of repetitions) are measured. Target behaviors can be derived from the PHODA items, and in most cases the behavioral tests can be considered as a variant of the exercise tolerance test described by Fordyce.[40] To assess the extent to which avoidance occurs, patients are asked to perform the activity "... until pain, weakness, fatigue or any other reason causes you to wish to stop", quoted in Fordyce[40] (page 170). Behavioral tests have the advantage that anticipatory anxiety and the fear during exposure can be measured separately. In addition, they provide a more objective measure of avoidance behavior.

EDUCATION

The first session of graded exposure *in vivo* always consists of unambiguously educating the patient in a way that the patient views their pain as a common condition that can be self-managed, rather than as a serious disease or a condition that needs careful protection. The aim is to correct the misinterpretations and misconceptions that have occurred early on during the development of the pain-related fear. Each patient is given a careful explanation of the fear-avoidance model, using the patient's individual symptoms, beliefs, and behaviors to illustrate how vicious circles (pain → catastrophic thought → fear → avoidance → disability → pain) maintain the pain problem. In cases where the pain-related fear appears to be fuelled by having a ("positive") diagnostic test, it may be useful to review these tests together with a physician. It can be explained to patients that they probably have overestimated the value of these tests, and that in symptom-free people similar abnormalities can also be found. One of the effects of this education is that it increases the patient's willingness to finally engage in activities that they have been avoiding for a long time. Additionally, the provision of a more fluid, less localized understanding of pain could provide a greater sense of legitimacy for the pain in the absence of positive test results.[41]

EXPOSURE *IN VIVO*

Exposure

Current treatments of excessive fears and anxiety are based on the experimental psychological work of Wolpe,[42] who reported on systematic desensitization. In this keystone treatment method, individuals progress through increasingly more anxiety-provoking encounters with phobic stimuli while utilizing relaxation as a reciprocal inhibitor of rising anxiety. Because relaxation was intended to compete with the anxiety response, a graded format was chosen to keep anxiety levels as weak as possible. Later studies revealed that exposure to the feared stimuli appeared to be the most essential component of the systematic desensitization, and when applied without relaxation produced similar effects.[43] For a fearful patient, experiencing first-hand the results of changes in their behavior is far more convincing than rational argument; therefore, the most essential step consists of graded exposure to the situations that the patient has identified as "dangerous" or "threatening." Subsequently, individually tailored practice tasks are developed based on the graded hierarchy of fear-eliciting situations, thereby following the general principles for exposure. The patient agrees to perform certain activities or movements that they used to avoid. Patients are also encouraged to engage in these fearful activities as much as possible until anxiety levels have decreased. The therapist, who demonstrates how the activity can be performed in the most ergonomically efficient manner, first models each activity or movement. The presence of the therapist, who may initially encourage further exposures, is gradually withdrawn to facilitate independence and to create contexts that mimic those of the home situation.

Behavioral experiments

Following on from cognitive theory, which assumes that cognitive "errors" can be corrected through conscious reasoning, behavioral experiments have been developed for which the basis is a collaborative empiricism. The essence of a behavioral experiment is that the patient performs an activity to challenge the validity of his catastrophic expectations and misinterpretations. These interpretations take the form of "if … then …" statements, and are empirically tested during a behavioral experiment. Three steps can be distinguished. First, the patient formulates a hypothesis, for example a back pain patient may expect that jumping down from a stair will inevitably cause nerve damage in the spine and excruciating pain. Second, an alternative hypothesis is generated, for example after jumping down, I will be able to pursue my activity. Third, an experiment is designed, for example if the patient is convinced that jumping down is harmful then the therapist can further inquire about the minimal height that is needed to cause nerve injury. Finally, the experiment is carried out and evaluated. The therapist invites the patient to jump down from the stair and the consequences are assessed (see **Box 16.2**). In practice, behavioral experiments are difficult to separate from mere exposure, and they can best be used simultaneously.

Case illustrations

Although many patients with chronic musculoskeletal pain have similar fears (fear of physical activities that produce pain or that are assumed to cause reinjury), the origin of their fears may be different. Rachman[28] suggested three pathways for the acquisition of excessive fears: traumatic experience, observation of others in pain, and informational transmission. We will describe two patients, one of whom developed fear as a result of direct trauma and one as a result of informational transmission.

Ms X was a 40-year-old married woman who worked for a cleaning service. Her pain started five years before referral to the rehabilitation center while lifting a trash bag and throwing it into a big container. During this movement, she heard a "crack" in her lower back, immediately followed by a "shooting" pain. As she had never felt anything similar, and did not have an alternative explanation at hand, she interpreted this event as nerve damage and was afraid of becoming paralyzed. From then on, she experienced about four to six of these "cracks" a day. She could almost predict which movements provoked these frightening cracks, and tried to avoid them as much as possible.

The exposure part of the program consisted of nine sessions, each lasting about 60–90 minutes, spread over three weeks. During the educational part, it was made clear to the patient that "cracks" may occur without causing damage, and the vicious circle was explained with the message that she was suffering from excessive avoidance behavior because of her misbelief that "cracks" are dangerous. **Table 16.1** gives an overview of the graded hierarchy based on PHODA. One of the essential stimuli was bending forward, and we chose to start the exposure with simply bending at the knees and coming up again by putting small objects on the floor and picking them up. Before each trial, the patient's expectations of pain and harm were noted, and after the actual performance the experienced pain and harm were evaluated (**Table 16.2**). Gradually, the activities became physically more intense. During the last sessions, Ms X was bicycling over rough terrain, jumping from a 75-cm-high stool, playing badminton, and performing all of the daily household chores.

Box 16.2 Dialogue between Ms X and therapist during a behavioral experiment

Therapist: OK, today we'll start with the next activity. Why don't we try lifting this empty crate. What do you think?

Patient: [sighs] I don't think I can manage that.

Therapist: What do you think might happen?

Patient: I'm sure I'll get more pain. The disks in my back can't take such pressure. It may further damage the nerves there.

Therapist: How would you notice this?

Patient: My back will collapse, I won't be able to stand, and I may become paralyzed.

Therapist: How likely is it that this will happen when lifting this crate, on a scale 0 (not likely) to 100 (very likely)?

Patient: I am not sure, around 70.

Therapist: OK, well why don't we try and see what happens. I'll do it first, and then it's your turn. [At this point the therapist models the lifting task, and invites the patient to do the same, and while the patient is holding the case the therapist goes on inquiring about what happens.]

Therapist: Good. You're doing very well. How did it go?

Patient: OK, I guess. It did hurt somewhat, but my back could hold it quite well. It did not collapse.

Therapist: Right, despite the pain, you managed to lift this crate, right? Suppose we do this again, how would you rate the chances of your becoming paralyzed?

Patient: Well, I would say a 40, but there was no crack.

Therapist: Would the situation be different if you had felt a crack?

Patient: Oh yes, definitely.

Therapist: How could we induce such a crack.

Patient: When I was still working, I usually carried heavier weights than the one I just lifted.

Therapist: Shall we make this one a bit heavier?

Patient: [Laughs nervously] OK then.

Therapist: OK, go ahead and add more bottles. [The patient fills the whole case with bottles. After that, the therapist models the activity before the patient attempts it herself.]

Therapist: Did you feel a crack?

Patient: Not really, but, you know, suppose I should turn to this side [left] while lifting – that would make the situation much more dangerous.

Therapist: OK, is that worrying you more than lifting objects?

Patient: I think so, yes.

By doing this behavioral experiment, a new stimulus is introduced: rotating while lifting. At this point, the therapist invites the patient to show what she means by rotating. Thereafter, a new behavioral experiment is carried out incorporating this new stimulus, and the process of challenging expectations is repeated over again.

Because Ms X was included in a controlled outcome study, the exposure treatment was followed by a period of graded activity of equal length.

Ms Y was a 35-year-old married woman whose back and pelvic pain complaints started during her first pregnancy, six years ago, and increased after the delivery. After a second and third pregnancy, her pain complaints increased, and she remained unable to carry out a number of daily activities. An orthopedic assessment was performed and radiographs of the pelvis showed a ridged symphysis pubis and a pelvic instability. The visual confrontation with the radiographs was upsetting to her, and she became quite worried after hearing the diagnosis. She started worrying about the future because a relative who had received the same diagnosis finally became wheelchair bound. Her main belief was that during certain movements the tissue and nerves around the ridged symphysis pubis could be damaged or ruptured, possibly resulting in paralysis of the lower limbs.

During the educational part of the program, the rehabilitation physician explained to her that the so-called abnormal findings on the radiographs were, in fact, not unusual and were also seen in people without pain symptoms. Although Ms Y seemed reassured, she was not totally convinced. The therapist subsequently proposed to test the activity–harm assumption by exposing her to the activities that she had fearfully avoided. **Table 16.2** displays the graded hierarchy based on PHODA. Because Ms Y was included in a controlled outcome study, the exposure treatment was preceded by a period of graded activity of equal length. The treatment course was quite similar to that of Ms X, with a steep decrease in levels of fear and catastrophizing.

Complicating factors

PAIN INCREASES

Although patients have agreed that the treatment is not primarily aimed at reducing pain levels, it is very frightening to experience a sudden pain attack during the exposure treatment. This is what happened to Ms Z, a 46-year-old woman with CLBP. Before starting the fifth session, she complained of a severe, sharp pain that struck her in the morning while getting out of bed. She described this event as being very similar to the beginning of her pain problem. She was quite worried that this again was a sign of something being seriously wrong in her back. Her major concern was that too much movement would only worsen the situation, and she suggested that she should not take part in the program that day. The therapist briefly explored the circumstances of the pain attack and concluded with the patient that there was no reason for further medical examination. Ms Z did not think that this attack was caused by her increased activity level, and both she and the therapist decided to continue with the treatment and chose badminton for the activity as Ms Z liked it very much. As Ms Z experienced no substantial increase in her pain during this activity, she gradually became more confident, and the session was completed almost as planned. It is clear from **Figure 16.3**, which shows the patient's daily ratings of pain and fear, that after four days the ratings were back down again.

Maintenance of change

EXPANDING CONTEXTS

What is actually learned during exposure? Although some researchers assume that exposure leads to a disconfirmation of overpredictions of the aversive characteristics of fear stimuli, there is growing evidence that exposure cannot simply be equated with unlearning. Studies have demonstrated that a competition occurs

between the original threatening (excitatory) meaning of the stimuli and a new (inhibitory) meaning. In other words, during successful exposure, exceptions to the rule are learned rather than a fundamental change of that rule.[32] Crombez et al.[44] showed that, in CLBP patients, exposure to one movement (bending forward) did not generalize toward another dissimilar movement (straight leg raising). This pattern of results was only characteristic for high pain catastrophizers. The treatment implications of these findings are lengthy exposures to the full variety of contexts and natural settings in which fear has been experienced.[45] PHODA might be a useful tool in eliciting information about these contexts in chronic pain patients.

EFFECTIVENESS

Despite the fact that the importance of pain-related fear continued to be highlighted by behavioral theorists, empirical investigations including clinical outcome studies lagged behind theoretical thinking. We recently conducted two empirical studies to examine the effectiveness of a graded *in vivo* exposure treatment with behavioral experiments compared with the usual graded activity in reducing pain-related fears, catastrophizing, and pain disability in CLBP patients reporting substantial fear of movement/(re)injury.[46, 47] A replicated single-case crossover design was applied, one with four and one with six consecutive CLBP patients. Only patients who reported substantial fear of movement/(re)injury (TSK score > 40), and who were referred for outpatient behavioral rehabilitation, were included. After a no-treatment baseline measurement period, the patients were randomly assigned to one of two interventions. In intervention A, patients received the exposure first, followed by graded activity. In intervention B, the sequence of treatment modules was reversed. Daily measures of pain-related cognitions and fears were recorded using visual analog scales. Before and after the treatment, the following measures were taken: pain-related fear, pain catastrophizing, pain control, and pain disability.

Figure 16.4 displays the daily measures for fear of movement/(re)injury, fear of pain, and pain catastrophizing. Although the supplemental value of this "background" treatment program cannot be ruled out in this

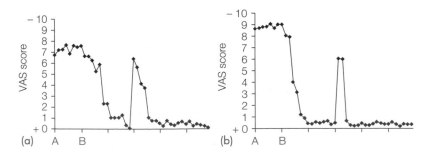

Figure 16.3 Daily measures of fear of pain severity: (a) visual analog scale; and movement/(re)injury (b) for subject Z across baseline and exposure *in vivo*. A, start baseline; B, start exposure *in vivo*.

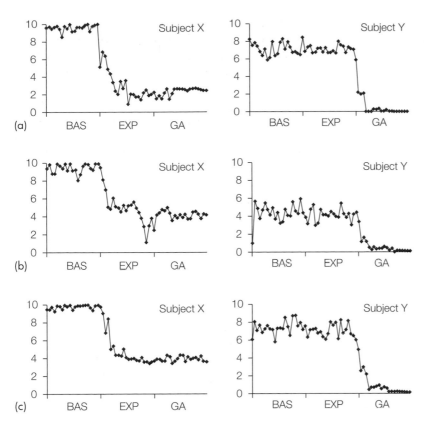

Figure 16.4 Daily measures of fear of movement/(re)injury for subjects X and Y across baseline (days 0–21) and both treatment modes (days 22–42 and days 43–63). (a) Fear of movement/(re)injury; (b) fear of pain; (c) pain catastrophizing. BAS, baseline; EXP, exposure *in vivo*; GA, graded activity. Redrawn from *Behaviour Research and Therapy*, **39**, Vlaeyen JW, de Jong J, Geilen M *et al.*, Graded exposure *in vivo* in the treatment of pain-related fear: a replicated single-case experimental design in four patients with chronic low back pain, 151–66, © Elsevier (2001).

study, the remarkable improvements that are observed whenever the graded exposure was initiated suggests that the therapeutic power of the graded exposure is much stronger. The crossover design gave us the opportunity to examine the differential effects of graded exposure and graded activity and also the additional treatment effect of the second treatment module. To tease apart the differential effects of the educational and the exposure components of the treatment, another study allocated fearful patients with CLBP randomly to two treatment conditions.[48] Both conditions started with a three-week baseline wait list period followed by one session of education, again followed by a three-week wait period. In one treatment, the second wait period was followed by exposure *in vivo*, while in the other treatment it was followed by graded activity. The results were striking. Subjective ratings of pain-related fear and pain catastrophizing decreased substantially after the educational part in all patients. However, self-reported difficulties in performing activities at home only decreased in the patients who received exposure *in vivo*. These results suggest that education may change patients' perceptions about the harmfulness of activity, but, alone, or in combination with graded activity, is not powerful enough to reverse avoidance and escape behaviors. Replications in other settings have also been carried out.[49, 50] These results, together with the initial studies, provide a basis for pursuing and further developing the exposure technique.

Although these first results are quite promising, there are a number of caveats to be considered. First, the preliminary evidence reported here is limited in that it included a small number of patients. On the other hand, single-case experimental designs were chosen with appropriate time series statistical analyses or randomization tests. More recently, two randomized controlled trials with large patient samples revealed that exposure *in vivo* is successful in reducing pain-related fear and pain catastrophizing, and to a lesser extent, pain disability.[51, 52]

SUMMARY

"Fear of pain and what we do about it may be more disabling than pain itself." According to this statement quoted by Waddell *et al.*[16] (page 164), the intuitively appealing idea that the lowered ability to accomplish tasks of daily living in chronic pain patients is merely the consequence of pain severity is refuted. The recent literature supports the early conjecture that chronic pain and phobia share important characteristics. Indeed, studies have shown that, during confrontation with feared movements, CLBP patients who are fearful of movement/(re)injury typically show behavioral (escape and avoidance), attentional (hypervigilance) and cognitive (worry) responses. It was not until recently that this line of thought was extended to the behavioral assessment and management of chronic pain. Specific pain-related fear measures, by which pain patients whose level of disability is likely to be controlled by pain-related fear, have been developed. As a result, a screening questionnaire that is aimed at the identification of acute back pain patients at risk has been developed for use in primary care and includes several items about fear and avoidance.[53, 54] In addition, the cognitive–behavioral assessment also includes the semistructured interview, the development of graded hierarchies, and the application of behavioral tests. This chapter describes an *in vivo* exposure treatment for the reduction of pain-related fear in CLBP patients. Preliminary outcome data show that an exposure *in vivo* consists of individually tailored practice tasks based on a graded hierarchy of fear-eliciting situations, and not just a physical training program or usual graded activity that does not take into account these essential and idiosyncratic fear stimuli. These data also show that exposure *in vivo* may help the patient to confront rather than avoid physical movement, and that a reduction in self-reported disability levels follows. Although cognitive–behavioral treatments for chronic pain are quite favorable,[55] there is an urgent need for further refinement of our treatments, including a better match between treatment modalities and patient characteristics. Although most of the research in pain-related fear was focused on musculoskeletal pain and back pain in particular, there is every reason to believe that fear processes are applicable to other pain problems as well. Indeed, the validity of the fear-avoidance model has been extended successfully to patients with osteoarthritis,[56] burn pain,[57] knee injury,[58] whiplash,[59] and neuropathic pain.[60] Exposure-based treatments for these pain problems have not been reported, but are likely to be developed in the near future. The approach described in this chapter may contribute to the process of customization of cognitive–behavioral treatments in the care of chronic pain patients.

ACKNOWLEDGMENTS

The authors wish to thank the staff of the Department of Pain Rehabilitation of the Hoensbroeck Rehabilitation Center and University Hospital Maastricht for their contribution in making the application of the exposure treatment possible. This contribution is supported by grant 904-65-090 and grant 96-06-006, both from the Council for Medical and Health Research of the Netherlands (ZonMW) to the first author.

REFERENCES

* 1. Lethem J, Slade PD, Troup JD, Bentley G. Outline of a fear-avoidance model of exaggerated pain perception. I. *Behaviour Research and Therapy.* 1983; **21**: 401–08.
* 2. Vlaeyen JW, Kole-Snijders AM, Boeren RG, van Eek H. Fear of movement/(re)injury in chronic low back pain and its relation to behavioral performance. *Pain.* 1995; **62**: 363–72.
3. Vlaeyen JWS, Kole Snijders AMJ, Rotteveel AM *et al.* The role of fear of movement/(re)injury in pain disability. *Journal of Occupational Rehabilitation.* 1995; **5**: 235–52.
* 4. Philips HC. Avoidance behaviour and its role in sustaining chronic pain. *Behaviour Research and Therapy.* 1987; **25**: 273–9.
5. Klenerman L, Slade PD, Stanley IM *et al.* The prediction of chronicity in patients with an acute attack of low back pain in a general practice setting. *Spine.* 1995; **20**: 478–84.
6. Linton SJ, Buer N, Vlaeyen JWS, Hellsing A-L. Are fear-avoidance beliefs related to the inception of an episode of back pain? A prospective study. *Psychology and Health.* 2000; **14**: 1051–9.
* 7. Kori SH, Miller RP, Todd DD. Kinesiophobia: a new view of chronic pain behavior. *Pain Management.* 1990; **3**: 35–43.
* 8. Asmundson GJ, Norton PJ, Norton GR. Beyond pain: the role of fear and avoidance in chronicity. *Clinical Psychology Review.* 1999; **19**: 97–119.
* 9. Vlaeyen JW, Linton SJ. Fear-avoidance and its consequences in chronic musculoskeletal pain: a state of the art. *Pain.* 2000; **85**: 317–32.
10. Sullivan MJL, Bishop SR, Pivik J. The pain catastrophizing scale: development and validation. *Psychological Assessment.* 1995; **7**: 524–32.
11. Crombez G, Eccleston C, Baeyens F, Eelen P. When somatic information threatens, catastrophic thinking enhances attentional interference. *Pain.* 1998; **75**: 187–98.
12. Leeuw M, Goosens ME, Linton SJ *et al.* The fear-avoidance model of musculoskeletal pain: current state of scientific evidence. *Journal of Behavioral Medicine.* 2007; **30**: 77–94.
13. Arntz A, Claassens L. The meaning of pain influences its experienced intensity. *Pain.* 2004; **109**: 20–5.
14. Cipher DJ, Fernandez E. Expectancy variables predicting tolerance and avoidance of pain in chronic pain patients. *Behaviour Research and Therapy.* 1997; **35**: 437–44.
* 15. Crombez G, Vlaeyen JW, Heuts PH, Lysens R. Pain-related fear is more disabling than pain itself: evidence on the role of pain-related fear in chronic back pain disability. *Pain.* 1999; **80**: 329–39.
* 16. Waddell G, Newton M, Henderson I *et al.* A Fear-Avoidance Beliefs Questionnaire (FABQ) and the role of fear-avoidance beliefs in chronic low back pain and disability. *Pain.* 1993; **52**: 157–68.
17. Swinkels-Meewisse IE, Roelofs J, Oostendorp RA *et al.* Acute low back pain: pain-related fear and pain catastrophizing influence physical performance and perceived disability. *Pain.* 2006; **120**: 36–43.
18. Bar-Haim Y, Lamy D, Pergamin L *et al.* Threat-related attentional bias in anxious and non-anxious individuals: a meta-analysis. *Psychological Bulletin.* 2007; **133**: 1–24.
19. Crombez G, Van Damme S, Eccleston C. Hypervigilance to pain: an experimental and clinical analysis. *Pain.* 2005; **116**: 4–7.
20. Crombez G, Vervaet L, Lysens R *et al.* Avoidance and confrontation of painful, back-straining movements in chronic back pain patients. *Behavior Modification.* 1998; **22**: 62–77.

* 21. McCracken LM. "Attention" to pain in persons with chronic pain: a behavioral approach. *Behavior Therapy.* 1997; **28**: 271–81.

22. Goubert L, Crombez G, Van Damme S. The role of neuroticism, pain catastrophizing and pain-related fear in vigilance for pain: a structural equations approach. *Pain.* 2004; **107**: 234–41.

23. Roelofs J, Peters M, Zeegers M, Vlaeyen J. The modified Stroop paradigm as a measure of selective attention towards pain-related stimuli among chronic pain patients: a meta-analysis. *European Journal of Pain.* 2002; **6**: 273.

24. Peters ML, Vlaeyen JW, van Drunen C. Do fibromyalgia patients display hypervigilance for innocuous somatosensory stimuli? Application of a body scanning reaction time paradigm. *Pain.* 2000; **86**: 283–92.

25. Eccleston C, Crombez G, Aldrich S, Stannard C. Attention and somatic awareness in chronic pain. *Pain.* 1997; **72**: 209–15.

26. Crombez G, Eccleston C, Baeyens F *et al.* Attention to chronic pain is dependent upon pain-related fear. *Journal of Psychosomatic Research.* 1999; **47**: 403–10.

27. Goubert L, Crombez G, Eccleston C, Devulder J. Distraction from chronic pain during a pain-inducing activity is associated with greater post-activity pain. *Pain.* 2004; **110**: 220–7.

28. Rachman S. The overprediction of fear: a review. *Behaviour Research and Therapy.* 1994; **32**: 683–90.

29. Crombez G, Vervaet L, Baeyens F *et al.* Do pain expectancies cause pain in chronic low back patients? A clinical investigation. *Behaviour Research and Therapy.* 1996; **34**: 919–25.

* 30. Fordyce WE, Brockway JA, Bergman JA, Spengler D. Acute back pain: a control-group comparison of behavioral vs traditional management methods. *Journal of Behavioral Medicine.* 1986; **9**: 127–40.

* 31. Lindstrom I, Ohlund C, Eek C *et al.* The effect of graded activity on patients with subacute low back pain: a randomized prospective clinical study with an operant-conditioning behavioral approach. *Physical Therapy.* 1992; **72**: 279–90; Discussion 291–3.

32. Bouton ME. Context and ambiguity in the extinction of emotional learning: implications for exposure therapy. *Behaviour Research and Therapy.* 1988; **26**: 137–49.

33. Roelofs J, McCracken L, Peters ML *et al.* Psychometric evaluation of the Pain Anxiety Symptoms Scale (PASS) in chronic pain patients. *Journal of Behavioral Medicine.* 2004; **27**: 167–83.

34. Jensen MP, Karoly P. Pain-specific beliefs, perceived symptom severity, and adjustment to chronic pain. *Clinical Journal of Pain.* 1992; **8**: 123–30.

35. Miller RP, Kori SH, Todd DD. *The Tampa Scale for Kinisophobia.* Unpublished report. 1991.

36. Roelofs J, Sluiter JK, Frings-Dresen MH *et al.* Fear of movement and (re)injury in chronic musculoskeletal pain: Evidence for an invariant two-factor model of the Tampa Scale for Kinesiophobia across pain diagnoses and Dutch, Swedish, and Canadian samples. *Pain.* 2007; **131**: 181–90.

37. Kirk J. Cognitive–behavioural assessment. In: Hawton K, Salkovskis PM, Kirk J, Clark DM (eds). *Cognitive behaviour therapy for psychiatric problems. A practical guide.* Oxford: Oxford University Press, 1989: 13–51.

38. Kugler K, Wijn J, Geilen M *et al. The Photograph series of Daily Activities (PHODA). CD-rom version 1.0.* Heerlen: Institute for Rehabilitation Research and School for Physiotherapy, The Netherlands, 1999.

39. Leeuw M, Goossens ME, Breukelen GJ *et al.* Measuring perceived harmfulness of physical activities in patients with chronic low back pain: the photograph series of daily activities-short electronic version. *Journal of Pain.* 2007; **8**: 840–9.

40. Fordyce WE. *Behavioral methods for chronic pain and illness.* St Louis, MO: Mosby, 1976.

41. Rhodes LA, McPhillips-Tangum CA, Markham C, Klenk R. The power of the visible: the meaning of diagnostic tests in chronic back pain. *Social Science and Medicine.* 1999; **48**: 1189–203.

42. Wolpe J. *Psychotherapy by reciprocal inhibition.* Stanford, CA: Stanford University Press, 1958.

43. Craske MG, Rowe MK. A comparison of behavioral and cognitive treatments of phobias. In: Davey GCL (ed.). *Phobias. A handbook of theory, research and treatment.* Chichester: Wiley & Sons, 1997: 247–80.

44. Crombez G, Eccleston C, Vansteenwegen D *et al.* Exposure to movement in low back pain patients: restricted effects of generalisation. *Health Psychology.* 2002; **21**: 573–8.

45. Goubert L, Crombez G, Lysens R. Effects of varied-stimulus exposure on overpredictions of pain and behavioural performance in low back pain patients. *Behaviour Research and Therapy.* 2005; **43**: 1347–61.

* 46. Vlaeyen JW, de Jong J, Geilen M *et al.* Graded exposure in vivo in the treatment of pain-related fear: a replicated single-case experimental design in four patients with chronic low back pain. *Behaviour Research and Therapy.* 2001; **39**: 151–66.

* 47. Vlaeyen JWS, de Jong J, Geilen M *et al.* The treatment of fear of movement/(re)injury in chronic low back pain: further evidence for the effectiveness of exposure in vivo. *Clinical Journal of Pain.* 2002; **18**: 251–61.

48. de Jong JR, Vlaeyen JW, Onghena P *et al.* Fear of movement/(re)injury in chronic low back pain: education or exposure in vivo as mediator to fear reduction? *Clinical Journal of Pain.* 2005; **21**: 9–17.

49. Linton SJ, Overmeer T, Janson M *et al.* Graded in vivo exposure treatment for fear-avoidant pain patients with functional disability: a case study. *Cognitive Behaviour Therapy.* 2002; **31**: 49–58.

50. Boersma K, Linton S, Overmeer T *et al.* Lowering fear-avoidance and enhancing function through exposure in vivo. A multiple baseline study across six patients with back pain. *Pain.* 2004; **108**: 8–16.

51. Woods MP, Asmundson GJ. Evaluating the efficacy of graded in vivo exposure for the treatment of fear in patients with chronic back pain: a randomized controlled clinical trial. *Pain.* 2008; **136**: 271–80.

52. Leeuw M, Goossens ME, van Breukelen GJ *et al.* Exposure in vivo versus operant graded activity in chronic low back pain patients: results of a randomized controlled trial. *Pain* (in press). http://dx.doi.org/10.1016/j.pain.2007.12.009.

53. Kendall NAS, Linton SJ, Main CJ. *Guide to assessing psychosocial yellow flags in acute low back pain: risk factors for long-term disability and work loss.* Wellington: Accident Compensation Corporation, 1997.

54. Linton SJ, Hallden K. Can we screen for problematic back pain? A screening questionnaire for predicting outcome in acute and subacute back pain. *Clinical Journal of Pain.* 1998; **14**: 209–15.

∗ 55. Morley S, Eccleston C, Williams A. Systematic review and meta-analysis of randomized controlled trials of cognitive behaviour therapy and behaviour therapy for chronic pain in adults, excluding headache. *Pain.* 1999; **80**: 1–13.

56. Heuts PH, Vlaeyen JW, Roelofs J *et al.* Pain-related fear and daily functioning in patients with osteoarthritis. *Pain.* 2004; **110**: 228–35.

57. Sgroi MI, Willebrand M, Ekselius L *et al.* Fear-avoidance in recovered burn patients: association with psychological and somatic symptoms. *Journal of Health Psychology.* 2005; **10**: 491–502.

58. Kvist J, Ek A, Sporrstedt K, Good L. Fear of re-injury: a hindrance for returning to sports after anterior cruciate ligament reconstruction. *Knee Surgery, Sports Traumatology, Arthroscopy.* 2005; **13**: 393–7.

59. Nederhand MJ, Ijzerman MJ, Hermens HJ *et al.* Predictive value of fear avoidance in developing chronic neck pain disability: consequences for clinical decision making. *Archives of Physical Medicine and Rehabilitation.* 2004; **85**: 496–501.

60. de Jong JR, Vlaeyen JW, Onghena P *et al.* Reduction of pain-related fear in complex regional pain syndrome type I: The application of graded exposure in vivo. *Pain.* 2005; **116**: 264–75.

Physical therapy and rehabilitation protocols

17

Transcutaneous electrical nerve stimulation

TIMOTHY P NASH

KEY LEARNING POINTS

- The gate theory of pain explained how skin stimulation could modulate pain, and led to the development of transcutaneous electrical nerve stimulation (TENS).
- TENS can help in the management of many types of chronic, and to a lesser extent acute, pain.
- It is a straightforward and inexpensive treatment.
- Electrodes are placed along the painful dermatome, or if necessary along the contralateral dermatome.
- Tolerance may develop from continuous therapy.

- There is little evidence that any particular type of stimulation is superior to any other.
- Care should be taken in patients with pacemakers.
- Complications and side effects are generally minor and reversible, provided simple precautions are observed.
- Treatment is dose dependent and should be for at least 30 minutes twice a day for at least a month for chronic pain.

INTRODUCTION

Man has been aware of the effects of electricity for thousands of years. A bas-relief in Egypt from 2750BC shows a Nile catfish (electric catfish) known as the "releaser of many" or the "shaker." About 400BC, Hippocrates used electric fish to treat headache and arthritis, and in 46BC Scribonius Largus described the use of the electric torpedo ray by the Romans for gout and headache. Baron Von Humboldt studied the electric eel of South America in 1800. He stood on one and experienced the development of a painful numbness up to his knees,

which left him with violent pain in his knees and the rest of his joints for the remainder of the day. He prophesied, "The discoveries that will be made on the electromotive apparatus of these fish will extend to all phenomena of muscular motion subject to volition. It will perhaps be found that in most animals every contraction of a muscle fiber is preceded by a discharge from the nerve to the muscle." He also predicted that electricity was the source of life and movement in all living things.[1]

The development of the Leyden jar in 1745–6 enabled electricity to become more readily available and portable, rather than requiring a wet fish at the seaside! This led to the development of magnetoelectric, electroanesthetic equipment. In 1759, John Wesley used his electrostatic machine to treat "rheumaticky pains" in a patient "made helpless like an infant." After the second shock, he felt some change; after the third he was able to raise himself; after two more he rose and walked about the room; and before noon he was quite well. In England in 1858, Althaus described the application of his apparatus to peripheral nerves. At the same time, in Philadelphia, Francis was producing analgesia for dental extractions. Oliver in Buffalo and Garratt in Boston were similarly producing dental analgesia, and developing its use at other sites. Garratt in particular used it for dental neuralgias, hyperalgesia, tic douloureux, toothache, and jaw ache. Oliver used it also for amputation of limbs and for childbirth. The Cataphoresis machine of 1925 was used for dental analgesia and can be seen in the Charles King Collection at the Association of Anaesthetists of Great Britain and Ireland. The modern equivalent is the H-wave and Ultracalm machines.

The "gate theory" of pain[2] attempted to explain how chronic stimulation of the nervous system could be used to treat nociceptive pain, and led to the development of percutaneous stimulation of peripheral nerves and dorsal column stimulation. TENS was initially introduced as a prognostic test prior to spinal cord stimulation.

Prolonged stimulation of peripheral nerves with percutaneous needle electrodes was shown in 1967 to modify the reaction of healthy human volunteers to acute noxious stimuli, without any ill effects,[3] and to inhibit the prolonged after-discharge in the tegmentum and medulla that normally follows electrical tetanic stimulation of a peripheral nerve.[4] This confirmed clinically the spinal gate control theory of Melzack and Wall.[2] Confirmation of this effect with brief, intense transcutaneous electrical stimulation at trigger points or acupuncture points on severe clinical pain was published in 1975.[5] Such stimulation produced a decrease in pain of 60–70 percent depending on the type of pain, significantly higher than the strong placebo contribution.

Many different electrical stimulation therapies have now been developed, all working on the same idea. Action potential stimulation therapy mimics the action potential in its electrical waveform. Interferential therapy is a static machine used by physiotherapists, and transcutaneous spinal electroanalgesia and transcutaneous cranial electrical stimulation are claimed to produce analgesia by percutaneously stimulating the spinal cord and brain, respectively. Cutaneous field stimulation uses a flexible plate with needle-like electrodes to electrically stimulate nerve fibers in the superficial skin, and has been developed to treat itch without damaging the skin.

APPLIED ANATOMY

The exact mechanism of TENS and acupuncture is still not clear. Both peripheral and central neural mechanisms are involved. Acupuncture and TENS for analgesia are now considered in the light of the type of stimulus used. Conventional TENS is a high-frequency, low-intensity stimulus, and acupuncture and acupuncture-like TENS is a low-frequency, high-intensity stimulus.

The low-intensity (TENS) stimulus is considered to activate large muscle (type I) and large skin (Aβ) fibers. This produces gating by segmental inhibition of the central afferents of the polymodal C pain fibers within the substantia gelatinosa, possibly through interneurons with γ-aminobutyric acid receptors. The Aβ-fibers pass in the dorsal columns to produce descending inhibition via the periaqueductal gray matter. The analgesia is often of rapid onset and short duration, and tolerance can develop from continuous therapy. At least part of TENS-mediated hypoalgesia is a consequence of a direct peripheral effect of TENS.[6]

Low-frequency, high-intensity stimulation (acupuncture) is considered to act by stimulating small muscle afferents (type III, Aδ-fibers) to produce both segmental and suprasegmental inhibition via endorphinergic and serotoninergic pathways. Segmental inhibition is produced by presynaptic inhibition via interstitial enkephalinergic fibers in the substantia gelatinosa. The central afferents of the Aδ-fibers pass in the spinothalamic tract to the hypothalamus, and again can produce suprasegmental inhibition via endorphinergic and serotoninergic pathways. The analgesia produced has slow onset and long duration, and 30-minute treatments do not produce tolerance. Animal evidence must be considered with caution, but both low- and high-frequency TENS has been shown to reduce the hyperalgesia of kaolin-carrageenan-induced knee joint inflammation in rats via activation of deep somatic large diameter primary afferents.[7]

INDICATIONS

TENS is used widely. In Canada, 93 percent of hospitals use it for acute pain, 43 percent for labor and delivery, and 96 percent for chronic pain, amounting to an estimated 450,000 hospital uses of TENS per year.[8]

TENS can be used for localized, mild, superficial pain of somatic or neurogenic origin, but is less useful for widespread, severe, deep-seated pain. It may be useful for visceral pain, especially angina pectoris.

Acute pain

Most acute pain is due to trauma, and settles sufficiently quickly to render TENS unnecessary. Sports injuries, however, including back sprains, torn ligaments, and pulled muscles, can respond usefully. Major trauma usually includes multiple injuries and will produce pain that is widespread and severe. TENS is unlikely to be of any value in this situation.

TENS may also be valuable for the pain of fractured ribs, acute orofacial inflammatory pain (periodontal infections and pulpal inflammation), acute rheumatoid arthritis, myalgia, and myofascial pain. Postoperative pain has also been treated, and the electrodes may be applied adjacent to the incision by the surgeon at the end of surgery. Postoperative nausea and vomiting can be reduced using TENS, which has been found to be as effective as commonly used antiemetic drugs.

Analgesia for procedures such as dental treatment and lancet-induced trauma to the fingertip can also be provided by TENS, and it has become popular for the pain of labor. During labor, two sets of electrodes are used: one pair at T10–L1 for the first stage and a second at S2–S4 for the second stage. Primary dysmenorrhea may also respond.

Chronic pain

TENS is associated with improvement on multiple outcome variables in addition to pain relief for chronic pain patients, and can be effective long term.

Myofascial/musculoskeletal/spasticity

Myofascial or muscular pain can respond to TENS, and it has been used instead of the Milwaukee brace in managing idiopathic scoliosis. It can also be effective in reducing spinal spasticity.

Neuropathic

The pain of peripheral diabetic neuropathy responds successfully to TENS, as does phantom limb pain, where it can be usefully applied to the contralateral leg. Other neuropathic pains, such as brachial plexus avulsion and postherpetic neuralgia, can also respond, provided the skin site for the electrodes has sufficient sensation for paresthesiae to be produced in the painful area.

Visceral

TENS is useful for angina pectoris, providing an increased work capacity, reduced frequency of anginal attacks, and reduced consumption of short-acting nitroglycerin, due to a decreased afterload resulting from systemic vascular dilatation. Lactate metabolism is reduced and there is less pronounced ST segment depression with an increased coronary flow to ischemic areas in the myocardium. Sympathetic activity may be decreased either directly or indirectly as a consequence of pain inhibition, and blood pressure can also be lowered. Tissue perfusion may also be improved by TENS, producing ulcer healing in peripheral vascular disease, leprosy, and in skin flaps with deficient circulation after reconstructive surgery, and it can also be useful in thrombophlebitis.

TENS may be a useful treatment for noncardiac chest pain of esophageal origin, and can decrease lower esophageal sphincter pressure in patients with achalasia. It can also reduce perception of gut distension without interfering with local and reflex gut responses. TENS has been shown to produce prompt onset of analgesia with no significant effect on uterine activity in patients with primary dysmenorrhea. It may also have a role in the treatment of detrusor instability and urinary urgency.

It has also been used successfully for antiemesis in cancer therapy and as an adjunct to other analgesic regimes.

CONTRAINDICATIONS

Contraindications include the following.

- Broken/dysaesthetic/numb skin. Application of the electrodes to broken or dysesthetic skin will be poorly tolerated, and application to numb areas will not stimulate the skin nerve fibers. It is essential that paresthesiae can be generated in the region of the pain or within the same or closely related dermatome.
- Application to the front of the neck should never be performed, as the laryngeal muscles and carotid sinus may be stimulated.
- Stimulation overt fetus. Except in labor, it is probably sensible to avoid stimulation over the pregnant uterus, and especially during the first trimester, as electrical fields may have an effect on the development of the fetus. If premature labor or miscarriage occurs while TENS is being used, the treatment is likely to be blamed, despite its application well away from the uterus. No reports exist in the literature, however.

CAUTION

Cardiac pacemaker

Caution should be exercised in the presence of a cardiac pacemaker, although it is not uncommon to use it in the presence of a fixed rate pacemaker, with the agreement of the cardiologist in charge of the patient. Patients with cardiac pacemakers should not be excluded from the use of TENS, but careful evaluation and extended cardiac monitoring should be performed.[9, 10] It is our practice to give the patient an initial trial in the day ward with electrocardiographic monitoring before discharging them with a unit. Even so, interaction can occur at a later date.[11]

Driving/operating machinery

Caution should be observed while driving or operating machinery, as transient disconnection of the electrodes can cause a surge of current on reconnection that could startle the patient and cause gross sudden movement, with the consequent dangers.

Senility/low intelligence quotient

It is unwise to use TENS in senile patients, children, or those with a low intelligence quotient (IQ), as they need a good understanding of how to apply and use the unit.

LIMITATIONS: FREQUENCY OF THERAPY

The use of TENS for acute pain depends on the availability to the patient of both the unit and education on its use.

For it to be effective in postoperative pain, sterile electrodes must be applied alongside the incision and underneath the dressings, preferably by the surgeon. The site of application must not have been denervated by the surgery.

For chronic pain, TENS must be used for at least 30 minutes twice a day and for at least one month before any effect may be felt. About half the patients using TENS can reduce their pain by more than 50 percent, and the analgesia is rapid both in onset (less than 30 minutes in 75 percent of patients) and in offset (less than 30 minutes in 51 percent of patients). One-third of patients generally use TENS for over 61 hours/week.[12]

EQUIPMENT

- TENS stimulator.
- Electrode leads.
- Electrodes:
  - carbon–rubber, with electrode gel and fixative;
  - disposable.

TENS is normally provided by a portable, battery-operated, semiconductor pulse generator connected via leads to electrodes applied to the skin. Generally, it has the following controls:

- combined on/off and amplitude (intensity) control;
- frequency control (from around 2 to > 100 Hz or even to 250 Hz);
- mode selector to select between continuous and pulsed stimulation, sometimes with a further choice to modulate the stimulation giving a slow increase then decrease in amplitude or frequency to produce a sensation similar to stroking. Modulated or pulsed output reduces the development of tolerance to the stimulation;
- width control (varying the width of the electrical pulse, usually between 40 and 500 μs);
- multichannel units will have a separate amplitude switch for each channel.

There are also stimulators that produce complex waveforms to achieve deeper stimulation (Likon) or further reduce the development of tolerance by utilizing multiple electrodes activated randomly (Codetron). Action potential stimulation therapy uses a waveform that mimics the action potential. It is generally used with below-threshold stimulation.

A pair of insulated wires with a small jack plug at one end connects to the stimulator, and separate plugs at the other end connect to the electrodes. The leads are the weakest link in the circuit, and frequently fracture at the junction with the plugs at either end. The more supple the leads, the less likely they are to fracture, and the more comfortable to wear.

The electrodes are generally either carbon–rubber (conductive) or disposable self-adhesive electrodes. The carbon–rubber electrodes require electrode gel applying between the electrode and the skin, and fixing in place with adhesive tape. Alternatively, karaya pads, made from conductive karaya gum and adhesive on both sides, may be used. The self-adhesive electrodes require no fixative or gel, becoming adhesive with wetting of the surface of the electrode that is applied to the skin.

Some older machines may have sponge or cotton wool pads that require wetting, and may be fixed in place with Velcro bands. Larger electrodes require greater voltage output, but less pulse-charge density than the smaller electrodes, and evoke significantly greater nonpainful and maximally tolerated painful muscle torques for high-threshold stimulation.[13]

Electrode position

The electrodes are used in pairs. To avoid short-circuiting between them, they should never be positioned with less than 1 cm between their edges. The electrodes should be positioned to lie over, and along the line of, the nerves supplying the area to be treated (**Figure 17.1**). Consequently, the electrodes should be applied longitudinally on the limbs, and along the main axis of the nerves or dermatomes on the trunk.

Connect the electrodes to the leads before applying to the skin. The skin should be clean and dry and free from grease or powder. If not, the electrical conductivity will be affected and self-adhesive electrodes will become soiled and lose their adhesiveness. Electrodes should not stay on the skin for more than 24 hours.

Carbon–rubber electrodes

Carbon–rubber electrodes are applied to the skin after smearing a layer of conductive gel over the skin surface of the electrode, and then placing it in the required position and fixing it in position with adhesive tape. Saline jelly (normally 2 percent sodium chloride and containing a bactericide) is advisable to give good electrical

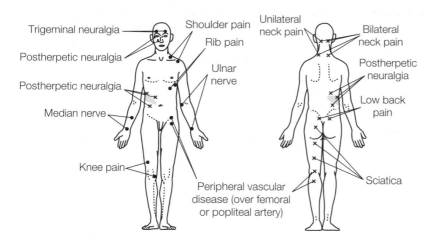

Figure 17.1 Useful transcutaneous electrical nerve stimulation electrode application points.

conductivity between the skin and the electrode. Electrocardiograph (ECG) jelly contains a much higher concentration of saline, which will irritate the skin if left on for the usual time for TENS therapy. It should therefore be avoided. KY jelly, although not an electrode gel, in practice does provide adequate conductivity, and may be useful when allergies develop to the normal electrode gels. Once applied, the electrode is fixed in position with adhesive tape. The most suitable is Micropore because it does not usually cause skin irritation and is easy to apply.

Self-adhesive electrodes

The electrode is normally stored on a backing sheet of either wax or polythene. It should be peeled off the backing sheet, moistened, and applied evenly to the skin. To remove it, it should be peeled off the skin from one corner and immediately applied to the backing sheet to prevent drying.

Connection to the stimulator

The electrodes are then connected to the stimulator via the leads. The stimulator must be switched off at the time of connection. The stimulator is then switched on and adjusted appropriately.

TYPES OF STIMULATION

TENS can be used in three different types of stimulation modality.

1. Continuous (conventional); high frequency (40–150 Hz); low intensity (10–30 mA).
2. Pulsed (burst); low frequency (bursts of 100 Hz at 1–2 Hz); low intensity (10–30 mA).
3. Acupuncture-like (Acu-TENS); low frequency (bursts of 100 Hz at 1–2 Hz); high intensity (15–50 mA).

Application

1. Clean skin well before application.
2. Check stimulator is switched off.
3. Apply electrodes to skin with normal sensation.
4. Position electrodes with their adjacent edges at least 2 cm apart.
5. Position along direction of nerves or dermatomes supplying the painful area.
6. Connect electrodes to stimulator.
7. Select stimulation mode (continuous, pulsed, modulated).
8. Turn stimulator on and increase amplitude to maximum comfortable.
9. Increase frequency to maximum comfortable.
10. Increase pulse width to maximum comfortable.
11. If using acupuncture-like TENS, increase amplitude to produce muscle twitches in muscles between electrodes.

SITE OF APPLICATION

The rationale of use is to apply the electrodes to the skin to stimulate along the general direction of the nerves supplying the area to be treated. Thus, when treating the limbs, the electrodes should be applied longitudinally; on the trunk, they should be placed along the course of the nerves or the dermatomes. Whichever stimulation modality is used, the stimulation sensation should be directed into the painful part and should be strong, but comfortable.

When conventional or pulsed stimulation is used, muscle twitching should not be produced, but acupuncture stimulation should be adjusted to be strong enough to produce muscle twitching. Large areas of pain will require two or more pairs of electrodes, by using either a double adaptor lead with a single channel unit or a dual channel stimulator with two leads.

In angina pectoris, the electrodes are applied to the dermatome where the pain is felt. Thus, stimulation of the cutaneous afferents from that dermatome will enter the cord at the same or closely related level as that of the visceral afferents producing the pain.

TRIAL

It is normal to have a trial period of treatment to ensure that the pain is not aggravated by TENS, to teach the patient how to use the system, and to give a guide as to the likelihood of the pain responding to treatment. However, initial poor response does not mean that long-term use will not achieve some benefit. At least one hour of stimulation is required in the first instance. It should then be used regularly for at least one hour three times each day for a minimum of 14 days. The frequency of use should be adjusted according to need and response. The patient should use TENS as much as they wish, and be encouraged to compare the effects of all modalities. This will enable them to choose the modality most effective for them, or the most effective at particular times, using all types of stimulation as necessary. They should be told that a period of poststimulation analgesia might occur.

The patient should be reviewed regularly over the first year, and thereafter as required, if they continue to use TENS.

SETTING THE STIMULATOR

Continuous (conventional) stimulation

All the controls should be set at zero, and the mode switch set at continuous. The amplitude should then be increased slowly to the maximum comfortable level, i.e. strong but comfortable, and then the pulse frequency increased to the maximum comfortable level. If there is a pulse width control, this should also be increased to again the maximum comfortable level. Increasing the pulse width may enable a reduced amplitude setting to be used, reflecting the power delivered by the unit and necessary to produce adequate stimulation.

Pulsed (burst) stimulation

All controls should be set at zero and the mode switch set to pulsed mode. The amplitude, pulse frequency, and pulse width are adjusted as in continuous stimulation.

Acupuncture-like TENS

Adjust the stimulator as for pulsed stimulation, but increase the amplitude to produce muscle twitches in the muscles beneath the electrodes. These muscle twitches should not be so strong that they are painful.

Sequential stimulation

Sequential TENS involves two periods of stimulation with different parameters. If conventional TENS is used initially, this may enable burst stimulation to be better tolerated, with the possibility of greater efficacy and more prolonged effect.[14]

Choice of stimulation modality

Patients will choose the most suitable settings for their own pain by trial and error. There is no evidence in favor of any particular settings for any particular condition.

COMPLICATIONS

Skin irritation occurs in 30 percent of patients and is usually due to inadequate application. The most common cause is failure to clean carbon–rubber electrodes after use; these must be removed from the skin at least once in every 24 hours. Electrodes should not be applied to the same area of skin every day, but an adjacent position on fresh skin should be used.

Allergic reactions are uncommon, but may occur to the electrode, the jelly, or the fixative (tape or gum). When this does occur, a different type of jelly, tape, or electrode should be used. Thus, carbon–rubber electrodes can be replaced by self-adhesive electrodes; TENS saline jelly can be replaced by KY jelly (KY jelly is theoretically not conductive, but in practice is satisfactory). Micropore tape can be replaced by some other suitable tape (even Sellotape!).

Electrical skin burns can occur, particularly if excessive current is applied to denervated or poorly innervated areas of skin that are numb or partially numb. Before using TENS, always check that there is normal sensation where the electrodes are being applied.

There may be failure of various parts of the equipment. The most common parts to fail are the leads, which may fracture where they connect to the plugs. The plugs themselves may become dirty, corroded, or heavily oxidized. The battery may fail, or be inserted incorrectly. If rechargeable batteries are used, the charger itself may be at fault.

Tolerance may develop to the analgesic effect and occurs in about 30 percent of patients, developing slowly over time. Apparent tolerance may be due to a worsening of the pain. This may be reversed by temporary withdrawal of TENS or by changing the pulse pattern (perhaps from continuous to pulsed).

A case of respiratory arrest, explained by the production of tetanic stimulation of the intercostal muscles of a patient using TENS for angina, has been described.[15]

SIDE EFFECTS

Only 47 percent of patients considered the TENS sensations to be consistently pleasant. Forty-six percent suffered side effects as follows:[16]

- sensations at the site of TENS application (18 percent), including:
  - pins and needles;
  - soreness;
  - tingling;
  - itching;
  - prickling;
  - numbness;
  - shaking;
  - burning;
  - stabbing;
  - a new "pulling" pain;
- sensations at a distance to site of application (12 percent);
- headaches (8 percent);
- increased pain (8 percent);
- muscle aches (6 percent);
- nausea (3 percent);
- bad temper (3 percent);
- dizziness (1 percent).

EVIDENCE FOR THE USE OF TENS

Experimental evidence

Evaluating TENS in randomized, double-blind trials is not easy. It is very difficult to blind patients to the fact that they are receiving TENS, as its effect depends on producing electrical sensation at the site of application. This leads to bias that can exaggerate the estimate of treatment effect by up to 17 percent. Trials that are not randomized or are inadequately randomized exaggerate the estimate of treatment effect by up to 40 percent.[17] This has to be taken into account when reviewing the evidence of efficacy of TENS or any of its stimulation modalities.

The effect of TENS appears to be similar to that produced by other nonpharmacological analgesic manipulations, such as counter-irritation and changes in attention.[18] Like counter-irritation, it needs to be felt to be effective, as shown by a trial where subthreshold TENS had no effect on myofascial pain syndromes when compared with placebo in a single-blind trial.[19] This confirms the need to produce paresthesiae within the painful area to provide analgesia.

TENS is associated with improvement on multiple outcome variables in addition to pain relief for chronic pain patients who are long-term users. Also, for some patients, long-term TENS use continues to be effective.[20]

Acupuncture and acupuncture-like TENS produce stimulation, either mechanical or electrical, at low frequencies (below 10 Hz) given at an intensity that produces muscle contractions which extend to the whole muscle group (high-intensity, low-frequency stimulation), with TENS producing high-frequency, low-intensity stimulation (**Table 17.1**).

Considerable experimentation has been performed in animals, human volunteers, and in the clinical arena. Despite this, no one stimulation modality (acupuncture-like or conventional) has been proven better than any other in any particular situation. Stimulation modality is therefore chosen on the basis of patient preference or prolongation of battery life.

There has been the suggestion from nonblinded studies that high-frequency TENS, continuous or pulsed, may be more effective than low-frequency TENS in rheumatoid arthritis patients with severe wrist pain.[21] Again, nonblinded studies have suggested that acupuncture-like TENS is more effective in neurogenic pain.[22] However, there was no significant difference in efficacy between continuous 100 Hz, pulsed 100 Hz, continuous 10 Hz, or pulsed 10 Hz in a randomized, double-blind study comparing the four different stimulation modalities in 200 patients (**Figure 17.2**). Combining the groups did not result in a significant difference between pulsed and continuous stimulation or low and high frequency, although there was a trend for a speedier response with pulsed high frequency acupuncture-like TENS. Half of the patients found TENS reduced their pain by more than 50 percent, and there was a steady increase in the number achieving a 50 percent reduction in pain with time (**Figure 17.3**).[23] Similar results were obtained in a shorter duration randomized controlled study comparing high-frequency, low-intensity TENS with high-frequency, high-intensity TENS or a control group where patients were free to select their own choice of intensity and duration of stimulus.[24]

Indeed, patients choose frequencies and patterns of stimulation according to reasons of comfort that may not be related to mechanisms specific to the pain system.[25] In

Table 17.1 The different qualities of conventional TENS and acupuncture/acupuncture-like TENS.

	TENS	**Acupuncture**
Frequency	40–100 Hz	1–4 Hz
Intensity	Low	High
Sensations	Tingling, vibration	Teh Chi, close to pain, beating
Induction time	Short	Long
Pain threshold effect	Transient	Long lasting
Distribution	Segmental	Segmental and nonsegmental

TENS, transcutaneous electrical nerve stimulation.

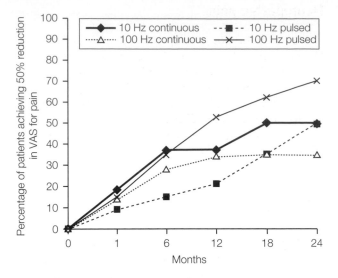

Figure 17.2 Percentage of patients over time achieving 50 percent reduction in visual analog scale for pain according to stimulation modality.

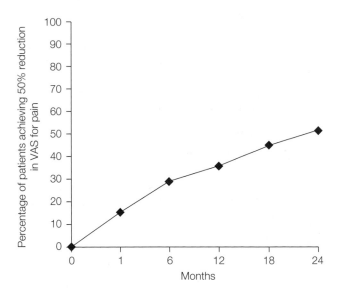

Figure 17.3 Total percentage of patients achieving 50 percent reduction in visual analog scale for pain over time.

one study, they preferred modulated stimulation modes, such as frequency modulation and burst, rather than conventional constant mode.[26, 27] A recent prospective continuous sample of 154 patients referred to the TENS clinic showed that 59 percent used conventional TENS as this gave the best reduction in patient's pain, and a 50 percent reduction in pain was found in 44 percent of patients. Those with neuropathic pain tended to have a greater effect ($p = 0.17$), and it was less beneficial in the over 60-year age group. The average time for those who gained benefit for TENS to start to reduce pain was 26 minutes, and relief continued for 77 minutes after switching off the machine.[14]

Acute pain

In a systematic review of TENS for acute postoperative pain,[28] TENS was judged by the reviewers to be no better than placebo in 15 out of 17 randomized studies. The two positive trials showed a reduced analgesic consumption, one after total hip replacement and the other after abdominal and thoracic surgery. However, a further systematic review of 21 randomized controlled trials involving 1350 patients showed that TENS reduced analgesic consumption by 26.5 percent,[29] and TENS has been shown to reduce the need to administer opioids, with improved respiratory function, during the five days following thoracotomy.[30] Applied after shoulder surgery, TENS reduced analgesic consumption in the first 72 hours.[31] A more recent study of TENS applied at the dermatomal level of the skin incision in a randomized controlled trial of hysterectomy or myomectomy patients found TENS to be as effective as Zusanli acupoint stimulation, and both treatments were more effective than stimulation at a nonacupoint (shoulder) location.[32]

Neither indometacin nor TENS reduced the postoperative opiate requirement after cholecystectomy.[33] However, TENS has been shown to significantly reduce the pain of lancet-induced trauma to the fingertip.[34] In a further study, 78 percent of children preferred electrodental anesthesia to local anesthesia for dentistry.[35] TENS has also been used to reduce postoperative nausea and vomiting, and was found to be equivalent to commonly used antiemetic drugs. The incidence of vomiting postoperatively was significantly less in the TENS-treated group than in the control group.[36] TENS has also been shown to be more effective than nonsteroidal anti-inflammatory drugs or placebo in patients with uncomplicated rib fractures, and has been shown to be useful in acute neck pain.[37, 38] Renal colic also responds to 100-Hz TENS.[39]

Pain of labor

TENS has not been shown to have any value in labor pain and the pain of delivery in any randomized controlled trials. Indeed, in one randomized controlled trial, intracutaneous sterile water injections were found to be more effective than standard care (back massage, bath, and mobilization) or TENS for relieving low back pain during labor. Randomized controlled trials provide no compelling evidence for TENS having any analgesic effect during labor. Weak positive effects in secondary (analgesic sparing) and tertiary (choosing TENS for future labors) outcomes may be the result of inadequate blinding causing overestimation of treatment effects.[40]

Chronic pain

TENS has been a successful analgesic treatment for 58.6 percent of 1582 patients attending a UK clinic over a period of ten years. TENS for chronic pain needs to be used for at least 30 minutes twice a day, and for at least one month before any effect may be felt. One-third of patients utilized TENS for over 61 hours/week.[41] Pulse frequencies between 1 and 70 Hz were utilized by 75 percent of patients, and 44 percent of patients benefited from burst mode stimulation.[12]

There is evidence that TENS should be used for at least 30 minutes twice a day for at least one month to obtain any effect and this effect may be progressive, with 51 percent of patients reducing their visual analog scale (VAS) score for pain by over 50 percent at two years.[20] None of the randomized trials used TENS for an equivalent duration to that of either Johnson et al.[41] or Nash et al.,[23] stimulation being for fewer than four weeks in 83 percent of the trials and for fewer than ten hours per week in 85 percent of the trials. Sixty-seven percent of the patients had fewer than ten total sessions of TENS. McQuay and Moore[42, 43] therefore concluded that TENS might be useful in chronic pain, although the evidence is not conclusive. More recent studies have shown efficacy in various specific pain states.

Myofascial/musculoskeletal/spasticity

One randomized controlled trial of acupuncture against TENS in elderly back pain patients in general practice showed TENS to be of similar efficacy for pain, but not for increased flexibility of the spine. Systematic reviews of acupuncture have shown an effect, which could suggest that TENS does have an effect in chronic pain, although several recent Cochrane reviews have suggested a lack of effect from acupuncture and TENS in low back pain and osteoarthritis.[43, 44, 45, 46, 47, 48] Vibratory stimulation and TENS are as efficient, or more efficient, than measures such as aspirin in myofascial or muscular pain, and TENS merits consideration in the choice of treatment of myofascial or musculoskeletal pain.[49] Both TENS and exercise have been shown to improve neck pain after six weeks.[50]

TENS also appears to be effective in reducing spinal spasticity, as measured clinically.[51] Repeated applications of TENS can reduce clinical spasticity and improve control of reflex and motor functions in hemiparetic subjects. Furthermore, the underlying mechanisms may be due partly to an enhancement in presynaptic inhibition of the spastic plantar-flexor, and partly to a possible "disinhibition" of descending voluntary commands to the paretic dorsi-flexor, motor neurons,[52] and has been recommended as a supplement to medical treatment in the management of spasticity.[53] Shoulder pain after stroke may not be influenced by TENS, but it does benefit passive humeral rotation.[54] Electrical stimulation has been shown to be similar to the Milwaukee brace in managing idiopathic scoliosis.[55]

Neuropathic pain

TENS is useful for neuropathic pain, including postherpetic neuralgia, painful peripheral neuropathies (especially if sufficient sensation is retained in the area of pain), and phantom limb pain. TENS applied to the contralateral leg in phantom limb pain has been shown to be significantly more effective than when applied to the outer ear, and skin conductance variations correlated well with stump sensations.[56]

Visceral

TENS has various visceral effects. It appears to reduce esophageal pain sensitivity and thus may be a useful treatment for noncardiac chest pain of esophageal origin.[57] There is also decreased lower esophageal sphincter pressure in patients with achalasia,[58] and somatic stimulation can reduce the perception of gut distension without interfering with local and reflex gut responses.[59]

TENS significantly increases uterine contractions when applied to postterm pregnant women.[60] However, high-frequency TENS has been shown to produce prompt onset of analgesia with no significant effect on uterine activity in several small studies of patients with primary dysmenorrhea, possibly by reducing uterine ischemia, or by spinal or supraspinal inhibition of pain transmission.[61, 62, 63, 64]

TENS may also have a role in the treatment of detrusor instability and urinary urgency.[65, 66, 67]

Intractable angina

TENS can be very useful in intractable angina. It produces an increased tolerance to pacing, improved lactate metabolism, and less pronounced ST depression. In the long term, there is an increase in work capacity, reduced frequency of anginal attacks, and reduced consumption of short-acting nitroglycerine, all due to a decreased afterload resulting from systemic vascular dilatation.[68, 69] There is also an increased coronary flow to ischemic areas in the myocardium. TENS has been shown to have an effect on lowering blood pressure at low frequencies (2 Hz). TENS may decrease the sympathetic activity either directly or indirectly as a consequence of pain inhibition. This hypothesis is supported by the fact that arterial levels of epinephrine and norepinephrine dropped during TENS in TENS responders.[70]

Peripheral ischemia

The subjective pain assessment and the maximum pain tolerance produced by ischemic pain after a submaximal effort tourniquet test were significantly modified by peripheral electrical stimulation at nonnoxious intensities.[71] There is also evidence that it can improve tissue perfusion and ulcer healing in peripheral vascular disease[72, 73] and leprosy.[74] The most useful stimulation modalities for ischemic pain, as for other pain states, are still under discussion. High-intensity, low-frequency TENS has been shown to prevent cooling of the hand in a controlled comparison with high-frequency, low-intensity stimulation and placebo.[75] Stimulation of 4 Hz had a significantly greater hypoalgesic effect on experimentally induced ischemic pain,[76] although in a further study, looking purely at femoral arterial blood flow in normal subjects, the flow rate was directly proportional to the frequency of stimulation.[77] TENS appears, therefore, to have a mild inhibitory action on the sympathetic nervous system and this is more apparent when the stimulation may be greater, as during isometric exercise.[78]

Blood flow in skin flaps with deficient circulation after reconstructive surgery can be significantly increased by TENS (p-value less than 0.001), but not by placebo TENS.[79, 80] TENS can also be useful in thrombophlebitis.[81]

Evidence in brief for TENS

Evidence for the use of TENS can be summarized as follows:

- reduction of opiate requirement for acute pain (with reduction in opiate side effects);
- not effective for labor pain;
- some evidence of efficacy in individual chronic pain states;
- no evidence in favor of any one type of stimulation;
- as good as aspirin in myofascial pain;
- some evidence for phantom limb pain;
- can reduce postoperative nausea;
- positive physiological effects in angina;
- can reduce health care costs by 55 percent for medication and 66 percent for physiotherapy or occupational therapy.

CONCLUSION

There is evidence that analgesic requirement can be reduced by TENS in postoperative pain, with a consequent reduction in opiate side effects. In chronic pain, there is evidence that TENS effectiveness increases slowly, and that its effect is dose dependent. Regular prolonged stimulation needs to be used for TENS to be useful in chronic pain. Treatment must be for at least 30 minutes twice a day for at least one month. The poor results with randomized controlled trials may well be due to such a protocol not being adhered to. There are an increasing number of studies showing benefits in myofascial and musculoskeletal pain, and dysmenorrhea, which begins to answer the criticism that there is a lack of evidence for the effectiveness of TENS in chronic pain, rather than

evidence for lack of efficacy.[82] Cost simulations of medication and physiotherapy or occupational therapy indicate that, with long-term TENS use, costs can be reduced by up to 55 percent for medications and by up to 69 percent for physiotherapy or occupational therapy.[83] TENS has, however, been shown not to be effective in labor pain.

REFERENCES

1. Nash TP. Development of medicine and stimulation produced analgesia. *Pain Clinic.* 1992; **5**: 181–5.
∗ 2. Melzack R, Wall PD. Pain mechanisms: a new theory. *Science.* 1965; **150**: 971–9.
3. Wall PD, Sweet WH. Temporary abolition of pain in man. *Science.* 1967; **155**: 108–09.
4. Shealy CN, Taslitz N, Mortimer JT, Becker DP. Electrical inhibition of pain: experimental evaluation. *Anesthesia and Analgesia.* 1967; **46**: 299–305.
∗ 5. Melzack R. Prolonged relief of pain by brief, intense transcutaneous somatic stimulation. *Pain.* 1975; **1**: 357–73.
6. Walsh DM, Lowe AS, McCormack K *et al.* Transcutaneous electrical nerve stimulation: effect on peripheral nerve conduction, mechanical pain threshold, and tactile threshold in humans. *Archives of Physical Medicine and Rehabilitation.* 1998; **79**: 1051–8.
7. Radhakrishnan R, Sluka KA. Deep tissue afferents, but not cutaneous afferents, mediate transcutaneous electrical nerve stimulation-induced antihyperalgesia. *Journal of Pain.* 2005; **6**: 673–80.
8. Reeve J, Menon D, Corabian P. Transcutaneous electrical nerve stimulation (TENS): a technology assessment. *International Journal of Technology Assessment in Health Care.* 1996; **12**: 299–324.
9. Chen D, Philip M, Philip PA, Monga TN. Cardiac pacemaker inhibition by transcutaneous electrical nerve stimulation. *Archives of Physical Medicine and Rehabilitation.* 1990; **71**: 27–30.
10. Rasmussen MJ, Hayes DL, Vlietstra RE, Thorsteinsson G. Can transcutaneous electrical nerve stimulation be safely used in patients with permanent cardiac pacemakers? *Mayo Clinic Proceedings.* 1988; **63**: 443–5.
11. Pyatt TJR, Trenbath D, Chester M, Connelly DT. The simultaneous use of a biventricular implantable cardioverter defibrillator (ICD) and transcutaneous electrical nerve stimulation (TENS) unit: implications for device interaction. *Europace.* 2003; **5**: 91–3.
∗ 12. Johnson MI, Ashton CH, Thompson JW. An in-depth study of long-term users of transcutaneous electrical nerve stimulation (TENS). Implications for clinical use of TENS. *Pain.* 1991; **44**: 221–9.
13. Alon G. High voltage stimulation. Effects of electrode size on basic excitatory responses. *Physical Therapy.* 1985; **65**: 890–5.

14. Sandkuhler J. Long-lasting analgesia following TENS and acupuncture: spinal mechanisms beyond gate control. In: Devor M, Rowbotham MC, Wiesenfeld-Hallin Z (eds). *Proceedings of the 9th World Congress on Pain, Progress in Pain Research and Management*, vol. 16. Seattle, WA: IASP Press, 2000.

15. Mann CJ. Respiratory compromise: a rare complication of transcutaneous electrical nerve stimulation for angina pectoris. *Journal of Accident and Emergency Medicine.* 1996; **13**: 68.

16. Richardson C, MacIver K, Wright M, Wiles JR. Patient reports of the effects and side-effects of TENS for chronic non-malignant pain following a four week trial. *Pain Clinic.* 2002; **13**: 265–76.

17. Deyo RA, Walsh NE, Schoenfeld LS, Ramamurthy S. Can trials of physical treatments be blinded? The example of transcutaneous electrical nerve stimulation for chronic pain. *American Journal of Physical Medicine and Rehabilitation.* 1990; **69**: 6–10.

18. Marchand S, Bushnell MC, Duncan GH. Modulation of heat pain perception by high frequency transcutaneous electrical nerve stimulation (TENS). *Clinical Journal of Pain.* 1991; **7**: 122–9.

19. Kruger LR, van der Linden WJ, Cleaton-Jones PE. Transcutaneous electrical nerve stimulation in the treatment of myofascial pain dysfunction. *South African Journal of Surgery.* 1998; **36**: 35–8.

☀ 20. Fishbain DA, Chabal C, Abbott A et al. Transcutaneous electrical nerve stimulation (TENS) treatment outcome in long-term users. *Clinical Journal of Pain.* 1996; **12**: 201–14.

21. Mannheimer C, Carlsson CA. The analgesic effect of transcutaneous electrical nerve stimulation (TNS) in patients with rheumatoid arthritis. A comparative study of different pulse patterns. *Pain.* 1979; **6**: 329–34.

22. Eriksson M, Sjolund B. Acupuncture-like electroanalgesia in TNS-resistant chronic pain. In: Zotterman Y (eds). *Sensory functions of the skin.* Oxford: Pergamon Press, 1976: 575–81.

☀ 23. Nash TP, Williams JD, Machin D. TENS: does the type of stimulus really matter? *Pain Clinic.* 1990; **3**: 161–8.

24. Koke AJ, Schouten JS, Lamerisch-Geelen MJ et al. Pain reducing effect of three types of transcutaneous electrical nerve stimulation in patients with chronic pain: a randomized crossover trial. *Pain.* 2004; **108**: 36–42.

☀ 25. Johnson MI, Ashton CH, Thompson JW. The consistency of pulse frequencies and pulse patterns of transcutaneous electrical nerve stimulation (TENS) used by chronic pain patients. *Pain.* 1991; **44**: 231–4.

26. Tulgar M, McGlone F, Bowsher D, Miles JB. Comparative effectiveness of different stimulation modes in relieving pain. Part I. A pilot study. *Pain.* 1991; **47**: 151–5.

27. Tulgar M, McGlone F, Bowsher D, Miles JB. Comparative effectiveness of different stimulation modes in relieving pain. Part II. A double-blind controlled long-term clinical trial. *Pain.* 1991; **47**: 157–62.

☀ 28. Carroll D, Tramèr M, McQuay H et al. Randomization is important in studies with pain outcomes: systematic review of transcutaneous electrical nerve stimulation in acute postoperative pain. *British Journal of Anaesthesia.* 1996; **77**: 798–803.

☀ 29. Bjordal JM, Johnson MI, Ljunggreen AE. Transcutaneous electrical nerve stimulation (TENS) can reduce postoperative analgesic consumption. A meta-analysis with assessment of optimal treatment parameters for postoperative pain. *European Journal of Pain.* 2003; **7**: 181–8.

30. Erdogan M, Erdogan A, Erbil N et al. Prospective, randomized, placebo-controlled study of the effect of TENS on post-thoracotomy pain and pulmonary function. *World Journal of Surgery.* 2005; **29**: 1563–70.

31. Likar R, Molnar M, Pipam W et al. Postoperative transcutaneous electrical nerve stimulation (TENS) in shoulder surgery. *Schmerz.* 2001; **15**: 158–63.

32. Chen L, Tang J, White PF et al. The effect of location of transcutaneous electrical nerve stimulation on postoperative opioid analgesic requirement: acupoint versus nonacupoint stimulation. *Anesthesia and Analgesia.* 1998; **87**: 1129–34.

33. Laitinen J, Nuutinen L. Failure of transcutaneous electrical nerve stimulation and indomethacin to reduce opiate requirement following cholecystectomy. *Acta Anaesthesiologica Scandinavica.* 1991; **35**: 700–5.

34. Webster DP, Pellegrini L, Duffy K. Use of transcutaneous electrical nerve stimulation for fingertip analgesia: a pilot study. *Annals of Emergency Medicine.* 1992; **21**: 1472–5.

35. teDuits E, Goepferd S, Donly K et al. The effectiveness of electronic dental anesthesia in children. *Pediatric Dentistry.* 1993; **15**: 191–6.

36. Fassoulaki A, Papilas K, Sarantopoulos C, Zotou M. Transcutaneous electrical nerve stimulation reduces the incidence of vomiting after hysterectomy. *Anesthesia and Analgesia.* 1993; **76**: 1012–14.

37. Oncel M, Sencan S, Yildiz H, Kurt N. Transcutaneous electrical nerve stimulation for pain management in patients with uncomplicated minor rib fractures. *European Journal of Cardio-Thoracic Surgery.* 2002; **22**: 13–17.

38. Vernon HT, Humphreys BK, Hagino CA. A systematic review of conservative treatments for acute neck pain not due to whiplash. *Journal of Manipulative Physiological Therapeutics.* 2005; **28**: 443–8.

39. Mora B, Giorni E, Dobrovits M et al. Transcutaneous electrical nerve stimulation: an effective treatment for pain caused by renal colic in emergency care. *Journal of Urology.* 2006; **175**: 1737–41.

☀ 40. Carroll D, Tramer M, McQuay H et al. Transcutaneous electrical nerve stimulation in labour pain: a systematic review. *British Journal of Obstetrics and Gynaecology.* 1997; **104**: 169–75.

☀ 41. Johnson MI, Ashton CH, Thompson JW. Long term use of transcutaneous electrical nerve stimulation at Newcastle Pain Relief Clinic. *Journal of the Royal Society of Medicine.* 1992; **85**: 267–8.

∗ 42. McQuay H, Moore A. Transcutaneous electrical nerve stimulation (TENS) in chronic pain. In: McQuay H, Moore A (eds). *An evidence-based resource for pain relief*. Oxford: Oxford University Press, 1998: 205–11.

∗ 43. Carroll D, Moore RA, McQuay HJ *et al*. Transcutaneous electrical nerve stimulation (TENS) for chronic pain. *Cochrane Database of Systematic Reviews*. 2000; CD003222.

∗ 44. van Tulder MW, Cherkin DC, Berman B *et al*. The effectiveness of acupuncture in the management of acute and chronic low back pain. A systematic review within the framework of the Cochrane Collaboration Back Review Group. *Spine*. 1999; **24**: 1113–23.

∗ 45. Milne S, Welch V, Brosseau L *et al*. Transcutaneous electrical nerve stimulation (TENS) for chronic low back pain. *Cochrane Database of Systematic Reviews*. 2001; CD003008.

∗ 46. Khadilkar A, Milne S, Brosseau L *et al*. Transcutaneous electrical nerve stimulation (TENS) for chronic low-back pain. *Cochrane Database of Systematic Reviews*. 2005; CD003008.

47. Khadilkar A, Milne S, Brosseau L *et al*. Transcutaneous electrical nerve stimulation (TENS) for chronic low back pain: a systematic review. *Spine*. 2005; **30**: 2657–66.

∗ 48. Osiri M, Welch V, Brosseau L *et al*. Transcutaneous electrical nerve stimulation for knee osteoarthritis. *Cochrane Database of Systematic Reviews*. 2000; CD002823.

49. Lundeberg T. The pain suppressive effect of vibratory stimulation and transcutaneous electrical nerve stimulation (TENS) as compared to aspirin. *Brain Research*. 1984; **294**: 201–09.

50. Chiu TT, Hui-Chan CW, Chein G. A randomized clinical trial of TENS and exercise for patients with chronic neck pain. *Clinical Rehabilitation*. 2005; **19**: 850–60.

51. Goulet C, Arsenault AB, Bourbonnais D *et al*. Effects of transcutaneous electrical nerve stimulation on H-reflex and spinal spasticity. *Scandinavian Journal of Rehabilitation Medicine*. 1996; **28**: 169–76.

52. Levin MF, Hui-Chan CW. Relief of hemiparetic spasticity by TENS is associated with improvement in reflex and voluntary motor functions. *Electroencephalography and Clinical Neurophysiology*. 1992; **85**: 131–42.

53. Aydin G, Tomruk S, Keles I *et al*. Transcutaneous electrical nerve stimulation versus baclofen in spasticity: clinical and electrophysiologic comparison. *American Journal of Physical Medicine and Rehabilitation*. 2005; **84**: 584–92.

54. Price CIM, Pandyan AD. Electrical stimulation for preventing and treating post-stroke shoulder pain. *Cochrane Database of Systematic Reviews*. 2000; CD001698.

55. Fisher DA, Rapp GF, Emkes M. Idiopathic scoliosis: transcutaneous muscle stimulation versus the Milwaukee brace. *Spine*. 1987; **12**: 987–91.

56. Katz J, France C, Melzack R. An association between phantom limb sensations and stump skin conductance during transcutaneous electrical nerve stimulation (TENS) applied to the contralateral leg: a case study. *Pain*. 1989; **36**: 367–77.

57. Borjesson M, Pilhall M, Eliasson T *et al*. Esophageal visceral pain sensitivity: effects of TENS and correlation with manometric findings. *Digestive Diseases and Sciences*. 1998; **43**: 1621–8.

58. Guelrud M, Rossiter A, Souney PF, Sulbaran M. Transcutaneous electrical nerve stimulation decreases lower esophageal sphincter pressure in patients with achalasia. *Digestive Diseases and Sciences*. 1991; **36**: 1029–33.

59. Coffin B, Azpiroz F, Malagelada JR. Somatic stimulation reduces perception of gut distention in humans. *Gastroenterology*. 1994; **107**: 1636–42.

60. Dunn PA, Rogers D, Halford K. Transcutaneous electrical nerve stimulation at acupuncture points in the induction of uterine contractions. *Obstetrics and Gynecology*. 1989; **73**: 286–90.

61. Milsom I, Hedner N, Mannheimer C. A comparative study of the effect of high-intensity transcutaneous nerve stimulation and oral naproxen on intrauterine pressure and menstrual pain in patients with primary dysmenorrhea. *American Journal of Obstetrics and Gynecology*. 1994; **170**: 123–9.

62. Kaplan B, Peled Y, Pardo J *et al*. Transcutaneous electrical nerve stimulation (TENS) as a relief for dysmenorrhea. *Clinical and Experimental Obstetrics and Gynecology*. 1994; **21**: 87–90.

63. Dawood MY, Ramos J. Transcutaneous electrical nerve stimulation (TENS) for the treatment of primary dysmenorrhea: a randomized crossover comparison with placebo TENS and ibuprofen. *Obstetrics and Gynecology*. 1990; **75**: 656–60.

64. Proctor ML, Smith CA, Farquhar CM, Stones RW. Transcutaneous electrical nerve stimulation and acupuncture for primary dysmenorrhoea. *Cochrane Database of Systematic Reviews*. 2002; CD002123.

65. Bower WF, Moore KH, Adams RD, Shepherd R. A urodynamic study of surface neuromodulation versus sham in detrusor instability and sensory urgency. *Journal of Urology*. 1998; **160**: 2133–6.

66. Okada N, Igawa Y, Ogawa A, Nishizawa O. Transcutaneous electrical stimulation of thigh muscles in the treatment of detrusor overactivity. *British Journal of Urology*. 1998; **81**: 560–4.

67. Nakamura M, Sakurai T, Tsujimoto Y, Tada Y. Bladder inhibition by electrical stimulation of the perianal skin. *Urologia Internationalis*. 1986; **41**: 62–3.

∗ 68. Mannheimer C, Carlsson CA, Emanuelsson H *et al*. The effects of transcutaneous electrical nerve stimulation in patients with severe angina pectoris. *Circulation*. 1985; **71**: 308–16.

∗ 69. Mannheimer C, Carlsson CA, Vedin A, Wilhelmsson C. Transcutaneous electrical nerve stimulation (TENS) in angina pectoris. *Pain*. 1986; **26**: 291–300.

∗ 70. Emanuelsson H, Mannheimer C, Waagstein F, Wilhelmsson C. Catecholamine metabolism during pacing-induced angina pectoris and the effect of transcutaneous electrical nerve stimulation. *American Heart Journal*. 1987; **114**: 1360–6.

∗ 71. Woolf CJ. Transcutaneous electrical nerve stimulation and the reaction to experimental pain in human subjects. *Pain*. 1979; **7**: 115–27.

72. Kaada B. Promoted healing of chronic ulceration by transcutaneous nerve stimulation (TNS). *VASA (Journal for Vascular Diseases)*. 1983; **12**: 262–9.

73. Debreceni L, Gyulai M, Debreceni A, Szabo K. Results of transcutaneous electrical stimulation (TES) in cure of lower extremity arterial disease. *Angiology*. 1995; **46**: 613–18.

74. Kaada B, Emru M. Promoted healing of leprous ulcers by transcutaneous nerve stimulation. *Acupuncture and Electro-therapeutics Research*. 1988; **13**: 165–76.

75. Scudds RJ, Helewa A, Scudds RA. The effects of transcutaneous electrical nerve stimulation on skin temperature in asymptomatic subjects. *Physical Therapy*. 1995; **75**: 621–8.

76. Walsh DM, Foster NE, Baxter GD, Allen JM. Transcutaneous electrical nerve stimulation. Relevance of stimulation parameters to neurophysiological and hypoalgesic effects. *American Journal of Physical Medicine and Rehabilitation*. 1995; **74**: 199–206.

77. Zicot M, Rigaux P. Effect of the frequency of neuromuscular electric stimulation of the leg on femoral arterial blood flow. *Journal des Maladies Vasculaires*. 1995; **20**: 9–13.

78. Sanderson JE, Tomlinson B, Lau MS *et al*. The effect of transcutaneous electrical nerve stimulation (TENS) on autonomic cardiovascular reflexes. *Clinical Autonomic Research*. 1995; **5**: 81–4.

79. Kjartansson J, Lundeberg T. Effects of electrical nerve stimulation (ENS) in ischemic tissue. *Scandinavian Journal of Plastic and Reconstructive Surgery and Hand Surgery*. 1990; **24**: 129–34.

80. Kjartansson J, Lundeberg T, Samuelson UE, Dalsgaard CJ. Transcutaneous electrical nerve stimulation (TENS) increases survival of ischaemic musculocutaneous flaps. *Acta Physiologica Scandinavica*. 1988; **134**: 95–9.

81. Roberts HJ. Transcutaneous electrical nerve stimulation in the symptomatic management of thrombophlebitis. *Angiology*. 1979; **30**: 249–56.

∗ 82. McQuay HJ, Moore RA, Eccleston C *et al*. Systematic review of outpatient services for chronic pain control. *Health Technology Assessment*. 1997; **1**: i–iv, 1–135.

∗ 83. Chabal C, Fishbain DA, Weaver M, Heine LW. Long-term transcutaneous electrical nerve stimulation (TENS) use: impact on medication utilization and physical therapy costs. *Clinical Journal of Pain*. 1998; **14**: 66–73.

Acupuncture

MIKE CUMMINGS

KEY LEARNING POINTS

- "Western medical acupuncture" principally involves dry needling of myofascial trigger points and segmental sensory neuromodulation.
- The specific analgesic effects of needling are mediated through stimulation of Aδ or type III afferent nerve fibers in muscle and other deep somatic tissues.
- Electroacupuncture at different frequencies can result in the release of four different endogenous opioids: enkephalin, β-endorphin, endomorphin, and dynorphin.

- The principal methodological difficulty in explanatory studies of acupuncture is in finding a physiologically inert control that facilitates subject blinding.
- Acupuncture is a very safe procedure, but adequate knowledge of anatomy and infection control procedures is essential.
- Serious adverse events are rare: pneumothorax is estimated to occur at a rate of 1:250,000 treatments.

INTRODUCTION

Historical perspective

Fossil evidence of trepanning indicates that man has used physical therapies in the treatment of disease since Neolithic times (circa 10,000 to 3500BC). Whilst the Chinese are reputed to have evidence of the use of acupuncture from bone etchings dating back to 1600BC, the recent discovery of Ötzi, the Tyrolean iceman, dates the use of a therapeutic needling technique in Europe to 3200BC.[1] It is clear that acupuncture-like therapies have developed independently in different civilizations around the world, and this is probably due to late evolutionary features in the mammalian nervous system, combined with intelligence, and the consequent use of tools, in humans.

Children learn at a very early age to rub energetically directly over the site of an acute pain to reduce the noxious sensation. In the case of a more chronic discomfort from aching, "knotted" muscle we tend to massage the local tissues more deeply and vigorously even though doing so may temporarily exacerbate the discomfort. With the development of stone tools it is easy to hypothesize a progression of therapeutic techniques which resulted ultimately in piercing the skin and muscle at a site of chronic pain.

Traditional theories

The development of acupuncture points probably resulted from clinical observation that certain places in the body were more likely to harbor tender points than others and that treating these points by pressure or piercing could relieve pain as well as various other nonpainful symptoms. Consistent patterns of pain referral from myofascial trigger points, together with the relief resulting from needling these and other muscle points, may have contributed to the development of acupuncture meridians. Radiation patterns of painful medical conditions such as sciatica, other radiculopathies, and possibly the consistent rashes of herpes zoster may also have contributed to the idea that certain points were connected in some way. These hypotheses do not explain the location of all acupuncture points, nor the paths of all the meridians, but there is clearly considerable overlap between myofascial trigger points and acupuncture points,[2] and between the pain referral patterns of the former and meridians (see **Figure 18.1**).

Acupuncture was probably used pragmatically by the Chinese and others for centuries before it became systematized within a documented form of medicine some 2000 years ago.[3] The theories which developed were influenced by rational observations imposed upon a limited clinical knowledge base and within the philosophical framework of Taoism. The tendency towards syncretism

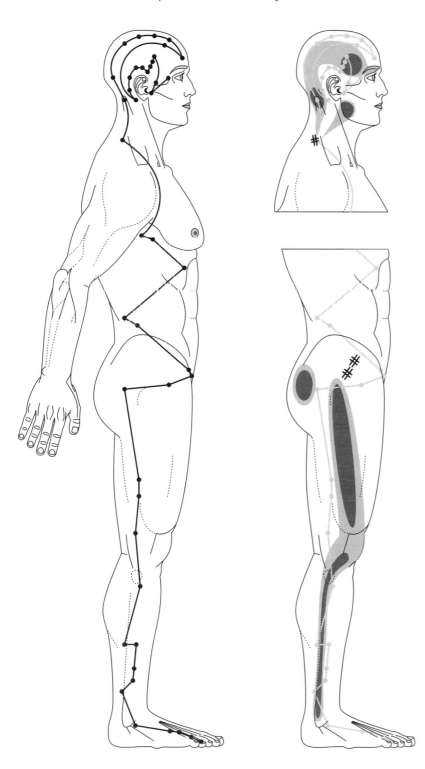

Figure 18.1 An example of the overlap between acupuncture points and meridians, and myofascial trigger points and their typical pain referral patterns. On the left-hand side is a representation of the Gallbladder meridian, and on the right are referral patterns from myofascial trigger points in upper trapezius and gluteus minimus.

resulted in the adoption and inclusion of many different theories, and over the centuries this has resulted in the development of a complex system of medicine. Whilst it can be initially unpalatable to the sceptical Western scientist, closer inspection reveals that traditional Chinese medicine is built on a series of logical assumptions, and although some of these are clearly wrong, many may still represent valid clinical observations.

Western medical acupuncture

Western medical acupuncture is a term with a variety of potential meanings. The most literal interpretation invokes thoughts of geographical boundaries, but the term was probably introduced to distinguish a developing system of needle therapy from its traditional philosophical roots which happened to be in the East.

Filshie and Cummings[4] interpret "Western medical acupuncture" as the scientific application of acupuncture as a therapy following orthodox clinical diagnosis. It is important to note that the scientific evaluation of acupuncture is not restricted to the West,[5] and therefore adherence to a geographical definition is inappropriate. Probably a more accurate description of "Western medical acupuncture" is a modern scientific approach to therapy involving dry needling of tissues, which has developed from the introduction and evaluation of traditional Chinese acupuncture in the West.

The key facets of Western medical acupuncture are myofascial trigger point needling,[6, 7, 8] and segmental acupuncture.[4]

RESEARCH

Methodological difficulties in acupuncture studies

The principal methodological difficulties in acupuncture research are concerned with controls and blinding in explanatory studies, i.e. studies of the efficacy of acupuncture beyond placebo.[9] For a placebo control to be credible, the subjects receiving it must believe that they have had an active treatment, identical to, or at least equivalent in potency to, the active intervention. Ideally, for any needling therapy, the control should involve an inactive form of needling, but it seems clear that a needle placed anywhere in the body is likely to have some neurophysiological effect.[10] Indeed, two large trials from Germany demonstrated that both real and sham acupuncture (minimal needling off classical acupuncture points) were significantly superior to guideline-based standard care,[11, 12] though not significantly different from each other.

Nonpenetrating "placebo" needles have been developed[13, 14] and whilst these are useful, they are also demonstrably superior to placebo pills.[15]

A convincing control procedure should result in blinding of the subject, but it is almost impossible to blind an experienced therapist who is performing both real and sham needling techniques. A common way of reducing bias in this situation is to use a blind assessor, although a double-blind needle has been developed.[16]

Evidence for needling in myofascial pain

A systematic review of 23 randomized controlled trials conclusively shows, when treating myofascial pain with trigger point injection, that the nature of the injected substance makes no difference to the outcome, and that there is no therapeutic benefit in wet over dry needling.[17] These conclusions are supported by all the high quality trials in the review.[18, 19, 20, 21, 22, 23, 24, 25, 26]

The authors of the review concluded: "The hypothesis that needling therapies have specific efficacy in the treatment of myofascial pain is not supported by the research to date, but this review suggests that any effect derived from these therapies is likely to be derived from the needle, rather than from either an injection of liquid in general, or any substance in particular. All groups in the review in whom trigger points were directly needled showed marked improvement in their symptoms; therefore further research is urgently needed to establish the specific effect of trigger point needling, with emphasis on the use of an adequate control for the needle."

Evidence for needling in other pain conditions

Systematic reviews provide evidence for the efficacy of acupuncture in osteoarthrosis of the knee,[27, 28] chronic low back pain,[29, 30] and chronic mechanical neck pain.[31] Acupuncture appears to be as effective as conventional medicine in chronic headache,[32, 33] but there are still questions over its efficacy beyond placebo.[32, 34]

Large pragmatic trials from Germany confirm clinically relevant effects and acceptable cost utility in osteoarthrosis,[35, 36] chronic low back pain,[37] chronic headache,[36, 38] and chronic neck pain.[39, 40]

MECHANISMS

Neurophysiology of needling

The therapeutic effects of needling are mediated through stimulation of the peripheral nervous system, and so can be abolished by local anesthetic.[41, 42] In particular, stimulation of Aδ or type III afferent nerve fibers has been implicated as the key component in producing analgesia.[43] The therapeutic effects of needling can be divided into four categories based on the area influenced: local, segmental, heterosegmental, and general.

LOCAL EFFECTS

Release of trophic and vasoactive neuropeptides including neuropeptide Y (NPY), calcitonin gene-related peptide (CGRP) and vasoactive intestinal peptide (VIP) has been demonstrated.[44, 45] It is likely that the release of CGRP and VIP from peripheral nerves stimulated by needling results in enhanced circulation and wound healing in rats,[46, 47] and equivalent sensory stimulation has proved effective in human patients.[48]

SEGMENTAL EFFECTS

Through stimulation of high threshold mechanoreceptors (possibly ergoreceptors) in muscle, needling can have a profound influence on sensory modulation within the dorsal horn at the relevant segmental level. C fiber pain transmission is inhibited via enkephalinergic interneurones in lamina II, the substantia gelatinosa (see **Figure 18.2**). Bowsher[49] reviews the basic science literature that supports this mechanism, and White[50] appraises both experimental and clinical evidence. Segmental stimulation appears to have a more powerful effect than an equivalent stimulus from a distant segment, in modulating pain,[51, 52] local autonomic activity,[53] and itch.[54] Aδ or type III afferent nerve fibers can be stimulated by superficial needling as well as by needling deeper tissues, but it seems that segmental stimuli from the latter (usually muscle) have a more powerful effect.[52, 54, 55]

HETEROSEGMENTAL EFFECTS

Whilst segmental stimulation appears to be the more powerful effect, needling anywhere in the body can influence afferent processing throughout the spinal cord. The needle stimulus travels from the segment of origin to the ventral posterior lateral nucleus of the thalamus, and projects from there to the somatosensory cortex. Collaterals in the midbrain synapse in the periaqueductal gray (PAG). This is the origin of descending inhibitory systems that run via the nucleus raphe magnus to influence afferent processing in the dorsal horn at every level of the spinal cord. Serotonin is the prominent neurotransmitter in the caudal stages of this descending pathway, and the fibers synapse with the enkephalinergic interneurones in lamina II (see **Figure 18.3**). A second descending system from the PAG travels via the nucleus raphe gigantocellularis; its fibers are noradrenergic, and their influence is mediated directly on lamina II cells, rather than via enkephalinergic interneurones. Diffuse noxious inhibitory controls (DNIC) is the term introduced by Le Bars et al.[56] to define a third analgesic system, which is induced by a noxious stimulus anywhere in the body. Heterosegmental needling exerts influence through all three mechanisms to different degrees,[49, 50] and possibly through others, as yet undefined.

GENERAL EFFECTS

These are more difficult to define, and there is clearly some overlap with heterosegmental effects. The latter term is used to denote effects mediated at every segment of the spinal cord, as opposed to effects mediated by humeral means or by influence on higher centers in the central nervous system (CNS) controlling general responses.

Acupuncture needling has proven efficacy in the treatment of nausea and vomiting,[57, 58] although the mechanism is not understood.

Electroacupuncture at different frequencies can result in the release of four different endogenous opioids: enkephalin, β-endorphin, endomorphin, and dynorphin.[59, 60] These may in part mediate the general responses observed in clinical practice, including short-term sedation and improved well-being following treatment.

Imaging studies are now demonstrating that real acupuncture may be associated with reduced activity in limbic structures,[61, 62] and this may correlate with the observation that acupuncture has a greater influence on the affective component rather than the intensity of pain.

Needling of trigger points

The mechanism of action of needling in the deactivation of trigger points is undetermined. The effect of vigorous direct needling techniques (described below under Needle technique) is most likely to be through mechanical disruption of motor end-plates or muscle fibers, but gentler needling techniques may work through segmental reflexes or target-directed expectation (i.e. regional placebo effects).[63, 64]

TECHNIQUE

Western medical acupuncture

SAFETY ASPECTS

Acupuncture involves the insertion of, usually stainless steel, needles into the body. Whilst it is often perceived by the general public as "natural" and "safe," along with many complementary therapies, it is neither natural nor completely safe. As with any needling therapy the serious risks are associated with the transmission of blood-borne infection, and direct trauma. Rampes and Peuker[65] categorize adverse events associated with acupuncture as follows:

- delayed or missed diagnosis;
- deterioration of disorder under treatment;
- pain;
- vegetative reactions;
- bacterial and viral infections
- trauma of tissues and organs;
- miscellaneous.

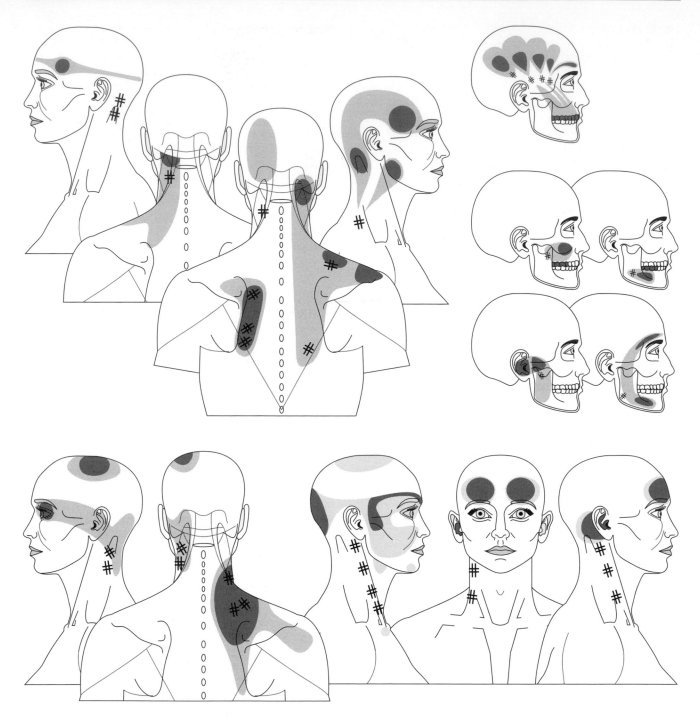

Figure 18.2 Some of the more common myofascial trigger point (TrP) sites (#) in the head and neck and their respective pain patterns. The top left group (left to right) represents TrPs in semispinalis capitis and cervicis, rhomboids and trapezius. The top right group (top down) represents TrPs in temporalis and masseter. The lower group (left to right) represents TrPs in splenius capitis and cervicis, levator scapulae and sternocleidomastoid (sternal and clavicular heads).

If acupuncture is performed as a therapy by an orthodox medical practitioner within his or her sphere of competence, the first two categories will be avoided.

Persistent pain attributed to acupuncture treatment is rare, but temporary exacerbation of the presenting complaint for a day or so is common.

Vegetative reactions include syncope and sedation. Syncope can be largely avoided by treating patients lying on an examination couch; however, very occasionally a profound sinus bradycardia will result in loss of consciousness of a patient who is lying down. In all such anecdotal case reports heard by the author, the patient has recovered spontaneously within a few minutes. Sedation is relatively common, and occurs in perhaps 20 percent of patients after their first two treatments. In maybe 5 percent of patients there is always some degree of sedation

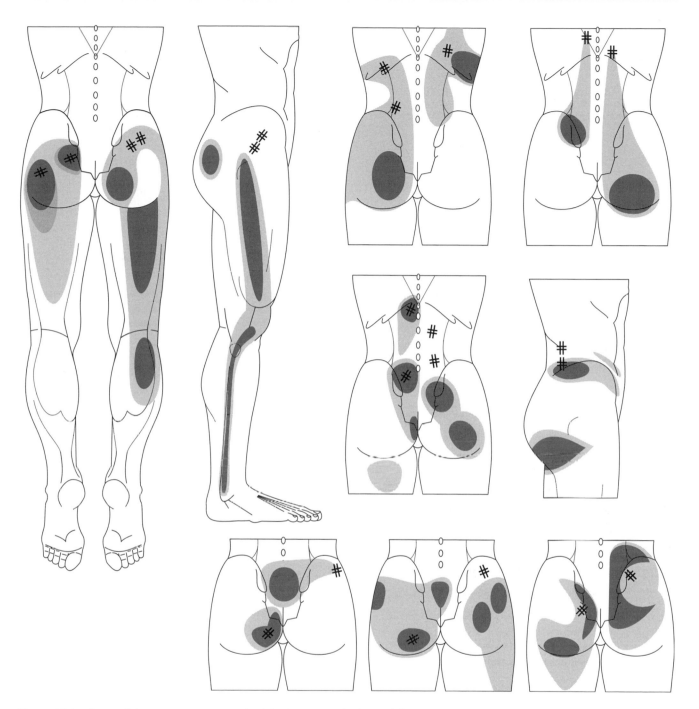

Figure 18.3 Some of the more common myofascial trigger point (TrP) sites (#) in the back and hip girdle and their respective pain patterns. The left-hand group (left to right) represents TrPs in piriformis and gluteus minimus. The top right group (left to right) represent TrPs in iliocostalis lumborum, iliocostalis thoracis, and longissimus thoracis. The middle right group (left to right) represents TrPs in multifidus at L1 and L5, and quadratus lumborum. The lower group represents TrPs in gluteus maximus (on the left of each diagram) and gluteus medius (on the right of each diagram).

associated with acupuncture treatment. Sedation is rarely seen as an adverse event by patients, and is only of concern in terms of driving home or operating machinery after treatment.

Apart from hepatitis B, infections associated with acupuncture treatment are uncommon and avoided by the use of sterile disposable needles and cleanliness.

Traumatic complications of acupuncture needling are avoidable, and on occasion they have been fatal.[66] White[67] has performed a useful review of the range and incidence of significant adverse events associated with acupuncture. The most frequent serious adverse event in the West is pneumothorax, and from prospective trials this is estimated to occur at a rate of 1:250,000 treatments.[67]

POINT SELECTION

The two main themes in Western medical acupuncture are dry needling of trigger points and segmental acupuncture. The latter is defined as the technique of needling an area of the soma innervated by the same spinal segment as the disordered structure under treatment. Based on neurophysiological and clinical evidence,[49, 50, 51, 52, 53, 54, 55] the main principle in point selection is to stimulate the soma as close as is practical to the seat of the pathology (without making it worse), or at least within the same segment. Local trigger points, tender points, or acupuncture points are chosen, and often these will overlap so that the key point to stimulate is a trigger point (which is tender by definition) at the site of an acupuncture point (see **Figures 18.2, 18.3** and **18.4** for examples of commonly used points, and **Table 18.1** for

acupuncture point locations). If the key element of the somatic pathology is a myofascial trigger point, this is arguably the only point that it is necessary to treat. In most other cases the analgesia afforded by local needling may be enhanced by using one or more points at a distance from the pathology, in addition to the relevant local points. Distant points are chosen because they stimulate the appropriate segment, or because they are conveniently located and known to generate strong needling sensation (heterosegmental acupuncture). In individual cases point selection may be modified by the need to avoid local conditions:

- skin infection;
- ulceration;
- moles and tumors;
- varicosities;

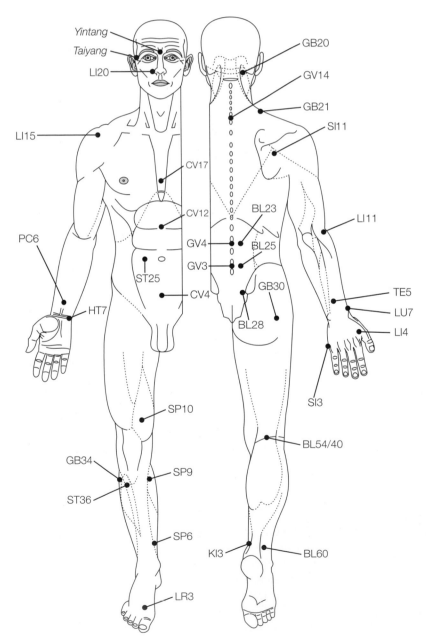

Figure 18.4 The point locations of 34 of the most commonly used points in Western medical acupuncture. Refer to **Table 18.1** for detailed descriptions of each point: location; angulation; target structure; indications; cautions; and innervation. Reprinted and modified with permission from the British Medical Acupuncture Society, *BMAS Foundation Course Notes*, 2007.

Table 18.1 Acupuncture point locations.

Name	Location of point / Angulation of needling / Indications	Target structure for needle	Dermatome	Myotome	Sclerotome
Yintang	Midpoint between the eyebrows Angulation: oblique inferior *Headache, hayfever, relaxation*	Target: procerus or periosteum	D Vi	M VII	S Vi
Taiyang	1 cun posterior to the midpoint between the lateral end of the eyebrow and the lateral canthus of the eye Angulation: perpendicular *Headache, eye symptoms*	Target: temporalis	D Vii	M Viii	S Vii
LI20	In the nasolabial groove, level with the widest part of the ala nasi Angulation: superiorly along groove *Hayfever, nasal symptoms*	Target: facial muscles	D Vii	M VII	S Vii
GB20	Below the occipital bone, in the depression between trapezius and sternomastoid and above splenius capitis Angulation: towards opposite eyebrow *Headache, neck pain and stiffness* **CAUTION – note the position of the vertebral artery**	Target: semispinalis capitis	D C2/C3	M C1/C2	S C1/C2
GB21	Midway between GV14 and tip of the acromion at the highest point of trapezius Angulation: tangential to ribs, posteriorly *Headache, neck pain and stiffness, anxiety* **CAUTION – note the proximity of the pleura between the 1st and 2nd ribs**	Target: upper trapezius	D C3	M C3/C4	S n/a
GV14	Between spinous processes C7 and T1 Angulation: transverse *Spinal neck pain, headache of cervical origin*	Target: interspinous ligament	D C4/C5/T1	M C8	S C8
LI15	Anterolateral and inferior to the anterior tip of the acromion, in the groove between the anterior and middle fibers of deltoid Angulation: perpendicular *Shoulder and arm pain*	Target: supraspinatus insertion	D C4	M C5	S C5
SI11	1/3 down a line from the midpoint of the scapular spine to the inferior angle of the scapula Angulation: perpendicular *Shoulder and arm pain*	Target: infraspinatus	D C4/T1/T2	M C5/C6	S C5/C6
LI11	At the radial end of the antecubital crease, halfway between the biceps tendon and the lateral epicondyle Angulation: perpendicular *Lateral epicondylalgia, forearm pain; immunomodulation*	Target: ECRL	D C5/C6	M C5/C6	S C6/C7
TE5	On the dorsal surface of forearm, 2 cun proximal to wrist joint, between radius and ulna, and between extensor indicis and extensor pollicis longus Angulation: perpendicular *Local pain; strong point for central effects*	Target: connective tissue plane	D C6/C7/C8	M C7/C8	S C7/C8
PC6	2 cun proximal to the distal wrist crease, between the tendons of flexor carpi radialis and palmaris longus Angulation: oblique proximal *Nausea, carpal tunnel syndrome* **CAUTION – note the position of the median nerve**	Target: flexor digitorum superficialis	D C6/C8/T1	M C7/C8	S n/a

(Continued over)

Table 18.1 Acupuncture point locations (continued).

Name	Location of point Angulation of needling Indications	Target structure for needle	Dermatome Myotome Sclerotome
LU7	On the radial aspect of the radial styloid, 1.5 *cun* from the wrist crease, between the tendons of abductor pollicis longus and brachioradialis Angulation: proximal oblique *Wrist and forearm pain*	Target: connective tissue space	D C6 M C7/C8 S C6
HT7	On the ulnar end of the distal volar crease of the wrist, at the radial side of the tendon of flexor carpi ulnaris, between the pisiform and the ulna Angulation: perpendicular *Classically used for anxiety and sedation* **CAUTION – the ulna artery and nerve are very close to this point**	Target: close to the ulnar nerve	D C8/T1 M C8 S C8
LI4	On the dorsal aspect of the hand, in the middle of the 1st web space, halfway along the second metacarpal bone Angulation: perpendicular *General point for pain; strong point for central effects* **CAUTION – the radial artery is at the apex of the 1st web space**	Target: 1st dorsal interosseous	D C6/C7 M T1 S n/a
SI3	On the palmar aspect of the neck of the 5th metacarpal, in the tissue plane between the metacarpal neck and the hypothenar muscles Angulation: perpendicular *Hand pain; also used for pain elsewhere especially spinal pain*	Target: connective tissue plane	D C8 M T1 S C8
CV17	In the center of the sternum at the 4th intercostal space (level with nipples in a man) Angulation: cranial oblique at 30 degree to the sternum *Chest pain; respiratory conditions* **CAUTION – a sternal foramen occurs at this point in 10% of men and 4% of women; never needle perpendicularly**	Target: periosteum of the sternum or sternalis	D T5 M C8/T1 or T5 S T5
CV12	On the midline of the upper abdomen, midway between the umbilicus and the lower border of the body of the sternum Angulation: perpendicular *Upper gastrointestinal disorders, including nausea and vomiting* **CAUTION – avoid needling through the abdominal wall**	Target: linea alba	D T8 M T8 S n/a
CV4	On the midline of the lower abdomen, 3 *cun* inferior to the umbilicus, and 2 *cun* superior to the pubic symphysis Angulation: perpendicular *Lower gastrointestinal, urological, and gynecological symptoms* **CAUTION – avoid needling through the abdominal wall**	Target: linea alba	D T11/T12 M T11/T12 S n/a
ST25	2 *cun* lateral to the umbilicus, halfway between the umbilicus and the linea semilunaris (SP15) Angulation: perpendicular or medial oblique *Abdominal pain; gastroenterological symptoms* **CAUTION – avoid needling through the abdominal wall**	Target: rectus abdominis	D T10 M T10 S n/a
GV3	Between spinous processes L4 and L5 Angulation: transverse *Spinal pain*	Target: interspinous ligament	D T11/T12 M L4 S L4
GV4	Between spinous processes L2 and L3 Angulation: transverse *Spinal pain*	Target: interspinous ligament	D T9/T10 M L2 S L2

(Continued over)

Point	Description	D	M	S
BL23	1.5 cun lateral to the midline, level with the lower border of L2 Angulation: oblique towards spine Target: erector spinae *Back pain*	T10/T11	T12/L1/L2	L2
BL25	1.5 cun lateral to the midline, level with the lower border of L4 Angulation: oblique towards spine Target: erector spinae *Back pain*	T11/T12	L2/L3/L4	L4
BL28	Level with the S2 posterior foramen, or the lower aspect of the posterior super or iliac spine Angulation: perpendicular Target: erector spinae or multifidus *Back pain*	S1/S2	L5	S2
GB30	1/3 of the way from the highest point of the greater trochanter to the sacral hiatus Angulation: towards symphysis Target: tensor fascia lata *Hip girdle pain, back pain, leg pain, sciatica* **CAUTION – avoid direct needling of the sciatic nerve**	L2/L3	L5/S1/S2	L4/L5/S1
GB34	In the depression just anterior and inferior to the head of the fibular Angulation: perpendicular Target: peroneus longus *Leg pain; general point for musculoskeletal pain* **CAUTION – avoid needling the common fibular nerve**	L5	L5/S1	L5
ST36	3 cun inferior to the knee joint, 1 fingerbreadth lateral to the lower border of the tibial tuberosity, in the middle of the upper third of the tibialis anterior Angulation: perpendicular Target: tibialis anterior *Knee pain, abdominal problems, strong point for central effects*	L4/L5	L4/L5	L4/L5
SP10	2 cun proximal to the superiomecial border of the patella, in the center of vastus medialis Angulation: perpendicular Target: vastus medialis *Knee pain (vastus medialis)*	L3	L2/L3/L4	L3
SP9	In a depression inferior to the medial condyle of the tibia and posterior to the medial border of the tibia, at the same level as GB34 Angulation: perpendicular Target: connective tissue space *Knee pain, gynecological and urological problems*	L3	L2/L3/L4	L3
SP6	3 cun superior to the most prominent part of the medial malleolus, on the medial border of the tibia Angulation: perpendicular Target: flexor digitorum longus *Gynecological problems; strong point for central effects*	L4/S1/S2	S1/S2	L4/L5
BL54/40	On the popliteal crease midway between the tendons of biceps femoris and semitendinosus, in the connective tissue space between the heads of gastrocnemius Angulation: perpendicular Target: connective tissue space *Local pain, sciatica* **CAUTION – note the popliteal artery and tibial nerve are deep to this point**	S1/S2	S1/S2	n/a
BL60	In the depression midway between the lateral malleolus and the Achilles tendor Angulation: perpendicular Target: connective tissue *Leg pain, Achilles tendon pain*	L5/S1	L5/S1	S1/S2
KI3	At the level of the most prominent part of the medial malleolus, half way between it and the Achilles tendon Angulation: perpendicular toward BL60 Target: connective tissue space *Ankle problems; urogenital problems; strong point for central effects*	L4/S2	S2	n/a
LR3	On the dorsum of the foot, in the 1st metatarsal space, in a depression distal to the junction of the bases of the 1st and 2nd metatarsals Angulation: perpendicular Target: 1st dorsal interosseous *Local pain; headache; abdominal problems; strong point for central effects* **CAUTION – the dorsalis pedis artery is at the apex of the 1st metatarsal space**	L4/L5	S2/S3	L5/S1

Cun, Chinese inch (a proportional measurement, e.g. the width of the interphalangeal joint of the thumb); I, ophthalmic; ii, maxillary; iii, mandibular divisions; V, trigeminal nerve.

or by the need to avoid regional conditions:

- lymphedema;
- anesthetic areas;
- hyperesthetic areas;
- ischemia.

As a general rule, therapeutic needling should be performed in healthy tissue.

POINT LOCATION

Precise point location is not thought to be particularly important from the Western neurophysiological perspective, apart from direct needling of trigger points in some individuals. Intensity of the stimulus is thought to be a more critical therapeutic factor. Despite this, there is still considerable interest in the concept of specific acupuncture points, and so-called "point detectors" are popular. These are devices that measure lowered skin impedance. Lowered skin impedance has not been found to correlate with traditional acupuncture points, and the devices concerned probably do not give reliable or reproducible results on the human skin surface.

NEEDLE TECHNIQUE

Sterile, single-use, disposable needles should always be used. In most cases acupuncture needling involves stimulation of muscle tissue. Needling of muscle produces a characteristic sensation, often described as a dull, diffuse ache, pressure, swelling, or numbness, which can be referred some distance from the point of stimulation. Needling of most other tissues of the soma, such as skin, ligament, tendon, periosteum, and fascial layers, produces relatively localized and often sharp sensations. If the aim is to stimulate a point in muscle, a rapid insertion through the skin and superficial layers minimizes discomfort for the patient. Practitioners who are learning the technique find that the use of an introducer facilitates a rapid, often painless insertion. If an introducer is not used, the practitioner will stretch the skin over the point during insertion. Once through the skin, the needle should be rapidly advanced to the desired position or muscle layer, and is then stimulated by rotation back and forth combined with a varying degree of "lift and thrust" (slight withdrawal and reinsertion) until the desired sensation is achieved. If constant stimulation of the needle is required, an electrical stimulator can be used. For the latter technique, usually a minimum of two needles are inserted and a specially designed electroacupuncture device is used to deliver the electrical stimulus.

Dry needling of trigger points involves a very similar procedure, although the practitioner will often lift and thrust the needle to a greater degree with alteration of the angle of insertion, aiming to hit the trigger point precisely. When the needle directly impinges on the trigger point, a local twitch is often seen or felt in the associated band of muscle, and the symptoms derived from that point are reproduced.

In clinical practice a wide variety of needling techniques have been described. These range from superficial needling to periosteal needling, with a variety of intermediate depths in muscle. Superficial needling of acupuncture points is common in Japanese forms of acupuncture, and Baldry[68] describes a superficial needling technique exclusively over trigger points. Periosteal needling was first described by Mann,[69, 70] although he, as most Western practitioners who came after him, uses a variety of techniques. As suggested above, muscle is the most common site of stimulation. Depth and strength of needling in this tissue ranges from brief, superficial stimulation of the muscle surface to deep, repetitive intramuscular stimulation. The latter is not uncommon in Chinese acupuncture, but is also promoted by some practitioners in the West, in particular by Gunn,[71, 72] who targets motor points and paraspinal muscles.

Moxibustion, the burning of a herb (moxa: *Artemesia vulgaris*; mugwort) on the handle of needles, or on its own direct at points, is common in traditional practice, however, the presence of smoke detectors limits its use in most orthodox clinical settings. The most intense form is known as scarification moxibustion. This involves direct application of the burning herb onto the skin, which causes a burn, and if repeated can result in sinus formation into deeper tissues. This is clearly a very intense stimulus, and may have been used historically in the East as a form of counterirritation in some cases of intractable pain.

CLINICAL ASPECTS

There is a range of different responses to acupuncture treatment, from no effect, in 5 or 10 percent of the population, at one end, to profound analgesia and improved well-being, in a similar proportion, at the other end. Empirical observation suggests that about 70 percent of the population have a useful response in primary care, although this is likely to be 50 percent or less for the pain population seen in secondary care. Patient selection will clearly influence success, and a healthy patient with a short-lived myofascial pain syndrome is much more likely to have a beneficial outcome than a debilitated patient with a chronic, ill-defined, and complex problem.

It is difficult to define a "dose" for acupuncture treatment, because on many occasions a judicious single needle insertion may have the same effect as ten or more needles left in place for 20 minutes; and similar strength, sequential treatments often have increasing potency in the early stages of a course of treatment. Experimental work does appear to support a type of dose–response relationship for sensory stimulation (Lundeberg, personal communication, 1997), but it is unlikely to be linear, and it is likely to be dependent on both individual genetic and environment factors.[73] There is probably a stepwise increase in potency of sensory stimulation down the following list:

- superficial, heterosegmental needling with minimal sensation;
- superficial, segmental needling with minimal sensation;
- deep, heterosegmental needling with strong sensation;
- deep, segmental needling with strong sensation;
- deep, segmental needling with electrical stimulation sufficient to cause muscle contraction.

Whilst acupuncture is likely to do more than simply offer pain relief, the standard pattern of effect from treatment is most easily appreciated in terms of analgesia. There may be little or no effect after the first session, as the practitioner will usually start with gentle treatment. This is to avoid aggravating the complaint in those most sensitive to needling. The initial response is seen within the first 72 hours after treatment, and its onset is often not perceived until the day after needling. Repeat treatments are performed either bi-weekly or weekly, and the interval can be lengthened with the response. Typically there is a progressive increase in the quality and duration of the effect following repeated sessions, and in chronic pain states, symptom control can be maintained for some patients with relatively infrequent treatments, perhaps every four to six weeks, or sometimes longer.

SUMMARY

Needling therapies have been applied to the treatment of pain disorders for thousands of years, and the techniques used today probably do not differ dramatically from those applied to Ötzi in 3200BC. Empirical evidence suggests that direct needling of trigger points is probably the most valuable needling technique, but definitive research to establish the specific action of the needle is still sought. All doctors who treat musculoskeletal dysfunction would find needling of trigger points and segmental acupuncture useful, but adequate knowledge of anatomy and infection control procedures is essential.

REFERENCES

1. Dorfer L, Moser M, Bahr F et al. A medical report from the stone age? Lancet. 1999; 354: 1023–5.
2. Melzack R, Stillwell DM, Fox EJ. Trigger points and acupuncture points for pain: correlations and implications. Pain. 1977; 3: 3–23.
3. Veith I. The Yellow Emperor's classic of internal medicine. Berkeley: University of California Press, 1972.

* 4. Filshie J, Cummings TM. Western medical acupuncture. In: Ernst E, White A (eds). Acupuncture – a scientific appraisal. Oxford: Butterworth Heinemann, 1999: 31–59.
* 5. Han JS, Terenius L. Neurochemical basis of acupuncture analgesia. Annual Review of Pharmacology and Toxicology. 1982; 22: 193–220.
6. Cummings M. Myofascial pain syndromes. In: Hazelman B, Riley G, Speed C (eds). Soft tissue rheumatology. Oxford: Oxford University Press, 2004: 509–22.
7. Cummings M. Acupuncture and trigger point needling. In: Hazelman B, Riley G, Speed C (eds). Soft tissue rheumatology. Oxford: Oxford University Press, 2004: 275–82.
8. Cummings M, Baldry P. Regional myofascial pain: diagnosis and management. Best Practice and Research. Clinical Rheumatology. 2007; 21: 367–87.
* 9. White AR, Filshie J, Cummings TM. Clinical trials of acupuncture: consensus recommendations for optimal treatment, sham controls and blinding. Complementary Therapies in Medicine. 2001; 9: 237–45.
10. Lund I, Lundeberg T. Are minimal, superficial or sham acupuncture procedures acceptable as inert placebo controls? Acupuncture in Medicine. 2006; 24: 13–15.
11. Haake M, Muller HH, Schade-Brittinger C et al. German Acupuncture Trials (GERAC) for chronic low back pain: randomized, multicenter, blinded, parallel-group trial with 3 groups. Archives of Internal Medicine. 2007; 167: 1892–8.
12. Scharf HP, Mansmann U, Streitberger K et al. Acupuncture and knee osteoarthritis: a three-armed randomized trial. Annals of Internal Medicine. 2006; 145: 12–20.
13. Streitberger K, Kleinhenz J. Introducing a placebo needle into acupuncture research. Lancet. 1998; 352: 364–5.
14. Kleinhenz J, Streitberger K, Windeler J et al. Randomised clinical trial comparing the effects of acupuncture and a newly designed placebo needle in rotator cuff tendinitis. Pain. 1999; 83: 235–41.
15. Kaptchuk TJ, Stason WB, Davis RB et al. Sham device v inert pill: randomised controlled trial of two placebo treatments. British Medical Journal. 2006; 332: 391–7.
16. Takakura N, Yajima H. A double-blind placebo needle for acupuncture research. BMC Complementary and Alternative Medicine. 2007; 7: 31.
17. Cummings TM, White AR. Needling therapies in the management of myofascial trigger point pain: a systematic review. Archives of Physical Medicine and Rehabilitation. 2001; 82: 986–92.
18. Mendelson G, Selwood TS, Kranz H et al. Acupuncture treatment of chronic back pain. A double-blind placebo-controlled trial. American Journal of Medicine. 1983; 74: 49–55.
19. Kuang X, Su Y, Guo H. [Study on combined acupunctural and general anesthesia in pneumonectomy]. Chung Kuo Chung Hsi I Chieh Ho Tsa Chih. 1996; 16: 84–6.
20. Lao L. Acupuncture techniques and devices. Journal of Alternative and Complementary Medicine. 1996; 2: 23–5.

21. Vilholm OJ, Moller K, Jorgensen K. Effect of traditional Chinese acupuncture on severe tinnitus: a double- blind, placebo-controlled, clinical investigation with open therapeutic control. *British Journal of Audiology*. 1998; **32**: 197–204.

22. Cooper RA, Henderson T, Dietrich CL. Roles of nonphysician clinicians as autonomous providers of patient care. *Journal of the American Medical Association*. 1998; **280**: 795–802.

23. McMillan AS, Nolan A, Kelly PJ. The efficacy of dry needling and procaine in the treatment of myofascial pain in the jaw muscles. *Journal of Orofacial Pain*. 1997; **11**: 307–14.

24. Tfelt-Hansen P, Lous I, Olesen J. Prevalence and significance of muscle tenderness during common migraine attacks. *Headache*. 1981; **21**: 49–54.

25. Tschopp KP, Gysin C. Local injection therapy in 107 patients with myofascial pain syndrome of the head and neck. *ORL; Journal for Oto-rhino-laryngology and its Related Specialties*. 1996; **58**: 306–10.

26. Wheeler AH, Goolkasian P, Gretz SS. A randomized, double-blind, prospective pilot study of botulinum toxin injection for refractory, unilateral, cervicothoracic, paraspinal, myofascial pain syndrome. *Spine*. 1998; **23**: 1662–6.

27. Manheimer E, Linde K, Lao L et al. Meta-analysis: acupuncture for osteoarthritis of the knee. *Annals of Internal Medicine*. 2007; **146**: 868–77.

∗ 28. White A, Foster NE, Cummings M, Barlas P. Acupuncture treatment for chronic knee pain: a systematic review. *Rheumatology (Oxford)*. 2007; **46**: 384–90.

29. Furlan AD, van Tulder MW, Cherkin DC et al. Acupuncture and dry-needling for low back pain. *Cochrane Database of Systematic Reviews*. 2005; **CD001351**.

30. Manheimer E, White A, Berman B et al. Meta-analysis: acupuncture for low back pain. *Annals of Internal Medicine*. 2005; **142**: 651–63.

31. Trinh KV, Graham N, Gross AR et al. Acupuncture for neck disorders. *Cochrane Database of Systematic Reviews*. 2006; **CD004870**.

32. Diener HC, Kronfeld K, Boewing G et al. Efficacy of acupuncture for the prophylaxis of migraine: a multicentre randomised controlled clinical trial. *Lancet Neurology*. 2006; **5**: 310–16.

33. Melchart D, Linde K, Fischer P et al. Acupuncture for idiopathic headache. *Cochrane Database of Systematic Reviews*. 2001; **CD001218**.

34. Linde K, Streng A, Jurgens S et al. Acupuncture for patients with migraine: a randomized controlled trial. *Journal of the American Medical Association*. 2005; **293**: 2118–25.

35. Witt CM, Jena S, Brinkhaus B et al. Acupuncture in patients with osteoarthritis of the knee or hip: a randomized, controlled trial with an additional nonrandomized arm. *Arthritis and Rheumatism*. 2006; **54**: 3485–93.

36. Witt C, Selim D, Reinhold T et al. Cost-effectiveness of acupuncture in patients with headache, low back pain and osteoarthritis of the hip and the knee. *FACT*. 2005; **10**: 57–8.

37. Witt CM, Jena S, Selim D et al. Pragmatic randomized trial evaluating the clinical and economic effectiveness of acupuncture for chronic low back pain. *American Journal of Epidemiology*. 2006; **164**: 487–96.

38. Jena S, Becker-Witt C, Brinkhaus B et al. Effectiveness of acupuncture treatment for headache – the Acupuncture in Routine Care study (ARC-Headache). *FACT*. 2004; **9**: 17.

39. Willich SN, Reinhold T, Selim D et al. Cost-effectiveness of acupuncture treatment in patients with chronic neck pain. *Pain*. 2006; **125**: 107–13.

40. Witt CM, Jena S, Brinkhaus B et al. Acupuncture for patients with chronic neck pain. *Pain*. 2006; **125**: 98–106.

∗ 41. Chiang CY, Chang CT, Chu HL, Yang LF. Peripheral afferent pathway for acupuncture analgesia. *Scientia Sinica*. 1973; **16**: 210–7.

42. Dundee JW, Ghaly G. Local anesthesia blocks the antiemetic action of P6 acupuncture. *Clinical Pharmacology and Therapeutics*. 1991; **50**: 78–80.

43. Chung JM, Fang ZR, Hori Y et al. Prolonged inhibition of primate spinothalamic tract cells by peripheral nerve stimulation. *Pain*. 1984; **19**: 259–75.

44. Dawidson I, Angmar-Mansson B, Blom M et al. The influence of sensory stimulation (acupuncture) on the release of neuropeptides in the saliva of healthy subjects. *Life Sciences*. 1998; **63**: 659–74.

45. Dawidson I, Angmar-Mansson B, Blom M et al. Sensory stimulation (acupuncture) increases the release of vasoactive intestinal polypeptide in the saliva of xerostomia sufferers. *Neuropeptides*. 1998; **32**: 543–8.

46. Jansen G, Lundeberg T, Kjartansson J, Samuelson UE. Acupuncture and sensory neuropeptides increase cutaneous blood flow in rats. *Neuroscience Letters*. 1989; **97**: 305–9.

47. Jansen G, Lundeberg T, Samuelson UE, Thomas M. Increased survival of ischaemic musculocutaneous flaps in rats after acupuncture. *Acta Physiologica Scandinavica*. 1989; **135**: 555–8.

48. Lundeberg T, Kjartansson J, Samuelsson U. Effect of electrical nerve stimulation on healing of ischaemic skin flaps. *Lancet*. 1988; **2**: 712–4.

∗ 49. Bowsher D. Mechanisms of acupuncture. In: Filshie J, White A (eds). *Medical acupuncture – a western scientific approach*, 1st edn. Edinburgh: Churchill Livingstone, 1998: 69–82.

50. White A. Neurophysiology of acupuncture analgesia. In: Ernst E, White A (eds). *Acupuncture – a scientific appraisal*. Oxford: Butterworth Heinemann, 1999: 60–92.

51. Chapman CR, Chen AC, Bonica JJ. Effects of intrasegmental electrical acupuncture on dental pain: evaluation by threshold estimation and sensory decision theory. *Pain*. 1977; **3**: 213–27.

52. Lundeberg T, Eriksson S, Lundeberg S, Thomas M. Acupuncture and sensory thresholds. *American Journal of Chinese medicine*. 1989; **17**: 99–110.

53. Sato A, Sato Y, Suzuki A, Uchida S. Neural mechanisms of the reflex inhibition and excitation of gastric motility elicited by acupuncture-like stimulation in anesthetized rats. *Neuroscience Research*. 1993; **18**: 53–62.

54. Lundeberg T, Bondesson L, Thomas M. Effect of acupuncture on experimentally induced itch. *British Journal of Dermatology*. 1987; **117**: 771–7.

55. Ceccherelli F, Gagliardi G, Visentin R, Giron G. Effects of deep vs. superficial stimulation of acupuncture on capsaicin-induced edema. A blind controlled study in rats. *Acupuncture and Electro-therapeutics Research*. 1998; **23**: 125–34.

56. Le Bars D, Dickenson AH, Besson JM. Diffuse noxious inhibitory controls (DNIC). I-Effects on dorsal horn convergent neurones in the rat; II-Lack of effect on non-convergent neurones, supraspinal involvement and theoretical implications. *Pain*. 1979; **6**: 305–27.

57. Lee A, Done ML. The use of nonpharmacologic techniques to prevent postoperative nausea and vomiting: a meta-analysis. *Anesthesia and Analgesia*. 1999; **88**: 1362–9.

58. Vickers AJ. Can acupuncture have specific effects on health? A systematic review of acupuncture antiemesis trials. *Journal of the Royal Society of Medicine*. 1996; **89**: 303–11.

59. Han JS. Acupuncture and endorphins. *Neuroscience Letters*. 2004; **361**: 258–61.

∗ 60. Han JS. Acupuncture: neuropeptide release produced by electrical stimulation of different frequencies. *Trends in Neurosciences*. 2003; **26**: 17–22.

61. Hui KK, Liu J, Makris N *et al*. Acupuncture modulates the limbic system and subcortical gray structures of the human brain: evidence from fMRI studies in normal subjects. *Human Brain Mapping*. 2000; **9**: 13–25.

62. Hui KK, Liu J, Marina O *et al*. The integrated response of the human cerebro-cerebellar and limbic systems to acupuncture stimulation at ST 36 as evidenced by fMRI. *Neuroimage*. 2005; **27**: 479–96.

63. Benedetti F, Arduino C, Amanzio M. Somatotopic activation of opioid systems by target-directed expectations of analgesia. *Journal of Neuroscience*. 1999; **19**: 3639–48.

64. Benedetti F, Mayberg HS, Wager TD *et al*. Neurobiological mechanisms of the placebo effect. *Journal of Neuroscience*. 2005; **25**: 10390–402.

65. Rampes H, Peuker E. Adverse effects of acupuncture. In: Ernst E, White A (eds). *Acupuncture – a scientific appraisal*. Oxford: Butterworth Heinemann, 1999: 128–52.

66. Peuker ET, White AR, Ernst E *et al*. Traumatic complications of acupuncture, therapists need to know human anatomy. *Archives of Family Medicine*. 1999; **8**: 553–8.

∗ 67. White A. A cumulative review of the range and incidence of significant adverse events associated with acupuncture. *Acupuncture in Medicine*. 2004; **22**: 122–33.

68. Baldry PE. *Acupuncture, trigger points and musculoskeletal pain*, 3rd edn. Edinburgh: Churchill Livingstone, 2005.

69. Mann F. A new system of acupuncture. In: Filshie J, White A (eds). *Medical acupuncture – a western scientific approach*, 1st edn. Edinburgh: Churchill Livingstone, 1998: 61–6.

70. Mann F. *Reinventing acupuncture: a new concept of ancient medicine*, 2nd edn. Oxford: Butterworth Heinemann, 2000.

71. Gunn CC. *Treating myofascial pain, intramuscular stimulation (IMS) for myofascial pain syndromes of neuropathic origin*. Seattle: University of Washington, 1989.

72. Gunn CC. Acupuncture and the peripheral nervous system. In: Filshie J, White A (eds). *Medical acupuncture – a western scientific approach*, 1st edn. Edinburgh: Churchill Livingstone, 1998: 137–50.

73. Wan Y, Wilson SG, Han J, Mogil JS. The effect of genotype on sensitivity to electroacupuncture analgesia. *Pain*. 2001; **91**: 5–13.

19

Physiotherapy

HARRIËT M WITTINK AND JEANINE A VERBUNT

KEY LEARNING POINTS

- The role of the physical therapist is to form a close partnership with patients, help patients set and attain self-directed goals at activities and participation level, and teach patients self-management skills.
- For assessment of a patient with chronic pain, the International Classification of Functioning, Disability and Health (ICF) framework is recommended.
- There is evidence for the efficacy of education, exercise, and cognitive–behavioral treatment. Passive modalities should only be used in conjunction with active treatment.
- Patients' beliefs influence treatment outcomes.
- Therapists' beliefs influence treatment.
- Patients should set measurable, realistic goals so that treatment can be time-limited and have an observable end point.

INTRODUCTION

To address the biopsychosocial nature of the problem of chronic pain, patients are ideally treated by an interdisciplinary team approach. As a result of this holistic approach, the interdisciplinary pain rehabilitation team consists of a diversity of health workers: physicians, psychologists, physical and occupational therapists, social workers, and nurses. In addition, the patient has an important role in his/her own treatment as an educated and active participant. Within this multidimensional focus of treatment, physical therapy emphasizes the performance of daily activities. Physical therapists help patients address and overcome physical and psychological obstacles, return to activities, and achieve personal goals.[1]

To achieve this, a comprehensive assessment of factors that may influence physical functioning is needed, and patient-centered, evidence-based physical rehabilitation focused on regaining optimal activity and participation levels.

In evidence-based practice, clinical decisions must include consideration of, first, the patient's clinical, physical, and psychosocial circumstances to establish what is wrong and what treatment options are available. Second, the latter need to be tempered by research evidence concerning the efficacy, effectiveness, and efficiency of the options. Third, given the likely consequences associated with each option, the clinician must consider the patient's preferences and likely actions (in terms of what interventions she or he is ready and able to accept). Clinical expertise is needed to bring these considerations together and recommend a treatment that the patient is agreeable to accepting.[2] Accordingly, it is important to identify patient expectations at the initial visit to prevent disappointment with referrals to pain management.

THE PATIENT'S CLINICAL, PHYSICAL, AND PSYCHOSOCIAL CIRCUMSTANCE

The purposes of a physical therapy evaluation are to exclude serious acute conditions (red flags), signal psychosocial "yellow flags" risk factors, establish a baseline from which to plan and begin interventions, assist in the selection of appropriate interventions, and evaluate the efficacy of interventions. To establish a baseline, a thorough inventory of all factors contributing to a patient's perceived level of disability is important. The International Classification of Functioning, Disability and Health (ICF) provides a holistic model that identifies three concepts described from the perspective of body systems, the individual, and society. Within the context of health, the ICF defined "bodily functions and structures" as physiological functions of body systems or anatomical elements, such as organs, limbs, and their components. "Activity" is defined as the execution of specific tasks or actions by an individual, while "participation" is envisioned as encompassing involvement in a life situation. In the ICF, "functioning" refers to all body functions, activities, and participation. Disability is the person's health condition (impairment, activity limitation, and participation restrictions) and contextual factors. Contextual factors are provided within the ICF framework, consisting of external environmental factors (such as significant others, employers, medications, and health-care providers) and personal factors (such as age, education, income, worry that activity will exacerbate pain, or injury resulting in avoidance of activity to prevent anticipated negative consequences).

Within the activity and participation classification of the ICF, a patient's inherent capacity to perform actions within a domain and actual performance in his or her environmental context can be separated.[3] Capacity refers to the environmentally adjusted inherent ability of the individual, or in other words, the highest probable functioning of a person in a given domain at a given point in time, in a standardized environment. Capacity can be measured by physical tests or by questionnaires that ask "can you?" Performance describes what a person actually does in her or his current environment and thus describes the person's functioning as observed or reported in the person's real-life environment with the existing facilitators and barriers.[4] Performance can be measured by direct observation. As this is often highly impractical, self-report measures can be substituted that ask "do you?"

The ICF model provides a useful framework for the selection of appropriate measurement tools to complete the patient's health profile. The health profile should include sociodemographic information, medical diagnosis, patient goals, symptoms and signs, the development and course of symptom and signs, previous episodes and treatment results, impairments, current level of activities and activity limitations, current level of participation in society and participation restrictions, environmental and personal factors. The relationships between these variables is then mapped out to arrive at a treatment plan. If, for instance, it appears from the health profile that a patient's activity limitations could, in large part, be determined by psychological factors, such as catastrophizing and fear avoidance, then these factors need to be targeted in treatment if the patient's goals include increasing his/her activity level. An overview of the assessment and measurement is provided in **Table 19.1**.

The use of measurement instruments for each of these domains will objectify patient information and is highly recommended. Pain assessment is discussed in Chapter 3, Selecting and applying pain measures. In addition, physical therapists focus on the interference of pain with activities and participation; the number of hours lying down because of pain during a day, activities of daily living such as housework, grocery shopping, getting around in the community, recreational and social activities, and ability to do work and sleep. Significant others, such as partners, parents, and children, may influence the patient's activity and participation levels in helpful and unhelpful ways.

Table 19.1 Measurement of International Classification of Functioning, Disability and Health domains.

ICF domain	Measurement
Impairments	Patient history (pain variables)
	Physical examination
	Diagnostic tests
	Questionnaires (depression/anxiety)
Activities	Patient history
Capacity	
Performance	
	Questionnaires – (can you?)
	Functional tests
	Patient history
	Questionnaires (do you?)
	Observation daily activities
Participation	Patient history
	Questionnaires
Environmental factors	Patient history
	Questionnaires
Personal factors	Patient history
	Questionnaires

Impairments

First, diagnostic procedures based on both history taking and physical examination should focus on the identification of potentially serious "red flag" conditions that require prompt medical evaluation. Physical impairments can be assessed through the traditional rehabilitation-oriented physical examination of joint range of motion (ROM), strength, neurological integrity, and gait. Aerobic fitness can be estimated from submaximal bicycle ergometer tests or measured using a treadmill test.[5] The main objective is to determine whether there is a relationship between pain reports and objective physical findings, or whether the patient presents with intractable pain (chronic pain syndrome). The latter group often presents with a discrepancy between objective findings during physical examination and their reported disability level in daily functioning. In the first group, rehabilitation might focus more specifically on impairments related to pain that interfere with the ability to function, while in the latter case rehabilitation might focus on improving physical functioning in general and have a more significant behavioral approach.

Activity limitations

Unfortunately, there are no perfect measures of activity limitations. Comparison measures include both "subjective" measures (based on self-report, usually questionnaires) and "objective" measures (based on direct measurement). Self-report measures can be self-administered or interviewer-administered, both in person or on the telephone. Self-reported status often involves outcomes of most relevance and importance to patients and their loved ones because they capture patient experience and perspective.[6] However, self-report of activity limitations can reflect a difference between how patients function and how they believe they function, resulting in a different reported activity limitation level compared to the actual observed active behavior.[7] In an experimental setting, it appears that patients in pain especially have difficulties judging their own performance.[8] In addition, there may be a discrepancy between what patients actually do (performance) and what they are capable of doing (capacity). Relatively few comparison studies have been performed between self-report and objective measures. The studies that are available seem to indicate a gap between self-report and objective measurement.[9, 10]

In rehabilitation practice, there is a tendency to use objective as well as self-report measures to assess activity limitations. Objective measures include functional tests, markers of movement (accelerometers), and observed or videotaped activity (direct observation).

For a further exploration of a patient's activity limitations, addressing changes in the level of physical activity over time will result in additional information. Some patients with pain report a physical activity level that fluctuates dramatically over time in reaction to pain. These patients are likely to persevere until increasing pain prevents further activity, then rest completely until the pain subsides or frustration over inactivity stimulates resumption of activity. Subsequently, they persevere again until increasing pain hinders further activity.[11] Murphy et al.[12] referred to this as "all or nothing" behavior, which has been observed in many chronic pain patients. Adequate registration of changes in the activity level over time could provide insight in the way in which a patient tries to cope with the limitations in daily life.

In addition to the above-mentioned exploration of daily activity limitations, physical performance can be evaluated by functional testing to complete the assessment of physical functioning. Two sets of functional tests that have been used in a chronic pain population include the Back Performance Scale[13, 14] and the physical performance test battery.[15] The Back Performance Scale is a condition-specific performance measure of activity limitation in patients with back pain. It includes five tests of daily activities requiring mobility of the trunk: sock test, pick-up test, roll-up test, fingertip-to-floor test, and lift test. This test is reliable, valid, and discriminative ability and responsiveness to important change have been demonstrated.[13, 14] The physical performance test battery is a generic test battery that includes nine physical performance tests: the time taken to complete various tasks (e.g. picking up coins, tying a belt, reaching up, putting on a sock, standing from sitting, a 50-foot fast walk, a 50-foot walk at preferred speed), the distance walked in six minutes, and the distance reached forward while standing. The test battery is reliable and has discriminant ability.

A number of studies have shown that self-report and functional tests, although related, appear to tap into different aspects of the activities domain.[16] For instance, patients with chronic low back pain (CLBP) showed considerable differences in limitations when comparing self-report, clinical examination, and functional testing for assessing work-related limitations. Professional health-care workers should be aware of these differences.[17, 18]

Participation restrictions

Participation restrictions are problems an individual may experience in involvement in life situations, meaning the social environment. Employment, community life, travel, recreation, and leisure activities are frequently assessed as an important part of patient functioning. Many questionnaires contain items on these domains and can be used to objectify the extent of participation restrictions.

An example of a questionnaire which specifically addresses the level of participation in society is the Impact on Participation and Autonomy (IPA) questionnaire.[19]

Environmental factors

Common environmental factors measured in patients with chronic pain include medication use, living environment (house, apartment, stairs, etc.), physical aids and appliances, attitudes of immediate family (e.g. solicitous spouse,[20] work tasks, and work environment). Attitudes of healthcare providers belong here too and may have a significant impact on treatment outcome (see below under Clinical expertise). The ICF core set for chronic widespread pain includes a number of these items.[21]

Personal factors

Yellow flags are risk factors associated with chronic pain or disability[22, 23] and have a significant psychosocial predominance. Examples include negative coping strategies, poor self-efficacy beliefs, catastrophizing, fear-avoidance behavior, and distress. A questionnaire, based on screening on yellow flags that can be used to identify patients in the (sub)acute phase of pain, having a high risk for future disability and sick leave, is the Orebro Musculoskeletal Pain Screening Questionnaire.[24] Psychological screening by means of history taking has shown to have low sensitivity and predictive value for identifying distressed patients, thus formal screening of some sort, such as with a questionnaire, is recommended.[25] Psychosocial factors contributing to a patient's disability level in pain that can be assessed by a questionnaire are, for instance, fear of movement (Tampa Scale of Kinesiophobia[26]) or catastrophizing.[27]

RESEARCH EVIDENCE

Many treatment modalities in physiotherapy and rehabilitation treatment address chronic pain.[28] However, not all treatment concepts are evidence-based. Below we attempt to outline what is currently known about the (in)effectiveness of different treatment modalities.

Education

Education on both the complexity of pain and the holistic treatment approach appears quite important to patients with chronic pain and may be considered a precondition for pain management success. A number of studies have shown that most patients expect an explanation or an improved understanding of their pain problem, a clear diagnosis of the cause of their pain, information, and instructions. Patients expect confirmation from the healthcare provider that their pain is real.[29, 30] For patients attending pain clinics, the explanation of their pain problem is rated as important as the cure or relief of their pain.[29] Unfortunately, the underestimation of patients' ability to understand currently accurate information about the neurophysiology of pain represent

barriers to reconceptualization of the problem in chronic pain within the clinical and lay arenas.[31] However, patients are quite capable of understanding the complexities of pain if explained well. The main goals of education are reassurance and empowerment. It is important that patients understand the holistic approach of the treatment of chronic pain. Studies that have employed an approach to education that emphasizes the cognitive, behavioral, and neurophysiological aspects of chronic pain have reported reduced disability, reduced healthcare utilization, normalization of pain cognitions, and increased self-efficacy.

Exercise

Clinical trials have provided strong evidence for the efficacy of muscle conditioning and aerobic exercise to lessen symptoms in people with osteoarthritis of the knee.[32, 33, 34] Others have reported that exercise is an important tool for reducing pain, stiffness, and joint tenderness in rheumatoid arthritis[35, 36] and fibromyalgia syndrome patients.[37] Exercise has been shown to be effective for short-term pain relief in patients with rotator cuff disease, and provides a longer-term benefit with respect to daily functioning measures.[38] Exercise may be helpful for patients with CLBP, enhancing return to normal daily activities and work.[39, 40] Supervised exercise therapy that consists of individually designed programs, including stretching or strengthening, may improve pain and function in chronic nonspecific low back pain.[41]

There is strong evidence that exercise therapy and multidisciplinary treatment programs are effective in chronic low back pain and moderate evidence that nonsteroidal anti-inflammatory drugs, back schools, and behavioral therapy are effective in CLBP.[42] Physical conditioning programs that include a cognitive–behavioral approach plus intensive physical training (specific to the job or not) that (1) includes aerobic capacity, muscle strength, endurance, and coordination; (2) are in some way work-related; and (3) are given and supervised by a physical therapist or a multidisciplinary team, seem to be effective in reducing the number of sick days for some workers with chronic back pain, when compared to usual care.[43]

Guzman[44] performed a Cochrane review on the efficacy of multidisciplinary treatment of chronic back pain and concluded there was strong evidence that intensive multidisciplinary biopsychosocial rehabilitation with a functional restoration approach improved function when compared with inpatient or outpatient non-multidisciplinary treatments. There was moderate evidence that intensive multidisciplinary biopsychosocial rehabilitation with a functional restoration approach improved pain when compared with outpatient non-multidisciplinary rehabilitation or usual care.

In summary, exercise therapy encompasses a heterogeneous group of interventions and although the previously cited studies found positive effects of exercise on pain and function, at the moment the most effective exercise approach is still unknown. In most studies there were insufficient data to provide useful guidelines on optimal exercise type or dosage, although some evidence exists that patients with a poorer prognosis for return to work may benefit from more intensive treatment. Haldorsen et al.,[45] for instance, showed that patients with poor prognosis for return to work returned to work at significantly higher rates when treated with a more intense multidisciplinary treatment program. On the contrary, patients with good return to work prognosis benefited equally from ordinary treatment as multidisciplinary treatment. Patients thus do not all benefit from the same exercise program. Exercise programs therefore need to be individually designed and tailored to the individual needs of the patient.

Passive modalities

At the moment, there is only little evidence that supports the use of passive modalities in the treatment of patients with chronic pain. Spinal manipulative therapy has no statistically or clinically significant advantage over general practitioner care, analgesics, physical therapy, exercises, or back school in patients with CLBP.[46] Massage, on the other hand, might be beneficial for patients with subacute and chronic nonspecific low back pain, especially when combined with exercises and education.[47] Locally applied thermal treatments (ice and heat packs) are commonly used in painful conditions and can be easily applied by the patient at home. There is no evidence to demonstrate that treatment by a practitioner is better than treatment by patients themselves. The evidence base to support the common practice of superficial heat and cold for low back pain is limited. There is insufficient evidence to evaluate the effects of cold for low back pain and conflicting evidence for any differences between heat and cold for low back pain.[43] Temperature modalities should rarely be used alone, but rather in conjunction with appropriate exercises, such as stretching, for increasing range of motion and for strengthening.[48]

The evidence base to support the common practice of superficial heat and cold for low back pain is limited. There is moderate evidence in a small number of trials that heat wrap therapy provides a small short-term reduction in pain and disability in a population with a mix of acute and subacute low back pain, and that the addition of exercise further reduces pain and improves function.[43]

Behavioral approaches

Operant behavioral therapy (OBT) refers to the group of interventions focused on the observed behavior of a patient. In the operant model, the reinforcing role of social and environmental factors in the development and maintenance of pain through observed pain behaviors is identified with the behaviors themselves being targeted for intervention. OBT techniques include pacing and graded activity (quota setting), positive reinforcement of "well" behaviors, and scheduling and tapering of pain medications. Cognitive–behavioral therapy (CBT) is directed towards changing patients' maladaptive responses to chronic pain by examining and posing alternatives to the thoughts, attitudes, and beliefs underlying them, as well as by encouraging the acquisition of new coping skills and techniques to take their place. The focus of CBT is on self-control and self-regulation.[49] It is still unknown what type of patients benefit most from what type of behavioral treatment, although a number of systematic reviews have demonstrated efficacy of behavioral treatment in patients with chronic pain.[50, 51, 52, 53] Recent evidence in patients with fibromyalgia suggests that OBT physical impairment responders display significantly more pain behaviors, physical impairment, physician visits, solicitous spouse behaviors, and level of catastrophizing compared with nonresponders. The CBT physical impairment responders, compared with nonresponders, reported higher levels of affective distress, lower coping, less solicitous spouse behavior, and lower pain behaviors.[54] Patients receiving OBT or CBT reported a significant reduction in pain intensity following treatment. In addition, the CBT group reported statistically significant improvements in cognitive and affective variables and the OBT group demonstrated statistically significant improvements in physical functioning and behavioral variables, compared with the control group (unstructured discussion).[55] Although OBT tends to be part of the standard repertoire of the physical therapist, CBT is not. Several studies suggest that brief training in CBT techniques may not be enough to bring about clinically significant change.[56, 57] For nonbehavioral therapists to incorporate CBT aspects into their treatment delivery with only a brief training program may not be realistic.[57] Although multidisciplinary programs have shown effectiveness in patients with chronic pain, which component is most effective and whether combining treatment approaches has a summative effect remains obscure. For example, in a recent study, Smeets et al.[58] studied the effectiveness of three rehabilitation interventions: an active physical, a cognitive–behavioral, and a combined treatment for nonspecific CLBP. The three interventions were compared to each other and to a waiting list control group. All three active treatments were effective in comparison to no treatment, but no clinically relevant differences between the combined and the single component treatments were found. For a subgroup of patients, those with a high level of pain-related fear, exposure in vivo treatment shows promising results.[59] In this treatment, patients are challenged to actually perform physical activities which they believe will harm them. Most of the time exposure treatment is performed in combined therapy with a physical therapist and a behavioral therapist. At this moment, most studies addressing the effect of exposure are only based on a small number of patients in a single case design.[60] Further research to confirm the effectiveness of exposure to *in vivo* treatment in chronic pain is warranted.

Self-management programs

The evidence regarding the effectiveness of self-management programs in reducing pain and disability is growing. To decrease the negative impact of chronic pain on functioning and health-related quality of life, patients must adopt self-management skills. For a good collaboration between the physical therapist and the patient, the patient must at least be planning to take an active orientation towards self-management and the therapist should support and encourage this. Positive results on health-related quality of life outcomes (self-reported, health distress, disability, activity limitation, global health, pain, and fatigue), health behaviors (practice of mental stress management, stretching and strength exercise, aerobic exercise), self-efficacy, and health-care utilization (physician visits and hospitalizations) have been reported with self-management programs.[61]

PATIENT'S PREFERENCES AND LIKELY ACTIONS

Increasingly, there is evidence that patient beliefs play a considerable role in treatment outcome. For instance, a patient who is looking for pain relief only and insists on medication management as the sole treatment for the pain is unlikely to be compliant with a rehabilitation program. As a result of this, a pretreatment evaluation of a patient's readiness for behavior change is essential. The stages of change model, presenting five different stages of readiness for behavioral change, seems to offer a tool to assess this.[62] Patients in the precontemplation stage are not motivated to adopt self-management skills; patients in the contemplation stage think about it and may see a reason to change; patients in the preparation stage are planning to change and are already trying some (parts) of the skills; patients in the action stage are actively learning to engage in self-management, whereas patients in the maintenance stage keep on working to stabilize the new behavior pattern. Further research to the applicability of this model in chronic pain is still warranted, however.

To enhance patients' perception of the importance of pain self-management and increase self-efficacy, motivational interviewing techniques can be used.[63] To win the collaboration of patients and their families further, physical therapists need to negotiate and agree on a definition of the problem they are working on with each patient (what goals are we going to work on?) The patient and therapist must then agree on how to achieve the goals (how are we going to work on the goals?) Studies have shown that high patient expectations about certain kinds of treatment may influence clinical outcome independently of the treatment itself.[64] In one study, patients who preferred one type of treatment and received another actually got worse during treatment.[65] Return to work or vocational rehabilitation should be part of the treatment plan when appropriate. A directive return to work approach has been shown to be successful in patients with chronic pain.[66]

CLINICAL EXPERTISE

The physical therapist should have the following.

- A dynamic, multidimensional knowledge base that is patient-centered. The focus of pain management is to help patients regain control over their lives by active participation in their pain management program and independent management of their pain. To achieve this, an active partnership is needed between the patient and the therapist.
- A clinical reasoning process that is embedded in a collaborative, problem-solving venture with the patient. Like other patients, patients with chronic pain want a confidence-based association that includes understanding, listening, respect, and being included in decision-making.[30]
- A central focus on movement assessment linked to patient function. Patients with chronic pain are not a homogeneous group and there is no magic bullet that fits all. Because each patient has a unique set of circumstances, psychosocial issues, and physical findings, treatment is individualized and based on the comprehensive assessment of the patient and the patient's individual goals.
- Consistent virtues seen in caring and commitment to patients as has been shown to be central to expert physical therapy care.[67]

Not only do patients bring expectations about treatment, providers do as well. Treatment decisions are often based on the beliefs of the provider. It has been shown that providers who scored high on biomedical orientation were more likely to use a pain-contingent treatment approach and focus on "curing" impairments.[68] Providers who scored high on biopsychosocial orientation were more likely to use a time-contingent treatment approach and focus on increasing activities. Linton *et al.*[69] concluded that some practitioners hold beliefs reflecting fear avoidance that may influence treatment practice. Their findings were recently studied by Coudeyre *et al.*,[70] confirming that provider fear-avoidance beliefs about lower back pain negatively influence their following guidelines concerning physical and occupational activities for patients with lower back pain.

ACHIEVEMENT OF PATIENT GOALS

During treatment, the use of goal-setting charts is recommended. Goals must be measurable so that treatment can be time-limited and have an observable end point to prevent confusion and disappointment on both sides. Having a definite end point increases patient adherence and provides a framework for the patient and the treatment team in which to achieve goals. A treatment contract that includes goals, the intensity and frequency of treatment and expected compliance with treatment can be helpful.

Return to a pain-free state is a good example of an unrealistic goal. Common (realistic) goals are associated with a reduction of the impact of pain on the patient's life (i.e. increased level of activities and participation), independent pain management, and the attainment of functional goals. Examples of functional goals are being able to walk for one hour, sitting through a meal or a movie, being able to carry and lift a certain amount of weight, playing with the children, going out with the family, and being able to perform essential job components. Patients set a target for activities each week, record their achievements on the chart, note the nature of any difficulties and how these will be tackled next time, and make other comments. Patients may comment on their performance or on the appropriateness of the goals they had set. In this manner, they can monitor their progress and improve their accuracy in goal setting. Goal attainment scaling, a technique to objectify and evaluate the achievement of patient-specific goals for treatment, can be used to evaluate treatment outcome in both clinical practice and research.[71] A second method to objectify and evaluate patient-specific treatment goals is the Canadian Occupational Performance Measure (COPM),[72] a generic tool to be used in conjunction with the visual analog scale (VAS) to facilitate comparison with other patients is recommended. Generic and disease-specific measurement tools have been developed over the past decades, many of which are discussed in Chapter 3, Selecting and applying pain measures. Evaluative or outcome measures, used at baseline, can help determine treatment efficacy.

FOLLOW UP AFTER TREATMENT

Limited information is available on the effect of planned follow up after interdisciplinary treatment. Planned follow up can be undertaken on an individual basis or in group settings, and serves to prevent crisis management. To date, there is no evidence as to the optimal frequency or duration of follow-up visits.

CONCLUSIONS

The assessment and treatment of patients with chronic pain is a challenging task that is best performed in an interdisciplinary team setting, since both biomedical and psychosocial aspects related to the pain problem have to be addressed. The collaborative goal of the team (which includes the patient) is to significantly increase the performance of daily activities regardless of pain and increase patients' self-reported ability to cope with pain. The role of the physical therapist is to form a close partnership with patients, help patients set and attain self-directed goals at activities and participation level, and teach patients self-management skills. Ultimately, patients should become experts in managing their own chronic pain in order to enjoy the best quality of life possible.

REFERENCES

* 1. Harding V, Simmonds MJ, Watson P. Physical therapy for chronic pain. *Pain: Clinical Updates*. 1998; **VI**: 1–2. Available from: http://www.iasp-pain.org/PCU98c.html.

   2. Haynes RB, Devereaux PJ, Guyatt GH. Physicians' and patients' choices in evidence based practice. *British Medical Journal*. 2002; **324**: 1350.

   3. Ustun TB, Chatterji S, Bickenbach J *et al*. The International Classification of Functioning, Disability and Health: a new tool for understanding disability and health. *Disability and Rehabilitation*. 2003; **25**: 565–71.

* 4. Stucki G, Cieza A, Ewert T *et al*. Application of the International Classification of Functioning, Disability and Health (ICF) in clinical practice. *Disability and Rehabilitation*. 2002; **24**: 281–2.

   5. Wittink HM. Physical fitness, function and physical therapy in patients with pain: clinical measures of aerobic fitness and performance in patients with chronic low back pain. In: Max M (ed.). *Pain 1999 – an updated review. Refresher course syllabus*. Seattle: IASP press, 1999: 137–45.

* 6. Patrick DL, Chiang YP. Measurement of health outcomes in treatment effectiveness evaluations: conceptual and methodological challenges. *Medical Care*. 2000; **38**: II14–II25.

   7. Fordyce WE, Lansky D, Calsyn DA *et al*. Pain measurement and pain behavior. *Pain*. 1984; **18**: 53–69.

   8. Schmidt AJ. Performance level of chronic low back pain patients in different treadmill test conditions. *Journal of Psychosomatic Research*. 1985; **29**: 639–45.

* 9. Verbunt JA, Westerterp KR, van der Heijden GJ *et al*. Physical activity in daily life in patients with chronic low back pain. *Archives of Physical Medicine and Rehabilitation*. 2001; **82**: 726–30.

  10. Wittink H, Rogers W, Gascon C *et al*. Relative contribution of mental health and exercise-related pain increment to treadmill test intolerance in patients with chronic low back pain. *Spine*. 2001; **26**: 2368–74.

  11. Harding VR, Williams AC. Activities training: integrating behavioural and cognitive methods with physiotherapy in

pain management. *Journal of Occupational Rehabilitation.* 1998; **8**: 47–61.

12. Murphy D, Lindsay S, Williams AC. Chronic low back pain: predictions of pain and relationship to anxiety and avoidance. *Behaviour Research and Therapy.* 1997; **35**: 231–8.

13. Magnussen L, Strand LI, Lygren H. Reliability and validity of the back performance scale: observing activity limitation in patients with back pain. *Spine.* 2004; **29**: 903–07.

14. Strand LI, Moe-Nilssen R, Ljunggren AE. Back Performance Scale for the assessment of mobility-related activities in people with back pain. *Physical Therapy.* 2002; **82**: 1213–23.

15. Simmonds MJ, Olson SL, Jones S et al. Psychometric characteristics and clinical usefulness of physical performance tests in patients with low back pain. *Spine.* 1998; **23**: 2412–21.

16. Wittink H, Rogers W, Sukiennik A, Carr DB. Physical functioning: self-report and performance measures are related but distinct. *Spine.* 2003; **28**: 2407–13.

17. Brouwer S, Dijkstra PU, Stewart RE et al. Comparing self-report, clinical examination and functional testing in the assessment of work-related limitations in patients with chronic low back pain. *Disability and Rehabilitation.* 2005; **27**: 999–1005.

18. van Heuvelen MJ, Kempen GI, Brouwer WH, de Greef MH. Physical fitness related to disability in older persons. *Gerontology.* 2000; **46**: 333–41.

19. Cardol M, de Haan RJ, van den Bos GA et al. The development of a handicap assessment questionnaire: the Impact on Participation and Autonomy (IPA). *Clinical Rehabilitation.* 1999; **13**: 411–19.

20. Flor H, Kerns RD, Turk DC. The role of spouse reinforcement, perceived pain, and activity levels of chronic pain patients. *Journal of Psychosomatic Research.* 1987; **31**: 251–9.

＊ 21. Cieza A, Stucki G, Weigl M et al. ICF Core Sets for chronic widespread pain. *Journal of Rehabilitation Medicine.* 2004; **44**: 63–8.

＊ 22. Kendall N, Linton SJ, Main CJ. *Guide to assessing psychosocial yellow flags in acute low back pain: Risk factors for long-term disabilty and work loss.* Wellington, New Zealand: Accident Rehabilitation and Compensation Insurance Corporation of New Zealand and the National Health Committee, 1997.

23. Linton SJ. A review of psychological risk factors in back and neck pain. *Spine.* 2000; **25**: 1148–56.

24. Linton SJ, Boersma K. Early identification of patients at risk of developing a persistent back problem: the predictive validity of the Orebro Musculoskeletal Pain Questionnaire. *Clinical Journal of Pain.* 2003; **19**: 80–6.

25. Grevitt M, Pande K, O'Dowd J, Webb J. Do first impressions count? A comparison of subjective and psychologic assessment of spinal patients. *European Spine Journal.* 1998; **7**: 218–23.

26. Vlaeyen JW, Kole-Snijders AM, Boeren RG, van Eek H. Fear of movement/(re)injury in chronic low back pain and its relation to behavioral performance. *Pain.* 1995; **62**: 363–72.

27. Sullivan MJL, Bishop SR, Pivik J. The Pain Catastrophizing scale: development and validation. *Psychological Assessment.* 1995; **7**: 524–32.

＊ 28. Wittink HM, Cohen LJ, Michel TH. Pain rehabilitation: physical therapy treatment. In: Wittink HM, Michel TH (eds). *Chronic pain management for physical therapists,* 2nd edn. Boston: Butterworth-Heinemann, 2002: 127–60.

29. Petrie KJ, Frampton T, Large RG et al. What do patients expect from their first visit to a pain clinic? *Clinical Journal of Pain.* 2005; **21**: 297–301.

30. Verbeek J, Sengers MJ, Riemens L, Haafkens J. Patient expectations of treatment for back pain: a systematic review of qualitative and quantitative studies. *Spine.* 2004; **29**: 2309–18.

31. Moseley L. Unraveling the barriers to reconceptualization of the problem in chronic pain: the actual and perceived ability of patients and health professionals to understand the neurophysiology. *Journal of Pain.* 2003; **4**: 184–9.

32. Brosseau L, MacLeay L, Robinson V et al. Intensity of exercise for the treatment of osteoarthritis. *Cochrane Database of Systematic Reviews.* 2003; **CD004259**.

33. Fransen M, McConnell S, Bell M. Exercise for osteoarthritis of the hip or knee. *Cochrane Database of Systematic Reviews.* 2003; **CD004286**.

34. Roddy F, Zhang W, Doherty M. Aerobic walking or strengthening exercise for osteoarthritis of the knee? A systematic review. *Annals of the Rheumatic Diseases.* 2005; **64**: 544–8.

35. Hakkinen A, Sokka T, Kotaniemi A, Hannonen P. A randomized two-year study of the effects of dynamic strength training on muscle strength, disease activity, functional capacity, and bone mineral density in early rheumatoid arthritis. *Arthritis and Rheumatism.* 2001; **44**: 515–22.

36. Hakkinen A, Sokka T, Kautiainen H et al. Sustained maintenance of exercise induced muscle strength gains and normal bone mineral density in patients with early rheumatoid arthritis: a 5 year follow up. *Annals of the Rheumatic Diseases.* 2004; **63**: 910–16.

37. Busch A, Schachter CL, Peloso PM, Bombardier C. Exercise for treating fibromyalgia syndrome. *Cochrane Database of Systematic Reviews.* 2002; **CD003786**.

38. Green S, Buchbinder R, Hetrick S. Physiotherapy interventions for shoulder pain. *Cochrane Database of Systematic Reviews.* 2003; **CD004258**.

39. van Tulder MW, Malmivaara A, Esmail R, Koes BW. Exercise therapy for low back pain. *Cochrane Database of Systematic Reviews.* 2000; **CD000335**.

40. Hayden JA, van Tulder MW, Malmivaara AV, Koes BW. Meta-analysis: exercise therapy for nonspecific low back pain. *Annals of Internal Medicine.* 2005; **142**: 765–75.

41. Hayden JA, van Tulder MW, Tomlinson G. Systematic review: strategies for using exercise therapy to improve outcomes in chronic low back pain. *Annals of Internal Medicine*. 2005; **142**: 776–85.

42. van Tulder MW, Koes BW, Assendelft WJ *et al*. [Chronic low back pain: exercise therapy, multidisciplinary programs, NSAID's, back schools and behavioral therapy effective; traction not effective; results of systematic reviews]. *Nederlands Tijdschrift voor Geneeskunde*. 2000; **144**: 1489–94.

43. French SD, Cameron M, Walker BF *et al*. A Cochrane review of superficial heat or cold for low back pain. *Spine*. 2006; **31**: 998–1006.

∗ 44. Guzman JE, Esmail R, Karjalainen K *et al*. Multidisciplinary bio-psycho-social rehabilitation for chronic low back pain. *Cochrane Database of Systematic Reviews*. 2002; **CD000963**.

45. Haldorsen EM, Grasdal AL, Skouen JS *et al*. Is there a right treatment for a particular patient group? Comparison of ordinary treatment, light multidisciplinary treatment, and extensive multidisciplinary treatment for long-term sick-listed employees with musculoskeletal pain. *Pain*. 2002; **95**: 49–63.

46. Assendelft WJ, Morton SC, Yu EI *et al*. Spinal manipulative therapy for low back pain. A meta-analysis of effectiveness relative to other therapies. *Annals of Internal Medicine*. 2003; **138**: 871–81.

47. Furlan AD, Brosseau L, Imamura M, Irvin E. Massage for low-back pain: a systematic review within the framework of the Cochrane Collaboration Back Review Group. *Spine*. 2002; **27**: 1896–910.

∗ 48. Watson PJ. Physical medicine and rehabilitation. In: Charlton JE (ed.). *Core curriculum for professional education in pain*, 3rd edn. Seattle: IASP Press, 2005: 1–5

49. Wooton RJ, Caudill-Slosberg MA, Frank JB. Psychotherapeutic management of chronic pain. In: Warfield CA, Bajwa ZH (eds). *Principles and practice of pain medicine*, 2nd edn. New York: McGraw-Hill, 2004: 157–69.

50. Schonstein E, Kenny D, Keating J *et al*. Physical conditioning programs for workers with back and neck pain: a cochrane systematic review. *Spine*. 2003; **28**: E391–5.

51. Schonstein E, Kenny DT, Keating J, Koes BW. Work conditioning, work hardening and functional restoration for workers with back and neck pain. *Cochrane Database of Systematic Reviews*. 2003; **CD001822**.

52. Ostelo RW, van Tulder MW, Vlaeyen JW *et al*. Behavioural treatment for chronic low-back pain. *Cochrane Database of Systematic Reviews*. 2005; **CD002014**.

53. van Tulder MW, Ostelo R, Vlaeyen JW *et al*. Behavioral treatment for chronic low back pain: a systematic review within the framework of the Cochrane Back Review Group. *Spine*. 2000; **25**: 2688–99.

54. Thieme K, Turk DC, Flor H. Responder criteria for operant and cognitive-behavioral treatment of fibromyalgia syndrome. *Arthritis and Rheumatism*. 2007; **57**: 830–6.

55. Thieme K, Flor H, Turk DC. Psychological pain treatment in fibromyalgia syndrome: efficacy of operant behavioural and cognitive behavioural treatments. *Arthritis Research and Therapy*. 2006; **8**: R121.

56. Jellema P, van der Windt DA, van der Horst HE *et al*. Should treatment of (sub)acute low back pain be aimed at psychosocial prognostic factors? Cluster randomised clinical trial in general practice. *British Medical Journal*. 2005; **331**: 84.

57. Johnson RE, Jones GT, Wiles NJ *et al*. Active exercise, education, and cognitive behavioral therapy for persistent disabling low back pain: a randomized controlled trial. *Spine*. 2007; **32**: 1578–85.

∗ 58. Smeets RJ, Vlaeyen JW, Hidding A *et al*. Active rehabilitation for chronic low back pain: Cognitive-behavioral, physical, or both? First direct post-treatment results from a randomized controlled trial [ISRCTN22714229]. *BMC Musculoskeletal Disorders*. 2006; **7**: 5.

59. Boersma K, Linton S, Overmeer T *et al*. Lowering fear-avoidance and enhancing function through exposure in vivo. A multiple baseline study across six patients with back pain. *Pain*. 2004; **108**: 8–16.

60. Vlaeyen JW, de Jong J, Geilen M *et al*. The treatment of fear of movement/(re)injury in chronic low back pain: further evidence on the effectiveness of exposure in vivo. *Clinical Journal of Pain*. 2002; **18**: 251–61.

∗ 61. Lorig K, Ritter PL, Plant K. A disease-specific self-help program compared with a generalized chronic disease self-help program for arthritis patients. *Arthritis and Rheumatism*. 2005; **53**: 950–7.

62. Dijkstra A. The validity of the stages of change model in the adoption of the self-management approach in chronic pain. *Clinical Journal of Pain*. 2005; **21**: 27–37.

63. Miller W, Rollnick S. *Motivational interviewing: preparing people to change*, 2nd edn. New York: Guilford Press, 2002.

64. Kalauokalani D, Cherkin DC, Sherman KJ *et al*. Lessons from a trial of acupuncture and massage for low back pain: patient expectations and treatment effects. *Spine*. 2001; **26**: 1418–24.

65. Klaber Moffett JA, Jackson DA, Richmond S *et al*. Randomised trial of a brief physiotherapy intervention compared with usual physiotherapy for neck pain patients: outcomes and patients' preference. *British Medical Journal*. 2005; **330**: 75.

66. Catchlove R, Cohen K. Effects of a directive return to work approach in the treatment of workers' compensation patients with chronic pain. *Pain*. 1982; **14**: 181.

67. Jensen GM, Gwyer J, Shepard KF. Expert practice in physical therapy. *Physical Therapy*. 2000; **80**: 28–43.

68. Houben RM, Ostelo RW, Vlaeyen JW *et al*. Health care providers' orientations towards common low back pain predict perceived harmfulness of physical activities and recommendations regarding return to normal activity. *European Journal of Pain*. 2005; **9**: 173–83.

69. Linton SJ, Vlaeyen J, Ostelo R. The back pain beliefs of health care providers: are we fear-avoidant? *Journal of Occupational Rehabilitation*. 2002; **12**: 223–32.

70. Coudeyre E, Rannou F, Tubach F *et al.* General practitioners' fear-avoidance beliefs influence their management of patients with low back pain. *Pain*. 2006; **124**: 330–7.

71. Fisher K, Hardie RJ. Goal attainment scaling in evaluating a multidisciplinary pain management programme. *Clinical Rehabilitation*. 2002; **16**: 871–7.

72. Walsh AD, Kelly JS, Johnson SP *et al.* Performance problems of patients with chronic low-back pain and the measurement of patient-centered outcome. *Spine*. 2004; **29**: 87–93.

20

Manual medicine

STEVE ROBSON AND LOUIS GIFFORD

KEY LEARNING POINTS

- Manual therapy is a treatment widely used for musculoskeletal pain and pain-related disability.
- Manual therapy assessment techniques can provide accurate details of patients' physical impairments and disability that can be addressed in a multidimensional management package.
- Manual therapy can be easily integrated into a multidimensional biopsychosocial model and approach.

- The chapter reviews the challenges in reasoning that are required for this integration and shifts the emphasis to a focus on central nervous system (CNS) processing changes that occur, rather than changes isolated in the tissues for the treatment of pain.
- The main emphasis is that manual therapy needs to be viewed as a potential component in management rather than being a centrally placed modality.

INTRODUCTION

Historically, manual medicine provides some of the oldest documented accounts of treatments for pain. It seems that a caring touch has always helped. Many manual therapy techniques continue to occupy a central and integral part of the clinical approaches adopted by many physiotherapists, osteopaths, and chiropractors. Although not exclusively the domain of these professions, most of the manual medicine carried out in western society today is provided by these three groups.

More recently, pain science has amassed substantial evidence outlining the biopsychosocial nature of pain.[1, 2, 3, 4] From this, a body of knowledge has emerged that sheds light on some of the mechanisms by which manual therapy may act to produce pain relief.[5, 6, 7] Interestingly, but perhaps unsurprisingly, this evidence indicates that the efficacy of manual therapy appears to be largely mediated by neurophysiological mechanisms and not via the correction of mechanical dysfunction, as is so often postulated by many traditional manual therapy theories.[8, 9, 10, 11]

MANUAL MEDICINE DEFINED

Manual medicine techniques can be broadly categorized into the following groups.

- **Joint mobilizations**, which are "passive movements performed in such a way that at all times they are within the control of the patient so that the patient can prevent the movement if they so choose."[9]

- **Joint manipulations** are small high velocity movements that force a joint beyond its presumed physiologic barrier and up to its anatomical barrier. Manipulation often produces an audible click or crack.[12]
- **Massage** techniques are usually applied to soft tissues such as skin, ligaments, tendons, and muscles, without causing movement or change of joint position.[12] Examples of common massage techniques used to treat pain include effleurage, kneading, petrissage, transverse or deep friction massage, and connective tissue massage.

Manual therapy is also characterized by a large variety of physical testing procedures whose sensitivity and specificity in relation to diagnostic inference (anatomy, biomechanics, and pathology) is questionable and needs urgent scrutiny.[13, 14, 15, 16] However, these same physical tests, regardless of hypothetical notions about the viability of the tissues they purport to test, reveal therapeutically useful observations and findings that can often be successfully addressed in treatment and management.

ASSESSMENT AND EXAMINATION

It should be emphasized that part of the training for manual therapy practitioners usually involves the acquisition of a high level of subjective and physical examination skills specific to inculpating or exculpating serious injury or pathology (i.e. assessment of red flags[2, 17]).

In response to the evidence surrounding the biopsychosocial nature of pain, manual medicine practitioners are starting to undertake additional training enabling them to assess for relevant psychosocial factors known to influence human pain states and predict outcome.[1, 2] Since psychosocial factors are now seen to be critical in modulating pain and influencing future disability, it is recommended that a full or modified psychosocial (yellow flag) assessment is always performed when initially examining all patients presenting with pain.[8] This not only flags those at risk of chronicity (which in itself may be an indicator for not doing manual therapy), but also allows vital psychosocial information to be entered into the clinical reasoning process alongside the findings gleaned from the physical examination procedures. The aim is to embrace best evidence and encourage a necessary shift for manual medicine away from untenable one-dimensional biological models,[1, 2, 4, 6] towards a much fuller integration of biopsychosocial factors.

A careful and comprehensive physical assessment of the patient is fundamental to the successful prescription of manual medicine interventions. When combined with information from the clinical history, manual therapy physical assessment tests can do the following.

- Help to find out, or hypothesize about, what is wrong in relation to the pain complaint.
- Help the practitioner make decisions about whether the musculoskeletal tissues involved are safe to start being loaded for a graded return to normal movement and function.
- Reveal a series of physical impairments and functional restrictions that can be addressed in the treatment and management process.
- Reveal the patient's level of physical confidence, physical capacity, and physical performance. It is emphasized that both physical and psychological components are always involved.
- Reveal a great deal of information about the patients' pain and its behavior and the extent of sensitivity involved.
- When used alongside nonthreatening explanations of the physical findings, a physical assessment provides a great deal of reassurance to the anxious patient.

Examples of physical tests include:

- simple active movements, passive movement and handling of limbs and joints through their available ranges;
- resisted tests for muscle power and willingness to move and tense against resistance;
- tests of joint play (accessory movement), palpation of anatomy and structural deformity, palpation in order to explore the regions of increased sensitivity;
- physical tests of peripheral nerve sensitivity and extensibility (e.g. the straight leg raise in the lower limb and the various upper limb neural tension tests in the arm).[18, 19]

CASE HISTORY: MANUAL MEDICINE WITHIN THE CONTEXT OF THE BIOPSYCHOSOCIAL MODEL

In order to demonstrate how the appropriate use of manual medicine can assist with the management of patients with painful neuromusculoskeletal conditions, we can consider the following case history.

John is a 42-year-old self-employed engineer who owns and runs a small engineering company. His work involves both assessing and costing engineering work and, to a lesser degree, working on-site with his team of engineers. He lives with his wife and their two children aged eight and six years. His interests include cycling, skiing, scuba diving, and hill walking.

He described low back pain beginning insidiously five weeks prior to attending clinic. Two weeks after it began, the pain became far more severe, radiating into his left buttock and over the posterior aspect of his left leg spreading distally to the level of his ankle. He also described numbness over the left buttock and at the lateral border of the left foot and lateral two toes (**Figure 20.1**).

Nine days before he presented in clinic, he had called his family doctor out after collapsing in pain at home. His doctor prescribed ibuprofen, paracetamol, and diazepam and recommended physiotherapy. At this juncture he had been unable to attend work for a week because of constant pain, which made it impossible for him to sit, stand, or walk for any significant length of time. He had not ventured beyond his home and reported high levels of pain that would wake him from sleep every two to three hours. This compelled him to get out of bed and walk for a few minutes which occasionally eased his pain enough to allow him to get back to sleep. He was spending most of each day resting on the settee at home, getting up occasionally to walk for a few minutes spurred on by increasing pain. He had not been participating in normal family life, was avoiding driving on the school run, going swimming or playing football with his children, and believed that these activities would cause more damage to his back.

Psychosocial factors

A yellow flag assessment was carried out using the standard A, B, C, D, E, and F format.[1, 2] This included the findings shown in **Table 20.1**.

Physical examination

During the physical examination, it became apparent that John was apprehensive about full weight bearing through his left leg, standing with his left hip and knee partially flexed creating a compensatory thoracolumbar scoliosis convex to the left. All lumbar spine movements were slow and very tense. There was a marked limitation into extension and moderate limitation of flexion; both of these movements increased lower back and left leg pain. End of range right and left side-flexion also increased his leg pain. During the assessment of his spinal movement he was viewed from the front as well as behind so that both visual and verbal communication could be maintained to assist with gathering information about his thoughts and feelings towards the movements being tested. This facilitated both the assessment of his range of movement and additional visual appraisal of his level of fear or confidence when performing each movement. Deep tendon reflexes revealed a sluggish response at the left ankle grading 1+. Selective neural tension tests applied to the left sciatic nerve revealed a painful response to the slump test, which elicited increased left leg and low back pain during the left knee extension component of this maneuver and straight leg raise (SLR),[18, 19] which was painful and limited to 20° as compared to 60° on the contralateral side. Manual muscle tests indicated marked weakness of the left knee flexors (grading 3) and weakness of the big toe extensors, ankle dorsiflexors, and evertors (grading 4). Skin sensation was diminished over the left L5/S1 dermatomes. Modest palpatory pressures over L3, 4, and 5 elicited pain and spasm locally and increased the pain in his left calf. Further surface palpation over the

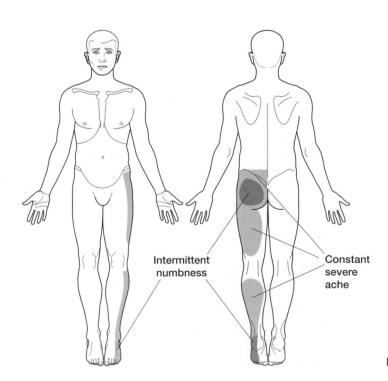

Intermittent numbness

Constant severe ache

Figure 20.1 Body chart.

Table 20.1 Findings from the yellow flag assessment.

	Findings	
A	Attitudes and beliefs	Fear avoidance, believing that activity will cause further injury
		Belief that pain must be abolished before returning to normal activity
		Catastrophizing, a negative outlook regarding his condition and future
		Belief that he had no control over his pain
B	Behaviors	Use of extended rest
		Reduced activity and withdrawal from activities of daily living
		Report of extremely high pain intensity
		Sleep quality reduced since onset of pain
C	Compensation issues	Nil
D	Diagnosis and treatment	Doctor diagnosed sciatica caused by a probable disk prolapse and suggested that this may require surgery
		Doctor was very worried about his level of pain and did not want to touch him
E	Emotions	Frightened of his pain and what it might signify
		Heightened awareness of his symptoms, particularly anxious about the numbness at his left buttock and foot
		Increased stress, related to not feeling capable of going to work and loss of control in the running of his company
		Totally frustrated and sometimes angry about his pain, disturbed sleep, and lack of progress/ineffectiveness of the management so far
F	Family	His wife had been supportive throughout; however, his children did not understand why he would not take them swimming or play sport
W	Work	He enjoyed his work, but was finding that even reduced duties consisting of desk-based administration still aggravated his pain
		He expressed a sense of guilt as regards letting his workforce down by refraining from work
		Worried about the detrimental financial effect his long-term absence would have on his company's revenue

route of the left sciatic nerve trunk (buttock and posterior thigh) increased pain locally and distally over the limb.

Management

EXPLANATION, REASSURANCE, AND SETTING THE RECOVERY AGENDA

John's clinical examination did not reveal any red flags indicating the possible presence of serious pathology. This information was conveyed to him via careful explanation of the various physical findings, emphasizing that there was "no evidence that anything was seriously wrong." Good explanations and reassurance cannot be underestimated in terms of their positive potential to influence a patient's attention, concerns, and beliefs about pain and their situation. If done well, good reassurance can have beneficial secondary effects on pain processing within the central nervous system (CNS), as well as on the patient's recovery behavior. Simply put, reduced concern and anxiety allows patients to shift from avoidance, high focus, and tension about the pain and their situation to a more confident and confrontational perspective.[20, 21, 22] The essence and emphasis of this part of management, we

believe, should be on positive findings once negative ones have been ruled out.

Once reassured from a seriousness perspective, John was then provided with a diagnosis and explanation about the nature of his problem, the recovery process, and the role of physiotherapy management – what could be done to help and his role in getting the best outcome. A provisional diagnosis of sciatica was explained to John in simple terms of the biomechanics, anatomy, and neurophysiology involved. This was carried out using a model of an articulated spine and basic diagrams sketched on a whiteboard. John was encouraged to appreciate the location of the nerve, the effects of movement on it, and the relative strength and toughness of the spine itself. The focus of the neurophysiology explanation was centered on how such a small area of nerve root injury could cause such persistent and widespread pain and sensitivity and also how modest nerve injury sometimes leads to the frequent findings of local muscle weakness and reflex changes. He was also reassured that sciatic nerve pain was common, that it gets slowly better, and that it is often out of proportion to the amount of strain or injury actually done and quite commonly comes on spontaneously, as in this case. Reassuring explanations are important for the simple reason that patients are hardly going to be happy to exercise, get going physically, or feel comfortable with manual therapy techniques if they are concerned about the structural vulnerability of their back. For patients, becoming comfortable with the view that hurt does not equate with harm can be the one factor that provides an appreciation that it is not only safe but also very helpful to gradually increase activity and exercise in order to improve their situation.[23] Also, accepting the notion that pain is a big part of the problem and that relieving pain plays an important early part of the recovery process can be very helpful. A great many patients worry that getting rid of pain will cause them to become overactive/less cautious which will in turn lead to further injury and thus prolonging their problem.

After the explanations and discussion of the problem, John stated that he was hugely relieved to have a better understanding of it and that even though it hurt a great deal, that it was not a serious condition. The positive clinical scenario was that he now felt reassured,[20, 22] he accepted the situation (it will take time but it will improve), and was pleased to get involved in helping his own recovery, as well as looking forward to being helped by physiotherapy input.

INITIAL PHYSIOTHERAPY INPUT

John now agreed that the first priority was to get better pain control and reduce the muscle spasm in his back. He also agreed that learning smoother more relaxed movements would be of great benefit too. After discussion of treatment options, gentle massage techniques were used with the aim of reducing muscle tension and improving movement quality. Clinical reasoning was influenced by the psychosocial and physical examinations that revealed high levels of reported pain, increasing psychosocial distress, and a great deal of observable tension during physical movement testing. Since the processing of pain is likely to be strongly influenced by an individual's sensitivity state in all dimensions, it was reasoned that strong forms of manual therapy would risk exacerbating his condition.[8, 24, 25]

Initially, he was asked to find his most comfortable position to receive the massage, choosing right side-lying. He was also asked to provide feedback regarding the massage and to feel comfortable with requesting more or less pressure with this or any other manual therapy technique that might be administered during treatment. Giving over an active degree of treatment control like this is unusual in traditional doctor/therapist encounters. Importantly, it fosters a successful therapeutic patient–clinician alliance.

Following the massage treatment, he reported reduced back pain and chose to remain side-lying, while treatment was progressed to include modified small amplitude accessory joint mobilization techniques akin to those described by Maitland[9] and Mulligan.[26] These techniques helped to reduce his leg pain, after which he was

encouraged to try some slow, smooth, and relaxed lumbar spine movements in various easy starting positions. After some experimentation, it was found that he was able to move best and with least tension and discomfort in crook lying (rotation), four-point kneeling (flexion, extension, and side flexion) and sitting (flexion and up into a small degree of extension). He was keen to practice these successful movements at home and agreed a baseline and goal amount for each. Advice regarding pacing up of exercises and other activities, such as walking, sitting, resting, and light administrative work, was also discussed and agreed.[27]

At one week review, he returned to clinic in a distressed state and recounted that as a result of feeling much better following treatment and the exercises, he had made a decision outside his treatment plan and returned to work full time. This had resulted in a major exacerbation of his pain, which was now preventing him from sleeping. Following a discussion with the patient and his GP, it was agreed that the addition of gabapentin to his medication might be helpful. Forty-eight hours after starting gabapentin and receiving further spinal massage and mobilization with the addition of relaxation techniques taught to him in clinic, his pain significantly decreased.

CONTINUING MANAGEMENT

This leap forward in getting better pain control enabled future treatment to be much more focused on improving his physical impairments. Larger amplitude joint mobilization techniques were progressed from side-lying to prone positions and further into range. The progress with pain relief was paralleled with graded increases in repetitions, range, and speed/confidence of spinal exercises, as well as walking and sitting-based activities. Manual therapy techniques, called sustained natural apophyseal glides (SNAG), were found to be helpful in facilitating further increases in painless lumbar spine flexion and extension.[26] Limitation of left leg movement/sciatic nerve sensitivity were addressed using neural mobilizations,[18, 19] these were performed as passive rhythmical mobilizations by the therapist in positions of SLR, as well as the base slump test. An active variation of the slump technique, whereby he performed smooth oscillatory repetitions of left knee flexion and extension was also included in his home exercise program because it helped to produce improvements in his pain-free flexion range (**Figure 20.2**). The specific program given for this exercise was carefully graded for the first few sessions to help prevent any flare up in nerve reactivity.

Specific strengthening exercises (e.g. using a latex resistance band over the foot) and more generalized strengthening exercises (e.g. tip-toe walking and bridging) were quickly introduced to facilitate recovery of power at the affected L5/S1 supplied muscles of the left lower limb. The notion of "work the muscle to work the nerve and help it to recover" can be very helpful. Being shown that

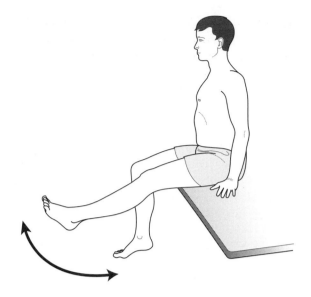

Figure 20.2 Active knee flexion and extension performed in the base slump position.

something is weak and then finding that working on it improves it, is a very powerful motivator, as well as promoting a more optimistic outlook. Throughout treatment, all manual therapy techniques and rehabilitation was centered on addressing the physical impairments identified during examination with the aim that gains made could be generalized to John's functional goals of returning to work, hill walking, cycling, and scuba diving. He was seen in clinic a total of six times over four months having successfully returned to normal work (two weeks after the flare up), exercise, and sporting activity (graded return of elements of these were started within seven to ten days). His only reported symptom on discharge was intermittent paresthesia affecting the little toe and lateral aspect of his left foot. This had diminished significantly at six-month follow up and resolved completely at 12 months.

SOME PROPOSED CNS-BASED MECHANISMS THAT MAY UNDERLIE THE PAIN RELIEVING ACTION AND EFFICACY OF MANUAL THERAPY

Current evidence indicates that pain relief related to manual medicine is in large part mediated by CNS mechanisms. Thus, when manual therapy techniques relieve pain they are most likely to do so via centrally mediated changes in pain processing rather than via changes in the tissues. It is the opinion here that the inclusion of the biopsychosocial model and reasoning into manual medicine requires therapists to harbor concurrent thoughts about mechanisms of action that embrace psychophysiological effects (so-called top-down effects), as well as those generated via manually produced somatic inputs (i.e. bottom-up effects). The two clearly

need to mesh well and work in tandem – which may go a long way to explaining why a given technique can be very successful when provided by one therapist but not by another! Knowledge of the powerful influence of top-down effects on outcome presses manual therapists to take time and care in making their treatments meaningful and appropriate to the patient. This applies not only to the techniques used, but also to the various tasks, goals, and exercises that may be given too.

Eight potential CNS-derived mechanisms are briefly reviewed below.

Gate control

Gate control theory proposes that manual stimulation of tissues and structures containing Aβ-fibers synapsing at second-order dorsal horn cells can have an inhibitory effect on the nociceptive output of these cells.[28, 29] However, manual therapists need to be aware that neurobiological changes, including death of dorsal horn neurons or changes in their structure, function, and synapsing resulting from the high input activity of damaged peripheral nerves, can lead to a loss of the normal gate control mechanism.[24] In these circumstances, manual therapy may lead to the facilitation of nociception and thus the exacerbation of pain.[8] This is one peripheral mechanism that may account for those patients who report a flare up of pain following manual therapy.

Descending inhibition

There is now quite strong evidence that descending top-down pathways from the brain and brain stem can exert an influence on the dorsal horn gate and hence on the sensitivity and plasticity of sensory processing here.[6, 7, 29, 30] For example, descending influences from the periaqueductal gray (PAG), nucleus cuneiformis, locus coeruleus (LC), nucleus reticularis gigantocellularis (NGC), nucleus reticularis dorsalis (NRD), and the rostral ventromedial medulla (RVM) area in the brain stem have been shown to be capable of contributing to manual therapy-induced hypoalgesia.[29, 30, 31, 32] Research indicates that inhibitory descending pain-off pathways utilize the neurotransmitters noradrenaline and serotonin (5HT),[5, 7, 29] but that there are excitatory, or pain-on pathways too. The clear but complex links of these nuclei and their descending pathways to the higher brain centers, and hence to areas involved in reasoning, emotions, and consciousness, has been emphasized for manual therapists by Zusman.[30]

Diffuse noxious inhibitory control

Historically, there are numerous recorded accounts of pain being used as a treatment to relieve pain.[33] Contemporary manual medicine includes many massage, mobilization, and manipulation techniques that can be applied to intentionally produce discomfort, yet yield subsequent relief via so-called counter-irritation effects.

Identification of close connections between ascending nociceptive pathways and the PAG–RVM–dorsal horn descending modulatory pathway described above has highlighted a potential mechanism via which intense noxious stimuli of tissues distant from a pathological focal point can bring about pain inhibition.[29] This inhibition appears to be mediated by the enkephalin group of endogenous opiates released at spinal and supraspinal levels.[33] Again, an aspect of this system that is of importance to manual therapists is the knowledge that vigorous peripheral stimulation can also activate the pain on-cells and inhibit the pain off-cells at the RVM, thus enhancing pain. A key factor when administering techniques capable of stimulating the diffuse noxious inhibitory control (DNIC) pathways may be to consider the meaning and context of the noxious stimulation to the patient. A suggestion is to get proficient at confidently and simply explaining how a proposed treatment works before applying it! Thus, acceptable/low fear of pain produced during treatment is more likely to be of benefit, while unacceptable/fear-producing pain or discomfort is less likely to!

Habituation

There is good evidence that rhythmical mechanical stimuli which can sometimes initially produce a degree of pain will, if continued, cause it to diminish or disappear via the process of habituation. Useful reviews of habituation with respect to underlying neurophysiological mechanisms and their relevance to manual therapy techniques and pain management can be found in Zusman[6] and Jastreboff and Hazell.[34]

Extinction

Under conditions of learning, the CNS develops novel synaptic connections between neurons. As a result, new pathways form which are thought to then represent specific memories. In pain states, this neurobiological learning process may well include the formation of pathways that represent pain.[6, 35] Memory and pain memory biology appear to share a process known as long-term potentiation (LTP). Conversely, and in a positive contrast for ongoing pain states, new learning, via the acquisition of new painless memories (again formed by synaptic learning and LTP) may be used to bring about extinction of the activity of an ongoing maladaptive pain pathway.

In clinical situations, extinction can be of significant therapeutic value if the mode of new learning and LTP is of functional relevance to the patient. An example of this was described in the case history, when the SNAG technique was administered to John's lumbar spine during his active movements of flexion and extension. Application of the technique with adequate explanation and reassurance produced immediate improvements in the pain-free range of lumbar spine movement. Thus, the imprinted memory circuit of painful flexion was challenged and could potentially go on to be replaced by the new memory of painless flexion. Just as in all learning, a degree of good quality practice and repetition is required. This manual therapy approach can be used to assist many spinal and peripheral joint movements by simply modifying the direction, force, and anatomical site of the applied technique. The goal is always to reassure the patient and to encourage them to explore restricted and/or feared directions of movement with or without the concurrent application of manually applied pressures. In order to maximize the success, the patient must understand what is expected, hence addressing the top-down aspects before the bottom-up technique is applied. From the practitioners perspective, a high degree of ingenuity and adaptability with the various manual therapy techniques that can be used to aid this process is paramount. In order to achieve significant levels of extinction (forgetting!), it is advised that therapists prescribe exercises that replicate and regularly reinforce the new pain-free movement, thus maximizing new synaptic learning and LTP.

Motor responses

The literature contains contradictory accounts of manual therapy producing both inhibitory and facilitatory effects on the motor system. At present, there appears to be no conclusive evidence either way.[7, 36, 37, 38, 39] There may be a number of factors influencing the variability of these study results, including the validity of the experimental models used, the effects of the patient's thoughts and beliefs regarding the intervention, and how these psychosocial factors might concomitantly modulate the PAG and the motor systems, thus providing the possibility for either facilitation or inhibition.[5, 40] Once again, just as for the other mechanisms discussed, any therapeutic effects on the motor system are just as likely to be influenced by top-down products and this needs consideration. Analysis of the studies performed indicates that the inhibitory effects of manual therapy are transient, lasting up to 60 seconds. Similarly, facilitation appears to occur for no more than two minutes following the applied techniques.[40] What seems uncertain is whether the effect of manual therapy on the motor system is sustained for any clinically meaningful length of time.

Sympathetic nervous system responses

Large, rhythmically produced mobilizations have been shown to elicit an excitatory sympathetic nervous system

(SNS) response producing sudomotor (increased body temperature) and cutaneous vasomotor (blood vessel dilation) responses for up to 20 minutes following mobilization.[41, 42] It is possible that mobilization techniques applied at appropriate stages of tissue healing may assist recovery by improving local tissue metabolism and perfusion. There is no conclusive evidence to indicate that manipulation techniques have any influence on the SNS.[5, 40]

Placebo response

Placebo responses have been consistently observed during both human and animal research. Inevitably and productively, manual medicine interventions will include varying levels of psychophysiological or placebo responses. As already argued, the reasons behind why a specific manual therapy (or any other) intervention appears to be efficacious for one patient but not another is likely to be due to more than variations in pure physical factors. Recognizing and respecting this goes some way towards understanding the potency and importance of the placebo response and, by inference, the importance of therapeutic interactions, alliances, and relations in the treatment of human disease and pain states.[43] Current evidence suggests that placebo responses are a complex, dynamic, and multidimensional mixture of biopsychosocial factors. For a detailed discussion of placebo analgesia, see Fields and Price.[44] The placebo response provides evidence for the need to embrace and understand psychophysiological mechanisms more fully.

CLINICAL TRIALS: THE EVIDENCE

Many problems arise when attempting to qualify and quantify the specific effects related to any therapeutic intervention. Even in placebo-controlled trials, a range of contextual factors may influence outcomes.[45] These include the mode of intervention and the healthcare setting in which it is delivered, the status and gender of the practitioner, and the models of explanation used by the practitioner, as well as their belief in the treatment they provide. Similarly, the patient's presenting condition, their understanding of this, and their beliefs related to treatment, and such variables as anxiety and adherence to treatment protocols, can also exert influence. Clinical trials scrutinizing manual medicine interventions have the added difficulty of providing a credible placebo group and in double blinding both patient and practitioner to recognition of the active or placebo intervention.

Most of the higher quality randomized trials, systematic reviews, and meta-analyses have looked at mobilization and/or manipulation techniques applied to the spine.[46, 47, 48, 49, 50, 51, 52] There appears to be a consensus of agreement that these manual therapy techniques applied in isolation provide little efficacy in the treatment of acute or chronic neck or low back pain.[47, 48, 49, 50, 52] However, there is an indication that they can provide short-term pain relief for acute and chronic low back pain.[46, 47] Furthermore, when combined with exercise therapy, patients with acute and subacute neck pain and chronic low back pain demonstrated better outcomes in both the short and long term.[46, 47, 48, 51] In contrast to the unimodal or bimodal methodology used in most of the clinical trials of manual medicine to date, it seems reasonable to suggest that multidimensional biopsychosocial pain presentations are likely to require multidimensional biopsychosocial treatment approaches that are capable of addressing as many known factors as possible. Future trials incorporating a biopsychosocial approach to examination and treatment, including elements of pain neurophysiology education, graded functional rehabilitation, and manual therapy, may prove to be far more efficacious in treating painful conditions.

In view of current evidence which includes observed changes both in the structure and function of the CNS of people with pain,[24] it seems apparent that manual therapy used in isolation is at best only likely to produce short-term improvements, particularly for those with persistent/chronic pain.[40, 47, 46, 51] Conversely, if manual therapy is used as part of a multidimensional approach and is administered alongside an understanding of normal tissue healing, recovery, and natural history, while supported by other key factors including skilled examination, reassurance, pain education, and graded rehabilitation, it can occupy a valuable place in preventing chronic pain and disability.[23, 53, 54]

In summary, there are levels of evidence indicating that manual therapy can help:

- reduce pain in acute and chronic pain states;
- assist with the restoration of physical impairments and normal movement patterns;
- overcome fear of movement (kinesophobia);
- assist recovery alongside other management including drug therapy, postural advice, activity pacing, and graded rehabilitation/exercise programs.

Recent evidence has helped to define more clearly the role of contemporary manual medicine in the treatment of pain. Full realization of the potential benefits of manual therapy will require a cultural change for many therapists and a shift to a new working paradigm rooted firmly within the biopsychosocial model.

REFERENCES

1. Linton SJ. *Understanding pain for better clinical practice: A psychological perspective.* Edinburgh: Elsevier, 2005: 19–52.

∗ 2. Waddell G. *The back pain revolution,* 2nd edn. Edinburgh: Churchill Livingstone, 2003.

3. Lederman E. *Fundamentals of manual therapy: Physiology, neurology and psychology*. Edinburgh: Churchill Livingstone, 1997.

4. Butler DS, Moseley GL. *Explain pain*. Adelaide: Noigroup publications, 2003.

* 5. Souvlis T, Vicenzino B, Wright A. Neurophysiological effects of spinal manual therapy. In: Boyling JD, Jull GA (eds). *Grieve's modern manual therapy – the vertebral column*, 3rd edn. Edinburgh: Churchill Livingstone, 2004: 367–79.

* 6. Zusman M. Mechanisms of musculoskeletal physiotherapy. *Physical Therapy Reviews*. 2004; 9: 39–49.

7. Wright A. Hypoalgesia post-manipulative therapy: a review of a potential neurophysiological mechanism. *Manual Therapy*. 1995; 1: 11–16.

* 8. Robson S, Gifford L. Manual therapy in the 21st century. In: Gifford L (ed.). *Topical issues in pain*, 5th edn. Falmouth: CNS Press, 2006: 3–34.

9. Maitland GD. *Vertebral manipulation*, 5th edn. Oxford: Butterworth Heineman, 1986.

10. DiGiovanna EL, Schiowitz S. *An osteopathic approach to diagnosis and treatment*. Philadelphia: JB Lippincot, 1991.

11. Keating JC, Charlton KH, Grod JP et al. Subluxation: dogma or science? *Chiropractic and Osteopathy*. 2005; 13: 17.

12. Haldeman S, Hooper PD. Mobilization, manipulation, massage and exercise for the relief of musculoskeletal pain. In: Wall PD, Melzack R (eds). *Textbook of pain*, 4th edn. Edinburgh: Churchill Livingstone, 1999: 1399–418.

13. Bogduk N. *Clinical anatomy of the lumbar spine and sacrum*, 3rd edn. Edinburgh: Churchill Livingstone, 1997: 81–100.

14. Van der Wurff P, Meyne W, Hagmeijer RHM. Clinical tests of the sacroiliac joint, a systematic methodological review. Part 1: Reliability. *Manual Therapy*. 2000; 5: 30–6.

15. Van der Wurff P, Meyne W, Hagmeijer RHM. Clinical tests of the sacroiliac joint, a systematic methodological review. Part 2: Validity. *Manual Therapy*. 2000; 5: 89–96.

16. Lee DG. *The pelvic girdle*, 2nd edn. Edinburgh: Churchill Livingstone, 1999.

* 17. Greenhalgh S, Selfe J. *Red flags: A guide to identifying serious pathology of the spine*. Edinburgh: Churchill Livingstone, 2000.

18. Butler DS. *The sensitive nervous system*. Adelaide: Noigroup Publications, 2000: 274–309.

19. Shacklock MO, Butler DS, Slater H. The dynamic central nervous system: structure and clinical neurobiomechanics. In: Boyling JD, Palastanga N (eds). *Grieve's modern manual therapy – the vertebral column*, 2nd edn. Edinburgh: Churchill Livingstone, 1994: 21–38.

20. Flor H. The modification of cortical reorganisation and chronic pain by sensory feedback. *Applied Psychophysiology and Biofeedback*. 2002; 27: 215–27.

21. Martin P. *The sickening mind*. London: Harper Collins, 1997: 45–80.

22. Sapolsky RM. *Why zebras don't get ulcers*. New York: WH Freeman, 1998: 126–58.

23. Moseley GL. Combined physiotherapy and education is effective for chronic low back pain: a randomised controlled trial. *Australian Journal of Physiotherapy*. 2002; 48: 297–302.

* 24. Woolf CJ, Salter M. Plasticity and pain: role of the dorsal horn. In: McMahon SB, Koltzenburg M (eds). *Wall and Melzack's textbook of pain*, 5th edn. Edinburgh: Churchill Livingstone, 2006: 91–105.

25. Devor M. Response of nerves to injury in relation to neuropathic pain. In: McMahon SB, Koltzenburg M (eds). *Wall and Melzack's textbook of pain*, 5th edn. Edinburgh: Churchill Livingstone, 2006: 905–27.

26. Mulligan BR. *Manual therapy; "nags", "snags", "mwm's" etc*, 4th edn. Wellington: Plane View Services, 1999.

27. Gifford L. Perspectives on the biopsychosocial model – part 3: Patient example – using the shopping basket approach and graded exposure. *In Touch*. 2003; 102: 3–15.

28. Wall PD. *Pain: the science of suffering*. London: Weidenfield & Nicholson, 1999: 32–48.

* 29. Fields HL, Basbaum AI, Heinricher MM. Central nervous system mechanisms of pain modulation. In: McMahon SB, Koltzenburg M (eds). *Wall and Melzack's textbook of pain*, 5th edn. Edinburgh: Churchill Livingstone, 2006: 125–42.

30. Zusman M. Forebrain-mediated sensitisation of central pain pathways: 'non-specific' pain and a new image for MT. *Manual Therapy*. 2002; 9: 80–8.

31. Casey KL. Forebrain mechanisms of nociceptors and pain: analysis through imaging. *Proceedings of the National Academy of Sciences of the United States of America*. 1999; 96: 7668–74.

32. Skyba DA, Radhakrishnan R, Rohlwing JJ et al. Joint manipulation reduces hyperalgesia by activation of monoamine receptors but not opioid or GABA receptors in the spinal cord. *Pain*. 2003; 106: 159–68.

33. Melzack R. Folk medicine and the sensory modulation of pain. In: Wall PD, Melzack R (eds). *Textbook of pain*, 3rd edn. Edinburgh: Churchill Livingstone, 1994: 1209–17.

34. Jastreboff PW, Hazell JWP. *Tinnitus retraining therapy*. Cambridge: Cambridge University Press, 2004: 16–62.

35. Le Doux J. *Synaptic self: How our brains become who we are*. New York: Penguin Books, 2002: 134–73.

36. Zusman M. Central nervous contribution to mechanically produced motor and sensory responses. *Australian Journal of Physiotherapy*. 1992; 38: 245–55.

37. Keller TS, Colloca CJ. Mechanical force spinal manipulation increases trunk muscle strength assessed by electromyography: a comparative clinical trial. *Journal of Manipulative and Physiological Therapeutics*. 2000; 25: 585–95.

38. Colloca CJ, Keller TS. Electromyographic reflex responses to mechanical force, manually assisted spinal manipulative therapy. *Spine*. 2001; 26: 447–57.

39. Dishman JD, Ball KA, Burke J. Central motor excitability changes after spinal manipulation: a transcranial magnetic stimulation study. *Journal of Manipulative and Physiological Therapeutics*. 2002; 25: 1–9.

40. Vicenzino B, Wright A. Physical treatments. In: Strong J, Unruh AM, Wright A, Baxter GD (eds). *Pain – a textbook for therapists*. Edinburgh: Churchill Livingstone, 2002: 187–206.

41. Souvlis T, Vicenzino B, Wright A. Dose of spinal manual therapy influences change in SNS function. Paper presented at the Musculoskeletal Physiotherapy Australia (MPA) Biennial Conference, Adelaide, 2001.

42. Vicenzino B, Cartwright T, Collins D, Wright A. An investigation of the stress and pain perception during manual therapy in asymptomatic subjects. *European Journal of pain*. 1999; **3**: 13–18.

43. Shapiro AK, Shapiro E. The placebo: is it much ado about nothing? In: Harrington A (ed.). *The placebo effect: an interdisciplinary exploration*. Cambridge, MA: Harvard University Press, 1999: 12–36.

∗ 44. Fields HL, Price DP. Placebo analgesia. In: McMahon SB, Koltzenburg M (eds). *Wall and Melzack's textbook of pain*, 5th edn. Edinburgh: Churchill Livingstone, 1999: 361–7.

∗ 45. Di Blasi Z, Harkness E, Ernst E *et al*. Influence of context effects on health outcomes: a systematic review. *The Lancet*. 2001; **357**: 757–62.

46. van Tulder MW, Waddell G. Conservative treatment of acute and subacute low back pain. In: Nachemson A, Jonsson E (eds). *Neck and back pain: the scientific evidence of causes, diagnosis and treatment*. Philadelphia, PA: Lippincott Williams & Wilkins, 2000: 241–69.

47. van Tulder MW, Goossens M, Waddell G, Nachemson A. Conservative treatment of chronic low back pain. In: Nachemson A, Jonsson E (eds). *Neck and back pain: the scientific evidence of causes, diagnosis and treatment*.

Philadelphia, PA: Lippincott Williams & Wilkins, 2000: 271–303.

48. UK BEAM Trial Team. United Kingdom back pain exercise and manipulation (UK BEAM) randomised trial: effectiveness of physical treatments for back pain in primary care. *British Medical Journal*. 2004; **329**: 1377.

49. Assendelft WJ, Morton SC, Yu El *et al*. Spinal manipulative therapy for low back pain. A meta-analysis of effectiveness relative to other therapies. *Annals of Internal Medicine*. 2003; **138**: 871–81.

50. Ernst E, Canter PH. A systematic review of systematic reviews of spinal manipulation. *Journal of the Royal Society of Medicine*. 2006; **99**: 192–6.

51. Harms-Ringdahl, Nachemson A. Acute and subacute neck pain: nonsurgical treatment. In: Nachemson A, Jonsson E (eds). *Neck and back pain: the scientific evidence of causes, diagnosis and treatment*. Philadelphia, PA: Lippincott Williams & Wilkins, 2000: 327–38.

52. van Tulder MW, Goossens M, Hoving J. Nonsurgical treatment of chronic neck pain. In: Nachemson A, Jonsson E (eds). *Neck and back pain: the scientific evidence of causes, diagnosis and treatment*. Philadelphia, PA: Lippincott Williams & Wilkins, 2000: 339–54.

53. van Griensven H. *Pain in practice: theory and treatment strategies for manual therapists*. Edinburgh: Butterworth Heinemann, 2005.

54. Moseley GL. Joining forces – combining cognition-targeted motor control training with group or individual pain physiology education; a successful treatment for chronic low back pain. *Journal of Manual and Manipulative Therapy*. 2003; **11**: 88–94.

SECTION D

Interventional procedures

21

Introduction to interventional procedures

WILLIAM I CAMPBELL AND HARALD BREIVIK

KEY LEARNING POINTS

- The interventions described in the following chapters are from current evidence, although some is based on the opinion of experienced pain experts alone.
- Detailed discussion with the patient prior to any intervention helps in carrying out the procedure, as well as preventing unrealistic expectations.
- The information on analgesic administration methods described in the following chapters, although intended

- primarily for acute pain, can be of value in other situations.
- Neuroablative interventions should not be undertaken by the novice practitioner.
- Chemical neurolysis is primarily reserved for the management of difficult cancer pain problems.
- The following chapters should be read in conjunction with related chapters in this and the other volumes to optimize outcome.

INTRODUCTION

Over the past few decades the management of pain has evolved to such an extent that physical interventions are now carried out mainly on a background of evidence-based practice. The following 16 chapters describe various pharmacological and thermotherapeutic (radiofrequency and cryotherapy) methods of managing acute, chronic nonmalignant and cancer pain. The first chapter (Chapter 22, Psychological aspects of preparation for painful procedures), however, deals with the psychological preparation of the patient prior to interventions and painful procedures. This is essential in preparing and advising the patient about realistic outcomes before any procedure. Such preparation will also help the intervention run more smoothly and may prevent later issues about expected outcome.

Although Chapter 24, Intravenous and subcutaneous patient-controlled analgesia and Chapter 25, Alternative opioid patient-controlled analgesia delivery systems – transcutaneous, nasal, and others deal with a wide variety of analgesic administration in the management of acute pain, the information and techniques utilized may be of interest to those dealing with cancer pain. These chapters go beyond the description of opioid use, including adjuvants that can be effectively deployed to obtain better pain control. Analgesic dosing issues at the extremes of age are described, as well as issues in renal failure, morbid obesity, and the opioid tolerant patient.

Chapter 23, Peripheral nerve blocks: practical aspects, is applicable prior to surgical procedures and acute postoperative pain. However, this chapter goes further to outline the various types of peripheral nerve block including neurolytic, cryotherapy, and radiofrequency lesioning, before describing the traditional approaches used to block peripheral nerves with local anesthetic. It will therefore be of value to those involved in the management of any type of pain.

Epidural analgesia is frequently deployed in the management of acute pain after major surgery as well as labor pain and Chapter 26, Epidural analgesia for acute pain after surgery and during labor, including patient-controlled epidural analgesia gives the rationale for appropriate levels of siting these, as well as the value of various adjuvants. The use of epidural and intraforaminal steroid injection in patients suffering from chronic low back and radiculopathic pain is put in context in Chapter 35, Epidural (intralaminar, intraforaminal, and caudal) steroid injections for back pain and sciatica. Chapter 36, Epiduroscopy and endoscopic adhesiolysis, describes the value of epiduroscopy in identifying the pathophysiology of lumbar radiculopathic pain in the more difficult cases of this type of pain, as well as how endoscopic adhesiolysis may be of value in its management. Additional methods to treat radiculopathic pain are described through spinal cord stimulation in Chapter 34, Spinal cord stimulation.

Chapter 29, Intra-articular and local soft-tissue injections, will be of special interest to the rheumatologist and pain clinician alike. The importance of meticulous injection and aseptic technique are emphasized to improve outcome and avoid complications. Chapter 31, Intrathecal drug delivery, covers the increasing level of sophistication of this means of drug delivery, including the different pump types that are available. Patient selection is essential for optimum outcome, and the importance of multidisciplinary team working is explained. Spinal cord stimulation is covered in Chapter 34, Spinal cord stimulation and although this method of pain control avoids the use of drugs, patient selection and meticulous aseptic technique are essential, as with intrathecal drug delivery.

Chronic spinal pain is a major issue worldwide leading to long-term suffering and considerable loss to the community through time lost from unemployment. Chapter 30, Facet (zygapophyseal) joint injections and medial branch blocks, describes the management of facetal pain whereas Chapter 37, Discogenic low back pain: intradiscal thermal (radiofrequency) annuloplasty and artificial disk implants, deals with low back pain of discogenic origin.

Radiofrequency (RF) lesions are a valuable technique for both chronic and cancer pain. If considered for the former situation they should only be considered after assessment of the biopsychosocial setting. As an alternative to microvascular decompression, RF lesions of the gassarian ganglion, or indeed retroganglion injection of glycerol, can radically change a patient's life for years by completely alleviating the pain of trigeminal neuralgia. An RF thermal lesion of the cervical spine (cordotomy) can be invaluable in managing certain types of unilateral cancer pain, for example mesothelioma. These procedures are described in detail within the following chapters, and although there may appear to be some overlap in content, readers are encouraged to read all the chapters pertinent to any particular technique as useful information will be derived from each, since each author has expertise in these techniques. Chapter 32, Cryoanalgesia, is included for completeness, since although this technique has become less popular in recent years, it does offer a means of blocking nociception for months without damaging the nerve axon, if a good technique is used.

Blockade of the sympathetic nervous system can be of value in various nonmalignant chronic pain states (sympathetically mediated pain), as well as in the management of certain types of cancer pain (Chapter 27, Sympathetic blocks and Chapter 28, Neurolytic blocks). The rationale for these blocks as well as the reasons for the so-called lack of evidence in the management of chronic pain is discussed in Chapter 27, Sympathetic blocks.

Finally, neurolytic blocks are covered in Chapter 28, Neurolytic blocks. The majority of the procedures discussed are for the management of cancer pain and, due to the high potential for morbidity associated with these techniques, they are best carried out by an experienced practitioner. When reading about any technique please do read related chapters, in this volume as well as in the other volumes, to optimize your pain management.

22

Psychological aspects of preparation for painful procedures

RACHAEL POWELL AND MARIE JOHNSTON

KEY LEARNING POINTS

- Many patients experience anxiety when faced with a painful procedure.
- Anxiety may adversely affect patients' ability to follow instructions, perception of pain, and recovery.
- Accurate assessment of anxiety and pain assists appropriate psychological preparation and assessment of whether preparation has been effective.
- Psychological preparation methods include giving information and instruction, teaching cognitive coping methods, and relaxation training.

- There is good evidence that psychological preparation reduces anxiety (before, during, and after procedures), reduces pain and pain medication, facilitates faster recovery, and reduces length of hospital stay.
- Psychological preparation for children needs to take account of the child's developmental level and of parental anxiety.

INTRODUCTION

The preparation of patients to undergo a painful procedure takes a range of forms. For example, their medical history is documented, they undergo physical examinations to ensure that they are fit for the procedure, they have consultations with specialists, such as anesthetists, and may be given preprocedure medication. Many aspects of preparation focus on the patient's biomedical status, but psychological aspects of preparation are also important.

Many patients experience fear and anxiety when faced with a procedure that they know may cause pain.

Examples of the potential effects of extreme anxiety are illustrated in the cases in **Boxes 22.1**, **22.2**, and **22.3**. If a patient is sufficiently afraid of a procedure, they may choose not to go ahead with it (e.g. **Box 22.1**). In such cases, not only is the patient's health put at risk, but the costs to the health service are increased when resources reserved for a particular patient are not utilized. A similar example is where a patient requires frequent blood tests to determine appropriate treatment. If a patient finds giving blood samples aversive and therefore does not attend regularly, treatment could suffer (**Box 22.2**). **Box 22.3** demonstrates how fear about a painful procedure may affect a patient's self-referral behavior, causing delay in

---

Box 22.1 Jack, a 59-year-old man hospitalized for hernia repair surgery

Jack experienced such extreme fear of surgery that he felt unable to go ahead with surgery and discharged himself after taking premedication. He was referred to a clinical psychologist who took him through a course of systematic desensitization (envisaging progressively more threatening scenarios, whilst practicing relaxation techniques until the prospect of surgery could be considered without excessive anxiety). With this psychological preparation, Jack was subsequently readmitted and successfully completed surgery.

Box 22.2 Annette, a 40-year-old woman with a hypothyroidism

Annette required regular blood tests to effectively manage her underactive thyroid condition.
However, because she had a needle phobia, she avoided going for these tests. By the time she saw a consultant, she was suffering serious symptoms. Thus, because of what might be considered a trivial needle phobia, what was an essentially controllable condition was not effectively managed.

Box 22.3 Euan, a 35-year-old man with toothache

Euan experienced anxiety about visiting the dentist when suffering toothache because of anticipated pain and fear of the drill. He therefore put off going for as long as possible, self-medicating with painkillers to cope with the discomfort. When he finally overcame the anxiety and visited the dentist, his condition had deteriorated and he needed six extractions.

---

seeking medical attention until the condition is more serious. Alternatively, in an extreme case, medical staff may decide that a patient is too distressed to be able to cope with a procedure.

Where people show extreme anxiety, support from specialist clinicians (e.g. psychologists) may be required (as in **Box 22.1**). This chapter focuses on the levels of anxiety found in more typical individuals undergoing painful procedures. For these patients, anxiety may be easily moderated by other health professionals. Effective preparation will enable patients to undergo procedures at an optimal time, with maximal effectiveness. Some procedures require the patient to take an active role in proceedings; a highly anxious patient will be less able to follow directions than a less anxious patient. Anxiety can also affect patients' perceptions of pain: for a highly anxious patient, procedures will be more painful than for less anxious patients.[1] This chapter considers the assessment of anxiety and pain, what psychological preparation can achieve, how preparation can be carried out and aspects of psychological preparation that are specific to children.

ASSESSING ANXIETY AND PAIN

Accurate assessment of anxiety and pain has three purposes: (1) to decide whether or not exceptional preparation is needed (e.g. referring a patient to a psychologist); (2) to determine when psychological preparation is needed; and (3) to assess whether or not preparation has been effective.

Anxiety

Patients' anxiety levels are not always accurately estimated by healthcare professionals. For example, fellow patients were found to more accurately describe surgical patients' worries than were nursing staff.[2] It is likely that, being in a similar situation, patients had a clearer understanding of what it was like for their fellow patients than did the nursing staff, but, additionally, they were able to ascertain the specific concerns of the individuals which suggests that concerns emerged through the course of general conversation. Ward staff may not have as much time to get to know patients as their fellow patients, but this may be a last opportunity to reduce anxiety and so identifying patient concerns is vital. Additionally, the level of trauma associated with a procedure is not directly associated with the patients' anxiety level[3] and the outcome of a procedure is concerning to patients, as well as the process of undergoing the procedure itself.[4, 5] Patients may also be concerned about the impact of a procedure on issues other than their own health.[4, 5] In a group of patients scheduled for elective surgery, 89.6 percent indicated that they were concerned about their family and 65.8 percent were worried about financial loss.[5] The worries reported by patients in these studies are shown in more detail in **Figure 22.1a,b**.

Thus, the level and source of anxiety may differ to those anticipated by healthcare providers. In addition, the time span of anxiety may exceed that anticipated. Surgical patients experience elevated anxiety before admission to hospital, between admission and surgery, and post-operatively; anxiety is therefore not restricted to the period immediately before the operation.[6, 7]

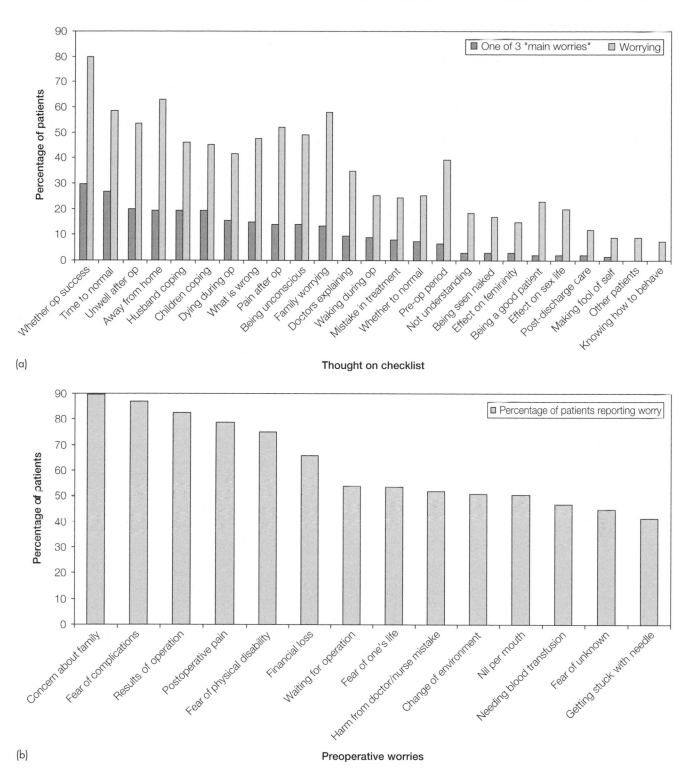

(a)

Thought on checklist

(b)

Preoperative worries

Figure 22.1 (a) Patients' worries before gynecological surgery: response to checklist of 25 preoperative thoughts. Compiled from data presented by Johnston[4]; (b) Patients' worries before elective surgery. Compiled from data presented by Jawaid et al.[5]

In order to address patients' anxiety, highly anxious patients need to be identified and methods of assessment are useful. Simple questionnaire items requesting patients to rate their level of anxiety and a checklist for them to indicate their worries are a quick way of gauging patients' concerns, allowing them to be effectively prepared for the procedure. For example, patients can be asked to indicate how worried they are feeling on a 10-cm line anchored with the words "not at all worried" and "extremely worried" (a visual analog scale, VAS).[8] For a more detailed assessment of anxiety, a standardized measure such as the State Trait Anxiety Inventory (STAI) can be used.[9] This scale contains 20 items assessing state anxiety and 20 to assess more general trait anxiety. When there is insufficient time available or when patients are not well enough to complete the full version, a six-item short form of the state scale of the STAI is useful.[10] A version of the STAI has also been specifically developed to assess anxiety in children. These standardized measures allow the comparison of patients with normative data. For example, mean scores for surgical patients the day before surgery are typically between 40 and 45 on the STAI. People who are not awaiting surgery would typically score lower, and individuals with generalized anxiety disorder would score higher on this scale.

Examples of items used in checklists for indicating worries are shown in **Figure 22.1a,b**. Johnston's 1987 25-item checklist[4] was developed both from items used in the literature and patients' spontaneous comments. These checklists assess what people are worried about, but not whether they catastrophize, exaggerating the risks of negative outcomes. Recent work using the Pain Catastrophizing Scale[11] has found that people who catastrophize about pain before undergoing surgical procedures experience worse postoperative pain.[12, 13] However, neither paper investigated catastrophizing independently of general anxiety, so general anticipation of negative outcomes could be responsible for this effect. Further research controlling for the effects of general anxiety is therefore necessary.

Pain

The healthcare provider's expectation or perception of pain might also differ from the patient's experience. Health professionals have consistently been shown to underestimate patients' pain, compared with patient reports (e.g. Refs 14, 15, 16, 17). Physicians in an emergency department have been found to rate patients' pain as lower than patients rated themselves.[14] This miscalibration was greater with expert physicians than with novices (students or residents undergoing training). Why this occurred is not clear. Pain was rated using a VAS anchored with "no pain" and "most intense pain imaginable." It could be that more experienced doctors have observed a wider range of pain experiences and their idea of "most intense pain imaginable" is more severe than the patient's. Alternatively, patients may try not to show emotion to physicians and so do not communicate their pain level effectively.

When asked to rate the pain of people with shoulder pain who were videotaped when undergoing physiotherapy assessment, health professionals (physiotherapists and occupational therapists), individuals with family experience of chronic pain, and control observers all underestimated patients' pain compared with patients' self-reports.[18] However, the health professionals underestimated pain more, and individuals with family experience underestimated less, than the control observers. Thus, it is not only experience with people in pain but the type of experience that seems to affect pain perceptions. The authors suggested that the health practitioners could be distancing themselves from the pain in order to be better able to cope, or their training might focus on solving the problem rather than focusing on the pain. In contrast, family members may be more aware of the consequences of pain in terms of activity restrictions than healthcare staff.

This mismatch between pain experienced by individuals and the pain perceived by health professionals has implications with respect to how pain is managed by health professionals, for example affecting the level of analgesia given. This communication problem can be tackled in two ways: first, during preparation, in discussing how to communicate pain with patients and, second, by enabling health professionals to more accurately assess pain level. As for anxiety measurement, pain can also be assessed using a quick VAS. A more detailed assessment of pain can be gained using a standardized measure such as the McGill Pain Questionnaire (MPQ), or the short form of this measure.[19, 20, 21] The MPQ includes both descriptors of the type of pain being experienced and short items about the level of current pain. Computerized methods of administering the MPQ have been developed which may facilitate its use in clinical settings.[22] In addition to giving information about pain, the type of pain reported may give useful diagnostic information. For example, different patterns of words are used by patients whose low back pain has identified "organic" causes as opposed to pain where the cause is unidentified.[21] However, the use of the MPQ in clinical settings has not been widely documented; it may be that such differentiations have not been found to be useful in the clinical context.

Thus, evidence suggests that there is a gap between patient experience and health professional perceptions for both anxiety and pain which needs to be bridged to achieve optimal patient outcomes. This can be achieved, for both pain and anxiety, first by health professionals being aware of the mismatch and having tools to facilitate assessment and, second, by enabling patients to communicate their anxiety and pain and, third, by using methods to reduce pain and anxiety.

WHAT DOES PSYCHOLOGICAL PREPARATION ACHIEVE?

There are three phases for which preparation for a painful procedure might be relevant for an individual patient: before the procedure, during the procedure, and after the procedure.

Before the procedure

Many patients are anxious when anticipating a procedure. They may be worried about the procedure itself (procedural stress) or worried about the outcome of the procedure (outcome stress).[23] It is important to address the anxiety caused by these stressors because not only is anxiety of itself an unpleasant state, but patients high in anxiety experience higher levels of pain during medical procedures and greater pain after surgery.[24] The type of procedure is likely to affect the extent to which each type of stress is relevant for an individual patient. For example, for 135 patients undergoing gynecological surgery, patients' main worries were not associated with the procedure itself, but with the outcome of surgery – whether it would be successful, how long it would take them to return to normal, and concern about being away from home.[4] In contrast, for a procedure such as dental restoration work, where the treatment is unpleasant but the benefits are apparent rapidly after treatment, patients' concerns are likely to be focused on the procedure, with the outcome being viewed positively.

In the case of preprocedure anxiety, it would be logical to assume that the more physical trauma involved in the procedure, or the more life-threatening the procedure, the more severe the patient's anxiety. However, this is not the case. An investigation of patients undergoing elective surgery found that extent of surgery did not affect patients' preoperative anxiety level, as assessed with the STAI. Patients undergoing minor surgical procedures, such as dilation and curettage, had equivalent levels of anxiety to those having more major procedures, such as cholecystectomy, carried out.[3] Many minor procedures are diagnostic, perhaps yielding more anxiety about the outcome of tests, whereas more major procedures are carried out as treatment leading to procedural stress, but possibly less outcome stress.

During the procedure

For some patients, such as those having surgery under general anesthetic, the procedure itself is not painful and patients are unaware of what is happening during the procedure (although the process of being anesthetized may cause some individuals anxiety). However, other procedures are themselves painful or uncomfortable and may require patients to actively participate in the procedure. Procedures fitting this category include diagnostic procedures, such as bone marrow aspiration, blood tests, and endoscopy, and also some treatments, such as dental restoration work and injections. These patients will require preparation which gives them skills to minimize their anxiety and perceptions of pain during the procedure. Not only is anxiety an aversive state but, where the participation of the patient affects the way a procedure is carried out, minimizing anxiety enables the patient to better attend to and follow instructions, enabling the procedure to be carried out more quickly and more effectively.

After the procedure

For patients under general anaesthetic, the procedure itself should not be painful, but postprocedure pain may be severe. Effective preparation will minimize the pain by enabling patients to carry out the behaviors that will minimize pain such as knowing how to obtain analgesia, how to use patient-controlled analgesia when appropriate, and requesting analgesia before pain becomes too severe. In addition, preparation will enable individuals to use cognitive and emotional strategies (managing thoughts and feelings) to minimize pain perception.

In contrast, some patients may experience little postprocedure pain, for example those who have undergone the diagnostic procedures of bone marrow aspiration or mammography. However, these patients may still experience anxiety after these diagnostic procedures out of concern about the results. Thus, giving patients techniques that help them to manage their anxiety after the procedure, as well as before and during the procedure, will be of benefit.

Good preparation involves giving patients enough information for them to anticipate what will happen and how they will feel after the procedure. For example, patients undergoing inguinal hernia repair may experience extensive bruising after the operation. This is not unusual but can be alarming for the patient who is then likely to seek medical advice and reassurance. Patients can be saved anxiety, and the health service the costs of follow-up visits, if they are adequately informed about what to expect beforehand.

Presurgical psychological preparation has benefits on a range of health outcomes. A meta-analysis has demonstrated that interventions, such as giving information, giving behavioral instruction, cognitive interventions and relaxation can lead to improved mood (negative affect), pain, lower use of pain medication, shorter stays in hospital, and higher scores on recovery and physiological indices (see **Figure 22.2**).[25] Clinical outcome was not significantly improved following intervention (the 95 percent confidence interval crosses the line of zero effect), but the wide confidence intervals are likely to result from the small number of studies available for inclusion for this outcome ($n = 3$). This work clearly demonstrates that psychological preparation not only makes the patient feel better in terms of mood and pain and facilitates their behavioral recovery but is also effective in reducing pain medication required and the length of time patients stay in hospital. Physiological indices, such as blood pressure, heart rate, cortisol and adrenaline levels, are also affected.

PSYCHOLOGICAL PREPARATION TECHNIQUES

Many individual studies have been carried out assessing particular preparation techniques with particular patient groups. A meta-analysis drew this research together in the context of surgery under general anesthetic (see **Table 22.1**).[25] These findings are not a comprehensive list of the effects of each intervention because not all interventions have been tested for all health outcomes.

However, it does demonstrate the range of outcomes that an intervention can affect. For example, giving procedural information not only affected patient reports of mood and pain, but also healthcare costs (pain medication and length of stay) and physiological measures.

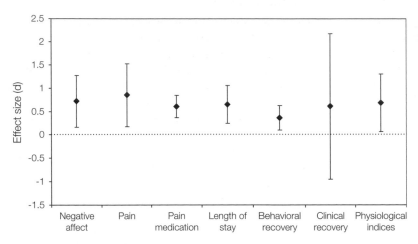

Figure 22.2 Pooled-effect sizes (*d*), ±95% confidence intervals, of psychological preparation interventions on health outcome measures. Compiled from data presented by Johnston and Vögele.[25] *Note*: Effect-size *d* = the difference between the means of two groups, divided by the pooled within-group standard deviation. A positive effect size indicates benefit for the intervention group compared with the control group. Individual study effect sizes were averaged to produce an estimate of the average population effect size for each outcome. Medium-effect size: *d* = 0.5; large effect size: *d* = 0.8.[26]

Table 22.1 Surgical outcomes improved by psychological preparation procedures.

Preparation type	Outcomes improved by procedure
Relaxation, e.g. breathing exercises	Pain Pain medication Length of stay Negative affect Physiological indices Clinical recovery
Information: procedural, e.g. "…you will then receive a local anesthetic…";	Pain Pain medication Length of stay Physiological indices Negative affect Clinical recovery
sensory, e.g. "…you will stop being able to feel sensations in the area of the anesthetic…"	Length of stay
Cognitive, e.g. reframing negative thoughts	Pain Pain medication Negative affect Clinical recovery
Behavioral instruction, e.g. training in use of analgesic equipment	Pain Pain medication Length of stay Physiological indices Negative affect Clinical recovery

Compiled from data presented by Johnston and Vögele.[25]

Types of preparation methods

INFORMATION GIVING

Patients can be given two types of preparatory information: procedural information and sensory information. Procedural information describes the process to the patient – what will happen, and when and how parts of the procedure will take place. Sensory information gives patients an insight as to the experiential aspect of the procedures and the postprocedure recovery time: what it will feel like to undergo the processes, what sensations they should expect. The rationale behind giving information is that patients become more aware of what to expect, making stimuli less anxiety-provoking,[27] and ensuring that the unusual sensations experienced are anticipated rather than being unexpected, leading patients to suspect that something might be wrong. Informing patients of what to expect also empowers them to prepare themselves, showing them the stages at which other techniques (e.g. cognitive preparation) might be of use, and enables them to actively participate in procedures, facilitating their successful completion.

It is important to consider whether or not information is given to patients in a way in which it will be understood. One study reported that, out of 100 surgical patients, 27 "informed" patients were unable to report the basic information of which organ had been operated on.[28] This communication problem was more common where patients were over 60 years old. It may be that patients struggle to recall the information they are given; patients undergoing surgery for skin cancer were found to recall 26.5 percent of a list of potential complications 20 minutes after the consultation and 24.4 percent one week later.[29] However, an evaluation of informed consent documentation has suggested that information given to patients may be inconsistent.[30] It is therefore important to ensure that full and consistent information is given to patients in a form in which they can understand and remember or refer to it (e.g. written information or audio/video recordings).

BEHAVIORAL INSTRUCTION

Behavioral instruction involves telling individuals what they should do to facilitate a procedure or their recovery.[31] For example, someone undergoing joint replacement surgery might be told how soon they should start walking after surgery to minimize muscle wastage and facilitate recovery.

COGNITIVE PREPARATION

Cognitive preparation techniques are designed to change the way that an individual thinks about negative aspects of a procedure. Patients are taught skills that they can then use in their own time, or during a procedure, to reduce their negative thinking and anxiety about the procedure. The two main methods are cognitive reframing and distraction, i.e. techniques which encourage a different way of thinking or thinking less about the procedure.

Reframing cognitions

Reframing cognitions involves taking a negative thought and developing a more positive perspective. For example, a cognitive reframing intervention, presented to patients in a manual, was developed by Ridgeway and Mathews.[27] Patients were first presented with common worries paired with more positive ways of looking at a situation (e.g. in response to worry about anesthesia, a given positive perspective was the high number of people who successfully undergo anesthesia). The patients were then asked to give a positive thought in response to a common worry, before being asked to supply their own negative thought along with a more positive reappraisal. Patients can also be encouraged to reevaluate the procedure, such that a threatening situation becomes a challenging situation (e.g. Cheung et al.[32]). For example, instead of feeling afraid of the pain associated with a procedure, patients can be encouraged to see it as a challenge to deal with and to feel proud when they successfully complete the procedure.

Distraction techniques

A second form of cognitive-coping strategy is distraction. Instead of finding a new way of viewing a positive thought, individuals are encouraged to focus on thoughts about other things. For example, a dentist who talks about the drill as sounding like an airplane may successfully distract a young person from worrying about the drill itself. Work with children has looked at using tools such as virtual reality systems to facilitate distraction during procedures (see below under Psychological preparation for children). Relaxation may also serve the function of distraction.

RELAXATION

These techniques can be used before a procedure, to increase relaxation, and reduce anxiety, but, once a technique has been learnt, a patient can also take it forward to use during procedures (simple relaxation may be a more useful technique than progressive muscle relaxation in this sense). When a relaxation technique is first learnt, it is helpful to be "talked through" the procedure by a caregiver/therapist, and patients can also be given an audio recording guiding them through the procedure to practice with. The more a relaxation technique is practiced, the easier it becomes for the individual to gain a relaxed state (and so teaching relaxation at a presurgical clinic allows individuals time to practice) but, even when a person is talked through the procedure at a single event (e.g. the morning of surgery), a more relaxed state can be achieved. Both techniques described below can be supported by asking patients to take slow, deep breaths.

Simple relaxation

Individuals are asked to systematically work round the body, relaxing each muscle group in turn.

Progressive muscle relaxation

This approach involves slowly tensing and then relaxing all the main muscle groups in the body. An example of a script to use while training individuals with this technique is found in Goldfried and Davidson.[33] Individuals who have difficulty in achieving simple relaxation of the body may prefer this technique, but the process of tensing and relaxing muscles can make this technique inappropriate to use during some medical procedures.

MODELLING

Modelling is the process during which an individual observes another person in a situation and learns, through watching that person, how to cope with the event themselves. Either mastery or coping models can be presented. For example, a patient might be presented with a video in which a calm, relaxed person undergoes the patient's procedure (a mastery model) or a video where the model patient is seen to find the procedure challenging, but manages to cope (a coping model). Modelling has been used most extensively in studies with children.[34]

COMMUNICATION

It is not always easy for a medical professional to accurately determine a patient's level of anxiety or pain perceptions. Yet, in order to properly prepare an individual to undergo a procedure with the optimum outcome, staff need to be able to assess anxiety and pain. Preprocedure preparation can enable a patient to communicate how they are feeling to staff. Many patients feel unwilling to bother staff and instead suffer in silence and so may need to be reassured that it really is appropriate for them to talk to staff about issues like anxiety and pain. They can also be shown how to use rating scales that are quick to complete and easy to interpret.

PSYCHOLOGICAL PREPARATION FOR CHILDREN

Many painful procedures are performed on children who, because of their developmental stage, may not understand what is happening to them in the same way that adults would.

The categories of techniques that are used with adults can also be used with children, but strategies should be adapted appropriately for the child's level of development. For example, when giving procedural and sensory information, discussion with health professionals and simple written or picture information may be helpful, but sessions involving structured play around the themes of the procedure can also be used, and hospital tours or computer programs also provide information in a way in which young people can absorb it.[35]

Distraction techniques, particularly during stressful procedures, have been found to be effective with children, for example the use of books, video games, and audiotapes (see LeRoy et al.[35] for review). The use of virtual reality as a distracter during painful procedures is also being developed.[36] Teaching relaxation techniques can be effective with children[35] and relaxation induced by slow, deep breathing can be encouraged by instructing children to "blow the pain away."[37]

Modelling of procedures by peers is an effective method for reducing anxiety in children although, where children have previous experience, it is less likely to be effective.[35]

Involving parents

An issue to be considered when preparing children for painful procedures is the extent to which parents should be involved. Children prefer their parents to be with them when they have to undergo a painful procedure or anesthesia,[37] but is having a parent stay through a procedure beneficial to the child?

For parents, watching a child undergo a painful procedure or undergo anesthesia induction is a highly stressful process; for parents of children undergoing minor surgery, the induction of anesthesia has been reported as the moment of greatest stress for 56 percent of parents.[38] In addition, evidence suggests that children are more anxious when undergoing procedures when accompanied by an anxious parent than when they are accompanied by a calm parent or, indeed, unaccompanied by any parent.[39, 40] Thus, to reduce parental distress and to protect children from parental distress, it is important for parents to be appropriately prepared to support their child through painful procedures. A video intervention giving parents procedural information about the procedure has been found to be effective in reducing parental anxiety.[41]

Children can be influenced not only by their parents' level of anxiety, but also by their parents' behavior. Counterintuitive as it seems, parents who reassure children can actually increase their distress.[42, 43] In a trial randomizing parents to training in reassurance, training in distraction or a control group, reassuring parents were found to be the most distressing for children on a range of measures, whereas the children of distracting parents showed the least distress.[43] This finding is also relevant to healthcare professionals. Even though reassuring children is intuitive and well-intentioned, distraction would appear to be a more effective method of enabling them to cope with procedures.

CONCLUSIONS

Psychological preparation can facilitate patient coping both before, during, and after painful procedures. Effective preparation improves health outcomes on a range of measures, including anxiety, pain, use of healthcare resources and physiological measures. Effective preparation not only affects how the patient thinks, feels, and behaves, but can also affect how they interact with others, such as health professionals and family members. In particular, parent–child interactions can greatly affect how a procedure is received by the child.

ACKNOWLEDGMENTS

Thanks to Dr Julie Bruce for her comments on a draft of this chapter. RP was supported by a Research Training Fellowship from the Chief Scientist Office of the Scottish Government Health Directorates.

REFERENCES

1. Tanq J, Gibson SI. A psychophysical evaluation of the relationship between trait anxiety, pain perception, and induced state anxiety. *Journal of Pain*. 2005; **6**: 612–19.
2. Johnston M. Recognition of patients' worries by nurses and by other patients. *British Journal of Clinical Psychology*. 1982; **21**: 255–61.
3. Domar AD, Everett LL, Keller MG. Preoperative anxiety: Is it a predictable entity? *Anesthesia and Analgesia*. 1989; **69**: 763–7.
4. Johnston M. Emotional and cognitive aspects of anxiety in surgical patients. *Communication and Cognition*. 1987; **2**: 245–60.
5. Jawaid M, Mushtaq A, Mukhtar S, Khan Z. Preoperative anxiety before elective surgery. *Neurosciences*. 2007; **12**: 145–8.
6. Johnston M. Anxiety in surgical patients. *Psychological Medicine*. 1980; **10**: 145–52.
7. Carr ECJ, Thomas VN, Wilson-Barnet J. Patient experiences of anxiety, depression and acute pain after surgery: A longitudinal perspective. *International Journal of Nursing Studies*. 2005; **42**: 521–30.
8. Broadbent EA, Petrie KJ, Alley PG, Booth RJ. Psychological stress impairs early wound repair following surgery. *Psychosomatic Medicine*. 2003; **65**: 865–9.
9. Spielberger C. *Manual for the state trait anxiety inventory STAI form Y*. Palo Alto, CA: Consulting Psychologists Press, 1983.
10. Marteau TM, Bekker H. The development of a six-item short-form of the state scale of the Spielberger State-Trait Anxiety Inventory STAI. *British Journal of Clinical Psychology*. 1992; **31**: 301–06.
11. Sullivan MJL, Bishop SR, Pivik J. The Pain Catastrophizing Scale: Development and validation. *Psychological Assessment*. 1995; **7**: 524–32.
12. Pavlin DJ, Sullivan MJL, Freund PR, Roesen K. Catastrophizing: A risk factor for postsurgical pain. *Clinical Journal of Pain*. 2005; **21**: 83–90.
13. Strulov L, Zimmer EZ, Granot M et al. Pain catastrophizing, response to experimental heat stimuli, and post-cesarean section pain. *Journal of Pain*. 2007; **8**: 273–9.
14. Marquié L, Raufast E, Lauque D et al. Pain rating by patients and physicians: Evidence of systematic pain miscalibration. *Pain*. 2003; **102**: 289–96.
15. Thomas T, Robinson C, Champion D et al. Prediction and assessment of the severity of post-operative pain and of satisfaction with management. *Pain*. 1998; **75**: 177–85.
16. Idvall E, Berg K, Unosson M, Brudin L. Differences between nurse and patient assessments on postoperative pain management in two hospitals. *Journal of Evaluation in Clinical Practice*. 2005; **11**: 444–51.
17. Sloman R, Rosen G, Rom M, Shir Y. Nurses' assessment of pain in surgical patients. *Journal of Advanced Nursing*. 2005; **52**: 125–32.
* 18. Prkachin KM, Solomon P, Hwang T, Mercer S. Does experience influence judgements of pain behaviour? Evidence from relatives of pain patients and therapists. *Pain Research and Management*. 2001; **6**: 105–12.
19. Melzack R. The McGill Pain Questionnaire: Major properties and scoring methods. *Pain*. 1975; **1**: 277–99.
20. Melzack R. The short form McGill Pain Questionnaire. *Pain*. 1987; **30**: 191–7.
21. Melzack R, Katz J. The McGill Pain Questionnaire: Appraisal and current status. In: Turk DC, Melzack R (eds). *Handbook of pain assessment*. New York: The Guilford Press, 2001: 35–52.
22. Huang HY, Wilkie DJ, Zong SP et al. Developing a computerized data collection and decision support system for cancer pain management. *CIN: Computers, Informatics, Nursing*. 2003; **21**: 206–17.
23. Weinman J, Johnston M. Stressful medical procedures: An analysis of the effects of psychological interventions and of the stressfulness of the procedures. In: Maes S, Spielberger CD, Defares PB, Sarason IG (eds). *Topics in health psychology*. Chichester: John Wiley & Sons, 1988: 205–17.
24. Katz J, Poleshuck EL, Andrus CH et al. Risk factors for acute pain and its persistence following breast cancer surgery. *Pain*. 2005; **119**: 16–25.
* 25. Johnston M, Vögele C. Benefits of psychological preparation for surgery: A meta-analysis. *Annals of Behavioral Medicine*. 1993; **15**: 245–56.
26. Cohen J. *Statistical power analysis for the behavioral sciences*, 2nd edn. Hillsdale, NJ: Lawrence Erlbaum, 1988.

27. Ridgeway V, Mathews A. Psychological preparation for surgery: A comparison of methods. *British Journal of Clinical Psychology.* 1982; **21**: 271–80.

28. Byrne DJ, Napier A, Cuschieri A. How informed is signed consent? *British Medical Journal.* 1988; **296**: 839–40.

29. Fleischman M, Garcia C. Informed consent in dermatologic surgery. *Dermatologic Surgery.* 2003; **29**: 952–5.

30. Issa MM, Setzer E, Charaf C *et al.* Informed versus uninformed consent for prostate surgery: The value of electronic consents. *Journal of Urology.* 2006; **176**: 694–9.

* 31. Mathews A, Ridgeway V. Psychological preparation for surgery. In: Steptoe A, Mathews A (eds). *Health care and human behaviour.* London: Academic Press, 1984: 231–59.

32. Cheung LH, Callaghan P, Chang AM. A controlled trial of psycho-educational interventions in preparing Chinese women for elective hysterectomy. *International Journal of Nursing Studies.* 2003; **40**: 207–16.

33. Goldfried MR, Davidson GC. *Clinical behavior therapy.* New York: Holt, Rinehart & Winston, 1976.

34. O'Halloran CM, Altmaier EM. The efficacy of preparation for surgery and invasive medical procedures. *Patient Education and Counseling.* 1995; **25**: 9–16.

* 35. LeRoy S, Elixson EM, O'Brien P *et al.* Recommendations for preparing children and adolescents for invasive cardiac procedures – A statement from the American Heart Association Pediatric Nursing Subcommittee of the council on cardiovascular nursing in collaboration with the council on cardiovascular diseases of the young. *Circulation.* 2003; **108**: 2550–64.

36. Gershon J, Zimand E, Lemos R *et al.* Use of virtual reality as a distractor for painful procedures in a patient with pediatric cancer: A case study. *Cyberpsychology and Behavior.* 2003; **6**: 657–61.

37. Kennedy RM, Luhmann JD. The "ouchless emergency department" – Getting closer: Advances in decreasing distress during painful procedures in the emergency department. *Pediatric Clinics of North America.* 1999; **46**: 1215–47.

38. Messeri A, Caprilli S, Busoni P. Anaesthesia induction in children: A psychological evaluation of the efficiency of parents' presence. *Pediatric Anesthesia.* 2004; **14**: 551–6.

39. Bevan JC, Johnston C, Haig MJ *et al.* Preoperative parental anxiety predicts behavioural and emotional responses to induction of anaesthesia in children. *Canadian Journal of Anaesthesia.* 1990; **37**: 177–82.

40. Kain ZN, Caldwell-Andrews AA, Maranets I *et al.* Predicting which child–parent pair will benefit from parental presence during induction of anesthesia: A decision-making approach. *Anesthesia and Analgesia.* 2006; **102**: 81–4.

41. Cassady JF, Wysocki TT, Miller KM *et al.* Use of a preanesthetic video for facilitation of parental education and anxiolysis before pediatric ambulatory surgery. *Anesthia and Analgesia.* 1999; **88**: 246–50.

42. Salmon K, Pereira JK. Predicting children's response to an invasive medical investigation: The influence of effortful control and parent behavior. *Journal of Pediatric Psychology.* 2002; **27**: 227–33.

43. Manimala MR, Blount RL, Cohen LL. The effects of parental reassurance versus distraction on child distress and coping during immunizations. *Children's Health Care.* 2000; **29**: 161–77.

23

Peripheral nerve blocks: practical aspects

DAVID HILL

KEY LEARNING POINTS

- The ability to perform peripheral nerve blocks is an essential skill in the comprehensive management of acute, chronic, and cancer pain.
- A peripheral nerve stimulator (PNS) is not a substitute for anatomical knowledge and should not be used to hunt blindly for nerves.

- Ultrasound is emerging as the technique of choice in aiding peripheral nerve blocks. A high resolution ultrasound probe can reliably identify nerves, vessels, and neighboring structures in the target region.
- Individual peripheral nerve blocks are described including continuous catheter techniques.

AGENTS AND TECHNIQUES FOR PERIPHERAL NERVE BLOCKS

Local anesthetics

Local anesthetics are sodium channel-blocking drugs that are unique in their ability to block nerve impulses conducted proximally (pain relief) and impulses conducted distally (motor blockade) in any peripheral nerve. Unlike neurolytic agents, local anesthetics produce a conduction block that is painless and completely reversible. Nerve fiber types vary in their sensitivity to local anesthetics, so that injection of differing concentrations selectively blocks different types of fiber. Differential blockade is a useful diagnostic tool and has several practical uses in pain management:

- attributing pain to a single nerve;
- differential block to identify the neural pathway that subserves the pain;

- permits precise targeting prior to a destructive procedure;
- allows the patient to experience the effects temporarily before permanent blockade;
- repeated at intervals, temporary blockade may have a long-lasting effect (e.g. scar neuromas or muscle trigger point injections).

Local anesthetic blocks are both diagnostic and therapeutic and may obviate the need for permanent neurolysis.

INDIVIDUAL AGENTS

Individual agents are detailed as follows.[1]

Lidocaine (lignocaine)

- Rapid onset and short duration (hours).
- Maximum recommended dose in an adult is 200 mg (data sheet), although doses of 4–7 mg/kg have been advocated.

- Lidocaine causes vasodilatation at the site of injection.
- Addition of 5 μg/mL (1:200,000) epinephrine (adrenaline) may slow systemic absorption and prolong duration of the block.
- Large doses (up to 35 mg/kg) combined with 1 μg/ml (1:1,000,000) epinephrine by subcutaneous infiltration have been used for liposuction.
- Available preparations with adrenaline may contain the preservatives sodium metabisulfite (antioxidant) and methylparahydroxybenzoate, both of which may cause nerve injury and allergic reactions.

Prilocaine

- Rapid onset and duration.
- Similar potency to lidocaine.
- Readily hydrolyzed, reducing risk of systemic toxicity.
- Aminophenol metabolites oxidize hemoglobin to methemoglobin.
- Maximum dose 10 mg/kg (total maximum adult dose 600 mg).
- Has no vasoactivity.
- Multidose vials contain methylparahydroxybenzoate as preservative.

Bupivacaine (racemic)

- Slow onset and long duration (lasts two to three times longer than lidocaine).
- Maximum recommended dose in adults 150 mg, dosage should not exceed 2 mg/kg.
- Epinephrine does not seem to prolong duration of block.
- Main disadvantage is low threshold for cardiotoxicity.
- Epinephrine-containing preparations contain sodium metabisulfite.
- Opioid–bupivacaine mixtures provide epidural analgesia in a synergistic manner.

Levobupivacaine

- This S-enantiomer of bupivacaine is less cardiotoxic.
- Equipotent to racemic bupivacaine by the epidural route.
- Still to be fully evaluated clinically in peripheral nerve blockade.

Ropivacaine

- Claims a greater degree of separation between sensory and motor nerve block (differential block).
- Claims of less toxicity may be secondary to its potency being lower than bupivacaine.
- Ropivacaine causes vasoconstriction and prolongation of nerve blockade compared with bupivacaine.
- The addition of epinephrine probably confers no additional benefit for peripheral nerve blocks.
- Maximum recommended dose 2 mg/kg.

Neurolytic agents and techniques for peripheral nerve blockade

Neurolysis of peripheral nerves by chemical, thermal, or cryogenic means is indicated for patients with limited life expectancy. Peripheral neurolysis has several disadvantages.[2][II]

- The analgesia is not permanent.
- It is associated with neuritis and deafferentation pain.
- It can produce unwanted motor blockade.
- It can damage surrounding tissues.

Therefore, it is usually performed under the following circumstances.

- The pain is severe and other methods have failed.
- The pain is in the distribution of an identifiable peripheral nerve.
- A trial block of local anesthetic has been successful.
- The effects of the local anesthetic block are acceptable to the patient.

The most undesirable complication of peripheral neurolysis is the onset of neuropathic pain. This has been reported following treatment in up to 28 percent of cases. Comparisons of different volumes and concentrations of neurolytic agents have not been reported. It would seem logical to use a small amount of agent to minimize damage to nontarget tissue; however, incomplete lesions may make neuropathic pain more likely. Repeat injections are often necessary to achieve success.

NEUROLYTIC AGENTS

Alcohol and phenol are the most commonly used agents. The incidence of neuropathic pain is believed to be greater following peripheral neurolysis with alcohol.

Alcohol

- Generally used undiluted for peripheral nerve blockade.
- Injection is immediately followed by burning pain along the distribution of the nerve, followed by warm numbness.
- Pain relief increases over a few days and is maximal by a week.

Phenol

- Various concentrations are available as an aqueous preparation or in glycerol. A maximum of 6.7 percent can be dissolved in water at room temperature.
- Aqueous phenol can be injected down smaller gauge needles.

- Following injection, an initial local anesthetic effect subsides to neurolysis, which may take three to seven days to become fully apparent.
- The density and duration of the block is felt to be less than that of alcohol; 5 percent phenol is equivalent to approximately 40 percent alcohol in neurolytic potency.

NEUROLYTIC TECHNIQUES

Cryoanalgesia

The basic principle is as follows:

- Freezing of a nerve segment to $-60\,°C$ with a 2-mm probe.
- Achieved by rapid expansion of carbon dioxide or nitrous oxide gas.
- The probe is left in contact with the nerve for one to two minutes and allowed to thaw before removal.
- An acute injury produces analgesia for 2–20 weeks.
- The basal lamina of the nerve is left intact, allowing eventual regeneration.

Although cryoanalgesia has its proponents, results can be disappointing. The technique requires accurate placement of a bulky probe, which is difficult to achieve when inserted percutaneously. Placement under direct vision is not usually a realistic option in pain management clinics. The main advantage of cryoanalgesia is the low risk of neuritis.

See Chapter 32, Cryoanalgesia, for further discussion of this topic.

Pulsed radiofrequency

- A pulsed radiofrequency (RF)[3] lesion is achieved by applying energy with a pulsed time cycle of 2.20 ms/second at temperatures not exceeding 42°C.
- The mechanism of neuromodulation is unclear, but the electromagnetic field energy may interrupt nerve transmission.
- Pulsed RF has been used with benefit for blockade of most peripheral nerves and ganglia.
- A typical lesion is 42°C for 120 seconds repeated three times.

See Chapter 33, Radiofrequency lesioning and treatment of chronic pain for further discussion of this topic.

Nerve location by peripheral nerve stimulation

A peripheral nerve stimulator (PNS) is not a substitute for anatomical knowledge and should not be used to hunt blindly for nerves.[4] Its main use is to place a needle close to the target nerve, especially when a nerve or plexus has a characteristic pattern of muscle movement in response to stimulation. The distinct endpoint is pulse-synchronous muscle movement or paresthesiae attributable to the target nerve.

PRINCIPLES OF NERVE LOCATION

- Use a PNS that has a variable current output up to 5 mA.
- Set for short duration of impulse (less than $100\,\mu s$) at a frequency of 1–2 Hz so that motor nerves are stimulated preferentially.
- Connect anode (+ve) to a large ground electrode well away from the site of the nerve block to ensure current flows through the target nerve.
- Initially set delivered current at 3 mA.
- Connect cathode (–ve) to the block needle.
- Using a standard approach to the nerve, advance needle until within the expected vicinity of nerve.
- When using a current of around 3 mA or less, the nerve will not be stimulated unless the needle tip is within 1 cm.
- Painful levels of stimulation will be needed if the nerve is more than 2 cm away.
- Look for pulse-synchronous muscle movement to indicate that the needle tip is close to the nerve.
- Carefully adjust the needle tip position so that "just discernible" muscle movement is seen with a current of 0.1–0.5 mA.
- Sudden pain or exaggerated muscle movement may indicate direct contact with the nerve.
- The exact current depends on the target nerve. Small nerves such as the median nerve require 0.1–0.3 mA whereas the sciatic nerve may require 2 mA.
- Elderly patients or the presence of neuropathy require greater current.
- Following injection of local anesthetic, muscle movement will increase because of increased current conduction and then fade as the nerve is displaced by the volume of the injection.

INSULATED OR NONINSULATED NEEDLES

- Insulated needles prevent current loss in surrounding tissue.
- Insulated needles require half the current of noninsulated needles.
- There is a greater variety and availability of noninsulated needles.
- For most uses, noninsulated needles are satisfactory.
- There is no evidence that one needle over another is more successful or minimizes the risk of neural damage.

Ultrasound-guided nerve blocks

Ultrasound is emerging as the technique of choice in aiding peripheral nerve blocks.[5] A high-resolution ultrasound probe can reliably identify nerves, vessels, and neighboring structures in the target region. The technique of real-time guidance during needle advancement can quickly localize nerves. Distinct patterns of local anesthetic spread observed on ultrasound can further confirm accurate needle location and significantly reduce the volume of local anesthetic solution. This results in a shortened onset time, improved quality, and longer duration of block.

Continuous peripheral nerve blockade

Continuous peripheral nerve blockade (CPNB)[6] allows prolonged analgesia both before and after surgery. In chronic pain patients, nerve targeted and regional analgesia is possible allowing physiotherapy, increased mobilization, and shorter hospitalization.

GENERAL PRINCIPLES

- Attention to asepsis is important as prolonged use is intended.
- Insertion point should be carefully chosen and catheter fixed to prevent dislodgement.
- Catheter needs to be accurately placed alongside nerve or plexus using real time ultrasound or stimulating catheter.
- Distension of tissue space with saline of local anesthetic aids catheter placement.
- Catheter should be flushed with saline to prevent obstruction by blood.
- Optimal regime is the combination of a basal background infusion (3–5 mL/h) with intermittent top-ups as required (3–5 mL).
- Levobupivacaine 0.125 percent, ropivacine 0.2 percent alone, or levobupivacaine 0.1 percent with fentanyl 2 µg/mL are usual solutions.
- Initial test-bolus through catheter must be large enough to exclude intravascular placement – often adrenaline-containing bolus is employed to increase sensitivity of test-bolus detection of intravascular injection.
- Duration should be no longer than necessary as myotoxicity may occur.

TECHNIQUES

- Cannula over needle with catheter through cannula.
- Inexpensive and needles generally small.
- Uncertainty of final position of catheter unless ultrasound used.
- Catheter is stiff and easily damaged by needle.

Catheter through Tuohy/Sprotte needle

- Needle tip angle aids threading of catheter.
- Uncertainty of final position of catheter unless ultrasound used.

- Inexpensive.
- Stimulating catheter.
- Accurate placement of catheter.
- Can be painful to place as tissue space must be distended with saline rather than local anesthetic.
- Catheter is stiff and may cause paresthesia.
- Expensive if using specially designed catheters.

General principles of practice

This chapter is essentially a "how to do it" guide, and detailed discussions of the indications and efficacy of the blocks for various pain conditions are not appropriate. This information can be found in the relevant chapters elsewhere or in the reference included with each block.

RESUSCITATION EQUIPMENT

- Infrequently, systemic toxicity from the administration of local anesthetic and neurolytic agents can occur.
- These techniques should not be performed without immediate availability of, and skill in using, airway and cardiovascular resuscitation facilities.

ASEPTIC TECHNIQUE

- All equipment should be sterile and preferably disposable.
- Cleaning fluids should be disposed of prior to drawing up local anesthetic solutions to avoid error.
- Both gloves and a mask should be worn.

NEEDLES

- Preliminary skin infiltration and wheals are performed with 23- or 25-gauge hypodermic needles.
- There is no consensus on which design of needle to use for peripheral nerve block, both long and short beveled needles have been shown to produce nerve trauma.
- Short, beveled needles (angle approximately 45°) offer more feedback to the operator.
- Pencil-point needles (side port) are designed to prevent intraneural injection and may yet prove to be beneficial.

NERVE BLOCKS OF THE HEAD AND NECK

Occipital nerve block

INDICATIONS

- Diagnosis and treatment of occipital neuralgia.
- Scalp anesthesia for surgical procedures.

As defined by the International Headache Society, occipital neuralgia is diagnosed by successful local anesthetic block of that nerve.[7][II] Chronic occipital neuralgia can be treated by repeated injections of local anesthetic and depot steroid.

RELEVANT ANATOMY

- The greater occipital nerves originate from the posterior rami of C2, often with a branch from C3.
- Interneuronal connections within the upper spinal cord may allow occipital pain to be referred to the trigeminal distribution.
- The nerve becomes subcutaneous inferior to the superior nuchal line, 3 cm lateral to the occipital protuberance, and lies immediately medial to the occipital artery.
- The lesser occipital nerve originates from the anterior rami of C2 and C3.
- The nerve runs upwards along the posterior border of the sternomastoid muscle to supply the lateral and posterior scalp.
- The lesser occipital nerve lies superficial to, and becomes lateral to, the occipital artery.

LANDMARKS

- Greater occipital protuberance.
- Mastoid process.
- Occipital artery.

PRACTICAL STEPS (FIGURE 23.1)

- Best position is sitting with the head flexed.
- Selection of nerve for block is based on reproduction of pain with nerve palpation.
- Identify the line between the occipital protuberance and the mastoid process.
- Insert a 25-gauge needle subcutaneously 2 cm lateral to the occipital protuberance, and medial to the pulsation of the occipital artery.
- Inject 4–5 mL of solution to block the greater occipital nerve.
- Redirect the needle along the line between the bony landmarks toward the mastoid process and inject a further 3–4 mL subcutaneously to block the lesser occipital nerve.

COMPLICATIONS

- The superficial nature of the block should make complications rare.

Peripheral branches of the trigeminal nerve

Blockade of the more peripheral branches (mental nerve, infraorbital nerve, supraorbital nerve, and supratrochlear nerve) has the advantage of a lower incidence of unwanted motor blockade and sensory disturbances than blockade of the Gasserian ganglion.[8]

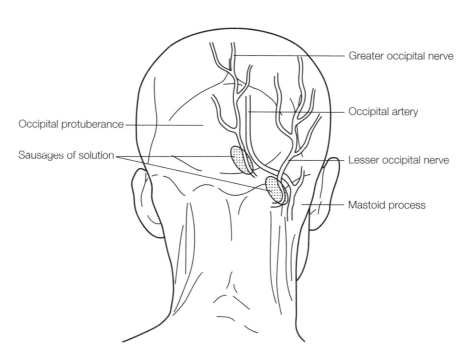

Figure 23.1 Occipital nerve block. Landmarks for blockade of the greater and lesser occipital nerves. Reproduced with permission from Pinnock CA, Fischer HBJ, Jones RP. *Peripheral nerve blockade.* Edinburgh: Churchill Livingstone, 1996.

INDICATIONS

See **Table 23.1**.

RELEVANT ANATOMY (FIGURE 23.2)

- The three foramina for the mental nerve, the infraorbital nerve, and the supraorbital nerve all lie in the same plane, which passes through the pupil in its resting position.
- The supratrochlear nerve lies medial to the supraorbital nerve.

Mental nerve block

The mental nerve can be blocked by an intraoral or an extraoral route. The extraoral route will be described.

LANDMARKS

- Mental foramen.

PRACTICAL STEPS

- Palpation to identify the mental foramen.
- Clean skin.
- A 25-gauge needle is inserted toward the foramen.
- To avoid nerve damage, the needle should not be placed in the canal.
- Aspirate for blood.
- Inject 2–3 mL of local anesthetic.
- Neurolysis can be achieved with incremental injections of 0.1 mL of glycerol or phenol in glycerol after trial block with local anesthetic. Cryoanalgesia can also be performed, but a small scar may occur.

Table 23.1 Indications for blockade of the peripheral branches of the trigeminal nerve.

Local anesthetic block	Local anesthetic and steroid block	Neurolytic block
Surgical anesthesia	Adjunct to pharmacological treatment of trigeminal neuralgia	Cancer pain
Differential neural block	Atypical facial pain	Trigeminal neuralgia
Trial block prior to neurolysis	Cluster headaches	Cluster headache
Palliation in acute emergencies	Facial trauma	
Palliation of acute shingles		

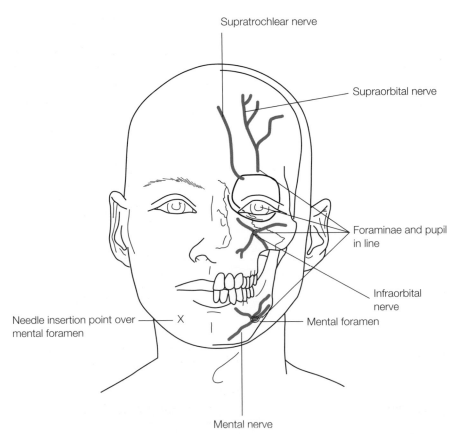

Figure 23.2 Peripheral branches of the trigeminal nerve. Landmarks for blockade of supraorbital, infraorbital, and mental nerves. Reproduced with permission from Pinnock CA, Fischer HBJ, Jones RP. *Peripheral nerve blockade.* Edinburgh: Churchill Livingstone, 1996.

Infraorbital nerve block

LANDMARKS

- Infraorbital foramen.

PRACTICAL STEPS

- Palpate infraorbital foramen (1 cm lateral to external nares and 1 cm below the lower border of the orbit).
- Insert a 25-gauge needle subcutaneously towards the foramen.
- Avoid entering the canal with the needle.
- Aspirate for blood.
- Inject 2–3 mL of local anesthetic.
- Neurolysis as above.

Supraorbital and supratrochlear nerve blocks

LANDMARKS

- Supraorbital notch.
- Bridge of nose.

PRACTICAL STEPS

- Palpate supraorbital notch.
- Clean skin, avoiding the eye.
- Move 25-gauge needle subcutaneously toward notch.
- Avoid entering foramen.
- Aspirate for blood.
- Inject 3–4 mL of local anesthetic.
- Redirect needle medially toward the bridge of the nose.
- Aspirate for blood.
- Inject a further 3–4 mL of local anesthetic.
- For bilateral block, insert the needle in the midpoint of the bridge of the nose.
- Neurolysis as above; avoid damaging hair follicles in the eyebrow with cryoanalgesia.

COMPLICATIONS

- Trauma to nerves (compression).
- Facial hematoma.
- Infection.
- Activation of herpes zoster.
- Postneurolytic dysesthesia.

Spinal accessory nerve block

Primarily, the spinal accessory nerve block[9] was advocated for the treatment of cervical dystonias. However, the efficacy and safety of botulinum toxin injections has largely made this block redundant.

INDICATIONS

- Diagnosis and treatment of spasm of sternomastoid or trapezius muscles (multiple sclerosis, posterior fossa tumors, collagen diseases, or myopathies).
- Neurodestruction of the nerve has been carried out by chemical, cryogenic, radiofrequency, or surgical lesions.

RELEVANT ANATOMY

- Origin – nucleus ambiguus.
- Exits the skull through the jugular foramen.
- The nerve traverses the posterior border of the sternomastoid muscle in the upper third of the muscle.
- Along with the cervical plexus, the nerve innervates the trapezius muscle.

LANDMARKS

- Posterior border of the sternomastoid.

PRACTICAL STEPS (FIGURE 23.3)

- Patient lies supine looking away from the side of the block.
- Patient lifts the head against resistance to outline the posterior border of the sternomastoid muscle.
- Insert a 25-gauge needle at the junction of the upper one-third with the lower two-thirds of the posterior border of the muscle.
- Direct the needle slightly anteriorly to a depth of approximately 2 cm.
- Aspirate for blood.
- Inject 10 mL of local anesthetic, which may be combined with steroid (up to 80 mg depot methylprednisolone).

COMPLICATIONS

- Inadvertent intravascular injection (jugular vessels).
- Hematoma (reduced by applying pressure or ice packs).
- Inadvertent block of phrenic, recurrent laryngeal, vagus, or glossopharyngeal nerves.
- Inadvertent central neural block.

Cervical plexus block

Cervical plexus block[10] can be deep or superficial; the deep block also provides muscle relaxation (motor block).

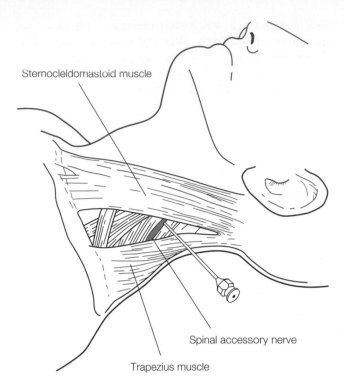

Sternocleidomastoid muscle

Spinal accessory nerve

Trapezius muscle

Figure 23.3 Spinal accessory nerve block. Landmarks for blockade of the spinal accessory nerve. Reproduced with permission from Cousins MJ, Bridenbaugh PO (eds). *Neural blockade in clinical anesthesia and management of pain.* Philadelphia: JB Lippincott, 1988.

INDICATIONS

- Surgery of the neck (usually carotid endarterectomy).
- Pharyngeal cancer pain.
- Occipital and posterior auricular neuralgia.

Superficial cervical plexus block

RELEVANT ANATOMY (FIGURE 23.4a)

- The superficial branches of the plexus (C2–4) are cutaneous and emerge from behind the posterior border of the sternomastoid muscle at its midpoint.
- They penetrate the cervical fascia and radiate out subcutaneously.
- Innervates the skin of the scalp and ear (lesser occipital and great auricular nerve).
- Innervates the skin of the submandibular area, the neck, top of the shoulders, and anterior chest wall (anterior cutaneous nerve and supraclavicular nerves).

LANDMARKS

- Posterior border of the sternomastoid.
- Cricoid cartilage.

PRACTICAL STEPS

- Position patient supine with head turned away from side of block.
- Single injection technique (**Figure 23.4b**):
  - A line drawn laterally from the cricoid cartilage usually crosses the middle of the posterior border of the sternomastoid muscle where the nerves emerge.
  - Insert a 22-gauge needle immediately behind the muscle at the midpoint and at right angles to the skin until it "pops" through the cervical fascia.
  - Inject 10 mL of local anesthetic solution, which if correctly placed will be seen flowing up and down the posterior border of the muscle.
- Superficial injection technique (**Figure 23.4c**):
  - Insert a 22-gauge needle subcutaneously and infiltrate along the middle one-third of the posterior border of the sternomastoid.
  - Inject 5–10 mL of local anesthetic.

Deep cervical plexus block (Labat method)

RELEVANT ANATOMY

- The cervical roots emerge from the intervertebral foraminae.
- They lie in the sulcus of the transverse processes before combining to form the plexus.
- A deep plexus block is in effect a cervical paravertebral block of C2–4.

LANDMARKS (FIGURE 23.5)

- Mastoid process.
- Chassaignac's tubercle (C6).
- Cricoid cartilage.

PRACTICAL STEPS (FIGURE 23.5)

- The patient lies supine with the head turned away from the side of the block.
- A line is drawn from the mastoid process to the anterior tubercle of C6 at the level of the cricoid cartilage.
- This line indicates the position of the cervical transverse processes.
- On this line, the transverse processes of C2–4 are palpated (approximately 1.5-cm intervals below the mastoid process).
- C3 lies at the level of the hyoid bone.
- C4 lies at the level of the upper border of the thyroid cartilage.
- The skin is infiltrated overlying the transverse processes of C2, 3, and 4.
- A 22-gauge, 3.5-cm needle is inserted medially and downwards onto the transverse processes at these three points (usually less than 2 cm deep, they become more superficial as they descend).

- The needle is then walked laterally off the transverse process.
- Aspirate for blood and cerebrospinal fluid (CSF).
- Inject 3–5 mL of local anesthetic.

The needle must locate the transverse process as far laterally as possible to avoid the vertebral artery. The downward direction of the needle avoids insertion into the intervertebral foramen, and reduces the risk of epidural or subarachnoid injection.

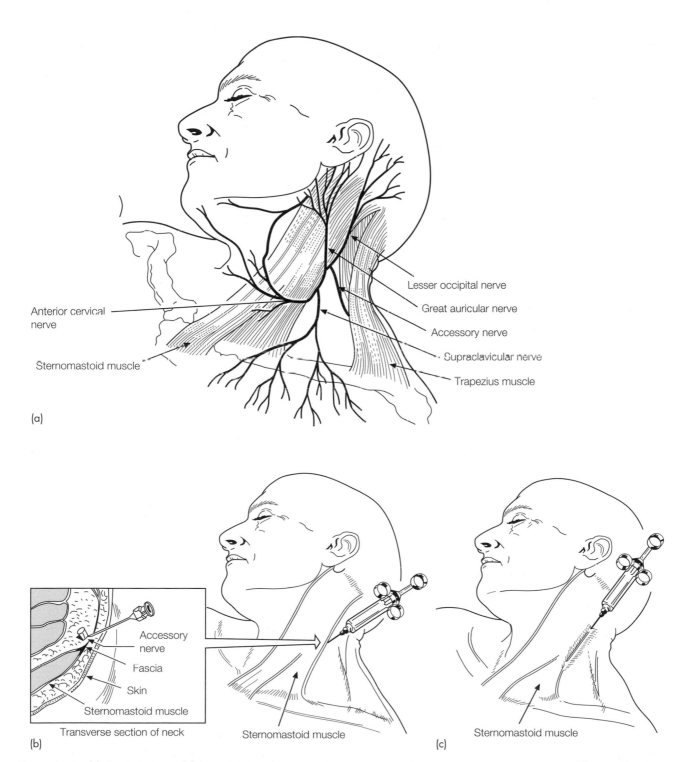

Figure 23.4 (a) Cervical plexus. (b) Superficial cervical plexus block; landmarks for the single-injection technique. (c) Superficial cervical plexus block; landmarks for the superficial injection technique. Reproduced with permission from Cousins MJ, Bridenbaugh PO (eds). *Neural blockade in clinical anesthesia and management of pain*. Philadelphia: JB Lippincott, 1988.

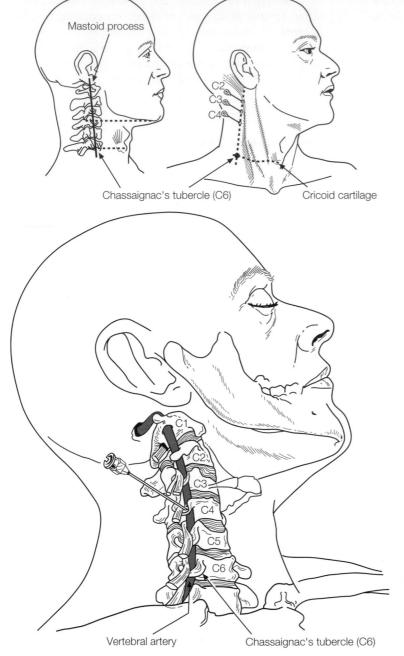

Mastoid process

C2
C3
C4

Chassaignac's tubercle (C6)

Cricoid cartilage

C1
C2
C3
C4
C5
C6

Vertebral artery

Chassaignac's tubercle (C6)

Figure 23.5 Deep cervical plexus block. Landmarks and needle insertion points for deep cervical plexus block. Reproduced with permission from Cousins MJ, Bridenbaugh PO (eds). *Neural blockade in clinical anesthesia and management of pain.* Philadelphia: JB Lippincott, 1988.

COMPLICATIONS

- Inadequate block for surgery.
- Intravascular injection of local anesthetic (vertebral artery, jugular veins).
- Hematoma (tear of vein).
- Compression of carotid sheath (large volumes of local anesthetic).
- Central neural blockade.
- Recurrent laryngeal nerve block (2 percent).
- Phrenic nerve block (50 percent).
- Hypoglossal nerve block.
- Injury of spinal cord.

NERVE BLOCKS OF THE UPPER LIMB

Brachial plexus block[11]

The literature describes over 40 different techniques, which fall into four approaches: interscalene, supraclavicular, infraclavicular, and axillary.

- No one technique is clearly better than another.
- The axillary approach is the easiest to learn with the fewest complications.
- The infraclavicular, the lateral, and sagittal approach (Klaastad's approach) is becoming popular as it is

usually successful, less painful than axillary blocks, and well suited for catheter infusion and prolonged analgesia.[12, 13, 14]

- The use of 40 mL of solution (in a healthy male patient) combined with digital pressure should produce a satisfactory block, whatever approach is used.
- Smaller volumes of solution are effective when ultrasound guidance is used, as volume to surround each root/cord can be visualized.
- The "immobile needle" technique is important. Using a 10- to 20-cm extension tube, the needle can be isolated from the movements of the syringe (aspiration, injection, and changing of syringes).
- A short, beveled needle may give better sensation when the brachial plexus sheath is breached.
- A peripheral nerve stimulator is often used to confirm the needle position, and pulse synchronous muscle movements are easily detected in the arm.
- Onset of block may take up to 40 minutes with bupivacaine.

INDICATIONS

- Surgical anesthesia of the shoulder, arm, or hand.
- Postsurgical analgesia employing continuous infusion.
- Chronic pain management employing intermittent bolus or continuous infusion:
  - Differential block.
  - Complex regional pain syndrome (to facilitate physical therapy).
  - Brachial plexus invasion by tumor.

RELEVANT ANATOMY (FIGURE 23.6)

(The ramifications and various junctions of the roots on their way to becoming peripheral nerves are not clinically relevant, only the anatomy of practical use will be described.)

- Roots arise from C4–T1.
- The radial nerve supplies all dorsal muscles in the upper arm below the shoulder.
- The musculocutaneous nerve supplies the muscles in the arm and skin sensation in the forearm.
- The median and ulnar nerves are nerves of passage in the arm, but result in motor function in the forearm and hand together with sensation in the hand.
- The median nerve is mainly responsible for forearm innervation, whereas the hand is more heavily innervated by the ulnar nerve.
- The four main peripheral nerves can be checked using the "four Ps" (**Table 23.2**).
- The vertebral arteries leave the brachiocephalic or subclavian arteries and travel upwards to enter a

bony canal in the transverse process of C6. It is important to be aware of needle tip position in this area.
- The phrenic nerve passes through the neck to the thorax on the ventral surface of the anterior scalene muscle. It is always blocked with the interscalene approach.

Interscalene block

- Best for shoulder analgesia.
- Often the ulnar nerve is spared.
- Can be performed with arm in any position.

LANDMARKS

- Cricoid cartilage.
- Posterior border of the sternomastoid muscle.
- Interscalene groove.

PRACTICAL STEPS (FIGURE 23.7)

- Position the patient supine with the head on a pillow, and turned away from the side of the block.
- Push patient's shoulder to lower the clavicle.
- A line drawn laterally from the cricoid cartilage crosses the midpoint of the sternomastoid.
- Locate the interscalene groove behind the midpoint of the posterior border of sternomastoid (roll fingers).
- The interscalene groove is at an oblique angle to the sternomastoid (it is not parallel to the sternomastoid).
- Asking the patient to sniff or inspire vigorously will relax the scalene muscles enough to feel the transverse process of C6.
- At this point, insert a 22-gauge, 3.5-cm needle aiming slightly caudad, posterior, and medially (an extension of the needle would exit the neck through the spinous process of T1).
- The plexus sheath will usually be breached at 1–2.5 cm deep; remember this should be a very superficial block.
- Advance the needle carefully until paresthesiae are elicited or there is a motor response with a nerve stimulator.
- Aspirate for blood or CSF.
- Inject slowly and incrementally.

An interscalene catheter can provide prolonged analgesia, particularly after shoulder surgery. Phrenic nerve palsy and respiratory problems have been reported, therefore the optimal infusion regime needs to be decided on an individual patient basis.

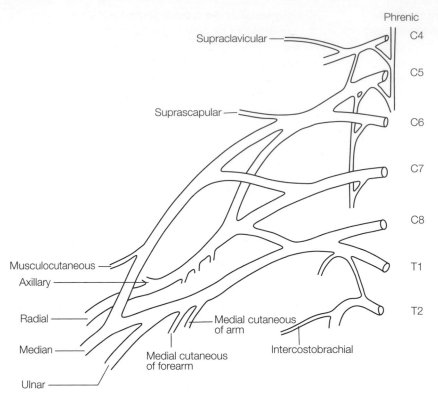

Figure 23.6 Brachial plexus. Basic anatomy of the brachial plexus. Reproduced with permission from Pinnock CA, Fischer HBJ, Jones RP. *Peripheral nerve blockade.* Edinburgh: Churchill Livingstone, 1996.

Table 23.2 Testing of four main peripheral nerves of the brachial plexus.

"Four Ps"	Action	Nerve checked
Push	Extend arm with triceps	Radial
Pull	Flex arm with biceps	Musculocutaneous
Pinch	Fifth digit	Ulnar
Pinch	Index finger	Median

Meier's approach

A different technique is required to place an interscalene catheter (Meier's approach).

LANDMARKS

- Posterior border of sternomastoid.
- Thyroid cartilage (C4).
- Subclavian artery.

PRACTICAL STEPS

- Place a mark at posterior border of sternomastoid at level of thyroid cartilage (C4).
- Draw a line from this mark to the subclavian artery above the clavicle and over the first rib.
- This line approximates to the interscalene groove.
- Insert catheter placement device caudally and parallel to the marked interscalene groove towards the subclavian artery.

- Stimulation of the deltoid muscle should occur at a depth of 3.5–5 cm.
- Real time ultrasound aids accurate catheter placement and allows visualization of the volume of solution to surround the plexus roots.

Supraclavicular block (subclavian perivascular technique)

- Best chance of blocking the entire arm.
- Delayed onset of pneumothorax may preclude use as an outpatient procedure.
- Block carried out at the "division" level of the plexus.

LANDMARKS

- Cricoid cartilage.
- Posterior border of the sternomastoid.
- Clavicle.
- Pulsation of subclavian artery.

PRACTICAL STEPS (FIGURE 23.8)

- Patient lies supine with a small pillow, head turned away from the side of the block.
- Locate the interscalene groove as above.
- Follow the interscalene groove distally until it meets the clavicle.
- The pulsation of the subclavian artery can be felt in the interscalene groove 1 cm superior to the clavicle at its midpoint.

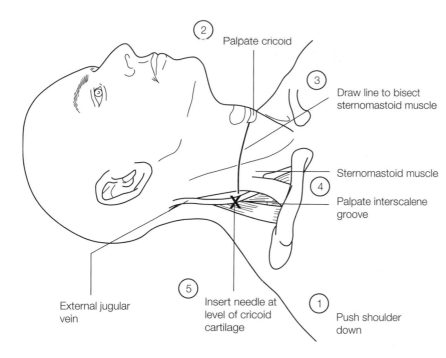

Figure 23.7 Interscalene block. Landmarks and steps for performing interscalene brachial plexus block. Reproduced with permission from Pinnock CA, Fischer HBJ, Jones RP. *Peripheral nerve blockade*. Edinburgh: Churchill Livingstone, 1996.

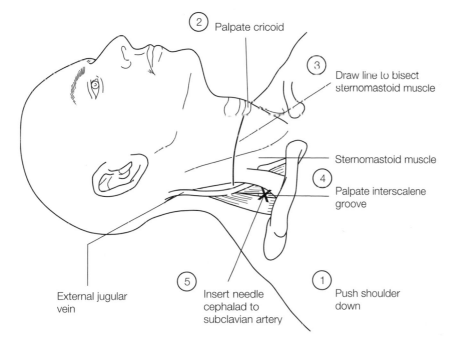

Figure 23.8 Supraclavicular block. Landmarks and steps for performing supraclavicular brachial plexus block. Reproduced with permission from Pinnock CA, Fischer HBJ, Jones RP. *Peripheral nerve blockade*. Edinburgh: Churchill Livingstone, 1996.

- The ideal position for needle insertion is just above the pulsation of the subclavian artery.
- Insert a 22-gauge, 3.5-cm needle caudally in the horizontal plane, parallel to the neck.
- The needle should pierce the plexus sheath 1–2 cm deep to the skin.
- Paresthesiae may occur immediately, and usually occur in the distribution of the superior trunk.
- A peripheral nerve stimulator may be used to confirm the needle position.
- Hold the needle in a steady position and aspirate for blood.

- Inject local anesthetic solution using digital pressure to encourage proximal or distal spread of local anesthetic as desired.
- Sheath should be seen distending.
- Subcutaneous swelling indicates an extrasheath injection.
- Continuous supraclavicular analgesia is not popular due to fear of pneumothorax. Real time ultrasound has been reported to be superior to nerve stimulation to aid catheter placement and should reduce fears of pleural puncture.

INFRACLAVICULAR, THE LATERAL AND SAGITTAL BLOCK (METHOD OF KLAASTAD[12, 13, 14])

The target is the plexus cords posterior to the pectoralis minor muscle.

LANDMARKS

- Lower border of clavicle.
- Medial aspect of coracoid process.
- Sagittal and coronal planes.

PRACTICAL STEPS (FIGURE 23.9)

- Patient lies supine with arm adducted and hand across abdomen.
- The junction of the medial aspect of the coracoid process and clavicle is marked.
- At this point a 22-gauge needle is inserted tangentially to the anteroinferior border of the clavicle and directed 15° posterior to the horizontal (coronal) plane.
- Cord contact is expected at a needle depth of 4–6.5 cm.
- A peripheral nerve stimulator is useful as it allows the patient to be sedated (needle insertion can be painful).
- Aspirate for blood (cephalic vein, axillary artery or vein), vascular puncture occurs infrequently.
- Real time ultrasound guidance reduces incidence of vascular puncture to 0.7 percent.
- Inject local anesthetic solution incrementally.

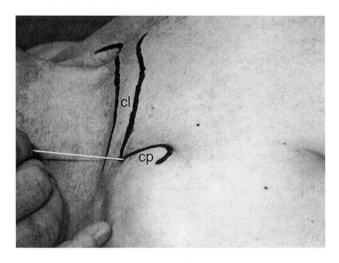

Figure 23.9 Right infraclavicular region. The coracoid process (cp) and the clavicle (cl) are marked in black. The white needle is directed approximately 15° posterior to the coronal plane. Cord contact is expected by a needle depth of 4–6.5 cm. Reprinted with permission from Klaastad Ø, Smith H-J, Smedby Ö *et al.* A novel infraclavicular brachial plexus block: the lateral and sagittal technique, developed by MRI studies. *Anesthesia and Analgesia.* 2004; **98:** 252–6.

Continuous infraclavicular block can prolong analgesia after distal arm surgery. Continuous infusion is not limited by the risks of phrenic nerve palsy. This technique has the advantage of an immobile insertion point limiting catheter dislodgment and aiding sterility. Real time ultrasound aids accurate catheter placement and optimal volume of solution to surround cords.

Axillary block

- Most effective for analgesia distal to the elbow.
- Risk of complications is low.
- Block can be single shot or continuous.
- Since the axillary artery lies at the center of a four-quadrant neurovascular bundle, some favor multiple injections to improve the quality of block.
- The block does not have to be performed high in the axilla, needle insertion in the mid to lower portion of the axillary hair patch may be easier and equally effective.
- The musculocutaneous nerve may be spared and require separate block.
- The intercostobrachial nerve is not part of the plexus and is blocked separately by subcutaneous infiltration in the medial axilla (prevents tourniquet pain).

LANDMARKS

- Axillary artery pulsation.
- Lateral border of pectoralis major.

PRACTICAL STEPS (FIGURE 23.10)

Position patient supine with arm abducted to 90° at the shoulder and the elbow flexed to 90° (overabduction may compress the axillary artery).

- Single injection or insertion of the cannula:
  - palpate the pulsation of the axillary artery at the level of the lateral border of the pectoralis major;
  - fix the artery with the palpating finger;
  - insert a 22-gauge, 3.5-cm needle or cannula just superior to the artery and parallel to it as if going to cannulate the artery;
  - as the plexus sheath is pierced, a change of resistance should be felt;
  - paresthesiae indicate correct needle placement;
  - a peripheral nerve stimulator can confirm the needle position;
  - aspirate for blood;
  - inject local anesthetic solution using digital pressure to encourage proximal spread of solution;
  - if the axillary artery is inadvertently entered, the needle can either be withdrawn or it can be advanced beyond the artery and the injection made deep to the artery (transarterial technique);

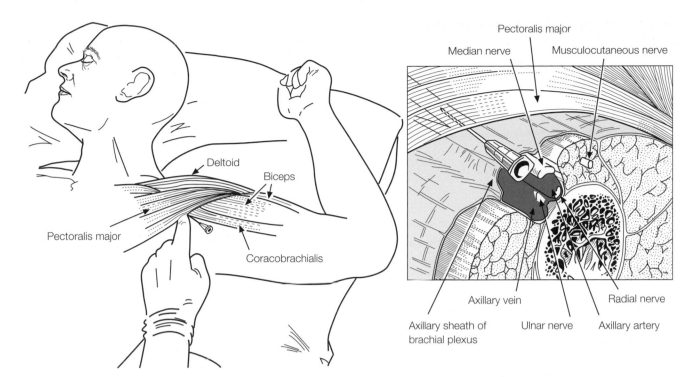

Figure 23.10 Axillary block. Landmarks for axillary brachial plexus block. Reproduced with permission from Cousins MJ, Bridenbaugh PO (eds). *Neural blockade in clinical anesthesia and management of pain.* Philadelphia: JB Lippincott, 1988.

- successful injection is indicated by a "sausage shaped" distension of the plexus sheath, whereas subcutaneous injection is indicated by a "hamburger-shaped" distension in the axilla.
- Multiple injections (**Figure 23.11**):
  - palpate and fix the axillary artery;
  - inject around the axillary artery in a "fan-like" manner;
  - divide the local anesthetic dose into four quadrant injections;
  - the median nerve is found in the 12-to-3 quadrant (as on a clock);
  - the ulnar nerve in the 3-to-6 quadrant;
  - the radial nerve in the 6-to-9 quadrant;
  - the musculocutaneous nerve in the 9-to-12 quadrant within the substance of the coracobrachialis muscle;
  - multiple stimulation has been reported as well tolerated in awake patients;
  - real time ultrasound aids accurate visualization of the nerves within these quadrants and optimal volume of solution to surround the nerves.

Continuous axillary block was one of the first perineural sites to be investigated. The ease of catheter placement and safety of infusion make this a popular technique. The main disadvantage is preventing catheter dislodgment and maintaining sterility of insertion site and catheter.

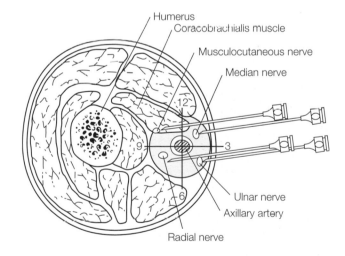

Figure 23.11 Axillary block: multiple injection technique. Needle insertion points for performing axillary brachial plexus block by multiple injection technique. Reproduced with permission from Cousins MJ, Bridenbaugh PO (eds). *Neural blockade in clinical anesthesia and management of pain.* Philadelphia: JB Lippincott, 1988.

COMPLICATIONS OF BRACHIAL PLEXUS BLOCK

For a description of possible complications, see **Table 23.3**.

Table 23.3 Complications of brachial plexus blocks.

	Axillary	Infraclavicular	Supraclavicular	Interscalene	
Vertebral artery injection	−	−	+/−	+ +	Rare but can be lethal
Subarachnoid/epidural injection	−	−	+	+ +	Rare but dangerous
Phrenic nerve palsy	+/−	+/−	+ +	+ + +	36–90% usually asymptomatic
Recurrent laryngeal nerve palsy	−	−	+	+	1.5–6% incidence
Stellate ganglion block	+	+	+ +	+ + +	50–90% incidence
Pneumothorax	+/−	+/−	+ + +	+	0.6–25% usually asymptomatic

Suprascapular nerve block

The suprascapular nerve can be blocked by the anterior, posterior, or superior approach.[15] Only the posterior approach will be described.

INDICATIONS

Local anesthetic block

- Postsurgical pain relief.
- Assessment of shoulder pain (differential block).
- Trial block prior to neurolysis.

Local anesthetic and depot steroid block

- To facilitate physical therapy of the shoulder joint (capsulitis, bursitis, tendonitis).
- Shoulder stiffness and pain secondary to complex regional pain syndrome.

Neurolytic block

- Cancer pain.

RELEVANT ANATOMY

- The suprascapular nerve is a branch of the brachial plexus (C4–6).
- The nerve passes under the coracoclavicular ligament through the suprascapular notch.
- The artery and vein accompany the nerve through the notch.
- The nerve supplies sensation of the shoulder joint.
- The nerve innervates infraspinatus and supraspinatus muscles.

LANDMARKS

- Spine of scapula.

PRACTICAL STEPS (FIGURE 23.12)

- The posterior approach is only suitable for conscious patients because the patient is sitting.
- Palpate the spine of the scapula and identify its midpoint.

- The suprascapular notch lies approximately 1 cm above.
- Insert a 22-gauge, short, beveled needle at right angles to the skin until bony contact is made (usually 2–3 cm).
- "Walk" the needle upwards to the edge of the suprascapular notch.
- Paresthesiae may occur.
- Avoid entering the notch too deeply and causing nerve damage or pneumothorax.
- Avoid angling the needle superiorly and passing over the top of the scapula.
- Aspirate for blood.
- Inject 10 mL of local anesthetic (+/− steroid).

COMPLICATIONS

- Intravascular injection.
- Pneumothorax.

Nerve blocks at the elbow[16]

- The ulnar, median, and radial nerves may be blocked at the elbow.
- This provides sensory loss to the hand and motor loss to forearm and hand muscles.
- Sensory loss to the forearm requires block of the lateral, medial, and posterior cutaneous nerves of the forearm.

INDICATIONS

- Minor surgery or postsurgery analgesia distal to the elbow.
- Supplementation of brachial plexus block.
- Localization of pain to a single nerve.

RELEVANT ANATOMY

- The ulnar nerve enters the forearm by passing behind the medial epicondyle of the humerus before passing down the ulnar side of the forearm.
- The median nerve lies immediately medial to the brachial artery just proximal to the flexor skin crease of the elbow. It lies just deep to the bicipital aponeurosis.

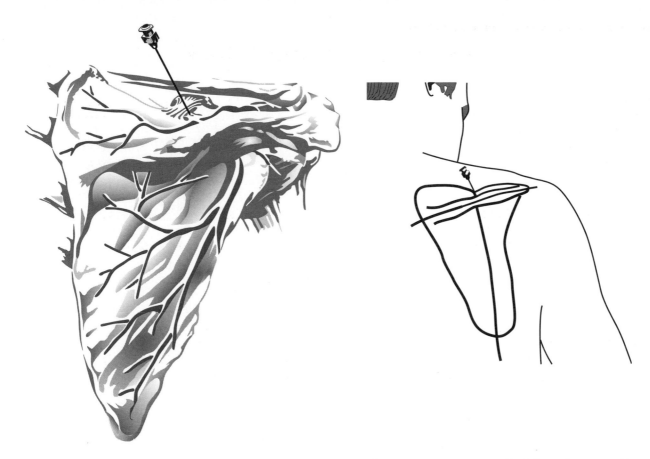

Figure 23.12 Suprascapular nerve block. Landmarks and needle insertion point for suprascapular nerve block (posterior approach). Reproduced with permission from Eriksson E (ed.). *Illustrated handbook in local anaesthesia.* Copenhagen: Munksgaard, 1969.

- The medial cutaneous nerve of the forearm lies subcutaneously above the bicipital aponeurosis.
- The radial nerve is the largest branch of the plexus. It crosses in front of the lateral epicondyle of the humerus, in a groove deep to the brachioradialis muscle and lateral to the biceps tendon to enter the forearm.
- The lateral cutaneous nerve of the forearm is the continuation of the musculocutaneous nerve and lies just below the deep fascia, lateral to the biceps tendon.
- The posterior cutaneous nerve of the forearm is a proximal branch of the radial nerve and lies subcutaneously over the lateral epicondyle of the humerus.

Ulnar nerve block

LANDMARKS

- Medial epicondyle of humerus.
- Ulnar sulcus.

PRACTICAL STEPS (FIGURE 23.13)

- Place the hand behind the head under a pillow.
- At the elbow, palpate the medial epicondyle.

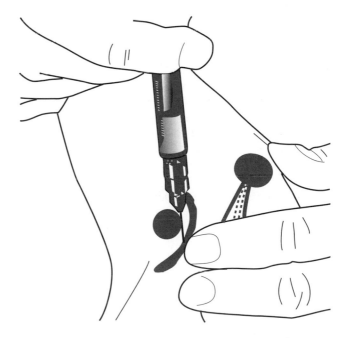

Figure 23.13 Ulnar nerve block. Landmarks and needle insertion point for ulnar nerve block. Reproduced with permission from Cousins MJ, Bridenbaugh PO (eds). *Neural blockade in clinical anesthesia and management of pain.* Philadelphia: JB Lippincott, 1988.

- Needle insertion site is 1 cm proximal to the epicondyle, where it may be possible to palpate the nerve.
- Insert a 25-gauge, 3.5 cm needle horizontally, 1–2 cm deep to the skin, until paresthesiae are elicited.
- If bone is contacted, reposition the needle.
- Nerve is superficial.
- Take care not to inject into nerve.
- Inject 5 mL of local anesthetic solution.
- Avoid the ulnar nerve sulcus within the epicondyle as the nerve is fixed and easily damaged by a needle or compression by local anesthetic.

Median nerve and medial cutaneous nerve of the forearm blocks

LANDMARKS

- Antecubital fossa.
- Pulse of brachial artery.
- Medial border of biceps tendon.
- Head of pronator teres.

PRACTICAL STEPS (FIGURE 23.14)

- With the arm abducted to 45°, palpate the intermuscular groove between the biceps tendon and pronator teres.
- Locate the brachial pulse within this groove.
- At this point, insert a 25-gauge, 3.5-cm needle just medial to the artery and just proximal to the elbow crease, angled at 45° to the skin.
- Piercing of the biceps aponeurosis may be felt.
- Once paresthesiae are elicited, inject 5 mL of local anesthetic solution slowly.
- On completion of the median nerve block, withdraw the needle until subcutaneous.
- Redirect proximally along intermuscular groove, injecting a "sausage" of local anesthetic (5–7 mL of solution).

Radial nerve and lateral cutaneous nerve of the forearm blocks

LANDMARKS

- Antecubital fossa.
- Lateral epicondyle of humerus.
- Lateral border of biceps tendon.
- Medial border of brachioradialis muscle.

PRACTICAL STEPS (FIGURE 23.14)

- Palpate the intermuscular groove between the biceps and brachioradialis muscles just proximal to the flexor skin crease of the antecubital fossa.

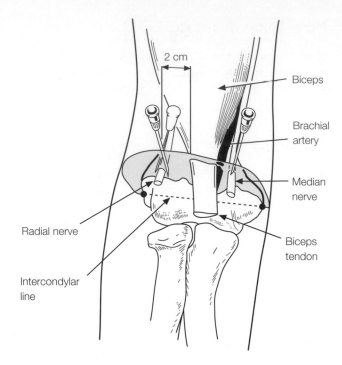

Figure 23.14 Median and radial nerve blocks. Landmarks and needle insertion point for median and radial nerve blocks at the elbow. Reproduced with permission from Cousins MJ, Bridenbaugh PO (eds). *Neural blockade in clinical anesthesia and management of pain.* Philadelphia: JB Lippincott, 1988.

- The nerve runs deep to the brachioradialis at this point.
- A nerve stimulator is useful as nerve location can be difficult.
- Insert a 25-gauge, 3.5-cm needle directed proximally to reach the anterior aspect of the lateral epicondyle.
- After contact with bone, inject 5 mL of local anesthetic solution.
- While withdrawing the needle, inject a further 5 mL of solution to block the lateral cutaneous nerve, which lies just deep to the fascia lateral to the biceps tendon.

Posterior cutaneous nerve of forearm block

- Flex arm across the chest of the patient.
- Inject a subcutaneous "sausage" over the lateral epicondyle toward the olecranon process.
- Inject 5 mL of local anesthetic solution.

COMPLICATIONS

- Risk of nerve damage with intraneural injection.
- Compression of nerve with a large volume of local anesthetic.
- Hematoma.

Nerve blocks at the wrist

Nerve blocks at the wrist[17] produces sensory block of the hand and motor block of the intrinsic hand muscles. The flexor and extensor muscle of the forearm are left intact.

INDICATIONS

- Minor surgery of all or part of the hand.
- Complex hand surgery where ability to use forearm muscles is required.
- Postsurgical analgesia (after brachial plexus block, to regain control of arm).
- Localization of pain in the territory of a single nerve.

RELEVANT ANATOMY

- The median nerve lies superficially at the level of the proximal skin crease, between the tendon of palmaris longus and the tendon of flexor carpi radialis.
- The ulnar nerve is lateral and deep to the flexor carpi ulnaris tendon, medial to the artery.
- The radial nerve emerges deep to the brachioradialis tendon and winds round the radius onto the dorsum of the wrist.

Ulnar nerve block (medial approach)

- The ulnar nerve divides into a dorsal and a palmar branch, both branches need to be blocked.
- The nerve can be blocked by a ventral or a medial approach. The medial approach allows both nerve branches to be blocked from the same needle insertion site. The medial approach is less likely to damage the artery.

LANDMARKS

- Flexor carpi ulnaris tendon.
- Ulnar artery pulse.
- Pisiform bone.

PRACTICAL STEPS (FIGURE 23.15)

- Position arm supine and abducted.
- At 1 cm proximal to the pisiform bone at the wrist, insert a 25-gauge needle at 90° to the skin immediately deep to the flexor carpi ulnaris.
- Advance the needle to a depth of 1–2 cm and aspirate for blood.
- Inject 4 mL of local anesthetic solution.
- Withdraw the needle until subcutaneous and redirect both dorsally and ventrally to block the dorsal and palmar branches with 2 mL of solution.

Median nerve block

LANDMARKS

- Flexor carpi radialis tendon.
- Palmaris longus tendon (if present).

PRACTICAL STEPS (FIGURE 23.16)

- Ask the patient to flex their wrist against resistance to outline the tendon of palmaris longus.
- If present, insert a 25-gauge needle just lateral to the tendon.
- If not present, insert needle 1 cm medial to the ulnar border of the flexor carpi radialis tendon.
- The flexor retinaculum should be encountered at a depth of less than 1 cm.

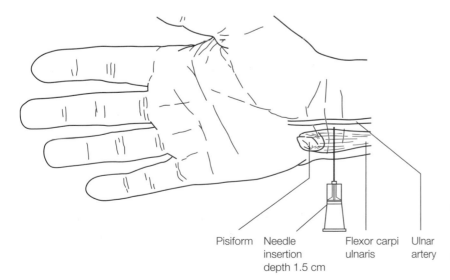

Pisiform   Needle insertion depth 1.5 cm   Flexor carpi ulnaris   Ulnar artery

Figure 23.15 Ulnar nerve block. Landmarks and needle insertion point for ulnar nerve block at the wrist. Reproduced with permission from Pinnock CA, Fischer HBJ, Jones RP. *Peripheral nerve blockade.* Edinburgh: Churchill Livingstone, 1996.

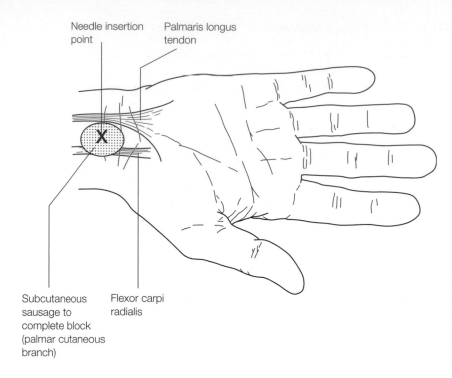

Figure 23.16 Median nerve block. Landmarks and needle insertion point for median nerve block at the wrist. Reproduced with permission from Pinnock CA, Fischer HBJ, Jones RP. *Peripheral nerve blockade*. Edinburgh: Churchill Livingstone, 1996.

- Advance the needle a further 2–3 mm as the nerve lies immediately deep to the retinaculum.
- Move needle fanwise to elicit paresthesiae.
- Immobilize needle and inject 3 mL of local anesthetic solution.
- Resistance to injection should not occur (withdraw to prevent intraneural injection).
- Withdraw needle until subcutaneous, and inject a further 2 mL to block the palmar cutaneous branch.

Radial nerve block

LANDMARKS

- "Anatomical snuff box."
- Radial styloid.
- Ulnar styloid.

PRACTICAL STEPS (FIGURE 23.17)

- At the level of the "anatomical snuff box," the radial nerve is superficial.
- Insert a 25-gauge needle and raise a subcutaneous "sausage" of local anesthetic solution in a ring from across the base of the anatomical snuff box toward the ulnar border of the wrist in a line joining both styloid processes together.
- Inject 7–10 mL of local anesthetic solution.
- This technique more resembles a "field block."

COMPLICATIONS

- Nerve blocks at the wrist are superficial and complications are few.
- Risk of nerve damage if intraneural injection occurs.
- Hematoma.

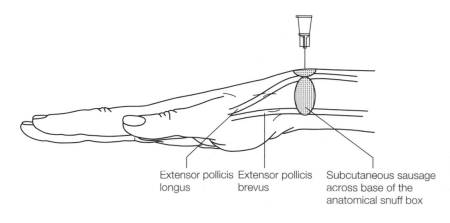

Figure 23.17 Radial nerve block. Landmarks and needle insertion point for radial nerve block at the wrist. Reproduced with permission from Pinnock CA, Fischer HBJ, Jones RP. *Peripheral nerve blockade*. Edinburgh: Churchill Livingstone, 1996.

NERVE BLOCKS OF THE THORAX AND ABDOMEN

Thoracic paravertebral block[18]

INDICATIONS

Local anesthetic block

- Analgesia following thoracotomy or nephrectomy.
- Fractured ribs.
- Thoracic vertebral collapse or compression fracture.
- Acute herpes zoster.
- Differential block for evaluation of chest wall, upper abdominal, and thoracic spinal pain.
- Prognostic block prior to neurolysis.

Local anesthetic and steroid block

- Postthoracotomy pain.
- Postherpetic neuralgia.
- Rib fractures.

Neurolytic block (phenol, cryoneurolysis, or radiofrequency)

- Cancer of thoracic spine, ribs, chest wall, and abdominal wall.

RELEVANT ANATOMY

- The spinal cord gives rise to 12 pairs of thoracic nerves (T1–12).
- The thoracic paravertebral nerves pass below the transverse process of the vertebra after leaving their intervertebral foramina.
- A branch loops back through the intervertebral foramina to supply the spinal ligaments, meninges, and vertebra.
- Within the paravertebral space, the thoracic nerve communicates with the sympathetic nervous system and then divides into a posterior and anterior primary division.
- The posterior division supplies the interfacetal joints, muscles, and skin of the back.
- The anterior division passes into the subcostal groove beneath the rib to become the intercostal nerve.
- The 12th thoracic nerve lies beneath the 12th rib and becomes the subcostal nerve.
- The intercostal and subcostal nerves supply skin, muscles, ribs, parietal pleura, and parietal peritoneum.

LANDMARKS

- Thoracic vertebral spinous processes.

PRACTICAL STEPS (FIGURE 23.18)

- Patient may be positioned prone or lateral.
- Identify the spinous process of the vertebra above the nerve to be blocked.

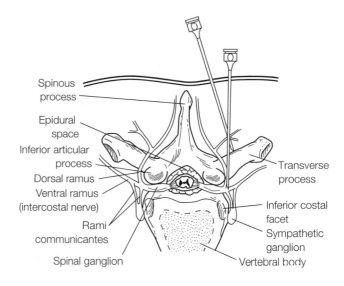

Figure 23.18 Thoracic paravertebral block. Landmarks and needle insertion point for thoracic paravertebral block. Reproduced with permission from Cousins MJ, Bridenbaugh PO (eds). *Neural blockade in clinical anesthesia and management of pain.* Philadelphia: JB Lippincott, 1988.

- Mark a point 3 cm lateral to the upper (cephalad) border of the spinous process.
- At this point, insert a 22-gauge, 8-cm spinal needle perpendicular to the skin and advance the needle aiming for the transverse process (usual depth 3–4 cm).
- Withdraw the needle slightly and redirect upwards (cephalad) so that the needle tip "walks off" the upper border of the transverse process.
- Once bony contact is lost, advance the needle a further 2–3 cm.
- Avoid directing the needle too medial as an epidural or intrathecal injection may occur.
- Avoid directing the needle too lateral as an intercostal or interpleural injection may occur.
- As the needle is advanced beyond the transverse process, a loss of resistance may be felt as the costotransverse ligament is crossed.
- Loss of resistance to saline can be used to confirm the needle position.
- Occasionally, paresthesiae may occur.
- A nerve stimulator can be used, when pulse synchronous movement of the rectus muscle will be seen.
- Aspirate for CSF or blood.
- Inject 5 mL of local anesthetic solution to block three or four dermatomes.
- If continuous analgesia is planned, the procedure can be performed using a peridural kit, leaving behind a catheter in the paravertebral space.

COMPLICATIONS

- Pneumothorax (up to 20 percent incidence).
- Epidural, subdural, or intrathecal injection.
- Trauma to nerve roots.
- Hematoma.
- Infection (immunocompromised patients).

Intercostal nerve block[19][I]

INDICATIONS

Local anesthetic block

- Rib fractures.
- Chest wall contusion.
- Pleurisy.
- Fractured sternum.
- Insertion of chest drain.
- Analgesia after thoracic or abdominal surgery.
- Diagnostic block in visceral versus somatic pain.

Local anesthetic and steroid

- Acute herpes zoster.
- Postherpetic neuralgia.
- Postthoracotomy pain.

Neurolytic block

- Rib or chest wall invasion by tumor.

RELEVANT ANATOMY

- Intercostal nerves are the continuation of the anterior primary division of thoracic nerves. T1 contributes to the brachial plexus; T2–3 form a cutaneous branch to the arm (intercostobrachial nerve); T12 forms the subcostal nerve, which descends in the abdominal wall and communicates with L1.
- The classic vein, artery, and nerve pattern below each rib only occurs in 17 percent of people. The nerve varies from midcostal (73 percent) to supracostal (10 percent). Intercostal nerves may split into two distinctive bundles, which may later rejoin.
- Each intercostal nerve usually gives off four branches (**Table 23.4**).

Table 23.4 Branches of the intercostal nerves.

Branch	Innervation
Gray rami communicantes	Sympathetic ganglion
Posterior cutaneous branch	Paravertebral muscles and skin
Lateral cutaneous division	Anterior and lateral skin sensation
Anterior cutaneous branch	Midline chest and abdominal skin

LANDMARKS

- Angle of rib.
- Midaxillary line.

PRACTICAL STEPS (FIGURE 23.19)

Posterior approach

The block is performed posteriorly at the angle of the rib, just lateral to the sacrospinous muscles (usually 8 cm lateral to the spinous process).

- Count ribs upwards from 12th rib and identify angle of required rib.
- Retract skin and subcutaneous tissues upwards.
- Insert a 25-gauge, 3.5-cm needle onto the rib.
- Withdraw the needle and redirect to "walk off" the lower border of the rib.
- Aspirate for blood.
- Inject 3–4 mL of local anesthetic solution.
- Multiple blocks are often carried out together and can be painful.

Midaxillary approach

- This block is performed in the midaxillary line. The lateral cutaneous branch may be missed, but this can be blocked by infiltrating subcutaneously on withdrawal of the needle.
- Suitable for supine patients that cannot be turned.
- Upper intercostal nerves can be blocked by raising the patient's arm to access the axilla.

Anterior approach

- The intercostal nerves can be blocked anterior to the midaxillary line.
- Parasternal blocks may be used after sternotomy or rectus sheath blocks for abdominal wall analgesia.

COMPLICATIONS

- Pneumothorax (related to the experience of the operator and failure to control the depth of the needle).
- Systemic toxicity.
- Hypotension (central spread of local anesthetic).
- Respiratory depression (effective nerve block after systemic opioids).

Interpleural block

The exact mechanism of action for an interpleural block[20] is not understood, but it has been shown that sensory and autonomic fibers are blocked, and often a unilateral block has bilateral effects. Interpleural block should not be attempted bilaterally as the risk of pneumothorax is too great.

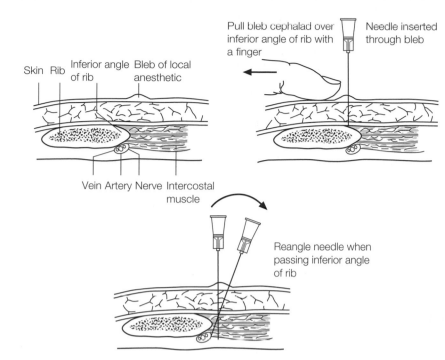

Figure 23.19 Intercostal nerve block. Landmarks and needle insertion point for intercostal nerve block. Reproduced with permission from Pinnock CA, Fischer HBJ, Jones RP. *Peripheral nerve blockade.* Edinburgh: Churchill Livingstone, 1996.

INDICATIONS

Postsurgical analgesia

- Unilateral subcostal analgesia after surgery.
- Breast surgery.
- Renal surgery.
- Multiple rib fractures.
- Cardiac surgery.

Chronic pain

- Chronic pancreatitis.
- Postherpetic neuralgia.
- Complex regional pain syndrome.

Cancer pain

- Pancreatic cancer.
- Upper abdominal cancer.
- Breast cancer.
- Chest wall cancer.

RELATIVE CONTRAINDICATIONS

- Significant respiratory disease (pneumothorax would be disastrous).
- Bronchopleural fistula.
- Prior pleurodesis.

RELEVANT ANATOMY

- The pleural space is 10–20 μm wide and 2000 cm^2 in area (in an adult male).
- The interpleural space lies between the visceral pleura lining the heart and lungs and the parietal pleura covering the thoracic cage.
- Interpleural pressure varies from −12 cmH$_2$O at the lung apices to −5 cmH$_2$O at the lung bases.

LANDMARKS

- Angle of sixth or seventh rib.

PRACTICAL STEPS (FIGURE 23.20)

The patient's position is determined by the requirement of the block.

- Sensory block of intercostal nerves: position the patient with affected side down with head down tilt (20°) to block T1–9.
- Sympathetic block: affected side up with head down tilt for cervical sympathetic chain.
- Combined sensory and sympathetic block: initially, affected side up, then turn patient supine:
  - with the patient in the lateral position, identify the angle of the sixth or seventh rib;
  - insert an 18-gauge Tuohy needle attached to a "loss-of-resistance" device (either a syringe of saline or a 500-mL bag of saline);
  - aim the needle at 45° toward the upper edge of the rib;
  - once contact has been made with the rib, walk the needle off the upper border of the rib and advance into the pleural space;
  - at this point, the saline will run easily or can be injected easily;
  - hold needle immobile with one hand and either insert a catheter or slowly inject 20 mL of local anesthetic solution;
  - the technique can be refined using one of several commercially available devices. Special "closed

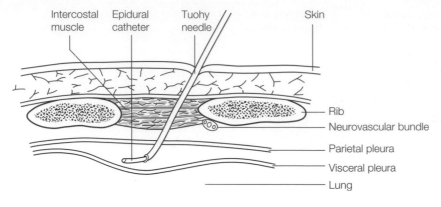

Intercostal muscle · Epidural catheter · Tuohy needle · Skin · Rib · Neurovascular bundle · Parietal pleura · Visceral pleura · Lung

Figure 23.20 Interpleural block. Landmarks and needle insertion point for interpleural block. Reproduced with permission from Pinnock CA, Fischer HBJ, Jones RP. *Peripheral nerve blockade.* Edinburgh: Churchill Livingstone, 1996.

system" kits are available with "one-way valves" to prevent the entrainment of air;
- the needle is best inserted at the end of expiration to minimize risk of lung damage;
- a postblock chest radiograph is advised, particularly after catheter insertion.

COMPLICATIONS

- Pneumothorax (5 percent).
- Pleural effusion (0.4 percent).
- Systemic toxicity of local anesthetic.
- Malposition of catheter.
- Infection.
- Bronchopleural fistula.

Ilioinguinal, iliohypogastric, and genitofemoral nerve blocks[21]

INDICATIONS

- Inguinal hernia surgery.
- Postsurgical analgesia.
- Ilioinguinal–iliohypogastric neuralgia.
- Genitofemoral neuralgia.
- Chronic testicular pain.
- Neuroma.

RELEVANT ANATOMY

- The iliohypogastric nerve (L1) runs between transversus abdominus and internal oblique muscles reaching the lower abdomen 4 cm medial to the anterior superior iliac spine to supply the skin above the inguinal ligament.
- The ilioinguinal nerve (L1) runs parallel to, but deep to, the iliohypogastric nerve. The nerve passes through the external inguinal ring and gives branches to the scrotum (labia majora).
- The genitofemoral nerve (L1 and L2) splits into two on the psoas muscle just above the inguinal ligament to give the genital and femoral branches. The genital branch follows the spermatic cord and supplies the cremasteric muscle and skin of the scrotum (labia

majora), while the femoral branch supplies the skin overlying the femoral triangle.

LANDMARKS

- Anterior superior iliac spine (ASIS).
- Pubic tubercle.
- External inguinal ring.

PRACTICAL STEPS (FIGURE 23.21)

Iliohypogastric and ilioinguinal nerve blocks

- Position the patient supine.
- Identify the ASIS.
- Mark a point 2 cm medial and inferior to the ASIS.
- Insert a 22-gauge, 3.5-cm needle at this point, advancing until the resistance of the aponeurosis of the external oblique muscle is felt.
- The needle is advanced slowly until the aponeurosis is pierced, the iliohypogastric nerve lies just deep to the aponeurosis.
- Aspirate for blood, and inject 5 mL of local anesthetic solution.
- Advance the needle further through the internal oblique muscle (1–2 cm) and inject a further 5 mL of solution to block the ilioinguinal nerve.

Genitofemoral nerve block

- Invaginate the skin of the scrotum through the external ring to exclude hernia contents in the canal.
- Palpate the line between the ASIS and the pubic tubercle; 1 cm above its midpoint, the deep inguinal ring can be felt – place a finger at this point.
- Insert a 22-gauge, 3.5-cm needle parallel to the canal, 1 cm distal to the finger overlying the deep ring.
- Often a loss of resistance is felt as the needle pierces the external oblique aponeurosis to enter the inguinal canal.
- Aspirate for blood and inject 5 mL of local anesthetic solution.
- The femoral vessels and nerve lie immediately deep to the canal; therefore, the needle depth should be controlled.

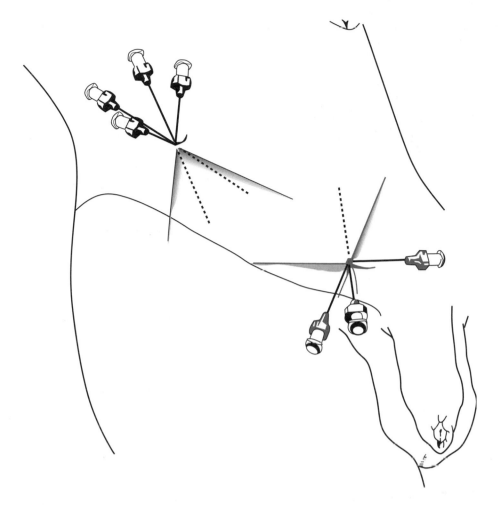

Figure 23.21 Ilioinguinal, iliohypogastric, and genitofemoral nerve blocks. Landmarks and needle insertion positions for ilioinguinal, iliohypogastric, and genitofemoral nerve blocks. Reproduced with permission from Eriksson E (ed.). *Illustrated handbook in local anaesthesia.* Copenhagen: Munksgaard, 1969.

COMPLICATIONS

- Hematoma.
- Damage to the spermatic cord.
- Damage to the bowel.
- Inadvertent femoral nerve block.

NERVE BLOCKS OF THE LOWER LIMB

The more easily accomplished central nerve blockade is often preferred to peripheal nerve blocks for surgical anesthesia.[22] However, in those patients in which central nerve blockade is contraindicated or patients who cannot tolerate the cardiovascular effects, peripheral nerve blocks still have a place. Discrete nerve blockade always has a place in diagnosis and treatment of chronic pain syndromes.

The nerve supply to the lower limb comprises two plexus and five major terminal branches.

Lumbar plexus block

The lumbar plexus can be blocked by two proximal techniques: a paravertebral technique which blocks the nerve roots and the lumbar plexus block or psoas compartment block which blocks the loops of the plexus.[23] A distal technique has also been advocated, referred to as either the "Winnie three-in-one block" the "inguinal paravascular block," or the "fascia iliaca block."

INDICATIONS

- Surgery of hip, thigh, or upper leg.
- Postsurgical analgesia.
- Cancer of hip or upper femur.

Blockade of the lower limb is not achieved without also blocking the sacral plexus.

RELEVANT ANATOMY

- The lumbar plexus is formed by the anterior divisions of L1–4; T12 is included in 50 percent and occasionally L5.
- The plexus is formed in front of the lumbar transverse processes and then lies as deep loops within a "compartment" deep in the psoas muscle at the medial border of quadratum lumborum.
- The individual nerves then course to their site of innervation.
- The lumbar sympathetic chain is closely related: it lies on the anterolateral surface of the lumbar and sacral bodies medial to the anterior foramina.
- There are connections between the lumbar plexus and the sympathetic chain, despite being separated anatomically.
- Lumbar spinous processes are nearly horizontal and are usually 3–4 cm deep.
- Lumbar transverse processes are short (3 cm). The average depth of a transverse process to skin is 5 cm.

LANDMARKS

- Spinous process of lumbar vertebrae.

PRACTICAL STEPS (FIGURE 23.22)

The classical technique describes multiple paravertebral injections; however, single injection techniques between L2 and L5 have been advocated (psoas compartment block).

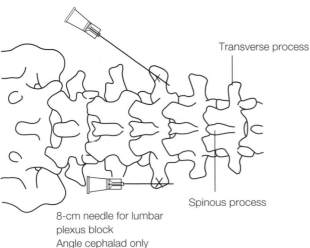

8-cm needle for paravertebral block
Angle medially and cephalad

Transverse process

Spinous process

8-cm needle for lumbar plexus block
Angle cephalad only

Figure 23.22 Lumbar plexus block. Landmarks and needle insertion points for the "paravertebral" and "psoas compartment" techniques. Reproduced with permission from Pinnock CA, Fischer HBJ, Jones RP. *Peripheral nerve blockade.* Edinburgh: Churchill Livingstone, 1996.

- Position the patient with the side of the block uppermost or, alternatively, prone with a pillow under the abdomen.
- Identify spinous process of L3 and mark a point 3 cm lateral.
- At this point, insert a 22-gauge, 8-cm spinal needle, at right angles to the skin until the tip contacts the transverse process (usually 5 cm deep).
- Withdraw needle slightly and redirect.

Paravertebral technique

Redirect the needle cephalad and medially so that the tip just passes above and 2–3 cm deep to the transverse process. Paresthesiae may occur. Aspirate for blood or CSF and inject local anesthetic solution: either 5-mL boluses at multiple levels or a single injection of 15–20 mL.

Lumbar plexus (psoas compartment) technique

Redirect needle cephalad only. Advance the needle until parallel to the midline about 2 cm deep to the transverse process. Entry into the psoas compartment will be indicated by a loss of resistance, which can be confirmed with a syringe of saline. Aspirate for blood and inject local anesthetic solution (15–20 mL).

Distal technique (Winnie three-in-one, or inguinal paravascular block or fascia iliaca block)

- Position patient supine.
- Mark a point just lateral to the femoral artery and just below the inguinal ligament.
- At this point, insert a 22-gauge, 8-cm needle or a 20-gauge cannula at an angle of 20° to the skin. Direct the needle cephalad and parallel to the artery – a distinct give will be felt as the needle penetrates the fascia lata and then the fascia iliaca around the nerve.
- Needle position can be confirmed by a syringe of saline demonstrating a "loss of resistance" or a nerve stimulator causing pulse-synchronous movement of the sartorius muscle.
- Aspirate for blood.
- Inject 20–30 mL of local anesthetic solution, which should block the femoral, obturator, and lateral cutaneous nerve of the thigh.

This distal approach to the lumbar plexus is not always reliable. The lateral cutaneous nerve of the thigh is frequently missed. The block may also spill over to involve the sacral plexus and the sciatic nerve may be blocked.

COMPLICATIONS

- Inadvertent epidural or intrathecal injection (proximal techniques).
- Inadvertent puncture of major vessels (needle too deep).

- Nerve trauma.
- Infection.

Continuous lumbar plexus block has been advocated for prolonged analgesia after hip, knee, and femoral shaft surgery. It is commonly combined with continuous sciatic nerve blockade when excessive doses of local anesthetic must be avoided. A proximal catheter can be inserted blindly using the psoas compartment technique to place 3–5 cm of catheter after distension of the tissue space with 20–30 mL of solution. A real time ultrasound technique employs the fascia iliaca approach where the catheter placement needle is advanced into the plane deep to the fascia iliaca and approximately 1 cm lateral to the femoral nerve. Correct needle position is confirmed by observing distribution of solution in the plane of the fascia iliaca towards the femoral nerve. After distension with 30 mL of solution the catheter is left in place. Catheter dislodgment and maintenance of sterilty at the groin can be problematic.

Sacral plexus block

This is a paravertebral block which, when combined with the lumbar plexus block, anesthetizes the lower limb; S1–3 contribute to the sciatic nerve.

INDICATIONS

- Temporary relief of sciatica.
- Cancer pain in the distribution of sacral nerve roots.
- In combination with lumbar plexus block for surgery of leg, thigh, or hip.

RELEVANT ANATOMY

- The sacral plexus comprises L4–5 and S1–3 nerves and part of S4.
- It lies on the anterior surface of the sacrum on top of the piriformis muscle.
- It is covered by pelvic fascia and anterior to the plexus and fascia lie the ureter, bowel, and iliac vessels.
- The plexus divides into two branches.
- The collateral branches supply the pudendal plexus, the hip joint, and gluteal, adductor, and hamstring muscles.
- The terminal branches supply the greater and lesser sciatic nerves.
- The sacrum has two rows of openings on its posterior surface (posterior sacral foramina).
- These rows of foramina are not parallel to the edges of the sacrum – they angle less steeply to the midline as they descend.
- The transacral canal is narrow, being 2.5 cm deep at S1 and 0.5 cm deep at S4.

LANDMARKS

- Posterior superior iliac spine.
- Sacral cornu.

PRACTICAL STEPS (FIGURE 23.23)

- Position patient prone with a pillow under the pelvis.
- Draw a line from a point 1 cm medial and 1 cm below the posterior superior iliac spine to a point 1 cm lateral and 1 cm above the sacral cornu. A third point is marked at the midpoint of this line. This identifies the foramina of S2–4.
- Soft tissues overlying the foramina are greatest over the upper foramina, but the S2 foramina is often easiest to identify.
- A 22-gauge, 8-cm needle is inserted toward the posterior surface of the sacrum until it contacts bone.
- The needle is withdrawn slightly and adjusted medially until it enters the foramina.
- Advance the needle 2 cm into the upper foramina and less than 0.5 cm for the lowest foramina.
- A peripheral nerve stimulator can be helpful for confirming the needle position.
- Aspirate for blood and CSF.
- Inject 5 mL of local anesthetic solution.
- Repeat at several foramina if blocking the entire plexus.

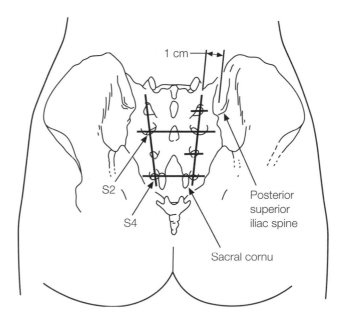

Figure 23.23 Sacral plexus block. Landmarks and needle insertion points for sacral nerve blocks. Reproduced with permission from Cousins MJ, Bridenbaugh PO (eds). *Neural blockade in clinical anesthesia and management of pain.* Philadelphia: JB Lippincott, 1988.

COMPLICATIONS

- Loss of parasympathetic function to bladder and bowel.
- Inadvertent intrathecal injection.
- Inadvertent vascular injection.
- Inadvertent puncture of bowel.

Peripheral branches of the lumbosacral plexus

The lumbar and sacral plexuses have five peripheral branches: femoral, obturator, lateral cutaneous, sciatic, and posterior cutaneous nerves.[24]

The femoral, obturator, and lateral cutaneous nerves can be blocked simultaneously by the "three-in-one block" or "fascia iliaca block" and are described above under Lumbar plexus block. In this section, blocks of the individual nerves will be described.

Femoral nerve block

INDICATIONS

- Analgesia after femoral fracture.
- Surgery or postsurgical analgesia of the knee (along with sciatic, obturator, and lateral cutaneous nerve block).

RELEVANT ANATOMY

- The femoral nerve is the largest branch of the plexus.
- It enters the leg below the inguinal ligament lateral to the femoral vessels.
- It is covered in its own fascial sheath (iliopectineal fascia) and lies deep to the fascia lata.
- It has an anterior and posterior division.

- The anterior division is motor to sartorius and sensory to the anterior and medial skin of the thigh, including the knee.
- The posterior division is motor to quadriceps femoris, sensory to the knee, and ends as the saphenous nerve.

LANDMARKS

- Inguinal ligament.
- Femoral artery.

PRACTICAL STEPS (FIGURE 23.24)

- Identify and mark a point 1 cm lateral to the femoral artery 1 cm below the inguinal ligament.
- Insert a 22-gauge, 3.5-cm needle to a depth of 3 cm (deeper than the artery).
- A peripheral nerve stimulator, showing pulse-synchronous movement of the sartorius muscle, can confirm needle placement.
- Aspirate for blood.
- Inject 10 mL of local anesthetic solution.
- Withdraw the needle, redirect it 3 cm lateral to the artery, and inject a further 5 mL of solution as often the nerve has already divided into two.
- If the artery is punctured, pressure should be applied for at least five minutes to minimize the hematoma.

COMPLICATIONS

- Hematoma.
- Nerve trauma.
- Pain at site of injection.
- Infection.

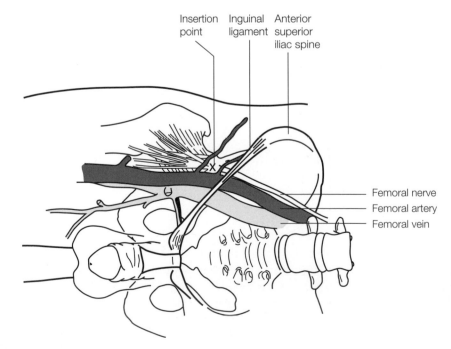

Insertion point   Inguinal ligament   Anterior superior iliac spine

Femoral nerve
Femoral artery
Femoral vein

Figure 23.24 Femoral nerve block. Landmarks and needle insertion point for femoral nerve block. Reproduced with permission from Pinnock CA, Fischer HBJ, Jones RP. *Peripheral nerve blockade.* Edinburgh: Churchill Livingstone, 1996.

Obturator nerve block

The obturator nerve can be blocked by either a direct or an indirect approach (Winnie three-in-one block). The Winnie three-in-one block may not reliably block the obturator nerve, and has been described above.

INDICATIONS

- Surgery or postsurgical analgesia of the knee (in conjunction with sciatic, femoral, and lateral cutaneous block).
- To abolish stimulation by diathermy during bladder surgery.
- Diagnosis of obturator nerve entrapment.
- Neurolytic block in adductor muscle spasticity (phenol or radiofrequency).

RELEVANT ANATOMY

- The obturator nerve enters the leg through the obturator foramen.
- It divides into two branches, the anterior and posterior branch, which are separated by the adductor brevis muscle.
- The anterior branch is sensory to the hip and medial aspect of the thigh and is motor to the anterior adductor muscles.
- The posterior branch is sensory to the capsule of the knee and is motor to the deep adductor muscles.

LANDMARKS

- Pubic tubercle.

PRACTICAL STEPS (FIGURE 23.25)

- The direct approach blocks the nerve as it passes through the obturator foramen below the superior ramus of the pubic bone.
- Position the patient supine with the leg to be blocked abducted.
- Protect the genitalia from cleaning solutions.
- Mark a point 1–2 cm below and 1–2 cm lateral to the pubic tubercle.
- At this point, insert a 22-gauge, 8-cm needle vertically downwards onto the pubis bone. Redirect the needle laterally and superiorly to enter the obturator foramen below the superior ramus.
- The needle should only be advanced 2–3 cm into the obturator foramen to avoid bladder damage.
- A peripheral nerve stimulator is helpful and pulse-synchronous movement of the adductor muscles confirms needle placement.
- Aspirate for blood.
- Inject 10 mL of local anesthetic solution.

COMPLICATIONS

- Hematoma.
- Nerve trauma.

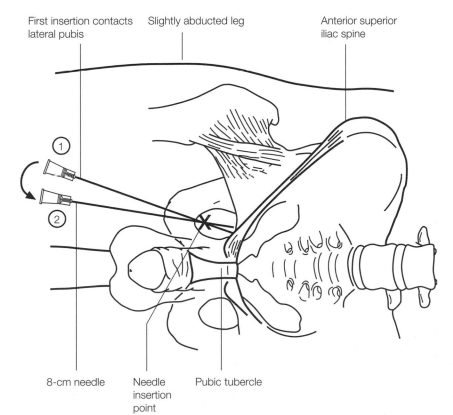

First insertion contacts lateral pubis Slightly abducted leg Anterior superior iliac spine

8-cm needle Needle insertion point Pubic tubercle

Figure 23.25 Obturator nerve block. Landmarks and needle insertion point for obturator nerve block. Reproduced with permission from Pinnock CA, Fischer HBJ, Jones RP. *Peripheral nerve blockade.* Edinburgh: Churchill Livingstone, 1996.

- Bladder damage.
- Infection.
- Pain at site of injection.

Lateral cutaneous nerve of the thigh

INDICATIONS

- Diagnosis and treatment of meralgia paresthetica.
- Postsurgical analgesia after hip surgery.
- Anesthesia for skin graft harvesting or muscle biopsy.

RELEVANT ANATOMY

- The nerve emerges at the lateral border of the psoas muscle below, passing obliquely under the iliac fascia to enter the thigh either deep to or through the inguinal ligament 2 cm medial to the anterior superior iliac spine.
- The course of the nerve varies as it crosses the inguinal ligament.
- Beyond the inguinal ligament, the nerve divides into anterior and posterior branches.
- The anterior branch becomes superficial approximately 10 cm distal to the anterior superior iliac spine and supplies the anterior and lateral thigh down to the knee.
- The posterior branch becomes superficial before the anterior branch and supplies the lateral thigh from the greater trochanter to mid-thigh.

LANDMARKS

- ASIS.
- Inguinal ligament.

PRACTICAL STEPS (FIGURE 23.26)

- Position patient supine.
- Mark a point 2–3 cm medial and 2–3 cm inferior to the ASIS.
- At this point, insert a 22-gauge, 3.5-cm needle at right angles to the skin.
- Direct the needle downwards until it lies deep to the fascia lata. A "give" should be felt in the needle.
- Fan-wise injection of 10 mL of local anesthetic is deposited above and below the fascia lata by moving the needle "in and out."
- If this block is supplementing a sciatic and femoral block, the total dose of local anesthetic must be controlled.
- A nerve stimulator may be used to confirm paresthesiae in the skin of the thigh, but patients with nerve entrapment may not be able to distinguish this.

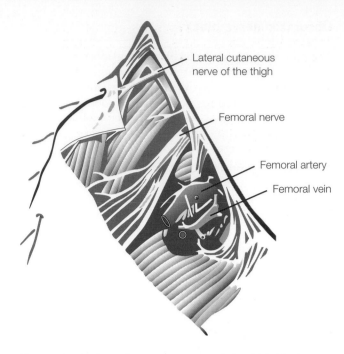

Figure 23.26 Lateral cutaneous nerve of the thigh block. Landmarks for the lateral cutaneous nerve of thigh and its relationship to the femoral nerve. Reproduced with permission from Eriksson E (ed.). *Illustrated handbook in local anaesthesia.* Copenhagen: Munksgaard, 1969.

COMPLICATIONS

- Nerve trauma.
- Local anesthetic toxicity (see above).
- Inadvertent femoral nerve block (needle too medial and deep).
- Hematoma.
- Infection.

Sciatic nerve block

As the nerve is deep, a peripheral nerve stimulator makes success more likely and avoids multiple needle redirections in a conscious patient. Because the nerve is large, high concentrations of local anesthetic are used (e.g. 0.75 percent bupivacaine) and the block may take 45–60 minutes to develop completely.

The following approaches have been advocated for this block:

- The posterior (classical) approach is the most proximal and is the most likely to produce a complete block of all the branches of the sciatic nerve. It is also the best route for a sciatic nerve catheter.
- The lithotomy approach is the easiest to learn as the nerve is at its most superficial, and the landmarks are identifiable in an obese limb. Assistance is needed to support the leg, and this position may be difficult if the patient has painful joints.

- The anterior and lateral approaches do not require the patient to be moved. Some find the lateral approach difficult to locate the nerve.

INDICATIONS

- Postsurgical analgesia of the knee (in combination with femoral, obturator, and lateral cutaneous blocks), ankle, and foot.
- Analgesia for fractures and amputations below the knee.
- Complex regional pain syndromes of leg.
- Ischemic pain of leg.

RELEVANT ANATOMY

- Sciatic nerve supplied by L4–S3.
- Largest nerve in body (2 cm wide as it exits the pelvis).
- Divides into peroneal and tibial branches anywhere from the sciatic foramen to the lower thigh.
- The sciatic nerve supplies the hip joint and hamstring muscles.
- The tibial nerve supplies the knee and ankle joint, the muscles of the calf, and plantar muscles of the foot. Cutaneous innervation is via the sural nerve, which supplies the posterolateral skin of the lower leg.
- The peroneal nerve supplies the knee and skin of the proximal and lateral part of the lower leg and the dorsum of the foot.

Sciatic nerve block: posterior approach

LANDMARKS

- Posterior superior iliac spine (PSIS).
- Sacrococcygeal joint.
- Greater trochanter.

PRACTICAL STEPS (FIGURE 23.27)

- Position the patient in the lateral position, with the side to be blocked uppermost.
- Flex the top leg to 90° to stabilize the patient ("recovery position").
- Draw a line from the greater trochanter to the PSIS.
- Draw a second line from the greater trochanter to the sacrococcygeal joint (1–2 cm below the sacral cornu).
- Draw a third line at 90° from the midpoint of the first line.
- Where this line bisects the second line represents a point overlying the sciatic nerve as it leaves the sciatic foramen.
- At this point, insert a 22-gauge, 8-cm needle perpendicular to the skin and advance through the gluteal muscles.
- If bone is contacted (5–6 cm deep), redirect the needle until it passes through the sciatic foramen.
- At this stage, connect the peripheral nerve stimulator and advance the needle until pulse-synchronous dorsiflexion and eversion of foot are produced (usually at a depth of 6–8 cm).
- In obese patients, a 10-cm needle may be necessary.
- Aspirate for blood and inject 10–15 mL of local anesthetic solution.

Sciatic nerve block: lithotomy approach

LANDMARKS

- Greater trochanter.
- Ischial tuberosity.

PRACTICAL STEPS (FIGURE 23.28)

- Position the patient supine with the leg to be blocked in the lithotomy position (knee and hip at 90°).

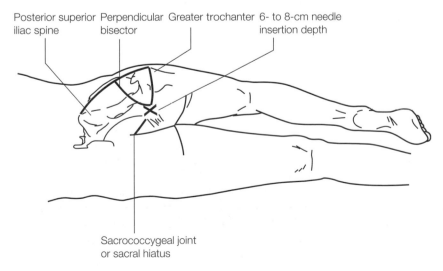

Posterior superior iliac spine Perpendicular bisector Greater trochanter 6- to 8-cm needle insertion depth

Sacrococcygeal joint or sacral hiatus

Figure 23.27 Sciatic nerve block: posterior approach. Landmarks and needle insertion point for a posterior approach to the sciatic nerve block. Reproduced with permission from Pinnock CA, Fischer HBJ, Jones RP. *Peripheral nerve blockade*. Edinburgh: Churchill Livingstone, 1996.

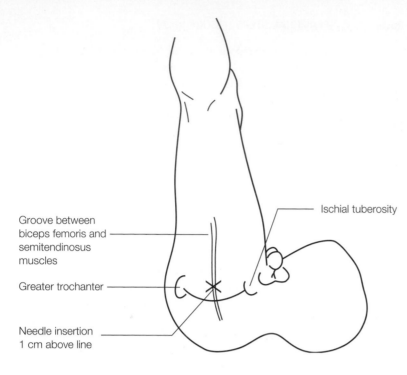

Groove between biceps femoris and semitendinosus muscles

Greater trochanter

Needle insertion 1 cm above line

Ischial tuberosity

Figure 23.28 Sciatic nerve block: lithotomy approach. Landmarks and needle insertion point for a lithotomy approach to the sciatic nerve block. Reproduced with permission from Pinnock CA, Fischer HBJ, Jones RP. *Peripheral nerve blockade*. Edinburgh: Churchill Livingstone, 1996.

- Draw a line between the greater trochanter and the ischial tuberosity.
- Mark a point 1 cm above the midpoint of this line.
- At this point, insert a 22-gauge, 8-cm needle perpendicular to the skin.
- Advance the needle through the intermuscular septum between biceps femoris and semitendinosus muscles.
- The nerve lies 5–7 cm deep to the skin.
- If bony contact is made, redirect the needle medially to miss the greater trochanter.
- A nerve stimulator will produce pulse-synchronous muscle movement of either the tibial (plantar flexion and inversion of foot) or peroneal (dorsiflexion and eversion of foot) nerve.
- Painful stiff joints may prevent this approach.

Sciatic nerve block: anterior approach

LANDMARKS

- Greater trochanter.
- Inguinal ligament.

PRACTICAL STEPS (FIGURE 23.29)

- Position the patient supine (leg slightly abducted).
- Draw a line the length of the inguinal ligament and divide it into three equal parts.
- Mark the junction between the middle and medial third.
- Draw a second line, parallel to the inguinal ligament from the greater trochanter across the anterior thigh.

- Draw a third line perpendicular to both lines. Starting from the junction, mark on the first line to a point where it bisects the second parallel line.
- At this point, insert a 22-gauge, 10-cm needle vertically downwards through the skin to pass medial to the femur.
- Bony contact is frequently made (femur) – correct by redirecting the needle more medial.
- The nerve lies just deep to the lesser trochanter behind the adductor magnus.
- A "give" may be felt as the needle enters this space (usually 8–10 cm deep).
- A nerve stimulator may confirm the needle position by demonstrating pulse-synchronous muscle movement (see above).
- Aspirate for blood.
- Inject 10–15 mL of local anesthetic solution.

Sciatic nerve block: lateral approach

LANDMARKS

- Lateral prominence of the greater trochanter.
- Inferior border of femur.

PRACTICAL STEPS (FIGURE 23.30)

- Position the patient supine.
- Mark a point on the inferior border of the femur 3 cm from the lateral tuberosity of the greater trochanter.
- Insert a 22-gauge, 15-cm needle perpendicular to the skin until it contacts the femoral shaft.

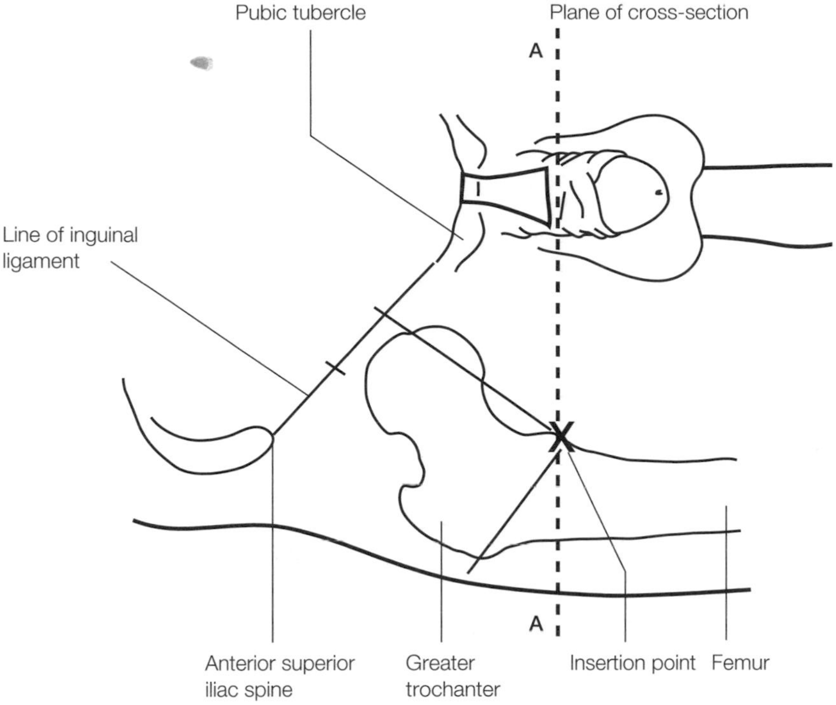

Pubic tubercle   Plane of cross-section

A

Line of inguinal
ligament

A

Anterior superior   Greater   Insertion point Femur
iliac spine   trochanter

Figure 23.29 Sciatic nerve block: anterior
approach. Landmarks and needle insertion
point for an anterior approach to the sciatic
nerve block. Reproduced with permission from
Pinnock CA, Fischer HBJ, Jones RP. *Peripheral
nerve blockade*. Edinburgh: Churchill
Livingstone, 1996.

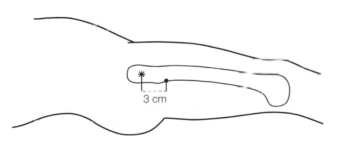

3 cm

Figure 23.30 Sciatic nerve block: lateral approach. Landmarks
and needle insertion point for a lateral approach to the sciatic
nerve block. Reproduced with permission from Cousins MJ,
Bridenbaugh PO (eds). *Neural blockade in clinical anesthesia
and management of pain*. Philadelphia: JB Lippincott, 1988.

- Withdraw the needle and redirect to pass beneath the
  femur.
- Connect the needle to a peripheral nerve stimulator
  and advance to a depth of 8–12 cm, when pulse-
  synchronous muscle movements should occur (see
  above).
- Aspirate for blood and inject 15 mL of local
  anesthetic solution.

COMPLICATIONS OF SCIATIC NERVE BLOCK

- Procedure may be painful in the conscious patient.
- Nerve trauma.
- Vasoconstriction in contralateral leg.
- Hematoma.
- Infection.

Posterior cutaneous nerve of the thigh

- The posterior cutaneous nerve (S1–3) innervates the
  posterior aspect of the thigh and upper part of calf.
- The nerve exits the greater sciatic foramen alongside
  the sciatic nerve and is inevitably blocked with the
  sciatic nerve.
- Continuous sciatic nerve block can be performed
  proximally or distally (see below under Nerve blocks
  around the knee: popliteal fossa block (distal sciatic
  nerve block). Prolonged analgesia can be provided
  after lower limb surgery. Commonly, the posterior
  approach is used employing a stimulating catheter,
  real time ultrasound or both. Ultrasound
  visualization in some adults may be difficult due to
  depth of the sciatic nerve, making the distal popliteal
  approach more popular in adults.

Nerve blocks around the knee

Four nerve blocks are commonly performed at the knee:
saphenous nerve block, tibial and peroneal nerve blocks
(popliteal fossa block), and intra-articular block within
the knee itself.

INDICATIONS

- Postsurgical analgesia for knee surgery (intra-
  articular block) or surgery on the foot (saphenous,
  tibial, and peroneal block).
- Chronic pain syndromes of the knee (intra-articular
  block).

RELEVANT ANATOMY

- The saphenous nerve is the continuation of the femoral nerve and supplies the medial half of the lower leg from above the knee to the ball of the great toe. The nerve becomes subcutaneous at the medial side of the knee, immediately below the sartorius muscle.
- The peroneal and tibial nerves are the continuation of the sciatic nerve.
- The tibial nerve arises at the upper border of the popliteal fossa and is the larger branch.
- The peroneal nerve enters the popliteal fossa at its upper border and exits by winding round the head of the fibula (prone to damage).

Nerve blocks around the knee: saphenous nerve block

LANDMARKS

- Medial tibial condyle.
- Tibial tuberosity.

PRACTICAL STEPS (FIGURE 23.31)

- Position the patient supine.
- Identify the medial border of the medial tibial condyle where the nerve lies subcutaneously.
- At a point 2 cm posteromedial to the medial condyle, insert a 22-gauge, 3.5-cm needle and, keeping the needle subcutaneous, inject a ring of local anesthetic solution (10 mL) inferiorly toward the posterior border of the condyle.

COMPLICATIONS

- Nerve trauma.
- Intravenous injection (beware varicose veins).
- Hematoma.
- Infection.

Nerve blocks around the knee: popliteal fossa block (distal sciatic nerve block)

Both the tibial and peroneal nerves can be blocked by a single injection in the upper triangle within the "diamond-shaped" popliteal fossa.

LANDMARKS

- Diamond-shaped popliteal fossa.
- Femoral condyles.
- Popliteal artery pulse.

PRACTICAL STEPS (FIGURE 23.32)

- Position the patient prone.
- Draw a line between the femoral condyles (posterior skin crease).
- Identify the popliteal artery pulse along this line.
- Mark a point just lateral to the pulse and 6–8 cm above the intercondyle line.
- At this point, insert a 22-gauge, 3.5-cm needle.
- Advance the needle 2–3 cm deep to locate the nerve by paresthesiae in the foot or pulse-synchronous movement of the foot (peripheral nerve stimulator).
- Aspirate for blood.
- Inject 10–15 mL of local anesthetic solution which should flow easily.

COMPLICATIONS

- Nerve trauma.
- Painful procedure.
- Intravenous injection.
- Hematoma.
- Infection.

Continuous popliteal nerve block is used for prolonged analgesia after ankle and foot surgery. A catheter can be placed using stimulation or real time ultrasound. With ultrasound the catheter placement needle is directed between the biceps femoris and semimembranosus/tendinosus muscles approximately 1 cm medial to the sciatic nerve. Following distension with local anesthetic solution the catheter is left in place. In the majority of persons the sciatic nerve divides within 10 cm of the popliteal crease, this can be visualized with ultrasound.

Nerve blocks around the knee: intra-articular block

This block has become popular for providing postsurgical analgesia following arthroscopy and depends on peripheral opioid receptors within the knee joint.

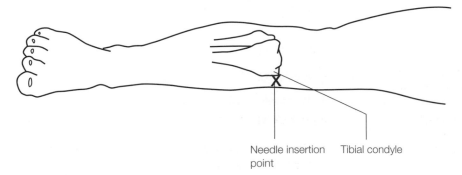

Needle insertion point   Tibial condyle

Figure 23.31 Saphenous nerve block. Landmarks and needle insertion point for a saphenous nerve block. Reproduced with permission from Pinnock CA, Fischer HBJ, Jones RP. *Peripheral nerve blockade.* Edinburgh: Churchill Livingstone, 1996.

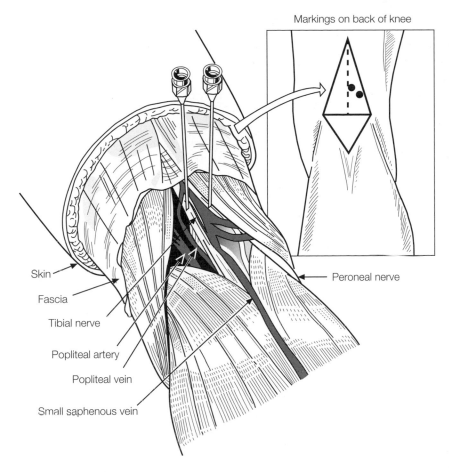

Markings on back of knee

Skin
Fascia
Tibial nerve
Popliteal artery
Popliteal vein
Small saphenous vein

Peroneal nerve

Figure 23.32 Tibial and peroneal nerve blocks. Landmarks and needle insertion points for the tibial and peroneal nerve blocks. Reproduced with permission from Cousins MJ, Bridenbaugh PO (eds). *Neural blockade in clinical anesthesia and management of pain.* Philadelphia: JB Lippincott, 1988.

INDICATIONS

- Postsurgical analgesia.
- Chronic pain syndromes of the knee (local anesthetic and steroid).

LANDMARKS

- Medial border of the patella.
- Groove between the patella and femur.

PRACTICAL STEPS (FIGURE 23.33)

- With the patient's leg extended, identify the groove between the medial border of the patella and the femur.
- Insert a 25-gauge, 3.5-cm needle into the knee joint along this groove.
- Avoid impaling the needle tip into the articular cartilage.
- Inject local anesthetic solution into the knee, up to 30 mL (with epinephrine (adrenaline)) may be injected.
- The injection should meet little resistance.
- Methylprednisolone may be injected for chronic pain syndromes or morphine 1–2 mg for postsurgical analgesia.

- This block does not cause any sensory or motor effects that would prevent ambulation.
- Careful asepsis must be followed to avoid an infected joint.

COMPLICATIONS

- Painful procedure.
- Damage to articular cartilage.
- Infection.
- Local anesthetic toxicity.

Nerve blocks at the ankle

The nerve supply to the foot is provided by five terminal nerves: superficial and deep peroneal, saphenous, sural, and tibial (**Figure 23.34**).

INDICATIONS

- Anesthesia for surgery of the foot.

RELEVANT ANATOMY

- The skin of the dorsum of the foot is supplied by the superficial and deep peroneal nerves.

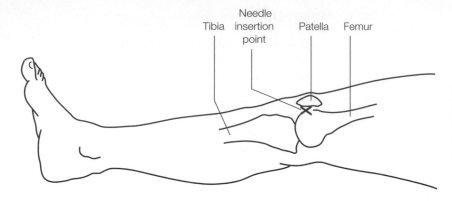

Figure 23.33 Intra-articular block of the knee. Landmarks and needle insertion point for an intra-articular block of the knee. Reproduced with permission from Pinnock CA, Fischer HBJ, Jones RP. *Peripheral nerve blockade*. Edinburgh: Churchill Livingstone, 1996.

- The lateral border of the fifth toe is supplied by the sural nerve.
- The superficial and deep nerves are blocked in combination because of their overlapping skin innervation.
- The saphenous nerve supplies the medial surface of the foot. It divides into two branches at the medial malleolus.
- The sole of the foot is supplied by four branches of the tibial nerve: medial calcaneal, medial plantar, lateral plantar, and sural nerves.
- The sural nerve branches off the tibial nerve in the popliteal fossa and passes between the lateral malleolus and calcaneum to supply the lateral border of the foot.

Sural nerve block (Figure 23.34)

LANDMARKS

- Achilles tendon.
- Lateral malleolus.

PRACTICAL STEPS

- Traditionally, the patient is positioned prone, alternatively the patient can lie supine with the foot inverted.
- Insert a 25-gauge, 3.5-cm needle immediately posterior to the lateral malleolus, and direct the needle tip toward the lateral border of the Achilles tendon.
- Inject a subcutaneous sausage of local anesthetic solution (5–7 mL) between the lateral malleolus and the Achilles tendon.

Saphenous nerve block (Figure 23.34)

LANDMARKS

- Medial malleolus.
- Long saphenous vein.

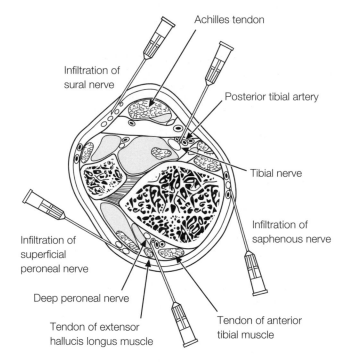

Figure 23.34 Nerve blocks at the ankle. Landmarks and needle insertion points for nerve blocks at the ankle. Reproduced with permission from Cousins MJ, Bridenbaugh PO (eds). *Neural blockade in clinical anesthesia and management of pain*. Philadelphia: JB Lippincott, 1988.

PRACTICAL STEPS

- Position the patient supine and externally rotate the foot.
- Identify a point 1 cm proximal and 1 cm anterior to the medial malleolus.
- Identify the long saphenous vein, which lies in close proximity to the nerve.
- At this point, insert a 25-gauge, 3.5-cm needle and inject 5 mL of local anesthetic solution around the long saphenous vein.
- Avoid intravenous injection.

Tibial nerve block (Figure 23.34)

LANDMARKS

- Posterior tibial artery.
- Medial malleolus.

PRACTICAL STEPS

- Traditionally, the patient is positioned prone, alternatively the patient can remain supine.
- Identify the posterior tibial artery.
- Insert a 25-gauge, 3.5-cm needle immediately inferior to this point at 45° to the skin parallel to the long axis of the tibia and advance toward the bone.
- Paresthesiae may be elicited before contacting bone.
- Inject 5 mL of local anesthetic solution.

Superficial and deep peroneal nerve block (Figure 23.34)

LANDMARKS

- Dorsalis pedis artery.

PRACTICAL STEPS

- Position patient supine, with the foot supported in extension.
- Palpate the dorsalis pedis pulse.
- Insert a 25-gauge, 3.5-cm needle immediately medial to the artery.
- Advance the needle 1 cm cephalad and deep.
- If the needle contacts bone or tendon, withdraw tip slightly.
- Aspirate for blood.
- Inject 5 mL of local anesthetic solution.
- Withdraw the needle to the subcutaneous plane and deposit a sausage of local anesthetic solution laterally toward the lateral malleolus (blocks superficial branch).

COMPLICATIONS OF ANKLE BLOCKS

- Nerve trauma.
- Hematoma.
- Vascular occlusion if local anesthetic volume too great.
- Infection.

NERVE BLOCKS OF THE PELVIS

Pudendal nerve block

This block provides analgesia of the lower vagina and perineum, and can be carried out via a transvaginal or a transperineal approach.[25, 26] The transvaginal approach is preferred as it is more reliable. Many would consider a caudal block more straightforward, with better effect.

INDICATIONS

- Analgesia for childbirth (second stage).
- Analgesia for episiotomy.
- Analgesia for suturing perineum.

RELEVANT ANATOMY

- The pudendal nerve is a branch of the sacral plexus.
- It runs lateral and posterior to the ischial spin and sacrospinous ligament.
- It has two branches: the dorsal nerve and the perineal nerve.
- The dorsal branch passes under the symphysis pubis to supply the clitoris/penis.
- The perineal branch supplies the inferoposterior aspect of the scrotum or the labia majora.
- The pudendal nerve is blocked as it passes the ischial spine.

LANDMARKS

- Ischial spine.
- Sacrospinous ligament.

PRACTICAL STEPS (TRANSVAGINAL APPROACH) (FIGURE 23.35)

- Position patient supine in the lithotomy position.
- Palpate the ischial spine and sacrospinous ligament transvaginally with the index and middle finger of one hand.

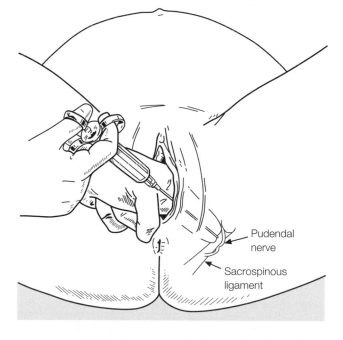

Figure 23.35 Pudendal nerve block. Landmarks and needle insertion point for a pudendal nerve block. Reproduced with permission from Cousins MJ, Bridenbaugh PO (eds). *Neural blockade in clinical anesthesia and management of pain.* Philadelphia: JB Lippincott, 1988.

- Guide a 20-gauge, 14-cm needle attached to a 10-mL syringe to the ligament just below the ischial spine.
- Advance the needle tip just through the ligament.
- Aspirate for blood (pudendal vessels run near the nerve).
- Inject 10 mL of local anesthetic solution.
- The procedure is repeated for the opposite nerve.
- Special needle guides (Kobak needle) have been advocated to limit the penetration of the needle.

COMPLICATIONS

- Inadvertent intravenous injection of local anesthetic.
- Hematoma.
- Nerve trauma.
- Infection.

CONCLUSIONS

Successful neural blockade is one of the most satisfying skills in the practice of pain medicine and anesthesia. A working knowledge of anatomy combined with training in the ultrasound location of nerves is the key to this goal. Once this skill has been acquired it is relatively easy to apply it to the practice of most neural blocks, allowing reduced doses of local anesthetic and minimizing the damage to nontarget tissue. Imaging is the norm in many areas of pain medicine and is now an exciting technique in the future of peripheral neural blockade.

REFERENCES

* 1. de Jong RH. Local anesthetics in clinical practice. In: Waldman SD (ed.). *Interventional pain management*. Philadelphia, PA: WB Saunders, 2001: 201–19.
2. Ramamurthy S, Walsh NE, Schoenfeld LS, Hoffman J. Evaluation of neurolytic blocks using phenol and cryogenic block in the management of chronic pain. *Journal of Pain and Symptom Management*. 1989; **4**: 72.
* 3. Cahana A, Van Zundert J, Macrea L *et al*. Pulsed radiofrequency: current clinical and biological literature available. *Pain Medicine*. 2006; **7**: 411–23.
4. Pither CE, Raj PP, Ford DJ. The use of peripheral nerve stimulators for regional anesthesia. A review of experimental characteristics, technique, and clinical applications. *Regional Anesthesia*. 1985; **10**: 49–58.
* 5. Marhofer P, Greher M, Kapral S. Ultrasound guidance in regional anaesthesia. *British Journal of Anaesthesia*. 2005; **94**: 7–17.
* 6. Klein S, Evans H, Nielsen K *et al*. Peripheral nerve blocks for ambulatory surgery. *Anesthesia and Analgesia*. 2005; **101**: 1663–76.
7. Bovim G, Sand T. Cervicogenic headache, migraine without aura and tension-type headache: diagnostic blockade of greater occipital and supra-orbital nerves. *Pain*. 1992; **51**: 41–8.

8. Waldman SD. Trigeminal nerve block. In: Weiner RS (ed.). *Innovations in pain management*, vol. I. Orlando, FL: PMD Press, 1990: 10–15.
9. Katz J. Vagus nerve block. In: Katz J (ed.). *Atlas of regional anesthesia*. Norwalk, CT: Appleton-Century-Crofts, 1995: 52–3.
10. Pappas JL, Warfield CA. Cervical plexus blockade. In: Waldman SD (ed.). *Interventional pain management*. Philadelphia: WB Saunders, 2001: 342–61.
11. Brown DL. Brachial plexus block: an update. *ASA Refresher Lectures*. 2000; **153**: 1–7.
12. Klaastad Ø, Smith H-J, Smedby Ö *et al*. A novel infraclavicular brachial plexus block: The lateral and sagittal technique, developed by MRI studies. *Anesthesia and Analgesia*. 2004; **98**: 252–6.
13. Klaastad Ø, Dodgson MS, Stubhaug A, Sauter AR. Lateral sagittal infraclavicular block (LSIB). *Regional Anesthesia and Pain Medicine*. 2006; **31**: 86.
14. Koscielniak-Nielsen ZJ, Rasmussen H, Hesselbjerg L *et al*. Infraclavicular block causes less discomfort than axillary block in ambulatory patients. *Acta Anaesthesiologica Scandinavica*. 2005; **49**: 1030–4.
15. Bonica JJ. Musculoskeletal disorders of the upper limb. In: Bonica JJ (ed.). *The management of pain*, 2nd edn. Philadelphia, PA: Lea and Febiger, 1990: 891–3.
16. Pinnock CA, Fischer HBJ, Jones RP. Nerve blocks at the elbow. In: Pinnock CA, Fischer HBJ, Jones RP (eds). *Peripheral nerve blockade*. London: Churchill Livingstone, 1996: 118–25.
17. Lofstrom B. Nerve block at the wrist. In: Eriksson E (ed.). *Illustrated handbook in local anaesthesia*. London: Lloyd-Luke, 1979: 90–2.
18. Richardson J, Lonqvist PA. Thoracic paravertebral block. *British Journal of Anaesthesia*. 1998; **81**: 230–8.
19. Moore D, Bush W, Scurlock J. Intercostal nerve block: a roentgenographic anatomic study of technique and absorption in humans. *Anesthesia and Analgesia*. 1980; **59**: 815.
20. Murphy DF. Interpleural analgesia. *British Journal of Anaesthesia*. 1993; **71**: 426–34.
21. Racz GB, Hagstrom D. Iliohypogastric and ilioinguinal nerve entrapment: diagnosis and treatment. *Pain Digest*. 1992; **2**: 43–8.
22. Bridenbaugh PO. The lower extremity: somatic blockade. In: Cousins MJ, Bridenbaugh PO (eds). *Neural blockade in clinical anesthesia and management of pain*. Philadelphia, PA: JB Lippincott, 1988: 417–36.
23. Chayen D, Nathan H, Chayen M. The psoas compartment block. *Anesthesiology*. 1976; **45**: 95–9.
24. Tagariello V. Sciatic nerve blocks: approaches, techniques, local anaesthetics and manipulations. *Anaesthesia*. 1998; **53**: 15–17.
25. Englesson S. Pudendal nerve block. In: Eriksson E (ed.). *Illustrated handbook in local anaesthesia*. London: Lloyd-Luke, 1979: 98–100.
26. Englesson S. Paracervical block. In: Eriksson E (ed.). *Illustrated handbook in local anaesthesia*. London: Lloyd-Luke, 1979: 96–7.

24

Intravenous and subcutaneous patient-controlled analgesia

STEPHAN LOCHER AND MICHELE CURATOLO

KEY LEARNING POINTS

- Technological advances have improved the safety of patient-controlled analgesia (PCA).
- Coherent prescriptions and monitoring of the use of PCA are essential and should be supervised by a specialized acute pain service.
- No one opioid is superior to another.

- The routine use of adjuvants is supported by only little evidence.
- PCA can be used in a variety of conditions, including patients with concurrent diseases, children, and elderly patients.

INTRODUCTION

Patient-controlled analgesia (PCA) implements the "what you need is what you get" concept in pain management.[1] This concept takes into account patients' individual variability in pain sensitivity and inter-individual pharmacological variability.[2] This individualizing of pain treatment highlights the role of psychological factors in the efficacy of PCA. The use of a PCA is intended to provide the patient with a direct sense of control over his or her pain, rather than being reliant upon another agent, such as a nurse or doctor to provide pain relief, and locus of control (LOC) is an important concept in health care.[3,4] The influence of LOC on pain levels is controversial.[3] Nevertheless, PCA has been shown to provide better pain control and greater patient satisfaction than conventional parenteral as-needed analgesia,[4] suggesting that LOC may be the important factor in conferring the advantage to PCA drug delivery.

The goal of this chapter is to demonstrate the safe and efficient use of intravenous and subcutaneous patient-controlled analgesia in daily practice.

TECHNIQUES

Routes of delivery

The most common route of delivery is the intravenous route. Additional options are the transdermal, intranasal, peroral, epidural, and intrathecal route. Inserting a fine

23-gauge indwelling cannula in the subcutaneous tissue, e.g. in the forearm or in the deltoid region, is quick, atraumatic, and easy to perform – especially in children – with neither interference with daily activity nor adverse local reactions. A bolus volume of 1 mL is used.[5]

Delivery systems

INFUSION SYSTEMS AND VALVES

A low-volume "Y"-connector is attached to the cannula. The branch to the infusion is secured with an antireflux valve to avoid drug accumulation in the infusion set and bag during an intravenous obstruction.

The branch to the pump device should contain an antisiphon valve. This prevents leaks in the drug cartridge, with entrainment of air, which may lead to a free flow of drug into the patient when the pump is above the patient's heart.[6]

INFUSION DEVICES

Disposable devices for PCA consist of two components: a balloon-reservoir constant infusion device and a patient-control module. The patient-control module contains a small bladder with a capacity of 0.5 mL. A button must be pressed that releases a clamp, thus emptying the bladder. Refilling of the bladder takes six minutes as the infusion device delivers 5 mL per hour. This system is simple and thus less prone to user error. However, lack of flexibility can be a disadvantage. If a larger bolus is required, a new infusion device with a higher concentration of the delivered drug must be prepared. Furthermore, neither the amount of bolus demanded nor the total dose delivered can be recorded precisely. Patients' acceptance of disposable devices was similar to that of the electronic device.[7]

The latest generation of electronic devices is based on sophisticated technology. Cleverly designed interfaces between user and machine allow easy handling with little training. The pump mechanism is highly precise with only little deviation from presser values. Tamper protection includes different lock levels, each accessible by different codes. Fail-safe mechanisms prevent free flow with alarms and include sensors for upstream and downstream occlusions.

Syringe drivers are usually larger pole-mounted systems that offer more sophisticated guidance and are often multifunctional. Ambulatory-style pumps are usually smaller peristaltic pumps that deliver fluid from a wide range of fluid containers (vials, syringes) in small bags or cassettes with emphasis on portability and simplicity of programming. The pumps are protected with different lock levels and codes to prevent unauthorized tampering.[8]

Advanced error-reduction features are available for PCA pumps to avoid incorrect programming and overmedication. Today, there are three types of advanced error-reduction features in use:

- bar coding;
- dose error reduction systems;
- computer-based pump-programming software.

Bar coding allows the clinician to scan a drug vial bar without manually entering the information in the pump. Furthermore, this information will be automatically compared to populated dosing protocols and dosing limits. Dose error reduction systems check manually input programming against preset drug and application limits stored in the pump. Using computer-based pump-programming software, the clinician sends a protocol via a wired connection from a computer to the pump. Complex safety software is housed and updated in the computer that populates the PCA pump. Ideally, all PCA pumps would provide an onboard bar-code reader that works in conjunction with a good dose error reduction system.[6]

MANAGEMENT OF PCA

PCA modes and parameters

PCA can be administered in different modes:

- on-demand fixed-size bolus dose;
- on-demand fixed-size bolus dose, plus background infusion or fixed-rate infusion.

Other programmable parameters include:

- bolus dose, ideally providing good pain relief with minimal or no side effects;
- lockout time, which uses a minimum time unit between two consecutive boluses delivered, even if the patient should press the button;
- dose maximums over a certain time period, usually one or four hours.

Basically, the PCA therapy is a maintenance therapy. The initial loading dose can be used to titrate towards an effective analgesic concentration. This dose should be delivered either preoperatively by the anesthesiologist or in the post-anesthesia care unit by the nurse. The patient can administer the on-demand dose or bolus dose via a button linked to the pump device.

Prescriptions and monitoring

Prescriptions, as simple standard orders for postoperative analgesia, should be available on the ward. Clarity, relevance to best practice and ease of use through comprehensive and stepwise approach are important features of these orders.

Each standard order should include:

- medication with detailed programmed parameters;
- monitoring needed;
- description of side effects and their treatment options;
- short guidelines for serious side effects, their acute treatment, and an emergency phone number.

Monitoring and documentation of the patient in fixed periods of time (for example, every two hours until six hours after surgery, then every four hours) includes:

- medication dose delivered;
- pain intensity at rest and during deep breathing and coughing using validated scales (e.g. visual analog scale (VAS), numeric rating scale (NRS));
- respiratory rate, sedation score;
- side effects (nausea, vomiting, pruritus, urinary retention, constipation, confusion);
- blood pressure, heart rate, oxygenation.

Acute pain services

PCA management run by an acute pain service (APS), rather than surgeons, provide more opioids with fewer side effects, patients are more likely to receive a loading dose, and PCA settings are adjusted more frequently.[9] APS members are familiar with the equipment and its daily use. Therefore, workshops to educate nurses on the ward is an important part of their continuing education.

Additional tips

If the number of trials is far beyond the number of boluses received, pain relief is often inadequate. If so, examine the doses delivered and adjust the bolus dose; a bedside bolus dose titration may be necessary. Lockout time and number of boluses per hour are seldom altered. An interdisciplinary approach in complex cases should be kept in mind.

DRUGS

Opioids

Morphine is widely used as standard medication. There seems to be no evidence in favor of one opioid over any other in terms of effects and side effects.[10] Following the concept of an individual minimum effective concentration (MEC),[11] **Table 24.1** presents a summary of common doses.

Since life-threatening complications occur more often with background infusion when using PCA, this technique should not be part of normal practice.[26]

Adjuvants

NALOXONE, PHYSOSTIGMINE, CLONIDINE, MAGNESIUM

These substances can be used in the PCA mixture or as separate infusions. Current data on PCA concerning the reduction of opioid requirements or the incidence of opioid side effects is limited or conflicting. Thus, no conclusion for practical use can be drawn.

KETAMINE

A qualitative and quantitative systematic review about perioperative ketamine for acute postoperative pain[27] concluded that ketamine in subanesthetic doses is effective in reducing morphine requirements and reduction of postoperative nausea and vomiting. The studies used for this meta-analysis were heterogeneous using small numbers of patients. In a study with 1026 patients, the combination of ketamine with morphine was demonstrated to be safe.[28] The same group did not demonstrate any benefit for the combination of morphine-ketamine compared to morphine alone in 352 orthopedic patients.[29] Additional evidence is required before this combination can be recommended.

PARACETAMOL

In two meta-analyses,[30, 31] there was no evidence that after major surgery the incidence of the opioid-related

Table 24.1 A summary of common opioid doses.

Opioid	Bolus dose	Lockout time (minutes)	No. of boluses per hour
Morphine[11, 12, 13, 14]	0.75–2 mg	8	4–6
Fentanyl[15, 16]	15–50 µg	8	4–6
Remifentanil[16, 17, 18]	15–40 µg (0.25–1.0 µg/kg)	2–10	6–30
Tramadol[14, 19]	20–30 mg	10	3–6
Oxycodone[20, 21]	0.03 mg/kg	10	3
Piritramide[22, 23]	0.75–1.5 mg	5	4–6
Hydromorphone[24, 25]	0.3–0.6 mg	2[a]	4
Pethidine[12, 13, 18]	9–18 mg	2–10	6–10

[a]With background infusion.

side effects are decreased due to the opioid-sparing effect of the combination with paracetamol. Currently, the routine use of paracetamol with an opioid PCA is not supported by evidence.

NONSTEROIDAL ANTI-INFLAMMATORY DRUGS

Nonsteroidal anti-inflammatory drugs (NSAIDs) given continuously and in multidose regimen reduces pain intensity significantly.[30] These drugs can reduce the risk of nausea and vomiting with a morphine PCA, the number needed to treat (NNT) was 15 patients. To decrease sedation with a morphine PCA, the NNT was 37. Slightly different numbers were calculated in an earlier meta-analysis: the NNT to prevent an episode of postoperative nausea and vomiting (PONV) was 12, the NNT to prevent sedation in one patient was 27.[32] Concerning the side effects of a renal failure, the number needed to harm was 73 and for a surgical bleeding the number was 65.[30] The clinical relevance of the side effects does not justify standard use, together with a morphine PCA.

METAMIZOLE SODIUM

This medication is not available in many countries, due to the risk of the side effect of agranulocytosis, although this seems to be rare.[33] Data on metamizole as an adjuvant is unclear in terms of efficacy for the reduction of pain and opioid consumption.[24, 34, 35]

The above-mentioned adjuvants can be used as base medication when PCA is stopped, which is normally the case at postoperative day 2 to 3. If the requirement during the previous 24 hours is less than the equivalent of 30 mg morphine, the PCA can be stopped as sufficient analgesia can be delivered with a maximal daily dose of adjuvants (paracetamol 4 g per day, metamizole 4 g per day, or NSAIDs). As a rescue medication, oral opioids permit mobilization of a patient without an intravenous line.

PATIENTS AND PROCEDURES

Patient selection

The ideal PCA patient:

- is informed orally and in writing;
- undergoes major surgery;
- is not younger than five years;
- is not confused due to medication, dementia, or psychiatric disorders.

Preoperative information

Psychological measures are important predictors of pain and PCA use. Higher anxiety levels and less social support correlates with higher postoperative pain and PCA requests. However, those with high anxiety levels experienced the greatest reduction in pain with PCA.[36] Although older patients preferred less information about and involvement in health care than young patients, the groups did not differ in concerns about pain relief and adverse drug effects, including opioid addiction and equipment use or malfunction.[37] Providing patients with adapted written information in advance is recommended.[38]

Management of side effects

After major surgery, the tolerability of the analgesic technique has direct implications for patient satisfaction. PCA is associated with the highest incidence of nausea (25 percent), while emesis was 20 percent for all examined analgesic techniques (intramuscular, PCA, and epidural analgesia). There were no differences between these techniques concerning mild (23.9 percent) or excessive sedation (2.6 percent), pruritus (14.7 percent), and urinary retention requiring catheterization (23 percent). The APS should aim to reduce these incidences with targeted measures.[39] In cases of nausea and vomiting associated with PCA, a reduction of the bolus dose may be helpful. If analgesia is insufficient, a combination with a non-opioid medication (NSAID, metamizole) is an alternative. If the problem of nausea and vomiting remains, a change to a different opioid can be considered.

To discriminate between PONV and adverse effects related to PCA remains a clinical challenge. The treatment of PONV following the guidelines published by an expert group includes the use of small doses of 5-HT$_3$-receptor antagonists in combination with drugs from different classes like droperidol, dexamethasone, or promethazine (**Table 24.2**).[40]

Another method is to add antiemetics to the PCA solution. High-dose ondansetron was compared to droperidol and showed no clinical advantage, but was more expensive.[41] While additional droperidol was significantly more effective than placebo with a NNT of 2.7,[42] its optimal antiemetic dose is unclear. Due to the side effect of sedation of droperidol, its dose recommendations vary between 10 and 50 µg/mg morphine.[43] No extrapyramidal symptoms or cardiac adverse events were noted in this work; in a case report of two adolescents, an extrapyramidal hypertonic syndrome happened with a PCA using a concentration of droperidol of 80 µg/kg.[44]

Special applications

CHILDREN

There are significant differences in pharmacokinetic, pharmacodynamic, and monitoring parameters in this

Table 24.2 Guidelines for the treatment of postoperative nausea and vomiting.

Drugs	Dose	Time of administration
5-HT$_3$-receptor antagonist		
Ondansetron	4–8 mg	End of surgery
Dolasetron	12.5 mg	
Granisetron	0.35–1 mg	
Tropisetron	5 mg	
Droperidol	0.625–1.25 mg	End of surgery
	10–50 µg/mg morphine	In the PCA solution
Dexamethasone	5–10 mg	Before induction of anesthesia
Promethazine	12.5–25 mg	End of surgery
Cyclizine	50 mg	End of surgery

Reprinted from *Anesthesia and Analgesia*, **97**, 2003, 62, Consensus guidelines for managing postoperative nausea and vomiting, with permission from Lippincott, Williams & Wilkins.

group, given by the great variety in age. Anxiety and coping styles are different compared to adults. A strategy to help children and adolescents to cope effectively with acute postoperative pain may be through targeted preoperative information. Although postoperative pain did not differ between the group with a standard educational program and the group with routine education, the children and parents reported the standard educational program to provide invaluable information about the use of PCA, the drugs, and their side effects.[45]

Children as young as five years are reported to have the cognitive ability to understand a patient-controlled pump.[46]

Generally, children of eight or more years can use VASs. For three- to eight-year-olds, self-reported measures such as face scales or color analog scales can be used. Behavioral observations including facial expression, limb and trunk motor response, verbal response, and physiological indexes are primary methods in neonates, children until four years, or children with developmental disabilities.[47]

A concurrent opioid infusion with PCA did not provide any clinically significant advantages over intermittent bolus doses in different types of surgery (scoliosis surgery, appendectomy).[48, 49]

Additional drugs for PCA-associated side effects are discussed in the current literature, but no conclusion can be drawn for the effect of the following drugs added to the morphine solution in the PCA: a small dose naloxon infusion of 0.25 µg/kg per hour,[50] the prophylactic intraoperative administration of tropisetron 0.1 mg/kg to a maximum of 5 mg,[51] ondansetron 0.1 mg/kg, or droperidol 0.01 mg/kg.[52] Although low-dose ketorolac in conjunction with morphine PCA improved the quality of analgesia and reduced morphine requirements compared to placebo in posterior spinal fusion surgery,[53] evidence-based analyses for children are lacking.[30]

OPIOID-TOLERANT PATIENTS

The anesthesiologist will come across two groups of opioid-tolerant patients. One group consists of chronic pain patients, as the percentage of patients to whom opioid analgesics are prescribed has substantially increased.[54] A second group of patients are opioid abusers, some of whom receive methadone in drug maintenance programs.

In either group, apprehensions about inadequate postoperative pain control or relapse of previous opioid dependency should be discussed in advance. This includes developing a realistic protocol to alleviate and not abolish postoperative pain. Co-dependency with other drugs (benzodiazepines) and alcohol is often linked to emotional psychological behaviors that demand an interdisciplinary management.

In addition to neuraxial blocks and nonopioid analgesic as adjuvants, the PCA is an option. Our discussion is limited to this feature, although in these patients there is no single solution to solve the problem.

While in standard PCA prescription, background infusion is better avoided in the opioid-tolerant patient, this can be used to deliver the equivalent of the patient's basal opioid dose.[55] Basal infusion may not be necessary in patients receiving the opioid via a transdermal system. Peroral drugs, as sustained-release formulations, can be taken preoperatively, if swallowing is allowed, and possibly 12 hours after surgery. PCA can be used successfully in matched bolus doses (**Table 24.3**).

Theoretically[56] and from experimental data,[57] a cross-tolerance to the antinociceptive effects of morphine in methadone-maintenance patients is possible. While higher morphine doses may achieve some pain relief, this may be at the cost of unacceptable respiratory depression.[58] Switching to another opioid to activate different subtypes of µ-receptors to which tolerance has not developed is an alternative.[59] As methadone is described as having *N*-methyl-D-aspartate (NMDA) receptor

Table 24.3 Matched bolus doses.

Opioid	Loading dose	Bolus dose	Lockout interval (minutes)
Morphine	5–20 mg	3–5 mg	6–10
Fentanyl	100–250 µg	50–100 µg	6–10
Hydromorphone	2–5 mg	0.5–1 mg	6–10
Sufentanil	25–75 µg	10–20 µg	6–10

Reprinted from *Anesthesiology*, **101**, 2005, 212, Perioperative management of acute pain in the opioid-dependent patient, with permission from Lippincott, Williams & Wilkins.

antagonistic and α-adrenergic agonistic properties in mice, this drug is the opioid of choice in case of ineffective opioid therapy.[60] These findings are confirmed in the clinical use of methadone, even when administered by PCA,[61] though the main clinical application was in cancer patients (**Table 24.4**).[62]

Nonopioid analgesics should be considered as an alternative. NSAIDs play a relevant role in opioid sparing.[32] Ketamine in subanesthetic doses yielded promising results in animal experiments. Earlier case reports with low dose (0.5 mg/kg) ketamine as a co-analgesic were promising.[63] Although co-analgesic ketamine is safe and useful, its clinical role remains unclear.[64] Clonidine can be used to reduce withdrawal symptoms,[65] although its clinical efficacy as peri- and postoperative co-analgesic is not yet determined.

PATIENTS WITH RENAL DISORDER

Caution is required among patients with renal disorders. Multiple morphine doses bear the risk of intoxication in patients with preexisting renal insufficiency or postoperative acute renal failure. Case reports describe a range of symptoms from profound unconsciousness to respiratory depression ending in ventilatory arrest.[66, 67] Accumulation can be avoided by using an opioid with pharmacokinetics independent of renal elimination and therefore no active metabolites. Drugs such as fentanyl, sufentanil, or buprenorphine meet this standard. Although buprenorphine (bolus doses 40–80 µg)[68, 69] and sufentanil (bolus dose 6 µg)[70] are suitable, they are rarely used in patient-controlled analgesia. Therefore, a fentanyl-PCA is recommended in patients with renal disorders.

MORBIDLY OBESE PATIENTS AND PATIENTS WITH OBSTRUCTIVE SLEEP APNEA

PCA is a valuable tool in morbidly obese patients when used with caution: no continuous infusion, limitation of the dose to one or four hours, monitoring of the patients closely in the first 24 hours.[71] Compared to epidural analgesia, PCA was found to be an acceptable strategy for pain management.[72] As 25 percent of these patients were affected by severe obstructive sleep apnea,[73] PCA can be used in this group as well, if the same restrictions are followed (**Table 24.5**).[74]

ELDERLY PATIENTS

In the elderly patient, postoperative pain management can be complicated by concomitant disease states and physiological changes that influence pharmacodynamic and pharmacokinetic properties. Pain assessment in elderly patients is sometimes difficult as they are reluctant

Table 24.4 Methadone.

Opioid-dependent patient	Loading dose	Bolus dose (mg)	Lockout time (minutes)
Maintenance program	Daily dose p.o. or s.c./i.m. (ratio oral to s.c./i.m. = 2:1)	1.25–2.5	5–10
No maintenance program	20–40 mg p.o. 10–20 mg s.c./i.m.	1.25–2.5	5–10

Reprinted from *Anesthesiology*, **101**, 2005, 212, Perioperative management of acute pain in the opioid-dependent patient, with permission from Lippincott, Williams & Wilkins.

Table 24.5 Morphine.

Bolus dose	Lockout time (minutes)	4 hour-limit
1–2 mg (20 µg/kg of ideal body weight)	8–10	20–80% of calculated dose

Reprinted from *Obesity Surgery*, **10**, 2000, 154, Efficacy and safety of patient-controlled analgesia for morbidly obese patients following gastric bypass surgery with kind permission of Springer Science and Business Media.

to request analgesia. Both conditions can be potentially alleviated with PCA. It offers the possibility to self-administer medications and to titrate according to the individual needs. Older patients use fewer opioids via PCA, but report a comparable pain relief and high satisfaction.[75, 76] As older patients expect less pain and even prefer less information and involvement in their medical management,[37] preoperative selection helps to identify patients who are unwilling or are incapable of using the device. Caution is required among patients with respiratory, renal, and hepatic insufficiency.[77] Under these circumstances, incremental doses of morphine 1–1.5 mg with a lockout time of five to seven minutes[76] is recommended. Continuous background infusion is contraindicated.[77] In cases of severe renal insufficiency use, an opioid without active metabolites, e.g. fentanyl, is indicated.

Close postoperative monitoring will increase the safety profile of PCA with less confusion and fewer pulmonary complications.[75] In a systematic review, no significant difference for postoperative delirium or cognitive decline was seen among commonly used opioids (morphine, fentanyl, hydromorphone).[78] However, pethidine (meperidine) was consistently associated with an increased risk of delirium and is best avoided for PCA use in the elderly surgical patients. The work of Vaurio et al.[79] may lead to an interesting debate as to whether elderly patients benefit from oral opioid management, as these patients showed a decreased risk for developing delirium in comparison to the PCA group.

CONCLUSIONS

PCA is an effective therapy for acute pain, while PCA prescription and monitoring in a standardized form increases safety. The knowledge and experience of an acute pain service can optimize this system for use after major surgery in a wide clinical spectrum.

ACKNOWLEDGMENTS

This chapter is adapted and expanded from Barrett R. Intravenous and subcutaneous patient-controlled analgesia: practical points and protocols. In: Breivik H, Campbell W, and Eccleston C (eds). *Clinical Pain Management: Practical Applications and Procedures*, 1st edn. London: Hodder Arnold, 2003: 393–400.

REFERENCES

1. Lehmann KA. Recent developments in patient-controlled analgesia. *Journal of Pain and Symptom Management.* 2005; **29**: S72–89.
2. Chou WY, Wang CH, Liu PH *et al.* Human opioid receptor A118G polymorphism affects intravenous patient-controlled analgesia morphine consumption after total abdominal hysterectomy. *Anesthesiology.* 2006; **105**: 334–7.
3. Snell CC, Fothergill-Bourbonnais F, Durocher-Hendriks S. Patient controlled analgesia and intramuscular injections: a comparisons of patient pain experiences and postoperative outcomes. *Journal of Advanced Nursing.* 1997; **25**: 681–90.
4. Hudcova J, McNicol E, Quah C *et al.* Patient controlled opioid analgesia versus conventional opioid analgesia for postoperative pain. *Cochrane Database of Systematic Reviews.* 2006; **CD003348**.
5. Dawson L, Brockbank K, Carr EC, Barrett RF. Improving patients' postoperative sleep: a randomized control study comparing subcutaneous with intravenous patient-controlled analgesia. *Journal of Advanced Nursing.* 1999; **30**: 875–81.
6. Southern DA, Read MS. Overdosage of opiate from patient controlled analgesia devices. *British Medical Journal (Clinical research ed.).* 1994; **309**: 1002.
7. Robinson SL, Rowbotham DJ, Mushambi M. Electronic and disposable patient-controlled analgesia systems. A comparison of the Graseby and Baxter systems after major gynaecological surgery. *Anaesthesia.* 1992; **47**: 161–3.
* 8. Anonymous. Patient-controlled analgesic infusion pumps. *Health Devices.* 2006; **35**: 5–35.
9. Stacey BR, Rudy TE, Nelhaus D. Management of patient-controlled analgesia: a comparison of primary surgeons and a dedicated pain service. *Anesthesia and Analgesia.* 1997; **85**: 130–4.
10. Chou R, Clark E, Helfand M. Comparative efficacy and safety of long-acting oral opioids for chronic non-cancer pain: a systematic review. *Journal of Pain and Symptom Management.* 2003; **26**: 1026–48.
11. Woodhouse A, Mather LE. The minimum effective concentration of opioids: a revisitation with patient controlled analgesia fentanyl. *Regional Anesthesia and Pain Medicine.* 2000; **25**: 259–67.
12. Plummer JL, Owen H, Ilsley AH, Inglis S. Morphine patient-controlled analgesia is superior to meperidine patient-controlled analgesia for postoperative pain. *Anesthesia and Analgesia.* 1997; **84**: 794–9.
13. Sinatra RS, Lodge K, Sibert K *et al.* A comparison of morphine, meperidine, and oxymorphone as utilized in patient-controlled analgesia following cesarean delivery. *Anesthesiology.* 1989; **70**: 585–90.
14. Stamer UM, Maier C, Grond S *et al.* Tramadol in the management of post-operative pain: a double-blind, placebo- and active drug-controlled study. *European Journal of Anaesthesiology.* 1997; **14**: 646–54.
15. Castro C, Tharmaratnam U, Brockhurst N *et al.* Patient-controlled analgesia with fentanyl provides effective analgesia for second trimester labour: a randomized controlled study. *Canadian Journal of Anaesthesia.* 2003; **50**: 1039–46.
16. Gurbet A, Goren S, Sahin S *et al.* Comparison of analgesic effects of morphine, fentanyl, and remifentanil with intravenous patient-controlled analgesia after cardiac

surgery. *Journal of Cardiothoracic and Vascular Anesthesia*. 2004; **18**: 755–8.

17. Kucukemre F, Kunt N, Kaygusuz K *et al*. Remifentanil compared with morphine for postoperative patient-controlled analgesia after major abdominal surgery: a randomized controlled trial. *European Journal of Anaesthesiology*. 2005; **22**: 378–85.

18. Blair JM, Dobson GT, Hill DA *et al*. Patient controlled analgesia for labour: a comparison of remifentanil with pethidine. *Anaesthesia*. 2005; **60**: 22–7.

19. Silvasti M, Svartling N, Pitkanen M, Rosenberg PH. Comparison of intravenous patient-controlled analgesia with tramadol versus morphine after microvascular breast reconstruction. *European Journal of Anaesthesiology*. 2000; **17**: 448–55.

20. Silvasti M, Rosenberg P, Seppala T *et al*. Comparison of analgesic efficacy of oxycodone and morphine in postoperative intravenous patient-controlled analgesia. *Acta Anaesthesiologica Scandinavica*. 1998; **42**: 576–80.

21. Tanskanen P, Kytta J, Randell T. Patient-controlled analgesia with oxycodone in the treatment of postcraniotomy pain. *Acta Anaesthesiologica Scandinavica*. 1999; **43**: 42–5.

22. Dopfmer UR, Schenk MR, Kuscic S *et al*. A randomized controlled double-blind trial comparing piritramide and morphine for analgesia after hysterectomy. *European Journal of Anaesthesiology*. 2001; **18**: 389–93.

23. Morlion B, Ebner E, Weber A *et al*. Influence of bolus size on efficacy of postoperative patient-controlled analgesia with piritramide. *British Journal of Anaesthesia*. 1999; **82**: 52–5.

24. Lehmann KA, Paral F, Sabatowski R. [Postoperative pain therapy with hydromorphone and metamizole. A prospective randomized study in intravenous patient-controlled analgesia (PCA)]. *Der Anaesthesist*. 2001; **50**: 750–6(in German).

25. Rapp SE, Egan KJ, Ross BK *et al*. A multidimensional comparison of morphine and hydromorphone patient-controlled analgesia. *Anesthesia and Analgesia*. 1996; **82**: 1043–8.

26. Sidebotham D, Dijkhuizen MR, Schug SA. The safety and utilization of patient-controlled analgesia. *Journal of Pain and Symptom Management*. 1997; **14**: 202–09.

27. Bell RF, Dahl JB, Moore RA, Kalso E. Peri-operative ketamine for acute post-operative pain: a quantitative and qualitative systematic review (Cochrane review). *Acta Anaesthesiologica Scandinavica*. 2005; **49**: 1405–28.

28. Sveticic G, Eichenberger U, Curatolo M. Safety of mixture of morphine with ketamine for postoperative patient-controlled analgesia: an audit with 1026 patients. *Acta Anaesthesiologica Scandinavica*. 2005; **49**: 870–5.

29. Sveticic G, Farzanegan F, Zmoos P *et al*. Is the combination of morphine with ketamine better than morphine alone for postoperative intravenous patient-controlled analgesia?. *Anesthesia and Analgesia*. 2008; **106**: 287–93.

* 30. Elia N, Lysakowski C, Tramer MR. Does multimodal analgesia with acetaminophen, nonsteroidal antiinflammatory drugs, or selective cyclooxygenase-2 inhibitors and patient-controlled analgesia morphine offer advantages over morphine alone? Meta-analyses of randomized trials. *Anesthesiology*. 2005; **103**: 1296–304.

* 31. Remy C, Marret E, Bonnet F. Effects of acetaminophen on morphine side-effects and consumption after major surgery: meta-analysis of randomized controlled trials. *British Journal of Anaesthesia*. 2005; **94**: 505–13.

* 32. Marret E, Kurdi O, Zufferey P, Bonnet F. Effects of nonsteroidal antiinflammatory drugs on patient-controlled analgesia morphine side effects: meta-analysis of randomized controlled trials. *Anesthesiology*. 2005; **102**: 1249–60.

33. Ibanez L, Vidal X, Ballarin E, Laporte JR. Agranulocytosis associated with dipyrone (metamizol). *European Journal of Clinical Pharmacology*. 2005; **60**: 821–9.

34. Grundmann U, Wornle C, Biedler A *et al*. The efficacy of the non-opioid analgesics parecoxib, paracetamol and metamizol for postoperative pain relief after lumbar microdiscectomy. *Anesthesia and Analgesia*. 2006; **103**: 217–22.

35. Montes A, Warner W, Puig MM. Use of intravenous patient-controlled analgesia for the documentation of synergy between tramadol and metamizol. *British Journal of Anaesthesia*. 2000; **85**: 217–23.

36. Perry F, Parker RK, White PF, Clifford PA. Role of psychological factors in postoperative pain control and recovery with patient-controlled analgesia. *Clinical Journal of Pain*. 1994; **10**: 57–63; discussion 82–5.

37. Gagliese L, Jackson M, Ritvo P *et al*. Age is not an impediment to effective use of patient-controlled analgesia by surgical patients. *Anesthesiology*. 2000; **93**: 601–10.

38. Chumbley GM, Hall GM, Salmon P. Patient-controlled analgesia: what information does the patient want? *Journal of Advanced Nursing*. 2002; **39**: 459–71.

* 39. Dolin SJ, Cashman JN. Tolerability of acute postoperative pain management: nausea, vomiting, sedation, pruritis, and urinary retention. Evidence from published data. *British Journal of Anaesthesia*. 2005; **95**: 584–91.

40. Gan TJ, Meyer T, Apfel CC *et al*. Consensus guidelines for managing postoperative nausea and vomiting. *Anesthesia and Analgesia*. 2003; **97**: 62–71.

41. Dresner M, Dean S, Lumb A, Bellamy M. High-dose ondansetron regimen vs droperidol for morphine patient-controlled analgesia. *British Journal of Anaesthesia*. 1998; **81**: 384–6.

42. Tramer MR, Walder B. Efficacy and adverse effects of prophylactic antiemetics during patient-controlled analgesia therapy: a quantitative systematic review. *Anesthesia and Analgesia*. 1999; **88**: 1354–61.

43. Culebras X, Corpataux JB, Gaggero G, Tramer MR. The antiemetic efficacy of droperidol added to morphine patient-controlled analgesia: a randomized, controlled, multicenter dose-finding study. *Anesthesia and Analgesia*. 2003; **97**: 816–21.

44. Park CK, Choi HY, Oh IY, Kim MS. Acute dystonia by droperidol during intravenous patient-controlled analgesia in young patients. *Journal of Korean Medical Science.* 2002; **17**: 715–7.

45. Kotzer AM, Coy J, LeClaire AD. The effectiveness of a standardized educational program for children using patient-controlled analgesia. *Journal of the Society of Pediatric Nurses.* 1998; **3**: 117–26.

46. Birmingham PK, Wheeler M, Suresh S *et al.* Patient-controlled epidural analgesia in children: can they do it? *Anesthesia and Analgesia.* 2003; **96**: 686–91.

∗ 47. Berde CB, Sethna NF. Analgesics for the treatment of pain in children. *New England Journal of Medicine.* 2002; **347**: 1094–103.

48. Weldon BC, Connor M, White PF. Pediatric PCA: the role of concurrent opioid infusions and nurse-controlled analgesia. *Clinical Journal of Pain.* 1993; **9**: 26–33.

49. Yildiz K, Tercan E, Dogru K *et al.* Comparison of patient-controlled analgesia with and without a background infusion after appendicectomy in children. *Paediatric Anaesthesia.* 2003; **13**: 427–31.

50. Maxwell LG, Kaufmann SC, Bitzer S *et al.* The effects of a small-dose naloxone infusion on opioid-induced side effects and analgesia in children and adolescents treated with intravenous patient-controlled analgesia: a double-blind, prospective, randomized, controlled study. *Anesthesia and Analgesia.* 2005; **100**: 953–8.

51. Allen D, Jorgensen C, Sims C. Effect of tropisetron on vomiting during patient-controlled analgesia in children. *British Journal of Anaesthesia.* 1999; **83**: 608–10.

52. Munro FJ, Fisher S, Dickson U, Morton N. The addition of antiemetics to the morphine solution in patient controlled analgesia syringes used by children after an appendicectomy does not reduce the incidence of postoperative nausea and vomiting. *Paediatric Anaesthesia.* 2002; **12**: 600–03.

53. Munro HM, Walton SR, Malviya S *et al.* Low-dose ketorolac improves analgesia and reduces morphine requirements following posterior spinal fusion in adolescents. *Canadian Journal of Anaesthesia.* 2002; **49**: 461–6.

54. Caudill-Slosberg MA, Schwartz LM, Woloshin S. Office visits and analgesic prescriptions for musculoskeletal pain in US: 1980 vs. 2000. *Pain.* 2004; **109**: 514–9.

∗ 55. Macintyre PE. Safety and efficacy of patient-controlled analgesia. *British Journal of Anaesthesia.* 2001; **87**: 36–46.

∗ 56. Mitra S, Sinatra RS. Perioperative management of acute pain in the opioid-dependent patient. *Anesthesiology.* 2004; **101**: 212–27.

57. Mao J. Opioid-induced abnormal pain sensitivity: implications in clinical opioid therapy. *Pain.* 2002; **100**: 213–17.

58. Athanasos P, Smith CS, White JM *et al.* Methadone maintenance patients are cross-tolerant to the antinociceptive effects of very high plasma morphine concentrations. *Pain.* 2006; **120**: 267–75.

59. Pasternak GW. Insights into mu opioid pharmacology and the role of mu opioid receptor subtypes. *Life Sciences.* 2001; **68**: 2213–19.

60. Davis AM, Inturrisi CE. d-Methadone blocks morphine tolerance and *N*-methyl-ᴅ-aspartate-induced hyperalgesia. *Journal of Pharmacology and Experimental Therapeutics.* 1999; **289**: 1048–53.

61. Fitzgibbon DR, Ready LB. Intravenous high-dose methadone administered by patient controlled analgesia and continuous infusion for the treatment of cancer pain refractory to high-dose morphine. *Pain.* 1997; **73**: 259–61.

62. Santiago-Palma J, Khojainova N, Kornick C *et al.* Intravenous methadone in the management of chronic cancer pain: safe and effective starting doses when substituting methadone for fentanyl. *Cancer.* 2001; **92**: 1919–25.

63. Clark JL, Kalan GE. Effective treatment of severe cancer pain of the head using low-dose ketamine in an opioid-tolerant patient. *Journal of Pain and Symptom Management.* 1995; **10**: 310–14.

∗ 64. Subramaniam K, Subramaniam B, Steinbrook RA. Ketamine as adjuvant analgesic to opioids: a quantitative and qualitative systematic review. *Anesthesia and Analgesia.* 2004; **99**: 482–95.

65. O'Connor PG, Carroll KM, Shi JM *et al.* Three methods of opioid detoxification in a primary care setting. *A randomized trial. Annals of Internal Medicine.* 1997; **127**: 526–30.

66. Angst MS, Buhrer M, Lotsch J. Insidious intoxication after morphine treatment in renal failure: delayed onset of morphine-6-glucuronide action. *Anesthesiology.* 2000; **92**: 1473–6.

67. Richtsmeier Jr AJ, Barnes SD, Barkin RL. Ventilatory arrest with morphine patient-controlled analgesia in a child with renal failure. *American Journal of Therapeutics.* 1997; **4**: 255–7.

68. Lehmann KA, Grond S, Freier J, Zech D. Postoperative pain management and respiratory depression after thoracotomy: a comparison of intramuscular piritramide and intravenous patient-controlled analgesia using fentanyl or buprenorphine. *Journal of Clinical Anesthesia.* 1991; **3**: 194–201.

69. Torres LM, Collado F, Almarcha JM *et al.* [Treatment of postoperative pain with intravenous PCA system. Comparison with morphine, metamizole, and buprenorphine]. *Revista Española de Anestesiología y Reanimación.* 1993; **40**: 181–4.

70. Lehmann KA, Gerhard A, Horrichs-Haermeyer G *et al.* Postoperative patient-controlled analgesia with sufentanil: analgesic efficacy and minimum effective concentrations. *Acta Anaesthesiologica Scandinavica.* 1991; **35**: 221–6.

71. Levin A, Klein SL, Brolin RE, Pitchford DE. Patient-controlled analgesia for morbidly obese patients: an effective modality if used correctly. *Anesthesiology.* 1992; **76**: 857–8.

72. Charghi R, Backman S, Christou N *et al*. Patient controlled i.v. analgesia is an acceptable pain management strategy in morbidly obese patients undergoing gastric bypass surgery. A retrospective comparison with epidural analgesia. *Canadian Journal of Anaesthesia*. 2003; **50**: 672–8.

73. Resta O, Foschino-Barbaro MP, Legari G *et al*. Sleep-related breathing disorders, loud snoring and excessive daytime sleepiness in obese subjects. *International Journal of Obesity and Related Metabolic Disorders*. 2001; **25**: 669–75.

74. Choi YK, Brolin RE, Wagner BK *et al*. Efficacy and safety of patient-controlled analgesia for morbidly obese patients following gastric bypass surgery. *Obesity Surgery*. 2000; **10**: 154–9.

75. Egbert AM, Parks LH, Short LM, Burnett ML. Randomized trial of postoperative patient-controlled analgesia vs intramuscular narcotics in frail elderly men. *Archives of Internal Medicine*. 1990; **150**: 1897–903.

76. Macintyre PE, Jarvis DA. Age is the best predictor of postoperative morphine requirements. *Pain*. 1996; **64**: 357–64.

77. Mann C, Pouzeratte Y, Eledjam JJ. Postoperative patient-controlled analgesia in the elderly: risks and benefits of epidural versus intravenous administration. *Drugs and Aging*. 2003; **20**: 337–45.

* 78. Fong HK, Sands LP, Leung JM. The role of postoperative analgesia in delirium and cognitive decline in elderly patients: a systematic review. *Anesthesia and Analgesia*. 2006; **102**: 1255–66.

79. Vaurio LE, Sands LP, Wang Y *et al*. Postoperative delirium: the importance of pain and pain management. *Anesthesia and Analgesia*. 2006; **102**: 1267–73.

Alternative opioid patient-controlled analgesia delivery systems – transcutaneous, nasal, and others

GUNNVALD KVARSTEIN

KEY LEARNING POINTS

- A new iontophoretic, transdermal, on-demand system for fentanyl administration and transmucosal sprayers which can be used for different opioids has been shown to provide postoperative pain relief with adverse effects similar to those of i.v. patient-controlled analgesia (PCA) administration.
- The bioavailability and onset time is equivalent to intramuscular and better than oral administration.

- Buccal fentanyl sticks ("lollipop") and fentanyl tablets can be used to treat "breakthrough pain" in cancer patients treated with controlled-release opioids.
- The new alternative PCA systems are more patient-friendly, they do not require expensive pumps or i.v. lines, and the risk of medication errors is low.
- Do remember that a bedside reservoir of analgesics (oral bedside PCA) may also provide autonomy and adequate analgesia in the later postoperative period.

INTRODUCTION

Worldwide, intramuscular opioid administration is the mainstay in the management of postoperative pain.[1] Drug absorption from muscular tissue is, however, highly dependent on local perfusion. The drug concentration in the central nervous system (CNS) becomes unpredictable with undesirable peaks and troughs. For the individual patient, a preset dose may just as easily represent an overdose as an underdose. Intravenous patient-controlled opioid analgesia (i.v. PCA) with computerized pumps, allows the patient to titrate the drug concentration until a desired level of analgesia is reached and has gained wide popularity in several western countries. The pumps, however, are expensive and require considerable time for training of nurses and programming. Recent advances in pharmaceutical technology and in the understanding of mucosal and dermal physiology have opened the way for less invasive and more patient-friendly opioid administration systems. The products are still in their infancy, but may in the future become more convenient than i.v. PCA (**Table 25.1**). Patient-controlled epidural analgesia is discussed in Chapter 26, Epidural analgesia for acute pain after surgery and during labor, including patient-controlled epidural analgesia.

Table 25.1 Alternative patient-controlled analgesia delivery systems.

Transdermal	Transmucosal
Iontophoretic devices for drug administered through skin	Nasal aerosol sprays
	Drug-impregnated lollipops[2]
	Buccal tablets

APPLIED ANATOMY

Transdermal route

The skin is not only an important protective barrier, but can also function as an effective and noninvasive route for drug administration. The transdermal route escapes presystemic hepatic elimination (the first-pass effect). Changes in skin blood flow are, under normal conditions, not a clinical problem.[3] Demographic characteristics, such as age, gender, ethnicity, body weight, and various anatomic locations do not interfere with the transdermal absorption of, for instance, fentanyl.[4]

Oral and nasal transmucosal route

High permeability to drugs and abundant blood flow make mucosal opioid administration highly promising.[5] The bioavailability is determined by patient-related factors like mucosal blood flow, secretion, ciliary activity, site of drug deposition, and head position, but also drug-related determinants, such as drug concentration, dose volume, molecular size, ionization, pK, and pH of the solution.[3,6] The drugs are transported by nonspecific diffusion through mucosal aqueous channels. The bioavailability is inversely correlated with the droplet size,[3] but in contrast to previous belief independent on lipid solubility.[6] There is no hepatic first-pass effect and despite a high activity of drug metabolizing enzymes (cytochrome P_{450}) in the nasal mucosa, a mucosal first-pass drug metabolism has not been demonstrated.[5,7] Interestingly, there is intimate contact between the olfactorial mucosa and the subarachnoidal space. It has been speculated whether compounds administered intranasally may circumvent the blood–brain barrier and reach the CNS directly.[5]

Inhalation route

The vascular tracheal mucosa has the potential of being an effective route for drug administration. Studies on tracheal administration of fentanyl have shown useful analgesia despite low serum concentrations. Inhalation as a different mode of analgesia compared with i.v. administration has therefore been suggested,[8] but the reports are not conclusive. Other studies suggest that inhalation of fentanyl is not more effective than other parenteral routes.[9]

Oral/gastrointestinal route

Most opioids are highly ionized in acid environments and unable to penetrate gastric mucosa. The absorption is facilitated in the more alkaline environment as in the small intestines, but a large portion is metabolized in the liver (the first-pass effect). Thus, the bioavailability of orally administered opioids is low or unpredictable. For drugs that are metabolized into more potent substances, such as morphine, codeine, or tramadol, the first-pass effect may be an advantage (particularly in rapid metabolizers).

TRANSDERMAL OPIOID DELIVERY

Fentanyl is the prototypical drug for transdermal administration, providing plasma concentration as stable as that for intravenous infusion.[10] It has been found to improve respiratory function and reduce the need for supplementary opioids.[11] Some clinical data indicate that transdermal fentanyl is an effective and safe method for controlling moderate to severe postoperative pain.[12] Within the first generation of transdermal delivery systems (Duragesic™, Jansen Pharmaceuticals, Titusville, NJ, USA), fentanyl was stored in a gel matrix and separated from the patient by a rate-controlling membrane. In the second generation of fentanyl patches, the gel is replaced by a matrix from which fentanyl cannot be extracted for intended abuse. The stable plasma concentration is, however, not optimal for controlling acute pain where intensity varies over time. When the pain subsides, the patient may easily be overdosed. Thus, fentanyl patches have not been recommended in the management of postoperative pain.

Patient–controlled transdermal system

A new iontophoretic, on-demand system with fentanyl hydrochloride is now commercially available (**Figure 25.1**). The first generation E-TRANS™ (model 4502; Alza, Palo Alto, CA, USA) or TRANSFENTA™ (Jansen Pharmaceuticals), is replaced by the patient-controlled transdermal system (PCTS) or iontophoretic transdermal system (ITS); IONSYS™ (Ortho-McNeil Pharmaceutical, Raritan, NJ, USA) and Janssen Pharmaceuticals, Titusville, NJ, USA. By an electrical field-promoted delivery (iontophoresis), the charged fentanyl molecules are transferred from the gel reservoir across the epidermal stratum corneum into systemic circulation. The system

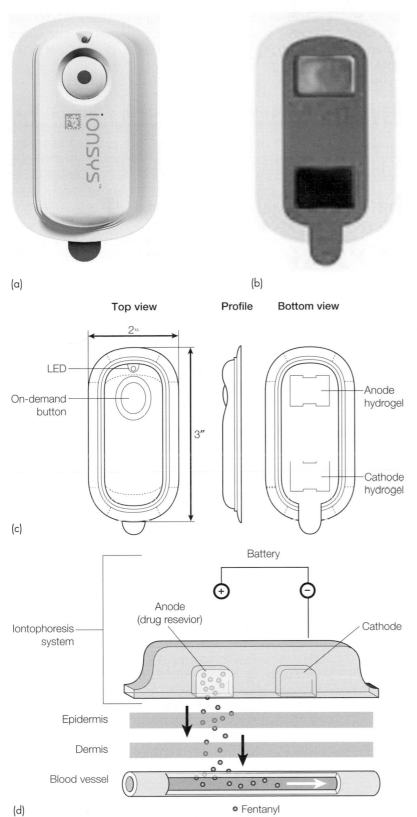

(a)

(b)

Top view   Profile   Bottom view

2"

LED

On-demand button

3"

(c)

Battery

Anode (drug resevior)

Cathode

Iontophoresis system

Anode hydrogel

Cathode hydrogel

Epidermis

Dermis

Blood vessel

(d)

○ Fentanyl

Figure 25.1 A new iontophoretic, on-demand system with fentanyl hydrochloride; IONSYS, Ortho-McNeil and Janssen Pharmaceuticals. (a,b) To initiate a bolus dose, the on-demand button is pressed twice. (c,d) The charged fentanyl molecules are transferred from the gel reservoir across the epidermal stratum corneum into the systemic circulation by an electrical field-promoted delivery (d).

combines the benefit of transdermal patches with those of a PCA pump.

Postoperatively, after the patient has been given adequate doses of i.v. analgesia, the PCTS can be initiated. It is applied to the skin like a fentanyl patch. To initiate a bolus dose, the on-demand button is pressed twice, then an audible beep appears, and a red light-emitting diode (LED) flashes. Fentanyl is not absorbed without an applied current. One flash represents one to five doses (40–200 µg) administered, two flashes six to ten doses (240–400 µg), and 16 flashes 76 to 80 doses (3040–3200 µg).[13] The bolus dose of fentanyl is fixed at 40 µg. Thus, when more analgesia is needed, the patient has to adjust the frequency of dosing (**Box 25.1**).

The amount of fentanyl which is absorbed increases with time and the amount of current delivered.[12] A current of 100 µA will give a controlled infusion of fentanyl 40 µg over ten minutes, which is needed to provide adequate serum levels (1–3 ng/mL).[12] With a current of 170 µA, however, 40 µg fentanyl is absorbed independently of the delivery time.[14] The patient can initiate six boluses per hour or a total of 240 µg fentanyl per hour. Each patch provides medication for up to 80 doses and should be replaced after 24 hours at a different skin site.

In three large randomized controlled trials (RCTs) on patients undergoing major surgery, PCTS fentanyl has been found to be superior to placebo and equivalent to i.v. PCA morphine.[15, 16, 17] Withdrawal due to inadequate pain relief was less frequent in the group who received fentanyl as compared with placebo (25–28 versus 40–60 percent),[16, 17] but not when compared with i.v. PCA morphine.[15] No respiratory depression was reported for the PCTS.[15] Thus, a 40-µg fentanyl dose seems to be safe. Nausea was the most frequently reported side effect (26–40[15, 16, 17] versus 26 percent in the placebo group[16]). Skin reactions were rare (<5 percent).[16] Most of the patients (86 percent) found fentanyl HCl PCTS convenient and easy to use.[17] In the future, fentanyl HCl PCTS may possibly be used in pediatric populations.

TRANSMUCOSAL OPIOID DELIVERY

Opioids have been effectively administered intranasally. The onset time is in general rapid and the bioavailability equivalent to intramuscular and better than oral administration (no hepatic first-pass effect).[18] Intranasal and i.v. PCA give equivalent pain control and patient satisfaction[19] with an onset of action that is nearly as fast as that for i.v. therapy.[19, 20, 21]

Most opioid products are formulated as liquids which can be delivered by metered spray pumps. The drug should be administered in volumes of less than 150 µL; otherwise, it will bypass the nasal mucosa and enter the pharynx or the lungs.[5, 22, 23] Nasal irritation and a bitter aftertaste are frequent (25 percent), and in one study only one-quarter of patients preferred patient-controlled intranasal analgesia (PCINA) to i.v. injection.[24] Other side effects include euphoria (3.6 percent), dizziness (1.4 percent), nausea (1.4 percent), vomiting (0.7 percent), and pruritus (0.7 percent), but the incidences are no higher than for i.v. PCA.[13]

Sufentanil

Sufentanil is a synthetic opioid. Given intermittently, the duration of action is shorter than morphine. The high lipophilicity makes sufentanil an ideal drug for intranasal administration with an onset time of ten minutes and bioavailability averaging 70 percent.[25] Postoperatively, titrated doses of 0.5 µg/kg sufentanil have been found to provide adequate pain relief in 80 percent of patients.[26]

Based on experience in acute pain management, intranasal administration of sufentanil has now been extended into the palliative care field to treat breakthrough pain. The bolus doses of sufentanil vary from 4.5 to 36 µg, the dose is repeated after 10 or 20 minutes.[27]

Fentanyl

Fentanyl is pharmacokinetically quite similar to sufentanil and well suited for intranasal administration. Fentanyl has no active metabolites. The most common fentanyl dose for adults is 25 µg (0.4–0.5 µg/kg). Significant pain reduction has been reported after ten minutes and within 20 minutes the efficacy equals that of i.v. fentanyl.[19] With a bioavailability of around 70 percent, an equipotent intranasal dose is 1.3–1.5 times the i.v. dose. In an RCT, repeated dosages of fentanyl 25 µg were equally effective and safe as intravenous doses of 17.5 µg.[21] PCINA fentanyl (bolus of 25 µg/kg) has been applied successfully in children as young as six years old. In patients with chronic pain, intranasal fentanyl administration has been reported to improve quality of life.[28]

Pethidine

Pethidine (meperidine) administered by an intranasal PCA device provides better postoperative analgesia than similar s.c. doses and is equally as effective as i.v.

Box 25.1 IONSYS characteristics

- An electrical field promotes transdermal delivery of the drug; standard electrical current: 170 µA over ten minutes (may vary).
- Bolus dose: 40 µg and lock-out time ten minutes.
- The patch provides 80 doses and should be replaced after 24 hours at a different skin site.
- No fentanyl is absorbed when current is not applied.
- Pain control equivalent to i.v. PCA.
- Global satisfaction assessment score is high.
- Side effects are similar to i.v. PCA and tolerable.

pethidine.[29] To achieve the same degree of pain relief, the intranasal dose has to be 1.36 times the i.v. dose.

Butorphanol

Butorphanol is a mixed agonist/antagonist and is rapidly absorbed into the vascular nasal mucosa. The bioavailability after intranasal administration varies from 48 to 70 percent,[30] but is low after oral (5 percent), sublingual (19 percent), and buccal (29 percent) administration.[31, 32] Equivalent analgesic efficacy compared with i.v. butorphanol is achieved within 15 minutes, but the onset is slower (15 versus 5 minutes), and the duration longer (4.5 versus 3 hours).[33] Two milligrams of butorphanol seems to be the optimal dose, but it is better tolerated when divided into 1 mg increments given one hour apart.[34] The metabolite hydroxybutorphanol may accumulate due to the long half-life (15 hours),[35] and in patients with renal hepatic impairment the dose intervals should be increased. Age- and sex-related changes, however, are not large enough to necessitate dosage differences.[30] Intranasal butorphanol is used to manage migraine attacks, although the abuse problems are considerable.[36]

Diamorphine (heroin)

Intranasal patient-controlled diamorphine (boluses of 0.5 mg) given postoperatively has been associated with high rates of satisfaction (69 percent).[37] In an RCT on young patients with bone fractures, intranasal diamorphine gave more rapid analgesia as compared with intramuscular administration,[38] but after orthopedic surgery, patient-controlled intranasal dosages of diamorphine 1.0 mg has been found to be less effective than 0.5 mg given intravenously.[20]

Methadone

In volunteers, intranasal methadone 10 mg (100 μL sprays in each nostril by a Pfeiffer BiDose sprayer) provided maximum plasma concentrations within seven minutes.[39] Maximum pain relief occurred after 30 minutes, compared with 15 minutes and 2 hours respectively for intravenous and oral administration. The duration was 10 hours for the intranasal methadone dose, and respectively 24 and 8 hours for the intravenous and oral doses. Properties of the ideal transdermal and transmucosal drug are shown in **Box 25.2**.

Patient-controlled intranasal analgesia devices

The Baxter PCINA on-demand system is a modification of the Baxter PCA system for intravenous administration; it consists of a mechanically driven infusor, a flow

---

> ### Box 25.2 Properties of the ideal transdermal and transmucosal drug
>
> - Highly potent;
> - Highly water and lipid soluble;
> - Not irritating to skin, mucosa, or cilia;
> - Unaffected by enzymes in the epidermis and mucosa;
> - Stable at room temperature.[3]

---

restrictor tube, and a patient-controlled module for bolus administration. A bolus volume of 0.5 mL (25 μg fentanyl) is injected through a 26-gauge plastic cannula with the needle tip removed. The flow restrictor provides a flow rate of 2 mL/hour or 5 mL/hour and lock-out interval at 6 or 15 minutes.[40] The delivered bolus volume is not exact and may vary from 87 to 135 percent of the intended volume.[19]

Go Medical has developed an inexpensive, low-tech, sprayer device (Therapeutic Goods Administration approval No. 54005; Go Medical, Subiaco, Western Australia) (**Figure 25.2**).[28] The small droplets (80 μm) improve the bioavailability and reduce, for instance, the incidence of bitter and burning taste after pethidine administration. The bottle is filled with 4 mL of a drug solution (fentanyl 200 μg or pethidine 200 mg). The bolus volume is 0.18 mL (9 μg fentanyl or 9 mg pethidine).[28] As it takes four minutes to refill the dose chamber (0.18 mL), the maximum hourly dose cannot exceed 2.85 m (142.5 μg fentanyl or 142.5 mg pethidine). In a recent pilot study, a more concentrated base was applied to provide fentanyl boluses of 54 μg.[24] The safety features are much like those of intravenous PCA. The Go Medical PCINA device should be stored in a locked cupboard (**Table 25.2**). A special screw top demonstrates whether the bottle has been opened or tampered with.

To facilitate the penetration into the mucosa, different vehicles are added, such as polyethylene glycols, glycofurol, ethylenediaminetetraacetic acid (EDTA), surfactant, bile salts, cyclodextrins, and chitosan.[5] Added microspheres make the solution more bioadhesive, while polymers increase the viscosity and slow clearance.[5] Local toxicity of such formulations should be considered.

Some companies (Pfeiffer, Radolfzell, Germany and Valois, Marly-Le-Roi, France) offer hand-held pump sprayers, bidose nasal sprayers, or disposable drug units.[5] The sprayers have a special activation system and deliver dose volumes of 100 μL or 2 × 100 μL. The variation in the given dose is small, less than 2 percent. A new bidirectional nasal delivery system has demonstrated improved drug distribution.[41] It takes advantage of the posterior connection between the nasal passages when the

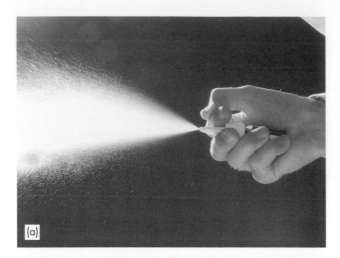

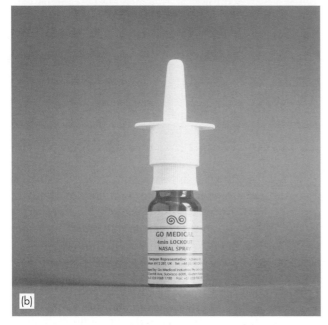

Figure 25.2 Patient-controlled intranasal analgesia (PCINA) gives equivalent pain control and patient satisfaction to i.v. administration. PCINA devices are now commercially available. Figure courtesy of Go Medical, Subiaco, Australia.

Table 25.2 Patient-controlled analgesia system characteristics.

Baxter PCINA device	Go Medical PCINA device
Bolus volume: 0.5 mL (= 25 μg fentanyl)	Bolus volume: 0.18 mL (9 μg fentanyl, 9 mg pethidine)
Lock-out interval: 6 or 15 minutes	Lock-out interval: 4 minutes
To avoid cross-infection the device is for single-patient use only	Repeated doses are required for pain control
The bottle must be kept vertical for 5 minutes after use to ensure refilling	

PCINA, patient-controlled intranasal analgesia.

velum closes during oral exhalation, but has so far not been applied for opioid administration.

Buccal delivery systems

Conventional short-acting opioids usually do not provide the rapid onset of analgesia required for breakthrough pain, and new delivery systems for buccal administration have been introduced.

Oral transmucosal fentanyl citrate (OTFC) ("lollipop") acts like a PCA treatment for breakthrough pain in cancer patients treated with controlled-release opioids (**Figure 25.3**).[42] The active drug is incorporated into a dissolvable matrix on a stick which is rubbed against the buccal mucosa. Doses of 0.5–1 mg or 15–20 μg/kg provide rapid and noninvasive analgesia with an onset time of 5–15 minutes. Bioavailability is greater than with oral administration.[43] One milligram of OTFC is equivalent to 5 mg of morphine i.v.[43] OTFC is commercially available in units containing 200, 400, 600, 800, 1200, or 1600 μg of fentanyl citrate (Oralet[TM] and Actiq[TM]).

New fentanyl buccal tablets (FBT) are designed to manage breakthrough pain in cancer patients treated with long-acting opioids.[44] The tablet formulation initiates a shift in pH that enhances absorption across the buccal mucosa. The bioavailability of fentanyl is higher with the use of FBT than OTFC. Single FBT doses of 100–800 μg are generally well tolerated and provide effective pain control from 15 to 60 minutes.[45] Caution should be used in prescribing FBT to patients with a history of substance abuse. A difficulty with buccal (and sublingual) administration is to know how much is absorbed, and how much is being swallowed and hence subjected to first-pass metabolism.

A new sublingual tablet technology allowing very fast dissolution of the tablet and rapid absorption of fentanyl for breakthrough pain, was registered in 2008 (Abstral[®], ProStrakan, Malmö, Sweden).[46]

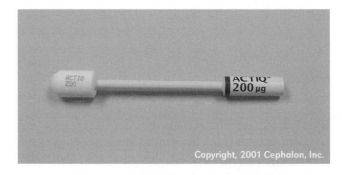

Figure 25.3 A delivery system for oral transmucosal fentanyl administration (Actiq[TM]). The active drug is incorporated into a dissolvable matrix on a stick. Reprinted from *Journal of Perianesthesia Nursing*, **20**, Miaskowski C, Patient-controlled modalities for acute postoperative pain management, 255–67, Copyright (2005), with permission from the American Society of PeriAnesthesia Nurses.

Box 25.3 Adverse reactions to and complications of transdermal, intranasal, and oral transmucosal opioid administration

- The incidence of adverse events is similar to that of i.v. opioid therapy.[19]
- Skin reactions after transdermal administration are mild and seem to be well tolerated.[12]
- Clinically relevant respiratory depression is rare.[12]
- Higher doses of intranasal pethidine are associated with a bitter taste,[29] but no significant changes in nasal mucosa are observed.[48]
- The most important side effects include pruritus, nausea, vomiting, dizziness, dry mouth, and respiratory depression.

ORAL BEDSIDE PCA

The issues of autonomy and control are equally important for patients receiving traditional oral opioids. A bedside reservoir of analgesics (oral bedside PCA) may provide more autonomy and improved analgesia for selected patients in the late postoperative period.[47]

CONTRAINDICATIONS AND LIMITATIONS

Previous allergic and serious adverse reactions exclude transdermal and transmucosal delivery. To minimize the risk of intentional and accidental overdose, the monitoring should be the same as for i.v. PCA. Whether an intravenous line is necessary is controversial (**Box 25.3**).[49] It is essential to ensure that Actiq™ and lollipop-like devices are kept out of the reach of children.

REFERENCES

1. Lehmann KA, Henn C. Status of postoperative pain therapy in West Germany. Results of a representative survey. *Anaesthesist*. 1987; **36**: 400–06.
2. Stanley TH. New routes of administration and new delivery systems of anesthetics. *Anesthesiology*. 1988; **68**: 665–8.
3. Biddle C, Gilliland C. Transdermal and transmucosal administration of pain-relieving and anxiolytic drugs: a primer for the critical care practitioner. *Heart and Lung*. 1992; **21**: 115–24.
4. Gupta SK, Hwang S, Southam M, Sathyan G. Effects of application site and subject demographics on the pharmacokinetics of fentanyl HCl patient-controlled transdermal system (PCTS). *Clinical Pharmacokinetics*. 2005; **44** (Suppl. 1): 25–32.
* 5. Dale O, Hjortkjaer R, Kharasch ED. Nasal administration of opioids for pain management in adults. *Acta Anaesthesiologica Scandinavica*. 2002; **46**: 759–70.
6. McMartin C, Hutchinson LE, Hyde R, Peters GE. Analysis of structural requirements for the absorption of drugs and macromolecules from the nasal cavity. *Journal of Pharmaceutical Sciences*. 1987; **76**: 535–40.
7. Hadley WM, Dahl AR. Cytochrome P-450-dependent monooxygenase activity in nasal membranes of six species. *Drug Metabolism and Disposition*. 1983; **11**: 275–6.
8. Worsley MH, MacLeod AD, Brodie MJ et al. Inhaled fentanyl as a method of analgesia. *Anaesthesia*. 1990; **45**: 449–51.
9. Higgins MJ, Asbury AJ, Brodie MJ. Inhaled nebulised fentanyl for postoperative analgesia. *Anaesthesia*. 1991; **46**: 973–6.
10. Duthie DJ, Rowbotham DJ, Wyld R et al. Plasma fentanyl concentrations during transdermal delivery of fentanyl to surgical patients. *British Journal of Anaesthesia*. 1988; **60**: 614–18.
11. Rowbotham DJ, Wyld R, Peacock JE et al. Transdermal fentanyl for the relief of pain after upper abdominal surgery. *British Journal of Anaesthesia*. 1989; **63**: 56–9.
12. Gupta SK, Bernstein KJ, Noorduin H et al. Fentanyl delivery from an electrotransport system: delivery is a function of total current, not duration of current. *Journal of Clinical Pharmacology*. 1998; **38**: 951–8.
* 13. Miaskowski C. Patient-controlled modalities for acute postoperative pain management. *Journal of Perianesthesia Nursing*. 2005; **20**: 255–67.
14. Nimmo WS. Fentanyl, absorption from Transfenta on-demand doses delivered by various currents in healthy volunteers. Annual Scientific Meeting of the American Pain Society, San Diego, 1998 (abstract).
* 15. Viscusi ER, Reynolds L, Chung F et al. Patient-controlled transdermal fentanyl hydrochloride vs intravenous morphine pump for postoperative pain: a randomized controlled trial. *Journal of the American Medical Association*. 2004; **291**: 1333–41.
* 16. Chelly JE, Grass J, Houseman TW et al. The safety and efficacy of a fentanyl patient-controlled transdermal system for acute postoperative analgesia: a multicenter, placebo-controlled trial. *Anesthesia and Analgesia*. 2004; **98**: 427–33.
* 17. Viscusi ER, Reynolds L, Tait S et al. An iontophoretic fentanyl patient-activated analgesic delivery system for postoperative pain: a double-blind, placebo-controlled trial. *Anesthesia and Analgesia*. 2006; **102**: 188–94.
18. Bell MD, Murray GR, Mishra P et al. Buccal morphine – a new route for analgesia? *Lancet*. 1985; **1**: 71–3.
19. Striebel HW, Pommerening J, Rieger A. Intranasal fentanyl titration for postoperative pain management in an unselected population. *Anaesthesia*. 1993; **48**: 753–7.

20. Ward M, Minto G, Alexander-Williams JM. A comparison of patient-controlled analgesia administered by the intravenous or intranasal route during the early postoperative period. *Anaesthesia*. 2002; **57**: 48–52.

21. Toussaint S, Maidl J, Schwagmeier R, Striebel HW. Patient-controlled intranasal analgesia: effective alternative to intravenous PCA for postoperative pain relief. *Canadian Journal of Anaesthesia*. 2000; **47**: 299–302.

22. Gizurarson S. The relevance of nasal physiology to design of drug absorption studies. Review. *Advances in Drug Delivery*. 1993; **11**: 329–47.

23. Schwagmeier R, Oelmann T, Dannappel T, Striebel HW. [Patient acceptance of patient-controlled intranasal analgesia (PCINA)]. *Anaesthesist*. 1996; **45**: 231–4; (in German).

24. Paech MJ, Lim CB, Banks SL et al. A new formulation of nasal fentanyl spray for postoperative analgesia: a pilot study. *Anaesthesia*. 2003; **58**: 740–4.

25. Stanley TH. The history and development of the fentanyl series. *Journal of Pain and Symptom Management*. 1992; **7**: S3–7.

26. Mathieu N, Cnudde N, Engelman E, Barvais L. Intranasal sufentanil is effective for postoperative analgesia in adults. *Canadian Journal of Anaesthesia*. 2006; **53**: 60–6.

27. Jackson K, Ashby M, Keech J. Pilot dose finding study of intranasal sufentanil for breakthrough and incident cancer-associated pain. *Journal of Pain and Symptom Management*. 2002; **23**: 450–2.

28. O'Neil G, Paech M, Wood F. Preliminary clinical use of a patient-controlled intranasal analgesia (PCINA) device. *Anaesthesia and Intensive Care*. 1997; **25**: 408–12.

29. Striebel HW, Bonillo B, Schwagmeier R et al. Self-administered intranasal meperidine for postoperative pain management. *Canadian Journal of Anaesthesia*. 1995; **42**: 287–91.

30. Shyu WC, Morgenthien EA, Pittman KA, Barbhaiya RH. The effects of age and sex on the systemic availability and pharmacokinetics of transnasal butorphanol. *European Journal of Clinical Pharmacology*. 1994; **47**: 57–60.

31. Shyu WC, Mayol RF, Pfeffer M et al. Biopharmaceutical evaluation of transnasal, sublingual, and buccal disk dosage forms of butorphanol. *Biopharmaceutics and Drug Disposition*. 1993; **14**: 371–9.

32. Gillis JC, Benfield P, Goa KL. Transnasal butorphanol. A review of its pharmacodynamic and pharmacokinetic properties, and therapeutic potential in acute pain management. *Drugs*. 1995; **50**: 157–75.

33. Abboud TK, Zhu J, Gangolly J et al. Transnasal butorphanol: A new method for pain relief in post-cesarean section pain. *Acta Anaesthesiologica Scandinavica*. 1991; **35**: 14–18.

34. Chu CC, Chen JY, Chen CS et al. The efficacy and safety of transnasal butorphanol for postoperative pain control following lower laparoscopic surgery. *Acta Anaesthesiologica Taiwanica*. 2004; **42**: 203–07.

35. Vachharajani NN, Shyu WC, Greene DS, Barbhaiya RH. The pharmacokinetics of butorphanol and its metabolites at steady state following nasal administration in humans. *Biopharmaceutics and Drug Disposition*. 1997; **18**: 191–202.

36. Loder E. Post-marketing experience with an opioid nasal spray for migraine: lessons for the future. *Cephalalgia*. 2006; **26**: 89–97.

37. Hallett A, O'Higgins F, Francis V, Cook TM. Patient-controlled intranasal diamorphine for postoperative pain: an acceptability study. *Anaesthesia*. 2000; **55**: 532–9.

38. Kendall JM, Reeves BC, Latter VS. Multicentre randomised controlled trial of nasal diamorphine for analgesia in children and teenagers with clinical fractures. *British Medical Journal*. 2001; **322**: 261–5.

39. Dale O, Hoffer C, Sheffels P, Kharasch ED. Disposition of nasal, intravenous, and oral methadone in healthy volunteers. *Clinical Pharmacology and Therapeutics*. 2002; **72**: 536–45.

40. Striebel HW, Romer M, Philippi W, Schwagmeier R. A device for patient-controlled intranasal analgesia (PCINA). *Schmerz*. 1995; **9**: 84–8.

41. Djupesland PG, Skretting A, Winderen M, Holand T. Breath actuated device improves delivery to target sites beyond the nasal valve. *Laryngoscope*. 2006; **116**: 466–72.

42. Portenoy RK, Payne R, Coluzzi P et al. Oral transmucosal fentanyl citrate (OTFC) for the treatment of breakthrough pain in cancer patients: a controlled dose titration study. *Pain*. 1999; **79**: 303–12.

43. Stanley TH, Hague B, Mock DL et al. Oral transmucosal fentanyl citrate (lollipop) premedication in human volunteers. *Anesthesia and Analgesia*. 1989; **69**: 21–7.

44. Webster LR. Fentanyl buccal tablets. *Expert Opinion on Investigational Drugs*. 2006; **15**: 1469–73.

45. Blick SK, Wagstaff AJ. Fentanyl buccal tablet : in breakthrough pain in opioid-tolerant patients with cancer. *Drugs*. 2006; **66**: 2387–3.

46. Lennernäs B, Hedner T, Holmberg M et al. Pharamcokinetics and tolerability of different doses of fentanyl following sublingual administration of a rapidly dissolving tablet to cancer patients: a new approach to treatment of incident pain. *British Journal of Clinical Pharmacology*. 2005; **59**: 249–53.

47. Litman RS, Shapiro BS. Oral patient-controlled analgesia in adolescents. *Journal of Pain and Symptom Management*. 1992; **7**: 78–81.

48. Hermens WA, Merkus FW. The influence of drugs on nasal ciliary movement. *Pharmaceutical Research*. 1987; **4**: 445–9.

49. Joly LM, Lentschener C, Benhamou D. Patient-controlled intranasal analgesia. *Anesthesia and Analgesia*. 1997; **85**: 465.

Epidural analgesia for acute pain after surgery and during labor, including patient-controlled epidural analgesia

HARALD BREIVIK

KEY LEARNING POINTS

- Thoracic epidural analgesia reduces risks of cardiopulmonary complications after thoracic and upper and major abdominal surgery.
- Lumbar epidural anesthesia for pelvic surgery and orthopedic surgery of the lower extremities, when prolonged after surgery, does not decrease cardiopulmonary risks and causes urinary retention and weak legs.
- Epinephrine, when added to a local anesthetic and fentanyl, decreases the doses needed and increases effectiveness and safety of thoracic epidural for postoperative pain relief.
- Epidural epinephrine does not decrease spinal cord blood flow; it does decreases epidural blood flow, systemic absorption of local anesthetic and opioid, and

therefore decreases opioid side effects (nausea, itching, urinary retention, respiratory depression).
- Effective and safe epidural analgesia for postoperative and obstetric analgesia is primarily spinal cord analgesia and requires appropriate segmental placement of the catheter, an infusion of low concentrations of a local anesthetic, a lipophilic opioid, and epinephrine; a robust monitoring regime where ward nurses observe and record at least every fourth hour, upper and lower segmental analgesic level using an ice cube, or alcohol swab, any leg weakness, pain intensity at rest and when moving, deep breathing, or coughing – on a 0–10 numeric scale. Inquire about any new backache, leg weakness, and leg numbness. A high preparedness for detecting early signs of epidural infection or bleeding,

for verifying diagnosis with magnetic resonance (MR) or computed tomographic (CT) scan and surgical preparedness for urgent laminectomy should spinal cord ischemia/compression occur.

- A prerequisite for a successful postoperative epidural practice is a well-organized acute pain team with well-trained pain nurses, anesthesiologist availability, and ongoing educational program for ward nurses, anesthesiologists, surgeons, and patients.
- Lumbar epidural analgesia after abdominoperineal or lower limb surgery gives good analgesia, but urinary retention, requiring catheter emptying, and leg weakness occur frequently when meaningful local anesthetic concentrations are used. This makes early mobilization, as well as monitoring of spinal cord functions and early detection of epidural hematoma or abscess, more difficult.

- Epidural analgesia for vaginal delivery is the "gold standard" for relief of severe pain during childbirth. When combined with subarachnoid (spinal) injection of low, analgesic doses of local anesthetic and lipophilic opioid early, the first stage of labor is shortened, and rates of cesarean section and instrumental deliveries are decreased. The risk of postpartum back pain is not increased.
- Alternative epidural analgesic mixtures containing sufentanil, diacetylmorphine, or morphine are effective as well, but the latter two may cause more respiratory depression, nausea, itching, and urinary retention.

INTRODUCTION: WHY USE EPIDURAL ANALGESIA?

The outcome after major surgery can be improved by relieving dynamic pain, i.e. pain during mobilization of the patient. The intense pain provoked by deep breathing, coughing, or moving a body part affected by surgery can be relieved effectively only with continuous neuraxial or peripheral nerve blocks. This enables patients to breathe deeply and cough, thereby preventing retention of secretions and development of atelectasis, pneumonia, and sepsis. Reducing dynamic pain will also enable the patients to perform active movements of limbs after orthopedic surgery, hastening rehabilitation of normal function. Thus, continuous cervical/brachial plexus blockade with catheter techniques and infusions of local anesthetics provides excellent analgesia and improves circulation and mobility of the upper extremity after shoulder, arm, or hand surgery.[1, 2] Epidural or continuous femoral nerve block enables patients to move their lower limbs more during the early days after major knee surgery.[3] This results in a more rapid rehabilitation than with intravenous (i.v.) patient-controlled analgesia (PCA) with morphine.[3] Epidural analgesia, as well as intercostal and paravertebral spinal nerve blocks, improve pulmonary function and reduce pulmonary complications after thoracic and upper abdominal surgery.[4, 5]

Epidural analgesia with a local anesthetic, with or without an opioid, decreases the risk of developing postoperative pulmonary complications, such as atelectasis and pneumonia, by 50–70 percent compared with systemic opioids.[4] Epidural opioids alone do not always reduce the risk of postoperative pulmonary complications.[4, 5] Thus, it is important to realize that a local anesthetic is needed in an epidural infusion in order to improve pulmonary function after major surgery.

This is also true for improved gastrointestinal motility after abdominal surgery: an epidural local anesthetic (and an epidural local anesthetic with an opioid) shortens the time of intestinal paralysis after surgery compared with i.v. morphine PCA or epidural morphine alone.[5, 6, 7, 8, 9, 10]

Epidural analgesia for vaginal delivery is the "gold standard" for relief of severe pain during childbirth. When combined with subarachnoid (spinal) injection of low, analgesic doses of local anesthetic and lipophilic opioid early, the first stage of labor is shortened and the rates of cesarean section and instrumental deliveries are decreased.

THORACIC EPIDURAL IMPROVES CARDIOPULMONARY OUTCOME AFTER SURGERY, LUMBAR EPIDURAL DOES NOT

It is now well established that a thoracic epidural is beneficial for patients who are at high risk of cardiac or pulmonary complications after thoracic or major abdominal surgery.[5, 11, 12, 13, 14, 15, 16] Postoperative myocardial infarction, respiratory and renal failure, and stroke were reduced by perioperative thoracic epidural analgesia,[6] but not by lumbar anesthesia and analgesia.[11, 12, 13, 14, 15, 16] In recent studies, mortality is not significantly different, most likely due to improved effectiveness and safety of general anesthesia and intensive care of patients suffering complications after surgery.[5, 16] Only thoracic epidural analgesia, segmentally tailored to the surgical wound area, containing an appropriate concentration of a local anesthetic and a low amount of an opioid, will improve cardiopulmonary outcome, as well as comfort for the high-risk patient during mobilization.[12] Thus, a double-blind comparison of low thoracic epidural (bupivacaine plus high-dose fentanyl) with i.v. fentanyl PCA did not find any differences in dynamic pain nor in outcome after abdominal aortic aneurysm surgery, but nor did it document (owing to the blinding procedure) that the catheter remained in the epidural space.[17] Even in the best of hands, there is at least a 10 percent catheter failure rate, which may be as high as

50 percent during the first few days after surgery.[18] Moreover, they used low thoracic position (T10–11) of the epidural catheter, which does not give optimal myocardial protection.[11]

Thoracic epidural analgesia containing a local anesthetic:[11, 19, 20]

- dilates stenotic coronary arteries and increases myocardial oxygen supply;
- decreases myocardial oxygen consumption;
- decreases myocardial ischemic events and postoperative myocardial infarction;
- improves lung function and oxygenation;
- improves gastrointestinal motility.

On the other hand, lumbar epidural analgesia with a local anesthetic:[11]

- dilates arteries of the lower part of the body;
- causes compensatory constriction of the upper part of the body, including the coronary arteries;
- decreases myocardial oxygen supply;
- causes leg weakness and urinary retention;
- does not improve gastrointestinal motility, nor pulmonary functions.[9, 10, 11]

Thus, a lumbar epidural may even increase the cardiac risk and does not improve either pulmonary function or gastrointestinal motility. Lack of awareness of these important differences between thoracic and lumbar epidural analgesia is one reason for the confusion and conflicting opinions regarding the effects of epidural analgesia on outcome after surgery.[12]

RISKS TO THE PATIENT FROM EPIDURAL ANALGESIA

Even with the epidural catheter in a low thoracic or thoracolumbar area, if an excessive dose of a local anesthetic is administered epidurally, the patient may develop:

- orthostatic hypotension, making mobilization difficult;
- motor blockade and weak legs, making mobilization difficult and risky;
- urinary retention, increasing risk of urinary tract infections.

If an excessive dose of an opioid is administered epidurally, the following may occur:

- sedation and respiratory depression (immediate, as well as late);
- increased incidence and severity of:
  - itching;
  - nausea and vomiting;

Rare, but potentially catastrophic complications are:[21]

- epidural bleeding;
- epidural infection.

Leg weakness and back pain are early warning symptoms of impending catastrophic complications. It is essential to have a robust monitoring regime to detect changes in leg weakness. Excessive doses of local anesthetic should be avoided, especially in the lumbar or thoracolumbar epidural segments as motor blockade will occur, concealing early signs of spinal cord compression/ischemia.[22, 23]

OPTIMIZING EFFICACY AND SAFETY OF EPIDURAL ANALGESIA

The efficacy and safety of epidural analgesia is optimized by exploiting the principle of synergy[24, 25] in combining two or more drugs with different mechanisms of analgesia and different dose-related side effects. For almost two decades we have had a successful regime for postoperative epidural analgesia using a combination of the following low concentrations of drugs:[26]

- a local anesthetic (bupivacaine 1 mg/mL);
- an opioid (fentanyl 2 μg/mL);
- an adrenergic agonist (epinephrine 2 μg/mL).

These three drugs cause spinal cord analgesia by three separate mechanisms acting on the pain impulse transmission process in the spinal cord. Fentanyl acts on pre- and postsynaptic opioid receptors and epinephrine (like clonidine) acts on α_2-receptors in the dorsal horn. These effects increase inhibition of pain impulse transmission from the primary afferent nociceptive neurons to the interneurons and transmission neurons in the dorsal horn of the spinal cord. Subanesthetic doses of bupivacaine inhibit excitatory synaptic mechanisms in the same area of the spinal cord.

Exploiting their synergistic antinociceptive effects, concurrent administration of these three pain-inhibiting drugs allows a reduction in the dose of each drug (**Figures 26.1** and **26.2**).[27, 28, 29] The three drugs have different dose-related side effects. Therefore, the overall risks of adverse effects are reduced. This is true for respiratory depression, nausea, itching, gastrointestinal motility, sedation, hypotension, urinary retention, motor blockade, and leg weakness.[22, 23, 24, 25, 26, 27, 28, 29]

- Nurses on the surgical wards titrate the infusion rate of the epidural analgesic mixture to ensure segmental sensory block of the wound area, aiming for no pain at rest and only mild pain during coughing.
- Patients, when awake, with stable cardiorespiratory functions, are allowed to use the dose administration button of the patient-controlled infusion pump to give themselves boluses, when needed, e.g. before mobilization and pulmonary physiotherapy.

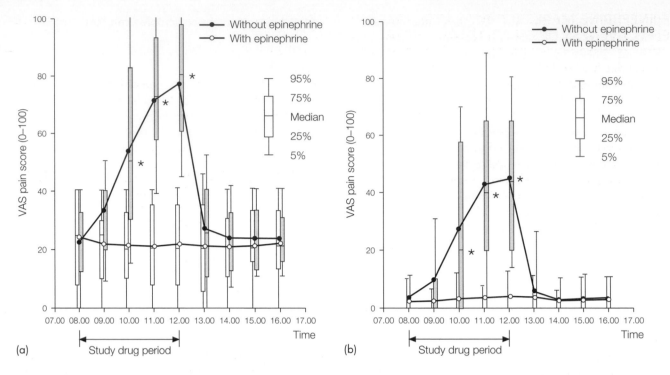

Figure 26.1 Double-blind, crossover study documenting the marked increase in epidural analgesia when epinephrine was added to bupivacaine and fentanyl. Visual analog scale (VAS) scores of pain intensity when coughing (a) and pain at rest (b) after major thoracic or abdominal surgery during infusion of epidural analgesic mixture containing bupivacaine 1 mg/mL and fentanyl 2 μg/mL with or without epinephrine 2 μg/mL. Redrawn with permission from Niemi and Breivik.[27]

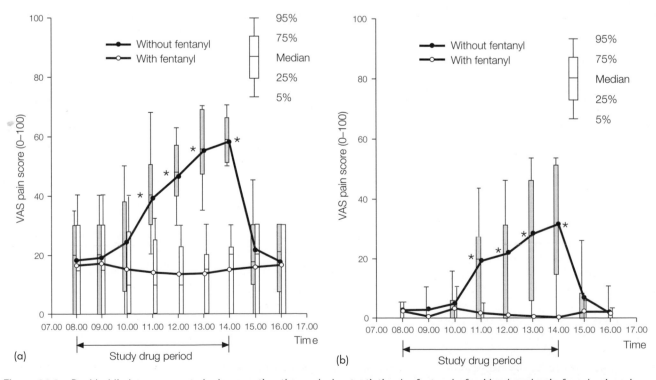

Figure 26.2 Double-blind, crossover study documenting the marked potentiation by fentanyl of epidural analgesia from bupivacaine and epinephrine (adrenaline). Visual analog scale (VAS) scores of pain intensity when coughing (a) and pain at rest (b) after major thoracic or abdominal surgery during infusion of epidural analgesic mixture containing bupivacaine 1 mg/mL and epinephrine 2 μg/mL with or without fentanyl 2 μg/mL. Redrawn with permission from Niemi and Breivik.[28]

EPINEPHRINE MARKEDLY INCREASES THE EFFECTIVENESS OF EPIDURAL ANALGESIA

Epinephrine has been administered with opioids and local anesthetics for epidural analgesia for vaginal deliveries and after surgical deliveries.[30] For more than two decades we have used epinephrine in our standard epidural regime to reduce the doses needed of local anesthetic and fentanyl. In a randomized, double-blind, crossover study, we documented the powerful effects of epinephrine in this regard.[27] Pain intensity was practically zero during rest after major abdominal or thoracic surgery with the triple mixture of bupivacaine, fentanyl, and epinephrine (**Figure 26.1**). When epinephrine was removed from the mixture, pain increased and, in spite of more patient-administered bolus epidural doses, i.v. rescue morphine was needed. When our standard mixture with epinephrine was reintroduced, pain relief again became optimal.[27]

Similarly, pain during coughing was only mild after major thoracic and upper abdominal surgery when the triple mixture was infused (**Figure 26.1**). When epinephrine was removed from the mixture, pain during deep breathing and coughing increased to severe intensity, but adding epinephrine again reduced cough-provoked pain to only mild pain (**Figure 26.1**).[27] In a study to establish optimal doses, we documented that epinephrine 0.5 and 1.0 μg/mL had less effect on the efficacy of the analgesic mixture than did 1.5 μg/mL, which had almost the same effect as 2.0 μg/mL.[31]

Exactly the same findings have been reproduced in a randomized, double-blind, crossover study of thoracic epidural analgesia with ropivacaine 1 mg/mL with fentanyl 2 μg/mL with or without epinephrine 2 μg/mL.[32]

EPINEPHRINE MARKEDLY INCREASES SAFETY OF EPIDURAL ANALGESIA WITH BUPIVACAINE AND FENTANYL

Epinephrine is important for the safety of prolonged epidural infusion of the analgesic mixture because absorption of fentanyl (and bupivacaine) into the systemic circulation is reduced. This is shown by a significantly lower serum concentration of fentanyl when epinephrine is added to the epidural infusion. With epinephrine 2 μg/mL, fentanyl is almost undetectable in serum.[27] When epinephrine is removed from the epidural infusion, the serum fentanyl concentration increases and patients experience adverse effects from systemic absorption: sedation, nausea, and pruritus.[27, 30]

An illustrative event was impressive in demonstrating the wide safety margins of this epidural regime: a human error in programming the epidural infusion pump occurred, with ten times the prescribed infusion rate (80 instead of 8 mL per hour) being administered to a patient for about three hours before the error was detected. Beside a profound analgesia and weak legs, no systemic

adverse effects occurred (Niemi and Breivik, personal communication).

Epinephrine, unlike the more specific α_2-receptor agonist clonidine, does not cause sedation or hypotension.[33] Furthermore, again unlike clonidine, it causes epidural vasoconstriction and less systemic absorption of concurrently administered drugs.[27, 34]

EPIDURAL EPINEPHRINE DOES NOT DECREASE SPINAL CORD BLOOD FLOW

Spinal cord and cerebral arterioles do not respond to adrenergic drugs with vasoconstriction.[35, 36] Therefore, epidural epinephrine 2 μg/mL at 5–15 mL per hour does not decrease spinal cord blood flow; even much larger doses of epinephrine directly into the cerebrospinal fluid (CSF) do not reduce spinal (or cerebral) blood flow.[35, 36, 37, 38] The potent constrictive action of epinephrine on vessels outside the central nervous system has led to misunderstanding and unfounded concern about the blood supply to the spinal cord when administering epinephrine-containing epidural infusions. There are, however, no human data supporting this concern,[39, 40] only misinterpreted case histories in which a temporal association with epidural or subarachnoidal administration of epinephrine has been interpreted as the cause of spinal cord ischemia.[41]

Epinephrine has been used with spinal anesthetics for decades without any clinical spinal cord dysfunction being observed.[39, 41] In 20 patients undergoing gynecological laparoscopy under selective spinal anesthesia with lidocaine 10 mg and sufentanil 10 μg with and without epinephrine 50 μg, spinal cord functions (spinothalamic, dorsal column, and motor) were well preserved, with or without epinephrine.[40] Several animal studies have shown that administering subarachnoid epinephrine (up to 200 μg bolus) does not decrease spinal cord blood flow in cats or dogs.[35, 37, 38] A study in dogs using a spinal-window preparation demonstrated a modest reduction (10.6 percent) in spinal pial vessel diameter produced by epinephrine 5 μg/mL – a small change that did not lead to a critical decrease in spinal cord blood flow.[36]

On the other hand, epinephrine administered epidurally reduces the epidural blood flow markedly,[37] but concentrations of epinephrine from 0.5 to 5 μg/mL have been found to be safe in epidural infusions.[42, 43, 44, 45]

An additional, possibly very important advantage of epinephrine infusion into the epidural space is the effect on platelets, increasing their adhesiveness, reducing any bleeding that may follow a vessel injury in the epidural space.

In a dose-determining study, we documented that epinephrine concentrations of 0.5 or 1 μg/mL were less effective than 1.5 and 2 μg/mL in potentiating epidural analgesia from bupivacaine and fentanyl.[31] Therefore, we chose a concentration of epinephrine of 2 μg/mL so that any oxidative inactivation (about 10 percent after several

---

Box 26.1 Epinephrine interacts pharmocokinetically and pharmacodynamically with bupivacaine and fentanyl to improve efficacy and safety of epidural analgesia

There are several positive interactions which occur between epinephrine and the two other components:

1. Pharmacokinetic interactions between epinephrine and the local anesthetic reduce systemic absorption, decreasing the systemic adverse effects of the latter two and allow higher passage from the epidural space to the cerebrospinal fluid (CSF) and spinal cord, where pharmcodynamic interactions between the α_2-agonist effects of epinephrine with the opioid agonist and the synaptic inhibition of the local anesthetic synergize to cause strong analgesic effects with low doses of each of the three drugs. This allows further reduction in the doses of each drug, reducing dose-related side effects.[47]
2. Epinephrine increases stickiness of platelets, potentially reducing any bleeding from needle/catheter injury of epidural vessels.

---

months shelf life[46]), would still leave sufficient epinephrine for the desired effect.

With this background and our extensive clinical experience over two decades, we are convinced that the minute dose of epinephrine (about 20 μg per hour) is not only advantageous for its analgesic effect but is also very safe (**Box 26.1**).[25, 26]

PRESCRIPTION FOR SAFE AND EFFECTIVE EPIDURAL ANALGESIA AND PATIENT-CONTROLLED EPIDURAL ANALGESIA FOR POSTOPERATIVE AND OBSTETRIC PAIN RELIEF

Our prescriptions for safe and effective epidural and patient-controlled epidural analgesia, which we have practiced now for two decades at the University Clinic Pain Services of Rikshospitalet, Oslo, Norway, and Inselspital, Berne, Switzerland, are summarized here. More detail and background can be found in several key references.[25, 26, 48]

Epidural analgesia for postoperative pain relief

- Indications:
  - ideal for relief of severe dynamic pain on moving, deep breathing, and coughing after thoracotomies, upper abdominal surgery, major abdominal surgery;

- because of motor blockade of lumbosacral nerve roots, causing weak legs and urinary retention, lumbar epidural analgesia is less than ideal after pelvic surgery and major orthopedic surgery on hips and lower extremities.
- Contraindications/relative contraindications:
  - any increased risk of bleeding into the spinal canal:
    - hereditary or aquired hematologic abnormalities;
    - international normalized ratio (INR) above 1.6;
    - platelets below 100,000;
    - potent platelet inhibitors, discontinued less than five days previously;
    - low molecular weight heparin (LMWH) in more than thromboprophylaxis doses, less than 24 hours previously;
    - fondaparinux less than 36 hours previously;
    - heparin less than four hours previously, or abnormal activated partial thromboplastin time (APTT).
  - infection in the skin area for epidural catheter insertion.
  - abnormal anatomy of the spine making epidural catheterization difficult.

Epidural analgesia with local anesthetic, opioid, and epinephrine is mainly spinal cord analgesic effects, but also spinal nerve root local anesthetic effects. Therefore, the following procedure should be followed: place the epidural catheter at the appropriate segmental level before surgery, test for bilateral sensory block before induction of general anesthesia, and continue epidural analgesic infusion during surgery to obtain a "flying start" of postoperative analgesia.

The recommended segmental level for the tip of the epidural catheter is as follows:

- thoracotomy: Th4–7;
- upper abdominal surgery: Th7–9;
- major abdominal surgery: Th8–11;
- low abdominal/pelvic surgery: Th10–L1;
- hip/knee surgery: L1–3.

We use a triple-component analgesic mixture with low concentrations of a local anesthetic, an opioid, and an adrenergic agonist. Our hospital pharmacy makes stock solutions, and bags containing 550, 275, or 110 mL are prepared with the following content:[46]

- bupivacaine 1 mg/mL;
- fentanyl 2 μg/mL;
- epinephrine 2 μg/mL.

This is an intentionally weak epidural analgesic mixture, intended to reduce severe dynamic pain to mild pain, but not aiming for complete pain-free movements. This enables patients to feel pathological pain (caused by surgical complication or epidural bleeding/infection). Because the systemic absorption of fentanyl is almost nil (with the epinephrine added), any pain outside the segmental areas covered with the epidural can be relieved with i.v. morphine or similar potent opioid given intravenously.

We use a closed system with a 550-mL bag (enough for about three days after major surgery) and a remote administration set in an electronically controlled and driven, tamper-proof infusion pump with patient-controlled bolus option (**Figure 26.3**).

Nurses or doctors on the surgical ward adjust the epidural analgesia infusion rates of between 5 and 10 mL per hour, adjusted to an area of cutaneous cold hyposensitivity (ice cube in glove) covering the wound.

When the patient is alert and has stable cardiorespiratory functions, patients are allowed patient-controlled bolus infusion (3–5 mL, lock-out time 30 minutes) to increase analgesia before mobilization or deep breathing and coughing exercises. The infusion rate and catheter site determine the segmental spread of the epidural analgesia. Epidural bolus doses will deepen and strengthen the intensity of analgesia.

The robust and vigilant monitoring regime is as follows. Nurses on the surgical wards monitor and record the following every four hours:

- sensory levels – upper and lower, bilateral, using cold stimuli, e.g. ice cube in plastic glove or alcohol swab;
- motor function: is there any leg weakness or increasing leg weakness?
- pain intensity during rest and during movement, using a 0–10 numeric rating scale (NRS) for pain intensity;
- sedation, on a 0–3 categorical scale;

- respiratory rate;
- systolic blood pressure;
- drug consumption, total since start;
- occurrence of any side effects, e.g. itching, nausea;
- need for urinary bladder catheterization?

When nursing time is limited (e.g. during night shifts), the following three questions must be answered.

- Can the patient be easily awakened?
- Is the patient pain free at rest and has only mild pain when deep breathing or coughing?
- Can the patient move the feet as easily as before?
- If all are affirmatively answered, the epidural is working as it should and there are no major complications.

Attention should be paid to sterile techniques in caring for epidural catheters and tube connections. The system should be kept closed, with no tube changes needed, unless there is contamination.

Once every 24 hours, examine for tenderness at the catheter entry site. If there is tenderness, inspect for rubor at the catheter entry site. If there are local signs of catheter channel infection, remove the catheter, culture for bacteria, and consider antibiotics if there are signs of systemic infection.

Discontinuing epidural analgesia should be undertaken as follows.

- Reduce infusion rate by about 30 percent every three hours.
- Start oral opioid and nonopioid analgesic at the appropriate dose (e.g. oral oxycodone 10–20 mg + paracetamol 1 g for adult patients above 50 kg in weight).

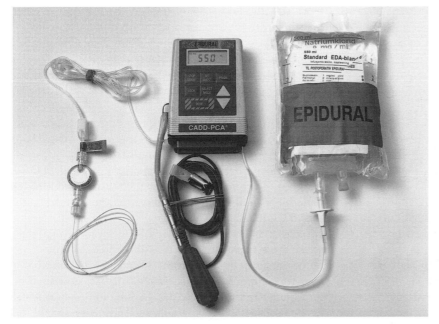

Figure 26.3 A closed system for delivering the epidural analgesic mixture. A 550-mL bag prepared by our hospital pharmacy and Fresenius-Kabi, Halden, Norway, contains bupivacaine 1 mg/mL, fentanyl 2 µg/mL, and epinephrine (adrenaline) 2 µg/mL. This solution is stable for several months.[46] The epidural analgesic mixture is delivered at a constant infusion rate of 5–10 mL per hour, titrated by the nurses on the surgical ward through a Deltec CADD pump (Deltec, Saint Paul, MN, USA). If more analgesia is required, the patient is allowed to self-administer a rescue analgesic bolus dose of usually 4 mL, up to twice per hour. This is possible only when the patient is awake, clear-headed, and has stable cardiorespiratory vital signs.

- Leave epidural catheter in place for at least three hours in order to be able to restart epidural infusion, if necessary.

EPIDURAL ANALGESIA IN CHILDREN

The same general precautions as for adults are needed in children. Epidural catheterization with the patient heavily sedated or under general anesthesia without muscle relaxants is accepted by many pediatric anesthesiologists, but the author feels that extreme caution should be exercised: spinal cord damage from needle trauma or epidural bleeding is possible and will not be easily detected in a child under deep general anesthetic.

The infusion rate of our standard epidural mixture (see above under Epinephrine markedly increases safety of epidural analgesia with bupivacaine and fentanyl) is 0.3–0.5 mL/kg per hour. Bolus dose administered by the patient is one-third of the hourly infusion rate.

EARLY DETECTION AND URGENT HANDLING OF EPIDURAL HEMATOMA OR ABSCESS

With our reliable, closed infusion pump system, the ongoing educational program for nurses, pump malfunctions, and programming errors are practically eliminated. With thoracic catheter position and low infusion rates of the low-concentrations standard epidural mixture, hypotension (in normovolemic patients), respiratory depression, and significant motor blockade occur infrequently. However, epidural bleeding and infection are always potential risks,[21, 22, 23, 25, 26, 48] and therefore everyone involved in the care of patients having epidural analgesia:

- must be vigilantly looking for early signs of infection or hematoma in the epidural space, including new backache, leg weakness, or increasing leg weakness;
- must have a high awareness for the need of urgent MR or CT scan to verify suspected spinal canal bleeding or infection;
- have high preparedness for urgent surgical decompression should spinal cord compression from bleeding or abscess be verified.

There is only a period of about ten hours from initial symptoms of increasing leg weakness until the spinal cord is irreversibly damaged by an epidural hematoma. The time of grace is longer when an epidural abscess is slowly increasing in size: averaging about three days.[22, 23]

EPIDURAL ANALGESIA AFTER ABDOMINOPERINEAL OR LOWER LIMB SURGERY

Prolonged epidural analgesia after lower abdominal or abdominoperineal surgery or major orthopedic surgery of the lower limb requires balancing the composition of the epidural analgesic mixture with segmental siting of the epidural catheter. A lumbar epidural catheter with a local anesthetic-containing epidural infusion will easily cause cauda equina nerve root anesthesia with motor blockade and leg weakness. For opioid and adrenergic components to affect dorsal horn pain transmission, the catheter has to be placed above L2 for a low-dose infusion to reach the spinal cord.

With our standard triple-component epidural solution, we have obtained the best results (best analgesia with least leg weakness) for perineal pain by placing the catheter at the thoracolumbar or upper lumbar levels.[29]

EPIDURAL ANALGESIA IN PATIENTS IN THE INTENSIVE CARE UNIT

If for any reason the postoperative patient becomes an intensive care unit patient, heavily sedated, or on the respirator, reliable monitoring of effects of the epidural and of spinal cord functions is not possible. Consider discontinuing the epidural and removing the epidural catheter, if no bleeding problems are present.

EPIDURAL ANALGESIA IN LABOR IS GOLD STANDARD OF OBSTERIC ANALGESIA

Epidural analgesia for vaginal delivery is the "gold standard" for relief of severe pain during childbirth. When instituted early during the first stage, combined with spinal analgesia, delivery may be shortened and outcome for mother and child improved, compared with systemic analgesics – and compared with epidural analgesia started later.[49, 50]

During the first stage of delivery, pain impulses enter the spinal cord at segmental levels Th10–L1-2; during the second stage pain impulses enter at low lumbar and sacral segments as well. The ideal regime may be a low dose of bupivacaine (1–1.25 mg) plus fentanyl (20 µg), or sufentanil (4 µg) given subarachnoidally at the start of painful contractions, and with an epidural catheter placed at the same time. Epidural low rate infusion 4–6 mL per hour (of bupivacaine (or ropivacaine) 1 mg/mL + fentanyl 2 µg/mL + epinephrine 2 µg/mL) is activated after one to two hours when the effects of the subarachnoid injection are weaning. The parturient may be allowed to administer patient-controlled epidural boluses of the same mixture (3–5 mL) up to twice per hour.

This, and similar regimes, results in specific spinal cord analgesia with minimal motor blockade, minimal systemic, fetal, and postpartum effects on the newborn, shortened first and second stages of labor, decreased or unchanged rates of cesarean section and instrumental deliveries (**Box 26.2**).[49, 50]

Box 26.2 Epidural (neuraxial) analgesia in labor

1. Spinal puncture at L3–4 with a 27-gauge spinal needle or combined spinal epidural when contractions are painful.
2. Subarachnoid injection of bupivacaine (1–1.25 mg) plus fentanyl (20 μg), or sufentanil (4 μg).
3. Place epidural catheter, aiming tip of catheter at L1–2.
4. Activate epidural infusion when painful contractions are recurring at 4–6 mL per hour of bupivacaine (1 mg/mL) plus fentanyl (2 μg/mL) and epidnephrine (2 μg/mL).
5. Allow patient-controlled epidural bolus 4–5 mL up to every 30 minutes.

REQUIREMENTS FOR A SUCCESSFUL POSTOPERATIVE PAIN MANAGEMENT PROGRAM

One important lesson from the last two decades of experience with acute postoperative pain relief, using epidural analgesia as well as intravenous opioid patient-controlled analgesia and upgraded "low-technology" traditional pain relief,[25, 26] is that in order to have a successful postoperative epidural pain management service, the following factors need to be in place.

- A minimum number of dedicated pain personnel: at least one pain nurse covering daytime activities, supported by an anesthesiologist who is able to spend most of his/her time on postoperative pain management.
- Through an educational program, the nurses on the surgical wards learn, and relearn, how to monitor and manage pain. The educational program has to be ongoing, to reach all new personnel and part-time and night-time nurses.
- There should be standard orders on how to adjust treatment, how to look out for early symptoms of potentially harmful adverse effect, and how to prevent and treat such adverse effects.
- The monitoring regime and educational program are instruments for continuous quality improvement, and will result in all patients having better pain control, i.e. not only those who benefit from high-skill, high-technology, postoperative epidural analgesia or i.v. opioid PCA, but also those who require only low-technology approaches.[25]

ALTERNATIVE EPIDURAL ANALGESIC MIXTURES

There are many alternative recipes for postoperative epidural analgesia. Ropivacaine is an alternative to bupivacaine, being less cardiotoxic.[32] When co-administering bupivacaine with fentanyl and epinephrine for epidural infusion analgesia, very low doses are required so that cardiotoxicity of bupivacaine is not an issue.[25]

Sufentanil is more potent than fentanyl; it is well documented and approved for epidural administration in several countries. With epinephrine and bupivacaine, sufentanil appears to function as well as fentanyl.[51] It is more expensive than fentanyl and our hospital pharmacy is still not able to obtain sufentanil (or ropivacaine) in dry form for our triple-component epidural mixture.

Morphine or diamorphine and bupivacaine, with or without epinephrine, may be a bit less sensitive to optimal segmental siting of the epidural catheter, but nausea and pruritus often reduce the quality of analgesia, and they may have a higher risk of respiratory depression.[18]

SUMMARY

Thoracic epidural analgesia reduces risks of cardiopulmonary complications after thoracic and upper and major abdominal surgery. Lumbar epidural anesthesia for pelvic surgery and orthopedic surgery of the lower extremities, when prolonged after surgery, does not decrease cardiopulmonary risks and causes urinary retention and weak legs. Epinephrine, when added to a local anesthetic and fentanyl, decreases the doses needed and increases effectiveness and safety of epidural analgesia for postoperative pain relief. Epidural epinephrine does not decrease spinal cord blood flow; it does decrease epidural blood flow, systemic absorption of local anesthetic and opioid, and therefore decreases opioid side effects (nausea, itching, urinary retention, respiratory depression).

Effective and safe epidural analgesia for postoperative and obstetric analgesia is primarily spinal cord analgesia and requires:

- appropriate segmental placement of the catheter;
- an infusion of low concentrations of a local anesthetic, a lipophilic opioid, and epinephrine;
- a robust monitoring regime where ward nurses observe and record at least every fourth hour:
  - upper and lower segmental analgesic level using an ice cube, or alcohol swab;
  - any leg weakness;
  - pain intensity at rest and when moving, deep breathing or coughing – on a 0–10 numeric scale;
  - any new backache, leg weakness, and leg numbness;
- a high preparedness for detecting early signs of epidural infection or bleeding, for verifying diagnosis

with MR or CT scan and surgical preparedness for urgent laminectomy should spinal cord ischemia/compression occur.

A prerequisite for a successful postoperative epidural practice is a well-organized acute pain team with well-trained pain nurses, anesthesiologist availability, and ongoing educational program for ward nurses, anesthesiologists, surgeons, and patients (see Chapter 47, Organization and role of acute pain services and Chapter 48, Acute pain services and organizational change).

Epidural analgesia after abdominoperineal or lower limb surgery gives good analgesia, but urinary retention, requiring catheter emptying, and leg weakness occur frequently when meaningful local anesthetic concentrations are used. This makes early mobilization, as well as monitoring of spinal cord functions and early detection of epidural hematoma or abscess, more difficult.

Epidural analgesia for vaginal delivery is the "gold standard" for relief of severe pain during childbirth. When combined with subarachnoid (spinal) injection of low, analgesic doses of a local anesthetic and a lipophilic opioid early, the first stage of labor is shortened, rates of cesarean section and instrumental deliveries are decreased. The risk of postpartum back pain is not increased.

Alternative epidural analgesic mixtures, instead of fentanyl, containing sufentanil, diacetylmorphine, or morphine are effective as well, but the latter two may cause more respiratory depression, nausea, itching, and urinary retention.

REFERENCES

1. Brown DL, Bridenbaugh LD. The upper extremity. Somatic block. In: Cousins MJ, Bridenbaugh PO (eds). *Neural blockade in clinical anesthesia and management of pain*, 3rd edn. Philadelphia, PA: Lippincott-Raven, 1998: 345–71.

2. Klaastad O, Smith HJ, Smedby O et al. A novel infraclavicular brachial plexus block: the lateral and sagittal technique, developd by magnetic resonance imaging studies. *Anesthesia and Analgesia*. 2007; **105**: 295–7.

3. Capdevila X, Barthelet Y, Biboulet P et al. Effects of perioperative analgesic technique on the surgical outcome and duration of rehabilitation after major knee surgery. *Anesthesiology*. 1999; **91**: 8–15.

* 4. Ballantyne JC, Carr DB, deFerranti S et al. The comparative effects of postoperative analgesic therapies on pulmonary outcome: cumulative meta-analyses of randomized, controlled trials. *Anesthesia and Analgesia*. 1998; **86**: 598–612.

* 5. Nishimori N, Ballantyne JC, Low JHS. Epidural pain relief versus systemic opioid-based pain relief for abdominal aortic surgery. *Cochrane Database of Systemic Reviews*. 2006; **CD005059**.

6. Park WY, Thomson JS, Lee KK. Effect of epidural anesthesia and analgesia on perioperative outcome. A randomized, controlled veterans affairs cooperative study. *Annals of Surgery*. 2001; **234**: 560–71.

7. Wattwil M, Thoren T, Hennerdal S, Garvill J-E. Epidural analgesia with bupivacaine reduces postoperative paralytic ileus after hysterectomy. *Anesthesia and Analgesia*. 1989; **68**: 353–8.

8. Liu SS, Carpenter RL, Meal JM. Epidural anesthesia and analgesia: their role in postoperative outcome. *Anesthesiology*. 1995; **82**: 1474–506.

9. Liu SS, Carpenter RL, Mackey DC et al. Effects of perioperative analgesic technique on rate of recovery after colon surgery. *Anesthesiology*. 1995; **83**: 757–65.

10. Steinbrook RA. Epidural anesthesia and gastrointestinal motility. *Anesthesia and Analgesia*. 1998; **86**: 837–44.

* 11. Van Aken H, Gogarten W, Rolf N. Epidural anesthesia in cardiac risk patients. *Anesthesia and Analgesia*. 1999; **89** (Review Course Suppl.): 104–10.

12. Breivik H. Postoperative pain management: why is it difficult to show that it improves outcome? *European Journal of Anaesthesiology*. 1998; **15**: 748–51.

13. Rodgers A, Walker N, Schug S, Kehlet H. Reduction of postoperative mortality and morbidity with epidural or spinal anaesthesia: results from overview of randomised trials. *British Medical Journal*. 2000; **321**: 1493–7.

14. Beatty WS, Badner NH, Choi P. Epidural analgesia reduces postoperative myocardial infarction: a meta-analysis. *Anesthesia and Analgesia*. 2001; **93**: 853–8.

15. Scott NB, Turfrey DJ, Ray DAA et al. A prospective randomized study of the potential benefits of thoracic epidural anesthesia and analgesia in patients undergoing coronary artery bypass grafting. *Anesthesia and Analgesia*. 2001; **93**: 528–35.

* 16. Gulur P, Nishimori M, Ballantyne JC. Regional anaesthesia versus general anaesthesia, morbidity and mortality. Best Practice and Research. *Clinical Anaesthesiology*. 2006; **20**: 249–63.

17. Norris EJ, Beattie C, Perler BA et al. Double-masked randomized trial comparing alternative combinations of intraoperative anesthesia and postoperative analgesia in abdominal aortic surgery. *Anesthesiology*. 2001; **95**: 1054–67.

18. Wheatley RG, Schug SA, Watson D. Safety and efficacy of postoperative epidural analgesia. *British Journal of Anaesthesia*. 2001; **87**: 47–61.

19. Stenseth R, Bjella L, Berg EM et al. Thoracic epidural analgesia in aortocoronary bypass surgery: hemodynamic effects. *Acta Anaesthesiologica Scandinavica*. 1994; **38**: 826–33.

20. Stenseth R, Berg EM, Bjella L et al. Effects of thoracic epidural analgesia on coronary hemodynamics and myocardial metabolism in coronary artery bypass surgery. *Journal of Cardiothoracic and Vascular Anesthesia*. 1995; **9**: 503–09.

* 21. Moen V, Dahlgren N, Irestedt L. Severe neurological complications after central neuraxial blockades in Sweden 1990–1999. *Anesthesiology*. 2004; **101**: 950–9.

22. Breivik H. Neurological complications in association with spinal and epidural analgesia – again. *Acta Anaesthesiologica Scandinavica*. 1998; **42**: 609–13.

* 23. Breivik H. Infectious complications of epidural anaesthesia and analgesia. *Current Opinion in Anaesthesiology*. 1999; **12**: 573–7.

24. Berenbaum MC. What is synergy? *Pharmacological Reviews*. 1989; **41**: 93–141.

* 25. Breivik H. High-tech versus low-tech approaches to postoperative pain management. In: Devor M, Rowbotham MC, Wiesenfeld-Hallin Z (eds). *Progress in Pain Research and Management 16*. Seattle: IASP-Press, 2000: 787–807.

* 26. Breivik H, Curatolo M, Niemi G *et al.* How to implement an acute postoperative pain service: an update. In: Breivik H, Shipley M (eds). *Pain – best practice and research compendium*. London: Elsevier, 2007: 255–70.

* 27. Niemi G, Breivik H. Adrenaline markedly improves thoracic epidural analgesia produced by a low-dose infusion of bupivacaine, fentanyl and adrenaline after major surgery. *Acta Anaesthesiologica Scandinavica*. 1998; **42**: 897–909.

* 28. Niemi G, Breivik H. Epidural fentanyl markedly improves thoracic epidural analgesia in a low-dose infusion of bupivacaine, adrenaline and fentanyl. A randomized, double-blind crossover study with and without fentanyl. *Acta Anaesthesiologica Scandinavica*. 2001; **45**: 221–32.

29. Breivik H, Niemi G, Haugtomt H, Högström H. Optimal epidural analgesia: importance of drug combinations and correct segmental site of injection. *Baillière's Clinical Anaesthesiology*. 1995; **9**: 493–512.

30. Cohen S, Armar D, Pantuck CB *et al.* Epidural patient-controlled analgesia after cesarean section buprenorphine–0.015% bupivacaine with epinephrine versus fentanyl–0.015% bupivacaine with and without epinephrine. *Anesthesia and Analgesia*. 1992; **74**: 226–30.

* 31. Niemi G, Breivik H. The minimally effective concentration of adrenaline in a low-dose thoracic epidural infusion of bupivacaine and fentanyl after major thoracic and abdominal surgery. A randomised, double-blind dose-finding study. *Acta Anaesthesiologica Scandinavica*. 2003; **47**: 439–50.

32. Niemi G, Breivik H. Epinephrine markedly improves thoracic epidural analgesia produced by a small-dose infusion of ropivacaine, fentanyl, and epinephrine after major thoracic or abdominal surgery: a randomized, double-blind crossover study with and without epinephrine. *Anesthesia and Analgesia*. 2002; **94**: 1598–605.

33. Paech MJ, Pavy TJ, Orlaikowski CE *et al.* Postoperative epidural infusion: a randomized, double-blind, dose-finding trial of clonidine in combination with bupivacaine and fentanyl. *Anesthesia and Analgesia*. 1997; **84**: 1323–8.

34. Verborgh C, Van der Auwera C, Noorduin H, Camu F. Epidural sufentanil for postoperative pain relief: effects of adrenaline. *European Journal of Anaesthesiology*. 1988; **5**: 183–91.

* 35. Porter SS, Albin MS, Watson WA *et al.* Spinal cord and cerebral blood flow responses to subarachnoid injection of local anesthetics with and without epinephrine. *Acta Anaesthesiologica Scandinavica*. 1985; **29**: 330–8.

36. Iida H, Ohata H, Iida M *et al.* Direct effects of alpha1- and alpha2-adrenergic agonists on spinal and cerebral pial vessels in dogs. *Anesthesiology*. 1999; **91**: 479–85.

37. Kozody R, Palahniuk RJ, Wade JG *et al.* The effect of subarachnoid epinephrine and phenylephrine on spinal cord blood flow. *Canadian Anaesthetists' Society Journal*. 1984; **31**: 503–08.

* 38. Dohi S, Takeshima R, Naito H. Spinal cord blood flow during spinal anesthesia in dogs: the effects of tetracaine, epinephrine, acute blood loss, and hypercapnia. *Anesthesia and Analgesia*. 1987; **66**: 599–606.

39. Hodgson PS, Neal JM, Pollock JE, Liu SS. The neurotoxicity of drugs given intrathecally (spinal). *Anesthesia and Analgesia*. 1999; **88**: 797–809.

* 40. Vaghadia H, Solylo MA, Henderson CL, Mitchell GW. Selective spinal anesthesia for outpatient laparoscopy. II. Epinephrine and spinal cord function. *Canadian Journal of Anaesthesia*. 2001; **48**: 261–6.

* 41. Bromage PR. Neurologic complications of epidural and spinal techniques. *Baillière's Clinical Anaesthesiology*. 1994; **7**: 793–815.

42. Baron CM, Kowalski SE, Greengrass R *et al.* Epinephrine decreases postoperative requirements for continuous thoracic epidural fentanyl infusions. *Anesthesia and Analgesia*. 1996; **82**: 760–5.

43. Lysak SZ, Eisenach JC, Dobson CE. Patient-controlled epidural analgesia during labor: a comparison of three solutions with a continuous infusion control. *Anesthesiology*. 1990; **72**: 44–9.

44. Sakaguchi Y, Sakura S, Shinzawa M, Saito Y. Does adrenaline improve epidural bupivacaine and fentanyl analgesia after abdominal surgery? *Anaesthesia and Intensive Care*. 2000; **28**: 522–6.

45. Breivik H, Högström H, Niemi G *et al.* Safe and effective post-operative pain-relief: introduction and continuous quality-improvement of comprehensive post-operative pain management programmes. *Baillière's Clinical Anaesthesiology*. 1995; **9**: 423–60.

46. Kjønniksen I, Brustugun J, Niemi G *et al.* Stability of an epidural analgesic solution containing adrenaline, bupivacaine and fentanyl. *Acta Anaesthesiologica Scandinavica*. 2000; **44**: 864–7.

* 47. Collins JG, Kitahata LM, Suzukawa M. Spinally administered epinephrine suppresses noxiously evoked activity of WDR neurons in the dorsal horn of the spinal cord. *Anesthesiology*. 1984; **60**: 269–75.

* 48. Breivik H. Benefits, risks and economics of post-operative pain management programmes. *Baillière's Clinical Anaesthesiology*. 1995; **9**: 403–22.

49. Marucci M, Cinella G, Perchiazzi G *et al.* Patient-requested neuraxial analgesia for labor. *Anesthesiology*. 2007; **106**: 1035–145.

* 50. Wong CA, Scavone BM, Peaceman AM *et al.* The risk of cesarean delivery with neuraxial analgesia given early versus late in labor. *New England Journal of Medicine*. 2005; **352**: 655–65.

51. Cohen S, Armar D, Pantuck CB *et al.* Postcesarean delivery epidural patient-controlled analgesia. Fentanyl or sufentanil? *Anesthesiology*. 1993; **78**: 486–91.

Sympathetic blocks

HARALD BREIVIK

KEY LEARNING POINTS

- Sympathetic efferent fibers are involved in nociception and transmission of pain impulses.
- Sympathetic efferent nerve impulses can modify functions of sensory nerves after injury or infection, causing sympathetically maintained pain as part of a neuropathic pain condition. However, only approximately one-third of complex neuropathic pain conditions have a sympathetically maintained pain component.
- The anatomy of the autonomic nervous system allows specific blocks and interference of sympathetic outflow so that sympathetically maintained pain can be diagnosed and treated specifically.
- Selective sympathetic blocks of the upper and lower extremities can be performed effectively with low risk of complications.
- The evidence-base for long-term effects of sympathetic blocks on chronic complex pain conditions is limited: negative studies are often flawed by not selecting patients with proven sympathetically maintained pain, whereas the reported long-term positive outcomes in the hands of experts is considered weak evidence.

INTRODUCTION

The sympathetic nervous system maintains a constrictor tone in blood vessels of the skin. The classic indication for sympathetic neural blockade and surgical sympathectomy has been to help in the healing of ischemic cutaneous ulcers and to relieve ischemic foot pain at rest.[1] Although vascular surgery may help such patients, rest pain due to ischemic conditions of the lower extremity is still an appropriate indication for lumbar sympathetic neural blockade.[1]

Sympathetically maintained pain is indicated by pain relief in complex regional pain syndromes subsequent to either systemic alpha blockade (intravenous phentolamine test;[2] see Chapter 5, Pharmacological diagnostic tests) or regional sympathetic block. This can be with repeated local anesthetic blocks, neurolytic sympathetic blocks, or radiofrequency (Chapter 33, Radiofrequency lesioning and treatment of chronic pain) or surgical neurolysis. A common indication for sympathectomy has been hyperhidrosis. However, this is now recognized as a significant cause of persistent pain: approximately 10 percent of patients develop postsympathectomy pain after open or endoscopic sympathectomy for hyperhidrosis.[3]

Sympathetic afferent and efferent pain impulses are stopped by brachial plexus, spinal, or epidural local anesthetic blocks. These effects are exploited with continuous brachial plexus blocks, obstetric epidurals, and postoperative epidurals using local anesthetic for the relief of visceral pain. Visceral sympathetic inhibition increases gastrointestinal motility after surgery (see Chapter 26, Epidural analgesia for acute pain after surgery and during labor, including patient-controlled epidural analgesia). It is, however, the more specific sympathetic blocks, made possible by the separation in peripheral anatomy of sympathetic and somatic nervous structures, which will be described in this chapter.

Specific sympathetic blockade is possible at the cervicothoracic and lumbar areas as well as at the celiac and hypogastric sympathetic plexa. Specific interruption of sympathetic afferent or efferent nerves at these three vertebral areas is possible because the sympathetic ganglia and plexa are sufficiently anatomically separated from somatic nerves that it is possible to achieve sympathetic blockade without blocking sensory or motor functions (**Figure 27.1**).

Lumbar sympathetic block for rest pain of the legs and celiac plexus block for abdominal visceral pain from cancer are two of the most beneficial neural blockade techniques available.[1]

Celiac plexus blockade, superior hypogastric plexus block, and ganglion impar block are described in Chapter 28, Neurolytic blocks.

ANATOMY OF THE SYMPATHETIC NERVOUS SYSTEM

The peripheral sympathetic nervous system originates in efferent neurons in the intermediolateral column of the spinal cord, with preganglionic fibers through the ventral roots from T1 to L2 leaving the spinal canal as the white rami communicantes to the sympathetic chain (**Figure 27.2**). The sympathetic chain lies at the anterolateral aspect of the vertebral bodies in the cervical region. In the thorax, it is adjacent to the neck of the ribs, relatively close to the somatic nerve roots, whereas in the lumbar region the sympathetic chain again lies anterolateral to the bodies of the vertebrae and is separated from the somatic nerve roots by the psoas muscle and psoas fascia. The preganglionic fibers run a variable distance within the sympathetic chain to ganglia in the chain up or down from the segment of the spinal cord where they originate, or they may pass to peripherally located ganglia in the gastrointestinal or urogenital tracts (**Figure 27.2**).

This variable level of relay between the preganglionic and the postganglionic neurons within the sympathetic chain is one reason for variable results from an apparently technically successful block, and also for regeneration of sympathetic function after a successful sympathetic block and gradual recurrence of symptoms.

There are three or four cervical sympathetic ganglia, 12 thoracic, four or five lumbar, and four sacral sympathetic ganglia. There is one coccygeal sympathetic ganglion – the ganglion impar.

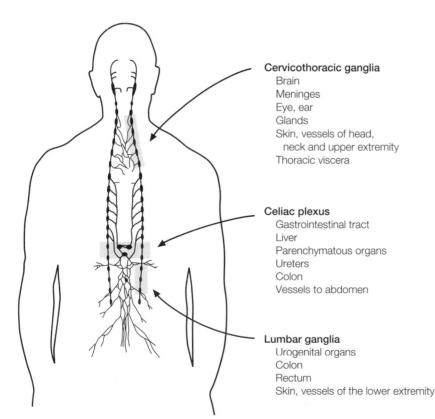

Cervicothoracic ganglia
Brain
Meninges
Eye, ear
Glands
Skin, vessels of head,
   neck and upper extremity
Thoracic viscera

Celiac plexus
Gastrointestinal tract
Liver
Parenchymatous organs
Ureters
Colon
Vessels to abdomen

Lumbar ganglia
Urogenital organs
Colon
Rectum
Skin, vessels of the lower extremity

Figure 27.1 Sympathetic nervous system outlined. Redrawn with permission from Breivik H, Cousins MJ, Löfström JB, *Neural Blockade in Clinical Anesthesia and Management of Pain*, 3rd edn, Cousins MJ, Bridenbaugh PO (eds), Lippincott-Raven Publishers, 1998.

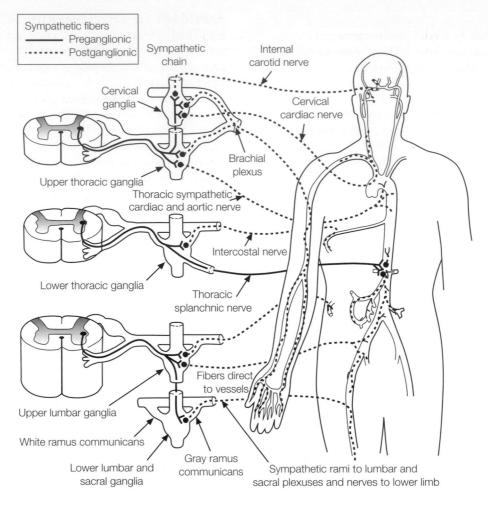

Figure 27.2 Sympathetic nerve supply to blood vessels. Redrawn with permission from Breivik H, Cousins MJ, Löfström JB, *Neural Blockade in Clinical Anesthesia and Management of Pain*, 3rd edn, Cousins MJ, Bridenbaugh PO (eds), Lippincott-Raven Publishers, 1998.

The postganglionic fibers from the sympathetic ganglion cells are widely distributed to join peripheral nerves via the gray rami communicantes and also to join blood vessels to various organs.

The sympathetic chain receives efferent preganglionic fibers from the spinal cord as well as afferent visceral fibers carrying pain impulses from the extremities, the head and neck, and the abdominal and pelvic viscera, including the urogenital system. The carotid arteries, aorta, and vena cava receive direct postganglionic nerves from nearby sympathetic ganglia and plexuses (**Figure 27.2**). Sympathetic nerve fibers may arrive at the vessel wall from adjacent ganglia, via postganglionic fibers passing in somatic nerves to the vessels, and postganglionic fibers that pass up or down the sympathetic chain, or fibers synapsing in the prevertebral plexuses before they pass to the vessels. All these sympathetic vascular nerves and filaments meet in extensive perivascular and adventitial sympathetic networks. Local anesthetic blockade using perivascular brachial plexus approaches will inhibit sympathetic nervous functions very effectively in the upper extremity, a fact exploited

well by continuous brachial plexus block after reimplantation surgery of the extremity.

The roles of the sympathetic nervous system in chronic pain are described in Chapter 27, Complex regional pain syndromes in the *Chronic Pain* volume of this series, and are reviewed by Breivik *et al.*[1] and Jänig and Stanton-Hicks.[4] A comprehensive review of functions and roles of the autonomic nervous system in health and disease is given by Jänig.[5]

INDICATIONS FOR SYMPATHETIC NEURAL BLOCKADE

The following clinical conditions may benefit from interruption of sympathetic efferent and afferent nerves.[1, 3, 4, 6]

Acute pain

- Acute pancreatitis.
- Renal colic.

- Cardiac pain.
- Visceral pain from uterine contractions.
- Acute ischemic pain from accidental intra-arterial injections of irritating drugs such as thiopental (thiopentone).
- Frostbite.
- Vascular surgery and reimplantation surgery (to reduce postoperative pain and improve postoperative blood flow).
- Acute exacerbation of Raynaud's disease.

Chronic pain

- Obliterative arterial disease causing rest pain in the lower extremities (when vascular surgery is not indicated).
- Complex regional pain syndromes (CRPS types I and II, without (I) or with (II) obvious nervous tissue injury).[4]
- Phantom limb pain.
- Central neuropathic pain.
- Chronic pancreatitis.
- Cancer pain from upper abdominal viscera.
- Cancer pain from pelvic viscera.

There is considerable disagreement on whether CRPSs are indications for sympathetic blockade.[4] This was formerly called reflex sympathetic dystrophy (RSD), but the diagnosis was often made without ascertaining whether sympathetic block relieved the pain.[4] Clearly, patients with a picture of what clinically was called "reflex sympathetic dystrophy" did not always have pain relief after sympathetic blocks. It is now realized that sympathetically maintained pain is present in only about one-third of patients with a clinical presentation of "reflex sympathetic dystrophy," now more correctly called complex regional pain syndrome (CRPS type I or type II, without or with obvious major nervous tissue damage, respectively).[1, 4]

Only an intravenous phentolamine test (see Chapter 5, Pharmacological diagnostic tests) or a specific diagnostic sympathetic block will indicate with some certainty whether the patient has a component of sympathetically maintained pain in the CRPS. Only one in three or one in four CRPS patients have sympathetically maintained pain.[1, 2, 3]

Studies on the pain-relieving effects of sympathetic neural blockade, in which patients with the clinical presentation of "RSD" or "CRPS" were included without documenting that they had sympathetically maintained pain, obviously must have had a low sensitivity: any beneficial effects on the few patients with sympathetically maintained pain would have disappeared among the majority of nonresponding patients included who did not have sympathetically maintained pain (60–75 percent of all with CRPS-like pain conditions). Such studies will have a high risk of false-negative results. Unfortunately, negative publications of "randomized controlled trials" with such obvious flaws have created a conviction among many that blockade of sympathetic nerves is obsolete treatment.[7] Experienced clinicians continue to carry out these blocks because we have seen otherwise intractable patients in whom repeated sympathetic blocks give significant relief.[1, 6, 8, 9, 10, 11]

However, long-standing CRPS with a component of sympathetically maintained pain do not often have long-lasting pain relief after sympathethic blockades alone. Clearly, long-standing CRPS most often has developed into a biopsychosocial complex. Sympathetic blocks can only be a part of the management of these complex patients. Some patients who initially had good pain relief with sympathetic blockade gradually, after several years, lost their component of sympathetically maintained pain.[8]

It is worrisome that sympathectomy by radiofrequency destruction, or by surgical removal of parts of the sympathetic chain, can produce new neuropathic pain problems in some unfortunate patients.[3, 6] This does not happen after sympathetic blockade performed with traditional local anesthetic drugs, nor after regional intravenous guanethidine sympathetic blockade (**Figure 27.3**).

TESTING FOR COMPLETENESS OF SYMPATHETIC BLOCKADE

In patients with a reasonably healthy vascular system, a clear-cut, objective, easily documented peripheral vasodilatation occurs after a sympathetic block. An increase in skin temperature of several centigrades can be felt and measured.

TESTS OF SYMPATHETIC FUNCTION, BLOOD FLOW, AND PAIN

Sympathetic function

- Skin conductance response.
- Sweat test.
- Skin plethysmography and ice response.[1]

Blood flow

- Plethysmography.
- Laser Doppler flowmeter.
- Pulse wave changes.
- Temperature.

Pain

- Subjective pain intensity score (numeric rating scale (NRS), visual analog scale (VAS), verbal categorical scale (VRS)).
- Subjective pain relief score.
- Analgesic drug consumption.

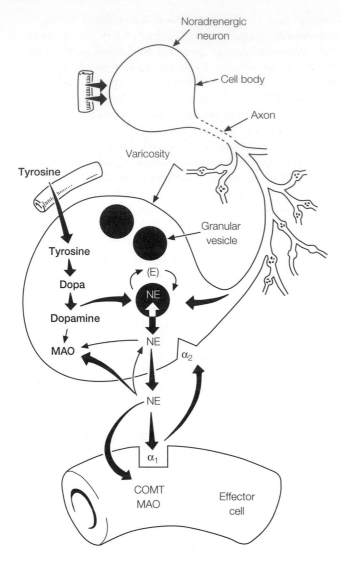

Figure 27.3 Sympathetic nerve endings and receptors. Norepinephrine (NE, noradrenaline) is released as the transmitter substance on depolarization of the presynaptic neuron. This is inhibited by local anesthetic blocking drugs. Reuptake of NE back into the presynaptic nerve terminals is blocked for several days by guanethidine. MAO, monoamine oxidase. Redrawn with permission from Breivik H, Cousins MJ, Löfström JB, *Neural Blockade in Clinical Anesthesia and Management of Pain*, 3rd edn, Cousins MJ, Bridenbaugh PO (eds), Lippincott–Raven Publishers, 1998.

Function

Improved functions that were inhibited by pain (e.g. claudication distance).

Skin temperature measurements

These can be carried out quite simply and reliably in clinical practice by measuring skin temperature with a thermocouple probe and a telethermometer. Reliable results are obtained by measuring the distal part of the extremity at ten different points (below each toe, in the middle of the sole, on the dorsum pedis; or similar points on the upper extremity) on each side.

At an appropriate time after the block has been performed (at least 30 minutes), expose both extremities to cold air. This will cause the temperature to drop on the unblocked side and remain unchanged or increase up to several degrees, depending on the state of the vessels of the patient, on the blocked side.

Skin conductance response and skin potential response

These two tests are reasonably reliable, they require some special equipment, and the results depend on the degree of arousal of the central nervous system. Sedation, drugs that alter sympathetic activity, anticholinergic drugs, and steroids all interfere with these tests.[1]

Pain assessment

Whenever the indication for sympathetic block is acute or chronic pain, a VAS or NRS of present pain intensity should be used before and after the block, as well as a categorical scale of pain relief.

Duration of any pain relief, and its effects on functions that have been inhibited by the pain, must be documented in a pain diary.

Contraindications

Patients with an increased bleeding tendency and those who are anticoagulated cannot have any of the major sympathetic blocks performed. The risk of deep-sited bleeding, which cannot be stopped by compression, is significant. For these patients, intravenous regional sympathetic block with guanethidine, where available, may be an alternative to sympathetic blocks of the sympathetic chain.

Bilateral sympathetic blocks should *not* be performed on the same day because of the risk of orthostatic hypotension (lumbar blocks) and airway problems and bilateral pneumothorax (stellate ganglion blocks). Bilateral lumbar sympathetic block may cause loss of ejaculation.

Sympathetic blockade with local anesthetic drugs

For diagnostic and prognostic sympathetic blocks, lidocaine, mepivacaine, bupivacaine, or ropivacaine can all be used. Carrying out a double-blind block with either a short-acting or a long-acting local anesthetic may help to evaluate any placebo effect in the response to the block.

Mepivacaine and lidocaine should have a sympathetic block duration of 1.5–3 hours, bupivacaine and ropivacaine 3–10 hours.[1]

A double-blind, true placebo-controlled block is usually not feasible. However, Tenicela and coworkers[12] performed a saline-controlled trial of stellate ganglion blocks for herpes zoster of the trigeminal nerve, providing evidence for a prophylactic effect on postherpetic neuralgia. For a review of effects of sympathetic blockades with local anesthetic drugs, see Cepeda et al.[13]

Image intensifier and contrast enhancement for verification of location of blocking solution

For those who have radiographic image intensifier facilities to visualize the procedure, the local anesthetic should be mixed with a small amount of iohexol (Omnipaque[TM]).[1] Imaging is essential when neurolytic blocks are used.

For neurolytic blocks

- Phenol 6 percent (60 mg/ml) in water or dissolved in Omnipaque.
- Ethanol 50–100 percent may be used for celiac plexus block.

Major complications due to neurolytic sympathetic blocks:

- For the sympathetic ganglion chain (cervical or lumbar), ethanol carries a risk of inducing new neuropathic pain.[1, 6] Phenol is a little safer in this respect.
- One can never completely eliminate the risk of injecting into the wall or lumen of a radicular artery supplying the spinal cord, or injection into a peripheral epidural sleeve. The risk is lower in the cervical and lumbar segments than in the thoracic segments, but it is never zero. These accidents result in permanent, major neurological sequelae.

STELLATE GANGLION BLOCK

The cervicothoracic sympathetic chain is located in the space between the fascia overlying the prevertebral muscles and the carotid sheath (**Figure 27.4**).

The sympathetic preganglionic fibers supplying the head, neck, and the upper extremities emerge from the spinal cord segments T1–T6. They converge and pass to the cervicothoracic sympathetic chain of ganglia, the upper thoracic and lower cervical ganglion in front of the neck of the first rib forming the stellate ganglion. Immediately below the stellate ganglion lies the cupula of the pleura, and directly posterior to the stellate ganglion lies the vertebral artery. The intermediate cervical ganglion lies in front of the medial part of the transverse process of C7, the middle cervical ganglion on the medial part of the transverse process of C5. The superior cervical ganglion is at the level of C2–C3.

The safe approach to the cervicothoracic sympathetic chain of ganglia is to aim for the transverse process of C6 (Chassaignac's tubercle) and inject a sufficient volume of the local anesthetic solution, with radio-opaque contrast medium added if a radiographic record of the spread is desired. Aiming directly toward the stellate ganglion risks causing pneumothorax or even injuring the vertebral artery. Injection into the vertebral artery results in major grand mal seizures as an immediate consequence.

Technique of cervicothoracic sympathetic ganglion (stellate ganglion) block

With the patient supine, head resting on a thin pillow the following procedure is undertaken.

- The neck should be slightly extended at the atlanto-occipital joint. This stretches the esophagus and moves it away from the needle path.
- Slightly opening the mouth relaxes some neck muscles.
- The carotid pulse is palpated lateral to the trachea at the level of the cricoid cartilage. The artery and sternocleidomastoideus muscle are gently moved laterally and the resistance of the prominent transverse process of C6 (Chassaignac's tubercle) is felt and placed between the index and the ring finger on the left hand.
- A fine needle (25 gauge) on a 20-mL syringe filled with the chosen local anesthetic solution (plus radiographic contrast medium if desired) is gently advanced toward the Chassaignac's tubercle.
- When bone is met, the needle is retracted slightly (approximately 2 mm); the needle and syringe are fixed with the left hand.
- Aspiration is performed and a small test dose of approximately 0.5 mL is injected while the patient's face is continuously monitored by the anesthesiologist performing the block, preferably maintaining eye contact with the patient.
- Another 0.5-mL test dose is injected slowly, and may be repeated three times at about ten-second intervals.
- When no reaction occurs, slightly larger injections are performed repeatedly, until the desired volume (up to 20 mL) has been injected.

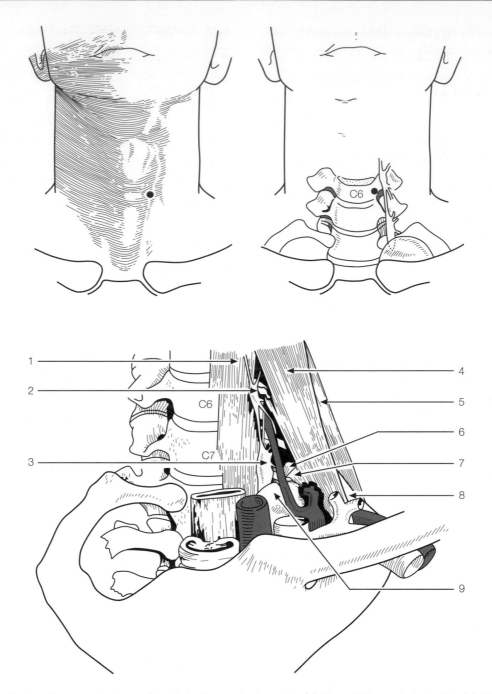

Figure 27.4 Cervicothoracic sympathetic ganglion chain. Prevertebral muscles (1). The middle cervical ganglion (2). The ganglion stellatum (3) is located on the neck of the first rib (6–8), extending up to the transverse process of C7. At this level, the vertebral artery is lateral and anterior to the ganglion; at the C7 level, the artery has dived posteriorly, safely into the foramen intertransversarium. The top of the pleura (9) is also well below the transverse process of C6 (Chassaignac's tubercle). Anterior (4) and middle (5) scalene muscles (see text). Redrawn with permission from Breivik H, Cousins MJ, Löfström JB, *Neural Blockade in Clinical Anesthesia and Management of Pain*, 3rd edn, Cousins MJ, Bridenbaugh PO (eds), Lippincott-Raven Publishers, 1998.

- The patient is then helped into a sitting position so that the injected local anesthetic solution may gravitate downwards toward the stellate ganglion.
- The patient will usually feel a "lump in the throat" and should be warned in advance that the voice may become hoarse.

An alternative technique is a two-operator technique, with one operator concentrating on placing the needle correctly in front of Chassaignac's tubercle while the other aspirates and injects the solution via an extension tube. The author would recommend a one-operator technique as the safest, but it requires more manual dexterity.

Signs of cervicothoracic sympathetic ganglion block

Within seconds to a couple of minutes, the patient feels the eyelid drooping and:

- ptosis can be observed;
- miosis (a shrinking pupil) develops;
- sinking of the eyeball (enophthalmos) develops.

These signs and dry, warm, pinkish skin on the blocked side of the face are the signs of Horner syndrome. The patient experiences a feeling of a blocked nose because of swelling of the nasal mucosa from vasodilatation, and the conjunctiva becomes reddish from vasodilatation.

The temperature of the hand and fingers should be measured, with cold exposure if possible to accentuate the skin temperature differences between the blocked and unblocked side (see above under Skin temperature measurements).

Horner syndrome alone does not confirm a sympathetic block of the upper extremity. Increased temperature and a warm and dry skin of the palm on the blocked side are indications that the sympathetic fibers to the upper extremity are blocked.

Complications

LIFE-THREATENING COMPLICATIONS

A stellate ganglion block is a simple block to learn and to perform (unless the patient has a short and obese neck). However, unintentional intra-arterial (vertebral artery or carotid artery) and intrathecal injections are easily done and are dangerous. The practitioner must therefore be prepared to treat such complications immediately. No one should attempt a stellate ganglion block without studying the anatomy closely, and this block should never be performed by anyone who is not experienced in resuscitation techniques. Injection of even a 0.5- to 1-mL volume directly into the vertebral artery will cause immediate grand mal seizures, leading to a situation which is dramatic and difficult to treat. The seizures may last for many minutes.

Clearly, stellate ganglion blockade should not be performed without having an intravenous catheter in place, together with drugs and resuscitation equipment immediately available for the treatment of such complications.

An intrathecal injection into a dural sleeve will cause more gradual onset of a high spinal anesthetic block, with respiratory muscle paralysis and hypotension. Again, expert anesthesiologic resuscitation skills, drugs, and equipment must be at hand.

LESS DRAMATIC ADVERSE EFFECTS

- Local anesthetic block of the recurrent laryngeal nerve causes temporary vocal cord paralysis, hoarseness, and a feeling of a lump in the throat. This can be unpleasant but is not dangerous, however, bilateral stellate ganglion blocks should not be performed for this reason.
- Some patients experience Horner syndrome as unpleasant. Eye drops with phenylephrine will reduce the pupillary changes as well as the enophthalmos and the red eye.
- A cervical hematoma may occur, but is usually not dramatic unless the patient is anticoagulated or has another reason for increased bleeding (which are contraindications for this block).
- Some patients have a feeling of paresthesiae along the chest wall and on the inside of the upper arm. This is transient.
- The brachial plexus may be blocked, in which case the patient does not have an isolated sympathetic block and the diagnostic value of the block is unreliable.
- Phrenic nerve block may occur; this is one reason why bilateral blocks should not be performed and care should be taken in patients with chronic obstructive lung disease.
- Pneumothorax may occur, another reason why bilateral stellate ganglion block should never be performed.

Neurolytic stellate ganglion block

Phenol 6 percent (60 mg/mL) in water or x-ray contrast medium, in a volume of 2 mL in front of the transverse process of C6, will cause incomplete cervicothoracic sympathetic block. This block may cause a persistent Horner syndrome, and if sympathetic blockade of the upper extremity is intended, the results are not reliable.

THORACIC SYMPATHETIC BLOCK

The chain of sympathetic ganglia in the thoracic region is located close to the neck of the ribs and quite close to the somatic nerve roots and their epidural sleeves (**Figure 27.5**). This is different from the cervical region, where the sympathetic ganglia are separated from the somatic roots by the longus colli and the anterior scalene muscles, and it is also different from the lumbar region, where the psoas major muscle separates the sympathetic ganglia from the somatic nerve roots. The close proximity to the pleura is a concern.

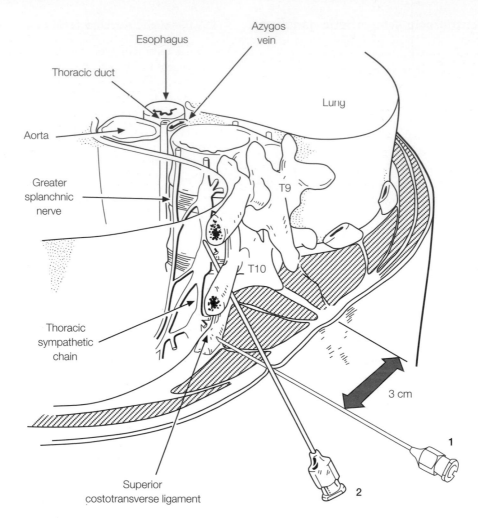

Figure 27.5 Thoracic sympathetic ganglia are lying close to spinal nerve roots and their dural sleeves. The pleura is very close anteriorly. The needle is positioned correctly for a thoracic sympathetic ganglion block, but proximity to these structures means that this block has a high risk of complications (see text). Redrawn with permission from Breivik H, Cousins MJ, Löfström JB, *Neural Blockade in Clinical Anesthesia and Management of Pain*, 3rd edn, Cousins MJ, Bridenbaugh PO (eds), Lippincott-Raven Publishers, 1998.

Indications

In order to obtain complete interruption of the sympathetic outflow to the upper extremity, the upper thoracic ganglia (down to T6) must be blocked. Because of the risk of damaging somatic nerve roots and the risk of intrathecal injections, blind (or even image intensifier) techniques using neurolytic agents have now generally been replaced by thoracoscopic techniques and radiofrequency denervation.[1]

Pain from coronary circulatory insufficiency can be treated with continuous stellate ganglion and upper thoracic sympathetic ganglion blocks. Even for these indications thoracic sympathetic block has been replaced by alternative techniques, such as epidural spinal cord stimulation and epidural or intrathecal local anesthetic and opioid drug infusions.

Technique

A needle enters the skin approximately 3 cm from the midline of the upper thoracic spinous processes and is advanced medially toward the vertebral body. A superficial contact with bone means that the rib has been hit, and the needle will have to be placed a little higher or lower to enter the intercostal space and advanced toward the body of the vertebra in the paravertebral space. At this point, 2 mL of a local anesthetic is deposited approximately 1 cm behind the crest of the vertebral body. A warm, dry hand indicates correct siting of the injection. Formerly, 6 percent (60 mg/mL) aqueous phenol (2 mL) or a similar amount of phenol dissolved in Omnipaque® was occasionally employed for neurolytic blocks, but the risks of neurological complications are considerable (see above).

Complications

Somatic nerve root injury and spinal cord damage from intrathecal (or injection into a radicular artery gong to the anterior spinal artery) injections of neurolytic solutions, as well as pneumothorax, are high-risk complications of specific thoracic sympathetic chain blockade.

LUMBAR SYMPATHETIC BLOCK

The ganglia of the sympathetic chain lie close to the anterior part of the lateral side of the lumbar vertebral bodies, being separated from the somatic nerves by the psoas fascia and the psoas muscle (**Figure 27.6**). One injection of approximately 20 mL of local anesthetic solution at the level of L2 or L3 in the correct fascial plane will spread upwards and downwards and achieve an adequate longitudinal spread for a complete sympathetic block of the lower extremity. For diagnostic and prognostic blocks, this may be a sufficiently precise technique; however, if neurolytic agents, such as phenol, are used, separate needles at levels L2, L3, and L4 are required.

Technique of lumbar sympathetic block

The spinous processes of L1 and L4 should be marked as reference points: L1 is at the level where the 12th ribs meet the lateral sides of the erector spina muscles. The L4 spinous process is at the level of the posterior superior iliac crests (**Figure 27.7**).

- A 12-cm-long, 20- to 22-gauge needle is introduced 8–10 cm lateral to the middle of the spinous process of L4 and another one at L2.
- Place a marker (piece of rubber or plastic) on the needle before entering the skin. The needle is then advanced medially towards the body of the vertebrae (of L2 and L4).
- If bone is met after about 4–5 cm from the skin, this will be the transverse process. The transverse process is approximately half the distance from the skin to the depth of the sympathetic chain on the anterolateral part of the vertebral body.
- If the transverse process is used as a marker of depth, the rubber marker should be placed (after withdrawing the needle to the subcutaneous tissue) about twice the distance from the tip of the needle (about 10 cm from the tip of the needle).
- Redirect the needle in a cranial or caudad direction to avoid the transverse process, and advance until contact with bone is made again.
- Withdraw the needle to the subcutaneous tissue (to avoid bending the needle) before changing direction to advance it to the depth of the rubber marker, or until the needle tip slides off the anterolateral part of the vertebral body.
- In thin patients with less back muscle tissue, the distance is less than 10 cm; in bigger patients with more back muscle tissue, the distance is more than 10 cm from the skin.
- The correct position of the needle tip is indicated by a loss-of-resistance as the needle penetrates the psoas fascia.
- If the needle at L2 is placed first, the second needle at L4 will usually have to be introduced slightly deeper.
- Aspiration for blood and cerebrospinal fluid (CSF) before a test dose.
- Resistance to injection means that the needle is in a wrong place, for example the wall of the aorta or vena cava, an abdominal viscus, or inside an intervertebral disk.
- Radiographic confirmation with a local anesthetic mixed with a contrast medium allows verification of the correct needle tip position.[14]

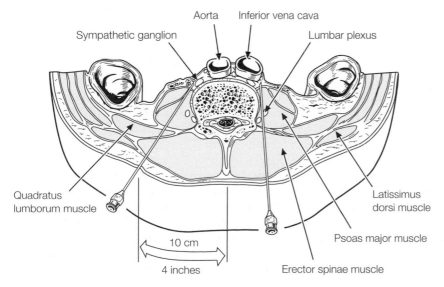

Sympathetic ganglion

Aorta   Inferior vena cava

Lumbar plexus

Quadratus lumborum muscle

Latissimus dorsi muscle

Psoas major muscle

Erector spinae muscle

10 cm

4 inches

Figure 27.6 Lumbar sympathetic block of ganglia at L2, L3, and L4, which are lying on the anterolateral aspect of the vertebral bodies well separated from other nervous tissues and blood vessels (see text). Redrawn with permission from Breivik H, Cousins MJ, Löfström JB, *Neural Blockade in Clinical Anesthesia and Management of Pain*, 3rd edn, Cousins MJ, Bridenbaugh PO (eds), Lippincott-Raven Publishers, 1998.

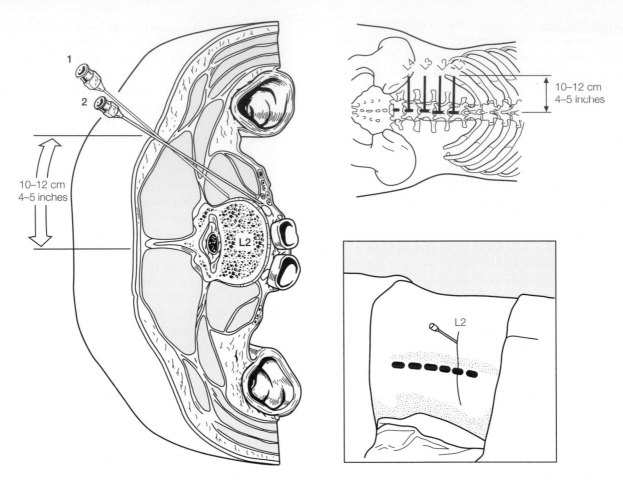

Figure 27.7 Lumbar sympathetic ganglion block. Redrawn with permission from Breivik H, Cousins MJ, Löfström JB, *Neural Blockade in Clinical Anesthesia and Management of Pain*, 3rd edn, Cousins MJ, Bridenbaugh PO (eds), Lippincott-Raven Publishers, 1998.

Dose of local anesthetic

If the indication for the block is to relieve visceral pain, such as renal colic, 20–30 mL of bupivacaine 2.5 mg/mL (0.25 percent) at L2 will eradicate the pain. If the indication for the block is to evaluate or prognosticate the effect of a possible neurolytic block, then 5 mL of a local anesthetic mixed with contrast medium is injected at L2 and at L4.

Continuous lumbar sympathetic blockade

This is possible by placing an 18-gauge long epidural needle at L2 and one at L4, positioning a catheter through each needle and injecting bupivacaine 2.5 mg/mL 5 mL in each catheter every six hours for up to several days. However, the catheters tend to shift with vertebral body movement. Verification of the position of the catheters is needed (with radiographic contrast) if the block becomes less effective.

Single needle injection technique

The tip of the 12th rib indicates the lower border of L2. A needle is placed 2–3 cm below and medial to the tip of the

12th rib and directed medially until the vertebral body of L3 is encountered at a depth of approximately 10 cm. Sufficient solution (15–25 mL) with radiographic contrast medium is added, and image intensifier control will indicate whether the most important ganglia of L2, L3, and L4 are covered by the solution.[15]

Neurolytic blocks of the lumbar sympathetic ganglia

When vascular surgeons refer patients who cannot be helped by vascular surgery for neurolytic lumbar sympathectomy, the indications are usually severe ischemic rest pain, an ulcer that does not heal, or the desire to obtain a demarcation between viable and nonviable tissue before leg amputation. These patients are usually quite ill, have a high incidence of ischemic heart disease, and often have chronic pulmonary disease, diabetes mellitus with complications, and other ailments of old age. There is less risk with a neurolytic sympathectomy, or radiofrequency neurolysis (see Chapter 33, Radiofrequency lesioning and treatment of chronic pain) than with surgical sympathectomy, which hardly will be tolerated by such ill patients.[1]

Agents for lumbar sympathetic blocks

Phenol 6 percent (60 mg/mL) in water, or up to 10 percent phenol in iohexol (Omnipaque) when an image intensifier is available.

Technique

- With the image intensifier[1] or biplanar image intensifier, lateral and anteroposterior views are obtained, tilting the patient ventrally and dorsally to thoroughly check the position of the needle.
- A 1-mL test dose of local anesthetic followed by 0.5-mL boluses (up to 3–4 mL of the phenol-containing contrast medium) with image intensifier verification of correct positioning is injected.
- The injected neurolytic solution with radiographic contrast should cover each level (L2, L3, and L4) in the correct anterolateral position.[1]
- Before withdrawing the needles, 0.5 mL of a local anesthetic is injected through the needle to avoid leaving neurolytic solution on somatic nerve roots or spinal nerves during the removal of the needle.
- The patient should remain on their side for approximately five minutes to prevent the solution from spreading laterally.
- The patient remains supine for 30–60 minutes while the skin temperature of the lower extremities, blood pressure, and heart rate are monitored.
- After about one hour, the patient is mobilized slowly and blood pressure is checked for orthostatic hypotension.
- Most patients are able to leave the pain clinic after a few hours. Unstable elderly patients should be monitored as inpatients for at least 24 hours after the block.
- The block can be repeated on the other side after a day, depending on the reaction to the first block.

Complications

Provided needle placement is executed carefully and verified by a local anesthetic test dose and/or radiographic contrast with image intensifier, complications are infrequent. However, injection of local anesthetic or neurolytic drugs into the cerebrospinal fluid, adjacent to spinal nerve roots or spinal nerves, and intravascularly is always possible.

- Transient postsympathectomy neuropathic pain occurs in up to 50 percent of patients in the anterolateral proximal part of the lower extremity.
- Neurolytic agents may reach the genitofemoral nerve (**Figure 27.8**). Genitofemoral neuralgia is infrequent when phenol is employed (5–10 percent),

and in most cases it is transient. However, when alcohol is used, more severe and protracted pain in the groin from genitofemoral ethanol neuritis occurs.

- The ureter may be damaged by phenol or alcohol.
- If bilateral upper level lumbar sympathectomy is performed, ejaculatory failure may follow.
- Postsympathectomy hyperesthesia (allodynia), most frequently occurring in the L1 dermatomal area, may be due to genitofemoral nerve damage from a neurolytic agent, but it may also result from a postsympathectomy denervation hyperesthesia. This occurs more frequently in younger patients having surgical sympathectomy for hyperhidrosis than with phenol sympathetic blocks. This neuropathic-type pain persists after cervicodorsal and lumbar surgical sympathectomy (also radiofrequency ablation) in 10–15 percent of patients.[3] Hyperesthetic burning discomfort in the groin and anterolateral part of the thigh may persist for two to five weeks after phenol sympathetic blocks.[16]

INTRAVENOUS REGIONAL SYMPATHETIC BLOCK

A technique that provides a simple and efficient means of producing long-term sympathetic blockade was described by Hannington-Kiff using guanethidine (Ismeline®) in an intravenous regional sympathetic functional block.[17] Its value has been reconfirmed by several pain clinicians and clinical neurophysiologists.[1, 2, 8, 9, 10, 18, 19, 20, 21, 22]

Unfortunately, a "randomized controlled trial" with three major flaws has been influential in weakening the reputation and widespread use of this valuable technique.[7] That study included a group of patients with "reflex sympathetic dystrophy" without documented sympathetically maintained pain. In such a group of pain patients, any positive effect of sympathetic blockade will disappear among confounding factors.

The second flaw in such studies has been diluting the guanethidine with a local anesthetic solution. The local anesthetic inhibits the release of norepinephrine (noradrenaline) from the sympathetic nerve endings. The sympathetic functional blocking effect of guanethidine occurs as a result of inhibition of reuptake of released norepinephrine back into the sympathetic nerve endings (**Figure 27.3**). The presence of a local anesthetic will therefore markedly reduce or prevent the effect of guanethidine.

Even a third flaw is possible in studies dissolving the guanethidine in a local anesthetic solution. The systemic, central nervous system, effects of lidocaine (and other sodium channel-blocking local anesthetic drugs) on neuropathic pain are well documented. When guanethidine dissolved in a lidocaine solution was compared with a lidocaine solution as "placebo," this "placebo-treatment"

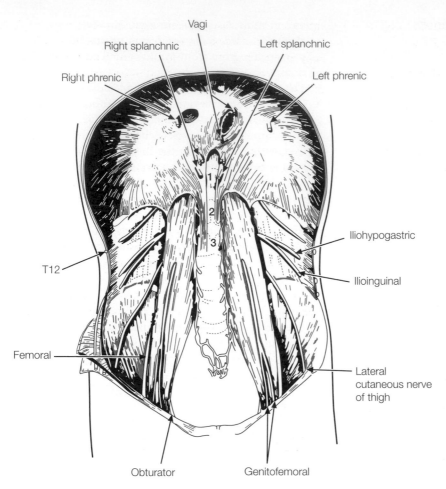

Vagi

Right splanchnic

Left splanchnic

Right phrenic

Left phrenic

T12

Iliohypogastric

Ilioinguinal

Femoral

Lateral
cutaneous nerve
of thigh

Obturator

Genitofemoral

Figure 27.8 Illustration of position of genitofemoral nerve making spread of neurolytic solutions from a posterior sympathetic ganglion blockade to this nerve possible, causing neuritis and neuropathic pain. Redrawn with permission from Breivik H, Cousins MJ, Löfström JB, *Neural Blockade in Clinical Anesthesia and Management of Pain*, 3rd edn, Cousins MJ, Bridenbaugh PO (eds), Lippincott-Raven Publishers, 1998.

was effective therapy for neuropathic pain in about one-third of patients. No wonder there was no demonstrable difference between guanethidine in lidocaine and lidocaine alone.

Unfortunately, such flawed publications seem to have led to the unavailability of guanethidine for sympathetic blocks in some countries. Fortunately, it is still available in western Europe. Alternatives to guanethidine for i.v. regional sympathetic blocks (e.g. bretyllium, phentolamine, clonidine) do not seem to result in prolonged functional sympathetic blockades.

Duration of guanethidine sympathetic functional block

Compared with stellate ganglion block with lidocaine, which results in vasodilatation lasting for about one hour, a regional intravenous sympathetic block with guanethidine increases the temperature of the cold extremity for as long as three days after block.[20]

Arnér[2] showed that intravenous phentolamine predicts the long-term effect of regional intravenous sympathetic block with guanethidine. Olsson *et al.*[9] documented the excellent, often curative, clinical effect on complex regional pain syndrome in adolescents.

Regional intravenous sympathetic block with guanethidine

This is less stressful than the alternative techniques, which are more invasive and carry more risks. Anticoagulation or bleeding disorders are not contraindications to a regional intravenous sympathetic block. The technique should therefore still be available as it remains a valuable alternative in pain clinics treating patients with complex regional pain syndromes, where sympathetically maintained pain is a component of the patients' pain condition.[10, 21]

Technique of regional intravenous block

- Normal saline should be used to dilute 10 mg of guanethidine (10 mg for the first block, up to 30 mg for repeat blocks).
- Approximately 25 mL of normal saline is used for the upper limb and approximately 40 mL for the lower limb.
- An intravenous cannula is placed in the affected limb, as close to the painful area as possible.
- A second cannula is placed in a vein on a nonaffected limb for analgesia and sedation if needed during the procedure.

- It is important not to use a local anesthetic to dilute the guanethidine (see above under Intravenous regional sympathetic block).
- A wide cuff of appropriate size is placed around the upper arm or thigh, the extremity lifted to drain as much venous and capillary blood as possible.
- The cuff is then inflated to approximately 50 mmHg above systolic blood pressure.
- The diluted guanethidine is injected intravenously in the affected limb, keeping the cuff inflated for a minimum of 20 minutes.
- It is often necessary to give the patient intravenous opioid with rapid onset (e.g. alfentanil), in titrated doses to make the patient comfortable during the procedure.
- When the blood pressure cuff is released and circulation reestablished in the treated extremity, norepinephrine released from sympathetic nerve endings by guanethidine will flood into the systemic circulation.
  - This creates a transient increase in blood pressure and heart rate.
  - During the block procedure, soon after injection of the guanethidine solution, the patient's sympathetically maintained painful sensation will often increase because of the same mechanism of norepinephrine release.
  - This should be treated with intravenous rapidly acting opioid rather than injecting a local anesthetic with the guanethidine, which may reduce or prevent the beneficial effect of the guanethidine (see above under Intravenous regional sympathetic block).

Adverse effects

- Some patients will have a stuffy nose due to the systemic distribution of guanethidine after release of the cuff.
- Occasionally, orthostatic hypotension occurs during the first one to two days after an intravenous regional sympathetic guanethidine block. Patients should be warned to take proper precautions, such as getting out of bed slowly, sit or lie down when dizzy.
- Patients with paroxysmal atrial cardiac arrhythmias may occasionally have an episode of cardiac arrhythmia precipitated by the guanethidine, when norepinephrine released from the sympathetic nerve endings circulates after release of the tourniquet. A betablocker may be given to prevent this side effect in patients with a history of such cardiac dysrythmias.

CONCLUSIONS

Sympathetic efferent fibers are involved in nociception and transmission of pain impulses. After injury or infection, sympathetic efferent nerve impulses can modify functions of afferent sensory nerves causing sympathetically maintained pain. Probably less than one-third of complex neuropathic pain conditions have a sympathetically maintained pain component.

The anatomy of the autonomic nervous system allows specific blocks of sympathetic outflow so that sympathetically maintained pain can be diagnosed and treated specifically. Selective sympathetic blocks of the upper and lower extremities can be performed effectively with low risk of complications, using local anesthetic drugs. Guanethidine intravenous regional block causes a functional interference of sympathetic noradrenergic transmission for a few days. In selected patients with sympathetically maintained pain as a significant part of their chronic pain condition, such reversible sympathetic blocks can give significant pain relief.

The evidence-base for long-term effects of sympathetic blocks on chronic complex pain conditions is limited: negative studies are often flawed by not selecting patients with proven sympathetically maintained pain, whereas the reported long-term positive outcomes in the hands of experts is considered weak evidence.

REFERENCES

* 1. Breivik H, Cousins MJ, Löfström JB. Sympathetic neural blockade of upper and lower extremity. In: Cousins MJ, Bridenbaugh PO (eds). *Neural blockade in clinical anesthesia and management of pain*, 3rd edn. Philadelphia, PA: Lippincott-Raven Publishers, 1998: 411–45.

* 2. Arnér S. Intravenous phentolamine test: diagnostic and prognostic use in reflex sympathetic dystrophy. *Pain*. 1991; **46**: 17–22.

* 3. Furlan AD, Mailis A, Papagapiou M. Are we paying a high price for surgical sympathectomy? A systematic literature review of late complications. *Journal of Pain*. 2000; **1**: 245–57.

4. Jänig W, Stanton-Hicks M (eds). *Reflex sympathetic dystrophy: a reappraisal. Progress in pain research and management*. Seattle, WA: IASP Press, 1996: 1–249.

* 5. Jänig W. The integrative action of the autonomic nervous system. *Neurobiology of homeostasis*. Cambridge: Cambridge University Press, 2006.

* 6. Cousins MJ, Walker S. Chronic pain: management strategies that work. *Anesthesia and Analgesia*. 2001; **92**: 15–25.

7. Kaplan R, Claudio M, Kepes E, Gu XF. Intravenous guanethidine in patients with reflex sympathetic dystrophy. *Acta Anaesthesiologica Scandinavica*. 1996; **40**: 1216–22.

* 8. Wahren LK, Gordh T, Torebjörk E. Effects of regional intravenous guanethidine in patients with neuralgia in the hand; a follow-up study over a decade. *Pain*. 1995; **62**: 379–85.

* 9. Olsson GL, Arnér S, Hirsch G. Reflex sympathetic dystrophy in children. In: Tyler DC, Krane EL (eds). *Advances in pain research and therapy.* New York, NY: Raven Press, 1990: 323–31.

* 10. Jørum E, Ørstavik K, Schmidt R *et al.* Catecholamine-induced excitation of nociceptors in sympathetically maintained pain. *Pain.* 2007; **127**: 296–301.

* 11. Burton AW, Lubenow TR, Raj PP. Traditional interventional therapies. In: Wilson PR, Stanton-Hicks M, Harden RM (eds). *CRPS: current diagnosis and therapy.* Seattle: IASP Press, 2005: 217–34.

  12. Tenicela R, Lovasik D, Eaglstein W. Treatment of herpes zoster with sympathetic blocks. *Clinical Journal of Pain.* 1985; **1**: 63–7.

  13. Cepeda MS, Carr DB, Lau J. Local anesthetic sympathetic blockade for complex regional pain syndrome. *Cochrane Database of Systemic Reviews.* 2005; **CD004598**.

  14. Walker SM, Cousins MJ. Complex regional pain syndromes: including "reflex sympathetic dystrophy" and "causalgia." *Anaesthesia and Intensive Care.* 1997; **25**: 113–16.

  15. Hatangdi VS, Boas RV. Lumbar sympathectomy: a single needle technique. *British Journal of Anaesthesia.* 1985; **57**: 285–90.

* 16. Cousins MJ, Reeve TS, Glynn CH *et al.* Neurolytic lumbar sympathetic blockade: duration of denervation and relief of rest pain. *Anaesthesia and Intensive Care.* 1979; **7**: 121–5.

  17. Hannington-Kiff JG. *Pain relief.* London: Heinemann Press, 1974: 68.

  18. Holland AJC, Davies KH, Wallace DH. Sympathetic blockade of isolated limbs by intravenous guanethidine. *Canadian Anaesthetists' Society Journal.* 1977; **24**: 597–602.

  19. McKain CW, Bruno JU, Goldner JL. The effects of intravenous regional guanethidine and eserpine. A controlled study. *Journal of Bone and Joint Surgery.* 1983; **6**: 808–15.

  20. Bonelli S, Conoscente F, Movilia PG *et al.* Regional intravenous guanethidine vs. stellate ganglion block in reflex sympathetic dystrophies: a randomized trial. *Pain.* 1983; **16**: 297–305.

* 21. Breivik H. Chronic pain and the sympathetic nervous system. *Acta Anaesthesiologica Scandinavica.* 1997; **41**: 131–4.

  22. Livingstone JA, Atkins RM. Intravenous regional guanethidine blockade in the treatment of post-traumatic complex regional pain syndrome type I (algodystrophy) of the hand. *Journal of Bone and Joint Surgery. British volume.* 2002; **84**: 380–6.

28

Neurolytic blocks

WILLIAM I CAMPBELL

KEY LEARNING POINTS

- Chemical neurolysis is primarily reserved for the management of difficult cancer pain problems.
- The patient must be made aware of the frequency of risks and benefits to ensure that a balanced, informed consent is obtained.
- Careful patient selection and appropriate timing of intervention is critical for best outcome.
- Intrathecal neurolysis is ideal for intense pain in one to two dermatomes, which is not well controlled by oral or parenteral medication.

- Neurolysis of the celiac plexus can provide excellent pain relief in pain due to carcinoma of upper abdominal viscera.
- Use of the smallest volume of neurolytic, targeted as accurately as possible, provides the best results with the lowest rates of complication.
- The use of contrast media with radiological imaging is essential for all but peripheral injection of neurolytics.
- Chemical neurolysis is not appropriate for the occasional practitioner.

INTRODUCTION

Procedures directed towards nerve destruction have been in use for the management of pain for many decades. These have included physical destruction, such as the application of thermal devices, cutting nerves, and the application of neurolytic substances. The aim of this chapter is to explore the indications and techniques of injecting neurolytics, such as phenol or alcohol in close proximity to nerves, as well as the potential hazards associated with this practice.

The most frequently used agents are aqueous phenol (7 percent) or phenol (5 percent) in glycerol preparation, alcohol (ethanol, 96 percent) or pure glycerol. Maher[1]

recommended phenol in glycerol for intrathecal neurolysis, and although he advocated the use of chlorocresol or silver nitrate, in cases refractory to phenol, this is no longer considered safe practice.[2]

Phenol is considered to have its action through protein coagulation.[3] The addition of glycerol to phenol, to render it a hyperbaric solution for intrathecal use, is thought to delay the release of phenol and render it less destructive than the aqueous preparation.[4] The neurolytic action of alcohol is considered to be due to lipid extraction and protein precipitation within the nerve.[5] These agents cause both motor and sensory nerve destruction, and their use can be hazardous, especially when administered intrathecally. Both agents can cause a neuralgia after administration, this being more common following the peripheral administration of alcohol.[6, 7] Toxic levels of phenol associated with cardiac failure can occur when more than 600 mg/70 kg is administered.[8] Pure glycerol tends only to be used within the cerebrospinal fluid (CSF), as described below under Trigeminal ganglion, as intraneural injection of this hypertonic solution will result in neurolysis similar to that seen following injection of 7 percent aqueous phenol.[9]

Neurolytic procedures tend to be reserved for patients who suffer from cancer pain where opioid administration has failed to be effective.[10] In these situations, patient selection is critical, as is the timing of the procedure.[11] Both intrathecal neurolysis and celiac plexus blocks may only provide pain relief for a few months, partly due to some nociceptive pathway recovery and extension of the disease.[12, 13] Even if neurolysis is technically successful, other sites of less intense pain may be unmasked and found to become a new major problem, such as muscle or joint pain.

A practical point to consider is that a syringe which locks (Luer lock) on to the needle for injection is advised, as disconnection can occur, resulting in uncontrolled ejection of neurolytic solution. Those in close vicinity to the procedure should therefore wear eye protection.

Some of the patients requiring neurolysis may be using anticoagulants. The risk of stopping this therapy prior to neurolysis must be taken into consideration. In some cases, stopping an anticoagulant even for a few days could be disastrous, yet this must be balanced against the risk of hematoma formation – especially if adjacent to the spinal cord.

PERIPHERAL

There is the potential to block the source of any nociception, but this should not be at the expense of motor blockade. Nerves with a mixed motor and sensory function should be avoided and especially any large somatic nerve plexus where such a mix is likely to be present.

Indications

Peripheral neurolytic blocks tend to have a limited value. They only provide analgesia for several months, but the resulting anesthesia can be permanent, generally rendering them unsuitable for the management of chronic nonmalignant pain. Pain from locally invasive facial cancers and areas of intense local pain, supplied by a clearly defined sensory nerve (such as an isolated pathological rib fracture) may be effectively managed by peripheral neurolysis. Large areas of pain may be difficult to control with peripheral neurolytic blockade, as there may well be more than a single nerve supplying the area.

A detailed discussion with the patient is necessary, to convey what one is attempting to achieve, together with potential hazards that may occur, i.e. informed consent, preferably written. A peripheral nerve block with local anesthetic prior to neurolysis may permit the patient to experience the type of sensation that is likely to occur in the long term, as well as helping the clinician to confirm that the appropriate nerve is blocked. However, the result of a neurolytic block is only similar (not identical) to blockade with local anesthetic, i.e. often the perceived paresthesia has a different quality following neurolysis.

The procedure is carried out using an aseptic technique, and the nerve located as in Chapter 23, Peripheral nerve blocks: practical aspects. A sound knowledge of surface anatomy is necessary, and one should be aware of any important structures adjacent to the nerve to be blocked, such as pleura or major blood vessels. The use of a peripheral nerve stimulator may be valuable for more precise nerve identification, especially if the nerve to be blocked is deeper than a few centimeters or not close to bony landmarks. The dose of neurolytic to be injected should be kept to a minimum (generally less than 1 mL) to limit local tissue destruction and ulceration. The aqueous formulation of phenol is the most destructive. Phenol injection tends to be painless, followed by warmth, pain relief, and paresthesia. The ultimate effect of the block cannot be truly evaluated for a further 48 hours.[14] Peripheral nerve blockade using alcohol generates an immediate burning paresthesia which increases in intensity over ten minutes and gradually fades over several hours, followed by pain relief over 24 hours. The peripheral use of alcohol (96 percent) now tends to be restricted to the management of trigeminal neuralgia, since its use can be associated with peripheral neuritis.

Technique

- Obtain informed written consent.
- Position the patient comfortably.
- Identify landmarks as appropriate.
- Cleanse the skin.
- A 23-gauge needle, is inserted to reach the nerve.
- Paresthesia should be established, before attempting injection.
- Attach a 1-mL Luer-lock syringe containing either pure alcohol or 7 percent aqueous phenol.
- Inject a 0.1-mL aliquot – this should result in a burning or warm sensation, this is followed by paresthesia in the distribution of nerve to be blocked.
- Continue with further aliquots up to 1 mL – until pain relief is obtained. Whilst holding the needle stationary, replace the syringe with a clean one, and inject air to clear the needle of neurolytic, before needle removal. (This is to clear the needle of

neurolytic and prevent a phenol track to the skin surface, where skin sloughing may occur, or in the case of alcohol, a painful neuritis of superficial nerves.)

Complications

The following complications should be considered:

- neuritis resulting from incomplete blockade;
- skin ulceration which results when the injectate is too close to the skin surface;
- deep tissue necrosis and possible abscess formation, if more than 1 mL of injectate is used;
- other complications as outlined in Chapter 23, Peripheral nerve blocks: practical aspects, specific to the nerve block carried out.

NEURAXIAL

Neuraxial neurolysis is indicated if nerve root blockade is required. It is segmental and usually unilateral in effect, obtunding nociceptive conduction. If the lesions are adjacent to the ventral roots, ventral root damage may occur, resulting in motor dysfunction. Lesioning is therefore intended for intense, somatic pain, which is unlikely to extend outside one to two dermatomes in a patient with a life expectancy of six months or less. Repeat blockade may therefore be necessary in three or four months, if the block becomes ineffective or the area of pain extends beyond the segments blocked.[7, 13] The procedure tends to be less effective in cases where the pain has been present for many weeks.[14] There is a narrow risk–benefit ratio associated with neurolytic neuraxial blockade, and it is inappropriate for the occasional practitioner. Typically, this procedure is used for trunk or limb pain, due to bone metastasis adjacent to a nerve root. Neuraxial blockade is unsuitable for visceral pain, but other forms of neurolysis may be effective (see below under Celiac plexus).

As with all of the blocks described in this chapter, neuraxial neurolysis should not be considered as an isolated treatment, but rather as a component of a care pathway.[15]

Intrathecal

INDICATIONS

When neurolysis is considered for pain covering a descrete area, in one or two dermatomes, intrathecal (subdural) administration of hyperbaric (phenol 5 percent in glycerol) or hypobaric (absolute alcohol) solutions permit good control of neurolysis.[1, 2, 14, 16] Hyperbaric solutions are utilized mainly in the low thoracic and lumbar areas, where it is relatively easy to control the flow of injectate, and it is slower to fix to nerve tissue.[14] Some practitioners use alcohol in this area to block the lower sacral roots, avoiding S1 and S2.[17] Generally, if neurolysis is required in the upper thoracic or low cervical areas, a hypobaric solution (alcohol) is preferable, as it is easier to position the patient for the solution to rise to the appropriate roots. However, there is less room for error with alcohol as it fixes very rapidly and it is impossible to make adjustments if the wrong level is selected.[14] Phenol tends to be used much more frequently than alcohol.[2] Motor dysfunction can be minimized during intrathecal neurolysis by careful technique and patient positioning.[2, 14, 16] Pain relief is good in 80 percent of cases, if referral is within the first four months of pain presentation. Late referral (after eight months) leads to much poorer results – only 25 percent achieving good relief.[14] Intrathecal phenol generally tends to give in excess of two months benefit, but the procedure can be repeated.

In a very large review of 5020 patients, pain relief following intrathecal ethanol was established as good in 60 percent, fair in 22 percent, and poor in 18 percent. In addition, benefit following intrathecal phenol (1982 patients) was noted to be good in 58 percent, fair in 16 percent and poor in 25 percent.[18]

TECHNIQUE

- Obtain fully informed written consent from the patient.
- A full aseptic technique is necessary: mask, hat, gown, gloves, and drape, together with an aseptic skin preparation.
- Position the patient on a level operating table, lying on the painful side (hyperbaric phenol to be used).
- Place an x-ray c-arm (image intensifier) over the appropriate region.
- The appropriate region is identified clinically followed by radiological confirmation, taking into account that the appropriate nerve root to be blocked confirms to the dermatome and associated intervertebral foramina.
- Infiltrate the subcutaneous tissues with local anesthetic to the depth of the interspinous ligaments.
- Insert an 18- or 20-gauge short bevel needle until cerebrospinal fluid is obtained.
- Slowly roll the patient to a semi-supine position (**Figure 28.1**).
- Withdraw the needle slowly until CSF flow is much slower or almost stops.
- Attach a 1-mL Luer-lock syringe containing 5 percent phenol in glycerol.
- Inject 0.2 mL of the solution.
- A warmth and tingling should be perceived in the area of pain within 30 seconds.

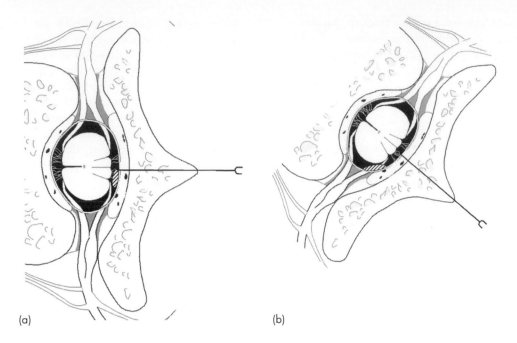

Figure 28.1 Intrathecal neurolysis using a hyperbaric solution, such as phenol in glycerol. (a) Needle just within the subarachnoid space and (b) the patient rolled to a semi-supine position to allow neurolytic just to come into contact with the dorsal nerve roots. (The hatched area indicates phenol flow.)

- If the level is incorrect, tilt the table so that the hyperbaric solution runs to the appropriate root. This can only be one root higher or lower.
- When the warmth and tingling correspond to the area of pain, further aliquots of 0.1 mL of neurolytic are slowly injected, up to 0.5 mL – until the pain is absent, usually several minutes. (If the patient is already incontinent and bedridden, up to 1 mL can be injected in the lumbar region.)
- Up to 1 mL of neurolytic can be injected in the thoracic or low cervical area.
- The needle is then withdrawn until 1–2 cm below the skin and a clean syringe with 1-mL air attached.
- Inject the air just before withdrawing the needle from the skin, to clear the needle of neurolytic.
- The patient is then kept in the semi-supine position, supported by pillows, for at least a further 30 minutes, followed by a further one hour in the supine position.
- If the perineal area is to be blocked, the needle should be inserted at the L5/S1 level, with the patient lying on his/her side, and the needle withdrawn until there is minimal CSF flow. Phenol 7 percent in glycerol 0.75 mL is injected, the needle immediately withdrawn, and the patient immediately but carefully rolled to the supine position. After a minute the patient is gradually aided to a sitting position, leaning slightly forward. The patient is kept in this position for at least half an hour.[14]
- T1–9 are difficult dermatomes to block using intrathecal neurolysis. There is also a high risk of direct cord damage.[14] Needle insertion is therefore

usually at a lower level than for the intended exiting nerve root, with the intention of injecting 1–3 mL of hyperbaric solution (phenol in glycerol) and running it up to the desired level by tilting the patient.

Phenol 5 percent in glycerol and contrast media may be used to confirm the position of the neurolytic. Normally, if the solution is injected at more than one root away from that intended, the procedure should be repeated, adjacent to the correct root to minimize the volume of neurolytic used, excluding special situations such as mid or high thoracic blocks. If the needle is not withdrawn until CSF flow just stops, the tip and therefore the neurolytic may pass over more caudal roots, or the cord itself, resulting in sphincter disturbance.

Intrathecal alcohol is hypobaric in CSF and some clinicians can use this to good effect for thoracic nerve root neurolysis – bearing in mind that the dorsal nerve roots must be positioned uppermost, and with the head at a lower level. This requires considerable skill, and since the alcohol has an immediate effect on the nerve, precise positioning is essential. Initial contact with the incorrect nerve root or the cord will result in immediate damage.[19]

COMPLICATIONS

The following complications should be considered:

- dysesthesia, together with loss of touch and proprioception;
- motor weakness;

- incontinence – risk much higher if the low lumbar roots are blocked;
- irreversible cord damage – with alcohol[19] or phenol;[20]
- alcohol, when used for upper thoracic or cervical pain, may result in paralysis of the upper limb or occasionally cranial nerve dysfunction.

In a review of complications, Gerbershagen[21] noted the risk of temporary paresis or paralysis was 4 percent (1 percent permanent), whereas transient bladder dysfunction occurred in 6 percent (1 percent permanent) and transient bowel dysfunction occurred in 0.5 percent (0.1 percent permanent).[21]

Extradural

This route of neurolytic administration is used infrequently now. The volume needed for a nerve root block is large and results tend to be unreliable[14] and is not recommended.

COMPLICATIONS

Motor weakness, dural puncture, and paralysis may occur, due to accidental intrathecal administration, or the thrombotic effect of phenol on feeder blood vessels – especially in the region of the thoracic cord, causing spinal cord infarction.

CELIAC PLEXUS

The celiac plexus is constructed of loose nerve fibers forming a ganglion of 4×3 cm, which lies between the two celiac ganglia, on either side of the aorta at the level of the T12 and L1 vertebral bodies. The inferior vena cava lies anterior and to the right side of the celiac plexus. Although 90 percent of patients with cancer pain may obtain moderate to good pain relief from oral or parenteral medications, some will require interventional techniques to control their pain.[22] Neurolysis of the sympathetic axis has been shown to be an effective and safe approach to manage visceral pain in such patients.[23] These procedures require fluoroscopy to demonstrate the level of needle insertion and the use of contrast media helps prevent injection into major vessels or organs.[24] Although ultrasonic guidance has been described for celiac plexus block,[25] most procedures are carried out using x-ray or computed tomography (CT).

Approximately 85 percent of patients with pain due to pancreatic cancer can expect good pain relief, with up to 75 percent having this relief for their remaining life.[26] Sharfman and Walsh[27] carried out a critical review of the available literature in 1990 and concluded at that time

that there were only 15 published series since 1964 and that there were many deficiencies in the reports, to the extent that they considered that there was insufficient evidence for the efficacy of this procedure. There have been many well-controlled clinical trials illustrating the benefits of this procedure in pain due to upper abdominal malignancy, where opioid use has been unsatisfactory.[28, 29, 30, 31, 32] The successful relief of pain due to pancreatic cancer and other abdominal malignancies can be expected in 85 and 73 percent of patients, respectively.[12] Staats et al.[29] noted a significant positive effect on life duration and mood scores, and this was associated with an increase in life expectancy. Wong et al.,[31] however, did not find such encouraging results in their double-blind, randomized trial of 100 patients.[31] They noted that although neurolytic celiac plexus block provided better pain relief than opioids, it did not affect quality of life measures or survival.

A unilateral approach to blockade of the celiac plexus has been successfully illustrated,[33] but the potential for inadequate neurolytic spread may be higher.[34] On reviewing the contrast spread during CT, De Cicco et al.[34] noted that the results following celiac plexus block were much improved if the contrast spread to all four quadrants. They concluded that by using a single needle approach, neurolytic spread is highly hampered by regional anatomical alterations.

Indications

Celiac plexus block is indicated for pain due to upper abdominal neoplasm, especially the pancreas and liver.[12] Although celiac plexus block can be a highly effective means of controlling pain due to chronic pancreatitis,[35] the procedure is associated with serious complications for such a nonmalignant condition. If pain due to pelvic disease is present, it is more appropriate to consider some of the sympathetic blocks mentioned later in this chapter (see below under Miscellaneous).

Technique

The aim of the block is to deposit a sufficient volume of neurolytic to destroy the plexus which covers a large area, adjacent to major organs and blood vessels. Since the volume of injectate needed is large, alcohol is used.

- Obtain informed written consent.
- Place the patient prone on a radiotranslucent operating table.
- With full asepsis, clean the low thoracic and upper lumber areas of the back.
- Mark the spinous processes of T12 and L1, together with the medial boarder and tip of each 12th rib, after confirmation by x-ray.

- Sedation is used for the initial phase of the procedure.
- A 12-cm, 22-gauge needle is inserted 5–6 cm lateral to the upper border of the spinous process of L1 (depending on the angle of the 12th rib).
- The needle is directed medially, at a 40° angle to the skin, to strike the vertebral body of L1. This should be at approximately 8 cm – if less it may be hitting the transverse process (**Figure 28.2**, needle position A).
- Place a marker on the needle 4 cm from the skin. Withdraw the needle to within a few centimeters of the skin and redirect the point at a 25–30° angle. Advance the needle until the marker is very close to the skin. The needle tip should be within the immediate vicinity of the celiac plexus, and adjacent to the aorta (**Figure 28.2**, needle position B).
- Repeat on the contralateral side.
- Aspirate for blood. Inject 5 mL of lidocaine 20 mg/mL (with epinephrine 5 μg/mL) plus radiocontrast media via each needle. This will exclude intrathecal and intravascular injection and should render the patient pain free.
- Potent analgesia and sedation are administered now, as injection of the neurolytic causes very intense abdominal pain.
- If the needle tips are correctly placed, 25 mL of the following neurolytic is injected on each side. (Dilute 25 mL ethanol 96 percent with 18 mL lidocaine 1 mg/mL and 7 mL radiocontrast.)
- The needles are flushed with 1 mL of 0.9 percent saline, to clear them of alcohol, and withdrawn.

- The patient is taken to a recovery area, where additional analgesia together with further intravenous fluids and possibly intravenous ephedrine may be needed.
- Support stockings are provided and care taken when initial ambulation takes place, as postural hypotension within the first few days can lead to syncope.

Complications

Most side effects tend to pass in a few days.[23] These include:

- postural hypotension;
- hematoma;
- visceral damage, especially the kidney;
- pneumothorax;
- diarrhea;
- somatic nerve lesions/neuritis, if solution comes in contact with somatic nerve;
- rarely, paraplegia.[36, 37]

SUPERIOR HYPOGASTRIC PLEXUS

The superior hypogastric plexus lies anterior to the lower aspect of the vertebral body of L5 and the upper promontory of the sacrum. Major iliac blood vessels lie immediately in front of the plexus, which innervates the bladder, rectum, prostate, uterus, and cervix.

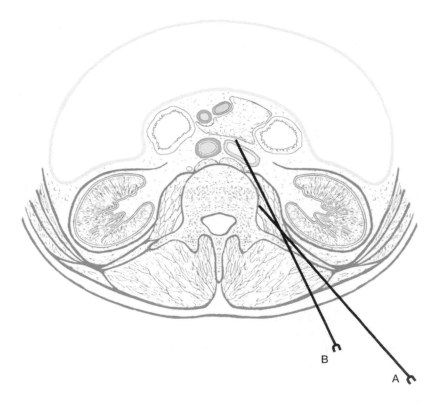

Figure 28.2 Celiac plexus block. Needle position after initial insertion (A), and (B), after redirection, so that the needle tip is at the celiac plexus.

Indications

Pain from pelvic cancer, such as colorectal or genitourinary.[38] In a study of 26 patients with pelvic cancer, in which pain was poorly controlled by opioids, de Leon-Casasola et al.[39] achieved good results in 69 percent of patients, although three required a second block. The good response continued over a six-month follow up without complications. Plancarte et al.[40] studied 227 patients and achieved similar results in 79 percent of patients, with a 43 percent reduction in opioid needs in 72 percent of patients. The results tend to be poor if there is extensive retroperitoneal disease.

Technique

- Obtain informed written consent.
- Place the patient prone on a radiotranslucent operating table.
- With full asepsis, clean the lumber and sacral areas of the back.
- Mark the spinous processes of L3–5, together with the medial border of each iliac crest and confirm anatomy with x-ray.
- Light sedation may be used for the procedure, but the patient should be able to respond coherently to sensations perceived.
- A 12-cm 22-gauge needle is inserted 5–6 cm lateral to the L4/5 interspace, after subcutaneous injection of local anesthetic.
- The needle is inserted and directed medially at a 30–40° and in a caudal direction, to strike the side of the vertebral body of L5. (The iliac crest can cause difficulty in directing the needle, requiring the needle to be withdrawn to the skin and reinserted at an appropriate angle.)
- The needle tip should be advanced to a point just 1 cm in front of the anterior border of L5.
- A click or pop is felt as the psoas fascia is pierced, at a point approximately 10 cm from skin entry. Needle tip will be adjacent to interior iliac vessels.
- Aspirate to ensure needle tip is not in a blood vessel. Inject 2–3 mL of contrast media to confirm injectate location on x-ray. There should be little resistance to injection and contrast media should spread across the anterior body of L5.
- The same procedure is carried out on the opposite side (if male, see below under Complications).
- Local anesthetic (5 mL) is injected on each side.
- If pain relief is achieved within five to ten minutes, proceed to inject aqueous phenol 7–10 percent made up in radiocontrast media, to confirm safe spread of injectate.
- The needles are flushed with 1 mL of 0.9 percent saline, to clear them of phenol, and withdrawn.
- Return patient to recovery area.

Complications

Complications include:

- back pain;
- hematoma;
- intravascular injection;
- somatic nerve;
- intrathecal block;
- sexual dysfunction in males, especially if bilateral block.

Although phenol is frequently employed,[39] alcohol can also be used, the success being related to the volume used – 10–20 mL.[41]

TRIGEMINAL GANGLION

The trigeminal ganglion lies just within the cranial cavity with the three divisions (ophthalmic, maxillary, and mandibular) supplying the face, including cornea, tongue, and teeth. Destructive lesions can therefore result in profound lack of sensation on the ipsilateral side of the face. Selective lesioning through the choice of an appropriate neurolytic can limit neuronal dysfunction yet permit good pain relief.

Indications

Trigeminal neuralgia is one of the few nonmalignant pain states where chemical neurolysis may be considered appropriate. It can generally be managed through the regular use of appropriate anticonvulsants, such as carbamazepine. Some clinicians will also carry out blockade of peripheral nerves to prevent triggering of the pain. If these measures are ineffective or not tolerated, interventions, such as microvascular decompression or radiofrequency lesioning, provide an excellent drug-free alternative.[42, 43] Although radiofrequency thermocoagulation offers the highest rate of complete pain relief,[43] microvascular decompression is the preferred treatment for younger healthy patients, with a long life expectancy.[44] Should these procedures be declined by the patient, or when the pain involves the ophthalmic or several divisions, the clinician may consider retroganglion injection of pure glycerol, as first described by Hakanson.[45] This does not regularly result in loss of sensation, as seen when phenol is used, and is particularly suited to the frail or elderly patient.[46, 47, 48, 49, 50]

Technique

- Informed written consent is obtained.
- The procedure may be carried out under general anesthesia or light sedation, with the patient supine,

with the table 10–15° head up, on a radiotranslucent operating table. Alternatively, a dental chair in the semi-recumbent position can be used.

- The key landmarks are indicated in **Figure 28.3** and are best marked prior to starting the procedure – these are a point 3 cm lateral from the corner of the mouth on the side of pain and 3 cm anterior to the external auditory meatus (**Figure 28.3**).
- It is useful at this stage to radiologically identify the foramen ovale, by tilting the head back slightly, and rotating it 10–15° away from the side of pain.
- Prophylactic antibiotic cover against staphylococcal infection is administered intravenously (cefuroxime).
- A full aseptic technique is necessary: mask, hat, gown, gloves, and drape, together with an aseptic skin preparation.
- A 100-mm, 20-gauge needle is inserted 3 cm lateral to the corner of the mouth on the side associated with pain (**Figure 28.3**, insertion at point B).
- The needle is directed towards the center of the pupil of the ipsilateral eye, but also directed backwards at the same time, as if to a point behind the eye, corresponding to point A in **Figure 28.3**.

- The needle should strike the base of skull at this point. Confirm the needle tip position in relation to the foramen ovale with x-ray.
- It is often necessary to withdraw the needle partly and reinsert it, directing the tip with the aid of fluoroscopy.
- When the foramen ovale is entered, the needle stylette is removed and the needle advanced just until CSF is obtained.
- A lateral x-ray view of the skull should confirm that the needle tip is just past the clivus.
- Radiocontrast media 0.1 mL may be injected and should show as a clearly defined bead.
- Pure sterile glycerol 0.2–0.4 mL is injected over 10–15 seconds, without moving the needle tip (injecting this hypertonic solution into the ganglion or a nerve root will cause permanent sensory loss).
- Recovery takes place in the position of injection, with minimal head movement over the following 15–20 minutes.
- Headache, face pain, and bruising are common, as is altered facial sensation which generally resolves within 24–48 hours.

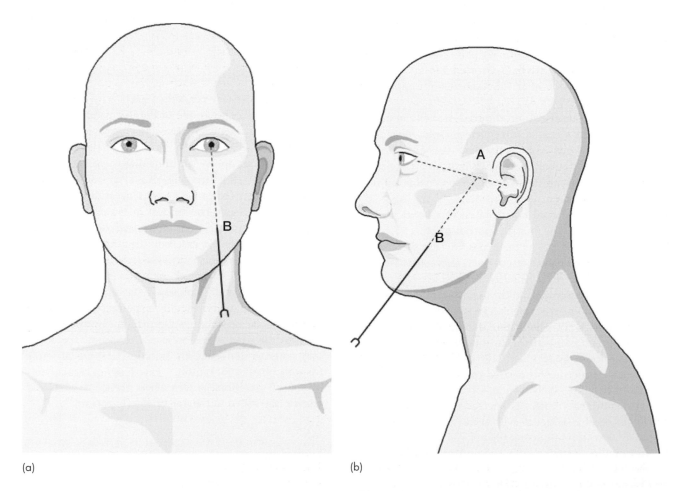

(a)　　　　　　　　　　　　　　　　　　　　(b)

Figure 28.3 Needle position to locate the foramen ovale. Insertion at (a) 3 cm lateral to the corner of the mouth, the needle is then directed towards the ipsilateral pupil, but backwards to a point 3 cm anterior to the external auditory meatus (b).

Complications

Complications include:

- preoperative vasovagal reaction;
- hematoma;
- meningitis – aseptic or septic;
- ipsilateral self-terminating circumoral herpetic eruption;
- sensory loss (any part of face, including cornea or lips);
- anesthesia dolorosa (rare);
- hearing deficit;
- tinnitus.

Results

Of the 75 cases observed by Hakanson, 86 percent were pain free after treatment.[45] Similar results have been noted by others.[48, 49] Saini[47] studied 552 cases 59 percent of whom were pain free at two years. In a study of 1174 patients, Kondziolka and Lunsford[50] concluded that retroganglion injection of glycerol had advantages over radiofrequency lesioning, avoiding the need for intraoperative sensory testing. Other studies have shown efficacy for up to three years in 50 percent of patients.[51, 52] Patients experiencing continuous pain are less likely to have an excellent outcome.[51] In studying 53 patients, Pickett et al.[52] noted that facial sensory loss was associated with a higher likelihood of pain relief and for a prolonged period. Side effects tend to be common, but are mostly mild and nondisabling.[53] The procedure should be considered in patients with disabling trigeminal pain requiring urgent pain relief, but other procedures such as gamma knife radiosurgery[54] or microvascular decompression are better long-term options.[42, 55]

MISCELLANEOUS

Pain due to malignancy in the face, head, upper limb, or upper thorax may well respond to sympathetic block of the region. Since the ipsilateral stellate ganglion supplies all of these areas, it is worth considering a local anesthetic block of this ganglion.[56, 57] If a desirable result ensues, a neurolytic block with phenol may be considered appropriate.

See Chapter 27, Sympathetic blocks, for more information in relation to this procedure. It is important to take into account the permanent effect of using a neurolytic in this region. In addition, the hazards of the solution entering the CSF or a blood vessel must be considered and hence the resultant need for the addition of contrast media to the phenol and the mandatory use of x-ray control.

Paravertebral

The use of neurolytic agents in this area may seem less hazardous than when administered by the intrathecal or extradural route. This is not the case. In a study of 31 patients, Purcell-Jones et al.[58] noted that the injectate was confined to the paravertebral area in only 18 percent of cases, when assessed by radiology or computed tomography. Indeed, spread was extradural in 70 percent of cases and exclusively so in 31 percent. They concluded that neurolytic and diagnostic paravertebral injections performed without the aid of radiological imaging and contrast media should be regarded as hazardous and interpreted with extreme caution. Paravertebral blockade with neurolytic is of limited use, such as in some cancer patients with a poor prognosis and pain restricted to a small number of thoracic segments. The injectate is rarely (18 percent) confined to the paravertebral area.[58]

Ganglion impar

As mentioned earlier, visceral pain due to cancer can often be managed by sympathetic blockade, if opioids are ineffective or not tolerated. Pain in the rectum or perineum is amenable to sympathetic block of the ganglion of impar, a tiny sympathetic plexus which lies just anterior to the sacrococcygeal junction.[23] The benefit of this procedure over the superior hypogastric block for pain in the perineum is that a much smaller volume of neurolytic is needed and the injectate is not administered in such close proximity to major blood vessels. The approach to the ganglion is usually through the use of a curved hypodermic needle, inserted lateral to the anococcygeal ligament, and the needle tip directed round to the anterior aspect of the sacrococcygeal junction. Care must be taken not to perforate the rectum and that the needle tip ends just in contact with bone. Fluoroscopy with contrast media is necessary. A diagnostic block with 0.5 mL local anesthetic may be desired before a definitive neurolytic block with 0.3–0.5 mL aqueous phenol 7 percent, or alcohol. Another approach has been described recently which may be less difficult to carry out.[59, 60] This involves inserting a needle under fluoroscopy perpendicular to the sacrococcygeal junction, just passing through it and confirming that the needle tip is within the retroperitoneal space. Contrast media 0.2 mL when injected produces a "comma sign."[60] The risk of rectal perforation should be less than with the curved needle technique. However, the use of an excessive volume of neurolytic may result in rectal ulceration.

Sphenopalatine

Extreme facial pain from cancer can be very difficult to control. The use of stellate blockade may be required or selective peripheral neurolytic blocks.[61] It may be necessary to carry out gassarian ganglion blockade with a neurolytic agent.[61] Any form of chemical neurolysis of this ganglion, especially if phenol or alcohol are used (even in fractions of a milliliter), can result in corneal and oral insensitivity. This, together with its consequences, must be discussed in detail with the patient prior to undertaking such a procedure. An alternative procedure to managing this type of pain is a neurolytic sphenopalatine ganglion block. Twenty-two patients with pain due to advanced head and neck malignancy were successfully managed with a sphenopalatine block by Varghese and Koshy,[62] with 17 patients obtaining immediate good relief, after injection of 6 percent phenol.

CONCLUSIONS

Although patients with cancer frequently experience pain in the terminal phases of the disease, approximately 90 percent can expect good pain control through the use of standard and adjuvant analgesics.[20] Intrathecal delivery systems using opioids and local anesthetics can provide excellent pain relief for most of the remaining situations, where pain is below the neck. Chemical neurolysis is an alternative method of pain control, where a continuous intrathecal delivery system is unavailable or unwanted by the patient. Intrathecal neurolysis is, however, limited to a few dermatomes, usually on one side of the trunk or a limb. Upper abdominal, visceral pain, however, is best managed by celiac plexus blockade. These procedures can provide excellent analgesia for many months but careful patient selection is essential for optimum results. A skilled practitioner who frequently carries out these procedures, supported by medical imaging, are also key factors in achieving good results with the least morbidity. Chemical neurolysis is not normally carried out for nonmalignant pain any longer, but is one of several treatment options for trigeminal neuralgia, especially in the frail, elderly patient. Any neurolytic procedure requires a detailed discussion with the patient. Simplified written information of the procedure, together with the potential benefits and risks are desirable when obtaining informed consent. In particular, the risk of functional side effects, such as motor weakness or incontinence, must be explained and balanced against any potential benefits. For these reasons, chemical neurolysis is unsuitable for the infrequent practitioner.

REFERENCES

* 1. Maher RM. Relief of pain in incurable cancer. *Lancet.* 1955; **268**: 18–20.
* 2. Swerdlow M. Intrathecal neurolysis. *Anaesthesia.* 1978; **33**: 733–40.
* 3. Wood KM. The use of phenol as a neurolytic agent: a review. *Pain.* 1978; **5**: 205–29.
4. Wood KM. Peripheral nerve and root chemical lesions. In: Wall PD, Melzack R (eds). *Textbook of pain*, 1st edn. Edinburgh: Churchill Livingstone, 1984: 577–80.
5. Rumsby MG, Finean JB. The action of organic solvents on the myelin sheath of peripheral nerve tissue. II. Short-chain aliphatic alcohols. *Journal of Neurochemistry.* 1966; **13**: 1509–11.
6. Lamacraft G, Molloy AR, Cousins MJ. Peripheral nerve blockade and chronic pain management. *Pain Reviews.* 1997; **4**: 122–47.
7. Lipton S. Useful nerve blocks. In: Lipton S (ed.). *Relief of pain in clinical practice.* Oxford: Blackwell Scientific Publications, 1979: 306–66.
8. Justins DM, Rubin AP. Pain and autonomoc blocks. In: Wildsmith JAW, Armitage EN (eds). *Principles and practice of regional anaesthesia*, 2nd Edn. Edinburgh: Churchill Livingstone, 1993: 233–47.
9. Westerlund T, Vuorinen V, Roytta M. Same axonal regeneration rate after different endoneurial response to intraneural glycerol and phenol injection. *Acta Neuropathologica.* 2001; **102**: 41–54.
* 10. Lamer TJ. Treatment of cancer-related pain: when orally administered medications fail. *Mayo Clinic Proceedings.* 1994; **69**: 473–80.
11. Ferrer-Brechner T. Anesthetic techniques for the management of cancer pain. *Cancer.* 1989; **63**(11 Suppl.): 2343–7.
* 12. Mercadante S, Nicosia F. Celiac plexus block: a reappraisal. *Regional Anesthesia and Pain Medicine.* 1998; **23**: 37–48.
13. Swerdlow M. Pain relief therapy for cancer pain. *Bulletin du Cancer.* 1980; **67**: 217–21.
* 14. Maher R, Mehta M. Spinal (intrathecal) and extradural analgesia. In: Lipton S (ed.). *Persistent pain: modern methods of treatment*, vol. 1. London: Academic Press, 1977: 61–99.
15. Kongsgaard UE, Bjorgo S, Hauser M. Neurolytic blocks for cancer pain – still a useful therapeutic strategy. *Tidsskr Nor Laegeforen.* 2004; **124**: 481–3.
* 16. Mehta M. Intrathecal injections for chronic pain. *Anaesthesia.* 1978; **33**: 838–9.
17. Porges P, Zdrahal F. Intrathecal alcohol neurolysis of the lower sacral roots in inoperable rectal cancer. *Anaesthesist.* 1985; **34**: 627–9.
* 18. Butler SH, Charlton E. Neurolytic blockade and hypophysectomy. In: Loeser JD, Butler SH, Chapman CR, Turk DC (eds). *Bonica's management of pain*, 3rd edn. Philadelphia: Lippincott, Williams and Wilkins, 2000: 1967–2006.
19. McGarvey ML, Ferrante FM, Patel RS *et al.* Irreversible spinal cord injury as a complication of subarachnoid ethanol neurolysis. *Neurology.* 2000; **54**: 1522–4.
20. Hughes JT. Thrombosis of the posterior spinal arteries. A complication of an intrathecal injection of phenol. *Neurology.* 1970; **20**: 659–64.

∗ 21. Gerbershagen HU. Neurolysis. Subarachnoid neurolytic blockade. *Acta Anaesthesiologica Belgica*. 1981; **32**: 45–57.

22. Sloan PA. The evolving role of interventional pain management in oncology. *Journal of Supportive Oncology*. 2004; **2**: 491–500, 503.

∗ 23. de Leon-Casasola OA. Critical evaluation of chemical neurolysis of the sympathetic axis for cancer pain. *Cancer Control*. 2000; **7**: 142–8.

24. Fischer MV, Schmidt M. [Diagnostic and therapeutic blockade of the celiac ganglia]. *Anästhesie, Intensivtherapie, Notfallmedizin*. 1987; **22**: 99–104.

25. Kirvela O, Svedstrom E, Lundbom N. Ultrasonic guidance of lumbar sympathetic and celiac plexus block: a new technique. *Regional Anesthesia*. 1992; **17**: 43–6.

26. Brown DL, Bulley CK, Quiel EL. Neurolytic celiac plexus block for pancreatic cancer pain. *Anesthesia and Analgesia*. 1987; **66**: 869–73.

∗ 27. Sharfman WH, Walsh TD. Has the analgesic efficacy of neurolytic celiac plexus block been demonstrated in pancreatic cancer pain? *Pain*. 1990; **41**: 267–71.

28. Mercadante S. Celiac plexus block versus analgesics in pancreatic cancer pain. *Pain*. 1993; **52**: 187–92.

∗ 29. Staats PS, Hekmat H, Sauter P, Lillemoe K. The effects of alcohol celiac plexus block, pain, and mood on longevity in patients with unresectable pancreatic cancer: a double-blind, randomized, placebo-controlled study. *Pain Medicine*. 2001; **2**: 28–34.

30. Suleyman Ozyalcin N, Talu GK, Camlica H, Erdine S. Efficacy of coeliac plexus and splanchnic nerve blockades in body and tail located pancreatic cancer pain. *European Journal of Pain*. 2004; **8**: 539–45.

∗ 31. Wong GY, Schroeder DR, Carns PE *et al.* Effect of neurolytic celiac plexus block on pain relief, quality of life, and survival in patients with unresectable pancreatic cancer: a randomized controlled trial. *Journal of the American Medical Association*. 2004; **291**: 1092–9.

∗ 32. Eisenberg E, Carr DB, Chalmers TC. Neurolytic celiac plexus block for treatment of cancer pain: a meta-analysis. *Anesthesia and Analgesia*. 1995; **80**: 290–5.

33. Prasanna A. Unilateral celiac plexus block. *Journal of Pain and Symptom Management*. 1996; **11**: 154–7.

34. De Cicco M, Matovic M, Bortolussi R *et al.* Celiac plexus block: injectate spread and pain relief in patients with regional anatomic distortions. *Anesthesiology*. 2001; **94**: 561–5.

35. Akinci D, Akhan O. Celiac ganglia block. *European Journal of Radiology*. 2005; **55**: 355–61.

36. De Conno F, Caraceni A, Aldrighetti L *et al.* Paraplegia following coeliac plexus block. *Pain*. 1993; **55**: 383–5.

37. Abdalla EK, Schell SR. Paraplegia following intraoperative celiac plexus injection. *Journal of Gastrointestinal Surgery*. 1999; **3**: 668–71.

38. Plancarte R, Amescua C, Patt RB, Aldrete JA. Superior hypogastric plexus block for pelvic cancer pain. *Anesthesiology*. 1990; **73**: 236–9.

39. de Leon-Casasola OA, Kent E, Lema MJ. Neurolytic superior hypogastric plexus block for chronic pelvic pain associated with cancer. *Pain*. 1993; **54**: 145–51.

∗ 40. Plancarte R, de Leon-Casasola OA, El-Helaly M *et al.* Neurolytic superior hypogastric plexus block for chronic pelvic pain associated with cancer. *Regional Anesthesia*. 1997; **22**: 562–8.

41. Cariati M, De Martini G, Pretolesi F, Roy MT. CT-guided superior hypogastric plexus block. *Journal of Computer-Assisted Tomography*. 2002; **26**: 428–31.

42. Pollock BE, Ecker RD. A prospective cost-effectiveness study of trigeminal neuralgia surgery. *Clinical Journal of Pain*. 2005; **21**: 317–22.

∗ 43. Lopez BC, Hamlyn PJ, Zakrzewska JM. Systematic review of ablative neurosurgical techniques for the treatment of trigeminal neuralgia. *Neurosurgery*. 2004; **54**: 973–82.

∗ 44. Jannetta PJ. Observations on the etiology of trigeminal neuralgia, hemifacial spasm, acoustic nerve dysfunction and glossopharyngeal neuralgia. Definitive microsurgical treatment and results in 117 patients. *Neurochirurgia*. 1977; **20**: 145–54.

∗ 45. Hakanson S. Trigeminal neuralgia treated by the injection of glycerol into the trigeminal cistern. *Neurosurgery*. 1981; **9**: 638–46.

∗ 46. Cappabianca P, Spaziante R, Graziussi G *et al.* Percutaneous retrogasserian glycerol rhizolysis for treatment of trigeminal neuralgia. Technique and results in 191 patients. *Journal of Neurosurgical Sciences*. 1995; **39**: 37–45.

∗ 47. Saini SS. Retrogasserian anhydrous glycerol injection therapy in trigeminal neuralgia: observations in 552 patients. *Journal of Neurology, Neurosurgery, and Psychiatry*. 1987; **50**: 1536–8.

48. Young RF. Glycerol rhizolysis for treatment of trigeminal neuralgia. *Journal of Neurosurgery*. 1988; **69**: 39–45.

49. Sahni KS, Pieper DR, Anderson R, Baldwin NG. Relation of hypesthesia to the outcome of glycerol rhizolysis for trigeminal neuralgia. *Journal of Neurosurgery*. 1990; **72**: 55–8.

∗ 50. Kondziolka D, Lunsford LD. Percutaneous retrogasserian glycerol rhizotomy for trigeminal neuralgia: technique and expectations. *Neurosurgery Focus*. 2005; **18**: E7.

51. Pollock BE. Percutaneous retrogasserian glycerol rhizotomy for patients with idiopathic trigeminal neuralgia: a prospective analysis of factors related to pain relief. *Journal of Neurosurgery*. 2005; **102**: 223–8.

52. Pickett GE, Bisnaire D, Ferguson GG. Percutaneous retrogasserian glycerol rhizotomy in the treatment of tic douloureux associated with multiple sclerosis. *Neurosurgery*. 2005; **56**: 537–45.

53. Blomstedt PC, Bergenheim AT. Technical difficulties and perioperative complications of retrogasserian glycerol rhizotomy for trigeminal neuralgia. *Stereotactic and Functional Neurosurgery*. 2002; **79**: 168–81.

54. Henson CF, Goldman HW, Rosenwasser RH *et al.* Glycerol rhizotomy versus gamma knife radiosurgery for the treatment of trigeminal neuralgia: an analysis of patients

treated at one institution. *International Journal of Radiation Oncology, Biology, Physics.* 2005; **63**: 82–90.

✳ 55. Barker 2nd FG, Jannetta PJ, Bissonette DJ *et al.* The long-term outcome of microvascular decompression for trigeminal neuralgia. *New England Journal of Medicine.* 1996; **334**: 1077–83.

56. Arter OE, Racz GB. Pain management of the oncologic patient. *Seminars in Surgical Oncology.* 1990; **6**: 162–72.

57. Chaturvedi A, Dash HH. Sympathetic blockade for the relief of chronic pain. *Journal of the Indian Medical Association.* 2001; **99**: 698–703.

58. Purcell-Jones G, Pither CE, Justins DM. Paravertebral somatic nerve block: a clinical, radiographic, and computed tomographic study in chronic pain patients. *Anesthesia and Analgesia.* 1989; **68**: 32–9.

59. Basagan Mogol E, Turker G, Kelebek Girgin N *et al.* Blockade of ganglion impar through sacrococcygeal junction for cancer-related pelvic pain. *Agri: The journal of the Turkish Society of Algology.* 2004; **16**: 48–53.

60. Munir MA, Zhang J, Ahmad M. A modified needle-inside-needle technique for the ganglion impar block. *Canadian Journal of Anaesthesia.* 2004; **51**: 915–7.

61. Iwade M, Fukuuchi A, Kawamata M *et al.* Management of severe pain after extended maxillectomy in a patient with carcinoma of the maxillary sinus. *Masui.* 1996; **45**: 82–5.

62. Varghese BT, Koshy RC. Endoscopic transnasal neurolytic sphenopalatine ganglion block for head and neck cancer pain. *Journal of Laryngology and Otology.* 2001; **115**: 385–7.

29

Intra-articular and local soft-tissue injections

MICHAEL SHIPLEY AND VANESSA MORRIS

KEY LEARNING POINTS

- Always obtain informed consent.
- Explain that steroid injections may cause local subcutaneous atrophy and depigmentation.
- Use scrupulous aseptic technique.
- If an effusion is present, aspirate and examine it before injecting steroid.
- Never inject into an infected lesion with corticosteroid.

- Never inject directly into a tendon (Achilles) as this may cause rupture.
- Resting the knee after injecting it improves outcome.
- It is best not to inject any joint more than two or three times a year and then only if the outcome is good and other treatments contraindicated as there is some evidence of an increased risk of tendon or joint damage.

INTRODUCTION

Local injection into peripheral joints and soft tissues are a central part of the management of many musculoskeletal diseases and pain syndromes. Corticosteroids are the most commonly used agents. Other techniques include dry needling, (acupuncture), injection of local anesthetic, sclerosants or autologous blood into soft tissue, or products derived from hyaluronan into joints. Although frequently used, the evidence-base for their use is not as good as it might be. This chapter reviews the literature and provides a practical approach to their use according to the evidence-base if it exists or to normal practice. There is scope for more and better-designed research. Injections require scrupulous sterile technique but do not need to be undertaken in an operating theater and therefore are ideal for the outpatient or general practice setting. They are, in general, not difficult but are best learnt initially under the guidance of an expert.

CORTICOSTEROID INJECTIONS

The use of steroid hormones in rheumatoid arthritis was first undertaken following the isolation of the agent "compound E" or cortisone by Hench and his colleagues in the late 1930s and 1940s. Cortisone was discovered during research into the mechanisms leading to disease remission in approximately 70 percent of women with rheumatoid arthritis (RA) during pregnancy. It was first used to treat patients with RA in 1948.[1] They rapidly relieved pain, stiffness, and swelling and improved function. It soon became clear that side effects were a major problem. Attempts to find safer agents, safer dosing techniques, and different means of using the agents were investigated but side effects remain a significant limitation to their use in regular oral doses.

Intra-articular and local soft tissue administration was first undertaken in the 1950s and remains important in the treatment of inflammatory arthritis and local soft tissue lesions including bursitis, tendonosis, and peripheral nerve entrapment syndromes.[2] With careful and appropriate application they are safe and effective (**Table 29.1**). There is evidence supporting their use in many specific clinical situations, the benefit is often rapid but may be short-lived unless combined with other therapeutic approaches. The benefit in practical terms to the patient who is unable to work or function normally because of pain which does not responded to analgesic and/or nonsteroidal anti-inflammatory agents (NSAID) is dramatic. It is important, however, to also address local causes and to give appropriate advice about short-term rest and altered activity as part of a rehabilitation program to reduce the risk of recurrence.

Usually, a local steroid injection is used for its powerful anti-inflammatory effect. Steroids act through a variety of mechanisms including the inhibition of cytokines, chemokines, and enzymes and by effects on transcription and translation processes. They also have a local anesthetic effect on nerves or nociceptive nerve endings.[3] Their mechanism of action in lesions such as tendonosis, where there is little evidence of a local inflammatory reaction, is not clear.

The mention of the word "steroid" may instill unreasonable fear because of the widely known side effects of long-term oral medication. This fear must be addressed positively and the different implications of one or a small number of local injections against the daily use of oral steroids discussed. Steroid preparations used for local injection reduce their systemic effects. Some do occur, particularly with high doses administered intra-articularly, and the patient should be warned, especially if they are diabetic, as their glucose levels may rise briefly. Informed consent after discussing the potential risks is advisable. Intra-articular or intralesional injections into infected lesions are absolutely contraindicated and may lead to severe local infections and occasionally to septicemia. Medicolegally this is considered a negligent act. If infection is suspected or possible, all care must be taken to detect or exclude it before any steroid is injected.

INTRA-ARTICULAR INJECTIONS OF CORTICOSTEROIDS

The hot swollen joint – is it septic arthritis?

The management of a hot swollen joint is a common medical problem. The least common but most serious cause is septic arthritis, which must be treated as a medical emergency and the patient given intravenous antibiotics. The patient usually presents with a short history of an increasingly painful joint and is feverish and unwell. The joint is hot, inflamed, and intensely painful. If immunosuppressed for therapeutic reasons such as a malignancy or an autoimmune disease, or as part of an infection with human immunodeficiency virus (HIV) or if they are frail and elderly, the systemic symptoms and signs may be less. A septic arthritis complicating rheumatoid arthritis should be considered if there is a single joint flare. The causative organism can be cultured from the aspirate and from blood cultures – septic arthritis is usually secondary to septicemia with a source of infection in the skin, genitourinary track, or gastrointestinal track. It may occasionally be the result of direct infection by trauma or rarely after an intra-articular injection. Septic arthritis is an absolute contraindication to the use of intra-articular steroids (and other agents). If during a planned intra-articular injection procedure the aspirate is cloudy or purulent or if sepsis is suspected, cultures of the fluid and blood and any other site of infection are obligatory and the steroid must not be injected until all cultures are negative.

Other causes of a hot swollen joint are trauma, the first onset of, or a flare of, a preexisting inflammatory arthritis such as RA or seronegative spondyloarthropathy, crystal arthritis, such as gout, pseudogout, or sickle cell disease.

Table 29.1 Indications for intra-articular corticosteroids.

Indications	
Posttraumatic synovitis with an effusion	Meniscal tear (think about arthroscopic management)
	Complicating osteoarthritis
	Hemarthrosis
Osteoarthritis with an acute effusion	Possibly osteoarthritis with no effusion
Acute inflammatory monoarthritis	Seronegative spondyloarthropathy
	Acute monoarticular flare of RA or spondyloarthropathy
	Crystal arthritis (gout or pseudogout)

PROCEDURE FOR INTRA-ARTICULAR INJECTIONS

Make the patient comfortable and adjust the couch height. Have everything ready – different size needles and syringes, alcohol swabs, gauze pads, and adhesive plaster. Draw up the local anesthetic (lidocaine 1 or 2 percent or bupivicaine 0.25 percent) in one syringe and the steroid preparation in another (see **Table 29.2**). Have an aspirating syringe ready and a sterile pot for the aspirate. Scrupulous sterile technique is obligatory. Many wear sterile gloves although this is not essential as long as the hands are well washed and rings and watches removed. Cleanse the skin and insert the needle (some use a prior spray of ethyl chloride). Inject the local anesthetic as the needle is inserted. Entering the joint is usually detectable as a fall in the injection pressure. Attempt to aspirate as much fluid as possible. Examine the fluid. If it is clear, the effusion is traumatic or complicating osteoarthritis (OA). Slightly cloudy fluid is obtained from inflamed joints. Very cloudy and opaque fluid could be due to crystal synovitis or septic arthritis. If in any doubt about the possibility of an infection, do not inject the steroid, end the procedure and send the fluid for Gram staining, polarizing light microscopy (for crystals of sodium urate or calcium pyrophosphate) and culture. If the patient is unwell or frail, seek the advice of a microbiologist about antibiotic treatment, take blood cultures and cultures from urine or any skin wounds, and admit the patient as a medical emergency.

Once satisfied that there is no infection or once the culture is sterile, inject the steroid. Ask the patient to rest the joint for a day or so, particularly if injecting a weight-bearing joint. This improves the outcome.[4] Warn them that there may be a flare of pain for approximately 24 hours and ask them to report back urgently should the joint become hot or inflamed or should they become unwell.

Depressingly, a recent study has shown that only 10 percent of intra-articular injections were placed correctly into the joint, even by experts.[5] For this reason, the use of ultrasound-guided injection is becoming popular. Further research is needed to evaluate the efficacy of injections under ultrasound guidance.

The shoulder joint

The movement of the shoulder comprises extension, flexion, abduction, and internal and external rotation. The shoulder girdle itself comprises three joints: the sternoclavicular, acromioclavicular, and glenohumeral joints. They combine with the scapulothoracic articulation to allow the large range of movement, moved by the rotator cuff muscles and deltoid. OA of the shoulder joint occurs in heavy workers (builders, farmers), athletes, and musicians. The shoulder joint is also affected in RA with lesions of the rotator cuff and long head of biceps leading to tears. Later, erosion of the humeral head and glenoid fossa occur. The shoulder joint is injected to ease pain in inflammatory and degenerative joint conditions.

INJECTING THE SHOULDER JOINT

Seat the patient with the arm hanging down.

ANTERIOR APPROACH

Place the arm in external rotation. Mark medial to humeral head and below and lateral to the coracoid process. Introduce the needle pointing upwards and laterally (**Figure 29.1**).

POSTERIOR APPROACH

Place the arm in neutral. Introduce the needle 2–3 cm below the posterolateral corner of the acromion and pointing forwards towards the coracoid process.

Injecting the acromioclavicular joint

Acromioclavicular (AC) joint pain is localized to the joint, which is tender. Reaching the arm across the front of the body is painful. Identify the AC joint by palpating the clavicle and feeling the depression at the joint with the patient seated. Insert the needle from above pointing down (**Figure 29.2**).

Table 29.2 Steroid preparations for intra-articular or soft tissue injection.

Steroid	Dose	Method of administration
Hydrocortisone acetate	25 mg/mL	Soft-tissue injections
Prednisolone acetate	25 mg/mL	Soft-tissue injections
Triamcinolone acetonide	40 mg/mL	Intra-articular – up to 2 mL
Triamcinolone hexacetonide	20 mg/mL	Intra-articular – up to 2 mL
Methylprednisolone depot	40 mg/mL	Intra-articular – up to 2 mL

The volume varies with the size of joint – 0.2 mL for an MCP, 0.5–1 mL for elbow or wrist, 1 mL for shoulder, 1–2 mL for knee.

The elbow and radiohumeral joints

There are three articulations at the elbow: the radio-humeral, humeroulnar, and radioulnar joints. The humeroulnar joint allows flexion and extension, the others pronation and supination. The elbow joint is injected in OA, RA, and crystal arthropathies.

INJECTING THE ELBOW JOINT

Seat the patient with the arm supported and the elbow at right angles. Palpate the radial head, the lateral olecranon, and the lateral epicondyle. Introduce the needle from a lateral approach between the radial head and lateral epicondyle, aiming towards the medial epicondyle. Attempt aspiration. Easy flow of the injectate suggests the needle is in the joint.

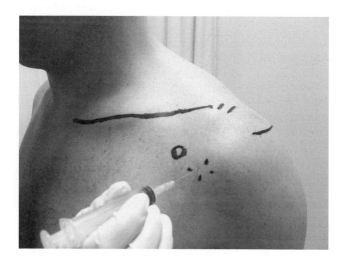

Figure 29.1 Anterior injection approach to the shoulder joint.

The wrist joint

The wrist joint is complex and is commonly affected in inflammatory arthritis. Injection reduces synovitis and pain.

INJECTING THE WRIST JOINT

Place the wrist in 15° of flexion. Mark next to the extensor tendon of the thumb, distal to the radius and on the ulnar side of the anatomical snuff box. Direct the needle towards the distal ulna (**Figure 29.3**). There is no evidence-base for immobilizing the wrist after steroid injection.[6]

The first carpometacarpal joint

The first carpometacarpal joint is prone to OA causing pain and poor grip. The joint appears "squared." As it stiffens, pain lessens for most. Even if the joint is injected under radiological imaging there is no evidence for a good outcome.[7]

INJECTING THE FIRST CARPOMETACARPAL JOINT

Palpate the joint line with the thumb flexed into the palm. Introduce the needle lateral to the abductor pollicis longus tendon and towards the fourth metacarpal base.

Metacarpophalangeal and interphalangeal joints

The metacarpal and interphalangeal joints are affected in inflammatory arthritis. Synovitis causes synovial bulging dorsally. OA can affect these joints. Find the joint line and inject local anesthetic as the needle is introduced from either side of the joint under the extensor tendon.

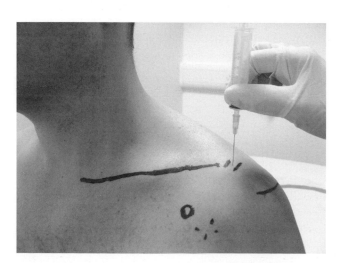

Figure 29.2 Injecting the acromioclavicular joint.

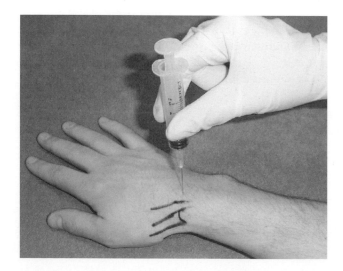

Figure 29.3 Injecting the wrist.

The hip joint

The hip is a ball and socket joint between the femoral head and the acetabulum. The glenoid labrum, an extension of the acetabular rim, the capsule, and ligaments provide support. The hip joint is also supported by strong muscles. It is affected in OA, RA, and seronegative spondyloarthropathy. The hip is rarely injected without fluoroscopic or ultrasound guidance. From a nonrandomized study there is evidence that ultrasound (US)-guided injection of 80 mg depot methylprednisolone in OA of the hip is effective with an improvement lasting 12 weeks compared with only six weeks when 40 mg was injected.[8]

INJECTING THE HIP JOINT (UNDER FLUOROSCOPY)

There are two approaches: Anterior approach – with the patient lying supine extend and externally rotate the hip. Insert local anesthetic 2–3 cm below the anterior superior iliac spine and 2–3 cm lateral to the femoral pulse. Then use a larger bore needle and inject anesthetic as it is introduced pointing backwards and medially at a 60° angle. Aspirate any synovial fluid before injecting the steroid. Lateral approach – the patient is supine with the hip internally rotated. After skin anesthesia, insert the needle anterior to the greater trochanter and directed medially and upwards towards the inguinal ligament. The tip of the needle may be felt entering the joint.

The knee joint

The knee comprises the tibiofemoral and patellofemoral joints. Knee pain is common and may be articular or periarticular. There is evidence for a short-term benefit in OA from a corticosteroid for up to 24 weeks.[9] The knee is routinely aspirated and injected in inflammatory and crystal arthropathies. After a knee injection, resting for up to 24 hours increases the benefit in RA.[4] It was assumed

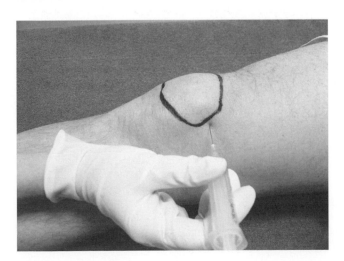

Figure 29.4 Injecting the knee joint.

that this retarded the systemic absorption of steroid leading to increased local concentrations. Weitoft and Ronnblom,[10] however, demonstrated an equal alteration in the hypothalamic-pituitary-adrenal axis in rested patients compared with those who mobilized after 20 mg of triamcinolone hexacetonide (THA), reflecting the same amount of systemic steroid absorption.

INJECTING THE KNEE JOINT

Place the patient lying comfortably on a couch. Relaxing the quadriceps is essential or the patella presses against the femur making joint aspiration and injection difficult. Extend the knee and feel the patella, femur, and tibia. Insert the needle with anesthetic medially and posterior to the patella and directed slightly backwards. Attempt to aspirate, pressing gently on the suprapatellar pouch (**Figure 29.4**). When in the joint space, the steroid flows freely. The knee can also be injected laterally. If the knee is fixed in flexion, inject with the patient sitting with the knee at 90°, inserting the needle to either side of the patellar tendon and just above the tibial plateau. Rest improves the outcome.

The ankle joint

The ankle is a hinged joint formed by the distal tibia and fibula with proximal part of the talus. The movement of this joint is plantar flexion and extension. Inversion and eversion occur at the subtalar joint.

INJECTING THE ANKLE

Place the leg and foot at right angles. Insert the needle medial to the tibialis anterior tendon and lateral to the medial malleolus, directed posteriorly.

Metatarsophalangeal and interphalangeal joints

The reasons to inject these joints are as for the hand and the techniques are similar. The needle is introduced dorsally and beside the extensor tendons.

PROCEDURE FOR INTRALESIONAL OR SOFT TISSUE INJECTIONS

The procedure is essentially the same as for intra-articular injections (see above under Procedure for intra-articular injections). There may be fluid to aspirate if there is bursitis or an abscess. The injection is best made under low pressure either into a cavity or adjacent to a tendon. For enthesitis, injection under slightly greater pressure is sometimes necessary.

SOFT-TISSUE INJECTIONS FOR TENOSYNOVITIS, TENDONOSIS, ENTHESITIS, AND BURSITIS

A caution about injecting into superficial soft-tissue lesions is that the steroid can produce local subcutaneous atrophy and depigmentation, which is more noticeable in those with dark skin. Distracting the skin to close the track helps but the patient should be forewarned.

The shoulder

ROTATOR CUFF SYNDROMES

Tendonosis usually of the supraspinatus tendon, sometimes with a partial tear or small complete tear of the rotator cuff, or subacromial bursitis, causes pain in the upper arm, which is made worse when the arm is abducted through the middle range. Pain may limit abduction above 90° although the passive range is often better. The pain is less if the arm is elevated in flexion, reducing impingement against the acromion. Rotator cuff pathology may be due to direct injury following a fall onto the outstretched arm, to working with the hands above the head or to impingement against the acromion and/or an osteoarthritic or un-stable acromio-clavicular joint. Eventually the supraspinatus muscle wastes and this increases impingement because it helps to hold the humeral head down as it rotates under the acromion against the strong upward pull of deltoid.

A calcific deposit in the tendon is visible on x-ray, lying adjacent to its insertion into the greater tuberosity. The material is crystalline and may rupture into the adjacent subacromial bursa causing severe pain and swelling due to calcific bursitis. This is visible on x-ray as cloudy radio-opacity in the bursa. Diagnostic ultrasound in skilled hands is probably the best way of specifically diagnosing the underlying cause(s).[11] Whether specific differential diagnosis of these different pathologies affects the decision to treat or the outcome is unclear.[12] Initially use simple analgesics or NSAIDs but the pain, which may be very disabling, is reduced rapidly by a local corticosteroid injection into the subacromial bursa.[12] Even specialists may not place an injection accurately into the subacromial bursa (29 percent) and this significantly correlates with outcome.[13] The relevance of a partial thickness tendon tear in deciding whether to inject or not is unclear. There is probably a slight risk of converting a partial to a full tear but the natural history, treated or untreated, is unclear. A full tear can be disabling, reducing active but not passive abduction of the arm. The patient learns to lift the arm with the other or prop it against something. Elevation in flexion is often possible. Pain can be the main limiting factor for movement and is difficult to manage.

SUBACROMIAL INJECTION TECHNIQUE

Approach from the side with the patient sitting with their arm hanging relaxed by their side. Clean the skin, palpate for the edge of the acromion and insert a green (21 gauge) needle just below it, injecting lignocaine as it is advanced (**Figure 29.5**). There is a fall in pressure when the needle enters the bursa. The acromion varies from almost horizontal to tilted – the needle may need repositioning and this is when local anesthetic is appreciated. Once in the bursa, attempt to aspirate any fluid (rarely possible), change the syringe, and inject steroid. The outcome of blind or ultrasound guided injections for bursitis at one week does not differ significantly.[14] If a diagnosis is unclear, a diagnostic ultrasound examination followed by injection is warranted.

PROXIMAL BICIPITAL TENDONOSIS

Proximal bicipital tendonosis is uncommon. It causes pain in front of the humeral head, which increases during flexion and supination of the elbow against resistance. It is difficult to diagnose clinically but is seen on ultrasound or magnetic resonance imaging (MRI). There may be swelling (tendonosis), inflammation of the tendon sheath, or rupture of the retaining ligament, allowing the tendon to dislocate. Rest and pain relief usually suffice. A corticosteroid injection alongside the tendon in the bicipital groove helps but is best performed under ultrasound guidance. Rupture of the long head of the biceps tendon occurs in older patients and causes sudden shoulder pain and bruising in the upper arm. Tensing the muscle causes a variable, painless swelling in the biceps muscle. Once the pain has settled there is little residual disability.

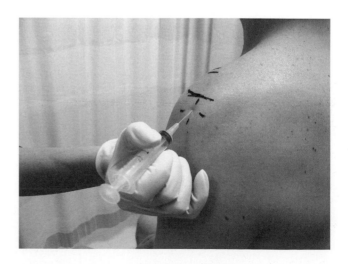

Figure 29.5 Injecting the subacromial bursa.

ADHESIVE CAPSULITIS

Adhesive capsulitis or true frozen shoulder causes intense, diffuse shoulder pain. It is rare and warrants secondary referral.[15, 16] The pain persists and the joint stiffens over a few weeks or months leading to complete loss of all movements, including internal and external rotation with the arm by the side. (Loss of rotation also occurs in shoulder arthritis but in rotator cuff syndromes is retained unless there is severe pain and spasm.) Rotator cuff tendonosis, injury, stroke, or myocardial infarction may precede adhesive capsulitis. Poorly controlled insulin-dependent diabetes is a risk factor for developing it. The etiology is not clear. The pain gradually lessens over a few months but the stiffness remains for up to 18 months. Thereafter the shoulder may be a bit stiff but is rarely disabling. Capsulitis is poorly visualized on MRI which can exclude other causes, however. NSAIDs and analgesics help but the pain is difficult to control. Oral corticosteroids reduce pain but do not prevent stiffening or speed recovery. A combined intra-articular and subacromial injection plus physiotherapy is more effective at six weeks in reducing pain and improving range of movement than either a subacromial or an intra-articular injection plus physiotherapy. There is no difference at 16 weeks.[17] Manipulation under anesthetic or arthroscopic release of the fibrous tissue in the rotator interval is undertaken during the fibrotic phase but the evidence-base is poor.

The elbow

LATERAL EPICONDYLITIS

Lateral epicondylitis or "tennis elbow" is an enthesitis causing pain at the insertion of the common extensor tendon at the lateral epicondyle and in the proximal forearm. It often resolves with rest. The lateral epicondyle is tender. Making a fist and dorsiflexing against resistance typically worsens the pain.

MEDIAL EPICONDYLITIS

Medial epicondylitis or "golfer's elbow" is an enthesitis and causes pain at the insertion of the common wrist flexor muscles at the medial epicondyle. Resisted flexion of the wrist with the elbow straight worsens the pain.

Epicondylitis is frequently self-limiting. If it persists and becomes disabling, a local corticosteroid injection at the site of maximum tenderness improves the pain but does not alter the long-term outcome when compared with physiotherapy.[18] The pain may worsen for a couple of days after the injection and the patient should be warned. It is best to avoid gripping and carrying for a week. These are common sites for developing subcutaneous fat atrophy and skin depigmentation. Acupuncture may help lateral epicondylitis.[19]

OLECRANON BURSITIS

Olecranon bursitis is usually traumatic. It causes pain, tenderness, and swelling over the point of the elbow. If traumatic, the aspirated fluid is clear, slightly cloudy, or blood stained. It is occasionally due to an inflammatory arthritis or gout when the fluid is cloudy. If it is bacterial there is usually cellulitis and the fluid is purulent. If infection has been excluded, a local corticosteroid injection directly into the cavity helps. Infective bursitis requires antibiotics.

The wrist and hand

DE QUERVAIN'S STENOSING TENOSYNOVITIS

De Quervain's stenosing tenosynovitis causes pain and swelling at the radial styloid where the abductor policis longus and extensor policis brevis tendons run under a retaining band. The pain extends proximally or towards the thumb. There is local tenderness and swelling over the tendons. The pain is worsened by passively flexing the thumb into the palm. Resting the thumb and wrist in a spika helps, as may therapeutic ultrasound or NSAID gels. A corticosteroid injection alongside the tendon under low pressure, not into the tendon, at the point of maximum tenderness, brings rapid relief for most although a second injection may be necessary. Failure to respond to injection may be due to the presence of a separate compartment for the extensor pollicis brevis tendon.[20, 21]

EXTENSOR TENOSYNOVITIS

Extensor tenosynovitis of the common extensor compartment causes an hourglass-shaped swelling from the back of the hand to just proximal to the wrist with constriction by the extensor retinaculum. (Synovitis of the wrist joint causes more diffuse swelling distal to the radius and ulna.) It is caused by repetitive wrist movements at work or in the home and causes forearm pain in keyboard workers who hold their wrists in excessive extension without a wrist support. A work station review is helpful. If rest does not help, a corticosteroid injection into the tendon sheath is straightforward.

FLEXOR TENOSYNOVITIS

Flexor tenosynovitis affects one or several fingers and follows repeated tight gripping at work or home. It causes finger stiffness in the morning and pain in the palm and along the dorsum of the finger. There is palpable tendon thickening and sometimes a tendon nodule in the palm. Passive extension of the finger is painful. The primary lesion is tenosynovitis leading eventually to fibrosis and constriction of the tendon sheath. It is common in RA and seronegative spondyloarthropathy. Nodular flexor tenosynovitis is more common in diabetic individuals and less responsive to treatment.[22] The thickened tendon may catch at the A1 pulley overlying the metacarpophalangeal (MCP) joint in the palm and cause a trigger finger on waking or during tight gripping. The finger is flexed into the palm and has to be forcibly extended with a sudden painless or painful click, palpable in the palm. A corticosteroid injection alongside the tendon nodule in the palm under low pressure helps.[23] If persistent, surgical release is indicated.

THUMB FLEXOR TENOSYNOVITIS AND TRIGGER THUMB

Thumb flexor tenosynovitis and trigger thumb are due to local trauma, for example opening a tight jar, or overuse. Thumb movements are painful and stiff. The sesamoid bone in the flexor pollicis brevis tendon over the volar aspect of the first MCP joint is tender. Triggering causes the interphalangeal joint either to stick in flexion or the thumb cannot be flexed. A low pressure local corticosteroid injection at the site of maximal tenderness adjacent to the sesamoid bone helps.[23]

The hip

TROCHANTERIC BURSITIS AND TEARS OF THE TENDON OF GLUTEUS MEDIUS

Trochanteric bursitis and tears of the tendon of gluteus medius cause lateral hip pain and tenderness when walking and running and on stairs, and lying on the affected side. The pain radiates to the lateral thigh as far as the knee but is not associated with paresthesia or numbness (compare meralgia paresthetica). A disk lesion at L2 can also cause lateral hip pain, usually with sensory symptoms. If rest and stretching do not help, an injection of steroid onto the trochanter at the point of maximum tenderness often does.

ISCHIAL BURSITIS AND ENTHESITIS

Ischial bursitis and enthesitis (hamstring tear) cause pain in the buttock and tenderness over the ischial tuberosity. If rest does not help, an injection is given onto the tuberosity with the patient semiprone and the affected hip flexed and internally rotated.

ADDUCTOR TENDONOSIS

Adductor tendonosis causes pain in the lower medial groin and is caused by injury or over use. The tendon is tender approximately 2 cm distal to its insertion or there may be an enthesitis with tenderness at the adductor tubercle. If rest does not help, an injection can be given alongside the tendon or at its insertion.

ILIOPSOAS BURSITIS

Iliopsoas bursitis presents as a tender swelling lateral to the neurovascular bundle in the groin. The pain is worsened by hyperextension and resisted flexion of the hip. It is clearly seen on MRI and can be injected with corticosteroid under ultrasound guidance.

RECTUS FEMORIS ENTHESITIS

Rectus femoris enthesitis occurs in athletes. The pain localizes to the upper pubic ramus and lower abdomen. Inflammation is clearly seen on MRI. Conservative measures and rest help. The tendon may rupture close to its insertion and require surgical repair.

The knee

MEDIAL KNEE PAIN

Medial collateral ligament strain

Medial collateral ligament strain causes pain and tenderness at its insertion into the medial tibia after an injury and in the overweight with valgus knees. Pain is increased by exerting a valgus stress on the knee.

Anserine bursitis and pes anserinus tendonosis

Anserine bursitis and pes anserinus tendonosis produce tenderness behind the line of the medial ligament and more distally. Rest helps, as does a local corticosteroid injection.

LATERAL KNEE PAIN

Iliotibial band friction syndrome

Iliotibial band friction syndrome (runner's knee) is the most common cause of overuse knee pain in runners and cyclists. It causes pain and tenderness over the lateral femoral condyle. It can be injected with steroid if rest and shoe-wear adjustment do not help.

ANTERIOR KNEE PAIN

Pain in front of the knee usually arises from the patellofemoral joint.

Prepatellar bursitis

Prepatellar bursitis causes fluctuant swelling in front of the patella. Aspiration and injection of a corticosteroid helps if infection has been ruled out. The deep infrapatellar bursa lies between the patellar tendon and the tibia and is locally tender when inflamed.

The superficial infrapatellar bursa lies over the patellar tendon at its insertion into the tibial tubercle. Ultrasound-guided aspiration and injection with corticosteroid helps.

Patellar tendonosis

Patellar tendonosis (jumper's knee) causes pain at the junction of the tendon and the inferior patella. Rest usually helps.

THE ANKLE AND FOOT

Achilles tendonosis

Achilles tendonosis[24] occurs during sport or with a change from heels to flat shoes or no shoes. It causes pain and a tender fusiform swelling approximately 2 cm proximal to the insertion. It is worse in the morning and when walking. A heel raise and rest are often helpful. When the pain has reduced, stretching exercises prevent recurrence. Local corticosteroid injections are contra-indicated as they may precipitate rupture of the tendon. Achilles tendon rupture occurs after the age of 50. Conservative management in plaster is usual although in the younger athlete, surgical repair is feasible.[25]

Achilles tendon enthesitis

Achilles tendon enthesitis causes pain at its insertion into the calcaneum and is due to overuse or occasionally to seronegative spondyloarthropathy. Rest and a heel raise help. Occasionally a low-pressure corticosteroid injection near the insertion is used.

Plantar fasciitis

Plantar fasciitis[26] is an enthesitis which causes pain under the heel when weight bearing in the overweight, middle-aged joggers, and those with flat feet. It also occurs in seronegative spondyloarthropathy. It is always worse in the morning or after nonweight bearing. There is local tenderness in front of the calcaneum. Approximately 30 percent have a plantar spur on a lateral x-ray – plantar spurs do not always cause pain. Inferior heel pain may also be due to subcalcaneal bursitis (policeman's heel) and fat pad disruption. MRI is rarely indicated but demonstrates the specific pathology clearly. A heel cup, an arch support, and thick-soled shoes help. Systematic reviews show no significant long-term benefit from corticosteroid injection versus placebo in plantar fasciitis and symptoms often settle spontaneously.[27] Local corticosteroid injections, with or without local anesthetic or tibial nerve blockade are painful.[28] The evidence-base for injection is weak.[29]

Tibialis posterior tendonosis

Tibialis posterior tendonosis causes pain and swelling behind the medial malleolus during running and dancing, especially with a flat foot. Longitudinal splits in the tendon sometimes lead to a tear which is disabling and causes sudden flattening of the foot. There may be tenosynovitis adjacent to the malleolus. Rest helps and a surgical boot may be needed. An arch support is often necessary. Ultrasound or MRI clearly demonstrates the pathology and tenosynovitis can be treated with a local corticosteroid injection. This is best avoided if there is significant tendon splitting as it may lead to a full tear.

Tarsal tunnel syndrome

Tarsal tunnel syndrome is an entrapment neuropathy of the posterior tibial nerve as it rounds the medial malleolus – see below under Tarsal tunnel syndrome.

Peroneus longus and brevis tendonosis

Peroneus longus and brevis tendonosis cause pain and tenderness posterior to the lateral malleolus. Rest helps but corticosteroid injections are occasionally necessary.

Tibialis anterior tenosynovitis

Tibialis anterior tenosynovitis is caused by unaccustomed walking or running or tight shoes. It causes pain and crepitus in front of the ankle and over the dorsum of the foot with swelling which extends across the joint (unlike synovitis of the ankle joint which bulges to either side of the extensor tendons). Rest and looser shoes help. A corticosteroid injection is sometimes necessary.

INJECTIONS FOR PERIPHERAL NERVE ENTRAPMENT SYNDROMES

Carpal tunnel syndrome

Carpal tunnel syndrome is the most common peripheral nerve entrapment syndrome and is usually associated with flexor tenosynovitis. It is common in inflammatory arthritis and in late pregnancy. Repetitive wrist and hand activity increases the risk of developing carpal tunnel syndrome. Its status as a work injury is controversial.[30] Pain, tingling, and numbness affect the thumb, index, middle, and radial side of ring fingers (median nerve distribution) and typically waken the patient or are present on wakening. The fingers feel more swollen than they appear. There is often intense forearm aching. During the day it is precipitated by holding a book or newspaper. Weakness and numbness cause clumsiness. The patient's description of the symptoms is often diagnostic.[31] When long-standing, there is wasting of the thenar eminence affecting flexor pollicis and opponens pollicis and weakness of abduction of the thumb when it is adducted towards the fifth digit. Tinel's sign, tapping the median nerve at the wrist, and Phalen's test, holding the wrist in forced dorsiflexion, both produce tingling in the fingers. Ultrasound or MRI demonstrates the carpal tunnel and median nerve well but is rarely necessary. A useful first approach, which is also diagnostic, is to use a wrist splint at night. If this relieves or reduces the symptoms, use for a few weeks may suffice. It is usual to perform nerve conduction studies if the diagnosis is in doubt and to check for nerve damage. Slowing of median nerve conduction at the wrist suggests demyelination. A reduced or absent action potential is due to nerve fiber damage and needle electromyography detects denervation.

INJECTING THE CARPAL TUNNEL

A corticosteroid injection into the carpal tunnel is indicated for mild to moderate carpal tunnel syndrome although it may recur and some patents opt for surgery. Insert a blue needle just to the ulnar side of the palmaris longus tendon (approximately 0.5 cm to the ulnar side of flexor carpi radialis if palmaris longus is absent) at the distal wrist skin crease at an angle of 45° pointing towards the middle finger. Inject local anesthetic superficially, but not into the carpal tunnel (**Figure 29.6**). Change syringe and advance the needle and insert 0.1 mL corticosteroid. If this causes pain in the fingers, the needle is in the nerve – withdraw slightly and test again. One milliliter of corticosteroid (usually hydrocortisone acetate 25 mg or depot methylprednisolone 40 mg) is injected slowly and may cause tingling due to a volume effect in an already tight carpal tunnel.[32, 33] Persistent symptoms or significant nerve damage require day-case surgical decompression or endoscopic surgery.[34] Incomplete recovery of sensation and/or strength occurs if the lesion is severe and longstanding. Median nerve compression occurs less commonly as it passes through pronator teres in the proximal forearm. The symptoms are different and rarely bad in the morning. Nerve conduction studies localize the site of compression, which may need surgical release.

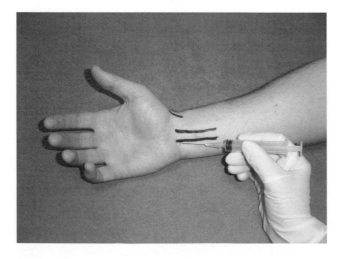

Figure 29.6 Injecting the carpal tunnel.

Tarsal tunnel syndrome

Tarsal tunnel syndrome is an entrapment neuropathy of the posterior tibial nerve as it rounds the medial malleolus. It causes burning pain and pins and needles in the toes, sole, and heel on waking. Tinel's sign is positive behind the medial malleolus and nerve conduction studies are diagnostic. Injecting steroid just behind the medial malleolus into the tibialis posterior tendon sheath helps.

Meralgia paraesthetica

Meralgia paresthetica is an entrapment neuropathy of the lateral femoral cutaneous nerve (LFCN) and produces burning pain, dysesthesia, and numbness of the anterolateral thigh from the trochanter to just above the knee. It is made worse by sitting and sudden weight increase. There is no weakness or muscle wasting. It may develop after pelvic or inguinal surgery, or a direct injury. The LFCN usually runs under the lateral inguinal ligament close to the anterior superior iliac spine and superficial to sartorius. Compression occurs in sartorius or as it emerges through the fascia lata approximately 10 cm distal to the anterior superior iliac spine. A lateral L2/3 disk compressing the L2 nerve root mimics the syndrome, although there is usually also back pain and may be wasting of vastus lateralis. Electrostimulation to localize the nerve precisely helps more accurate injection of local corticosteroid. Avoidance of local causes of pressure and rest are also helpful. Patients often live with it, especially when numbness is the only symptom.[35]

ACUPUNCTURE – DRY NEEDLING

Dry needling techniques using the classical Chinese approach or a westernized variant which involves needling of tender or "trigger" points are extremely popular. Two percent of adults in the UK and two million people in the USA use it annually. It is regarded as safe, although not without risk, and there is evidence that it has a small but significant and cost-effective benefit in chronic low back pain when compared with usual physiotherapy treatment.[36, 37] No sham acupuncture was used so that the recognized placebo effect of acupuncture cannot be fully excluded. A recent Cochrane review of acupuncture in back pain suggests that there is short- to medium-term pain relief with acupuncture which is greater than that seen with sham acupuncture.[38] In a recent systematic review and meta-analysis of the use of acupuncture in OA of peripheral joints, sham-controlled studies support the use of acupuncture for pain control.[39] The strongest data are for knee OA.[40] There is also evidence of a significant placebo effect from sham acupuncture. The adverse effects of acupuncture are lower than for many standard drug treatments but mild problems may arise in up to 7 percent.[41] Nonetheless, its favorable safety profile and small but proven effect on painful OA of the knee suggest that it is worthy of consideration.

RADIOACTIVE AND CHEMICAL KNEE SYNOVECTOMY

In some institutions radioactive synovectomy is carried out using yttrium (^{90}Y).[42] This form of treatment has been used for many years for the treatment of inflammatory and degenerative joint diseases. Other radiopharmaceuticals introduced recently are dysprosium-165 (^{165}Dy), holmium-166 (^{166}Ho), samurium-153 (^{153}Sm), rhenium-188 (^{188}Re), and lutetium-177 (^{177}Lu).[43] It is used after failure of conventional therapy, including corticosteroid injections, and reduces synovitis. Contraindications include pregnancy, breastfeeding, local skin infection, and a ruptured popliteal cyst. Relative contraindications are being under 20 years old, extensive joint instability, and advanced joint disease. It is usually combined with an intra-articular dose of steroid. Adverse effects are injection site necrosis, joint infection, and thrombosis of the immobilized limb.

Osmic acid has also been used as a treatment for chronic synovitis unresponsive to other forms of treatment[44] but may not be as good a treatment as radioactive synovectomy.[45]

HYALURONAN INJECTIONS

Hyaluronic acid (HA) is a natural component of synovial fluid. A variety of different preparations is available for intra-articular use in OA (viscosupplementation). Intra-articular injections of hyaluronan are used to reduce osteoathritic symptoms in the knee. There is evidence that injections give relief for up to six months, but repeat courses may not be beneficial.[46] The HA may act on inflammation as well as be a chondroprotectant.[47]

REFERENCES

1. Hench PS, Kendall EC, Slocumb CH *et al*. The effect of a hormone of the adrenal cortex (17-hydroxy-11-dehydrocorticosteroine: Compound E) and of pituitary adrenocorticotrophic hormone on rheumatoid arthritis: preliminary report. *Proceedings of Staff Meeting of the Mayo Clinic.* 1949; **24**: 181–97.

2. Haslock I, Macfarlane D, Speed C. Intra-articular and soft-tissue injections: a survey of current practice. *British Journal of Rheumatology.* 1995; **34**: 449–52.

3. Paget SA. Clinical use of corticosteroids: an overview. In: Lin AN, Paget SA (eds). *Principles of corticosteroid therapy.* New York: Arnold Publishers, 2002: 6–16.

 * 4. Chakravarty K, Pharoah PDP, Scott DGI. A randomized controlled study of post-injection rest following intra-articular steroid therapy for knee synovitis. *British Journal of Rheumatology.* 1994; **33**: 464–8.

5. Eustace JA, Brophy DP, Gibney RP *et al*. Comparison of the accuracy of steroid placement with clinical outcome in shoulder symptoms. *Annals of the Rheumatic Diseases.* 1997; **56**: 59–63.

6. Weitoft T, Rönnblom L. Randomised controlled study of post injection immobilization after intraarticular glucocorticoid treatment for wrist synovitis. *Annals of the Rheumatic Diseases.* 2003; **62**: 1013–15.

7. Meenagh GK, Patton J, Kynes C, Wright GD. A randomised controlled trial of intraarticular corticosteroid injection of the carpometacarpal joint of the thumb in osteoarthritis. *Annals of the Rheumatic Diseases.* 2004; **63**: 1260–3.

 * 8. Robinson P, Keenan A-M, Conaghan PG. Clinical effectiveness and dose response of image-guided intra-articular corticosteroid injection for hip osteoarthritis. *Rheumatology.* 2007; **46**: 285–91.

9. Aroll B, Goodyear-Smith F. Corticosteroid injections for osteoarthritis of the knee. *British Medical Journal.* 2004; **328**: 869.

10. Weitoft T, Ronnblom L. Glucocorticoid resorption and influence on the hypothalamic-pituitary-adrenal axis after intra-articular treatment of the knee in resting and mobile patients. *Annals of the Rheumatic Diseases.* 2006; **65**: 955–7.

11. Roberts CS, Walker JA, Seligson D. Diagnostic capabilities of shoulder ultrasonography in the detection of complete and partial rotator cuff tears. *American Journal of Orthopaedics.* 2001; **30**: 159–62.

12. Speed C, Hazleman B. Shoulder pain. *Clinical Evidence.* 2002; **7**: 1122–39.

13. Eustace JA, Brophy DP, Gibney RP *et al*. Comparison of the accuracy of steroid placement with clinical outcome in patients with shoulder symptoms. *Annals of the Rheumatic Diseases.* 1997; **56**: 59–63.

 * 14. Chen MJ, Lew HL, Hsu TC *et al*. Ultrasound-guided shoulder injections in the treatment of subacromial bursitis. *American Journal of Physical Medicine and Rehabilitation.* 2006; **85**: 31–5.

15. Warner JJ. Frozen shoulder; diagnosis and management. *Journal of the American Academy of Orthopaedic Surgeons.* 1997; **5**: 130–40.

16. Hay EM, Paterson SM, Lewis M *et al*. Pragmatic randomised controlled trial of local corticosteroid injection and naproxen for treatment of lateral epicondylitis of elbow in primary care. *British Medical Journal.* 1999; **319**: 964–8.

17. Ryans I, Montgomery A, Galway R *et al*. A randomized controlled trial of intra-articular triamcinolone and/or physiotherapy in shoulder capsulitis. *Rheumatology.* 2005; **44**: 529–35.

✱ 18. Bisset L, Beller E, Jull G *et al.* Mobilisation with movement and exercise, corticosteroid injection, or wait and see for tennis elbow: randomised trial. *British Medical Journal.* 2006; **333**: 939.

19. Trinh KV, Phillips SD, Ho E, Damsma K. Acupuncture for the alleviation of lateral epicondyle pain: a systematic review. *Rheumatology.* 2004; **43**: 1085–90.

20. Witt J, Pess G, Gelberman RH. Treatment of de Quervain's tenosynovitis: a prospective study of the results of injection of steroid and immobilization in a splint. *Journal of Bone and Joint Surgery.* 1991; **73**: 219–22.

21. Rankin ME, Rankin EA. Injection therapy for management of stenosing tenosynovitis (de Quervain's disease) of the wrist. *Journal of the National Medical Association.* 1998; **90**: 474–6.

22. Stahl S, Kanter Y, Karnelli E. Outcome of trigger finger treatment in diabetes. *Journal of Rheumatology.* 1997; **24**: 931–6.

23. Lambert MA, Morton RJ, Sloan JP. Controlled study of the use of local steroid injection in the treatment of trigger finger and thumb. *Journal of Hand Surgery.* 1992; **17**: 69–70.

✱ 24. Maffulll N, Sharma P, Luscombe KL. Achilles tendinopathy: aetiology and management. *Journal of the Royal Society of Medicine.* 2004; **97**: 472–6.

25. Jarvinen TAH, Kannus P, Paavola M *et al.* Achilles tendon injuries. *Current Opinion in Rheumatology.* 2001; **13**: 150–5.

26. Buchbinder R. Plantar fasciitis. *New England Journal of Medicine.* 2004; **350**: 2159–67.

27. Crawford F. Plantar heel pain (including plantar fasciitis). *Clinical Evidence.* 2002; **7**: 1091–100.

28. Crawford F, Atkins D, Young P *et al.* Steroid injection for heel pain: evidence of short term effectiveness. A randomised controlled trial. *Rheumatology.* 1999; **38**: 974–7.

✱ 29. Crawford F, Atkins D, Edwards J. Interventions for heel pain (Cochrane review). *Cochrane Database of Systematic Reviews.* 2000; **CD000416**.

30. Yagev Y, Carel RS, Yagev R. Assessment of work-related risk factors for carpal tunnel syndrome. *Israel Medical Association Journal.* 2001; **3**: 569–71.

31. Pal B, O'Gradaigh D, Merry P. Diagnosis of carpal tunnel syndrome. *Rheumatology.* 2001; **40**: 595–7.

✱ 32. Wong SM, Hui ACF, O'Gradaigh D, Merry P. Corticosteroid injection for the treatment of carpal tunnel syndrome. *Annals of the Rheumatic Diseases.* 2001; **60**: 897.

33. Singh VAR, Sachdev A, Shekhar WS, Goel D. A prospective study of the long term efficacy of local methyl prednisolone acetate in the management of mild carpal tunnel syndrome. *Rheumatology.* 2005; **44**: 647–50.

34. Trumble TE, Gilbert M, McCallister WV. Endoscopic versus open surgical treatment of carpal tunnel syndrome. *Neurosurgery Clinics of North America.* 2001; **12**: 255–66.

35. Grossman MG, Ducey SA, Nadler SS, Levy AS. Meralgia paresthetica: diagnosis and treatment. *Journal of the American Academy of Orthopaedic Surgeons.* 2001; **9**: 336–44.

✱ 36. Thomas KJ, MacPherson H, Thorpe L *et al.* Randomised controlled trial of a short course of traditional acupuncture compared with usual care for persistent non-specific low back pain. *British Medical Journal.* 2006; **333**: 623–6.

✱ 37. Ratcliffe J, Thomas KJ, MacPherson H, Brazier J. A randomised controlled trial of acupuncture care for persistent non-specific low back pain: cost effectiveness analysis. *British Medical Journal.* 2006; **333**: 626–8.

38. Furlan AD, van Tulder MW, Cherkin DC *et al.* Acupuncture and dry-needling for low back pain. *Cochrane Database of Systematic Reviews.* 2005; **CD001351**.

✱ 39. Kwon YD, Pittler MH, Ernst E. Acupuncture for peripheral joint osteoarthritis. *Rheumatology.* 2006; **45**: 1331–7.

40. Witt C, Brinkhaus B, Jena S *et al.* Acupuncture in patients with osteoarthritis of the knee: a randomised trial. *Lancet.* 2005; **366**: 136–43.

41. Melchart D, Weidenhammer W, Strong A *et al.* Prospective investigation of adverse effects of acupuncture in 97733 patients. *Archives of Internal Medicine.* 2004; **164**: 104–5.

42. Kampen WU, Voth M, Pinkert J, Krause A. Therapeutic status of radiosynviothoresis of the knee with Yittrium [^{90}Y] in rheumatoid arthritis and related indications. *Rheumatology.* 2007; **46**: 16–24.

43. Valotassiou V, Wozniak G, Demakopoulos N, Georgoulias P. Radiosynoviothesis – indications, side effects. *Hellenic Journal of Nuclear Medicine.* 2006; **9**: 187–8.

44. Bessant R, Steuer A, Rigby S, Gumpel M. Osmic acid revisited: factors that predict a favourable response. *Rheumatology.* 2003; **42**: 1036–43.

45. Molho P, Verrier P, Stieltjes N *et al.* A retrospective study on chemical and radioactive synovectomy in severe haemophilia patients with recurrent haemarthrosis. *Haemophilia.* 1999; **5**: 115–23.

✱ 46. Bellamy N, Campbell J, Robinson V *et al.* Viscosupplementation for the treatment of osteoarthritis of the knee. *Cochrane Database of Systematic Reviews.* 2006; **CD005321**.

47. Moreland L. Intra-articular hyaluronan (hyaluronic acid) and hyalans for the treatment of osteoarthritis: mechanisms of action. *Arthritis Research and Therapy.* 2003; **5**: 54–67.

30

Facet (zygapophyseal) joint injections and medial branch blocks

RON COOPER

KEY LEARNING POINTS

- Facet joint pain is a common cause of axial spinal pain.
- Diagnostic blocks are necessary to establish the diagnosis.
- Standardized meticulous techniques should be used in every case.

- Radiological imaging is necessary to identify target and needle location.
- Review patients for complications, especially after neurolysis.

INTRODUCTION

Chronic spinal pain, especially involving the lumbar and cervical regions, is commonly encountered in pain clinic practice. It has been estimated that 60–70 percent of the adult population will experience it at some time in their lives.[1]

The exact diagnosis of low back pain can be difficult. At the turn of the twentieth century, mechanical disorders of the sacroiliac joint, such as distraction or dislocation, were considered common causes for low back pain. In 1911, Goldthwait[2] suggested that zygapophyseal or facet joint disturbances were mainly responsible for low back pain and instability. Contemporary surgical practice focused on intervertebral disk herniation as a cause for low back pain and sciatica.[3] As laminectomy and nerve root decompression did not always relieve symptoms, interest was directed toward other causes for spinal pain.

In over 85 percent of patients with lumbar and cervical pain, no specific spinal pathology can be identified as the cause.[4] Both lumbar and cervical zygapophyseal joints have been considered a significant source of chronic low back and neck pain.

The term "facet joint syndrome" (lumbar spine) was first attributed to Ghormley[5] in 1933, when he described this pain syndrome as usually occurring after a sudden twisting injury to the lumbar spine, producing low back pain, usually without limb pain referral.

In 1976, Mooney and Robertson[6] demonstrated that the pain patterns resulting from lumbar zygapophyseal joint injections of hypertonic saline could be relieved by subsequent intra-articular injections of local anesthetic. Kaplan et al.[7] reported that pain associated with capsular distension of lumbar zygapophyseal joints was abolished by local anesthetic lumbar medial branch blocks. A similar pain syndrome can occur in the cervical spine. In 1990, Aprill and colleagues[8, 9] described pain patterns associated with cervical disease in studies on healthy volunteers and patients with chronic neck pain.

APPLIED ANATOMY

The reader is referred to the extensive work of Bogduk[10, 11] for a detailed description of the anatomy of the zygapophyseal joints, and only a brief outline will be given here. Any two consecutive vertebrae articulate to form three joints: the large joint between the two vertebral bodies and the two paired (right and left) zygapophyseal joints, which are formed between the superior articular process of one vertebra and the inferior articular process of the vertebra above. The term "facet joint" is used in clinical practice to describe these paired synovial joints, which are also referred to as the posterior intervertebral joints.

Posterolaterally, a firm fibrous capsule covers the joint, while anteriorly the softer ligament flavum contacts the synovium. Fatty tissue around the exiting spinal nerve is continuous with that in the superior recess of the joint providing a direct route to the epidural space. Zagopophyseal joint volume in the lumbar spine is in the order of 1–2 mL. If larger volumes are injected, this can produce capsular distension and spread directly into the epidural space, confounding any observed results from diagnostic blocks. Drugs injected on one side can spread contralaterally at that level, or to an adjacent level on the same side.[12] The zygapophyseal joints help to resist the associated shearing movements with forward flexion and the compressive forces with rotational spinal movements.

The nerve supply of the zygapophyseal joints is derived from the posterior primary ramus of the nerve root. The spinal nerve divides into anterior (ventral) and posterior (dorsal) rami as it emerges through the intervertebral foramen (**Figure 30.1**).

The medial branch of the posterior primary ramus is responsible for joint sensation. Innervation from the medial branch divides to supply the lower pole at its own level, and also the upper pole of the joint below. Terminal branches of the medial branch nerve supply the ligaments and periosteum of the vertebral arches posterior cervical muscles, as well as the multifidus and interspinalis muscles. Successive medial branches from above and below supply each joint. This dual-segment innervation has important implications for zygapophyseal nerve block and denervation procedures, as both branches need to be blocked to completely denervate a single joint.

The course of the medial branch of the posterior ramus is fixed anatomically at two points: at its origin near the superior aspect of the base of the transverse process and distally where it emerges from the canal formed by the mammilloaccessory ligament.

In the cervical spine, nerves supplying the zygapophyseal joints only make a small contribution to cervical posterior muscle sensation.[13]

INDICATIONS

The zygapophyseal facet joints are regarded as a common source of spinal pain, particularly in the lumbar and cervical regions.[10, 11, 13, 14, 15] The clinical diagnosis of zygapophyseal joint pain is poorly defined and nonspecific. Features of zygapophyseal joint pain include:

- deep, dull, aching pain;
- uni- or bilateral;
- paravertebral tenderness;
- associated muscle spasm;
- lateral bending or rotational movements increase pain intensity;
- extension rather than flexion movements increase pain intensity;
- Valsalva maneuver and straight-leg raising (SLR) do not affect pain intensity;

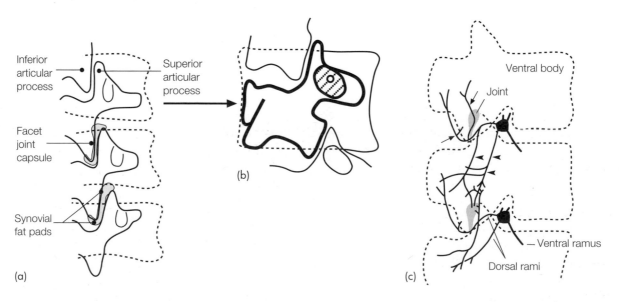

Figure 30.1 Zygapophyseal joint anatomy.

- segmental referral pattern in relation to the joint of origin.

Cervical zygapophyseal joint pain occurs in the following regions.

- occiput and behind ear C1/2;
- vertex and upper neck C2/3;
- posterolateral neck C3/4;
- supraclavicular fossa C4/5;
- deltoid C5/6;
- posterior scapular C6/7.

Lumbar zygapophyseal joint pain commonly occurs in the following regions.

- groin T12/L1;
- hips L1/2;
- buttocks L2/3;
- thighs L3/4.

Clinical history and examination, including radiological investigations such as computed tomography (CT) scans, are not particularly useful in its accurate diagnosis.[16, 17]

Relief of pain rather than provocation of pain is considered the more reliable test.[18] Either intra-articular injections at the suspected painful level, using 1–2 mL of local anesthetic, or medial branch nerve blocks using 0.5–1 mL of local anesthetic, are used to achieve this. Care should be taken to avoid false-positive results, which can confound the interpretation of the procedure, particularly if neurolysis is planned after diagnostic blocks. Excessive doses of local anesthetic can result in spread to other structures, such as the epidural space, producing a false-positive result. Vascular uptake of local anesthetic from the site of injection, by reducing the effective drug dose, can result in a false-negative result. Psychological factors associated with the block can form a false sense of expectation that their pain will be relieved. Some individual patients are therefore likely to have false-positive results. False-positive rates in patients undergoing diagnostic blocks have been reported to be between 25 and 50 percent.[19, 20][II], [21][II]

Repeat blocks using different local anesthetics with different duration of action, or placebo blocks with saline, are sometimes used to try and overcome these hurdles. This is particularly important in patients with suspected secondary gain phenomena. However, such methods are not without ethical problems and should be undertaken only after careful consideration and discussion with patients and their advisors.

Zygapophyseal joint blocks should be performed in a meticulous standardized manner to determine the site of pain generation and avoid the subjectivity associated with clinical assessment.

CONTRAINDICATIONS

The same contraindications apply to zygapophyseal blocks as for any other block used in pain management and include:

- coagulopathy;
- infection (systemic or local site);
- pregnancy (x-rays);
- allergy (contrast media or local anesthetics).

LIMITATIONS OF TREATMENT

Informed consent for the procedure should be obtained and the patient advised that the procedure is primarily diagnostic rather than therapeutic. It is important not to build up expectations or introduce bias before carrying out the procedure, which is ideally carried out using a placebo control. Patients should be advised to record the duration of any pain relief obtained.

The aim of any zygapophyseal joint block is either to anesthetize the target joint by intra-articular injection of a small dose of local anesthetic or to block the medial branch that innervates the joint. The practical preparation of the patient is similar for both lumbar and cervical spines, but differences in technique due to the anatomy of each region will be described.

PREPARATION FOR ZYGAPOPHYSEAL BLOCKS

The following should be available:

- resuscitation facilities;
- procedure room with C-arm fluoroscopy;
- needles, sterile basic pack;
- skin preparation solutions;
- local anesthetics;
- radiographic contrast media.

Patients should understand what to expect during and after the procedure. In particular, they should be aware that the procedures are carried out while awake, as cooperation and verbal contact are needed to determine provocation of pain and analgesia during and after the procedure. Skin infiltration with local anesthetics will reduce pain associated with needle passage during localization of the target joints, but care should be taken to avoid deep infiltration of anesthetic solution and interference with the block.

Fluoroscopy screening of needle insertions is mandatory. Skill is needed in the correct and safe use of a fluoroscopic C-arm, so as to direct the x-ray beam at variable angles to the identified target. Any changes in either depth or direction of the needle are immediately checked by screening. The use of a water-soluble contrast medium can assist this. A printed image showing positioning of the needle in two planes, with or without contrast, is desirable, particularly when a neurolytic procedure is being undertaken.

The procedure is performed aseptically after adequate skin preparation using an iodine-based solution, chlorhexidine, or alcohol-based antiseptic (e.g. chlorhexidine 0.5 percent in 70 percent alcohol). Sterile drapes for the patient and C-arm and a minimal-touch technique should be adhered to. Skilled radiographic assistance with a knowledge of the particular screening projections required is desirable and proper x-ray safety guidance should be followed for the protection of staff and patients. Special thin radioabsorbent sterile gloves and protective eyewear can be worn by the operator to reduce personal absorption of radiation during the procedure.

A 22–25-gauge spinal needle may be used for intra-articular injections, whereas medial branch blocks and radiofrequency procedures are generally carried out using a 22-gauge needle. Longer needles (100 mm) are generally required for lumbar procedures, whereas shorter needles are sufficient for cervical procedures. Obese patients may require longer needles and use of Luer-lock needles and extension T-connectors can help reduce both needle movements, and radiation exposure to the operator's hands, especially when contrast is being injected during screening. Verbal contact is maintained with the patient throughout the procedure and sedation is avoided. Staff familiar with the procedure should be present to assist the operator. Routine noninvasive monitoring of the patient should include electrocardiography, blood pressure, and heart rate during the procedure. This is particularly important during cervical procedures, during which sudden untoward cardiovascular changes or transient loss of consciousness could occur during injection of local anesthetics. Precision is required and screening with the C-arm should be carried out to check every change of needle position. Patients are usually discharged accompanied by an adult escort from the Day Procedure Unit between 30 and 60 minutes after the procedure, provided observations are satisfactory.

Lumbar zygapophyseal blocks

For lumbar procedures, the patient is initially placed prone, with a pillow under the upper abdomen and the legs slightly abducted.

INTRA-ARTICULAR BLOCKS

Patients must be positioned so that an oblique view of the lumbar spine is obtained (**Figure 30.2**). The patient either has to lie in a semi-prone position on the x-ray-translucent table with a pillow under the abdomen or, more commonly, the C-arm may be rotated to direct the beam obliquely through the target area. This view is necessary to visualize the joint cavity, which must be seen clearly at

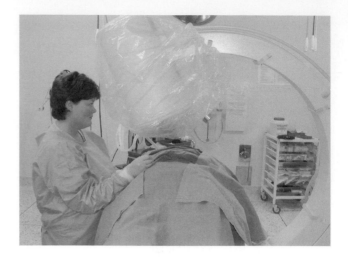

Figure 30.2 Positioning of C-arm for "line of vision" introduction of needle toward target in lumbar spine.

the target level and can require up to a 45° oblique projection from the sagittal plane. This angle decreases as the spine is ascended.

The joint to be blocked should be identified and marked. Following skin preparation, local anesthetic is infiltrated into the skin and deeper tissues over the joint. The block needle is inserted in the line of sight along the direction of the x-ray beam, with its target being the midpoint of the joint. Contact with bone should be achieved to allow a depth assessment of the target joint. The needle is then guided to the joint cavity, when some "give" is initially felt on entry, followed by a firmer gripping sensation on the needle tip. A small amount of contrast (not more than 0.3 mL) is injected to produce an arthrogram. This is seen as either a slit or dumb-bell shape in outline, and confirms intra-articular location of the needle. At this point the C-arm can be rotated in the sagittal plane to confirm that the needle is indeed located in an intra-articular position. Up to 1.5 mL of local anesthetic or a mixture of local anesthetic with steroid is injected.

MEDIAL BRANCH BLOCKS

Initially an anteroposterior view is used and the C-arm is rotated obliquely through 15° in order to visualize the target point of the medial branch nerves. The "Scottie dog" image is seen with the target point lying high on the "eye" of the "dog" (**Figure 30.1**).

The spinal needle or radiofrequency electrode is introduced in the line of sight along the direction of the x-ray beam. The skin entry point is at the junction between the upper edge of the transverse process and the lateral edge of the superior articular process. Contact is made with bone at this target junction, then the needle is redirected more cephalad and laterally until loss of bone contact occurs in this groove (**Figures 30.3** and **30.4**). Lateral x-ray views are taken to check the depth of the needle or electrode, which should lie level with a line joining the posterior intervertebral part of the intervertebral foramina. If it lies anterior to this line it should be withdrawn and rechecked on screening.

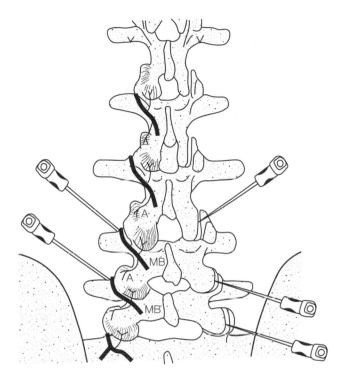

Figure 30.3 Needle positioning for lumbar intra-articular zygapophyseal and medial branch blocks. Medial branches (MB) of the dorsal rami, and articular branches (A) are shown on the left, with needles placed L3–4, L4–5, and L5 S1 on the right. Reproduced with permission from Bogduk N. Back pain: zygapophyseal blocks and epidural steroids. In: Cousins MJ, Bridenbaugh PO (eds). *Neural blockade in clinical anesthesia and management of pain*, 2nd edn. Philadelphia, PA: JB Lippincott 1998: 935–46.

The preferred technique is to use a radiofrequency electrode or insulated (Pole) needle to permit sensory threshold testing. Stimulation at 50 Hz to detect proximity to the medial branch nerve should be elicited below 0.5 V, and this is repeated at 2 Hz to exclude proximity to the emerging segmental spinal nerve. No motor stimulation should be detected at up to 2 V. When both sensory threshold testing and radiographic screening in oblique and lateral views indicate satisfactory electrode positioning, a small volume of contrast medium (0.2 mL) can be injected to exclude any vascular uptake. If this is satisfactory, 0.5–1.0 mL of local anesthetic is then injected to produce a diagnostic block. If performing radiofrequency neurolysis, a lesion can be made for 60 s at 80°C using a temperature-controlled electrode. Both medial branch nerves which supply the target joint are blocked separately (above and below the joint).

Cervical zygapophyseal blocks

For cervical procedures, the patient is placed in the supine position with the head and neck slightly extended.

INTRA-ARTICULAR BLOCKS

The neck is screened using a lateral view and adjusted until the outline of both the right and left articular pillars are superimposed (absence of double image). It is then necessary to rotate the C-arm slightly to separate the images. This is confirmed when the intervertebral foramina and associated zygapophyseal joints are easily seen. Preparation and draping can be carried out once the C-arm has been set up in the appropriate position. After infiltration of the skin with local anesthetic at the entry site, the block needle is directed toward the target joint, already identified by radiographic screening.

This is achieved by carefully observing the image during tilting of the beam from the lateral to oblique

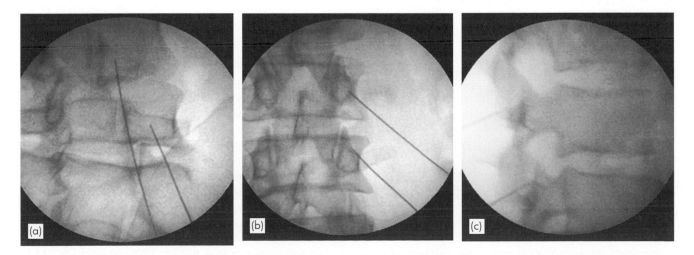

Figure 30.4 X-rays for lumbar medial branch blocks: showing needle positions in: (a) oblique; (b) AP; and (c) lateral views.

position while the needle is in contact with bone. The joint image will appear to move in the same direction as the needle, confirming the correct target image. The degree of C-arm tilt that gives the clearest image, with the widest joint cavity view, should be used before attempting to enter the joint. A true lateral view should be obtained to avoid the risk of passing the needle through the spinal canal toward the opposite side.

To assure safety during the procedure, the needle should be in contact with bone on either the superior or inferior articular process of the target joint, and then toward the joint edge and into the joint cavity, when it is felt to "give." An arthrogram using not more than 0.3 mL of contrast confirms positioning when a sigmoid shape can be seen. Up to 1.5 mL of local anesthetic or anesthetic and steroid is then injected into the joint.

For C2–3 joints the lateral view will not show the target joint cavity particularly well, and it is necessary to turn the patient's head from the neutral position into the table to give a better view of the joint cavity, which slopes downwards and medially.

MEDIAL BRANCH BLOCKS

The C-arm is initially positioned in the anterior–posterior projection and then rotated obliquely to approximately 20° and 10° caudocranially (**Figure 30.5**). This is to direct the x-ray beam parallel to the axis of the intervertebral foramen, and so the emerging segmental nerves will also be parallel to the x-ray beam.

As the posterior primary ramus traverses the base of the superior articular process, which is easily viewed in this projection, it allows the operator to safely judge the depth between the segmental nerve and the needle tip. The entry site is behind the posterior border of the facet column and slightly below the target joint. The needle or electrode is advanced anteriorly and cranially to make

bone contact with the posterior facetal column; the C-arm is then rotated to obtain an anteroposterior view. The tip of the needle should lie at the "waist" of the articular pillars on the target joint (**Figures 30.6** and **30.7**).

Electrical sensory threshold testing is then carried out as for the lumbar spine. Stimulation at 50 Hz should elicit sensation in the neck at below 0.5 V, and at 2 Hz there should be absence of motor stimulation at up to 2 V. A diagnostic block using 0.5–1.0 mL of local anesthetic is performed, after which a radiofrequency thermal lesion at 80°C for 60 s can be made if desired.

COMPLICATIONS OF ZYGAPOPHYSEAL BLOCKS

Most patients will experience nothing more than local muscular pain for several days after the procedure, but in addition the following have all been reported:

- motor block from spinal anesthesia;
- meningitis due to chemical irritation;
- hematoma around the injection site, particularly in cervical spine procedures;
- transient ataxia and disturbed gait after upper cervical blocks;
- postdenervation pain and dysesthesia;
- local anesthetic reactions;
- superficial skin infections;
- skin burns from faulty electrodes.

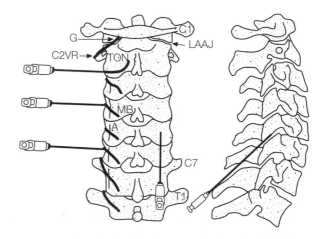

Figure 30.6 Needle placement for cervical medial branch and intra-articular zygapophyseal blocks. Posterior view showing C2 ganglion (G) location behind the lateral atlantoaxial joint (LAAJ), C2 anterior ramus C2 UR, courses of the medial branches (MB) of the cervical dorsal rami and articular branches (A), 3rd occipital nerve (TON). Needles show position for blocking. C4 and C6 medial branches and 3rd occipital nerve. Lateral view showing needle directed into C5–6 zygapophyseal joint. Reproduced with permission from Bogduk N. Back pain: zygapophyseal blocks and epidural steroids. In: Cousins MJ, Bridenbaugh PO (eds). *Neural blockade in clinical anesthesia and management of pain*, 2nd edn. Philadelphia, PA: JB Lippincott 1998: 935–46.

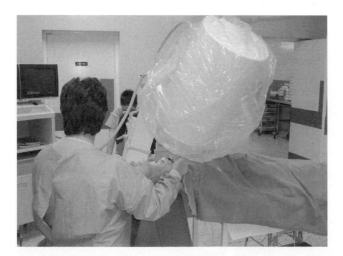

Figure 30.5 Positioning of C-arm for "line of vision" introduction of needle toward target in cervical spine.

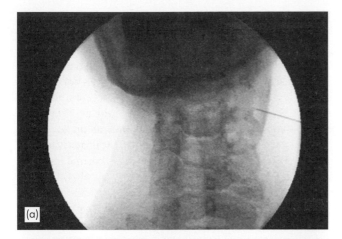

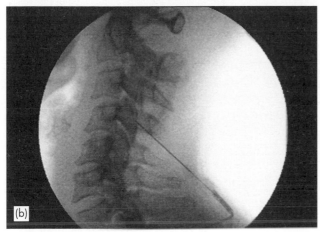

Figure 30.7 X-rays for cervical medial branch blocks: showing needle positions in (a) AP and (b) lateral views.

Complications from radiofrequency lumbar facet denervation are uncommon if the procedure is performed carefully and with precision. Postprocedure neuritis, which is often described as a deep sunburn-like feeling in the area of the lesion, can occur after radiofrequency neurolysis and is often distressing to patients. This usually resolves within six to eight weeks, and the majority of patients only require reassurance. The etiology is unknown but may be related to the denervation of the lateral branch, as well as the medial branch fibers. If it is particularly distressing, a short (two-month) trial of a membrane-stabilizing drug such as gabapentin or pregablin can be helpful. Regeneration of the medial branch nerve may be responsible for the return of pain in patients who initially achieved good pain relief after denervation.

Relying on these interventional procedures alone is not usually sufficient to achieve prolonged relief of pain. They are best carried out in conjunction with ongoing physiotherapy and pain management treatments in order to maintain any symptomatic improvements achieved from a reduction in spinal nociceptive input.

EVIDENCE FOR THE USE OF ZYGAPOPHYSEAL JOINT BLOCKS

The reported results from zygapophyseal joint blocks vary considerably. The results of cervical spine procedures tend to be more favorable than the results of procedures in the lumbar area (69–86 versus 16–69 percent effectiveness).[22] [V] Similar outcomes have been reported whether intra-articular or medial branch blocks have been carried out.[23] [II], [24][II] Manchiikanti et al.[25][III] reported effective management of chronic neck pain using cervical medial branch blocks in a prospective outcome study. Sluijter and Koetsveld-Baart[26][V] investigated radiofrequency lesioning of cervical zygapophyseal joints and/or the dorsal root ganglion in patients with chronic neck pain and cervicobrachalgia. They reported more than 40 percent pain relief in 60 percent of the patients treated. Lord et al.[27][II] observed that 70 percent of patients achieved effective pain relief following lower cervical denervations, compared with 44 percent who had upper cervical denervations in an open prospective study, with selection based on relief of pain after diagnostic medial branch nerve blocks. In a randomized, controlled, double-blind trial of chronic lower cervical spine pain after whiplash injury, Lord et al.[28][II] found that the duration of pain relief was greater when radiofrequency medial branch denervation was carried out compared with local anesthetic nerve blocks alone. The median time that elapsed before the pain returned to at least 50 percent of the preoperative level was 263 days in the active-treatment group and eight days in the control group.

In a population of patients with chronic low back pain who received intra-articular blocks with local anesthetics, Mooney and Robertson[6] demonstrated 60 percent initial relief, with 20 percent continuing to have complete relief at six months. Silvers[29] was unable to demonstrate any benefit from using blocks with dilute phenol compared with local anesthetic and steroid. In randomized-controlled trials, Carette et al.[30][II] demonstrated that zygapophyseal joint injections of corticosteroids were of no value in patients with low back pain, while Gallagher et al.,[20][II] on the efficacy of radiofrequency denervation in patients with chronic low back pain, reported a significant improvement in pain scores after denervation compared with placebo. Dreyfuss et al.[31][III] showed that, in patients who had been carefully selected by controlled diagnostic blocks, test sensory stimulation prior to lesioning of lumbar medial branch nerves was unnecessary to achieve a good outcome after radiofrequency lesioning. Lesion accuracy was demonstrated by multifidus muscle electromyography performed before and after lesioning. In this well-conducted study with experienced operators, careful electrode placement using fluoroscopy alone, without sensory testing, was associated with effective reduction of pain, with 60 percent of patients obtaining at least 90 percent relief of pain at 12 months, and 87 percent obtained at least 60 percent relief.

Recently, studies have focused on the use of ultrasound rather than fluoroscopy for lumbar medial branch blocks, but further studies are needed to detect intravascular uptake.[32, 33, 34]

CONCLUSIONS

There is good evidence that facet joint or medial branch blocks can alleviate chronic spinal pain of facet joint origin. These confirm the diagnosis, and longer pain relief can be achieved by denervation, usually with radiofrequency lesioning. Although these procedures are not overly difficult to perform, a standardized, meticulous technique, based on applied anatomy and supported by radiological imaging, should be used. Procedures should be carried out in an environment with immediately available resuscitation facilities.

REFERENCES

1. *Epidemiological evidence on back pain.* Report of a CSAG Committee on Back Pain. London: HMSO Publications Centre, 1994: 9–21.
2. Goldthwait JR. The lumbosacral articulation: an explanation of many cases of lumbago, sciatica and paraplegia. *Boston Medical and Surgical Journal.* 1911; **164**: 365.
3. Mixter WJ, Barr JS. Rupture of the intervertebral disc with involvement of the spinal canal. *New England Journal of Medicine.* 1934; **211**: 210–15.
4. Bardense GAM, Weber W, van Kleef M. Treatment of spinal pain by means of radiofrequency procedures – Part I: The lumbar area. *Pain Reviews.* 1999; **6**: 143–54.
5. Ghormley RK. Low back pain with special reference to the articular facet, with presentation of an operative procedure. *Journal of the American Medical Association.* 1933; **101**: 1773–7.
* 6. Mooney V, Robertson J. The facet syndrome. *Clinical Orthopaedics and Related Research.* 1976; **115**: 149–56.
7. Kaplan M, Dreyfuss P, Halbrook B *et al.* The ability of lumbar medial branch blocks to anesthetize the zygapophysial joint: a physiologic challenge. *Spine.* 1998; **23**: 1847–52.
* 8. Dwyer A, Aprill C, Bogduk N. Cervical zygapophyseal joint pain patterns. I. A study in normal volunteers. *Spine.* 1990; **15**: 453–7.
* 9. Aprill C, Dwyer A, Bogduk N. Cervical zygapophysial joint pain patterns. II. A clinical evaluation. *Spine.* 1990; **15**: 458–61.
10. Bogduk N. The lumbar vertebrae. In: *Clinical anatomy of the lumbar spine and sacrum,* 3rd edn. London: Churchill Livingstone, 1997: 1–11.
11. Bogduk N. The clinical anatomy of the cervical dorsal rami. *Spine.* 1982; **7**: 319–30.
12. McCormick CC, Taylor JR, Twang LT. Facet joint arthrography in lumbar spondylosis: anatomic basis for spread of contrast medium. *Radiology.* 1989; **171**: 193–6.
13. Bogduk N, Long DM. The anatomy of the so-called "articular nerves" and their relationship to facet denervation in the treatment of low back pain. *Journal of Neurosurgery.* 1979; **51**: 172–7.
14. Raymond J, Dumas J. Intra-articular facet block: diagnostic test or therapeutic procedure? *Radiology.* 1984; **151**: 333–6.
15. Bogduk N, Marsland A. The cervical zygapophysial joints as a source of neck pain. *Spine.* 1988; **13**: 610–17.
16. Schwarzer AC, Aprill CN, Derby R *et al.* Clinical features of patients with pain stemming from the lumbar zygapophysial joints. Is the lumbar facet syndrome a clinical entity? *Spine.* 1994; **19**: 1132–7.
17. Schwarzer AC, Wang S, O'Driscoll D *et al.* The ability of computed tomography to identify a painful zygapophysial joint in patients with chronic low back pain. *Spine.* 1995; **20**: 907–12.
18. Schwarzer AC, Derby R, Aprill CN *et al.* The value of the provocation response in lumbar zygapophysial joint injections. *Clinical Journal of Pain.* 1994; **10**: 309–13.
19. Barnsley L, Lord S, Wallis B, Bogduk N. False positive rates of cervical zygapophysial joint blocks. *Clinical Journal of Pain.* 1993; **9**: 124–30.
20. Gallagher J, di Vadi PLP, Wedley JR *et al.* Radiofrequency facet joint denervation in the treatment of low back pain: a prospective controlled double-blind study to assess its efficacy. *The Pain Clinic.* 1994; **7**: 193–8.
21. North RB, Kidd DH, Zahurak M, Pantiadosi S. Specificity of diagnostic nerve blocks: a prospective, randomized study of sciatica due to lumbosacral spine disease. *Pain.* 1996; **65**: 77–85.
22. Pawl RP. Headache, cervical spondylosis, and anterior cervical fusion. *Surgery Annual.* 1977; **9**: 391–408.
* 23. Marks RC, Houston T, Thulbourne T. Facet joint injection and facet nerve block. A randomised comparison in 86 patients with chronic low back pain. *Pain.* 1992; **49**: 325–8.
* 24. Barnsley L, Lord S, Wallis B, Bogduk N. Lack of effect of intraarticular corticosteroids for chronic pain in the cervical zygapophyseal joints. *New England Journal of Medicine.* 1994; **330**: 1047–50.
25. Manchikanti L, Manchikanti KN, Damron KS, Pampati V. Pain effectiveness of cervical medial branch blocks in chronic neck pain: A prospective outcome study. *Pain Physician.* 2004; **7**: 195–201.
26. Sluijter ME, Koetsveld-Baart CC. Interruption of pain pathways in the treatment of the cervical syndrome. *Anesthesia.* 1980; **35**: 302–07.
27. Lord SM, Barnsley L, Bogduk N. Percutaneous radiofrequency neurotomy in the treatment of cervical zygapophyseal joint pain: a caution. *Neurosurgery.* 1995; **36**: 732–9.
* 28. Lord SM, Barnsley L, Wallis BJ *et al.* Percutaneous radiofrequency neurotomy for chronic cervical

zygapophyseal joint pain. *New England Journal of Medicine*. 1996; **335**: 1721–6.

29. Silvers RH. Lumbar percutaneous facet rhizotomy. *Spine*. 1990; **15**: 36–40.

∗ 30. Carette S, Marcoux S, Truchon R. A controlled trial of corticosteroid injections into facet joints for chronic low back pain. *New England Journal of Medicine*. 1991; **325**: 1002–07.

31. Dreyfuss P, Halbrook B, Pauza K *et al*. Efficacy and validity of radiofrequency neurotomy for chronic lumbar zygapophysial joint pain. *Spine*. 2000; **25**: 1270–7.

32. Greher M, Scharbert G, Kamolz LP *et al*. Ultrasound-guided lumbar facet nerve block: A sonoanatomic study of a new methodological approach. *Anesthesiology*. 2004; **100**: 1242–8.

33. Greher M, Kirchmair L, Enna B *et al*. Ultrasound-guided lumbar facet nerve block: Accuracy of a new technique confirmed by computed tomography. *Anesthesiology*. 2004; **101**: 1195–200.

34. Jae-Kwang Shim, Jin-Cheon Moon, Kyung-Bong Yoon *et al*. Ultrasound-guided lumbar medial-branch block: A clinical study with fluoroscopy control. *Regional Anesthesia and Pain Medicine*. 2006; **31**: 451–4.

31

Intrathecal drug delivery

JON RAPHAEL AND KATE GRADY

KEY LEARNING POINTS

- Intrathecal drug delivery for chronic pain and spasticity is a scientifically rational and evidence-based therapy.
- A drug delivery mechanism and energy source is needed and increasing levels of sophistication are required for different circumstances.
- Selection for these therapies is crucial to optimal outcome and requires experienced multidisciplinary teams.

- Complications can be related to equipment, drugs, and comorbidities.
- Careful attention to operative detail reduces complications.
- Centers undertaking this therapy need to provide long-term aftercare to avoid drug withdrawal.

INTRODUCTION

Chronic spinal administration of selected analgesics and antispasmodics has advantages over systemic delivery for pharmacodynamic and pharmacokinetic reasons. Furthermore, there is a body of clinical research that supports this mode of delivery for certain agents (see Chapter 21, Spinal administration in the *Chonic Pain* volume of this series). This chapter describes the practical details of management of chronic intrathecal drug delivery.

TYPES OF INTRATHECAL DRUG DELIVERY SYSTEMS

Various types of chronic intrathecal administration are feasible.[1] From the least sophisticated to the most they are as follows.

1. Percutaneous systems with or without subcutaneous tunnelling (e.g. Portex® catheter). This might be injected periodically by bolus or connected to an external infusion device with programmable facilities (e.g. CADD micro™).
2. A totally implanted intrathecal catheter with a subcutaneous injection port which acts as an access port (e.g. PORT-A-CATH®).
3. A system that involves both a totally implanted catheter and implanted manually activated pump (e.g. AlgoMed™).
4. A totally implanted catheter and pump, with the pump providing continuous delivery (e.g. Infusaid™).
5. A totally implanted catheter with an implanted programmable infusion pump (e.g. Synchromed®).

The first two are more applicable where life expectancy is limited and the costs of implanted devices are an issue or where prolonged trialling is necessary before deciding on permanent drug delivery. This might be the case in some cases of chronic nonmalignant pain with psychological factors or when trialling of ziconotide is needed due to the slow titration necessary with this agent. In general, implanted pumps are preferred because of the reduced infection rate and lower maintenance.

IMPLANTATION EQUIPMENT

The primary objective of long-term intrathecal drug delivery of analgesics or antispasmodics is control of symptoms through maintenance of drug levels within an effective range. Totally implanted intrathecal drug delivery systems require a spinal catheter and a drug reservoir driven by an energy source.

The catheters are either silastic alone or with an additional reinforcement of coiled titanium wire to prevent kinking.

Since implantable drug pumps are designed for use in chronic conditions, the power source must be rechargeable or have a lifetime of adequate length so that surgical revision for battery replacement is infrequent. There are four types of pumps commercially available for implantation: two of these have programmable rates of delivery and two are constant flow rate devices.

Programmable pumps

The energy source is a battery and flow control is by means of a peristaltic method. These allow for additional operating control, sensing, recording, and disseminating information to a processing unit which allows for algorithms, to compensate for pressure and temperature changes. A patient-activated reservoir can be included. These devices permit noninvasive rate change and allow for the varying of rates with time through the day. It is also feasible to noninvasively stop the pump, provided there is access to the programmer.

Constant flow pumps

There are two types of constant flow pump: one gas-driven and the other reliant upon a polymeric diaphragm.

Gas-driven pumps

These have a flexible bellows which acts as the drug reservoir and is surrounded by a chamber of a volatile liquid. Body heat warms the liquid and generates a pressure. The vapor pressure of the volatile liquid then compresses the bellows. In effect, the systems driving

energy are replenished when the bellows is refilled with drug as this compresses the pump and so the vapor condenses. Flow restrictors convert a constant pressure into a constant flow as a function of capillary dimensions and viscosity. The latter is a function of temperature with modest reductions in viscosity and consequent increases in flow rate as temperature rises. This is of the order of a 2 percent decrease for every degree temperature increase. In comparison, vapor pressure changes are more significant (see **Box 31.1**).

The most common volatile agent used is N butane as its vapor pressure is less subject to changes in temperature; nevertheless at 41°C, flow rate would be predicted to rise by up to 20 percent.[2]

Diaphragmatic pumps

These are engineered to produce a constant force over the displacement range, unlike conventional diaphragms which generate a higher pressure at the beginning of the delivery stroke. In contrast to gas-driven pumps, in which the metallic reservoir shields the volatile liquid from ambient pressure, there is no such effect with diaphragmatic pumps. As a consequence, the reservoir pressure is independent of ambient pressure. Therefore, only viscosity is affected by temperature change (see **Box 31.2**).

Box 31.1

The pressure difference driving flow, $\delta P =$ capillary inlet pressure, P_i – capillary outlet pressure, P_o

$$P_i = P_r + P_a$$

where P_r is the reservoir pressure and P_a is the ambient pressure

$$P_o = P_{csf} + P_a,$$

where P_{csf} is cerebrospinal fluid pressure

$$\delta P = (P_r + P_a) - P_{csf} + P_a)$$
$$\delta P = (P_r + P_a) - P_a,$$

assuming P_{csf} is negligible.

For gas-driven pumps, the metallic case negates the effects of ambient pressure upon the volatile liquid. Therefore,

$$\delta P = P_r - P_a$$

and so falls in ambient pressure increase pressure differential and result in increased drug delivery.

Box 31.2

$$\delta P = (P_r + P_a) - (P_{csf} + P_a)$$
$$\delta P = (P_r + P_a) - P_a.$$

assuming P_{csf} is negligible.

For diaphragmatic pumps, ambient pressures equate. Therefore

$$\delta P = P_r$$

and so diaphragmatic pumps are independent of changes in ambient pressure.

Comparison of programmable and constant flow rate pumps

Constant flow pumps are simpler and cheaper than programmable pumps, even without taking account of the replacement costs of battery-operated programmable pumps; however, they are less sophisticated and it is necessary to alter drug concentration to change the dose per unit time. The patient with a gas-driven pump should be cautious in taking saunas or using sunbeds as the temperature increase may result in an increase in the rate of delivery of the drug. Both the reservoir and catheter of constant flow pumps need to be emptied for magnetic resonance imaging (MRI) investigations, as temperature rise could lead to increased drug delivery.

On the other hand, the sophistication of programmable pumps increases the complexity with risk of human error in programming and requires battery replacement with risks of infection from the need for reoperation.

The advantages and disadvantages of programmable and constant flow pumps are summarized in **Tables 31.1** and **31.2**.

PREIMPLANTATION TRIALLING

One of the advantages of spinal therapy is the ability to use it for a trial period, prior to permanent pump implantation. This gives the patient and clinical team the opportunity of assessing the effects of the therapy on both the level of pain or spasticity and the functional effects. Different techniques have been used for trialling; both epidural and intrathecal routes and by single bolus, repeated bolus, and continuous infusions of medications.[3] It is not possible to determine if trialling improves outcome since patients who fail the trial do not get implanted. Selection criteria differ between institutions with various types of neurosurgical and psychological

Table 31.1 Advantages and disadvantages of programmable pumps.

Advantages	Disadvantages
Noninvasive rate change	Expensive
Controllable (purging, titration)	Bulk
Vary rates through the day	Replacement cost
	Infection risk with replacement surgery
Interrogation	Human errors with programming
Easier to manage with MRI	Computer required for refill

Table 31.2 Advantages and disadvantages of constant flow pumps.

Advantages	Disadvantages
Cheaper	Cannot stop immediately
Simpler	Require refilling to titrate
No replacement (less infection risk)	Less information if troubleshooting
Larger volume	Cannot vary rate through the day
Higher flow rates	More difficult to manage with MRI

assessments. Nevertheless, a trial is valuable since a negative response may avoid an operation unlikely to benefit the patient. However, a positive response in the short term cannot be expected to determine long-term outcome alone and reliance of multidimensional assessment is advisable (see Chapter 21, Spinal administration, in the *Chronic Pain* volume of this series).

Where an objective physiological measure is available, such as in spasticity, or where pain produces a reversible functional deficit, then bolus tests are acceptable. However, the placebo effect should be borne in mind and repeated testing, either with different doses to look for a concordant response or with saline, is recommended.[4]

Infusions mimic the status postpump implant more closely and are preferred by some. However, there can be problems during the trial if placebo testing is required, as it is not possible to know when the active drug ceases to have an effect and placebo starts. Perhaps the most valuable use of infusions is to determine the dose requirements when the pump is implanted, although this can be estimated from daily bolus dose requirements.

THERAPEUTIC CONTEXT AND CONDUCT OF THE TECHNIQUE

The context and conduct of the technique must be carefully considered. Intrathecal drug delivery is one of pain medicine's more interventional methods. As such, it is a commitment on the part of patient and carers to discuss the pros and cons of this mode of drug delivery in keeping with best practice.[5, 6] Resources should be planned and funded. Intrathecal drug delivery should be undertaken in a multiprofessional context, with all team members having a role in selection, the delivery of ongoing care, and the management of complications. The implanter and technical members of the team, such as refillers, should have a sufficient caseload to maintain technical expertise.

The composition of the team would vary depending on the condition to be treated. For example, the clinicians caring for the patient's primary condition, i.e. the pain medicine team, together with those in the rehabilitation, neurology, or palliative care who are essential to decision-making and ongoing care. Psychology, physiotherapy, pharmacy, and microbiology expertise should be available. The patient's primary care physicians and members of the primary care team should be involved. The implanter and refiller should be specifically trained in these roles and other carers fully conversant with the technique. All staff should be educated in the day-to-day care and the recognition and management of complications. Networks and mentoring systems may provide support, education, and advice. Support should be in place for critical care if necessary.

Implanting centers should have adequate theater and postoperative care facilities, not only for implantation but also for the immediate management of complications. There should also be protocols for the immediate treatment of and referral of complications to appropriate centers, for example back to the implanting center and, if that center does not have it, access to neuroradiological and neurosurgical expertise. It should be recognized that intrathecal drug delivery can be delivered alongside other therapies and cognitive-behavioral therapy may be an adjunct.[7]

Informed consent planning and discussion

Patients should be made fully aware of the potential therapeutic outcome, the risks of the procedure, and the potential for failure of a successful outcome. The following should be discussed:

- reasonable expectation from the trialling should be planned as appropriate;
- the site of insertion and site of pump should be determined;
- information about programming, prescription adjustments, and attendance for refilling should all be made clear.

Patient information booklets from professional bodies are available (www.britishpainsociety.org).

The patient should undergo an assessment for general fitness for anesthesia. Preoperatively, analgesic drugs may need to be discontinued and provision made for pain control in the immediate preprocedure period. Plans should be made to discontinue anticoagulant and antiplatelet drugs as appropriate. Local guidelines should be followed for preprocedure infection screening and antibiotic prophylaxis.

OPERATIVE TECHNIQUE

Advice on the operative technique is derived from studies of complications and from views expounded by experienced physicians. The most frequent complications are infection and catheter dislodgement,[8] these dictating attention to detail.

Preoperative phase

During preoperative assessment, the patient's physical and neurological status is recorded, together with the pump and catheter system implantation operation in mind. Spinal deformity, previous surgery, abdominal surgery, present and future enterostomies, extreme obesity, or malnutrition all affect surgical planning. Preoperative spinal radiography and MRI is valuable, especially if there has been spinal pathology or spinal surgery.

Preoperative planning

The pump placement is dependent on several factors. Some determined by the physician, some by the patient. The pump is usually placed on one or other side of the anterior abdominal wall or in the upper half of the buttock. Factors to consider include patients' handedness with preference for the nondominant side, typically car seatbelt use depending on country of residence, and whether more commonly driver or passenger, whether a wheelchair is used, occupation, fashion, and trouser belt location. Body habitus is another factor and particularly small and emaciated individuals may require special planning and occasionally preimplantation plastic surgical procedures to make sufficient room for pump implantation. In any event, the lower ribs and iliac crest should be avoided to prevent discomfort.

Operation preparation

Antibiotic prophylaxis according to local microbiological advice is recommended. A full surgical scrub and skin preparation is recommended with sterile drapes. If there are risks for deep venous thrombosis, such as prolonged general anesthesia, immobility, excess weight, or previous venous thromboses, then subcutaneous fractionated heparin should be administered in advance of the operation.

Operation

CATHETER PLACEMENT

Entry to the cerebrospinal fluid (CSF) is generally advised below the level of the spinal cord if possible. A paramedian entry using a shallow plane should reduce the CSF leak and subsequent risk of postdural puncture headache.[8] A small paravertebral incision to the paraspinous fascia is made and a spinal needle passed into the subarachnoid space (**Figure 31.1**). It is advisable to undertake this in an awake patient under fluoroscopic guidance to minimize the risk of neurological injury. Once there is free flow of CSF, the catheter is passed through the needle and threaded cephalad (**Figure 31.2**). It should pass without resistance and be followed fluoroscopically (**Figure 31.3**).

There are competing demands on deciding the spinal level of the catheter. Generally, one prefers to thread a sufficient length of catheter into the intrathecal space to minimize the risk of migration of the catheter out of the spinal canal. Another consideration is the level of pain, especially if lipophilic agents are to be used, so as to place the catheter at the level of the relevant dermatome. There is a differential concentration between spinal and cerebal CSF levels when drug is delivered spinally which would favor lower level placement for lower body symptoms. In the light of the rare but important risks of granuloma formation, it may be considered preferable to avoid the cervical area if possible.[9]

The catheter should be anchored to the fascia to minimize migration.[8] Avoidance of catheter kinking is important. A purse string suture around the tissues where the catheter punctures the dura may minimize postdural puncture headache or development of CSF hygroma[6] (**Figure 31.4**). Free flow of CSF should be confirmed after the catheter is secured to check that there has not been any catheter kinking.

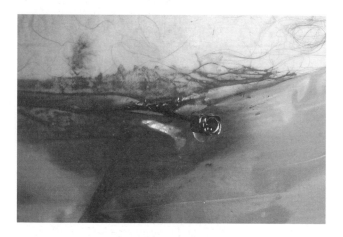

Figure 31.1   Spinal needle in cerebrospinal fluid.

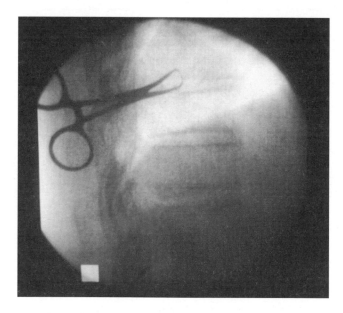

Figure 31.3   Fluoroscopy of spinal needle and catheter.

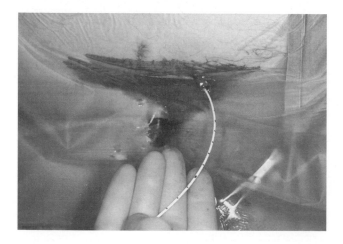

Figure 31.2   Spinal catheter through needle.

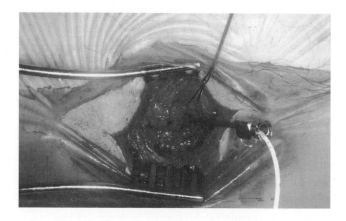

Figure 31.4   Purse string suture around catheter.

PUMP PLACEMENT

The spinal catheter itself, or a second one to which the spinal catheter is attached, is then tunnelled subcutaneously towards the site of pump implantation (**Figures 31.5, 31.6**, and **31.7**). This stage of the operation may be better tolerated by the patient under general anesthesia; however, with ready access to the subarachnoid space, a spinal anesthetic can be administered or alternatively a local tissue infiltration technique can be used.

The site of the pump will have been determined preoperatively with the patient sitting and standing. The pocket for the pump should be designed so that the incision does not overlie the refill port after the wound is closed. The catheter that connects to the pump should be of sufficient length that a few loops can form before attaching to the pump to minimize disconnection risk. These loops should be placed behind the pump to avoid puncture during refill. Further observation of CSF flow should occur before connecting the catheter to the pump to confirm that the catheter remains in the intrathecal space and that the integrity of the system is sound. Connections between the catheter and the pump are secured with strong, nonabsorbable sutures.

Different pumps have different filling regimes. Some are transported with water that needs removal. The pump should be filled with the drug and concentration as determined from the trial (**Figure 31.8**).

The pump may be placed on the fascia of the external oblique or rectus muscles, or in thin patients below this, but should be approximately 1–2 cm below the skin, superficial enough to allow easy refilling, and deep enough for minimal cosmetic effects (**Figure 31.9**). The closure of the pocket should result in security of the pump from turning. Some devices have anchoring sutures to reduce this possibility.

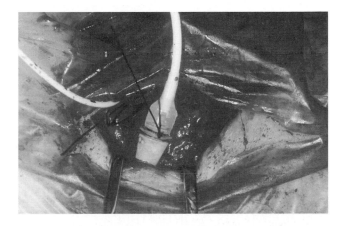

Figure 31.7 Connecting catheter to tunneller to pull through.

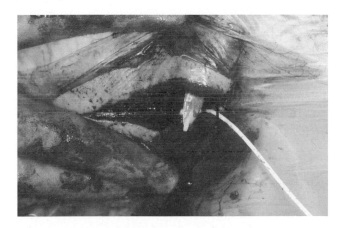

Figure 31.5 Subcutaneous tunnel for catheter.

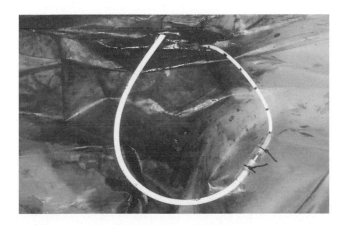

Figure 31.6 Connection between catheters (if two piece catheter).

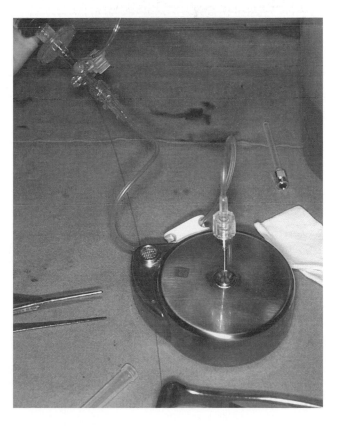

Figure 31.8 Filling pump.

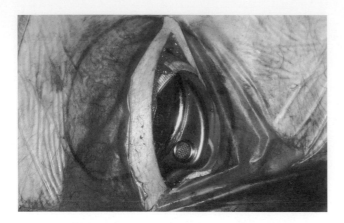

Figure 31.9 Placing pump in pocket.

Irrigation of wounds followed by closure in at least two layers should minimize infection.

It is possible to fill the catheter with active drug using a programmable pump that can calculate the catheter volume accurately so as to avoid a delay before drug effect. After closure of wounds, the patient will require close monitoring as the diffusion of drug to cerebral levels can be delayed and patients' responses are variable.

COMPLICATIONS OF INTRATHECAL DRUG DELIVERY AND SIDE EFFECTS OF DRUGS

Complications and side effects of drugs should be carefully considered as part of a risk–benefit analysis for each patient for whom intrathecal drug delivery may be a potential treatment (**Table 31.3**). They should be addressed in informed consent. Complications can be serious or minor. Minor complications are common; in a

population of cancer patients, procedure, equipment, and illness-related complications occurred at 0.45 events per patient per year.[10] Serious complications are rare. Failure or poor outcome must be a potential expectation. In cancer pain, analgesic failure rates are high at approximately 30 percent.[10] Complications can be categorized as discussed below.

Complications of the technique

Neurological deficits can occur directly from the procedure and from inflammatory mass development. In malignant disease, neurological complications can occur because of subsequent tumor or disease progression, but may also be precipitated by bleeding or CSF leak at the time of the procedure.[11] There have been more than 500 reported cases of intrathecal catheter tip inflammatory mass development to date. The estimated incidence is 0.05 percent and they occur mainly in the thoracic area. An inflammatory mass should be suspected if motor or sensory symptoms and signs develop or if there is failure of analgesia. The etiology is unknown. It is hypothesized that it may be due to an inflammatory reaction to the infused medication, or due to low-grade infection. Masses have been reported from using infusions of morphine, hydromorphone, and baclofen.

Infections, such as meningitis,[12] epidural abscesses, and pump pocket or reservoir infections can complicate the technique.[13]

CSF leaks can cause postdural puncture headaches, which are usually self-limiting, but hygromas can occur.[14]

Problems can arise from the pump pocket whereby the pump becomes uncomfortable or from thinning and discomfort from the scar.

Table 31.3 2007 Polyanalgesic algorithm for intrathecal therapies.

Line	Therapy				
Line 1	(a) Morphine	↔	(b) Hydromorphone	↔	(c) Ziconotide
Line 2	(d) Fentanyl	↔	(e) Morphine/hydromorphone+ziconotide	↔	(f) Morphine/hydromorphone +bupivacaine/clonidine
Line 3	(g) Clonidine	↔	(h) Morphine/hydromorphonc/fentanyl/ bupivacaine+/clonidine+ziconotide		
Line 4	(i) Sufentanil	↔	(j) Sufentanil bupivacaine+/ clinidine+ziconotide		
Line 5			(k) Ropivacaine, buprenophine, midazolam, meperidine, ketoralac		
Line 6			Experimental drugs: Gabapentin, octreotide, conopeptide, neostigmine, adenosine, XE2174, AM336, XEN, ZGX 160		

Morphine, fentanyl, bupivacaine, sufentanil, ropivacaine, buprenophine, midazolam, meperidine, ketoralac, and experimental drugs not licenced for intrathecal therapy in the UK.
Modified from Deer T, Krames, Hassenbush SJ *et al.* Polyanalgesic Consensus Conference 2007: Recommendations for the management of pain by intrathecal (intraspinal) drug delivery: report of an interdisciplinary expert panel. *Neuromodulation.* 2007; 10: 300–28, with permission.

Complications due to malfunction of equipment

- There can be problems from catheter kinking, disconnections, dislodgement of lines, or pump failure.
- Intrathecal diamorphine is used in the UK. There have been a small number of case reports of the precipitation of diamorphine in the Synchromed programmable pump when used in high concentrations. This causes malfunction of the pump. A UK Consensus group has recommended that it is inadvisable to use diamorphine in a programmable Synchromed pump.[15]

Complications due specifically to the drugs administered

Local and systemic effects of drugs can be problematic and complications can also occur from failure of delivery of drugs due to pump malfunction resulting in withdrawal, and refilling errors resulting in overdose or withdrawal.

OPIOIDS

The intrathecal delivery of opioids can cause centrally mediated side effects such as respiratory depression, nausea and vomiting, constipation, urinary retention, pruritus, and sedation.[16] Endocrine suppression can cause weight gain, loss of libido, excessive perspiration, hypogonadotrophic hypogonadism, hypocorticism, memory and mood changes, and headache.[17]

LOCAL ANESTHETICS

Intrathecal local anesthetic delivery can cause cardiovascular instability, sensory deficits, urinary retention, and motor impairment. At higher doses, fatigue and somnolence can occur. There are reports of neurotoxicity following intrathecal infusions of local anesthetics.[18]

BACLOFEN

Side effects from the continuous infusion of baclofen are rare; side effects are more likely following bolus doses. They include dizziness, drowsiness, and constipation. Overdose can cause weakness, ataxia, light headedness, confusion, and excessive hypotonia with consequent severe weakness and respiratory embarrassment. Withdrawal can cause rebound spasticity, motor hyperactivity, headaches, drowsiness, disorientation, hallucinations, rhabdomyolysis, seizures, and even death.[19]

CLONIDINE

Intrathecal delivery of clonidine can cause hypotension, bradycardia, and sedation.

ZICONOTIDE

Common side effects from the intrathecal delivery of ziconotide are dizziness, nausea, nystagmus, gait imbalance, confusion, and urinary retention.[20] They can be severe but can be limited by very careful titration of the drug.

Dealing with complications

Knowledge of potential complications, early recognition, and familiarity with equipment are key to the prevention and management of complications and drug side effects. Intrathecal drug delivery systems should only be used where there is an infrastructure trained, prepared, and equipped to deal with all potential complications at all times. This applies to the hospital setting, the hospice setting, and in the community. Immediate carers must be able to resuscitate and deal with the consequences of overdose or sudden withdrawal. There must be established routes of referral for expert opinion and treatment. Close monitoring should take place, particularly in the immediate period of starting intrathecal delivery.

Suspected neurological deficits, caused either by the procedure of the subsequent development of an inflammatory catheter tip mass, constitute an emergency and neuroradiological and neurosurgical expertise must be sought. Where inflammatory masses have occurred, turning off the infusion for a period of weeks to months may allow the catheter tip inflammatory mass to resolve. However, removal of the catheter may be necessary. If spinal cord compression has occurred, decompression and removal of the inflammatory mass may be necessary.

Microbiological and if necessary, neurosurgical expertise should be sought in the management of infections. Surgical expertise may be needed for revision of pockets or scars. Endocrine screening is recommended prior to undertaking the technique and at yearly intervals thereafter to provide early warning of developing endocrine suppression. Baclofen overdose, which results in excessive hypotonia, may require a period of artificial ventilation in the intensive care setting. Physostigmine is used in baclofen overdose.

Pump malfunction can result from MRI scanners; discussion should take place between the implanter, the radiologist, and the pump manufacturer.

REFERENCES

* 1. Williams JE, Louw G, Towlerton G. Intrathecal pumps for giving opioids in chronic pain: a systematic review. *Health Technology Assessment*. 2000; 4: iii–iv, 1–65.
  2. Cameron T, Wigness BD, Bedder MD. Operating principles and clinical implications of constant flow pumps. *Neuromodulation*. 2002; 5: 160–6.

3. Anderson VC, Burchiel K, Cooke B. A prospective randomised trial of intrathecal injection vs epidural infusion in the selection of patients for continuous intrathecal opioid therapy. *Neuromodulation*. 2003; **6**: 142–52.
4. Raphael JH, Gnanadurai TV, Southall JL *et al*. Placebo controlled single blind study of short term efficacy of spinal morphine in chronic non malignant pain. *Regional Anesthesia and Pain Medicine*. 2006; **31**: 47.
* 5. Deer T, Krames ES, Hassenbush SJ *et al*. Polyanalgesic Consensus Conference 2007: Recommendations for the management of pain by intrathecal (intraspinal) drug delivery: report of an interdisciplinary expert panel. *Neuromodulation*. 2007; **10**: 300–28.
* 6. British Pain Society. *Intrathecal drug delivery for the management of pain and spasticity in adults; recommendations for best clinical practice*. London: The British Pain Society, 2008. Available from: http://www.britishpainsociety.org/book_ittd_main.pdf.
* 7. Follett KA, Naumann CP. A prospective study of catheter related complications of intrathecal drug delivery systems. *Journal of Pain and Symptom Management*. 2000; **19**: 209–15.
8. Hassenbusch S, Burchiel K, Coffey RJ *et al*. Management of intrathecal catheter tip inflammatory masses: a consensus statement. *Pain Medicine*. 2002; **3**: 313–23.
9. Kulkarni AV, Drake JM, Lamerti-Pasculli M. Cerebrospinal fluid shunt infection, a prospective study of risk factors. *Journal of Neurosurgery*. 2001; **94**: 195–201.
10. Chrubasik J, Chrubasik S, Martin E. Patient controlled spinal opiate analgesia in terminal cancer. Has its time really arrived? *Drugs*. 1992; **43**: 799–804.
11. Appelgren L, Nordborg C, Sjoberg M *et al*. Spinal epidural metastasis: implications for spinal analgesia to treat 'refractory' cancer pain. *Journal of Pain and Symptom Management*. 1997; **13**: 25–42.
12. Devulder J, Ghys L, Dhondt W *et al*. Spinal analgesia in terminal care; risk versus benefit. *Journal of Pain and Symptom Management*. 1994; **9**: 75–81.
13. Byers K, Axlerod P, Michael S *et al*. Infections complicating tunnelled intraspinal catheter systems used to treat chronic pain. *Clinical Infectious Diseases*. 1995; **21**: 403–08.
14. Mercadante S. Problems of long term spinal opioid treatment in advanced cancer patients. *Pain*. 1999; **79**: 1–13.
15. Simpson KH. Report from a meeting to consider the use of diamorphine in totally impalantable intrathecal pumps. *The British Pain Society Newsletter*. 2004; Summer: 10–11.
16. Gregory MA, Brock-Utne JG, Bux S *et al*. Morphine concentration in the brain and spinal cord after subarachnoid morphine injection in baboons. *Anesthesia and Analgesia*. 1985; **64**: 929–32.
17. Abs R, Verhelst J, Maeyaert J *et al*. Endocrine consequences of long term intrathecal administration of opioids. *Journal of Clinical Endocrinology and Metabolism*. 2000; **85**: 2215–22.
18. Rigler ML, Drasner K, Krejcie TC *et al*. Cauda equina syndrome after continuous spinal anesthesia. *Anesthesia and Analgesia*. 1991; **72**: 275–81.
19. Sampathkumar P, Scanlon PD, Plevak DJ. Baclofen withdrawal presenting as multiorgan system failure. *Anesthesia and Analgesia*. 1998; **87**: 562–3.
20. Wallace MS, Charapata SG, Fisher R *et al*. Intrathecal ziconotide in the treatment of chronic non-malignant pain: a randomised controlled clinical trial. *Neuromodulation*. 2006; **9**: 75–86.

32

Cryoanalgesia

GUNNVALD KVARSTEIN AND HENRIK HÖGSTRÖM

KEY LEARNING POINTS

- Cryoanalgesia (cryoneurolysis) causes a temporary loss of axonal continuity, but the nerve is able to regenerate.
- The incidence of neuritis is low.
- The intensity and duration of analgesia correlate with the size and temperature of the thermic lesion.

- The tip of the cryoprobe should generally not be more than 4–5 mm away from the target nerve trunk.
- The technique can be applied in the treatment of localized acute and chronic pain conditions and may provide pain relief for several months.
- The evidence-base of cryoneurolysis is largely lacking.

INTRODUCTION

Applying cold to tissues to relieve pain has been recognized for thousands of years. In 1917, Trendelenberg[1] demonstrated that freezing a nerve leads to reversible nerve injury without neuroma formation. In 1967, Amoils and coworkers[2] introduced a hand-held device to freeze tissue, using carbon dioxide or nitrous oxide. Ten years later, Lloyd et al.[3] brought the cryoprobe into pain therapy. Cryoanalgesia, in the sense of cryoneurolysis or cryoablation of nervous tissue is an interventional technique with the ability of providing long-lasting pain relief. This chapter aims to cover the basic principles of this method, and some of its most common clinical applications.

PHYSICS AND TECHNICAL DATA

Cryoprobes of today are adaptations of Amoils' gas-expansion prototype. In a closed tubal system, pressurized N_2O or CO_2 is circulated through a small nozzle (0.002 mm) in the tip of the probe into an inner lumen where the gas rapidly expands[4] (**Figure 32.1**). According to the adiabatic principle (Joule–Thompson effect) gas expansion causes a sudden drop in pressure from 5516 to 69 kPa (800 to 10 psi) and temperature from room temperature to approximately $-60°C$.[5] As a consequence, the surrounding tissue is converted into an ice-ball. To limit the tissue lesion the probe is insulated with Teflon except for the tip which is left uncoated. Modern cryomachines have a built-in nerve stimulator, flow monitor, and

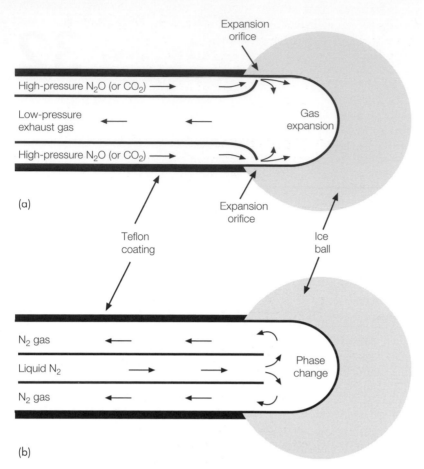

(a)

(b)

Figure 32.1 An adaptation of Amoils' gas-expansion cryoprobe. Inside the tip of the probe in a closed tubal system, pressurized N_2O or CO_2 is circulated through a small nozzle (0.002 mm) into an inner lumen where the gas rapidly expands. Cross-sections of: (a) the gas expansion type; (b) the change of phase type of cryogenic probe. Figures used courtesy of Thomas A Edell and Somayaji Ramamurphy.

thermistor, which help to localize the nerve and achieve the optimal tip temperature.

In the USA, two companies manufacture gas expansion cryomachines: Wallach Surgical Device with the Pain Blocker™ and Westco Medical Corporation with the Neurostat™. In Europe, Neurostat™ is produced by Spembly Medical (UK).

PHYSIOLOGY

Cryoneurolysis causes a loss of axonal continuity ("axonotmesis"), which is characterized by axonal disruption, Wallerian degeneration, and demyelination.[6] The endoneurium and basal lamina of the Schwann cells remain intact, and the nerve is able to regenerate completely.[7, 8] The exact mechanisms causing cell injury have not been established, but one theory involves crystal formation, rupture of the cell membranes, protein denaturation, and cellular dehydration (crystals remove water from the intra- and extracellular compartment).[6] Ice crystals, however, obliterating and damaging the vasa nervorum, may also cause ischemia.[4]

Cryoneurolysis generally provides pain relief for three months, although the nerve itself only seems to require two to three weeks for regeneration.[9] How can this be explained? Experimental studies have described long-lasting and reduced electrophysiological responses, as late as after 90 days and diminished axonal diameter after one year.[9] Some have speculated whether the block of peripheral nerve impulses and the subsequent modulation of the central sensitization, could be the reason.[10] A third possible mechanism could be autoimmune responses triggered by frozen and sequestered proteins.[11, 12, 13]

PHYSICAL DETERMINATORS FOR SUCCESSFUL CRYONEUROLYSIS

The following factors have been identified as essential for accomplishing effective cryoneurolysis.[14]

Probe temperature, duration, and number of freeze–thaw cycles

The intensity and duration of analgesia correlate with the size and temperature of the thermic lesion (ice-ball). A slow freezing rate (less temperature decrease due to low gas flow) causes ice crystal formation preferably in the extracellular space. This leads to intracellular dehydration and cell shrinkage, but not necessarily cell death. A rapid freezing rate (lower temperature due to high gas flow) forms ice crystals in both the intra- and extracellular space. This disrupts the cell membrane and causes cell death.

If the probe is in a suboptimal position, or close to highly vascularized tissue (acting like a heat sink), repeated freeze–thaw cycles may be favorable. Two to three freeze–thaw cycles have been shown to increase the ice-ball, but not more than 15 percent.[6] When the tissue has reached $-20°C$, there is no benefit in extending or repeating the freezing interval.[6] A larger ice-ball will act as insulation.[4]

Probe size and position

For gas expansion probes the ice-ball diameter (lesion size) is two to three times greater than the probe diameter itself. With a probe diameter of 1.4 mm, the ice ball diameter will reach 3.5 mm, with a probe diameter of 2 mm it will be 5.5 mm.[4] Thus, a thicker probe will more likely encounter the nerve trunk. Inside the ice-ball there is a sharp temperature gradient from the center to the surface, equivalent to 10°C/mm.[6] The cryoprobe should therefore not be more than 4–5 mm away from the target nerve trunk.

INDICATIONS

Cryoanalgesia does not provide a permanent block, and the pain relieving effect is of limited duration. On the other hand, one should bear in mind that even a temporary pain relief may open up for other therapeutic options, such as physiotherapy or physical exercise.

Patients considered for cryoablation should preferably be evaluated by a multispecialist pain team and try less invasive therapies. This is particularly important in patients with generalized pain disorders.

Cryoanalgesia may be considered for:

- **Chronic neuropathic pain** which does not respond to conventional treatment (antiepileptics, tricyclic antidepressants, topical lidocaine, etc).
- **Localized peripheral nerve lesion** (neuroma)[15] and entrapment neuropathies.[16]

One should be aware that neuropathic pain may be aggravated by the cryoneurotrauma.

Contraindications

There are no absolute contraindications to cryoanalgesia, but proper attention should be paid to the following aspects:

- Bleeding diathesis in previous history, particularly where bleeding may go unnoticed into large body cavities.
- Allergy to local anesthetic agents.
- Infected skin.
- Anxiety. Patients previously exposed to physical abuse (torture, rape, etc.) may not tolerate invasive procedures.

- Impeded communication by infancy, cognitive deficiency, or language barriers.
- Nociceptive, post-traumatic pain. Intercostal nerve cryotherapy has been applied postoperatively. Due to the risk of increased and chronic pain, it is no longer recommended.[17]

PATIENT PREPARATION

Cryoanalgesia should always be based on a mutual agreement between patient and therapist. Informed consent requires balanced information about the procedure including intra- and postprocedural pain, risks, complications, and anticipated long-term results. The patient must be warned of undue expectations.

RISKS AND COMPLICATIONS

- Sensory disturbances: Transient sensory disturbances such as allodynia and hyperalgesia may occur,[17, 18, 19, 20, 21] particularly if excessive freezing or a large cryoprobe is used. After intercostal nerve ablations, these symptoms have been reported to occur after six weeks and may last for two to four weeks.[18, 19] In some studies the incidence of neuralgia is 20–30 percent.[18, 19, 20] One case of neuroma formation has also been published.[22]
- Motor block can occur when neurolysis is performed in mixed nerves or in the immediate vicinity of a motor nerve. Cryolesions in the face can cause unintentional block of facial nerve branches with concomitant disfigurement lasting for days or weeks.[4]
- Infection is a rare complication. Deep tissue infection was registered in only two out of 2500 treatments (Högström, unpublished results).
- Bleeding: Unnoticed bleeding into thoracic, abdominal, or pelvic cavities is a serious complication. This calls for clear delineation of the postoperative follow up.
- Pneumothorax: The introducer or probe may penetrate into the lung during intercostal blocks.
- Other: Some patients develop depigmentation or hyperpigmentation of the lesion site. Alopecia of the eyebrow has been reported after a supraorbital cryolesion.

EQUIPMENT PREPARATION

- Check the machine and gas supply properly.
- The sterilized cryoprobe is purged/vented with a low gas flow (1–2 L/min) for two to four minutes to prevent obliteration of the probe lumina by water crystal formation.
- An introducer cannula (12 or 14 G cannula, depending on probe size) is recommended. It

functions as an extra protection in case of deficient Teflon coating and thereby prevents skin freezing and off-track neurostimulation.

DIFFERENT TECHNIQUES

Cryoneurolysis should always be performed under strictly aseptic conditions with sterile "prep and drape."

Peroperative ("open") technique

In 1974, Nelson *et al.*[23] described intraoperative (open) cryoneurolysis of intercostal nerves. Peroperatively, with direct vision and general anesthesia the neural structures are identified. Each nerve is frozen for 30–60 seconds.

Percutaneous ("closed") technique

The percutaneous closed technique is suited for chronic pain management in an outpatient setting.

Analgesia for procedural pain

Small amounts of a local anesthetic agent with epinephrine are infiltrated subcutaneously to provide pain relief and hemostasis. Epinephrine decreases local blood flow and limits the "heat sink" effect. It is important not to anesthetize the actual target nerve when stimulation is planned.

In some cases repeated intravenous doses of a short-acting opioid such as alfentanil 0.5–1 mg are required. Be aware that patients on chronic opioid medication will need higher doses.

If sedation is required, this can be accomplished with small incremental doses of midazolam 1–4 mg given intravenously, but appropriate communication with the patient (verbal, mimics, and body language) is essential for accurate probe placement, and will suffer if the sedation is too heavy.

Probe insertion

An introducer (or scalpel) is used to penetrate the skin. To counteract the "heat sink" from intercostal vessels, some recommend a 14 G cryoprobe as this generates a larger lesion (ice-ball). This advantage is, however, offset by a greater risk of hematoma and perforation into the lung. We therefore generally use a 18 G cryoprobe (round tip) inserted through a 14 G introducer. It is easier to manipulate and less painful to the patient. When close to the target nerve, the stylet is replaced with the cryoprobe.

Nerve localization

Mapping the peripheral nerve trunks and other structures relevant to the pain problem is crucial for the outcome.

Going ahead in a "trial-and-error" fashion without a proper plan will rarely result in success and could be detrimental to the global pain situation.

Palpation

Palpation is a reliable way of locating superficial nerve trunks, given well-defined landmarks. A good-quality anatomical atlas[24, 25] is helpful in planning the procedure, but not all textbooks are equally detailed, and some can be directly misleading.

Nerve stimulation

A nerve stimulator may increase the accuracy, but excessive stimulation is painful to the patient. Always use a grounding plate. When the probe is close to the nerve, start the stimulation with high-frequency current (100 Hz) at 2 volts to stimulate the sensory nerve, and decrease gradually down to 0.5 volts. Paresthesia should still be perceived in the area of maximal pain. Apply the same procedure with 2 Hz stimulation. If the muscle twitches, move the probe some millimeters to avoid damage to motor fibers.

Imaging techniques

Fluoroscopy or computed tomography (CT) is mandatory when aiming at deeper sensory nerves, particularly along the spine.[26] Ultrasound has been advocated to visualize peripheral nerves in the neck.[27, 28]

Diagnostic block

A diagnostic block should always be performed and pain relief assessed prior to cryoneurolysis. Small volumes of a local anesthetic agent, 0.2–0.8 mL (equivalent with the size of the ice-ball formed around the cryoprobe tip), will more precisely predict the effect of cryoablation.

Freezing

When the introducer is close to the target area, and the stylet replaced with the cryoprobe, the introducer is withdrawn a few millimeters to expose the tip of the cryoprobe. Gas flow is increased to 10–12 L/min (2.0 mm probe) or 8–10 L/min (1.4 mm probe) to achieve a probe tip temperature of approximately −60°C. The freezing interval varies from 1.5 to 3 minutes, and should be repeated once or twice.

Defrosting

After each freeze cycle the probe must be defrosted for 30 seconds. The cryoprobe should be withdrawn only after it has been defrosted to avoid avulsion of the nerve. Watch the "DEFROST" light on the panel.

CRYOANALGESIA IN THE TREATMENT OF ACUTE AND POSTOPERATIVE PAIN

Intercostal nerves

OPEN TECHNIQUE

The nerve is isolated by blunt dissection and visualized beneath the parietal pleura. Maiwand and Makey[29] recommended pleural retraction to ensure that the probe is accurately located on the nerve, proximal to the collateral branch. Because each rib has a nerve contribution from the rib below and above, additional lesions to adjacent intercostal nerves were recommended. Post-operative pain is no longer accepted as a good indication, due to risk of chronic neuropathic pain (see Indications).

PERCUTANEOUS (CLOSED) TECHNIQUE

See below under Cryoanalgesia of intercostal nerves.

Clinical efficacy

Two randomized studies on thoracotomized patients have reported better pain relief[30, 31] and respiratory function[30] after cryoanalgesia as compared with epidural, inter-pleural, or opioid analgesia. Intercostal cryoablation, however, does not block nociceptive signals from the pleura, ligaments, and muscles as these are transmitted by the phrenic, vagus, and sympathetic nerves. This may explain why cryoanalgesia in other studies has not been associated with improved respiratory function[32, 33] nor lower opioid consumption.[33, 34, 35] In one follow-up study, one-third of the patients reported increased pain after cryoanalgesia,[20] and other studies have shown an increased risk of chronic post-thoracotomy pain after cryotherapy.[17, 20, 21] Epidural is therefore preferred.[32, 34]

CRYOANALGESIA IN THE TREATMENT OF CHRONIC PAIN

Despite an early enthusiasm, the number of controlled randomized studies on cryoanalgesia is surprisingly low. The following text will pertain to the closed, percutaneous, or submucosal approach for cryoneurolysis of peripheral nerves. Where this method is used, only the most common pain syndromes will be addressed in detail. Different clinical applications for cryoanalgesia have been broadly reviewed by Trescott,[4] Saberski,[36] and Florete.[37]

Chronic pain syndromes in the head and neck area

- Occipital neuralgia.
- Cervicogenic headache (CGH).
- Whiplash-associated disorder (WAD).
- Facial pain.
- Trigeminal neuralgia.
- Temporomandibular joint dysfunction.

Occipital hyperalgesia is a frequent symptom in these syndromes (particularly in the first three) and involves the nerve roots C2 and C3 and their peripheral branches. The nerve roots C2 and C3 divide into the greater occipital nerve (GON), lesser occipital nerve (LON), third occipital nerve (TON), and the greater auricular nerve (GAN). There are considerable interindividual variations in the configuration of the main trunks and extensive anastomoses between the LON, GON, and TON. The anatomy of the occipital nerves has been reviewed in detail by Bogduk,[38, 39] Becser et al.,[40] and Tubbs et al.[41]

Facial hyperalgesia is more commonly observed in the three latter syndromes, in which one or more trigeminal nerve branches may be involved. The trigeminal nerve divides into the ophthalmic division with the supratrochlear and the supraorbital nerve, the maxillary division with the infraorbital nerve, and the mandibular division with the mental and auriculo-temporal nerve.

Trigeminocervical convergence involves afferent primary neurons from the occipital nerves and from the trigeminal nerve, descending into the upper cervical segments, converge on the same second-order neurons in the central nervous system (CNS). This explains coexisting occipital and facial hyperalgesia and referred pain patterns.[42] Central sensitization has been claimed to be a driving force behind these chronic pain states, and peripheral blocks with a reduction in nociceptive peripheral input may be a way of modulating it.[43]

Cryoanalgesia of the occipital nerves

In mixed trigeminocervical pain, a local anesthetic block can be used to rule out a cervical cause. Sjaastad et al.[44] included pain relief after an occipital nerve block as a criterion in the diagnosis of cervicogenic headache. Peripheral blocks (GON) seem to be equally effective as central blocks over the facet joint C2-3 (TON).[45] Transforming this diagnostic procedure into a long-term therapeutic modality by percutaneous cryoanalgesia of the occipital nerves, however, has so far caught little interest. There are no randomized control trial (RCT)-studies available supporting cryoneurolysis for occipital pain. From an ongoing randomized study we have gathered considerable clinical experience with the method, and the preliminary data are encouraging (Högström, unpublished results). Many patients report substantial pain relief and a reduction in autonomic, cognitive, and muscle dysfunction. In some patients we have observed an improved pain relief after repeated ablations, but the duration of pain relief remains unchanged, at three to six months.

TECHNIQUE

The patient is in the lateral recumbent position with the area to be treated upwards. No preoperative haircut is required. Skin and subcutaneous tissue is infiltrated with 1–2 mL of a local anesthetic agent with adrenaline (1:200,000) using a 25 or 27 G, 16–25 mm long needle depending on the size of the patient. If hyperalgesia is present, infiltration with local anesthetic is recommended all the way to the trunk before proceeding with cryoneurolysis.

Observe that branches of the same trunk may be found at different depths. Sticking to the coordinates and anatomic landmarks makes localization of the nerve trunk simple and the use of nerve stimulation mostly superfluous. Nerve stimulation may cause pain referred to the lower part of occiput. Two freeze–thaw cycles in one position are sufficient.

For more detailed procedural and anatomical description see **Figures 32.2**, **32.3**, and **Figure 32.4**.

The mastoid branch of the GAN traverses the upper part of the sternocleidomastoid (SCM) and is sometimes palpable in this position. Its clinical relevance and contribution to CGH is often doubtful. Cryoanalgesia of this nerve is demanding and causes considerable pain due to the muscle lesion. In our opinion, GAN is best left untreated.

COMPLICATIONS

We have not observed any serious complications. Puncture of an artery or vein accompanying the nerve trunk is quite common, but significant hematoma is rare unless the patient has a bleeding diathesis.

If the probe is inserted too far, it may theoretically puncture the dura mater, but complications related to the local anesthetic block, such as intravenous, intra-arterial, or intrathecal injection in cases of a cranial bone defect raise more concern.[48]

Cryoanalgesia of branches of the trigeminal nerve

Treatment of facial pain and trigeminal neuralgia with cryoanalgesia of the peripheral branches of the trigeminal nerve has been studied by several authors.[49, 50, 51]

TECHNIQUE

The supraorbital nerve is easily palpated at the supraorbital notch. The entry point is below the eyebrow. When in contact with the nerve, one to three lesions are performed with the needle in different directions

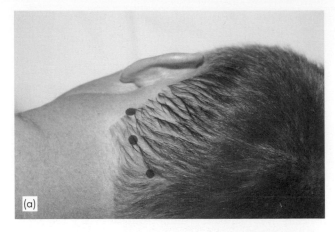

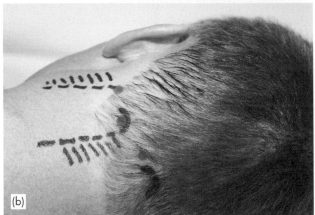

Figure 32.2 (a) The occipital entry points. (b) Anatomical landmarks. Palpable landmarks such as the superior nuchal line (SNL), the midline external occipital protuberance (EOP), the sterno-cleidomastoid (SCM), and trapezius muscles (TM) can be used to localize the main nerve trunks.[46] At the level of the SNL, both the GON and LON normally have two or sometimes even three branches.[47] (b) The nerve trunks can be palpated as three tender points on or slightly below the SNL. They correspond to the entry points for the probe: the lateral entry point for the lateral branch of the LON is located at the medial border of the SCM, 6–7 cm lateral of the EOP. The medial branch of LON can also be reached from the lateral entry point. It is palpated as a tender point between the lateral and intermediate entry point. The intermediate entry point for the main branch of GON is located at the crescent-shaped lateral edge of the cranial insertion of the TM, 4 cm lateral to the EOP. The medial entry point for the medial branch of GON is located at the rounded defect in the tendinous insertion of TM, 2 cm lateral to the EOP.

according to pain response or response to nerve stimulation.

The supratrochlear nerve is located more medially and treated similarly if indicated.

The infraorbital nerve and the mental nerve can be reached percutaneously or submucosally (orally), the alveolar nerves only orally. With the submucous approach, a small incision is inserted in the mucous membrane over the nerve to be neurolyzed, the tip of the

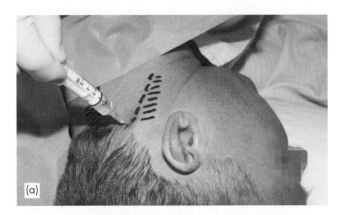

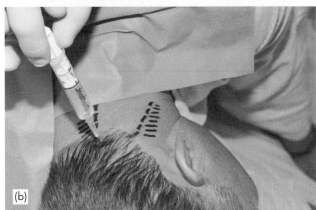

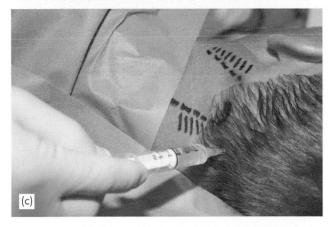

Figure 32.3 (a), (b), and (c) Local anesthetic block of the occipital nerves. The needle is advanced slightly cranially at a 45° angle to the sagittal plane at the lateral entry point, 30° angle at the intermediate entry point and parallel to the sagittal plane at the medial entry point. In this way, the planum nuchae will act as a backstop, and the nerve trunk is caught against the bone.

cryoprobe is inserted directly and the nerve exposed to one or two freeze–thaw cycles.

The auriculotemporal nerve, a sensory terminal branch from the mandibular nerve, becomes superficial and frequently palpable between the posterior edge of the mandible and the tragus. Opening the mouth gives access to the nerve. The risk of lesioning facial nerve trunks has to be kept in mind.

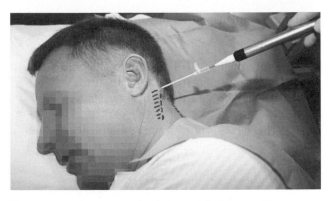

Figure 32.4 Cryoneurolysis of the occipital nerves. The introducer is held in the dominant hand while the index finger of the opposite hand palpates and fixates the tender nerve trunk, and is inserted from the entry points with a steady movement towards the nerve at the same angles as for the local anesthetic block (see above). To prevent too deep a penetration, it may be wise to support the probe with two fingers of the nondominant hand. The lateral branch of LON is encountered 1–2.5 cm from the lateral entry point. To reach the medial branch of LON the introducer is slightly retracted and redirected at 90° angle towards the sagittal plane. The nerve branch is reached at the same depth as for the lateral branch. The main branch of GON is found 1–2 cm from the intermediate entry point. The medial branch of GON is reached 0.5–1.5 cm from the medial entry point. The TON is reached 2–5 cm from the medial entry point with the probe in an inferior-medial direction along the medial portion of TM. TON can also be reached from a separate entry point close to the midline (0.3–0.5 cm) along the medial border of TM, 3–5 cm caudally from EOP.

Chronic pain syndromes in the thoracic and upper abdominal area

- Intercostal neuralgia.
- Postherpetic neuralgia.
- Cicatricial pain.

Patients exposed to thoracotomy,[52] mastectomy,[53] sternotomy,[54] laparotomy, nephrectomy, or laparoscopy may develop incapacitating chronic pain. The reasons could be neuroma or trapping of nerves in scar tissue.

Cryoanalgesia of intercostal nerves

Cryoablation of intercostal nerves can relieve pain in the chest and abdominal wall. When intercostal nerve cryoablation is considered:

- Palpate the scar, trigger points, neuroma, or the trapped nerve suspected of generating the pain.
- Define the intercostal nerves supplying the alleged pain origo. Be aware that laparotomy scars may cross the midline.

- Diagnostic local anesthetic blocks and cryoneurolysis should be limited to one side at a time due to the risk of pneumothorax.

TECHNIQUE

The procedure is easy to perform. In obese patients, however, x-ray guidance is useful. The patient is lying in the lateral or prone position. The skin is moved cranially before the probe is inserted. When the probe encounters the lower border of the costa, release the skin fold and redirect the probe. It is then possible to advance beneath and along the costa, for details see **Figure 32.5**.

CLINICAL EFFICACY

In a study of patients with postherpetic neuralgia or intercostal neuralgia, 50 percent noted significant pain

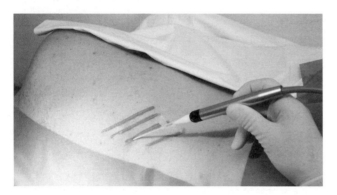

Figure 32.5 Cryoneurolysis of intercostal nerves. To prevent unintentionally deep penetration, it may be wise to support the probe with two fingers of the nondominant hand. The introducer is directed proximally parallel to the nerve near the angulus costae. This reduces the risk of pneumothorax and maximizes the length of nerve being frozen.

relief with a duration of three months outlasting the return of sensory function.[55] None of the patients developed neuritis. In another study on chest wall pain of different etiology, the effect of cryoneurolysis lasted from one week up to 12 months, and postherpetic neuralgia was associated with poorer response.[56]

COMPLICATIONS

Pneumothorax and hematoma and bleeding into the pleural cavity are potential and serious complications. A chest x-ray is recommended if in any doubt. Cryoanalgesia of the third and fourth intercostals can cause ipsilateral nipple anesthesia. Thus, freezing above the fifth intercostal nerve is not recommended by some authors.[57] Denervation of the intercostal muscles may reduce the tone of the external and internal oblique muscles and cause a subtle abdominal bulge which resolves within weeks.[29]

Chronic pain syndromes in the groin

- Ilio-hypogastric neuralgia.
- Ilio-inguinal neuralgia.

The ilio-hypogastric nerves (IHN) and ilio-inguinal nerves (IIN) are easily injured in connection with inguinal surgery or laparoscopic procedures.

TECHNIQUE

They can be reached at the lateral border of the quadratus lumborum muscle between the scapular and the posterior axillary line. For a detailed description of cryoneurolysis of IHN and IIN, see **Figure 32.6**.

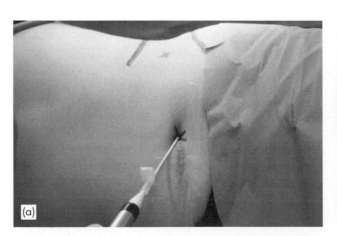
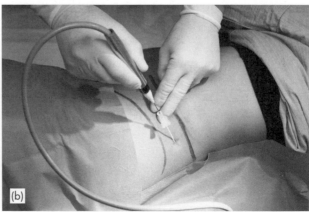

Figure 32.6 Cryoneurolysis of scar neuroma and the ilio-hypogastric nerve (IHN). The neuroma can be located by meticulous palpation and subsequently blocked with local anesthesia for diagnostic/prognostic purposes. The IHN can be approached midway between the costal arch and the iliac crest. The introducer is directed proximally parallel to the nerve trunk at the site where the IHN appears from the quadratus lumborum muscle (posterior axillary line).

COMPLICATIONS

Motor nerve blockade is usually short-lasting without clinical significance.

Chronic pelvic pain

- Coccygodynia.
- Perineal pain.

Chronic nonmalignant and cancer pain in the perineal area may constitute a considerable therapeutic problem. Sacral cryoanalgesia offers effective relief with little risk of motor block. The nerve roots are reached through the sacral foramina or the sacral hiatus. Note that the S4 root innervates the levator ani and coccygeal muscle, and that the rami of S5 root emerge through the sacral hiatus.

TECHNIQUE

Coccygodynia (S5)

The sacral hiatus is localized by palpation. Under fluoroscopic guidance the introducer is advanced cranially so that the tip of the probe lies between the sacral cornua and close to the coccygeal nerve. Nerve stimulation confirms adequate position and absence of motor involvement. Two freeze–thaw cycles, each of two to three minutes, are applied on each side.

Perineal pain (S4)

Under intermittent fluoroscopic guidance, the probe is advanced further to the level of the fourth sacral foramen. After a local anesthetic test block, lesions are made as for the coccygeal nerve or the S5 root. The technique provides good analgesia and minimal risk of sphincter dysfunction.[58]

REFERENCES

1. Trendelenberg W. Langdauernde Nervenausschaltung mit sicherer Regenerationsfähigkeit. *Zeitschrift fur die Gesamte Experimentelle Medizin.* 1917; **5**: 374.
2. Amoils SP. The Joule Thomson cryoprobe. *Archives of Ophthalmology.* 1967; **78**: 201–07.
3. Lloyd JW, Barnard JD, Glynn CJ. Cryoanalgesia. A new approach to pain relief. *Lancet.* 1976; **2**: 932–4.
* 4. Trescot AM. Cryoanalgesia in interventional pain management. *Pain Physician.* 2003; **6**: 345–60.
5. Garamy G. Engineering aspects of cryosurgery. In: Rand RW, Rinfret A, von Leden H (eds). *Cryosurgery.* Springfield, IL: Charles C Thomas, 1968.
* 6. Evans PJ. Cryoanalgesia. The application of low temperatures to nerves to produce anaesthesia or analgesia. *Anaesthesia.* 1981; **36**: 1003–13.
7. Myers RR, Powell HC, Heckman HM *et al.* Biophysical and pathological effects of cryogenic nerve lesion. *Annals of Neurology.* 1981; **10**: 478–85.
8. Sunderland S. *Nerves and nerve injuries.* Edinburgh and London: Livingstone, 1968: 180.
9. Kalichman MW, Myers RR. Behavioral and electrophysiological recovery following cryogenic nerve injury. *Experimental Neurology.* 1987; **96**: 692–702.
10. Curatolo M, Arendt-Nielsen L, Petersen-Felix S. Evidence, mechanisms, and clinical implications of central hypersensitivity in chronic pain after whiplash injury. *Clinical Journal of Pain.* 2004; **20**: 469–76.
11. Holden H. *Practical cryosurgery 2–3.* London: Pitman, 1975: 9.
12. Gander M, Soanes WA, Smith V. Experimental prostate surgery. *Investigative Urology.* 1967; **1**: 610.
13. Soanes WA, Ablin RJ, Gonder MJ. Remission of metastatic lesions following cryosurgery in prostatic cancer: immunologic considerations. *Journal of Urology.* 1970; **104**: 154–9.
14. Myers RR, Heckman HM, Powell HC. Axonal viability and the persistence of thermal hyperalgesia after partial freeze lesions of nerve. *Journal of the Neurological Sciences.* 1996; **139**: 28–38.
15. Caporusso EF, Fallat LM, Savoy-Moore R. Cryogenic neuroablation for the treatment of lower extremity neuromas. *Journal of Foot and Ankle Surgery.* 2002; **41**: 286–90.
16. Wang JK. Cryoanalgesia for painful peripheral nerve lesions. *Pain.* 1985; **22**: 191–4.
* 17. Richardson J. Chronic pain after thoracic surgery. *Acta Anaesthesiologica Scandinavica.* 2000; **44**: 220.
18. Detterbeck FC. Efficacy of methods of intercostal nerve blockade for pain relief after thoracotomy. *Annals of Thoracic Surgery.* 2005; **80**: 1550–9.
19. Roxburgh JC, Markland CG, Ross BA, Kerr WF. Role of cryoanalgesia in the control of pain after thoracotomy. *Thorax.* 1987; **42**: 292–5.
20. Conacher ID. Percutaneous cryotherapy for post-thoracotomy neuralgia. *Pain.* 1986; **25**: 227–8.
21. Mustola S *et al.* Intercostal nerve cryotherapy increases post-thoracotomy pain. Paper presented at 13th World Congress of Anaesthesiologists, Paris, 2004, S040.
22. Johannesen N, Madsen G, Ahlburg P. Neurological sequelae after cryoanalgesia for thoracotomy pain relief. *Annales Chirurgiae et Gynaecologiae.* 1990; **79**: 108–09.
23. Nelson KM, Vincent RG, Bourke RS *et al.* Intraoperative intercostal nerve freezing to prevent postthoracotomy pain. *Annals of Thoracic Surgery.* 1974; **18**: 280–5.
24. Waldman SD (ed.). *Atlas of interventional pain management,* 2nd rev edn. Philadelphia, PA: Elsevier, 2003.
25. Miller RD, Abram SE (eds). *Atlas of anesthesia,* vol. 6. Philadelphia, PA: Churchill Livingstone, 1998.
* 26. Ali NM, Zuniga R. Computed tomography-guided intercostal cryoanalgesia: a new technique. *Regional Anesthesia.* 1995; **20**: 356–7.
27. Eichenberger U, Greher M, Kirchmair L *et al.* Ultrasound-guided blocks of the ilioinguinal and iliohypogastric nerve: accuracy of a selective new technique confirmed by

anatomical dissection. *British Journal of Anaesthesia.* 2006; **97**: 238–43.

28. Eichenberger U, Greher M, Kapral S *et al.* Sonographic visualization and ultrasound-guided block of the third occipital nerve: prospective for a new method to diagnose C2-C3 zygapophysial joint pain. *Anesthesiology.* 2006; **104**: 303–08.

29. Maiwand O, Makey AR. Cryoanalgesia for relief of pain after thoracotomy. *British Medical Journal (Clinical Research Ed.).* 1981; **282**: 1749–50.

∗ 30. Moorjani N, Zhao F, Tian Y *et al.* Effects of cryoanalgesia on post-thoracotomy pain and on the structure of intercostal nerves: a human prospective randomized trial and a histological study. *European Journal of Cardio-thoracic Surgery.* 2001; **20**: 502–07.

31. Pastor J, Morales P, Cases E *et al.* Evaluation of intercostal cryoanalgesia versus conventional analgesia in postthoracotomy pain. *Respiration.* 1996; **63**: 241–5.

32. Miguel R, Hubbell D. Pain management and spirometry following thoracotomy: a prospective, randomized study of four techniques. *Journal of Cardiothoracic and Vascular Anesthesia.* 1993; **7**: 529–34.

33. Muller LC, Salzer GM, Ransmayr G, Neiss A. Intraoperative cryoanalgesia for postthoracotomy pain relief. *Annals of Thoracic Surgery.* 1989; **48**: 15–8.

34. Brichon PY, Pison C, Chaffanjon P *et al.* Comparison of epidural analgesia and cryoanalgesia in thoracic surgery. *European Journal of Cardiothoracic Surgery.* 1994; **8**: 482–6.

35. Hui J, Yi F, Ba-xian Y, Jun W. Comparison of epidural analgesia and intercostal nerve cryoanalgesia for post-thoracotomy pain control. *European Journal of Pain.* 2008; **12**: 378–84.

∗ 36. Saberski LR. Cryoneurolysis in clinical practice. In: Waldman SD (ed.). *Interventional pain management*, 2nd edn. Philadelphia: WB Saunders, 2000.

∗ 37. Florete OG. Cryoablative procedure for back pain. Jacksonville, FL, USA: Duval County Medical Society, last updated October, 1998. cited December 2007. Available from: www.coccyx.org/medabs/florete.htm

38. Bogduk N. The anatomy of occipital neuralgia. *Clinical and Experimental Neurology.* 1981; **17**: 167–84.

39. Bogduk N. The clinical anatomy of the cervical dorsal rami. *Spine.* 1982; **7**: 319–30.

40. Becser N, Bovim G, Sjaastad O. Extracranial nerves in the posterior part of the head. Anatomic variations and their possible clinical significance. *Spine.* 1998; **23**: 1435–41.

41. Tubbs RS, Salter EG, Wellons JC *et al.* Landmarks for the identification of the cutaneous nerves of the occiput and nuchal regions. *Clinical Anatomy.* 2006; **20**: 235–8.

42. Piovesan EJ, Kowacs PA, Oshinsky ML. Convergence of cervical and trigeminal sensory afferents. *Current Pain and Headache Reports.* 2003; **7**: 377–83.

43. Bogduk N. Cervicogenic headache: anatomic basis and pathophysiologic mechanisms. *Current Pain and Headache Reports.* 2001; **5**: 382–6.

44. Sjaastad O, Fredriksen TA, Pfaffenrath V. Cervicogenic headache: diagnostic criteria. The Cervicogenic Headache International Study Group. *Headache.* 1998; **38**: 442–5.

45. Inan N, Ceyhan A, Inan L *et al.* C2/C3 nerve blocks and greater occipital nerve block in cervicogenic headache treatment. *Functional Neurology.* 2001; **16**: 239–43.

46. Natsis K, Baraliakos X, Appell HJ *et al.* The course of the greater occipital nerve in the suboccipital region: a proposal for setting landmarks for local anesthesia in patients with occipital neuralgia. *Clinical Anatomy.* 2006; **19**: 332–6.

47. Madhavi C, Holla SJ. Triplication of the lesser occipital nerve. *Clinical Anatomy.* 2004; **17**: 667–71.

48. Okuda Y, Matsumoto T, Shinohara M *et al.* Sudden unconsciousness during a lesser occipital nerve block in a patient with the occipital bone defect. *European Journal of Anaesthesiology.* 2001; **18**: 829–32.

49. Barnard D, Lloyd J, Evans J. Cryoanalgesia in the management of chronic facial pain. *Journal of Maxillofacial Surgery.* 1981; **9**: 101–02.

50. Zakrzewska JM, Nally FF. The role of cryotherapy (cryoanalgesia) in the management of paroxysmal trigeminal neuralgia: a six year experience. *British Journal of Oral and Maxillofacial Surgery.* 1988; **26**: 18–25.

51. Pradel W, Hlawitschka M, Eckelt U *et al.* Cryosurgical treatment of genuine trigeminal neuralgia. *British Journal of Oral and Maxillofacial Surgery.* 2002; **40**: 244–7.

52. Perttunen K, Tasmuth T, Kalso E. Chronic pain after thoracic surgery: a follow-up study. *Acta Anaesthesiologica Scandinavica.* 1999; **43**: 563–7.

53. MacDonald L, Bruce J, Scott NW *et al.* Long-term follow-up of breast cancer survivors with post-mastectomy pain syndrome. *British Journal of Cancer.* 2005; **92**: 225–30.

54. Lahtinen P, Kokki H, Hynynen M. Pain after cardiac surgery: a prospective cohort study of 1-year incidence and intensity. *Anesthesiology.* 2006; **105**: 794–800.

55. Green CR. Long-term follow-up cryoanalgesia for chronic thoracic pain. *Regional Anesthesia.* 1993; **18**: 46.

56. Jones MJ, Murrin KR. Intercostal block with cryotherapy. *Annals of the Royal College of Surgeons of England.* 1987; **69**: 261–2.

57. Riopelle JM, Everson C, Moustoukos N *et al.* Cryoanalgesia; Present data status. *Seminars in Anesthesia.* 1985; **4**: 305–12.

58. Evans PJ, Lloyd JW, Jack TM. Cryoanalgesia for intractable perineal pain. *Journal of the Royal Society of Medicine.* 1981; **74**: 804–09.

33

Radiofrequency lesioning and treatment of chronic pain

BEN JP CRUL, JAN HM VAN ZUNDERT, AND MAARTEN VAN KLEEF

KEY LEARNING POINTS

- High success rates of radiofrequency lesioning in patients with refractory trigeminal neuralgia.
- Percutaneous cordotomy, often efficacious in cancer pain, resistant to all other pain therapies.
- Limited evidence about the clinical effectiveness of radiofrequency lesioning for spinal pain: with better evidence for percutaneous facet denervation than for the treatment adjacent to the dorsal root ganglion and heating of the intervertebral disk.
- Evidence about the effectiveness of pulsed radiofrequency needs further substantiation.
- In patients with chronic nonmalignant pain, radiofrequency lesioning should be imbedded in a biopsychosocial setting.

INTRODUCTION

Percutaneous current lesions were introduced by Kirschner[1] in 1931 for the treatment of patients with trigeminal neuralgia. The reliability and simplicity of thermocoagulation led to its widespread use in the USA and Europe. In 1953, Sweet and Mark[2] proposed the application of a high-frequency current with frequencies ranging from 300 to 500 kHz, as used in radiotransmitters. Radiofrequency (RF) lesions were far more predictable than lesions produced by the earlier direct current procedures.

Another milestone was the introduction of the percutaneous cordotomy in 1965.[3] By a lateral approach through the C1–C2 intervertebral space, a heat lesion was made in the spinothalamic tract of the spinal cord. This method is mainly used in cancer patients with severe unilateral pain and remains an established technique for this indication. In 1974, after Sweet and Wepsic[4] applied RF lesioning for patients with trigeminal neuralgia, Uematsu[5] also treated patients with spinal pain syndromes by RF lesioning. Sluijter and Metha[6] refined earlier techniques by introducing a small-diameter (22 gauge) temperature-monitoring electrode system.[7]

THEORETICAL ASPECTS OF RADIOFREQUENCY LESIONING AND PULSED RADIOFREQUENCY

In RF lesioning, heat is generated in the tissue which surrounds the electrode by the RF current generated by a lesion apparatus. The RF voltage from the generator is set up between the (active) electrode and the (dispersive) groundplate, which is placed on the arm or leg of the patient. The body tissues complete the circuit and RF current flows through the tissue, resulting in an electric field.

This electric field creates an electric force on the ions in the tissue electrolytes, causing them to move back and forth at a high rate. Frictional dissipation of the ionic current within the fluid medium causes tissue heating. This is the origin of the RF lesion. The temperature of the surrounding tissue will show a rapid decrease over the first few millimeters from the electrode tip. The size of the lesion also depends on the diameter of the electrode and the length of the uninsulated electrode tip.

The rationale for the application of RF denervation is the assumption that selectively heating nervous structures can impede nociceptive input. Practically, this is achieved by percutaneous application of small electrodes at target neural tissues, to produce size-controlled lesions. However, others have questioned the utility of thermal lesioning in chronic nonmalignant pain, which is essentially neurodestructive, in the presence of neuropathic pain, and have shown that application of continuous low temperature RF is equally effective as RF heat lesion.[8][II]

In 1998, Sluijter et al.[9] applied high voltage RF current in bursts of 20 ms per 500 ms, permitting during 480 ms "silent phase," to allow the generated heat to be washed out. This idea of applying high voltage energy near a nerve without subsequent heat-induced nerve injury with pulsed radiofrequency (PRF) was appealing. Initial clinical investigations had shown that PRF could be used safely as an alternative to heat lesions in patients suffering from refractory pain.[9, 10] However, today, it is still not clear what the differences are between PRF and RF in terms of clinical outcome and biological mechanisms involved.

CLINICAL APPLICATION OF RADIOFREQUENCY LESIONING IN PAIN

Before treatment by RF lesioning is considered, the patient is seen in a biopsychosocial setting where, in addition to physicians, a psychologist and physical therapist also participate. In general, RF lesioning is indicated only in patients in whom noninvasive means of pain treatment have failed. Especially in patients with chronic nonmalignant pain, it is necessary to combine RF lesioning with other measures aiming at a correction of the pain-provoking conditions. Otherwise, the beneficial effects of RF lesioning will be short-lasting. In most cases, ergonomic and psychological advice is needed. Changes in the life pattern and working habits of the patient are often necessary to prevent the recurrence of pain (Boxes 33.1 and 33.2).

PERCUTANEOUS CERVICAL CORDOTOMY

History

In 1965, Mullan et al.[3][IV] performed their first percutaneous cervical cordotomy by a lateral approach through the C1–C2 intervertebral space. A heat lesion was made in the spinothalamic tract in the spinal cord, at first using a direct current, but later an RF current. Other means of reaching the spinothalamic tract are an anterolateral approach through the intervertebral disk or a posterior approach, but these techniques have never had widespread popularity.

Applied anatomy

The spinothalamic tract, situated in the anterolateral quadrant of the spinal cord, consists of secondary nociceptive neurons conveying nociceptive stimuli from the

---

Box 33.1 General contraindications of radiofrequency lesioning

- Coagulopathy.
- Local infection.
- Insufficient cooperation by the patient.

Box 33.2 Equipment needed for RF lesioning

- RF lesion generator provided with impedance registration, stimulation facilities, and thermocouple lesion system.
- Appropriate electrode needle and corresponding electrodes.
- Radiographic C-arm image intensifier.

contralateral body half. Its origin is in the dorsal horn of the spinal cord and its destination is mainly situated in the ventral posterior lateral and the central lateral nucleus of the thalamus. At the level C1–C2, the column of facetal joints is interrupted, allowing an approach to the spinal cord by a laterally introduced needle electrode.

Indications

Percutaneous cervical cordotomy is indicated in unilateral, incident, and/or neurogenic pain in advanced cancer patients resistant to other therapy. In exceptional cases, remaining pain on the contralateral side following an earlier cordotomy can be treated by a second cordotomy on the opposite site. There should be a minimum interval of two weeks between the interventions.

Limitations

Popularity of the intervention has decreased considerably following the introduction of rational oral analgesic therapy. A further decline in the number of patients treated occurred because of the application of continuous spinal infusion techniques. Nevertheless, the treatment still deserves an important place in the treatment of severe and resistant neurogenic pain in patients with a life expectancy of not more than one to two years.

Technique

It is essential that the patient is fully informed about the procedure and the sensations that he/she may experience during it. It should be stressed that his/her full cooperation is necessary to obtain an optimal result. A full neurological assessment is performed with special attention to the sensory qualities (touch, pain, temperature) and motor power functions.

The patient should be in a dorsal recumbent position. Under direct lateral vision by use of a C-arm image intensifier, a marker rule is placed on a spot midway on the anteroposterior border of the spinal canal at the level C1–C2. A 22-gauge spinal needle is inserted and advanced to reach the anterior part of the intrathecal space. To gauge the depth of insertion of the needle, lateral views can be alternated with anteroposterior projections. Once the needle is inside the intrathecal space, 3 mL cerebrospinal fluid (CSF) is aspirated into a 5-mL glass syringe. After the addition of 2 mL of contrast dye (Lipiodol Ultrafluide, a fatty iodated ester, manufactured by Guerbet Laboratoires, Aulnay-sous Bois, France), the syringe is shaken well until an emulsion appears. After intrathecal injection of the mixture, three lines become visible: the most anterior line shows the delineation of the anterior border of the spinal cord, the second line represents the dentate ligament, and the third line is the projection of the posterior dura mater (**Figures 33.1** and **33.2**). The target for insertion of the

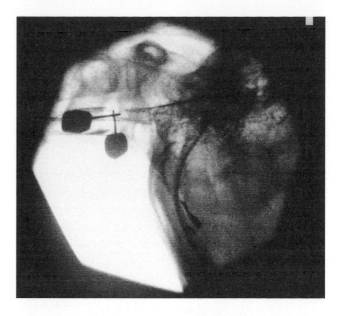

Figure 33.1 Percutaneous cordotomy, lateral view. After intrathecal injection through a 22-gauge spinal needle just ventral to the spinal cord of a mixture of iodated fatty acids (Lipiodol Ultrafluide) and aspirated CSF, three lines become visible: the most ventral line shows the delineation of the anterior border of the spinal cord, the second line represents the dentate ligament, and finally the third line is the projection of the dorsal dura mater. A second needle guiding the electrode is aimed at the target 1.0–1.5 mm ventral to the dentate ligament.

electrode is 1 mm anterior to the dentate ligament. A convenient trick is to introduce a small-bore hypodermic needle through the skin projecting just anterior to the dentate ligament as a marker. At this site, a 20-gauge electrode guiding needle is pierced through the skin and inserted in a direction perpendicular to the spinal cord. The trajectory of the needle is, therefore, in a horizontal plane. In the authors' experience, an upward (more ventral) direction carries the risk of pushing the spinal cord down by the electrode instead of the electrode entering it. During verification by alternating lateral and anteroposterior projections, the needle is advanced until the cervical dura is reached. This structure is usually rather resistant, and the utmost precaution has to be taken to prevent touching and subsequent damage of the spinal cord after an abrupt "give" of the dura. After the needle enters the intrathecal space, and after verification that its tip is just anterior to the dentate ligament, a Levin thermocouple electrode (Radionics, Burlington, MA, USA) is inserted through the needle. When the free tip of the electrode is inside the intrathecal space, the electrical impedance amounts to approximately 250–400 Ohm. After the needle tip has been introduced into the spinal cord, the impedance rises three- to four-fold. Stimulation with 2 Hz generally provokes contractions of the longus colli musculature at 0.5–1 V. Any other contractions are an indication that the tip of the electrode is in the corticospinal (motor) tract. A lesion here would provoke a paresis of the

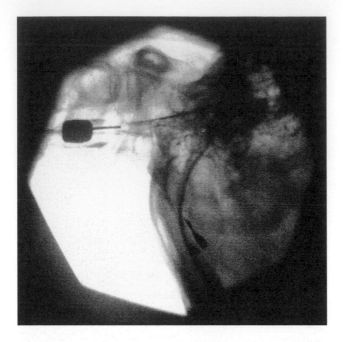

Figure 33.2 Percutaneous cordotomy, lateral view. The contrast needle is removed. The electrode-guiding needle is left in place and an RF lesion can be applied.

muscles situated within the projection of the interrupted nerve fibers. Repositioning of the needle more anteriorly is needed. Sensory tracts are identified by 50 Hz stimulation. When the tip of the electrode is inside the spinothalamic tract, intensities of 0.1–0.3 V can provoke temperature sensations (warmth or cold) in the corresponding part of the contralateral body half. After meticulous assessment of the correct position of the electrode tip by repeated stimulation, an RF lesion is made, resulting in a tip temperature of 90°C for ten seconds. Directly following the lesioning, pinprick tests are performed to assess the distribution of an analgesic area. Sometimes, one lesion is sufficient to attain freedom from pain. Mostly, two or three lesions are necessary with the needle tip in slightly different positions to reach this goal.

Complications

Complications are: paresis, 0.4–8 percent; urinary retention, 6–8 percent (mostly temporary); mirror pain, 6–54 percent; respiratory depression, 0–4 percent. Following a bilateral procedure, the occurrence of sleep apnea is reported.

Results

In approximately 70 percent of the patients treated by percutaneous cervical cordotomy (PCC), pain remains under control until death.[11][IV]

Side effects

The known side effects are changed body perception and loss of temperature sensation in segments under analgesia.

Discomfort of the procedure to the patient

This procedure can be very demanding for the patient, who has to be completely immobile in a supine position for 30–45 minutes. During assessment of the needle position and making the lesion, it is mandatory that the patient is fully aware of the procedure. Discomfort to the patient can be considerably alleviated by using repeated bolus injections or a continuous infusion of an ultra-short-acting opioid (e.g. remifentanil) during the procedure. Also, propofol can be used. Appropriate monitoring by pulse oximetry, electrocardiogram (ECG), and sphygmomanometry is mandatory.

RADIOFREQUENCY LESIONING OF THE GASSERIAN GANGLION

History

Percutaneous electric lesioning of the Gasserian ganglion has a long history, beginning in 1931 when Kirschner[1] first described the technique. Sweet and Wepsic[4] applied an RF current and improved the procedure. It is one of the techniques that has withstood the test of time. Together with microvascular decompression, RF lesioning of the Gasserian ganglion is one of the mainstays of nonpharmacological treatment of trigeminal neuralgia. Van Zundert et al.[10] used PRF treatment of the Gasserian ganglion in patients with idiopathic trigeminal neuralgia. A randomized controlled trial comparing the effect of RF with PRF of the Gasserian ganglion showed longer pain relief in the group treated with conventional RF.[12][II]

Applied anatomy

The Gasserian ganglion is situated in the middle cranial fossa, dorsal and cranial to the foramen ovale. The ophthalmic part is located medially and has the greatest distance to the foramen ovale. The maxillary cell bodies and nerve fibers are positioned centrally, whereas the mandibular section has the most lateral and superficial location. The position of the ganglion means that all parts can be reached by a needle entering through the foramen ovale.

The trigeminal nerve has a mixed composition. The motor fibers constitute the nervus intermedius, which accompanies the mandibular nerve and innervates the pterygoid, temporalis, and masseter muscles. The

Gasserian ganglion contains the cell bodies of the first-order sensory neurons of the trigeminal nerve. Medially, the Gasserian ganglion is next to the carotid artery and the cavernous sinus.

Indication

This technique is indicated for trigeminal neuralgia resistant to drug treatment. In young patients who want to avoid the risk of numbness of the face, and in patients with pain in the area innervated by the ophthalmic nerve, microvascular decompression may be considered.

Technique

The patient is placed in a horizontal recumbent position. The patient's head is fixed on a radiolucent head rest by an adhesive bandage. The intervention is performed under intermittent intravenous anesthesia with propofol. Great care must be taken to obtain an optimal picture of the foramen ovale. For this purpose, the C-arm of the image intensifier is placed in a caudal/cranial direction at an angle of approximately 45° to the horizontal plane and rotated 15–20° sideways. Consequently, a sub-orbital–occipital projection is obtained. The projection shows the ascending ramus and the angle of the mandible. The foramen ovale can be discerned medial to the ascending ramus. Subsequently, a marker ruler is placed on a spot on the skin overlying the projection of the foramen and an ink mark is made.

During the procedure, short periods of general anesthesia are necessary. Intermittent administration of propofol 1–1.5 mg/kg is a good choice. Under general anesthesia, a 22-gauge Sluijter–Metha (thermocouple) needle electrode with a 2-mm free tip (Radionics) is inserted at the ink-marked spot on the skin. The direction of the needle is the same as the direction of the radiation beam (tunnel-vision technique). The needle is guided through the musculature of the cheek by the left index finger, preventing piercing of the oral mucosa. If the oral mucosa is pierced, the needle has to be taken out and replaced by another sterile needle to avoid contamination of intracranial structures. Under fluoroscopic guidance, the needle is gradually pushed forward in the direction of the desired target within the foramen ovale (**Figure 33.3**). Once the needle enters the foramen, a clear "give" is perceived by the operator. During lateral fluoroscopy, the penetration of the needle into the skull base is verified when the end of the needle coincides with the intersection of the clivus and the os petrosum (**Figure 33.4**).

After the patient regains consciousness, electrical stimulation is applied. The patient should now feel paresthesiae in the painful area. Thresholds should be below 0.2 V. If stimulation yields a satisfactory outcome, the patient is anesthetized again and an RF lesion of 60–65°C

is made for a duration of 60 seconds. After awakening, a couple of minutes later, sensibility is tested by pinprick. Hyperesthesia should be present in the previously painful area. Special attention must be paid to verifying whether pain can still be elicited by tactile stimulation of the trigger area, related to the trigeminal neuralgia. If the test

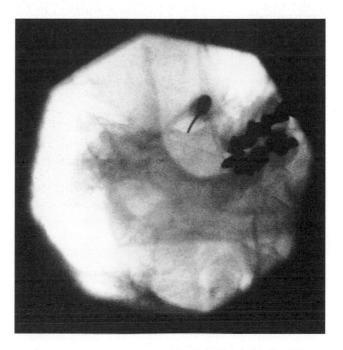

Figure 33.3 RF lesion of the Gasserian ganglion, suborbital–occipital projection. The ascending ramus and the angle of the mandible are visible. The electrode is inside the needle, which is placed in the central part of the foramen ovale.

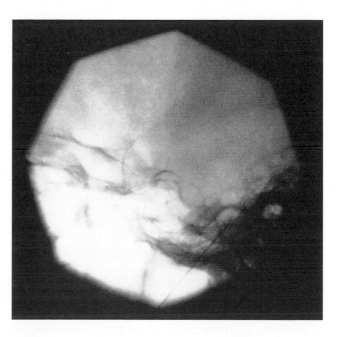

Figure 33.4 RF lesion of the Gasserian ganglion, lateral projection. The projection of the needle–electrode coincides with the intersection of the clivus and the os petrosum.

results are unsatisfactory, the needle position should be adjusted. It can be necessary to reintroduce the needle, changing its direction to enter the foramen ovale at a different angle. Some authors advocate the use of a curved electrode to produce a more selective lesion and a lower complication rate.

Results

Long-term (years) success rates vary from 80 to 90 percent. Sometimes, multiple treatments are necessary.[13, 14]

Side effects

Possible side effects include hyperesthesia of the treated trigeminal branch.

Complications and incidence

Complications include corneal anesthesia/hyperesthesia, 13.7 percent; dysesthesia in the treated area, 5–7 percent; masseter weakness, 1–2 percent.[13]

Discomfort of the procedure for the patient

The procedure can be performed during short-acting intravenous anesthesia on an outpatient basis. The procedure has a low morbidity; mortality has not been reported.

RADIOFREQUENCY LESIONING OF THE SPHENOPALATINE GANGLION

History

Neuroablation of the sphenopalatine ganglion for the treatment of cluster headache was first reported in the early 1970s. RF procedures were reported in 1988.[15]

Applied anatomy

The sphenopalatine ganglion is an autonomous ganglion containing parasympathetic and sympathetic fibers. The ganglion is situated within the fossa sphenopalatina, just lateral to the foramen sphenopalatina, and has close relationships with the maxillary nerve and its branches (nervi alveolares). The foramen sphenopalatinum connects the fossa sphenopalatinum with the cavum nasi. The fossa can be reached by a laterally placed needle entering through the triangle formed by the zygoma and the muscular and articular processus of the mandible.

Indications

This procedure is indicated by cluster headaches that are unreactive to conservative therapy (drugs, oxygen).[15]

Technique

The patient is placed in a horizontal recumbent position. The head is fixed on a radiolucent headrest by an adhesive bandage. Although the procedure can be carried out under local anesthesia, intermittent intravenous anesthesia is preferred because the introduction of the needle is painful.

Under lateral fluoroscopic projection, the projection of the sphenopalatine fossa can be seen in its narrow triangular form. A marker ruler is placed on the projection of the foramen sphenopalatinum and an ink dot made on the skin overlying the target.

The needle is inserted more caudally, just inferior to the zygoma, and directed medially. Often, several attempts are needed to direct the needle to the fossa, as bony structures can obstruct the passage. In our experience, it is virtually always possible to arrive at the desired target (**Figures 33.5** and **33.6**). It is important that the needle is not directed too far cranially as this risks the needle entering the dorsal part of the orbita. In the lateral fluoroscopic projection, this is at the cranial part of the fossa. In the anteroposterior fluoroscopic projection, the needle tip just projects over the ipsilateral os nasale. The target is localized approximately 6–7 cm under the skin.

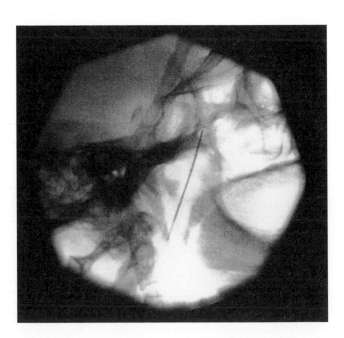

Figure 33.5 RF lesioning of the sphenopalatine ganglion, lateral projection. The projection of the sphenopalatine fossa can be seen in its narrow triangular form. The electrode tip is positioned in the foramen sphenopalatinum.

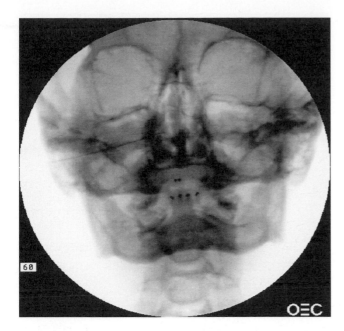

Figure 33.6 RF lesioning of the sphenopalatine ganglion, anteroposterior projection. The tip of the electrode is projected slightly medial to the right os nasale.

In the awake patient, stimulation is performed using a 50-Hz current. Paresthesiae should not be felt at <1.0 V. Otherwise, the tip of the electrode is too near to the maxillary nerve. Damage to this nerve can cause numbness and dysesthesia.

When the electrode is in the correct position, an RF lesion is made at 80°C for 60 seconds, concluding the procedure.

Indication

The indication for this procedure is cluster headache.

Results

In episodic cluster headache, complete pain relief has been achieved in 60 percent of patients. In chronic cluster headache, complete relief has been achieved in 30 percent of patients.[15]

Complications

The following complications have been observed: hyperesthesia due to involvement of the maxillary nerve (5 percent), epistaxis, cheek hematomas (10 percent), and bleeding of the nasal mucosa (needle entering the cavum nasi via the foramen sphenoplatimum).

Efficacy of treatment

Studies on the results of the technique are scarce. Controlled studies are not available. Sanders and Zuurmond[16]

[IV] reported on a series of 66 patients with cluster headache. RF lesioning of the sphenopalatine ganglion resulted in complete remission in 67 percent of patients, whereas partial relief was obtained in 18 percent.

RADIOFREQUENCY LESIONING FOR THE TREATMENT OF SPINAL PAIN

Applied anatomy of the spine

The innervation of the spine is complex and has been well described by Bogduk.[17] The spine can be divided into dorsal and ventral compartments.

Dorsal compartment

The dorsal compartment of the spine contains the facet joints (zygapophyseal joints), the dorsal part of the dura, and intrinsic neck/back muscles and ligaments. The dorsal compartment of the spine is innervated by the posterior primary ramus, which branches off the segmental nerve immediately after it exits from its foramen. It runs in a groove formed by the superior articular and transverse processes, where it divides into a medial and a lateral branch.

Ventral compartment

The ventral compartment contains the vertebral bodies, disks, anterior and posterior longitudinal ligaments, ventral dura, and prevertebral muscles. Innervation of the ventral compartment is not related to single nerves, but more to interconnected neural networks in the anterior and posterior longitudinal ligaments and ventral dura. Fibers from the nervous plexus in the posterior longitudinal ligament innervate the outer layer of the dorsal aspect of the annulus fibrosus. This plexus is mainly formed by branches from bilateral sinuvertebral nerves. The nervous plexus in the anterior longitudinal ligament, supplied with fibers from the sympathetic, the rami communicantes, and perivascular plexuses, innervates the anterior part of the annulus fibrosus bilaterally and multisegmentally.

RADIOFREQUENCY LESIONING IN THE CERVICAL AREA

RF treatment for cervical pain syndromes is utilized for the following main diagnostic categories:

- Cervical pain, defined as pain originating from the facet joints or from the intervertebral disk.[17, 18]
- Cervicobrachialgia, defined as pain originating from the cervical spine radiating from the neck beyond the

glenohumeral joint into the upper limb with referral to a particular spinal segment.

- Cervicogenic headache is a clinically defined headache syndrome hypothesized to originate from cervical nociceptive structures. The structures responsible for it have not been defined.[19] Each different pain syndrome may have more than one nociceptive source. As a consequence, more than one RF treatment modality may be required to relieve the patient's pain.

Two RF procedures in the cervical area are applied to reduce nociception:

1. Percutaneous cervical facetal joint denervation.
2. RF lesion of the dorsal root ganglion.

PERCUTANEOUS CERVICAL FACETAL JOINT DENERVATION BY RADIOFREQUENCY LESIONING

Indications

- Nociceptive pain emanating from the facetal joint.
- Clinical manifestations:
  - localized cervical pain;
  - cervicogenic headache.

Technique

For an RF lesion of the medial branch of the dorsal ramus in the upper and middle cervical area, the patient is positioned prone on the operating table. The C-arm is positioned slightly oblique so that the beam of radiation is parallel to the axis of the intervertebral foramen, which is upwards and slightly caudal. In this position of the C-arm, the segmental nerves exit parallel to the line of the radiation beam. Since the electrodes will be introduced from the posterolateral side, this projection will make it easy to maintain a safe distance between the electrode tip and the exciting segmental nerve. The dorsal ramus in this projection runs over the base of the superior articular process, which is clearly visible (**Figures 33.7** and **33.8**). Entry points are marked posterior to the posterior border of the facetal column and slightly caudal to the target point. A Sluijter–Metha (SMK), 22-gauge, C5 cannula with a 4-mm active tip (Radionics), or alternatively a TOP XE 6 needle (COTOP, Amsterdam, The Netherlands), is introduced and carefully advanced anteriorly and cranially until contact is made with the facetal column at the target point. The position of the C-arm is then changed to the anterior–posterior (AP) direction. This should confirm the position of the tip of the electrode adjacent to the "waist" of the articular pillars of the cervical spine at the corresponding level.

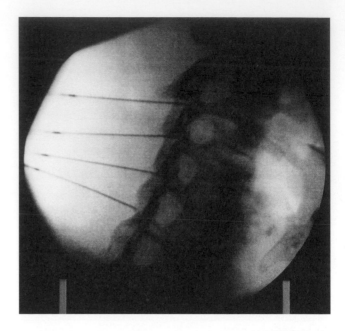

Figure 33.7 Percutaneous cervical facetal joint denervation by RF lesioning. Oblique view. In the transverse plane, the angle of the C-arm with the horizontal is about 30° and in the sagittal plane it is 75–80°. The needle tips are projecting on the base of the superior articular processes.

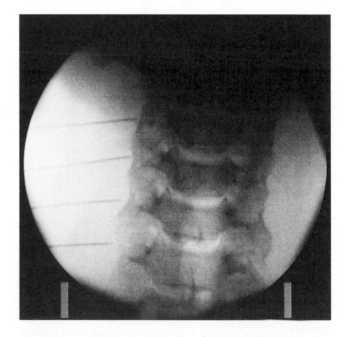

Figure 33.8 Percutaneous cervical facetal joint denervation by RF lesioning in the AP direction. The tips of the electrodes are adjacent to the "waist" of the articular pillars of the cervical spine at the corresponding levels.

At the C2 level, the electrode should be aimed at the small branches of the C2–C3 facet joint and not at the medial branch of C2, which is the greater occipital nerve. A suitable electrode placement is at the arch of C2 at the level of the upper border of foramen C3.

After this anatomical localization, electrical stimulation at a rate of 50 Hz should elicit a response (tingling sensation) in the neck at < 0.5 V. On motor stimulation at 2 Hz, there must be no muscle movements in the ipsilateral shoulder/arm. However, contractions of the multifidus muscles are often visible. After this physiological control, the medial branch of the dorsal ramus is anesthetized with 1–2 mL local anesthetic solution (lidocaine (lignocaine) 10 mg/mL), and an 80°C RF thermolesion is made for 60 seconds at each level. When a TOP XE needle is used, 20 V over 60 seconds is applied, resulting in a heating of the relevant tissue to a temperature of 80°C. When performing this technique, one should take care not to insert the needle too close to the mixed segmental nerve. A lesion should not be applied when muscle contractions occur at 2 Hz stimulation at a voltage less than 1.0 V.

Side effects

There have been no reports in the literature of complications from cervical facet joint denervation when the procedure is performed as described above. There may be some postoperative burning pain in 10–20 percent of patients that disappears spontaneously after some weeks.

Results

In 1996, Lord et al.[20][II] performed a randomized, double-blind, controlled trial in patients with chronic pain of the lower cervical facet joints after whiplash injury. They concluded that in patients with chronic facet joint pain, confirmed with double-blind, placebo-controlled local anesthetic blocks, percutaneous RF neurotomy with multiple lesions of target nerves can provide long-lasting pain relief. Another more recent study indicated that pain relief was observed in 71 percent of patients after the initial procedure. The median duration of pain relief was 219 days if failures are included, but 422 days when only successful cases are considered.[21]

PERCUTANEOUS RADIOFREQUENCY LESIONING OF THE CERVICAL DORSAL ROOT GANGLION

Indication

Percutaneous RF lesioning of the cervical DRG is indicated in nociceptive pain emanating from one segment in the cervical area. Most patients present with a cervicobrachial pain or cervicogenic headache.

The level involved in the pain syndrome is selected by means of diagnostic segmental nerve blocks.

Contraindication

Sensory deficit in the painful area.

Technique

DIAGNOSTIC ROOT BLOCKS

For the selection of the putative pain-conducting nerve root, a series of consecutive selective root blocks is performed. In this technique, the C-arm is positioned in such a way that the direction of the radiation beam is parallel to the axis of the foramen. In the transverse plane, this axis has an angle to the horizontal of 25–35°, and in the sagittal plane an angle of 75–80° to the horizontal. With the C-arm in this position, the entry point is found by projecting a metal ruler over the caudal part of the foramen. A 50-mm, 22-gauge neurography needle (Radionics) is inserted in the direction of the radiation beam and directed to the caudal part of the foramen (**Figure 33.9**). In this "tunnel-vision" projection, the needle should appear as a dot on the monitor screen. The direction of the radiation beam is than changed to anteroposterior, and the cannula is further introduced until the tip is projected just lateral from the facetal column. After identifying the segmental nerve root with 0.5 mL contrast dye (iohexol; Omnipaque 250),

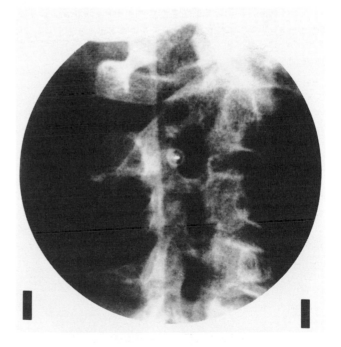

Figure 33.9 RF lesioning of the cervical dorsal root ganglion. The C-arm is positioned in such a way that the direction of the radiation beam is parallel to the axis of the foramen. In the transverse plane, the angle with the horizontal is approximately 30°, and in the sagittal plane is approximately 15–20°. In "tunnel-vision" projection, the needle is seen as a dot on the monitor screen.

0.5 mL of lidocaine 20 mg/mL is slowly injected. The position of the needle tip is critical because if the placement is too medial this results in epidural overflow, whereas if the placement is too lateral this can lead to spread of the local anesthetic into the nervous plexus, neither resulting in a selective block.[22]

RADIOFREQUENCY LESIONING AND PULSED RADIOFREQUENCY DORSAL ROOT GANGLION

After identification of the pain conduction nerve root, an RF lesion of the dorsal root ganglion (DRG) can be performed. The same viewing technique and entry point is used as described in the diagnostic segmental root block technique.

The cannula (Radionics SMK C5 with a 4-mm exposed tip) is introduced in the direction of the radiation beam and advanced until the electrode appears on the screen as a dot. In practice, this dot should lie directly over the dorsal part of the intervertebral foramen at the transition between the middle one-third and the most caudal one-third. This dorsal position is chosen in order to avoid possible damage to the motor fibers of the segmental nerve and to the vertebral artery which runs anterior to the ventral part of the foramen (**Figure 33.10**). The direction of the radiation beam is then changed to anteroposterior and the cannula is further advanced until the tip is projected over the middle of the facetal column (**Figure 33.11**).

The stylet is now replaced by the RF electrode probe. After checking the impedance, electrical stimulation is started at a rate of 50 Hz. The patient should feel a tingling sensation at voltages between 0.4 and 0.65 V. Next, the frequency is changed to 2 Hz, and the patient is observed for muscle contractions. These should not occur below a voltage of 1.5 times the sensory threshold. Afterwards, 0.5 mL of contrast medium (Omnipaque) is injected, to exclude an accidental intradural or intravascular position of the electrode, and 2 mL of local anesthetic solution (lidocaine 20 mg/mL) is administered. An RF current is applied through the electrode in order to increase the temperature at the tip slowly to 67°C for 60 seconds.

Pulsed RF lesioning of DRG has been studied recently. The PRF current is applied for 120 seconds.[9, 23]

Side effects

A side effect which is often seen after radiofrequency lesioning (40–60 percent) is a mild burning sensation in the treated dermatome, which subsides spontaneously after some weeks. This burning pain is probably the result of swelling in the vicinity of the segmental nerve. A slight hypoesthesia may occur, but usually disappears after several months. After pulsed radiofrequency, no neurologic complications have been mentioned up to now.

Efficacy of treatment

There are several publications in the literature evaluating the results of RF lesioning in chronic cervical pain and cervicobrachialgia using 22-gauge equipment.

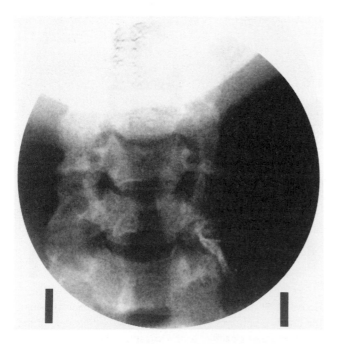

Figure 33.10 RF lesioning of the cervical dorsal root ganglion. C-arm in the anteroposterior direction. The cannula is introduced until the tip is projected midway to the facetal column. Injection of contrast dye makes the nerve root visible.

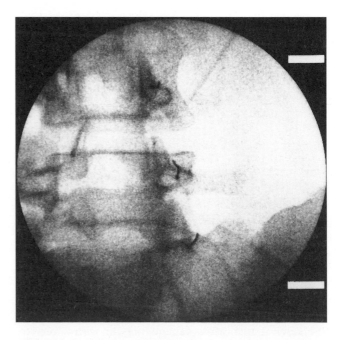

Figure 33.11 RF lesioning of the lumbar dorsal root ganglion. The tip of the electrode is placed in the craniodorsal part of the foramen.

In a prospective double blind randomized study of 20 patients with chronic intractable pain in the cervical region radiating to the head, shoulder, and/or arm, Van Kleef et al.[24][II] showed initial pain relief in 75 percent of patients after three months and in 50 percent of patients after six months.

A study comparing groups treated with 67°C and those treated with 40°C RF lesions could not demonstrate any difference.[25][II] A possible explanation given by the authors for lack of differences between the two groups is that a 40°C lesion is also an active treatment.

Studies about the efficacy of RF DRG in cervicogenic headache are not available.

The effect of PRF treatment patients with chronic cervical radicular pain was evaluated in a prospective audit that showed satisfactory pain relief for a mean period of 9.2 months, justifying a randomized sham controlled trial.

Twenty-three patients, out of 256 screened, met the inclusion criteria and were randomly assigned in a double-blind fashion to either receive PRF or sham intervention. The evaluation was carried out by an independent observer.

At three months, the PRF group showed a significantly better outcome with regard to the global perceived effect (>50 percent improvement) and visual analog scale (20 point pain reduction). The quality of life scales also showed a positive trend in favor of the PRF group but significance was only reached in the SF-36 domain vitality at three months. The need for pain medication was significantly reduced in the PRF group after six months. No complications were observed during the study period.

These study results are in agreement with the findings of a previous clinical audit that PRF treatment of the cervical DRG may provide prolonged pain relief in carefully selected patients with chronic cervical radicular pain.[26][II]

RADIOFREQUENCY LESIONING IN THE LUMBAR AREA

Spinal pain located in the lumbar area is frequently encountered in medical practice. Some studies indicate that 70–80 percent of the adult working population experience lumbar pain at some stage of their life. In less than 15 percent of patients, specific pathology is found such as disk herniation, spondylolisthesis, spinal stenosis, or infections. In the remaining patients, the pain resolves within a few weeks, and in approximately two months 80 percent of patients return to normal function. In about 5–12 percent of this population, the complaints last for a longer period; generally, after a duration of six months, spontaneous relief from pain is often not complete.

PERCUTANEOUS RADIOFREQUENCY LUMBAR FACETAL JOINT DENERVATION

Indication

Percutaneous RF lumbar facetal joint denervation is indicated in mechanical low back pain emanating from the facetal joints.

Patients are selected for the RF procedure after a positive response to a diagnostic block of the medial branch of the dorsal ramus.

Technique

With the patient prone on the operating table, the C-arm image intensifier is positioned in a slightly (10–15°) oblique position until the junction between the superior border of the transverse process and the lateral aspect of the superior articular process is clearly visible at the levels L4 and L5, and the junction of the ala of the sacrum and the articular process of the sacrum at level S1 is also visible. In these locations, the medial branches of the posterior primary rami of the L3, L4, and L5 segmental nerves run in a posterior direction on their way to the groove on the posterior aspect of the base of the transverse process or of the sacral ala, respectively. Entry points are marked overlying these junctions and the area is disinfected and draped. A 22-gauge SMK C10 cannula with a 5-mm active tip is introduced at each entry point in the direction of the radiation beam. Each of the three cannulas is carefully advanced, checking the proper direction following each step until the tip makes contact with bone at the posterior aspect of the junction. The cannula is then redirected in a slightly more cranial and lateral direction until contact with bone is lost. The position of the cannula is then checked on the lateral fluoroscopic projection. The depth is adjusted until the tip of the cannula is at the level of a line connecting the posterior aspects of the intervertebral foramina (**Figure 33.12**).

The stylet of the cannula is replaced by an RF probe and electrostimulation at 2 Hz is carried out to confirm the proximity of the electrode to the medial branch and to exclude inadvertent proximity to the exiting segmental nerve. When muscle contractions in the multifidus muscle do not occur below a voltage of 1.0 V, the cannula is repositioned. The absence of contractions of leg muscles is verified at 1.5 V. Once the position of the electrode is satisfactory, the RF probe is removed from the cannula and 1 mL of lidocaine 10 mg/mL is injected through each cannula. The RF probe is then reinserted and a 60-second 80°C lesion is made. When a TOP XE needle is used, 20 V for 60 seconds is applied to the electrode. PRF treatment of the lumbar facetal joints was recently studied, applying the PRF current over four minutes.[27][III]

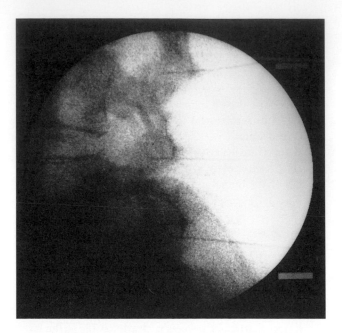

Figure 33.12 RF lesioning of the lumbar dorsal root ganglion. In the anteroposterior projection, the tip of the electrode should be projected on a line connecting the facetal joints.

Side effects

Although no side effects have been reported after RF lumbar facetal joint denervation, caution should be taken that the electrode is not too close to the segmental nerve (check lateral view).

Efficacy of treatment

The first prospective, controlled, double-blind randomized study to assess the efficacy of RF facet joint denervation was conducted by Gallagher *et al.*[28] After diagnostic blocks, 41 patients were randomized as they entered the study to undergo either RF facet joint denervation or a placebo procedure, which was identical in every way apart from the heat lesion. The study showed a significant improvement in pain scores following denervation at one and six months when compared with the placebo group. A recent randomized study indicated that RF lesioning of the medial branch of the primary posterior ramus results in a significant alleviation of pain and functional disability in a selected group of patients with chronic nonspecific low back pain.[29] Of the 42 patients who underwent RF treatment, 45 percent reported at least 50 percent pain relief two years after treatment or at the last follow up. This relief of pain was associated with an improvement in most activities in the patient's daily life. A randomized controlled trial comparing RF with PRF of the medial branches of dorsal rami in the treatment of facetal pain showed longer lasting pain relief with conventional RF.[27][III]

RADIOFREQUENCY LESION OF THE LUMBAR DORSAL ROOT GANGLION

Indication

RF lesion of the dorsal lumbar root ganglion is indicated in radicular pain without sensory motor function disturbances.

Nerve root pain is characterized by dermatomal spread, usually into the lower leg and often into the foot. The main clinical symptoms are irradiating pain in a dermatome, and pain on straight leg raising. The diagnosis is established by pain relief after a selective nerve root block. If there is no sensory deficit, an RF lesion of the dorsal ganglion has been proposed.[30]

Contraindication

Sensory deficit in the painful area.

Technique

DIAGNOSTIC ROOT BLOCKS

For the selection of the putative pain-conducting nerve root, a series of consecutive selective root blocks is performed. With the patient prone on the operating table, the C-arm is positioned in the AP direction. A 100-mm 22-gauge neurography needle (Radionics) is introduced at an entry point 8 cm from the midline and 4 cm caudal to the relevant transverse process. The electrode is carefully advanced in the direction of the caudal part of the corpus vertebrae until the tip is projected just lateral from the facetal column. After identifying the segmental nerve root with 0.5 mL contrast dye (Omnipaque 250), 0.5 mL of lidocaine 2 percent is slowly injected.

RADIOFREQUENCY LESION

An SMK C10 (100 mm) cannula with a 5-mm active tip is introduced at an entry point 8 cm from the midline and 4 cm caudal to the relevant transverse process. The electrode is carefully advanced to make contact with the junction of the lower border of the transverse process and the lamina. It is then manipulated slightly caudally and anteriorly until it slips into the craniodorsal part of the foramen. It is advanced until the tip is projected over the middle of the facetal column (**Figures 33.13** and **33.14**). Next, the posterior position in the foramen is confirmed on the transverse projection. The stylet is now replaced by an RF probe. After checking the impedance, electrical stimulation is started at 50 Hz. The patient should feel a tingling sensation at voltages between 0.4 and 0.65 V.

The frequency is then changed to 2 Hz and the patient is observed for muscle contractions. These should not

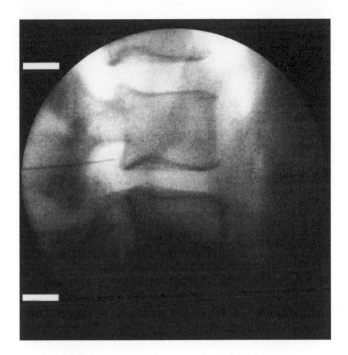

Figure 33.13 RF lesioning of the lumbar dorsal root ganglion, lateral projection. The tip of the electrode is visible in the craniodorsal part of the foramen.

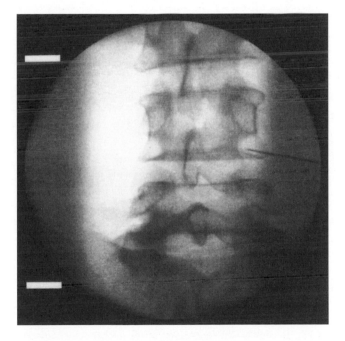

Figure 33.14 RF lesioning of the lumbar dorsal root ganglion, anteroposterior projection. The tip of the electrode is visible medial to the lateral border of the vertebra at a line connecting the openings of the facetal joints between the first and fourth lumbar vertebra.

occur below a voltage of 1.5 times the sensory threshold. Omnipaque (0.5 mL) is then injected in order to exclude an accidental intradural positioning of the electrode, and this is followed by 2 mL lidocaine 20 mg/mL.

RF current is then applied through the electrode (Radionics RFG 3) to increase the temperature at the tip to 67°C. The temperature is maintained for 60 seconds.

For L5, the approach may be more difficult owing to the iliac crest. The utilization of tunnel vision is then preferable. The dorsal root ganglion of S1 cannot be reached with a straight instrument. For an RF DRG at this level, a small hole has to be drilled with a Kirschner wire into the dorsal aspect of the sacrum.

Efficacy of treatment

A recent randomized trial using the reduction of pain, change in physical activities, and use of analgesics as its primary outcome criteria, could not demonstrate an efficacy of a 67°C RF lesion compared with placebo treatment.[30][II]

RADIOFREQUENCY LESIONING OF THE LUMBAR SYMPATHETIC GANGLIA

Indication

Diffuse pain in the leg with autonomic dysfunction. In patients with neuropathic radicular pain, autonomic symptoms are observed quite frequently. Patients present with a nonsegmental pain in the leg in combination with diffuse sensory loss and a cold extremity. The diagnosis of sympathetically maintained pain can be asserted by diagnostic sympathetic blocks. If temporary pain relief is achieved with these blocks, RF lesioning of the sympathetic chain may be considered.

Contraindication

Following a diagnostic block, only a temperature rise of the leg is observed without a concomitant pain reduction. Here, an RF lesion can result in an increase of pain.

Technique

This block is usually performed at the L3 and L4 levels. With the patient prone on the operating table, the C-arm is positioned in an oblique direction so that the spinous processes are projected over the facetal joint column of the opposite side. An entry point is selected overlying the side of the vertebral body at the junction of the lower and middle third of the vertebra. A 20-gauge SMK C15 cannula with a 10-mm active tip is introduced under tunnel vision. It is carefully advanced, passing cranial to the segmental nerve and avoiding contact with the periosteum of the vertebral body.

The position is then checked on the transverse and AP projections. The tip should lie level with the anterior margin of the vertebra and just medial to the middle of the facetal column. This is important to avoid damage to the ilioinguinal nerve. Injection of contrast should show the typical spread of contrast. To exclude the involvement of somatic nerve structures (e.g. nervus ilioinguinalis, nervus genitofemoralis), stimulation with 50 Hz is applied. During stimulation with an intensity up to 2 V, no sensations may be felt in the distribution areas of these nerves. Subsequently, 2 mL lidocaine 20 mg/mL is injected and an 80°C RF lesioning is applied for 60 seconds.

Side effects

Side effects include temporary swollen and hot foot on the treated side. The side effects subside in one to two weeks.

Complications

Complications include neuritis of the ilioinguinal or genitofemoral nerve and complaints of burning dysesthetic pain in the inguinal region and the inner side of the thigh.

Efficacy of treatment

More than in neurolytic blocks, the exact positioning of the needle (electrode) tip is of crucial importance. Only when the needle is in the direct vicinity of the sympathetic ganglion does a lesion result in neurolysis. A study comparing the results of RF lesioning or phenol injection showed a distinct superiority of the latter.[31][IV]

REFERENCES

1. Kirschner M. Zur Elektrochirurgie. *Langenbecks Archiv für Klinische Chirurgie*. 1931; **167**: 761–8.
2. Sweet WH, Mark VH. Unipolar anodal electrolytic lesion in the brain of man and cat: report of five human cases with electrically produced bulbar or mesencephalic tractotomies. *Archives of Neurology and Psychiatry*. 1953; 70: 224–334.
3. Mullan S, Hekmatpah J, Dobben G. Percutaneous intramedullary chordotomy utilizing the unipolar anodal electric lesion. *Journal of Neurosurgery*. 1965; **22**: 548–3.
4. Sweet WH, Wepsic JG. Controlled thermocoagulation of trigeminal ganglion and rootlets for differential destruction of pain fibers. Part I. Trigeminal. *Journal of Neurosurgery*. 1974; **39**: 143–56.
5. Uematsu S. Percutaneous electrocoagulation of spinal nerve trunk, ganglion and rootlets. In: Schmidel H, Sweet WH (eds). *Operative neurosurgical techniques: indications, methods and results*. New York: Grune and Stratton, 1982: 1171–98.
6. Sluijter ME, Metha M. Treatment of chronic back pain and neck pain by percutaneous thermal lesions. In: Lipton S (ed.). *Persistent pain, modern methods of treatment*, vol. 3. London: Academic Press, 1981: 141–79.
* 7. Stolker RJ, Vervest AC, Groen GJ. The management of chronic spinal pain by blockades: a review. *Pain*. 1994; **58**: 1–20.
8. Slappendel R, Crul BJ, Braak GJ *et al.* The efficacy of radiofrequency lesioning of the cervical spinal dorsal root ganglion in a double blinded randomized study: no difference between 40 degrees C and 67 degrees C treatments. *Pain*. 1997; **73**: 159–63.
9. Sluijter ME, Cosman ER, Rittman IIWB, van Kleef M. The effects of pulsed radiofrequency field applied to the dorsal root ganglion – a preliminary report. *Pain Clinic*. 1998; **11**: 109–17.
* 10. Van Zundert J, Brabant S, Van de Kelft E *et al.* Pulsed radiofrequency treatment of the Gasserian ganglion in patients with idiopathic trigeminal neuralgia. *Pain*. 2003; **104**: 449–52.
11. Crul BJP, Blok LM, Van Egmond J, Van Dongen RTM. The actual role of percutaneous cordotomy in cancer patients. *Journal of Headache and Pain*. 2005; **6**: 24–9.
12. Erdine S, Ozyalcin NS, Cimen A *et al.* Comparison of pulsed radiofrequency with conventional radiofrequency in the treatment of idiopathic trigeminal neuralgia. *European Journal of Pain*. 2007; **11**: 309–13.
13. Taha JM, Tew JM. Treatment of trigeminal neuralgia by percutaneous radiofrequency rhizotomy. *Neurosurgery Clinics of North America*. 1997; **8**: 31–9.
14. Kanpolat Y, Savas A, Bekar A, Berk C. Percutaneous controlled radiofrequency trigeminal rhizotomy for the treatment of idiopathic trigeminal neuralgia: 25-year experience with 1,600 patients. *Neurosurgery*. 2001; **48**: 524–32; discussion 532–4.
15. Sluijter ME, Vercruysse PJ, Sterk W. Radiofrequency lesions of the sphenopalatine ganglion neuralgia. *Schmerz/Pain/Douleur*. 1988; **9**: 56–9.
16. Sanders M, Zuurmond WWA. Efficacy of sphenopalatine ganglion blockades in 66 patients suffering from cluster headache: a 12- to 70-months follow-up evaluation. *Journal of Neurosurgery*. 1997; **87**: 876–80.
* 17. Bogduk N. The innervation of the lumbar spine. *Spine*. 1983; **8**: 286–93.
18. Dwyer A, Aprill C, Bogduk N. Cervical zygapophyseal joint pain patterns. I. A study in normal volunteers. *Spine*. 1990; **15**: 453–7.
19. Sjaastad O, Saunte C, Howdahl H *et al.* Cervicogenic headache. An hypothesis. *Cephalalgia*. 1983; **3**: 249–56.
20. Lord S, Barnsley L, Wallis B *et al.* Percutaneous radiofrequency neurotomy for chronic cervical zygapophyseal joint pain. *New England Journal of Medicine*. 1996; **335**: 1721–6.

21. McDonald GJ, Lord SM, Bogduk N. Long-term follow-up of patients with cervical radiofrequency neurotomy for chronic neck pain. *Neurosurgery.* 1999; **45**: 61–7.

22. Van Kleef M, Spaans F, Dingemans W *et al.* Effects and side effects of a percutaneous thermal lesion of the dorsal root ganglion in patients with cervical pain syndrome. *Pain.* 1993; **52**: 49–53.

23. Van Zundert J, Patijn J, Kessels A *et al.* Pulsed radiofrequency adjacent to the cervical dorsal root ganglion in chronic cervical radicular pain: a double blind sham controlled randomized clinical trial. *Pain.* 2007; **127**: 173–82.

∗ 24. Van Kleef M, Liem L, Lousberg R *et al.* Radiofrequency lesion adjacent to the dorsal root ganglion for cervicobrachial pain: a prospective double blind randomized study. *Neurosurgery.* 1996; **38**: 1127–32.

25. Slappendel R, Crul BJP, Braak GJJ *et al.* The efficacy of radiofrequency lesioning of the cervical spinal dorsal root ganglion in a double blind randomized study: no difference between 40 and 67 centigrade treatments. *Pain.* 1997; **73**: 159–63.

26. Van Zundert J, Lamé IE, de Louw A *et al.* Percutaneous pulsed radiofrequency treatment of the cervical dorsal root ganglion in the treatment of chronic cervical pain syndromes: a clinical audit. *Neuromodulation.* 2003; **6**: 6–14.

27. Tekin I, Mirzai H, Ok G *et al.* A comparison of conventional and pulsed radiofrequency denervation in the treatment of chronic facet joint pain. *Clinical Journal of Pain.* 2007; **23**: 524–9.

28. Gallagher J, Petricciore PL, Wedley JR *et al.* Radiofrequency facet joint denervation in the treatment of low back pain: a prospective controlled double-blind study to assess its efficacy. *Pain Clinic.* 1994; **7**: 193–8.

∗ 29. Van Kleef N, Barendse GAB, Kessel A *et al.* Randomized trial of radiofrequency lumbar facet denervation for chronic low back pain. *Spine.* 1999; **24**: 1937–42.

∗ 30. Geurts JWM, Van Wijk RMAW, Wynne HJ *et al.* Radiofrequency thermal lesion of the dorsal root ganglion for chronic lumbosacral radicular pain. A randomised, double blind sham-lesion controlled trial. In: Geurts JWM, Van Wijk RMAW (eds). *Minimally invasive procedures in the treatment of chronic low back pain.* Thesis. Utrecht: University of Utrecht, 2001.

31. Haynsworth RF, Noe CE. Percutaneous lumbar sympathectomy: a comparison of radiofrequency denervation versus phenol neurolysis. *Anesthesiology.* 1991; **74**: 459–63.

34

Spinal cord stimulation

SIMON THOMSON AND MALVERN MAY

KEY LEARNING POINTS

- Spinal cord stimulation (SCS) is indicated for the control of neuropathic pain of peripheral origin and of ischemia-related pain. Emerging indications include pain of visceral origin.
- The evoked paresthesiae must topographically map the affected pain region in order to have a pain-relieving effect.
- SCS is not a stand-alone treatment and should be applied within a multidisciplinary management setting in order to achieve good long-lasting results.
- SCS should be carried out by experienced (if not, then supervised) clinicians skilled in the implant technique.
- Care pathways and clinical networks should be developed to ensure that all patients who would benefit from SCS have access to it.
- The efficacy of SCS in reducing pain and disability is dependent on good patient selection. Explanation of the therapy to patients to produce appropriate patient expectation is essential.
- All implants should be carried out within an operating theater environment. Prophylactic antibiotics against skin commensal bacteria are given during the procedure.

- The stimulating electrodes can be implanted percutaneously through epidural needles under image intensifier assistance or under direct vision using a surgical laminotomy. The chosen method should be based upon the interests of the patient first and preferred choice of the implanter second.
- This reversible therapy allows the patient to be tested to see if the SCS effect is beneficial in the short term. Although this makes intuitive sense, there remains a debate as to whether long-term benefits can be accurately predicted from a short-term trial period and what the ideal trial period should be.
- Complications involving permanent neurological harm are very rare. However, biological and implant complications are quite common over the lifespan of the implant. Improvements in technology and implant technique will reduce these complications.
- The implanter has a duty of care to the patient for the period of implantation. It is essential that appropriate follow up and communication arrangements are made as the lifetime of the implant dictates.

INTRODUCTION

SCS (formerly known as dorsal column stimulation) has evolved considerably over the last four decades.[1, 2] Neuromodulation is a family of treatments with SCS the most common, and is defined as the reversible therapeutic interaction of activity of the central, peripheral, and autonomic nervous system with electrical or centrally applied pharmacological agents.

The Gate Control theory of pain in its simplest form explained how nociceptive information could be modulated peripherally and centrally by other nonnociceptive sensory activity.[3] This simple model, however, does not fully explain the pain-relieving qualities of SCS since experience and investigation have shown that SCS is not helpful in nociceptive pain but rather neuropathic pain of peripheral origin and ischemic pain. The mechanisms of action of SCS are discussed in Chapter 20, Neurostimulation techniques in the *Chronic Pain* volume of this series, but **Figure 34.1** summarizes some of our knowledge.[4, 5]

For pain relief using SCS it is crucial that the pleasant paresthesiae are felt by the individual in the area of their pain. The goal of both implanter and manufacturer is to achieve as near to 100 percent topographical paresthesiae coverage and to maintain this long term.[6]

This explains the emergence of multiple electrode systems with ever more programming ability so that, if necessary, multiple programs can be run simultaneously in order to achieve maximal paresthesiae coverage.[7, 8, 9, 10, 11, 12]

In order to power this and to stay cost effective, it has been necessary to develop rechargeable systems combining complexity of stimulation without reducing longevity (see Table 34.1).[13]

Within the broad indications of neuropathic pain of peripheral origin and ischemic pain, there are the following common clinical syndromes:

1. neuropathic back and leg pain following spinal root injury (often known as failed back surgery syndrome (FBSS));[14, 15, 16, 17, 18, 19, 20, 21, 22, 23, 24]
2. complex regional pain syndromes;[24, 25, 26, 27, 28, 29, 30, 31]
3. painful polyneuropathy;[32, 33, 34]
4. angina pectoris;[35, 36, 37, 38, 39, 40, 41, 42]
5. critical limb ischemia.[43, 44, 45, 46]

Together, these five diagnostic groups are the main indications for SCS but others, such as the visceral pain syndromes, are emerging indications.[47, 48, 49, 50, 51, 52, 53]

Historically, SCS tends to be positioned in most therapy algorithms as a treatment of late resort. Recent high quality randomized prospective comparison trials of clinical and cost effectiveness have suggested that SCS should be considered earlier in disease and symptom management. Two prospective trials in FBSS have compared SCS against a surgical comparator, such as is common practice in the USA, and against a package of best medical practice which is more common in other healthcare economies. In both studies, SCS has been shown to offer better outcomes for pain and downstream healthcare usage. In the latter study (PROCESS) which also measured quality of life in FBSS patients before and after treatment, it was highlighted just how poor self-assessed quality of life was in this patient group and how effective treatment (as seen with SCS) enhanced quality of life as well.[15, 17]

SCS appears to be a safe therapy with only rare reports of harm. Evidence and consensus is that SCS is best carried out in centers with experience in all aspects of clinical and resource management. This includes patient and device selection, implantation, troubleshooting, and audit.[54]

As chronic pain understanding and therapies have evolved, it has become more important to develop care pathways and treatment networks so that all patients who need SCS can have access, even if not provided by a single center.

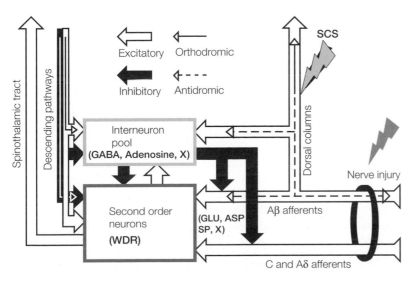

Dorsal horn   **Peripheral nerve**

Figure 34.1 Mechanisms of action of spinal cord stimulation. Redrawn from an original by B Linderoth, published in *Journal of Pain and Symptom Management*, **4**, Meyerson BA and Linderoth B, Mode of action of spinal cord stimulation in neuropathic pain. S6–S12, © Elsevier (2006).

Table 34.1 Comparison of three different rechargeable spinal cord stimulator systems.

Parameter	Medtronic "restore"	Advanced bionics "precision"	ANS "Eon™"
Number of electrical contacts	16	16	16
Vertebral segments covered	2	1	2
Battery fife (FDA labeling)	9 years (power level not defined by FDA)	5 years medium power	7 years high power
Battery strength (mA)	300	200	325
Zero-volt battery technology?	No	Yes	No
Battery warranty	1 Year	5 Year	1 year
Current delivery	Constant voltage for each array	Constant current independent for each electrical contact	Constant current for each array
Frequency range	Maximum = 260 pulse/ second Hz	Maximum = 1200 pulse/ second Hz	Maximum = 1200 pulse/ second Hz
Multiplexed channels per program	Up to 4 1 set at 130 Hz 2 sets at 130 Hz 4 sets at 65 Hz	Up to 4 1 set at 1200 Hz 2 sets at 130 Hz 4 sets at 80 Hz	Up to 8 1 set at 1200 Hz 2 sets at 600 Hz 4 sets at 300 Hz 8 sets at 150 Hz
Maximum pulse width (microseconds)	450	1000	500
Number of programs	1 to 32	1 to 4	1 to 24
Multistim®	4	4	8
Current steering	Manual	Automatic	Manual
Compatible percutaneous leads	6	1	5
Compatible surgical leads	4	1	10
Maximum implantation depth	2.5 cm	2.0 cm	2.5 cm
Size	72 gm/39 cc	36 gm/22 cc	75 gm/42 cc
Magnet option	No	No	Yes
Recharge time (after complete discharge)	6 hours (battery might not tolerate more than three complete drains)[a]	4 hours	4–5 hours
Charging mechanism	Portable charge available[b]	Portable charge with possible heat build up	AC plug required

[a]The statement "battery might not tolerate more than three complete drains" warrants clarification. If the battery has reached a level where recharge is required everyday, the patient will be prompted to begin recharging. Technically, if the device is over-discharged for longer than 60 days three separate times, the battery should be replaced. Medtronic writes, "If the patient is not motivated to recharge for three consecutive cycles of 60 days, there is a good chance that the therapy is not adequate and the stimulator should be explanted anyway".

[b]The Restore recharger by Medtronic contains a temperature sensor that will disable the recharger to ensure it stays below 41°C (a standard to ensure patient comfort and safety).

ANATOMY AND THE NEURAL INTERFACE

SCS electrodes are placed in the epidural space, either directly via a limited laminotomy using plate electrodes or percutaneously using cylindrical electrodes through modified epidural needles. An electrical field is generated that targets the exact spot within the dorsal columns that processes sensory information of the site that is to be treated. This represents an electrical challenge because of the variable distance between the dorsal columns and the cathode (thickness of cerebrospinal fluid (CSF)), as well as the conductivity of the bone, dura, blood vessels, and fat.

Holsheimmer[55, 56, 57] described this in detail and produced a computer model with relevance to electrode lead selection, current control technology, and voltage or current constancy.

The dorsal columns' sensory homunculus changes as the cord ascends. The spinal cord ascends from L1/2 with the sacral segments taking up position in the midline and sulcus with progressive layering of fibers from the lumbar region and thoracic and cervical region laterally.[58, 59] Barolat and Holsheimmer have described the probability of achieving stimulation in the various parts of the body at each spinal level (**Figure 34.2**). This knowledge helps the implanter to site the electrodes optimally.

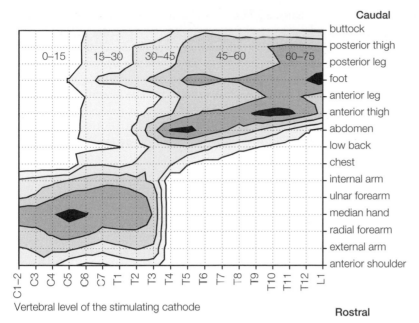

Caudal

buttock
posterior thigh
posterior leg
foot
anterior leg
anterior thigh
abdomen
low back
chest
internal arm
ulnar forearm
median hand
radial forearm
external arm
anterior shoulder

Vertebral level of the stimulating cathode

Rostral

Figure 34.2 Probability of paresthesia (percentage) in various body areas. Redrawn with permission from Ref. 60.

Some SCS implanters believe that most patients will have a "sweet spot," such that a single cathode placed in exactly the right place will evoke paresthesiae wherever the patient needs. In some this holds true but most now believe that multiple electrodes placed close together over two spinal levels with current splitting control and multiple simultaneous programs probably offers the best chance of 100 percent coverage maintainable without lead repositioning.

The developments of clinical technique and device technology are instrumental in the reduction in requirement for revision procedures of SCS due to loss of topographical paresthesiae or pulse generator exhaustion.

INDICATIONS

SCS is not a useful treatment for nociceptive pain such as musculoskeletal or joint pain.

SCS is used for neuropathic pain of peripheral origin and ischemic pain syndromes. New reports for its use accumulate, including visceral pain syndromes such as interstitial cystitis and irritable bowel syndrome.

The most common indications are:

- chronic neuropathic pain of radicular origin with or without previous spinal surgery (also known in the literature as FBSS);
- complex regional pain syndromes type 1 and 2;
- refractory angina pectoris;
- pain of critical limb ischemia secondary to occlusive and vasospastic disease.

PATIENT SELECTION

There are few absolute contraindications to SCS other than psychotic illness, dementia, local sepsis, continuing systemic infection, and titanium allergy. However, before recommending SCS, there are several relative contraindications which an experienced implanter will need to take into account, as described below.

Bleeding disorders

Anticoagulated patients receiving warfarin will need to be converted temporarily to heparin to enable more rapid reversal of anticoagulation during periods of surgery, the main risk being epidural hematoma. Patients with bleeding disorders should have this corrected before implantation.

Major anatomical abnormality of the spine

Scarring of the epidural space, kyphosis, scoliosis, or canal stenosis may make accurate lead placement difficult using percutaneous electrodes, but can be resolved occasionally using a surgical lead under direct vision.

Patients with implanted pacemakers or defibrillation devices

The advice of the manufacturer should be sought.

Morbid obesity

Technical factors may make lead placement or anchoring difficult. Also, the patient may not tolerate positioning such as the prone position for the duration of the procedure.

Unresolved psychological factors

Much has been written about the need for psychological assessment prior to a trial of SCS. We believe that it is important to make a multidimensional biopsychosocial assessment of a patient with chronic pain. This may require specialists within the pain team, such as a physiotherapist, with cognitive and behavioral training and counseling psychologist. There may be aspects of each patient's pain, disability, and suffering that are important and will not be affected by medical pain treatment alone and should, wherever possible, be identified in advance. This is common to all medical pain treatment and is not specific to SCS. If doubt exists, a formal psychological assessment (psychologist specializing in pain) should be sought. This may enable useful coping strategies such as pacing to be started, and unhelpful coping strategies, for example fear avoidance, to be challenged thus helping to achieve better long-term pain and disability improvements with SCS.

An understanding by the patient that SCS is "treating the pain itself" is essential. Cure seeking or unrealistic pain and disability improvement are not good prognostic signs before a trial of SCS. Patients with active psychotic illness, untreated nonpain-related depression, hysteria, somatoform disorders, and secondary behavioral gains are not likely to benefit from medical pain relieving interventions and should, whilst in existence, be regarded as a contraindication for SCS.[61, 62, 63, 64]

A TRIAL OF SCS OR FIRST STAGE OF PROCEDURE

SCS is an expensive and invasive therapy, although of low risk. The likelihood of worsening pain is extremely unlikely but morbidity, such as the need for revision procedures for lead migration or breakage or explantation due to nosoconial infection, are not uncommon.

The procedure can be divided into two stages so allowing a period for the patient to experience SCS with a temporary percutaneous system. The purpose of a trial is to ascertain whether the evoked paresthesiae can be maintained adequately to topographically match as much of the patient's pain as possible, to ensure that the paresthesiae are tolerated and finally to give an indication as to whether there are short-term reports of pain relief. The assumption being that if all these criteria are met then there is a good chance of long-term pain relief with SCS.

A trial of SCS involves the insertion of a specialized SCS lead into the epidural space. For the purposes of ascertaining whether SCS is efficacious a lead can be inserted, using the approaches referred to later, percutaneously. Simple fixation to the skin and coverage with a sterile dressing suffices during the period of trial. If the trial is successful, the lead can be removed by simply applying traction to it. This has the advantage of enabling a more simple insertion and removal for the trial to occur, but has the significant disadvantage that another definitive lead needs to be inserted at the same time as the permanent system, at a later date.

The technical aspects of conducting a trial are covered below under Implantation.

During a trial it is essential that goals are set for both physician and patient to achieve. For the physician, it is essential that stimulation covers the area which corresponds with the patient's pain (achieve topographic coverage). For the patient, improvements in pain and disability should be the aim. The literature frequently refers to a 50 percent reduction in pain intensity scores, which would indicate a successful trial. A clinically useful reduction in pain intensity of 30 percent with improvements in activity tolerance, sleep, and medication reduction would be further evidence of a successful trial.

Most patients are able to comment favorably on pain reduction within days of the start of a trial. An initial description of the paresthesiae invoking a "warm" or "pleasant" sensation is encouraging, as is the phenomenon of poststimulation analgesia. For patients who have significant axial back pain, recovery from the incisions may delay the ability to mobilize and comment. One week appears to be sufficient for the majority of cases. In some cases a longer trial period is advised. In some countries it is a requirement for reimbursement that the patient has a minimum of a four-week trial.[65, 66]

All superficial percutaneous implants will be at risk of infection with skin flora. The duration of the trial is just one factor of several that affects the incidence of hardware infection.

IMPLANTATION

The implantation procedure can be divided into the insertion and anchoring of SCS leads into the epidural space, and then the connection of the leads to an implanted pulse generator which is anchored in either the abdominal wall or "back pocket."

Both stages need to be performed in a sterile environment, with comparable cleanliness to that of any major implant surgery. Antibiotic prophylaxis against commensal skin bacteria is used at the beginning and end of the procedure.

Insertion of SCS leads

An image intensifier and an assistant for altering the test stimulation are needed. Patients may need sedation, and an anesthetist colleague may be needed in this case. Electro-cautery will be needed for hemostasis.

Most implanters position the patient in the prone position on a radiolucent table, with the spine slightly flexed. It is important for the patient to find the position comfortable, as they may need to remain in it for up to 90 minutes. Some may prefer the patient to be in the sitting position.

Anatomical sites in the epidural space have been mapped out so as to give the best probability in achieving topographical paresthesiae coverage (**Table 34.2** and **Figure 34.2**). To reduce lead motion after implantation, the epidural space should be entered approximately three vertebral levels below the intended site of the lead

Table 34.2 Anatomical sites in the epidural space.

Anatomical sites	
Upper limb pain	C4 to T1
Refractory angina	C6 to T2
Abdominal pain	T5 to T7
Low back pain	T8 to T9
Leg pain	T9 and T12

tip (i.e. for lower limb stimulation at T9 to T11, the entry point might be at L1/L2 – preferably L2/L3).

Plan the incision site and mark it on the skin before incision. This should be paravertebral at the lateral border of the vertebral bodies on an anteroposterior (AP) projection. Some implanters prefer to start with a percutaneous placement first and, when satisfied with the stimulation topography, cut around the needle to create the anchoring site. The authors prefer to create the anchoring site first and rarely have had to create a second site.

The patient may have a preference for which side they wish an abdominal implantable pulse generator (IPG) to be, for example contralateral to the side they sleep upon. If there is no particular preference, the authors advise that the IPG is placed on the left, particularly if the patient has not previously had an appendicectomy.

The superior end of the dorsal incision will be approximately 4 cm caudal to the entry point into the epidural space. The incision will need to be approximately 2–4 cm long.

Apply alcoholic skin preparation to include the incision site and as far as the projected exit site of the temporary extension lead laterally and cranially. Infiltrate the skin and deep tissues with lidocaine and epinephrine, to reduce bleeding and surgical pain.

Having incised the skin, obtain hemostasis and dissect through adipose tissue bluntly, using dissecting scissors. Eventually the adipose tissue, which is yellow/white ends, and anterior to it the thoracolumbar fascia (in this region), which is white, and is not easily parted with blunt instruments. This overlies the paraspinal muscles. If any doubt exists as to whether the thoracolumbar fascia has been reached, "scraping" it with a scalpel's blade will delineate the white tough surface better or a small (less that 5 mm) incision at a relevantly unimportant site will reveal the characteristic purple striated muscle appearance beneath it. Return the C arm, which is draped and sterile, to an AP position and image. The aim is to enter the mid line of the epidural space via a paramedial approach, with an acute, i.e. "flat," entry to the space so as to minimize any sharp deviations in the route of the lead. A midline approach is not recommended, and the puncture site of the thoracolumbar fascia should not be too lateral, again to minimize bends in the lead. The space is entered with an epidural needle using the familiar loss of resistance

technique. Once the epidural space has been entered, a soft blunt guide wire is inserted under imaging. This should pass painlessly and freely into the epidural space in the same direction as the loss of resistance needle. If sharp deviation occurs, this may be due to epidural septae or adhesions. Rotating the loss of resistance needle along its long axis will alter the position of the needle's bevel, and this may enable a better passage of the guide wire.

When easy passage of the guide wire occurs, a second needle to facilitate a second lead, if two leads are needed, can be inserted at the same level or one above or below. Sufficient anchoring space should be left for each lead.

The SCS lead has a removable stylet within it to provide rigidity and has a bent tip to facilitate steering of the lead in the epidural space. The SCS lead should be observed passing through the loss of resistance needle into the epidural space. The lead can then be advanced to the level required. This should require little force on the lead. Rotating the lead along its long axis will alter the direction of the bent tip, to enable steering to occur. The lead should not be allowed to deviate laterally, as this may result in anterior epidural space passage of the lead.

The lead can now be advanced cranially, and this should be ideally 1–2 mm lateral to the midline on an AP projection. This assumes the midline of the spinal column is the same as the electrophysiological midline, but this may not be the case in many patients, particularly if scoliosis is present.

It is common for the lead to be obstructed in its passage or be deviated by epidural adhesions, septae, or veins. It may be necessary to withdraw the lead several centimeters caudally and readvance it. Make sure that there is no sensation of snagging of the lead on the introducer needle. Ensure the lead has not deviated too laterally then returned medially.

When the tip of the lead has reached approximately the correct level, test stimulation can occur.

Screening for topographical paresthesiae coverage

Connect the terminals of the lead to the extension cable. The other end is passed to an assistant who connects it to an external pulse generator.

The most important factor in getting adequate topographic mapping will be the cathode position. It may be necessary to alter the pulse width and frequency of the stimulation to "fine tune," but 200–250 ms and 40–80 Hz are ideal starting values.

It is sensible to start with the middle electrodes of any lead as anode and cathode.

Start at zero voltage and gradually increase the amplitude. Some patients have a lag time of a few seconds before increases in amplitude have an effect. When paresthesiae are elicited they can be used to guide where lead placement ideally should be.

If the lead is at the electrophysiological midline, then bilateral stimulation will occur. As the lead moves more laterally from this point, stimulation will occur more in one side and reduce in the contralateral side until a point is reached where only unilateral stimulation occurs. If the lead is too lateral then painful chest wall paresthesiae occur due to dorsal root entry zone stimulation.

The site of the lead craniocaudally will determine which dermatomes are picked up preferentially and this often determines how proximal or distal stimulation in a limb is felt.

Agree with your assistant a numbering system of the electrodes on each lead beforehand. Automated systems have been developed to gradually change cathode arrays between all the electrodes so as to facilitate on table screening for topographical coverage.

For a single lead a typical series of stimulation would be to try the middle electrodes first (i.e. one and two). "Perfect" positioning of a four-electrode lead would be one where every pair of neighboring electrodes produces good topographic coverage. In general, the greater the number of electrodes combinations achieving coverage the better.

Although with a single lead it is possible to achieve bilateral stimulation, there is little margin for error and, if there is a small lateral migration of the lead, bilateral stimulation may be lost. If bilateral stimulation is required it is better to insert a pair of electrodes each side of the midline.

Anchoring of the SCS leads

Having achieved adequate lead positioning, the lead needs to be anchored in place. There are a variety of anchoring devices, and they will vary in their use. In general though, the same principles occur to all anchoring devices, as described below.

- Any anchoring sutures, which should be figure-of-eight sutures, should be inserted whilst the epidural needle is still in place; it will protect against inadvertently damaging the lead with the suture's needle tip.
- The anchor should be as close as possible to the entry point of the thoracolumbar fascia. If a silicone anchor is used, the proximal tip should be buried slightly in the thoracolumbar fascia. The anchoring device should provide adequate grip so as to avoid tracking in or out of the lead. Lead breakages often occur at any fulcrum where there is bodily movement. These are most often at the distal margin of the anchor.
- Prior to anchoring the lead, the loss of resistance epidural needle needs to be removed carefully. This needs to be performed whilst avoiding damaging the external covering of the lead and without disturbing the lead's position. A similar technique to that employed with an epidural catheter is used.

For a prolonged trial of SCS (days to weeks) a temporary extension cable can be passed under the skin laterally from the incision, approximately 20 cm or so to a convenient exit point, depending on the spinal level and subsequent care. Some prefer to exit at the same side as the incision to aid future implantation and others the opposite side to avoid potential abnormal skin flora contamination at future implantation.

Select the exit point and infiltrate with local anesthetic. The kit supplied with the lead will contain a tunneling device. The contacts of the SCS lead are cleaned with water, not saline, and are dried with a clean swab. The connection between the epidural lead and extension cable is typically covered with a plastic insulation cover (boot) device, which will need to be slid on to the lead prior to the contacts being connected. Ensure the contacts are in line visually or perform an impedance check, then secure the contacts with a torque wrench. If there is an insulation cover (boot), this can be slid over the connection and is sealed with two nonabsorbable sutures to prevent body fluids entering the connection and corroding it.

The connection is then placed within the dorsal incision. It is important that the run of the leads and extension cables avoids any sharp bends or twists. The whole system will have an intrinsic curve to it, and it should be buried in the incision pocket in this position. For this purpose, it may be necessary to slightly enlarge the incision pocket by dividing the fascial planes further as opposed to increasing the size of the skin incision.

The incision is then closed in two layers with absorbable suture material, and covered with an occlusive dressing.

At the exit point of the extension cable through the skin, it is important to adequately secure the exiting extension cable to avoid chafing on the skin edges (which might promote abnormal skin flora growth) and to be tug resistant. Minimal disturbance of the exit site wound during the trial is preferable. If possible, the dressings should be left undisturbed until definitive removal of the leads or full implantation occurs.

FULL IMPLANTATION OR SECOND–STAGE SCS PROCEDURE

This involves the connection of the SCS lead, or leads, to an IPG which has been placed in a subcutaneous pocket. Due to multiple incision sites and extensive subcutaneous tunneling, this is more comfortably performed under general anesthesia.

The IPG should be placed at a site that is potentially comfortable for the patient, usually the abdomen but sometimes "back pocket" or infraclavicular positions. Care should be taken to ensure positioning suits the patient and does not impinge on bony prominences or tent the skin. If the abdominal wall position is selected then the patient is positioned laterally, with the side into which the IPG is to be inserted uppermost. Sufficient space will be needed for the surgeon to operate on both the back and abdomen of the patient. The dressings that are covering the dorsal incision and the exit site of the temporary extension cable are taken down.

Antibiotic prophylaxis is needed. Antibiotic prophylaxis policy is best agreed with the infection control team in advance.

After preparing the skin with an alcoholic skin preparation, drape the patient to include the back incision, the patient's flank, and the abdomen as the projected site of the IPG. The exit site of a temporary extension cable is excluded from the sterile field; it needs to be accessible to an assistant.

An incision is made parallel to the skin folds of the abdomen, and by blunt dissection above and below the incision, a pocket of similar dimension to the IPG created. The pocket must not be too large, or the IPG may move later, causing traction on the extension, or flip over, such that communication with or recharging of the IPG is not possible. The IPG should lie in the pocket as if it were in the top pocket of a jacket; the incision should overly the superior margin of the IPG. Good hemostasis must be achieved. The posterior incision is reopened. If the patient has undergone a trial of stimulation, it is necessary to find the connection between the SCS lead and the temporary extension and disconnect it. Then, the temporary extension cable can be removed by an assistant by gently pulling them from their exit point. Permanent extension cables vary, but the basic principle is to place a cable subcutaneously from the abdominal pocket to the back incision.

In most patients, there is less tissue bruising if the tunneling is performed in two stages with a small incision at the apex of the body curve. Having cleaned the connectors with water and dried them, the SCS leads and IPG are connected via the extension cable. Make sure that the manufacturers' instructions are followed at this point as it is vital that electrical circuitry has been properly achieved. Some manufacturers merely recommend a visual check and others an impedance check. It is important that the contact screws are not over-tightened. A new boot, if this is required, will be needed to cover the connection between the SCS leads and the extension cable and made watertight with nonabsorbable sutures. The connection can usually be buried just lateral to the anchoring device with sufficient lead slack to allow for body movement. The anchoring device and connection device are both away from the midline bony prominences.

Some implanters prefer to use long SCS leads that can connect directly with the IPG (even in the abdominal area) so obviating the need for an extension device. In the authors' opinion this has the slight disadvantage of managing lead revision procedures should they be required at a future date.

The IPG can be gently anchored with nonabsorbable sutures to the abdominal musculature. If they are too tight, the IPG will be painful. The aim is to immobilize the IPG for a sufficient period for the pocket to heal, and a reasonable taut lining to form around the IPG.

All incisions are closed in two layers with absorbable sutures and dressed.

COMPLICATIONS OF SCS

Complications can be divided temporally into early and late and further divided into biological, disease-related, or device-related.[67, 68]

Early complications include all those of any surgery or epidural manipulation, including deep vein thrombosis or epidural hematoma. Specific biological early complications include:

- Dural tap. This may occur when attempting to enter the epidural space, or more rarely from inserting a guide wire or advancing a lead. Conservative management of the postdural puncture headache is preferable to an early epidural blood patch, but this may be necessary at a different level if symptoms do not settle.
- Infection. Superficial infection of the wound sites can be treated with antibiotics, but if deep infection of any of the sites occurs, it is usual to remove all implanted material, as infection in the presence of a foreign body is rarely cured. There is also the potential for meningitis or an epidural abscess to form if infection is left unchecked. However, these central neuraxial infections are very rare. It is important that each implanting center is aware of their infection rate and to ensure that appropriate efforts are made to keep it less than 2 percent of all full implants.[69]
- Serous collections. If possible these should be left to resolve spontaneously. If very uncomfortable, the pain from a seroma can be temporarily helped by wound aspiration under sterile conditions. If it occurs during a trial prior to implantation, it can be dealt with when the incision is reopened.
- Hematoma should be evacuated early. Good hemostasis will reduce this and serous collections.

An example of a specific early device-related complication would be early lead migration during the trial period resulting in loss of adequate topography of paresthesiae and requiring revision procedure or second SCS lead insertion.

Late complications are usually device- or disease-related. Most conditions for which SCS are used are relatively stable (e.g. medically refractory neuropathic pain), but other conditions, such as ischemia and degenerative spinal disease, may progress.

Device-related complications include:

- Lead failure. This will manifest as high impedance without stimulation and will either be due to breakage or corrosion of the internal wires or high impedance material around the electrode contacts. New leads will be necessary.[70]

- Lead migration. This will manifest as change of stimulation topography. Both lead fracture and migration can be reduced by optimal anchoring and routing techniques. Reprogramming the IPG to use different electrode combinations may return the stimulation to an acceptable site if migration occurs, but it may be necessary to open the back incision and manipulate the lead using the same techniques as used during the original lead insertion.[71]
- Lead migration and failure may occur in up to 20 percent of leads inserted over a four-year period. New technologies and implant techniques are expected to reduce these complications.[72]
- Late infection – usually during revision procedures or from hematogenous spread. Remove all components unless superficial.
- Pain at the connection site or IPG. This may be due to fluid ingress or movement of the IPG within the pocket or pressure over a bony prominence.
- IPG movement – it may need to be revised into a smaller pocket.
- Failure to relieve pain despite adequate topographic coverage – disease may progress or new disease may occur.
- Unpleasant stimulation. Reprogramming may reduce this. It is common for the level of stimulation to suddenly increase when the lumbar or cervical spine is extended; most patients come to anticipate this and will reduce their stimulation amplitude prior to these maneuvers.
- Adequate stimulation but failure to relieve pain. The cause of late failure in these circumstances is often unknown. However, the implanter should first consider disease progression, or indeed new disease, that may affect the same dermatome levels. Clearly there may be issues around initial patient selection or change in psychological factors. Other reasons might include withdrawal of coadministered pharmacological therapy.

PROGRAMMING

In some patients, it is surprising how wide the topographical map of evoked paresthesiae that can be achieved with a simple bipolar arrangement. In others, very complex arrays are needed to collect together sufficient paresthesiae coverage. For the latter patients, multiple electrode systems are required so as to be able to achieve and maintain this over time.

Continuous active stimulation is rarely needed by the patient as most will have some degree of poststimulation analgesia. Many patients prefer some sort of cycling whereby the IPG is programmed to be on for a few seconds and then off for some before gently ramping up

again. If using a nonrechargeable system, this energy-saving programming can be useful with respect to battery longevity.

Programming may take time to achieve best results. This can be aided by computer-generated drawings of pain sites and paresthesiae coverage.

EQUIPMENT SELECTION

External and internal battery SCS systems

This is a constantly developing field and it is likely that much of this information will change. Currently, three companies produce and market SCS systems. Two have a family of products, and the other a single product with broad capability. The pulse generator can either be powered by an external source that induces current in an implanted receiver; it may have its own long-lasting lithium oxide battery; or finally a rechargeable battery.

The rechargeable systems are the latest platform that the device companies have each designed in order to make SCS more clinically and, it is hoped, cost-effective. They each differ with various advantages and disadvantages which the reader can explore with the manufacturers in order to determine which system suits their practice best (see **Figure 34.2**).

Complications

The weakest parts of SCS are the electrodes and electrical junctions. Electrode migration is common to both percutaneous and surgical placement. Anchoring technique and technology is important to prevent inward or outward migration. Multiple electrode arrays have a role here as small degrees of migration should be salvageable with reprogramming. Electrode arrays can generate electrical fields over the dorsal columns that improve topographical coverage of pain with evoked paresthesiae.

Movements of the body may repetitively bend the leads, breaking their internal structure. Breaks occur at a fulcrum such as at the ligamentum flavum, muscle fascia, or anchoring point. Anchor technology that protects the lead through the fascia and displaces the fulcrum away from the point of fixation and internal lead technology improvements that allow free movement of the internal lead fibers around the central core are expected to improve lead durability.

RESEARCH, AUDIT, AND DEVICE REGISTRATION

Historically, SCS has been a treatment of curiosity offered by medical enthusiasts to patients for whom most other therapeutic strategies are unsatisfactory. Even now there are new indications that are emerging and being reported but cannot yet be regarded as a standard of practice.

However, there are now established indications (neuropathic, peripheral and ischemic pain) which are not just supported by thousands of patients in clinical reports but by well-conducted prospective randomized comparative studies of clinical and cost effectiveness. It is this degree of evidence quality that must be striven for in each clinical indication to make SCS for these indications a standard of practice.

It is a recommendation of the British Pain Society guidelines on best practice for SCS that each implanting center should audit the processes and outcomes of their work. It is also suggested that there should be a national registry of device implantation.

All device companies have to have a specific tracking number for all implant material, such that the center can be identified should there be a product recall. However, each implant center should ensure that they have a robust system with which to track to a specific patient.

There are many advantages in producing a national audit database, which include:

- patient safety;
- audit of clinical practice of center against a peer group;
- identification of clinical patterns of indication and outcomes;
- identification of patterns of complications including device-, disease-, or patient-related.

CONCLUSIONS AND SUMMARY

It has taken too long for SCS to be on the threshold of becoming a standard of practice for severe and disabling medically refractory neuropathic and ischemic pain.[73, 74, 75, 76] Compared to many other surgical and medical techniques of pain relief, the quality of evidence of efficacy and cost effectiveness of SCS in neuropathic pain and ischemia is really quite good although more is welcome.[29, 77, 78, 79, 80]

Evidence of cost effectiveness is vital to its more widespread accessibility by convincing health policymakers of its long-term worth.

Both intrinsic factors that relate to the design and functionality of the devices and extrinsic factors such as implant technique and complications are vital to optimize clinical and cost effectiveness.

Along with gene and stem cell therapies and gene-directed pharmacotherapy, neuromodulation is one of the most exciting developing themes of modern health care.

REFERENCES

1. Long DM, Erickson D. Stimulation of the posterior columns of the spinal cord for relief of intractable pain. *Surgical Neurology.* 1975; **4**: 134–41.

2. Shealy CN, Mortimer JT, Reswick JB. Electrical inhibition of pain by stimulation of the dorsal columns: preliminary clinical report. *Anesthesia and Analgesia.* 1967; **46**: 489–91.

3. Melzack R, Wall PD. Pain mechanisms: a new theory. *Science.* 1965; **150**: 971–9.

∗ 4. Meyerson BA, Linderoth B. Mode of action of spinal cord stimulation in neuropathic pain. *Journal of Pain and Symptom Management.* 2006; **31**: S6–12.

∗ 5. Krames ES. Mechanism of action of spinal cord stimulation. In: Waldman SD (ed.). *Interventional pain management,* 2nd edn. Philadelphia, PA: WB Saunders, 2001: 561–5.

∗ 6. Holsheimer J. Principles of neurostimulation. In: Simpson BA (ed.). *Pain research and clinical management, Vol. 15: Electrical stimulation and the relief of pain.* Amsterdam: Elsevier, 2003: 17–36.

7. North RB, Kidd DH, Olin JC, Sieracki JM. Spinal cord stimulation electrode design: prospective, randomized, controlled trial comparing percutaneous and laminectomy electrodes. Part I: technical outcomes. *Neurosurgery.* 2002; **51**: 381–9.

8. Oakley JC, Espinosa F, Bothe H *et al.* Transverse tripolar spinal cord stimulation: results of an international multicenter study. *Neuromodulation.* 2006; **9**: 192–203.

9. Sharan A, Cameron T, Barolat G. Evolving patterns of spinal cord stimulation in patients implanted for intractable low back and leg pain. *Neuromodulation.* 2002; **5**: 167–79.

∗ 10. Holsheimer J, Khan YN, Raza SS, Khan EA. Effects of electrode positioning on perception threshold and paresthesia coverage in spinal cord stimulation. *Neuromodulation.* 2007; **10**: 34–41.

11. Barolat G, Oakley JC, Law JD *et al.* Epidural spinal cord stimulation with a multiple electrode paddle lead is effective in treating intractable low back pain. *Neuromodulation.* 2001; **4**: 59–66.

12. North RB, Kidd DH, Petrucci L *et al.* Spinal cord stimulation electrode design: a prospective, randomized, controlled trial comparing percutaneous with laminectomy electrodes. Part II clinical outcomes. *Neurosurgery.* 2005; **57**: 990–6.

13. Van Buyten JP, Lazorthes Y, Spincemaille GH *et al.* Prospective outcomes study on the Restore® rechargeable neurostimulation system for neuropathic pain. *European Journal of Pain.* 2006; **10**: S160.

∗ 14. Taylor RS, Van Buyten JP, Buchser E. Spinal cord stimulation for chronic back and leg pain and failed back surgery syndrome: a systematic review and analysis of prognostic factors. *Spine.* 2005; **30**: 152–60.

∗ 15. North RB, Kidd DH, Farrokhi F, Piantadosi SA. Spinal cord stimulation versus repeated lumbosacral spine surgery for chronic pain: a randomized, controlled trial. *Neurosurgery.* 2005; **56**: 98–106.

∗ 16. Dario AM, Fortini G, Bertollo DM *et al.* Treatment of failed back surgery syndrome. *Neuromodulation.* 2001; **4**: 105–10.

∗ 17. Kumar K, Taylor RS, Jacques L *et al.* Spinal cord stimulation versus conventional medical management for neuropathic pain: a multicentre randomised controlled trial in patients with the failed back surgery syndrome. *Pain.* 2007; **132**: 179–88.

18. Ohnmeiss DD, Rashbaum RF. Patient satisfaction with spinal cord stimulation for predominant complaints of chronic, intractable low back pain. *Spine Journal: Official Journal of the North American Spine Society.* 2001; **1**: 358–63.

∗ 19. Spincemaille GH, Beersen N, Dekkers MA, Theuvenet PJ. Neuropathic limb pain and spinal cord stimulation: results of the Dutch prospective study. *Neuromodulation.* 2004; **7**: 184–92.

∗ 20. Ohnmeiss DD, Rashbaum RF, Bogdanffy GM. Prospective outcome evaluation of spinal cord stimulation in patients with intractable leg pain. *Spine.* 1996; **21**: 1344–50.

∗ 21. Burchiel KJ, Anderson V, Brown FD *et al.* Prospective, multicenter study of spinal cord stimulation for relief of chronic back and extremity pain. *Spine.* 1996; **21**: 2786–94.

22. Burchiel KJ, Anderson V, Wilson BJ *et al.* Prognostic factors of spinal cord stimulation for chronic back and leg pain. *Neurosurgery.* 1995; **36**: 1101–10.

∗ 23. North RB, Kidd DH, Olin J *et al.* Spinal cord stimulation for axial low back pain: a prospective, controlled trial comparing dual with single percutaneous electrodes. *Spine.* 2005; **30**: 1412–18.

∗ 24. Turner JA, Loeser JD, Deyo RA, Sanders SB. Spinal cord stimulation for patients with failed back surgery syndrome or complex regional pain syndrome: a systematic review of effectiveness and complications. *Pain.* 2004; **108**: 137–47.

∗ 25. Kemler MA, Barendse GA, van Kleef M *et al.* Spinal cord stimulation in patients with chronic reflex sympathetic dystrophy. *New England Journal of Medicine.* 2000; **343**: 618–24.

∗ 26. Kemler MA, De Vet HC, Barendse GA *et al.* Spinal cord stimulation for chronic reflex sympathetic dystrophy – five-year follow-up. *New England Journal of Medicine.* 2006; **354**: 2394–6.

27. Bennett DS, Aló KM, Oakley JC, Feler CA. Spinal cord stimulation for complex regional pain syndrome I [RSD]: a retrospective multicenter experience from 1995 to 1998 of 101 patients. *Neuromodulation.* 1999; **2**: 202–10.

28. Oakley JC, Weiner RL. Spinal cord stimulation for complex regional pain syndrome: a prospective study of 19 patients at two centers. *Neuromodulation.* 1999; **2**: 47–50.

∗ 29. Taylor RS, Van Buyten JP, Buchser E. Spinal cord stimulation for complex regional pain syndrome: a systematic review of the clinical and cost-effectiveness literature and assessment of prognostic factors. *European Journal of Pain.* 2006; **10**: 91–101.

30. Forouzanfar T, Kemler MA, Weber WE *et al.* Spinal cord stimulation in complex regional pain syndrome: cervical and lumbar devices are comparably effective. *British Journal of Anaesthesia.* 2004; **92**: 348–53.

31. Kumar K, Nath RK, Toth C. Spinal cord stimulation is effective in the management of reflex sympathetic dystrophy. *Neurosurgery.* 1997; **40**: 503–08.

∗ 32. Tesfaye S, Watt J, Benbow S *et al.* Electrical spinal cord stimulation for painful diabetic peripheral neuropathy. *Lancet.* 1996; **348**: 1698–701.

33. Daousi C, Benbow SJ, MacFarlane IA. Electrical spinal cord stimulation in the long-term treatment of chronic painful diabetic neuropathy. *Diabetic Medicine.* 2005; **22**: 393–8.

34. Kumar K, Toth C, Nath RK. Spinal cord stimulation for chronic pain in peripheral neuropathy. *Surgical Neurology.* 1996; **46**: 363–9.

∗ 35. Mannheimer C, Eliasson T, Augustinsson LE *et al.* Electrical stimulation versus coronary artery bypass surgery in severe angina pectoris: the ESBY study. *Circulation.* 1998; **97**: 1157–63.

∗ 36. Di Pede F, Lanza GA, Zuin G *et al.* Immediate and long-term clinical outcome after spinal cord stimulation for refractory stable angina pectoris. *American Journal of Cardiology.* 2003; **91**: 951–5.

∗ 37. TenVaarwerk IA, Jessurun GA, DeJongste MJ *et al.* Clinical outcome of patients treated with spinal cord stimulation for therapeutically refractory angina pectoris. The Working Group on Neurocardiology. *Heart.* 1999; **82**: 82–8.

∗ 38. Hautvast RW, DeJongste MJ, Staal MJ *et al.* Spinal cord stimulation in chronic intractable angina pectoris: a randomized, controlled efficacy study. *American Heart Journal.* 1998; **136**: 1114–20.

∗ 39. Yu W, Maru F, Edner M *et al.* Spinal cord stimulation for refractory angina pectoris: a retrospective analysis of efficacy and cost-benefit. *Coronary Artery Disease.* 2004; **15**: 31–7.

40. Buchser E, Durrer A, Albrecht E. Spinal cord stimulation for the management of refractory angina pectoris. *Journal of Pain and Symptom Management.* 2006; **31**: S36–42.

∗ 41. Armour JA, Linderoth B, Arora RC *et al.* Long-term modulation of the intrinsic cardiac nervous system by spinal cord neurons in normal and ischaemic hearts. *Autonomic Neuroscience – Basic and Clinical.* 2002; **95**: 71–9.

∗ 42. DeJongste MJ. Spinal cord stimulation for ischemic heart disease. *Neurological Research.* 2000; **22**: 293–8.

∗ 43. Amann W, Berg P, Gersbach P *et al.* Spinal cord stimulation in the treatment of non-reconstructable stable critical leg ischaemia: results of the European Peripheral Vascular Disease Outcome Study (SCS-EPOS). *European Journal of Vascular and Endovascular Surgery.* 2003; **26**: 280–6.

∗ 44. Klomp KHM, Spincemaille G, Steyerberg E *et al.* Spinal cord stimulation in patients with critical limb ischaemia: results of a randomised controlled multicentre study on the effect of spinal cord stimulation. *European Journal of Pain.* 2000; **4**: 173–84.

∗ 45. Ubbink D, Spincemaille G, Prins M *et al.* Microcirculatory investigations to determine the effect of spinal cord stimulation for critical limb ischaemia: the Dutch multicentre randomised controlled trial. *Journal of Vascular Surgery.* 1999; **30**: 236–44.

∗ 46. Horsch S, Schulte S, Hess S. Spinal cord stimulation in the treatment of peripheral vascular disease: results of a single-center study of 258 patients. *Angiology.* 2004; **55**: 111–18.

47. Meglio M, Cioni B, Amico ED et al. Epidural spinal cord stimulation for the treatment of neurogenic bladder. Acta Neurochirurgica. 1980; 54: 191–9.

48. Khan YN, Raza SS, Khan EA. Application of spinal cord stimulation for the treatment of abdominal visceral pain syndromes: case reports. Neuromodulation. 2005; 8: 14–27.

49. Ceballos A, Cabezudo L, Bovaira M et al. Spinal cord stimulation: a possible therapeutic alternative for chronic mesenteric ischaemia. Pain. 2000; 87: 99–101.

50. Meloy TS, Southern JP. Neurally augmented sexual function in human females: a preliminary investigation. Neuromodulation. 2006; 9: 34–40.

* 51. Simpson BA. Selection of patients and assessment of outcome. In: Simpson BA (ed.). Pain research and clinical management, vol 15: Electrical stimulation and the relief of pain. Amsterdam: Elsevier, 2003: 237–50.

52. Kapur S, Mutagi H, Raphael J. Spinal cord stimulation for relief of abdominal pain in two patients with familial Mediterranean fever. British Journal of Anaesthesia. 2006; 97: 866–8.

53. Krames ES, Mousad DG. Spinal cord stimulation reverses pain and diarrheal episodes of irritable bowel syndrome: a case report. Neuromodulation. 2004; 7: 82–8.

* 54. Simpson K, Stannard C. Spinal cord stimulation for the management of pain: recommendations for best clinical practice. London: British Pain Society, 2005.

55. Holsheimer J. Effectiveness of spinal cord stimulation in the management of chronic pain: analysis of technical drawbacks and solutions. Neurosurgery. 1997; 40: 990–6.

56. Holsheimer J. Computer modelling of spinal cord stimulation and its contribution to therapeutic efficacy. Spinal Cord. 1998; 36: 531–40.

57. Holsheimer J, Wesselink WA. Effect of anode-cathode configuration on paresthesia coverage in spinal cord stimulation. Neurosurgery. 1997; 41: 654–9.

58. Smith MC, Deacon P. Topographical anatomy of the posterior columns of the spinal cord in man. The long ascending fibres. Brain. 1984; 107: 671–98.

59. Alò KM, Varga C, Krames ES et al. Factors affecting impedance of percutaneous leads in spinal cord stimulation. Neuromodulation. 2006; 9: 128–35.

60. Holsheimer J, Barolat G. Spinal geometry and paresthesia coverage in spinal cord stimulation. Neuromodulation. 1998; 1: 129–36.

61. North RB, Kidd DH, Wimberly BS, Edwin D. Prognostic value of psychological testing in patients undergoing spinal cord stimulation: a prospective study. Neurosurgery. 1996; 39: 301–10.

62. Kumar K, Toth C, Nath RK, Laing P. Epidural spinal cord stimulation for treatment of chronic pain – some predictors of success. A 15-year experience. Surgical Neurology. 1998; 50: 110–20.

63. Gybels J, Erdine S, Maeyaert J et al. Neuromodulation of pain. European Journal of Pain. 1998; 2: 203–09.

64. Beltrutti D, Lamberto A, Barolat G et al. The psychological assessment of candidates for spinal cord stimulation for chronic pain management. Pain Practice. 2004; 4: 204–21.

65. Frank ED, Menefee LA, Jalali S et al. The utility of a 7-day percutaneous spinal cord stimulator trial measured by a pain diary: a long-term retrospective analysis. Neuromodulation. 2005; 8: 162–70.

66. Weinand ME, Madhusudan H, Davis B, Melgar M. Acute vs. prolonged screening for spinal cord stimulation in chronic pain. Neuromodulation. 2003; 6: 15–19.

67. Kumar K, Buchser E, Linderoth B et al. Avoiding complications from spinal cord stimulation: practical recommendations from an international panel of experts. Neuromodulation. 2007; 10: 24–33.

68. Kumar K, Wilson JR, Taylor RS, Gupta S. Complications of spinal cord stimulation, suggestions to improve outcome, and financial impact. Journal of Neurosurgery. Spine. 2006; 5: 191–203.

69. Torrens K, Stanley PJ, Ragunathan PL, Bush DJ. Risk of infection with electrical spinal-cord stimulation. Lancet. 1997; 349: 729.

70. Quigley DG, Arnold J, Eldridge PR et al. Long-term outcome of spinal cord stimulation and hardware complications. Stereotactic and Functional Neurosurgery. 2003; 81: 50–6.

71. Henderson JM, Schade CM, Sasaki J et al. Prevention of mechanical failures in implanted spinal cord stimulation systems. Neuromodulation. 2006; 9: 183–91.

* 72. May MS, Banks C, Thomson SJ. A retrospective, long-term, third-party follow-up of patients considered for spinal cord stimulation. Neuromodulation. 2002; 5: 137–44.

73. Meglio M, Cioni B, Rossi GF. Spinal cord stimulation in management of chronic pain. A 9-year experience. Journal of Neurosurgery. 1989; 70: 519–24.

74. Alò KM, Redko V, Charnov J. Four year follow-up of dual electrode spinal cord stimulation for chronic pain. Neuromodulation. 2002; 5: 79–88.

75. Sundaraj SR, Johnstone C, Noore F et al. Spinal cord stimulation: a seven-year audit. Journal of Clinical Neuroscience. 2005; 12: 264–70.

* 76. Van Buyten JP, Van Zundert J, Vueghs P, Vanduffel L. Efficacy of spinal cord stimulation: 10 years of experience in a pain centre in Belgium. European Journal of Pain. 2001; 5: 299–307.

* 77. Taylor RS, Van Buyten JP, Buchser E et al. The cost effectiveness of spinal cord stimulation in the treatment of pain: a systematic review of the literature. Journal of Pain and Symptom Management. 2004; 27: 370–8.

* 78. Andrell P, Ekre O, Eliasson T et al. Cost-effectiveness of spinal cord stimulation versus coronary artery bypass grafting in patients with severe angina pectoris – long-term results from the ESBY study. Cardiology. 2003; 99: 20–4.

* 79. Kumar K, Malik S, Demeria D. Treatment of chronic pain with spinal cord stimulation versus alternative therapies: cost-effectiveness analysis. Neurosurgery. 2002; 51: 106–15.

* 80. Ekre O, Eliasson T, Norrsell H et al. Electrical stimulation versus coronary artery bypass surgery in severe angina pectoris. Long-term effects of spinal cord stimulation and coronary artery bypass grafting on quality of life and survival in the ESBY study. European Heart Journal. 2002; 23: 1938–45.

35

Epidural (interlaminar, intraforaminal, and caudal) steroid injections for back pain and sciatica

IVAN N RAMOS-GALVEZ AND IAN D GOODALL

KEY LEARNING POINTS

- Epidural depot steroids relieve radicular pain caused by nerve root pathology, but not unspecific "low back pain."
- Transforaminal epidural injection of steroid is more effective, but also carries higher risk of major, irreversible complications than interlaminar or caudal epidural injection.
- Success depends on accurate steroid placement, and this is best achieved by the use of local anesthetic test dose and fluoroscopy.
- Multiple structures account for low back pain. Epidural steroids have evidence-based effects mostly on nerve

root pathology. The benefit of epidural steroid therapy depends on the contribution of nerve root factors to the back pain.
- Epidural steroid injections are generally safe in the hands of well-trained, experienced physicians, with experience in resuscitation routines, with adequate fluoroscopic equipment, and understanding of anatomic details and risk factors. However, even in the best of hands and with adequate precautions, tragic spinal cord complications may arise. Therefore, patients must be fully informed of possible benefits and risks.

INTRODUCTION AND HISTORICAL NOTES

The rationale for the use of corticosteroids in epidural injections stems from the hypothesis that there is a component of inflammation in the pathophysiology of low back pain. This inflammation is due to two sources: direct pressure from a prolapsed disk over the nerve roots and the chemicals released by the prolapsed nucleus pulposus.[1] Surgeons have remarked that, intraoperatively, the nerve root causing the problem can be easily identified by its edematous inflamed character,[2] although they have also stated that there is a normal vascularization of the dura covering the nerve roots, and the swelling of the nerves in the cauda equina is secondary to venous congestion from blocked venous drainage by the herniated disk. Nevertheless, pathologists have stepped into the surgical debate to see diffuse degenerative changes with regenerative areas and inflammatory infiltrates.[3, 4] Inflammatory changes were documented by Lindahl and Rexed[4] and are the rational for local steroid injection therapy.

The duration of depot methylprednisolone on cortisol depression is about two weeks.[5] However, some patients may benefit from these interventions several weeks after the procedure.[6, 7] Johansson et al.[8] documented a prolonged inhibition of C-fiber nociceptive transmission when these had been exposed to steroid. Nelson and Landau[9] believe that unspecific effects of the hypertonic injectates together with local anesthetics may impair the function of the small unmyelinated C-fibers.[9] Placebo and natural improvement with time may account for a variable proportion of the benefit of any intervention as Klenerman et al.[10] reported similar immediate relief rates in patients with sciatica treated with steroid injections compared to "dry needling."

INDICATIONS

Reviewing the evidence for epidural steroid injections, there are studies claiming success rates ranging from no better than placebo to 90 percent benefit.[11, 12, 13] One of the very few agreements with regards to epidural steroid injections is that the success depends greatly on accurate placement of the steroid, and this is best achieved with fluoroscopic control.[14, 15, 16] However, most of the studies in which the evidence for their success is based have been carried out without fluoroscopy, but with a local anesthetic, indicating that the origin of the pain has been reached by the injectate when the pain is immediately reduced.[17] The benefits of epidural local anesthetics alone are not different from the natural history of the process.[10, 18]

- Interlaminar epidural:
  - Diagnostic with local anesthetic alone:
    - no prognostic information can be obtained by this prior to spinal surgery.
  - Therapeutic with steroid:
    - radicular pain: level [II] evidence for short-term (<6 weeks) relief[7, 11, 12, 19] and level [IV] evidence for long-term (≥6 weeks) relief;[11, 12, 19]
    - failed back surgery syndrome: level [V] evidence;[12, 20]
    - spinal canal stenosis: level [V] evidence for short-term pain relief,[7, 11, 12, 21] no evidence for long-term relief;
    - discogenic: level [IV] evidence of long-term relief if end-plate changes on magnetic resonance imaging (MRI), and limited evidence of short-term relief.[22]
- Transforaminal epidural or selective nerve root block:
  - Diagnostic with local anesthetic alone – always problematic interpretations:
    - preoperative evaluation of patients with inconclusive or negative imaging and clinical findings suggestive of spinal root irritation. Level [III] evidence;[12]

    - to provide prognostic information prior to spinal surgery.[23]
  - Therapeutic with steroid:
    - radicular pain: level [II] evidence for short-term (<6 weeks) relief and level [III] evidence for long-term (≥6 weeks) relief;[11, 17, 24, 25]
    - failed back surgery syndrome: level [IV] evidence;[11, 26, 27]
    - spinal canal stenosis: level [IV] evidence of long-term relief and improvement in function;[11, 28, 29, 30]
    - discogenic: level [IV] evidence of long-term relief.[30]
- Caudal epidural:
  - Therapeutic with steroid:
    - radicular pain: level [II] evidence for short-term (<6 weeks) relief and level [III] evidence for long-term (≥6 weeks) relief;[11, 12, 31]
    - failed back surgery syndrome: level [II] evidence for short-term (<6 weeks) relief and level [III] evidence for long-term (≥6 weeks) relief;[11, 32]
    - spinal canal stenosis: level [IV] evidence.[33]

ANATOMICAL NOTES

The spine is anatomically divided into three columns.[34] The anterior column is formed by the vertebral bodies and intervertebral disks. The middle column is formed by the neurological structures surrounded by the meningeal membranes and the bony arch formed by pedicles, transverse processes, and laminae. In a normal spine, this middle column forms a perfectly aligned channel called the vertebral canal[35] which has defects at both sides called intervertebral foramina through which the spinal nerves and blood vessels to and from the spinal cord go. The posterior column is formed by the bony structures facetal line and spinous processes together with the ligamentous frame that holds the bony structures together. The dural sac is the meningeal envelope of the neural structures in the spinal canal. It normally extends down to S2[36, 37] and beyond through the external filum terminale that anchors it to the posterior aspect of the sacrum. It contains cerebrospinal fluid (CSF) and the neural spinal cord that, in an adult, ends with the conus medullaris at L1,[36, 37] although the lumbar and sacral nerve roots that comprise the cauda equina will extend beyond that limit together with the internal filum terminale.

The distal end of the bony spinal column is the sacrum and coccyx. The sacrum is formed by the fusion of the five sacral vertebrae. Its hollow cavity is the sacral canal that in an adult has an average volume of approximately 15 mL.[38] The space between these two bones is the sacral hiatus. This is a triangular bony defect with the sacral cornua at either side and it is covered by the sacrococcygeal membrane which is a functional part of the ligamentum flavum.[39]

Dorsal and ventral roots travel a variable distance caudally within the vertebral canal.[40] Then they join to form the spinal nerve that will exit the intervertebral foramen at the appropriate level. The exit is in an infero-lateral direction,[40] but the angle of exit is variable among different segments of the spinal columns.[40] L1 and L2 spinal nerves exit with an angle of 70–80°. L3 and L4 nerve roots exit with an angle of 60° and the L5 nerve root exits with an angle of 45°. The dural sleeves also vary in their origin.[41] L1 to L4 originate behind the body of the vertebra above in the foramen. However, the origin is increasingly higher to the point that L5 has its dural sleeve originating behind the intervertebral disc L4–5. Once exited, the spinal nerves will divide again into dorsal and ventral rami[17, 40] and the dural sleeve blends with the epineurium.[35]

PRACTICAL NOTES

There are multiple tissues in the lower back able to produce pain. These include bone, intervertebral disks, nerve roots, meningeal membranes, ligaments, muscles, fascias, and facet joints.[17, 42] Intervertebral disk herniation may evoke pain from the disk itself, but also from distension of the posterior longitudinal ligament, from radicular compression, from cord compression, and as time goes by from facet joint hypertrophy or from multifidus muscle spasm secondary to chemical irritation.[17] In addition, random MRI in the normal population shows that herniated intervertebral disks can be asymptomatic.[43] A large majority of patients that will be seen in a musculoskeletal clinic will have a complex low back pain that will be the response to several of the above structures. Since not all of the above respond to epidural steroid injections, the degree of response will vary depending on the proportions of all the relative components, as well as upon the concentration of active ingredient reaching the target site.

Epidural steroids can be administered via three routes.

1. The *interlaminar approach* that is directed to the assumed site of pathology[11] and accesses the epidural space through the ligamentum flavum. However, since the majority of causes of low back pain are located in the anterior epidural space, the concentration of active ingredient reaching the site of pathology will be variable, and hence the variable effect. Because of rostral migration of injectate, it is recommended that the injection be distal to the affected site.[44]

2. The *transforaminal approach* targets the affected site and uses the smallest volume to reach the anterior epidural space.[11] The access to the epidural space is through the intervertebral foramen, where a so-called "safety triangle" for injection has been described. This is the area limited by the horizontal base of the pedicle, exiting nerve root, and the lateral border of the vertebral body.[40, 45, 46] A needle placed on this "triangle" will lie above and lateral to the nerve root. Needle positioning has to be radiographically confirmed with lateral and anteroposterior views.[46] However, a classic neurogram is not always achieved, as this may depend on the presence and extent of local pathology.[45] It is common to provoke pain in the distribution of the injected nerve root as a response to chemical stimulation during injection. This is thought to be a sign of "foraminal stenosis"[15] and is normally followed by analgesia when the local anesthetic is active.[15, 45] An injection via this route will act on different structures depending on whether the injection is into the dural sleeve (selective subdural nerve root block) or outside the dural sleeve (transforaminal epidural).[15, 45] A selective subdural nerve root block will act upon the spinal nerve, the dorsal root ganglion, and via inhibition of nerve conduction on the ventral ramus.[15, 45, 47] A transforaminal epidural will have spread of steroid into the epidural fat, and it will also spread onto the dura, intervertebral disk, and posterior longitudinal ligament at the level of injection and one level above and two levels below.[15, 45, 47] A selective nerve root block targets the dural sleeve just outside the foramen and is a putative diagnostic procedure for radicular versus axial pain,[15, 45, 47] whilst a transforaminal epidural injection targets the safety triangle inside the inner interventricular foramen.[15, 45] A transforaminal epidural is said to have two advantages when compared to selective subdural nerve root block. One is that the risk of neural damage is smaller since the target is far away from the spinal nerve. Two is that the mixture will spread to all possible tissues that may contribute to the pain.[15, 45, 48] Some authors are starting to introduce the concept of "preganglionic" transforaminal epidural injections[49, 50, 51] and are claiming better success than when the "standard" transforaminal approach is used. The end point for these is the inferior aspect of the supra-adjacent neural foramen immediately dorsal to the posterior longitudinal ligament or herniated annulus.[51]

3. The *caudal approach* is the easiest and with least complications, but requires the largest volume to reach target areas.[11, 52, 53] However, in one randomized controlled trial (RCT) 20 mL of local anesthetic with 80 mg methylprednisolone (depot) was far superior to 20 mL of local anesthetic plus 60–80 mL of saline.[31]

Possible causes of failure of epidural steroid injection (ESI) are shown in **Table 35.1**.[54, 55, 56] One of the factors that can lead to failure of the injections is inaccurate placement of the needle. This can include both inaccurate tissue plane[14, 52, 53] and inaccurate level of injection.[57] To ensure the most accurate placement, the use of fluoroscopy is recommended as the gold standard.[14, 15, 16, 58] It is generally accepted that blindly performed single epidural injections through a needle will miss the target site in up to 50 percent of cases.[57] The use of contrast-enhanced fluoroscopy during the procedure ensures that the maximum concentration of mixture is delivered to the target site.[25] In view of the rising costs of health care, Fredman et al.[59] studied the practicalities of the routine use of fluoroscopy in the administration of epidural steroids. They concluded that loss of resistance is a reliable sign for locating the epidural space, although because of unreliable surface anatomy the actual space was not the intended space in 50 percent of cases, and subsequently the spread of steroid only reached the affected site in 26 percent of cases. There is no mention in this study of the treatment success, which should play a great part in the economical balance when a study is justified on those grounds.

Due to the toxicity of steroid preparations when administered intrathecally, some authors recommend the injection of a "test dose" of local anesthetic and wait for the development of a motor block suggestive of subarachnoid needle placement.[60]

Improvement of symptoms prior to discharge postinjection is suggestive of mixture being injected around the affected site. It would be normal to experience a transient deterioration of symptoms shortly after dissipation of the local anesthetic effect. This would tend to improve over the following days as the steroid effect starts to manifest itself.[60] If no improvement is experienced immediately after injection, it would be reasonable to repeat it at a later date as this may be the result of the mixture not reaching the target area.[60] The same principle applies to patients who experience short-lived improvement. However, the complications of repeated use of steroids are well known, are dose dependent, and include adrenal suppression, osteoporosis, and deterioration of diabetes.[60]

PHARMACOLOGICAL MIXTURES USED IN THE LITERATURE

Steroids

Drugs and doses used in studies are hydrocortisone 25 mg,[61] methylprednisolone 40 mg[62] or 80 mg,[61] triamcinolone 80 mg,[61] dexamethasone, betamethasone 12 mg,[18, 63] and prednisolone acetate 50 mg.[64]

Some advocate the use of nonparticulate steroid preparations, rather than the depot-formulations, on the rationale that should there be an accidental intra-arterial injection, there may be a smaller risk of spinovascular accident and a spinal cord infarction.

Local anesthetics

These are preservative-free lidocaine 5–20 mg/mL, bupivacaine 0.25 percent, mepivacaine 2.5 mg/mL.

EVIDENCE FOR RADICULAR LOW BACK PAIN

Interlaminar approach

Reports have claimed success in 20–100 percent of cases with an average of 67 percent, although on average this success has lasted less than three months. There have been several attempts to explain this disparity. Some authors believe that the nonstandard use of fluoroscopy is the cause. Figures of up to 50 percent have been quoted with regards to needle malpositioning when using blind techniques for single epidural injection through needle.[57] However, others believe that the anatomical barriers to anterior spread of the steroid mixture from the posterior epidural space are important.

The condition with the highest reported benefit is radicular pain secondary to disk herniation. There is good correlation between outcome and clinical features. However, there is poor correlation between outcomes and imaging.[60] The benefit is lower in patients who present with radicular symptoms postlaminectomy, as these will often have epidural fibrosis that prevents the spread of the local anesthetic mixture.

Table 35.1 Possible causes of failure of ESI.[54, 55, 56]

Pathology	Inadequate delivery	Noninjection factors
Multilevel	Wrong technique	Inappropriate level of activity postprocedure. Both extremes
Canal stenosis	Wrong tissue plane	Inappropriate type of activity postprocedure
Nonresponsive	Wrong level of procedure	Litigation factors
Wrong diagnosis		Pain-related unemployment
New postprocedure pathology		
Long history of pain		

Andersen and Mosdal[20] published the results of 16 patients with low back pain from axial, radicular, and postlaminectomy etiology. Their results suggest a very short-term benefit, but the sample had mixed etiologies and were all treated with the same intervention.

Klenerman et al.[10] assessed ESI against saline, local anesthetic, and dry needle. They analyzed data of 63 patients and concluded that all four groups improved at the same rate. They explained the findings as being due to the natural history of the process.

Koes et al.[13] looked at 12 RCTs to find that eight of them had poor methodological quality. Only four had acceptable methodology and of these, two reported a positive outcome. Overall, out of the 12 studies, six reported benefit from steroids. However, those trials included a multitude of indications treated via all possible routes and the use of fluoroscopy is not reported. They concluded that there is no indication that epidural injections may be effective for patients with low back pain without sciatica.

Watts and Silagy[65] studied 11 RCTs and found that steroids made a difference in pain levels and mobility in the short term, but after six weeks there was no difference between the treatment and the control groups.

McQuay et al.[61] analyzed the meta-analysis performed by Watts and Silagy[65] and established that the number needed to treat (NNT) for short-term efficacy (>75 percent pain relief within 60 days) was 7.3. For long-term efficacy (>50 percent pain relief within one year) NNT was 13, with no significant added benefit from mixing local anesthetic with steroid compared to local anesthetic alone when treating sciatica.

More recent studies that have included follow-ups to 12 months have concluded that the patients who had improved in the short term were actually further improved at 6 and 12 month follow-ups.[56]

Jamison et al.[66] identified several factors predictive of a poor outcome and these are shown in **Table 35.2**.

Valat et al.[64] studied the potential effect of a course of three epidural injections of steroid or saline in the management of sciatica secondary to disk herniation. They did not include a local anesthetic and the volume was only 2 mL in both arms. The improvement in both arms was significant, although the differences between the use of saline

or steroid were not. They concluded that there was no additional benefit from the use of steroids. With only 2 mL and no local anesthetic or fluoroscopic verification of correct placement of the injectate, this study is not informative.

The same is true of the study of Carette et al.[7] who looked into the potential effect of interlaminar steroids at reducing the need for surgery for disk herniation. The authors concluded that although ESI offers short-term improvement of symptoms, it offers no significant functional benefit and does not reduce the need for surgery. The authors of this study, however, did not use a local anesthetic in either arm and their epidural injections were placed without radiographic control.

Abdi et al.[11] tried to eliminate the bias in the Koes and Watts reviews and treated each approach as a different entity. They concluded that there is strong evidence for short-term benefit and limited benefit for long-term relief.[11][II], [IV] We agree with their conclusions.

Transforaminal approach

Radicular symptoms secondary to herniated nucleus pulposus is the condition with the highest reported success.

Kraemer et al.[67] compared translaminar with transforaminal approaches and paravertebral injection as placebo for radicular low back pain. They used steroid, local anesthetic, or saline, and the saline group received systemic steroid to avoid steroid bias. They concluded that the perineural approach with steroid was superior to any other technique.

Vad et al.[46] reported a success rate of 84 percent with a maximum benefit at six weeks of treatment in the group treated with transforaminal steroids when compared with placebo. Average follow up was 1.4 years and 1.7 injections. However, his study was not blinded and the placebo arm consisted of tender point injections administered in the outpatient department.

Riew et al.[18] went further to study the effect of selective nerve root blocks at reducing the need for surgery in radicular pain secondary to herniated disks or to spinal canal stenosis. They concluded that selective nerve root blocks with steroids can significantly reduce the need for decompression in more than 50 percent of candidates for surgery. They also found a statistically significant reduction in neurological symptoms in patients with spinal canal stenosis. The study consisted of a small sample (55) that may have been unable to detect small differences, followed up for 28 months. They also showed that the first injection has the greatest chance of success when compared to successive ones. The same results were reproduced by Yang et al.[23] in a similar study. Later, other studies have concluded that transforaminal epidural steroid injections are an effective nonsurgical treatment option once conservative treatments are not effective. They recommended that this intervention be considered prior to surgery.[25, 68]

Table 35.2 Factors predictive of a poor outcome.[66]

Factors at two weeks after onset of pain	Factors at one year after onset of pain
Greater number of previous treatments	Pain does not interfere with activities
Greater number of analgesic intake	Unemployment due to pain
Pain not increased by activity	Normal straight leg rising before treatment
Pain increased by coughing	Pain unaltered by medication

Derby et al.[69] studied the prognostic value of transforaminal epidural steroids as a predictor of success postsurgery. They concluded that patients with short duration of improvement following steroid injection were less likely to benefit from surgery.

Manchikanti et al.[70] compared the three routes of administration of epidural steroids in a randomly selected sample of 225 patients with low back pain. They concluded that epidural steroids are an effective way to treat low back pain by any of the three routes studied, although the order of efficacy would be transforaminal, caudal, and interlaminar. Although the authors emphasize the use of fluoroscopy,[17] they only applied this to caudal and transforaminal, allowing a blind technique for interlaminar epidural injections.

Caudal approach

Abdi et al.[11] published another systematic review in 2005. They tried to eliminate the bias in the Koes and Watts reviews and treated each approach as a different entity. They concluded that there is strong evidence for short-term and moderate evidence for long-term relief.[11][II], [III]

EVIDENCE FOR FAILED BACK SURGERY SYNDROME

The problem with failed back surgery syndrome (FBSS) is that it does not have a specific treatment because it does not have a specific cause.[26]

Transforaminal

Devulder[71] studied 20 patients with FBSS. Fifty-five percent of patients achieved more than 50 percent pain relief at one month, and 50 percent of those still at three months. However, he mixed hyaluronidase with the local anesthetic–steroid mixture.

Abdi et al.[11] concluded that there is limited (level IV) evidence for short-term or long-term relief.[11][IV]

Caudal

Abdi et al. concluded that there is strong evidence for short-term and moderate evidence for long-term relief after caudal epidural injection of local anesthetic and steroid.[11][II], [III]

Revel et al.[32] evaluated the efficacy of forceful epidural steroid injections in radicular pain secondary to postoperative spinal fibrosis. Twenty-nine percent had less pain after large volume compared with only 6 percent in the small volume groups. At 18 months, results were still in favor of the forceful group, although the proportion of patients returned to work was similar in both groups. The authors

admit that the results are not impressive, but given the simplicity of the procedure, caudal injections should have a role in the management of otherwise intractable FBSS.

EVIDENCE FOR SPINAL CANAL STENOSIS

Interlaminar

From Abdi et al. there is inconclusive evidence for short- or long-term relief.[11][V]

Fukusaki et al.[62] evaluated the effect of translaminar epidural steroid in pseudoclaudication. They found that epidural injection of local anesthetic with or without steroid was more effective than the saline injection used as control for short-term relief. However, the results were no different beyond the three months follow up of the study.

Buttermann[21] compared interlaminar epidural steroid injection with surgical intervention in patients with symptomatic spinal canal stenosis secondary to central intervertebral disk herniation who would be surgical candidates. They concluded that ESI was not as effective as discectomy at reducing pain and disability. On the critical side, the patients were not blinded to both therapeutic options and they did not use fluoroscopic control for the injections.

Transforaminal

Abdi et al. concluded that there is limited evidence for short- or long-term relief of pain from spinal stenosis.[11][IV]

Botwin et al.[28] examined radicular low back pain from degenerative spinal canal stenosis to find that in follow up one year later by an independent practitioner, 75 percent of patients reported pain relief of >50 percent. Sixty-four percent had also increased their walking tolerance and 57 percent their standing tolerance.

In an efficacy study, Riew et al.[18] concluded that transforaminal epidurals offer a significant reduction in neurological symptoms as well as a reduction in low back pain.

In a further one-arm efficacy study, Cooper et al.[29] assessed the use of transforaminal epidural steroids in 61 patients as treatment for radicular pain secondary to degenerative lumbar scoliotic spinal stenosis. Of these, 59.6 percent showed an improvement by two points in numeric rating score for pain and in disability scores at one week, 55.8 at one month, 37.2 at one year and 27.3 at two years. They therefore recommended that transforaminal ESI be considered before surgery.

Caudal

Barre et al.[33] looked at caudal ESI in 95 patients with lumbar spinal canal stenosis in a one-arm retrospective efficacy study. Thirty-five percent of patients had >50 percent improvement in pain scores, and 36 percent of patients had improvement by two points in disability scores. Thirty-five percent of patients had long-term improvement to the previously mentioned levels. However, 12 patients underwent surgery. This study identified the presence of spondylolisthesis as an independent positive predictive factor for successful outcome.

EVIDENCE FOR DISCOGENIC LOW BACK PAIN

Interlaminar

Buttermann[22] tried to determine the effect of steroid in discal pathology other than herniation. He compared intradiscal steroid injection with epidural steroid injection in terms of pain and function and concluded that epidural steroid injection was beneficial for patients with discogenic back pain and inflammatory end-plate changes on MRI. He included 232 patients for ESI and 171 for intradiscal injection. He also found that in a two-year follow up over 60 percent of patients had received further treatment.

Transforaminal

Abdi et al. concluded that there is indeterminate evidence for both short- and long-term relief.[11][V]

Caudal

Southern et al.[63] injected steroids caudally in 97 patients with axial low back pain and imaging consistent with disk pathology at L4–5 or L5-S1 without spinal canal stenosis. Only 23 percent of patients experienced pain relief at a one-year follow up. These patients had reported lower pain scores prior to injection. Previous studies of caudal interventions have mentioned that the key for success is a large volume of injectate. Although the authors of this study were very selective with the patients included with respect to the appropriate level of pathology, they only used 10 mL, and this may not have been enough to achieve adequate spread to the affected area, as suggested by previous studies on these injections.

COMPLICATIONS AND SIDE EFFECTS

Related to the procedure

During single injection procedures, malpositioning of the needle has been found in 25 to 52 percent of cases of transforaminal epidural injections.[46] Intraprocedural fluoroscopic confirmation of needle positioning with a suitable contrast medium is advisable.[16, 72] Botwin et al.[73] studied the radiation exposure from the use of fluoroscopy for the practice of these procedures, and they concluded that it was within safety limits and it did not

pose a danger to the clinician if minimal precautions were observed. These include minimizing exposure time, increasing the distance from hands to radiation source, and the use of shields.

These malpositions include the placement of the needle in the nonintended meningeal layer as well as subarachnoid, intravascular, intraneural, or intraligaments.

Transient exacerbation of symptoms lasting up to 48 hours after the initial improvement is common.[60]

The Australian National Health and Medical Research Council Advisory committee on ESI concluded that in view of the evidence for its use and the potential side effects associated with ESI, they could neither endorse nor proscribe their use. They advised patient's consent and hospital ethics approval prior to the procedure, and recommended that its use be restricted to radicular pain.[52]

Interlaminar approach

Needle malpositioning occurs in up to more than 50 percent of procedures carried out through this route. Up to 6 percent of those needle malpositions are inadvertent intrathecal injections. Furthermore, this is the route with the highest incidence of injection in a nonintended level due mainly to normal anatomical variations.

The epidural space is a virtual space that contains the spinal venous plexus. Hence, it is technically possible to damage these vessels.

Postdural puncture headache is a potential complication of dural penetration when inserting the needle. It is more frequent in cases where there has been previous spinal surgery.[60] Severe headaches may also be the consequence of air in the subdural space if air is used for loss of resistance.[11, 60]

There have been several reports of epidural abscesses, the risk being higher in diabetic patients,[60, 74] and in patients on systemic steroid medication. Two cases of meningitis have been reported in the literature.[74]

A rarer, but devastating adverse event is sudden onset of blindness shortly after the procedure.[75, 76] It appears to be related to the volume of injectate (up to 120 mL have been used in the literature) and to the speed of injection, causing a sudden rise in intracranial pressure that can compromise the retinal blood supply leading into hemorrhagic areas in the retina. In some cases the patients recovered some sight, but it never returned to the levels before the injury.

Transforaminal approach

The arterial supply to the spinal cord below T2 depends on direct blood supply from segmental spinal arterial tributaries from the aorta or iliac arteries that enter the spinal canal through the segmental spinal foramina. Although it is technically possible to lacerate these arteries through both interlaminar and transforaminal approaches, the risk is higher with transforaminal procedures because the needle is always close to the spinal cord radicular artery entering through the intervertebral foramen. A laceration or injecting air or particulate injectate at this level will risk spinal cord infarct or epidural hematoma with permanent spinal cord damage. Infarct of the medulla oblongata will result if the injury happens at a cervical level. Houten and Errico[77] reported three cases of paraplegia after computed tomography (CT) or fluoroscopy-guided transforaminal epidural. In all three cases the symptoms started immediately after injection and MRI showed lower thoracic spinal cord edema. The authors believe the reason for this complication was missed intra-arterial injection when the needle penetrated an aberrant artery of Adamkiewicz, arteria radicularis magna – the main radicular artery supplying the anterior spinal artery. Intrathecal administration of depot steroids and solvents can cause paraparesis. In this study the authors believe that accidental intrathecal injection was excluded by the use of contrast and fluoroscopy. Huntoon and Martin[78] reported a case of spinal infarct resulting in paraparesis and chronic pain following injection of 5 mL of triamcinolone and bupivacaine 0.125 percent. Glaser and Falco[79] reported a tragic case of paraplegia, in spite of injecting under fluoroscopic control and in the so-called "safe triangle."

Other reported risks are a 10 percent incidence of rash and pruritus, a 4 percent incidence of weight gain[70] and an 11.2 percent risk of intravascular penetration that was higher at S1 level at 21.3 percent. Blood aspiration was a highly specific (97.9 percent) but poorly sensitive (44.7 percent) sign for intravascular needle placement.[58]

Finn and Case[72] reported a case of intradiscal injection that reemphasizes the use of contrast-enhanced fluoroscopy to prevent complications.

Transforaminal steroid injections performed with fluoroscopy and local anesthetic injection to prevent intra-arterial injections are generally safe. However, major, devastating complications with tragic and permanent spinal cord damage can arise despite adhering to the safest techniques and precautions.

Caudal approach

Needle malpositioning is most common through this approach, with an incidence of up to 40 percent.[33]

The need to use larger volumes of injectate has been linked with complications from a sudden rise in intracranial pressure. These have included venous bleeding into the retina secondary to an increased presence of CSF around the optic nerve. Less dramatic complications from a sudden increment in intracranial pressure have included headache, nausea, dizziness, and spasm of back muscles. However, all case reports have used an excess of 40 mL.

Other less frequent complications include insomnia in 4.7 percent, transient non-postdural puncture headache (PDPH) 3.5 percent, increased back pain 3.1 percent, facial flushing 2.3 percent, vasovagal syncope 0.8 percent, nausea 0.8 percent, and 0.4 percent increased leg pain.[80]

Related to the injectate

Inadvertent intravascular injection of particulate steroids has been reported to cause cerebrovascular accidents, retinal infarcts, and deafness[81] from the formation of microembolae. Methylprednisolone acetate forms aggregates when dissolved in local anesthetics more than other depot steroids.[11]

Subarachnoid steroids were routinely used up until the late 1980s to prevent arachnoiditis reactive to the injection of contrast media during myelography. After several series of cases where patients developed arachnoiditis following the subarachnoid injection of methylprednisolone, it is widely accepted that up to 90 percent of patients will develop radiographic arachnoiditis, and up to 20 percent of such patients will progress to clinical arachnoiditis. This has been attributed to polyethylene glycol used as a vehicle in the preparations of methylprednisolone.[60] Other reported complications of subarachnoid steroids are chemical meningitis, convulsions, subarachnoid hemorrhage, and urinary incontinence. However, some authors still advocate their use as treatment for multiple sclerosis.

Epidural steroids have not been related to arachnoiditis.[60] However, there have been reports of encephalopathy, myelopathy, cauda equina syndrome, chemical meningitis, and epidural abscesses. The latter complications have resulted in para/tetraplegia and even death. There have been reports of activation of latent tuberculous or cryptococcal infections and of septicemia following epidural administration of steroids.

Some preservatives included in the steroid formulations may be potentially neurotoxic, as suggested by animal research.[9]

The depot steroids may produce a picture consistent with ACTH suppression that can last a few weeks.[11, 60] Patients with diabetes may experience a transitory rise in glycemic levels or in insulin requirements that may last several days.[11, 60] Other systemic problems reported from the use of steroids are osteoporosis, bone avascular necrosis, myopathy, truncal weight gain, and fluid retention.[11, 82] Within these lines, Manchikanti et al.[83] followed up patients for up to one year after epidural steroid injection and reported no incidence of bone mass density change or weight gain.

Lowell et al.[84] reported three cases of epidural abscess in patients who were injected with 40 mg of methylprednisolone intraoperatively after microdiscectomy.

CONTRAINDICATIONS

The number and doses of epidural steroid injections that a patient can have has not been determined. Existing studies do not offer injections any closer than two weeks apart since the systemic effect of the steroid may persist for at least two weeks, depending on dose of depot steroid.

Absolute

- Systemic infection or local infection at the site of the injection. There have been reports of tuberculosis being reactivated by epidural steroid injections.
- Any bleeding disorder, thrombocytopenia, potent platelet inhibitor, therapeutic doses of low molecular heparin, unfractionated heparin, pentasacharide, vitamin K-antagonist.
- History of allergic reaction to the injected solutions, including radiological contrast, local anesthetic, or steroids.
- Spinal canal stenosis of any cause: interlaminar epidural. A transforaminal injection of a small volume may carry less risk.
- Patient refusal.

Relative

- Unusual ("difficult") anatomy increases the risk of dural puncture and of intraspinal bleeding.
- Nonsteroidal anti-inflammatory drugs (NSAIDs) reduce platelet stickiness. Horlocker et al.[85] studied 1035 patients on NSAIDs receiving epidural steroids and found no epidural hematomas. However, they found that advanced age, needle gauge, approach, multiple passes, and accidental dural puncture were all related to increased incidence of blood in the needle, although there were no long-lasting complications.
- Steroids are relatively contraindicated in:
  - patients with congestive cardiac failure in whom a slight increase in circulating blood volume may pose a risk of decompensation;
  - insulin-dependent diabetics and patients on chronic steroid medication have increased risk of infection;
  - patients who are scheduled for surgery in the near future, as epidural depot steroid may cause adrenal suppression;
  - pregnancy: risk of intrauterine growth retardation with repeated steroid injections

REFERENCES

1. Saal JS, Franson RC, Dobrow R et al. High levels of phospholypase A2 activity in lumbar disc herniations. *Spine*. 1990; **15**: 674–8.
2. Haddox JD. Lumbar and cervical epidural steroid therapy. *Anaesthesiology Clinics of North America*. 1992; **10**: 179–203.
3. Lindblom K, Rexed B. Spinal nerve injury in dorso-lateral protrusions of lumbar discs. *Journal of Neurosurgery*. 1948; **5**: 413–32.
4. Lindahl O, Rexed B. Histologic changes in the spinal nerve roots of operated cases of sciatica. *Acta Orthopaedica Scandinavica*. 1951; **20**: 215–25.
5. Burn JM, Langdon L. Duration of action of epidural methylprednisolone. A study of patients with the lumbosciatic syndrome. *American Journal of Physical Medicine*. 1974; **53**: 29–34.
6. Dilke TFW, Burry HC, Grahame R. Extradural corticosteroid injection in the management of lumbar nerve root compression. *British Medical Journal*. 1973; **2**: 635–7.
7. Carette S, Leclaire R, Marcoux S et al. Epidural corticosteroid injections for sciatica due to herniated nucleus pulposus. *New England Journal of Medicine*. 1997; **336**: 1634–40.
8. Johansson A, Hao J, Sjolund B. Local corticosteroid application blocks transmission in normal nociceptive C-fibres. *Acta Anaesthesiologica Scandinavica*. 1990; **34**: 335–8.
9. Nelson DA, Landau WM. Intraspinal steroids, efficacy, accidentality and controversy with review of United States Food and Drug Administration reports. *Journal of Neurology, Neurosurgery, and Psychiatry*. 2001; **70**: 433–43.
10. Klenerman L, Greenwood R, Davenport HE et al. Lumbar epidural injections in the treatment of sciatica. *British Journal of Rheumatology*. 1984; **23**: 35–8.
* 11. Abdi S, Datta S, Lucas LF. Role of epidural steroids in the management of chronic spinal pain: A systematic review of effectiveness and complications. *Pain Physician*. 2005; **8**: 127–43.
* 12. Boswell MV et al. Interventional techniques in the management of chronic spinal pain: evidence-based practice guidelines. *Pain Physician*. 2005; **8**: 1–47.
* 13. Koes BW, Scholten RJPM, Mens JMA, Bouter LM. Efficacy of epidural steroid injections for low-back pain and sciatica: a systematic review of randomized clinical trials. *Pain*. 1995; **63**: 279–88.
14. Manchikanti L, Singh V, Bakhit C et al. Interventional techniques in the management of chronic pain: Part 1. *Pain Physician*. 2000; **3**: 7–42.
15. O'Neill C, Derby R, Knederes R. Precision injection techniques for the diagnosis and treatment of lumbar disc disease. *Seminars in Spine Surgery*. 1999; **11**: 104–18.
16. Manchikanti L, Bakhit CE, Pakanati RR et al. Fluoroscopy is medically necessary for the performance of epidural steroids. *Anesthesia and Analgesia*. 1999; **89**: 1326–7.
17. Manchikanti L. Transforaminal lumbar epidural steroid injections. *Pain Physician*. 2000; **3**: 374–98.
18. Riew KD, Yin Y, Gilula L et al. The effect of nerve-root injections on the need for operative treatment of lumbar radicular pain. *Journal of Bone and Joint Surgery. American volume*. 2000; **82**: 1589–93.
19. Buchner M, Zeifang F, Brocai D. Epidural corticosteroid injection in the conservative management of sciatica. *Clinical Orthopaedics and Related Research*. 2000; **375**: 149–56.

20. Andersen KH, Mosdal C. Epidural application of corticosteroids in low back pain and sciatica. *Acta Neurochirurgica*. 1987; **87**: 1–2.

21. Buttermann GR. Treatment of lumbar disc herniation: Epidural steroid injection compared with discectomy. A prospective, randomized study. *Journal of Bone and Joint Surgery. American volume*. 2004; **86-A**: 670–9.

22. Buttermann GR. The effect of spinal steroid injections for degenerative disc disease. *Spine Journal*. 2004; **4**: 495–505.

23. Yang SC *et al*. Transforaminal epidural steroid injection for discectomy candidates: An outcome study with a minimum of two-year follow-up. *Chang Gung Medical Journal*. 2006; **29**: 93–9.

24. Cahana A, Mavrocordatos P, Geurts JW, Groen GJ. Do minimally invasive procedures have a place in the treatment of chronic low back pain? *Expert Review of Neurotherapeutics*. 2004; **4**: 479–90.

25. Lutz GE, Vad VB, Wisneski RJ. Fluoroscopic transforaminal lumbar epidural steroids: an outcome study. *Archives of Physical Medicine and Rehabilitation*. 1998; **79**: 1362–6.

26. Mavrocordatos P, Cahana A. Minimally invasive procedures for the treatment of failed back surgery syndrome. *Advances and Technical Standards in Neurosurgery*. 2006; **31**: 221–52.

27. Devulder J. Transforaminal nerve root sleeve injection with corticosteroids, hyaluronidase, and local anaesthetic in the failed back surgery syndrome. *Journal of Spinal Disorders*. 1998; **11**: 151–4.

28. Botwin KP *et al*. Fluoroscopically guided lumbar transforaminal epidural steroid injections in degenerative lumber stenosis: An outcome study. *American Journal of Physical Medicine and Rehabilitation*. 2002; **81**: 898–905.

29. Cooper G, Lutz GE, Boachie-Adjei O, Lin J. Effectiveness of transforaminal epidural steroid injections in patients with degenerative lumbar scoliosis stenosis and radiculopathy. *Pain Physician*. 2004; **7**: 311–17.

30. Rosemberg SK, Grabinsky A, Kooser C, Boswell MV. Effectiveness of transforaminal epidural steroid injections in low back pain: a one year experience. *Pain Physician*. 2002; **5**: 266–70.

31. Breivik H, Hesla PE, Molnar I, Lind B. Treatment of low back pain and sciatica: Comparison of caudal epidural injections of bupivacaine and methylprednisolone with bupivacaine followed by saline. In: Bonica JJ, Albe-Fessard D (eds). *Advances in pain research and therapy*. Raven Press: New York, 1976: 927–32.

32. Revel M *et al*. Forceful epidural injections for the treatment of lumbosciatic pain with post-operative lumbar spinal fibrosis. *Revue du Rhumatisme (English ed.)*. 1996; **63**: 270–7.

33. Barre L, Lutz GE, Southern D, Cooper G. Fluoroscopically guided caudal epidural steroid injections for lumbar spinal stenosis: a retrospective evaluation of long term efficacy. *Pain Physician*. 2004; **7**: 187–93.

34. Bogduk N. The innervation of the lumbar spine. *Spine*. 1983; **8**: 286–93.

35. Bogduk N. *Clinical anatomy of the lumbar spine and sacrum*. New York: Churchill Livingstone, 1997: 55–6.

36. Brown DL. *Atlas of regional anaesthesia*. London: WB Saunders Company, 1992: 259.

37. Brown DL. *Atlas of regional anaesthesia*. London: WB Saunders Company, 1992: 261.

38. Crighton IM, Barry BP, Hobbs GJ. A study of the anatomy of the caudal space using magnetic resonance imaging. *British Journal of Anaesthesia*. 1997; **78**: 391–5.

39. Brown DL. *Atlas of regional anaesthesia*. London: WB Saunders Company, 1992: 264–5.

40. Bogduk N. *Clinical anatomy of the lumbar spine and sacrum*. New York: Churchill Livingstone, 1997: 127–44.

41. Bose K, Balasubramanian P. Nerve root canals of the lumbar spine. *Spine*. 1984; **9**: 16–18.

42. Manchikanti L, Singh V, Pampati V *et al*. Evaluation of the relative contributions of various structures in chronic low back pain. *Pain Physician*. 2001; **4**: 308–16.

43. Jensen MC, Bran-Zawadzki MN, Obukjowski N *et al*. Magnetic resonance imaging of the lumbar spine in people without back pain. *New England Journal of Medicine*. 1994; **331**: 69–73.

44. Hodgson PSA, Mack B, Kopacz D *et al*. Needle placement during lumbar epidural anaesthesiadeviates toward the non-dependent side. *Regional Anesthesia*. 1996; **21**: 26.

45. Derby R, Bogduk N, Kine G. Precision percutaneous blocking procedures for localising spinal pain. *Pain Digest*. 1993; **3**: 175–88.

46. Vad VB, Bhat AL, Lutz GE, Cammisa F. Transforaminal epidural steroids in lumbosacral radiculopathy. A prospective randomized study. *Spine*. 2002; **27**: 11–16.

47. Furman M. Is it really possible to do a selective nerve root block? *ISIS Scientific Newsletter*. 1999; **3**: 73–85.

48. Siddall P, Cousins M. Spinal pain mechanisms. *Spine*. 1997; **22**: 98–104.

49. Lee JW, Kim SH, Choi JY *et al*. Transforaminal epidural steroid injection for lumbosacral radiculopathy: preganglionic versus conventional approach. *Korean Journal of Radiology*. 2006; **7**: 139–44.

50. Sung MS. Epidural steroid injection for lumbosacral radiculopathy. *Korean Journal of Radiology*. 2006; **7**: 77–8.

51. Lew HL, Coelho P, Chou LH. Preganglionic approach to transforaminal epidural steroid injections. *American Journal of Physical Medicine and Rehabilitation*. 2004; **83**: 378.

52. Bogduk N, Christophidis N, Cherry D, et al. Epidural use of steroids in the management of back pain. Report of the working party on the epidural use of steroids in back pain. Camberra, Australia, National Health and Medical Research Council, 1994; 1–76.

53. White AH, Derby R, Wynne G. Epidural injections for diagnosis and treatment of low back pain. *Spine*. 1980; **5**: 78–86.

54. Saal JS, Saal JA. *Comprehensive cervical and lumbar intraspinal injection course*. Stanford, CA: Stanford University School of Medicine, July 11–12, 1998.

55. Hartrick CT. Screening instruments for the prediction of long-term response to epidural steroid injection in the treatment of lumbar radiculopathy. *Contemporary Neurology*. 1998; **1A**: 2–6.

56. Hopwood MB, Abram SE. Factors associated with failure of epidural steroids. *Regional Anesthesia*. 1993; **18**: 238–43.

57. Weinstein SM, Herring SA, Derby R. Contemporary concepts in spine care: Epidural steroid injections. *Spine*. 1995; **20**: 1842–6.

58. Furman MB, O'Brien EM, Zgleszewski TM. Incidence of intravascular penetration in transforaminal lumbosacralepidural steroid injection. *Spine*. 2000; **25**: 2628–32.

59. Fredman B *et al*. Epidural steroids for treating "Failed back surgery syndrome": Is fluoroscopy really necessary. *Anesthesia and Analgesia*. 1999; **88**: 367.

60. Abram SE. Treatment of lumbosacral radiculopathy with epidural steroids. *Anesthesiology*. 1999; **91**: 1937–41.

61. McQuay H, Moore A. Epidural steroids for sciatica. *Anaesthesia and Intensive Care*. 1996; **24**: 284–5.

62. Fukusaki M, Kobayashi I, Hara T, Sumikawa K. Symptoms of spinal canal stenosis do not improve after epidural steroid injection. *Clinical Journal of Pain*. 1998; **14**: 148–51.

63. Southern D, Lutz GE, Cooper G, Barre L. Are fluoroscopic caudal epidural steroid injections effective for managing chronic low back pain? *Pain Physician*. 2003; **6**: 167–72.

64. Valat JP, Giraudeau B, Rozenberg S *et al*. Epidural corticosteroid injections for sciatica: a randomised, double blind, controlled clinical trial. *Annals of the Rheumatic Diseases*. 2003; **62**: 639–43.

65. Watts RW, Silagy CA. A meta-analysis on the efficacy of epidural corticosteroids in the treatment of sciatica. *Anaesthesia and Intensive Care*. 1995; **23**: 564–9.

66. Jamison RN, VandeBoncouer T, Ferrante FM. Low back pain patients unresponsive to an epidural steroid injection: Identifying predictive factors. *Clinical Journal of Pain*. 1991; **7**: 311–17.

67. Kraemer J *et al*. Lumbar epidural perineural injection: a new technique. *European Spine Journal*. 1997; **6**: 357–61.

68. Weiner BK, Fraser RD. Foraminal injection for lateral lumbar disc herniation. *Journal of Bone and Joint Surgery*. 1997; **79**: 804–7.

69. Derby R, Kine G, Saal JA *et al*. Response to steroid and duration of radicular pain as predictors of surgical outcome. *Spine*. 1992; **17**: 176–83.

70. Manchikanti L, Pakanati RR, Pampati V. Comparison of three routes of epidural steroid injections inlow back pain. *Pain Digest*. 1999; **9**: 277–85.

71. Devulder J. Transforaminal nerve root sleeve injection with corticosteroid, hyaluronidase and local anaesthetic in the failed back surgery syndrome. *Journal of Spinal Disorders*. 1998; **11**: 151–4.

72. Finn K, Case J. Disk entry: a complication of transforaminal epidural injection. A case report. *Archives of Physical Medicine and Rehabilitation*. 2005; **86**: 1489–91.

73. Botwin KP, Thomas S, Gruber RD *et al*. Radiation exposure of the spinal interventionalistperforming fluoroscopically-guided lumbar transforaminal epidural steroid injections. *Archives of Physical Medicine and Rehabilitation*. 2002; **83**: 697–701.

74. Abram SE, O'Connor TC. Complications associated with epidural steroid injections. *Regional Anesthesia*. 1996; **212**: 149–62.

75. Young WF. Transient blindness after lumbar epidural steroid injection: a case report and literature review. *Spine*. 2002; **27**: 476–7.

76. Purdy EP, Ajimal GS. Vision loss after lumbar epidural steroid injection. *Anesthesia and Analgesia*. 1998; **86**: 119–22.

77. Houten JK, Errico TJ. Paraplegia after lumbosacral nerve root block: report of 3 cases. *Spine Journal*. 2002; **2**: 70–5.

78. Huntoon MA, Martin DP. Paralysis after transforaminal epidural injection and previous spinal surgery. *Regional Anesthesia and Pain Medicine*. 2004; **29**: 494–5.

79. Glaser SE, Falco F. Paraplegia following thoracolumbar transforaminal epidural steroid injection. *Pain Physician*. 2005; **8**: 1533.

80. Botwin KP, Gruber RD, Bouchlas CG *et al*. Complications of fluoroscopically-guided caudal epidural injections. *American Journal of Physical Medicine and Rehabilitation*. 2001; **80**: 416–24.

81. Cousins MJ. An additional dimension to the efficacy of epidural steroids. *Anesthesiology*. 2000; **93**: 565.

82. Latham JM, Fraser RD, Moore RJ *et al*. The pathologic effects of intrathecal betamethasone. *Spine*. 1997; **22**: 1558–62.

83. Manchikanti L, Pampati V, Beyer C *et al*. The effect of neuroaxial corticosteroids on weight and bone mass density: A prospective evaluation. *Pain Physician*. 2000; **3**: 357–66.

84. Lowell TD, Errico TJ, Eskenazi MS. Use of epidural steroids after discectomy may predispose to infection. *Spine*. 2000; **25**: 516–19.

85. Horlocker TT, Bajwa ZH, Ashraf Z *et al*. Risk assessment of haemorrhagic complications associated with non-steroidal antiinflammatory drugs in ambulatory pain clinic patients undergoing steroid epidural injection. *Anesthesia and Analgesia*. 2002; **95**: 1691–7.

36

Epiduroscopy and endoscopic adhesiolysis

JONATHAN RICHARDSON, JAN WILLEM KALLEWAARD, AND GERBRAND J GROEN

KEY LEARNING POINTS

- Epiduroscopy is a new development which may aid the understanding of complex pathophysiology of complex lumbar radiculopathy pain.
- Its main indication is chronic lumbar radiculopathic pain, particularly associated with previous back surgery or spinal stenosis.

- Two randomized controlled trials (RCTs) of endoscopic adhesiolysis show positive outcomes.
- Methods of improved adhesiolysis are under evaluation.
- Prospective well-designed and controlled studies are needed.

INTRODUCTION

Endoscopy has improved patient care in many areas of medicine, for example arthroscopic and laparoscopic surgery. Endoscopy of the spinal canal is still in an experimental developing stage and its future depends upon a number of factors, many of which are technical.

Epiduroscopy means endoscopic examination of the epidural space. The intrathecal space can be examined, but this is usually avoided as pathology and changes producing pain are thought to occur mainly within the epidural space.

HISTORY

Epiduroscopy is not a new subject. Seventy years ago, Elias Stern[1] anticipated that direct observation of the

contents of the spinal canal might be practically useful. Pathological changes of inflammation, adhesions of the spinal membranes, varicosities of the cord, and tumors were recognized soon afterwards.[2] The study of the blood supply of the cord and nerve roots both in normal and pathological conditions was anticipated.

Michael S Burman[3] is credited with carrying out the first cadaver spinal endoscopy and a few years later an American neurosurgeon, Pool,[4] published the largest case series ever of over 400 examinations. In the 1960s, Ooi et al.[5] published a case series of over 300 patient examinations. He studied the cessation of blood flow in the cauda equina during straight-leg raising[6] and the dynamic effects of posture on the vessels of the cauda equina in lumbar canal stenosis.[7]

Blomberg and Olsson[8] and Heavener et al.[9] published useful observations. In 1991, Shimoji et al.[10] made two very important points: for safety, patients must be examined awake and pain could be reproduced by gentle contact with affected nerve roots. Recently, Saberski and Kitahata[11] have popularized the caudal approach, thereby reducing the chances of inadvertent subarachnoid entry and neurological disturbance. Modern instruments are flexible, steerable, and have a saline irrigation port (**Figures 36.1** and **36.2**).

Areas in which epiduroscopy has contributed to patient care are living anatomy, its association with regional anesthesia, and the diagnosis and management of chronically painful conditions (see below under The role of epiduroscopy in chronic pain management).

EPIDURAL STRUCTURES

Epiduroscopy can provide views of the dura mater, nerve roots, fatty and fibrous connective tissue, the ligamentum flavum, and periosteum.

Fat exists in a segmental distribution between the laminae as previously shown by magnetic resonance imaging (MRI)[12] and cryomicrotomy.[13]

Epidural blood vessel trauma associated with the introduction of a Tuohy needle is seen in approximately one-quarter of patients.[14] It is reported that subsequent

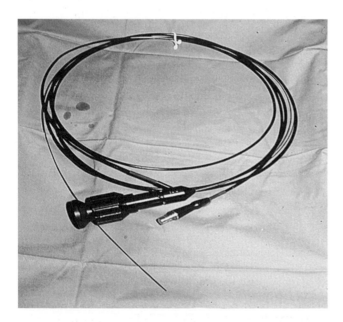

Figure 36.1 A modern epiduroscope.

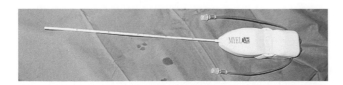

Figure 36.2 Outer steering sheath possessing two lumena: one for the scope and one for saline irrigation.

epidural anesthesia is unreliable, occasionally resulting in unilateral,[15] failed,[16] or insufficient analgesic spread.[17] Profound observations have been made by Igarashi and colleagues[17] with epiduroscopic examination revealing significant occlusive inflammatory changes.

The same authors have contributed to our knowledge in a number of other areas. The aging epidural space becomes readily widely patent following the injection of air, while at the same time there is a reduction in the amount of fatty tissue.[14] Fibrous connective tissue, the degree of vascularity, and susceptibility of blood vessels to trauma do not alter.

Fatty and fibrous connective tissue reduce rostrally compared to the lumbar space.[18] The thoracic epidural space is more distensible than the lumbar space, as shown by injection of air during epiduroscopy, and intrapleural pressures transmit to the epidural space.[19]

Epiduroscopy in pregnancy has revealed blood vessel engorgement in the first trimester with an increase in vascular network in the third trimester.[20]

THE ROLE OF EPIDUROSCOPY IN CHRONIC PAIN MANAGEMENT

Low back pain (LBP) is a major health resource consumer within the western world. At some time, 80 percent of the population will be affected and although most of these episodes settle, in many patients they recur. At 12 months most people are in pain and many are severely disabled.[21, 22] Chronic radiculopathic pain ensues in approximately 1 percent as defined by pain in the distribution of a lumbar nerve root accompanied by neurosensory and motor deficits.[23] Radiculopathic pain is probably the most painful and disabling condition in degenerative lumbar spine disease and is difficult to manage, as current treatments are only partially effective. Reliance upon traditional treatments (surgery, physiotherapy, and long-term pharmacotherapy) is expensive and often only partly effective.

The main indication for epiduroscopy is chronic lumbar radiculopathic pain, particularly in association with previous back surgery (failed back surgery syndrome (FBSS)) or spinal stenosis (SS). Other symptoms, for example numbness, may be an indication if this is thought to have arisen as part of a true radiculopathic syndrome, i.e. its cause is within the nerve root.

Pathophysiology of radiculopathy

Pain generation is complex and it is a gross simplification that compression of nerve roots alone causes pain. Nerve root alteration in morphology, along with injury leading to radiculopathy, can ensue without any mechanical cause being present.[24, 25, 26, 27, 28, 29, 30] Paresthesiae arise through compression but for the production of pain, inflammation of nerve roots in addition is required.

Human *in vivo* confirmatory evidence for this has come from volunteers undergoing back surgery under local anesthetic infiltration when only inflamed nerve roots which are in contact with (but not compressed by) herniated disks are pain sensitive.[31] The mechanisms involved in radiculopathy involve vascular, neurotoxic, immunological, and inflammatory reactions arising from the leakage of nucleus pulposus into the epidural space.

Nerve root properties

Nerve root (especially dorsal root) blood supply is poor with approximately 75 percent of its nutrition depending upon a flow of cerebrospinal fluid (CSF).[32, 33] In disease states, especially with adhesive arachnoiditis, nutrition becomes critical. This may occur not just through mechanical constriction of the vessels with intraneural edema, but also through thrombus formation in the intraneural capillaries which follows nucleus pulposus contact.[24, 25, 26, 27, 28, 29, 30] A compartment syndrome is effectively produced within the nerve root.[34]

Role of nucleus pulposus

Nucleus pulposus is chemically active, containing a host of potentially inflammatory chemicals.[24, 25, 26, 27, 28, 29, 30, 34] An annular tear of an intervertebral disk releases large amounts of phospholipase.[35] A direct pathway exists between degenerate disks and the epidural space, a feature well known to discographers, so that these chemicals can come into direct contact with the nerve root.[35] Pain generation occurs as cytokines present in the nucleus pulposis placed directly on intact nerves causes a painful neuropathy.[24, 25, 26, 27, 28, 29, 30, 34] Venous congestion and intraneural edema of the nerve root follows which is exacerbated by rapid thrombus formation.[24, 25, 26, 27, 28, 29, 30, 34] An impairment in intraneural blood flow is probably the final common pathway leading to abnormalities in nerve conduction (see below under Epidural fibrosis) and pain generation.[24, 25, 26, 27, 28, 29, 30, 34] For the reliable induction of abnormal pain behavior in experimental conditions, a combination of physical deformation of the nerve root is required, as well as chemical irritation from a herniated nucleus pulposus.[25] Either insult alone may be unreliable.

Demyelination with nerve conduction abnormalities ensue.[24, 25, 26, 27, 28, 29, 30, 34] Areas of demyelination become sources of ectopic discharge interpreted by higher centers as altered sensation and pain.[36] Extreme mechanical sensitivity develops, so that straight-leg raising leads to spontaneous discharge and pain.[37] Peripheral and central sensitization contribute to the overall process involved in chronic radicular pain and radiculopathy.

Epidural fibrosis

The overall events responsible for the production of an inflammatory process which leads to the development of fibrosis can be summarized as a chronic chemical radiculitis, neurogenic inflammation, probably an autoimmune response to nucleus puplosus and impaired fibrinolysis.[24, 25, 26, 27, 28, 29, 30, 31, 32, 33, 34, 35, 37, 38]

Spinal surgery is a potent source of fibrosis. Surgery for patients with sciatica can probably be expected to improve the mechanics of nerve compression, thereby possibly promoting a restoration of nerve root nutrition and circulation, but the potential risks include worsened direct, neurogenic and possible immunological inflammation, and further impairment of fibrinolysis through activation of the stress response to surgery.[39] Direct tissue trauma, bruising, bleeding, bacterial and possibly foreign body contamination encourage a further fibrous reaction. Stimulation of the nervous system through the process of intraoperative and postoperative pain generation, as well as any possible neurological damage, encourages the continuation of chronic pain.[36] The incidence of fibrosis in association with chronic radiculopathic pain is near to 100 percent of patients examined endoscopically.[40, 41]

Nerve root blood flow in the healthy situation is relatively poor with reliance upon a circulation of CSF. "Strangulation" of nerve roots due to epidural fibrosis has been described in terms of a compartment syndrome.[34] Dense fibrosis is usual following surgery. An overall quantitative relationship between epidural scar and radicular pain has been evaluated by MRI after lumbar laminectomy: subjects with extensive peridural scarring were three times more likely to experience radicular pain.[42]

In summary, the generation of chronic radiculopathic pain is complex, involving much more than nerve root compression. The main causes are biochemical and vascular. However, attention to physical abnormalities alone, for example disk prolapse, is unlikely to produce optimal results for many patients. Adhesiolysis, aimed at freeing nerves from tethering effects and allowing sufficient space around nerve roots for unimpeded flow of CSF and blood supply, may be beneficial, but needs to be studied in controlled trials.

PRACTICAL ENDOSCOPY

Most of the basic requirements for epiduroscopy will be available in most acute hospitals. These are listed in **Box 36.1**.

The requirements for a useful spinal endoscope are high quality optics, flexibility, steerability, a system for constant administration of a distending medium of saline (small volume air injection can be used for limited examinations), and of course safety. All this has to be made with as small an outside diameter as possible. It is only in the last decade that these requirements have been met.

A number of modern spinal endoscopes are in common use. Optics of between 10 and 15,000 pixels are the norm (**Figure 36.1**). The steering outer sheath produces an instrument with an outside diameter of approximately 2.5 mm (**Figure 36.2**).

The caudal route is the most appropriate entry for most examinations as a straight line up to the lumbar area is provided.

Consent

The following words should probably be included: *spinal endoscopy*, *headaches*, *sacral fluid leak of saline*, *tingling*, *numbness*, and *weakness of the legs*. Patients may also be consented for meningitis, nerve root avulsion, and paraplegia. To the best of our knowledge these complications have not so far been reported. Consent is also required for the drugs used, especially steroids. It may be appropriate to consent patients for unknown Creutzfeld–Jakob disease risk. Problems with vision have resulted from the transmission of saline pressure from the epidural space (ES) to the spinal space and thence by the hydraulics of the CSF to the brain. As the patient is prone, the eye is the most dependent part of the brain.

Exclusion criteria are listed in **Box 36.2**.

Box 36.1 Basic requirements for epiduroscopy

- Facilities for sterile patient management.
- Facilities for x-ray screening.
- A cold light source and a video display. An advantage is an image recording system, preferably digital (DVD).
- A saline flushing device.
- Equipment for entry into the epidural space.

Box 36.2 Exclusion criteria

- Lack of consent including difficulty with comprehension for any reason, for example language barrier, psychiatric disorder.
- Local infection at the entry site.
- The use of anticoagulants or a bleeding diathesis.
- Hypersensitivity to local anesthetic or contrast media (the procedure could be modified).
- Pregnancy.
- Marked obesity.
- Uncontrolled hypertension.
- Inability to lie prone for at least an hour due to any reason.
- Brain/eye disease.

Sterilization of the epiduroscope

A glutaraldehyde bath followed by careful rinsing is appropriate, but this can be modified according to local arrangements. Autoclaving is not possible as the delicate optical instrument is not made to withstand high temperatures.

The endoscope must be handled with great care to avoid fracture of fibers. Only gentle coiling should be attempted. Sudden uncoiling can easily cause contact with nonsterile surfaces. Careful storage is necessary to avoid damage. Training and interest of dedicated staff is optimal.

Observation of the epidural space

The room set up is shown in **Figure 36.3**. At least one and a half hours of operating time per patient should be allowed.

The side of the patient's pain and its approximate dermatomal level should be known to the operator. This allows confinement of the examination to the particular area in question, as opposed to an attempted examination of the entire lumbar spine. This substantially reduces the amount of operating time required. Dermatomal charts should be known.

Broad spectrum antibiotic prophylaxis (e.g. a cephalosporin) is generally used. Sedation is helpful but this should be light. Monitoring of blood pressures, oxygen saturations, and electrocardiograms are only helpful if excessive sedation has been used or if the patient has coexisting disease, otherwise the alarms are distracting.

With the patient positioned prone on the operating table, the skin of the back, especially around the sacral

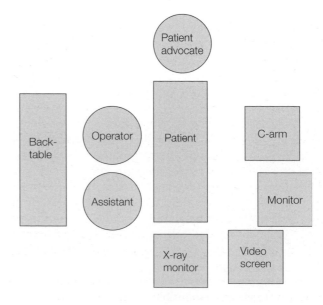

Figure 36.3 Procedure room set up.

hiatus, should be cleaned. A Seldinger technique is used for access to the sacral ES. An epidurogram (5–15 mL of nonionic water-soluble contrast medium) can delineate filling defects, indicating islands of epidural fibrosis which often correspond with the site of the patient's pain (**Figure 36.4**).

Gentle contact with nerve roots relevant to the patient's pain elicits a valuable response. Inflamed nerve roots are painful and will reproduce the pain, whereas noninflamed nerve roots produce mild discomfort only. It follows that maintenance of sensible verbal contact is essential for pain source location and safety.

A flow of saline is needed to lubricate the instrument and to push structures away from the lens in order to maintain vision. A continuous flow should be used, while pressures are kept low enough to prevent adverse symptoms (paresthesiae, pain in the back and legs, and sometimes headaches. If these symptoms occur, the procedure and the flow of saline must be temporarily suspended.

Patience is essential. With experience, the nerve root can be examined along its course up to the intervertebral foramen. Time and experience are necessary for orientation.

Adhesiolysis

If adhesions are found to be present on the nerve root, they can be mobilized with the tip of the instrument by sweeping it back and forth (neuroplasty). This procedure is only performed for "symptomatic" nerves. Adhesions attached to nerve roots not considered to be involved in the patient's pain should be left alone. This procedure must be carried out with great gentleness in a cooperative and sensible (albeit lightly sedated) patient. With a report

of paresthesiae it is essential to stop immediately. Flimsy adhesions can be hydrostatically mobilized via the saline flow. The success of adhesiolysis may be evaluated by pre- and postprocedure epidurography. In order to lessen the possibility of dural pucture, it is advisable to carry out this procedure as lateral and as close to the intervertebral foramen as possible (**Figures 36.5** and **36.6**).

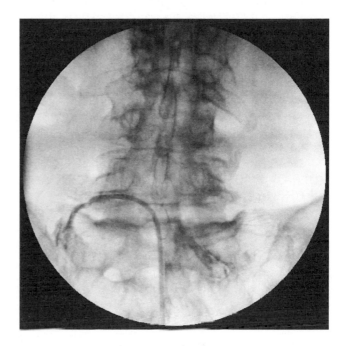

Figure 36.5 A "foramenogram" during a neuroplasty for the L5 nerve root.

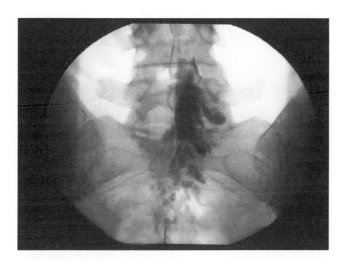

Figure 36.4 A preoperative epidurogram can delineate filling defects indicating islands of epidural fibrosis which often correspond with the site of the patient's pain.

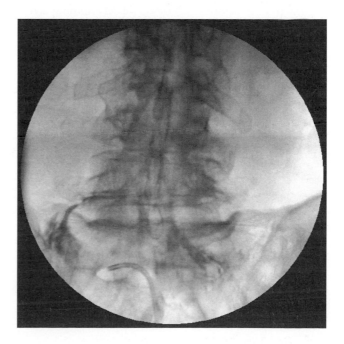

Figure 36.6 The endoscope is in place for an S1 neuroplasty.

Targeted therapy

Steroids, local anesthetic and other solutions, for example clonidine and hyaluronidase, at the end of the procedure can be deposited in exactly the correct area. This is one of the great advantages of spinal endoscopy over "blind" epidural placement (see below under Outcome studies).

Completion

Following completion, the instrument is removed and steristrips are placed across the sacral entry site. The patient is returned to the supine position and should rest for at least one hour before being allowed to go home on the same day or after an overnight stay. Postural hypotension is possible if local anesthetic/clonidine have been used.

ROLE OF EPIDUROSCOPY IN THE DIAGNOSIS OF CHRONIC RADICULOPATHIC PAIN

The accurate diagnosis of radicular pain is difficult. Imaging techniques provide superbly detailed views, but diagnostic usefulness for benign disease is disappointing. A major drawback is that they cannot distinguish the causes of pain from abnormalities related to trauma and aging. **Table 36.1** summarizes the differences between epiduroscopy and MRI scanning; the logical conclusion being that these investigations are mutually informative.

Spinal endoscopy is different to other imaging techniques in that it has a major interactive element with the patient.

Noninflamed healthy nerve roots appear as white or slightly pink structures with blood vessels running across their surface and they transmit a marked pulsation from the dural sac. Inflamed nerve roots on the other hand are red and edematous. Multiple adhesions may obscure the nerve, but nevertheless the area often remains very pain sensitive. Pathological nerve roots may be avascular structures (i.e. devoid of surface vessels) and nonpulsatile. Through interaction with the patient, by gently probing with the tip of the endoscope, the response elicited is diagnostically useful with the patient reporting if his typical pain has been reproduced.

POSSIBLE THERAPEUTIC USEFULNESS OF EPIDUROSCOPY IN RADICULOPATHY

As well as a neuroplasty, dilution or "washing-out" through intervertebral foraminae of chemicals leaked from damaged intervertebral disks and zygo-apophyseal joints[24, 25, 26, 27, 28, 29, 30, 31, 32, 33, 34, 35, 37] may also contribute to an improvement in symptoms.

The overall efficacy of epidural steroid administration is accepted to be positive in the treatment of chronic radicular pain.[43, 44, 45, 46, 47, 48]

Experimentally, the effects of injected nucleus pulposus cytokines can be blocked with topical lidocaine and methylprednisolone.[46] Epiduroscopy allows for highly accurate placement at the exact pain-generating neve root(s) while mechanical and hydrostatic adhesiolysis effectively forms a pocket for solution. The possible benefit from these medications is therefore optimized. An improvement in the ability of nerve roots to move and stretch with back movements and straight leg raising may ameliorate symptoms.[49, 50, 51, 52] Possible mechanisms of an improvement in symptoms through epiduroscopy are listed in **Table 36.2**.

From the point of view of complications of steroid injection, it is important that intrathecal injection is avoided[46] and this is readily achieved with the aid of direct vision.

Table 36.1 Suggested comparison of spinal endoscopy with MRI scanning in the management of LBP with radiculopathy.

	Spinal endoscopy	MRI scanning
Nerve root anatomy	+ (close up views only possible)	+ +
Nerve root vascularity	+ +	−
Nerve root inflammation	+ +	±
Nerve root sensitivity	+ +	−
Diagnostic localization of pain	+ +	−
Identification of fibrous tissue	+ +	+
Disc prolapse identification	− (anterior structure)	+ +
Assessment of spinal canal size	±	+ +
Exclusion of serious pathology	± (biopsy possible)	+ +
Therapeutic aspects	+ +	−

+ +, very helpful; +, helpful; ±, somewhat helpful; −, not helpful.
LBP, low back pain; MRI, magnetic resonance imaging.
Reprinted from Dolin SJ, Padfield NL (eds). *Pain medicine manual*, 2nd edn, 2004, by permission from Elsevier.

Table 36.2 Possible mechanisms of an improvement in symptoms through epiduroscopy.

Mechanism	References
Dilution or washing-out of the "chemical soup" leaking from damaged intervertebral discs and zygapophysial joints	24, 25, 26, 27, 28, 29, 30, 34, 35
Certain placement of epidural steroid containing medication into a pocket formed around the nerve root	40, 41
Adhesiolysis allowing freer nerve root stretching, slackening, excursion, and pendulum motion	49, 50
Nerve root and dura mater partial denervation	51, 52

Reprinted from Richardson J, Kallewaard JW, Groen GJ. Spinal endoscopy for chronic sciatica. *British Journal of Anaesthesia*. 2005; **95**: 275–6, by permission from Oxford University Press.

OUTCOME STUDIES

Low back pain with sciatica

The largest case series was one of the first publications on this subject by Pool[4] looking at 400 patients, Ooi and colleagues[5] reported on 300 patients.

Recent outcomes of three prospective case series,[40, 41, 53] two retrospective evaluations,[54, 55] and a randomized, double-blind controlled trial[56] have been positive for improvements in pain and physical function in patients with chronic LBP with radiculopathic leg pain who had previously obtained inadequate pain relief with traditionally placed caudal or lumbar epidural steroids.

Geurts and colleagues[40] prospectively evaluated whether abnormalities at the lumbar level as diagnosed by MRI are confirmed by epiduroscopy, and assessed if targeted epidural injection of medication alleviated sciatic pain. Nineteen of 20 patients studied showed adhesions via epiduroscopy. In eight patients, six of whom had never undergone surgery, these were not detected with earlier MRI. Six patients showed concomitant signs of active root inflammation. Out of 20 patients treated, 11 (55 percent) experienced significant pain relief at three months which was maintained at six, nine, and twelve months for eight (40 percent), seven (35 percent), and seven (35 percent) patients, respectively. Mean visual analog scores (VAS) at three months were significantly reduced (DeltaVAS = 3.55; $p < 0.0001$), and this persisted at 12 months (DeltaVAS = 1.99, $p = 0.0073$).

Richardson and colleagues[41] prospectively reported on all 38 patients listed for day-case epiduroscopy over a 12-month period (April 1998–April 1999), who had chronic severe LBP and radiculopathic pain. The mean (range) pain duration before treatment was 10.9 (2–26) years and 50 percent had an FBSS. In all patients in whom treatment was completed ($n = 34$), the pain-generating nerve roots were located through symptom interaction with the patient. All had epidural scar tissue, in 14 (41 percent) of whom this was dense. Neuroplasty was performed so that a pocket was formed for the subsequent placement of bupivacaine, Depomedrone®, and clonidine. No intraoperative complications occurred and side effects were minimal. Follow up over a 12-month period showed statistically significant reductions in pain scores and disability.

In a retrospective evaluation by Manchikanti *et al.*,[56] 112 epiduroscopies were studied in 85 consecutive patients who had failed to show a significant response of at least six weeks or longer from a single treatment that included epidural steroid injections. The procedure included visualization of adhesions, adhesiolysis, and deposition of corticosteroid and local anesthetic. Initial pain relief was greater than 50 percent in all patients (100 percent). The percentage of patients with substantial pain relief diminished to 94 percent at one to two months, to 77 percent at two to three months, and 7 percent after twelve months. Mean substantial pain relief in weeks per procedure was 19 ± 1.79. The total average cost per procedure was US2961 ± 139. Substantial relief was provided at a cost of $156 per one week improvement. For one year, substantial improvement would cost $8127.

In a prospective, randomized double-blind trial published by Manchikanti and colleagues,[56] all patients with chronic LBP of at least six months and having failed conservative modalities of management, including fluoroscopically directed epidural steroid injections and percutaneous adhesiolysis, were included. Group I ($n = 16$) served as a control with endoscopy to the sacral level without adhesiolysis, followed by injection of local anesthetic and steroid. Group II consisted of spinal endoscopy and appropriate adhesiolysis, followed by injection of local anesthetic and steroid. Outcome measures were pain, functional status, psychological, and behavioral status. In group II, 13 of 23 patients (57 percent) showed significant improvements in VAS scores of greater than 50 percent at one, three, and six months. Disability scores and ranges of motion were improved at one, three, and six months in group II, along with improved psychological and behavioral tests. No improvements were recorded in group I. The only adverse event was one patient with a subarachnoid block. The results clearly showed the value of adhesiolysis.

A prospective, randomized study recently published by Dashfield and colleagues[57] demonstrated negative results. Sixty patients with a 6–18-month history of sciatica were randomized to receive caudal epidural steroids versus epiduroscopic placement of steroid. No attempt was made with the epiduroscope to carry out adhesiolysis. Both groups demonstrated significant improvements compared to baseline in descriptive pain at six months. In the caudal epidural placement group, VAS scores improved at six weeks, three months, and six months. Present pain intensity (PPI) improved significantly at three and six months. Anxiety reduced significantly at six weeks, three months, and six months. Depression was less at six months. Overall there were fewer changes in epiduroscopy group: PPI reduced significantly at six weeks and six months; anxiety was less at six months only. The author's conclusion (with which we agree) was that putting a patient through the longer, more uncomfortable, more costly, and potentially more hazardous procedure of epiduroscopy (without adhesiolysis) is difficult to justify on symptomatic grounds. The reasons for the discrepancy in results between this study and other publications have been pointed out in a letter to the editor.[58]

Dashfield et al.'s study[57] examined different patients to those of other publications. None of their patients had an FBSS and symptom duration was a maximum of 18 months. Very little scar tissue was encountered. In the case series of Richardson and colleagues,[41] symptom duration was 10.9 years (range 2–26) and 19 out of 38 had had surgery. Epidural fibrosis was found in all patients and was dense in nine. In the study of Geurts et al.,[40] symptom duration was a mean of 5.5 years (range 2–10), with 12 out of 20 patients having had a total of 26 back operations between them. Adhesions were found in 19 patients, being dense in 14. Igarashi et al.[53] studied patients with SS, a significant amount of narrowing being caused by fibrous tissue encroachment on the spinal canal (see below under Epiduroscopy in spinal stenosis). Manchikanti et al.[54] published two studies, one involving postlumbar laminectomy patients and the other involving some patients who were postlaminectomy,[55] all of whom were nonresponsive to previous nonepiduroscopic percutaneous adhesiolysis. The majority of patients in Manchikanti et al's.[56] randomized, double-blind controlled trial had moderate or extensive epidural fibrosis and all had failed to obtain adequate pain relief from nonepiduroscopic percutaneous adhesiolysis.

Deliberate attempts were made in all these quoted publications to carry out adhesiolysis, indeed, this was felt to be an integral, important part of the procedure. Efficacy of adhesiolysis is hard to establish scientifically, but postoperative epidurography had improved (compared to preoperative epidurography) in approximately half the patients in the Richardson and Geurts case series. Positive effects of deliberately carried out adhesiolysis involving epiduroscopy have been found in all publications in terms of pain relief and physical function. The value of adhesiolysis was specifically studied in the Manchikanti et al.[56] randomized, double-blind controlled trial. Pain relief, physical function, psychological function, and behavioral

status all improved in a significant number of patients, without side effects. Only three patients in the Dashfield group underwent adhesiolysis.

Our conclusions, from the scientific studies so far carried out, are that in patients with short case histories with probably mild epidural chronic pathological changes, epiduroscopy may have little to offer over and above traditional steroid placement. If specific nerve roots require to be targeted, the simpler method of selective nerve root approach may be preferable and has been shown to be effective. For patients with more chronic symptoms, particularly with epidural fibrosis shown on MRI corresponding with the side and presumed site of symptoms, effective delivery of steroid to the required nerve roots is highly unlikely to be effective through nonspecific (caudal or translaminar lumbar) delivery. Epiduroscopy with neuroplasty is very useful for these patients.

Epiduroscopy in spinal stenosis

Igarashi et al.[53] recently published a case series of epidural adhesiolysis followed by injection of steroid and local anesthetic for the symptoms of SS. Patients with degenerative lumbar SS ($n = 58$, median age 71 years) were divided into two groups based on presenting symptoms: a monosegmental group ($n = 34$) and a multisegmental group ($n = 24$). Each patient underwent epiduroscopy and the findings were evaluated using VAS for LBP and leg symptoms. Epiduroscopy included adhesiolysis and instillation of steroid/local anesthetic. Epiduroscopy showed that the amount of fatty tissue and the degree of vascularity were greater in the monosegmental group than in the multisegmental group. Relief of LBP was observed up to 12 months after epiduroscopy in both groups. Relief of leg pain was evident up to 12 months after epiduroscopy in the monosegmental group, and up to three months in the multisegmental group. None of the patients showed deterioration of motor or sensory deficits during follow up. One patient was excluded from analysis because of accidental dural puncture during the procedure.

As well as an effect of adhesiolysis on radicular pain generation through biochemical means, as discussed above under Possible therapeutic usefulness of epiduroscopy in radiculopathy, it is possible that the amount of stretching, slackening, excursion, and pendulum motion needed by nerve roots in order to accommodate back flexion and extension[49] had improved. Nerve root blood flow even in health has been directly observed to cease with nerve traction.[6]

Conclusion from controlled studies

Spinal endoscopy is a safe undertaking, as demonstrated in these publications as well as others.[2, 4, 5, 6, 7, 9, 10, 11, 14, 17, 18, 19, 20, 47] A recent review of interventional outcomes concludes that the evidence is strong for short-term relief and moderate for long-term relief in chronic refractory LBP and leg pain secondary to postlumbar surgery syndrome.[48] Its usefulness in patients with chronic severe radiculopathic symptoms, especially in association with FBSS, appears to be established. Better and more scientific studies are required.

OTHER APPLICATIONS

Recovery of foreign bodies, for example sheered epidural catheter and targeted neurolytic substances for the management of terminal cancer pain, are potential applications. It has been suggested that the design of epidural and spinal needles could be aided by epiduroscopy.[59]

The ability to perform surgery with epiduroscopy will be exciting for the future. Animal studies seem promising.[60]

The ability to carry out adhesiolysis is highly important. Radiofrequency energy is being investigated. Raffaeli and Righetti[61] have recently reported on 14 patients with FBSS, having undergone a minimum of two operations and had previously done well with spinal endoscopy but had relapsed, who underwent epiduroscopic radiofrequency lesioning of adhesions. Patients were evaluated before, at one, three, and six months after the procedure. Pain relief of greater than 90 percent was found in eight, pain relief of between 60 and 70 percent was found in five, and less than 30 percent was reported in one. For a quarter of patients (five) the benefits lasted less than one month, for the others it was over 80 percent at six months. Surgical time was 35 minutes and no short term complications occurred.

REPORTED MORBIDITY

Potentially serious complications have arisen through over-pressurization of the epidural space with saline. Pressure transmitted centrally via the hydraulics of the CSF has lead to three cases of retinal hemorrhages producing temporary visual disturbance (personal communication) and two cases of serious medulla-radicular irritation, one involving dysesthesiae and diffuse spasms of the lower limbs, the other involving short intraoperative and repeated postoperative, tonic-clonic spasms of the lower limbs.[62] It is important to keep the flow of saline to the minimum that is required for reasonable views and to stop with any report of headache or shoulder pain. A head-up position is helpful. No deaths have been reported. To our knowledge, no case of severe persistent neurological damage has been described. No case of spinal infection has been reported. The greatest safety feature of all remains the patient's symptoms and it is essential to maintain sensible verbal contact at all times.

CONCLUSIONS

Epiduroscopy is a safe and remarkable development which aids understanding. Methods of improved adhesiolysis are under evaluation. Its future looks fascinating.

REFERENCES

1. Stern EL. The spinoscope: a new instrument for visualizing the spinal canal and its contents. *Medical Record.* 1936; **143**: 31–2.
2. Pool JL. Myeloscopy: diagnostic inspection of the cauda equina by means of an endoscope (Myeloscope). *Bulletin of the Neurological Institute of New York.* 1938; **7**: 178–89.
3. Burman MS. Myeloscopy or the direct visualisation of the spinal canal and its contents. *Journal of Bone and Joint Surgery.* 1931; **13**: 695–6.
4. Pool JL. Myeloscopy: intraspinal endoscopy. *Surgery.* 1942; **11**: 169–82.
5. Ooi Y, Morisaki N. Intrathecal lumbar endoscope. *Clinical Orthopaedic Surgery.* 1969; **4**: 295–7.
6. Ooi Y, Satoh Y, Inoue K et al. Myeloscopy, with special reference to blood flow changes in the cauda equina during Lasègue's test. *International Orthopaedics.* 1981; **4**: 307–11.
7. Ooi Y, Mita F, Satoh Y. Myeloscopic study on lumbar canal stenosis with special reference to intermittent claudication. *Spine.* 1990; **15**: 544–9.
8. Blomberg RG, Olsson SS. The lumbar epidural space in patients examined with epiduroscopy. *Anesthesia and Analgesia.* 1989; **68**: 157–60.
9. Heavner JE, Chokhavatia S, Kizelshteyn G. Percutaneous evaluation of the epidural and subarachnoid space with a flexible fiberscope. *Regional Anesthesia.* 1991; **15**: 85.
10. Shimoji K, Fujioka H, Onodera M et al. Observation of spinal canal and cysternae with the newly developed small-diameter, flexible fiberscopes. *Anesthesiology.* 1991; **75**: 341–4.
11. Saberski LR, Kitahata LM. Direct visualization of the lumbosacral epidural space through the sacral hiatus. *Anesthesia and Analgesia.* 1995; **80**: 839–40.
12. Westbrook JL, Renowden SA, Carrie LES. Study of the anatomy of the extradural region using magnetic resonance imaging. *British Journal of Anaesthesia.* 1993; **71**: 495–8.
13. Hogan QH. Epidural anatomy examined by cryomicrotome section. *Regional Anesthesia.* 1996; **21**: 395–406.
14. Igarashi T, Hirabayashi Y, Shimizu R et al. The lumbar extradural structure changes with increasing age. *British Journal of Anaesthesia.* 1997; **78**: 149–52.
15. Withington DE, Weeks SK. Repeat epidural analgesia and unilateral block. *Canadian Journal of Anaesthesia.* 1994; **41**: 568–71.
16. Korbon GA, Lynch 3rd C, Arnold WP et al. Repeated epidural anaesthesia for extracorporeal shock-wave lithotripsy is unreliable. *Anesthesia and Analgesia.* 1987; **66**: 669–72.
17. Igarashi T, Hirabayashi Y, Shimizu R et al. Inflammatory changes after extradural anaesthesia may affect the spread of local anaesthetic within the extradural space. *British Journal of Anaesthesia.* 1996; **77**: 347–51.

18. Igarashi T, Hirabayashi Y, Shimizu R et al. Thoracic and lumbar extradural structure examined by extraduroscope. *British Journal of Anaesthesia*. 1998; **81**: 121–5.

19. Igarashi T, Hirabayashi Y, Shimizu R et al. The epidural structure changes during deep breathing. *Canadian Journal of Anesthesia*. 1999; **46**: 850–5.

20. Igarashi T, Hirabayashi Y, Shimizu R et al. The fiberscopic findings of the epidural space in pregnant women. *Anesthesiology*. 2000; **92**: 1631–6.

21. Von Korff M, Deyo RA, Cherkin D, Berlow W. Back pain in primary care: outcomes at 1 year. *Spine*. 1993; **18**: 855–62.

22. Von Korff M, Saunders K. The course of back pain in primary care. *Spine*. 1996; **21**: 2833–9.

23. Frymoyer JW. Back pain and sciatica. *New England Journal of Medicine*. 1988; **318**: 291–300.

24. Olmarker K, Rydevik B, Nordborg C. Autologous nucleus pulposus induces neurophysiologic and histologic changes in porcine cauda equina nerve roots. *Spine*. 1993; **18**: 1425–32.

25. Olmarker K, Myers RR. Pathogenesis of sciatic pain: role of herniated nucleus pulposus, and deformation of spinal nerve root and dorsal root ganglion. *Pain*. 1998; **78**: 99–105.

26. Kayama S, Konno S, Olmarker K et al. Incision of the annulus fibrosus induces nerve root morphologic, vascular and functional changes. An experimental study. *Spine*. 1996; **21**: 2539–43.

27. Otani K, Arai I, Mao PG et al. Experimental disc herniation. Evaluation of the natural course. *Spine*. 1997; **22**: 2894–9.

28. Cornefjord M, Olmarker K, Rydevik B, Nordborg C. Mechanical and biochemical injury of spinal nerve roots. A morphological and neurophysiological study. *European Spine Journal*. 1996; **5**: 187–92.

29. Olmarker K, Nordborg C, Larsson K, Rydevik B. Ultrastructural changes in spinal nerve roots induced by autologous nucleus pulposus. *Spine*. 1996; **21**: 411–14.

30. Olmarker K, Blomquist J, Strömberg J et al. Inflammogenic properties of nucleus pulposus. *Spine*. 1995; **20**: 665–9.

31. Kuslich SD, Ulstrom CL, Michael CJ. The tissue origin of low back pain and sciatica: a report of pain response to tissue stimulation during operation on the lumbar spine using local anesthesia. *Orthopedic Clinics of North America*. 1991; **22**: 181–7.

32. Rydevik B, Brown MD, Lundborg G. Pathoanatomy and pathophysiology of nerve root compression. *Spine*. 1984; **9**: 7–15.

33. Rydevik B, Holm S, Brown MD, Lundborg G. Diffusion from the CSF as a nutritional pathway for spinal nerve roots. *Acta Physiologica Scandinavica*. 1990; **138**: 247–8.

34. Yabuki S, Onda A, Kikuchi S, Myers R. Prevention of compartment syndrome in dorsal root ganglia caused by exposure to nucleus pulposus. *Spine*. 2001; **26**: 870–4.

35. Saal JS. The role of inflammation in lumbar pain. *Pain*. 1995; **20**: 1821–7.

36. Devor M. Neuropathic pain and the injured nerve: peripheral mechanisms. *British Medical Bulletin*. 1991; **47**: 619–30.

37. Chen C, Cavanaugh JM, Song JM et al. Effects of nucleus pulposus on nerve root neural activity, mechanosensitivity, axonal morphology and sodium channel expression. *Spine*. 2004; **29**: 17–25.

38. Cooper RG, Mitchell WS, Illingworth KJ et al. The role of epidural fibrinolysis in the persistence of postlaminectomy back pain. *Spine*. 1991; **16**: 1044–8.

* 39. Kehlet H. Surgical stress: the role of pain and analgesia. *British Journal of Anaesthesia*. 1989; **63**: 189–95.

* 40. Geurts JW, Kallewaard JW, Richardson J, Groen GJ. Targeted methylprednisolone/hyaluronidase/clonidine injection after diagnostic epiduroscopy for chronic sciatica: a prospective, 1-year follow-up study. *Regional Anesthesia and Pain Medicine*. 2002; **27**: 343–52.

* 41. Richardson J, McGurgan P, Cheema S et al. Spinal endoscopy in chronic low-back pain with radiculopathy. A prospective case series. *Anaesthesia*. 2001; **56**: 447–84.

42. Ross JS, Robertson JT, Frederickson RC et al. Association between peridural scar and recurrent radicular pain after lumbar discectomy: Magnetic resonance evaluation. *Neurosurgery*. 1996; **38**: 855–63.

43. McQuay HJ, Moore RA (eds). Epidural corticosteroids for sciatica. In: *An evidence-based resource for pain relief*. Oxford: Oxford University Press, 1998; Chapter 27.

44. Watts RW, Silagy AC. A meta-analysis on the efficacy of epidural corticosteroids in the treatment of sciatica. *Anaesthesia and Intensive Care*. 1995; **23**: 284–5.

45. Koes BW, Scholten RJPM, Mens JMA, Bouter LM. Efficacy of epidural steroid injections for low-back pain and sciatica: a systematic review of randomized clinical trials. *Pain*. 1995; **63**: 279–88.

46. Olmarker K, Byrod G, Cornefjord M et al. Effects of methyl-prednisolone on nucleus pulposus nerve root injury. *Spine*. 1994; **19**: 1803–08.

47. Abram SE. Treatment of lumbosacral radiculopathy with epidural steroids. *Anesthesiology*. 1999; **91**: 1937–41.

48. Boswell MV, Trescot AM, Datta S et al. Interventional techniques: evidence-based practice guidelines in the management of chronic spinal pain. *Pain Physician*. 2007; **10**: 7–111.

49. Arbit E, Pannulo S. Lumbar stenosis: a clinical review. *Clinical Orthopaedics and Related Research*. 2001; **384**: 137–43.

50. Miyamoto H, Dumas GA, Wyss UP, Ryd L. Three-dimensional analysis of the movement of lumbar spinal nerve roots in non simulated and simulated adhesive conditions. *Spine*. 2003; **28**: 2373–80.

51. Cuatico W, Parker JC. Further observations on spinal meningeal nerves and their role in pain production. *Acta Neurochirurgica*. 1989; **101**: 126–8.

52. Cuatico W, Parker JC, Pappert E, Pilsl S. An anatomical and clinical investigation of spinal nerves. *Acta Neurochirurgica*. 1988; **90**: 139–43.

∗ 53. Igarashi T, Hirabayashi Y, Seo N *et al*. Lysis of adhesions and epidural injection of steroid/local anaesthetic during epiduroscopy potentially alleviate low back pain and leg pain in elderly patients with lumbar spinal stenosis. *British Journal of Anaesthesia*. 2004; **93**: 181–7.

∗ 54. Manchikanti MD, Pampati V, Bakhit CE *et al*. Non-endoscopic and endoscopic adhesiolysis in post lumbar laminectomy syndrome. A one-year outcome study and cost effective analysis. *Pain Physician*. 1999; **2**: 52–8.

∗ 55. Manchikanti L. The value and safety of epidural endoscopic adhesiolysis. *American Journal of Anesthesiology*. 2000; **27**: 275–8.

∗ 56. Manchikanti MD, Pampati V, Bakhit CE *et al*. Spinal endoscopic adhesiolysis in the management of chronic low back pain: a preliminary report of a randomized, double-blind trial. *Pain Physician*. 2003; **6**: 259–67.

∗ 57. Dashfield AK, Taylor MB, Cleaver JS, Farrow D. Comparison of caudal steroid epidural wilyh targeted steroid placement during spinal endoscopy for chronic sciatica: a prospective, randomized, double-blind trial. *British Journal of Anaesthesia*. 2005; **94**: 514–9.

58. Richardson J, Kallewaard JW, Groen GJ. Spinal endoscopy for chronic sciatica. *British Journal of Anaesthesia*. 2005; **95**: 275–6.

59. Holmström B, Rawal N, Axelsson K, Nydahl PA. Risk of catheter migration during combined spinal epidural block: percutaneous epiduroscopy study. *Anesthesia and Analgesia*. 1995; **80**: 747–53.

60. Monsivais JJ, Narakas AO, Turkof E, Sun Y. The endoscopic diagnosis and possible treatment of nerve root avulsions in the management of brachial plexus injuries. *Journal of Hand Surgery*. 1994; **19B**: 547–9.

61. Raffaeli W, Righetti D. Surgical radio-frequency epiduroscopy technique (R-ResAblator) and FBSS treatments: preliminary evaluations. *Acta Neurochirurgica*. 2005; **92**: 121–5.

62. Raffaeli W, Pari G, Visani L, Balestri M. Periduroscopy: preliminary reports. *Pain Clinic*. 1999; **11**: 209–12.

37

Discogenic low back pain: intradiscal thermal (radiofrequency) annuloplasty and artificial disk implants

GUNNVALD KVARSTEIN, LEIF MÅWE, AND AAGE INDAHL

KEY LEARNING POINTS

- Intradiscal thermal annuloplasty (thermal coagulation in the annulus fibrosus) has been restricted to patients who have low back pain, positive signs of disk degeneration (by magnetic resonance imaging (MRI)) and fulfilled the criteria for a positive low pressure provocative discography.
- The intradiscal electrothermal therapy (IDET) method with Spinecath[TM] and the alternative modality discTRODE[TM] both apply the energy from radiofrequency

- (RF) currency to heat the posterior annulus but by different techniques.
- IDET and discTRODE are still experimental treatment modalities.
- Artificial disk implants maintain more normal spinal motion.
- The clinical outcomes (pain and function) of artificial disk implantation are superior or equivalent to those of anterior lumbar interbody fusion surgery.

INTRODUCTION

Intervertebral disk degeneration has been considered a common cause of axial chronic low back pain (CLBP).[1] The condition is characterized by degradation of the nucleus pulposus, disruption of the circular lamella and radial tears in the annulus fibrosus.[2, 3] The theory is that proinflammatory nucleus material may leak through tears and stimulate annular nerve endings. Clinically, however, it is difficult to verify that the pain actually comes from an intervertebral disk. There is no accepted procedure that can ascertain the diagnosis discogenic pain.

CLBP patients with evidence of disk degeneration have been treated with fusion surgery, a risky procedure still associated with high morbidity. During the last decade, alternative and less invasive therapies have been introduced for relieving disk-related back pain. Some of the methods use RF energy, i.e. a high frequency, alternating current to perform disk lesions. In 1988, Sluijter suggested placing a straight RF electrode into the nucleus pulposus, but the method was later found ineffective.[4] This chapter will present and discuss RF-based intradiscal thermal annuloplasty (IDTA) as an option to treat back pain, possibly related to annular fissures. We will not cover percutaneous discectomy (chemonuclolysis and decompression techniques such as Nucleoplasty™, Coblation™) designed for herniated disks, but briefly review recent developments in implantation of artificial disks as a means of relieving discogenic pain.

RADIOFREQUENCY-BASED INTRADISCAL THERMAL ANNULOPLASTY

Intradiscal electrothermal therapy

In the late 1990s, Saal and Saal invented IDET.[5] Under x-ray vision with a 17 G straight introducer cannula, a navigable catheter (Spinecath; Smith and Nephew, Andover, MA) is inserted into the nucleus from a posterolateral approach and placed circumferentially within or along the inner side of the posterior annulus (see **Figure 37.1**). An electrically resistive heating element at the tip of the catheter converts RF energy into heat energy.[6] According to the protocol from Saal and Saal,[6] the catheter temperature is gradually increased to 90°C during a period of 13 minutes and is then maintained for four minutes to create a temperature in the annulus between 60 and 65°C.[6] The total lesion time is then 17 minutes.[6]

DiscTRODE

DiscTRODE is a monopolar RF system, developed by Radionics, now manufactured by Tyco Healthcare. From a posterolateral approach with a straight 17 G introducer cannula, the electrode is navigated between the lamellae of the posterior annulus under x-ray and electrical impedance control (see **Figure 37.2**). The small surface area of the active electrode leads to a high current density,[8] creating a thin cylindrically shaped heat lesion.[9] The electrically resistive tissue is heated in a step-wise manner (increasing by 5°C every two minutes) from 50°C and maintained for four minutes at 65°C. The total lesion time will therefore be ten minutes.

WHAT IS THE MECHANISM FOR PAIN RELIEF AFTER INTRADISCAL THERMAL ANNULOPLASTY?

The nature of discogenic pain is still not fully understood. Thus, the mechanism of possible pain relief following IDTA cannot be established. Several possibilities are suggested of which four deserve attention. Placebo effect and coagulation of nociceptors are the two most likely possibilities.

1. **The placebo response:** The placebo effect can be substantial, as it is in most invasive procedures. Only carefully and well-designed studies provide the answer.
2. **Thermal coagulation of nociceptors located in the annulus fibrosus:** Intervertebral disks are multisegmentally innervated by unmyelinated nerve fibers, normally ending in the outer third of the annulus. In degenerated disks the nerve fibers (and blood vessels) grow into the deeper layers of the annulus. Whether these ingrowths are involved in a pain process or simply are part of a repair response, has not been established, and we do not know whether the IDET and discTRODE system are able to coagulate sufficient nerve fibers to denervate the posterior annulus.[10] The radius

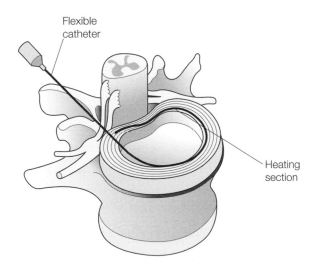

Figure 37.1 The Spinecath catheter placed along the inner side or within the inner lamellea of the annulus during IntraDiscal ElectroThermal annuloplasty (IDET). Redrawn from Pomerantz SR, Hirsch, JA. Intradiscal therapies for discogenic pain. *Seminars in Muskuloskeletal Radiology,* 2006; **2**: 125–36.

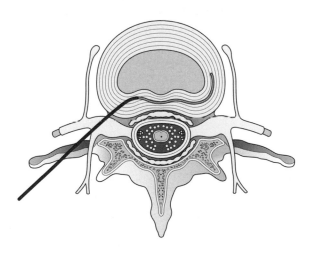

Figure 37.2 The discTRODE placed between the lamellae of the posterior annulus, as suggested by Finch.[7] The use of radiofrequency heat lesions in the treatment of lumbar discogenic pain. Redrawn from Pomerantz SR, Hirsch, JA. Intradiscal therapies for discogenic pain. *Seminars in Muskuloskeletal Radiology.* 2006; **2**: 125–36.

of the temperature zone where neurons are permanently injured is less than 6 mm with 90°C at the tip of the Spinocath catheter. Direct RF current applied for the discTRODE injures nerve tissue within a radius of 11 mm.[11]

3. **Denaturation of collagen fibers in the annulus fibrosus**:[12] Whether collagen denaturation is responsible for pain relief or not, is difficult to prove. Instability as a pain generating mechanism is controversial, and stability of a functional unit of the spine has not been defined. Furthermore, we do not know how instability is detected by the nervous system or sensed as pain.

4. **Altered sensorimotor control of the paraspinal muscles**:[13] Motion of a functional unit of the spine has a complex pattern where flexion, rotation, and translation occur simultaneously. Under experimental mechanical loading one has measured highly different pressure levels across the disk, which change uniquely under spinal motion (Indahl A *et al.*, unpublished results). The intervertebral disk seems to play an important role in the control of load transfer,[13] but the role of the intervertebral disk in the sensorimotor control of the paraspinal muscles is not clearly understood. Whether this sensory function is altered by IDTA, or how these pressure and motion patterns are affected by thermal coagulation, is completely unknown.

DIAGNOSTIC CONSIDERATIONS

Low axial back pain, which increases when the patient is sitting or standing, is considered typical, but not specific for disk-related pain. MRI (T2-weighted) can demonstrate disk degeneration characterized by reduced height and water content and high intensity zones (HIZ), and in a symptomatic population the HIZ closely correlate with the presence of annular tears.[14] The diagnostic problem is that these changes are nearly as prevalent in asymptomatic adults, the prevalence varies from 14 to 56 percent.[15, 16] Thus, MRI cannot predict whether disk pathology is the origin of the pain.

Provocative discography

Pain provocation discography is considered a more reliable tool for diagnosing discogenic low back pain.[16] The distension and chemical irritation of the annulus, following an injection of contrast dye in disrupted disks, may cause intensive pain, quite equivalent to the original back pain.[16, 17] Accordingly, several studies have demonstrated a close correlation between positive provocative discography and pronounced disk pathology and disruptions grade,[16][III], [18][IV] particularly when the fissures are located in the outer annulus.[17] Clinical findings and changes on MRI have been included in the Dallas quantitative scaled classification discogram system.[19]

CRITERIA FOR PROVOCATION DISCOGRAPHY

To perform provocation discography, the following four criteria should be fulfilled:[20, 21]

1. low axial back pain lasting for more than six months;
2. increased pain intensity when the patient is sitting or standing;
3. conservative treatment has failed;
4. evidence of disk degeneration on the MRI (T2-weighted) with either HIZ, decreased water content, or moderate height reduction <50 percent.

How provocative discography is performed

- A limited volume (<3.5 mL) of contrast dye is under manometrical pressure control injected into the nucleus pulposus of the suspected disk and at least one adjacent "normal" disk as a control.
- Pain intensity and concordance (equivalent to original pain) are assessed with increasing pressure up to 345 kPa (50 psi) above the opening pressure or until the numerical pain score reaches seven of a maximum ten.
- A postprocedural computed tomography (CT) scan is performed to assess the extent of disk disruption.

ADDITIONAL CRITERIA FOR INTRADISCAL THERMAL ANNULOPLASTY

To perform IDTA, three additional criteria should also be fulfilled:

1. radiological evidence of annular tears (CT discography);
2. intradiscal pressures <345 kPa (50 psi) above the opening pressure should reproduce intensive "concordant" back pain (≥7 on a ten-point scale);
3. injections into adjacent, apparently normal disks, should not elicit "concordant" pain.

RELATIVE AND ABSOLUTE CONTRAINDICATIONS FOR IDTA

Relative and absolute contraindications for IDTA include:[22]

- no painful disks or more than two painful disk levels on provocation discography;
- nerve root impingement with radicular pain, spinal stenosis with neurogenic claudication;
- more than 50 percent disk height reduction;

- spondylolisthesis or spinal instability;
- scoliosis;
- tumor, infection, or fracture.

Discography and controversies

Despite authoritative recommendations, the clinical value of discography is still under debate.

- Annular distension and stress following the injection of contrast dye during pain provocation discography is fundamentally different from the weight load under normal conditions.
- The disks are multisegmentally innervated which may preclude the assessment and evaluation.
- Disk injections may also elicit painful reactions in asymptomatic subjects.[23]

Some have argued that low pressure injections with a slow intradiscal injection rate <0.5 mL/s and intradiscal pressures within 103–138 kPa (15 or 20 psi) over opening pressure decrease the false-positive rate.[16, 24] In a recent study where low pressure discography was applied, however, Carragee et al.[25] found positive rates as high as 25 and 36 percent among patients with chronic pain, but no low back pain.[25] They consequently question the validity of the procedure.

Provocative discography as a diagnostic procedure should be interpreted cautiously, although it is probably the best diagnostic tool we have to distinguish asymptomatic from symptomatic disks. The study by Carragee et al.[25] points out some essential pitfalls and emphasizes how important it is to consider confounding factors before establishing a diagnosis and performing a treatment.

EFFECTIVENESS AND EFFICACY

Intradiscal electrothermal therapy

The early efficacy data on IDET (Spinecath), based on noncontrolled and case-controlled studies, were promising, showing substantial (60–80 percent) and long-lasting pain relief.[6, 26, 27] In a systematic review, including 11 prospective cohort studies and 256 patients,[28][II] the mean pain relief was 3.4 points on a 11 graded scale, and the change in Oswestry Disability Index (ODI) was 5.2 points (the index values varies from 0 to 100). In five retrospective studies,[28][III] including 379 patients, 13–23 percent of the patients dropped out of the study as they preferred back surgery instead.

The results from the first randomized controlled trial (RCT) were less impressive.[20] In the study by Pauza et al.[20] they found significantly larger pain reduction and improved ODI in the IDET group after six months.

However, there was no difference between the groups in overall pain (visual analog scale (VAS)) and SF 36 scores. One more recent investigation with a less rigorous patient selection found no difference between IDET and placebo.[29] The effect of IDET has consequently been questioned. The poor results may reflect that we are not able to select those patients who would respond to IDTA.

DiscTRODE

The efficacy data on discTRODE are more limited. A small noncontrolled study, including only 20 persons, was positive[30] and a case-controlled study reported significant pain reduction in the active group even after 12 months, compared with no change in the control group.[31] Another study, comparing the efficacy of discTRODE versus IDET (42 patients) showed lower pain (VAS) and Pain Disability Index scores in the IDET group compared with the RF group 3 and 12 months after treatment.[32] So far, no randomized controlled studies have been published. Preliminary results from a randomized, double-blinded study run by the authors do not show any difference between active and placebo treatment (Kvarstein G et al., personal communication). Therefore, the study has been stopped due to ethical reasons.

EMERGING INTRADISCAL MODALITIES

Accutherm

Smith and Nephew have designed a new electrothermal device; Accutherm™ in order to improve the IDET system. The catheter has a shorter heating coil with an integrated thermocouple. The system creates more focal lesions, and the electrode may probably be placed closer to the target and heated to higher temperatures.[33] No clinical data are so far available.

Biacuplasty™

A growing amount of data indicates that the small lesions generated by the IDET and discTRODE system do not adequately denervate the posterior part of the annulus fibrosus.[10, 11] To overcome this limitation a bipolar system, Transdiscal Annuloplasty or Biacuplasty™ (Baylis Medical Company, Montreal, Canada), has been introduced. With two electrodes, one in each posterior corner, the system can create large strip lesions covering most of the posterior part of the annulus. With an internal water cooling system the electrode temperature is kept at $55 \pm 5°C$,[34] in order to prevent injury of nerve tissue in the vertebral canal (Pauza, unpublished data). However, clinical efficacy data have not been published.

CONSIDERATIONS AND RECOMMENDATIONS

Percutaneous intradiscal annuloplasty with the Spinecath (IDET) is performed in an outpatient clinic with light sedation. The costs are calculated to be approximately US$8000, which is only 20 percent of what a lumbar fusion operation (US$45,000) costs,[28] the expenditures of complications and sick leave are then not included. Taking into account the relatively low risk and costs compared to surgery and possible positive effects in some selected patients, the IDET treatment has become widely used. According to the Smith and Nephew Company, 60,000 IDET procedures had been performed worldwide by June 2005.[28]

Although the procedure represents less tissue damage, shorter recovery time, and lower infection risk, various rare complications have been reported such as catheter breakages, nerve root injuries, post-IDET disk hernia-tion,[35] cauda equina syndrome,[36, 37, 38] vertebral body osteonecrosis,[39] discitis, radicular pain, cerebrospinal fluid leaks, and severe headache.[40] More importantly, the scientific evidence does not support the efficacy or effectiveness of percutaneous intradiscal thermocoagula-tion for discogenic low back pain.[41] We therefore cannot recommend IDTA with Spinecath (IDET) or discTRODE as treatment for discogenic pain. They are still experimental treatment modalities and patients offered this treatment should be included in RCTs or at least in carefully designed follow-up studies.[42]

ARTIFICIAL DISK IMPLANTS

Lumbar fusion surgery is being challenged by new implantable artificial disks. The disks are designed to restore and maintain normal motion and may possibly prevent degeneration of adjacent levels, which is a serious complication to the fusion surgery techniques. Some argue that it can be a solution to previously fused patients with adjacent segment degeneration. Four commercially available implants will be presented.

The Charité® artificial disk is the most widely used, with 7000 implants worldwide in 2004.[43] The device has a bi-convex metal on plastic design, and acts as a mobile core fixed with ventral and dorsal teeth.

In the ProDisc®,[43] which also has a metal on plastic design, the end plates are secured to the vertebral end plates by means of a central keel, spikes, and a porous coated surface. The first reports were encouraging with satisfaction rates as high as 92.7 percent. There does not seem to be any difference in outcome between one- and two-level implantations.

The MAVERICK™ artificial disk has a metal on metal design.[43] The device is based on a ball and socket joint and provides a fixed posterior center of rotation which resists anterior and posterior shear forces. The end plates are covered with hydroxyapatite. Different disk footprints and posterior disk heights open for adequate end plate coverage and appropriate lordoses. Wear particles, generated in testing, have been evaluated and do not seem to be toxic with regard to macrophage production.

The FlexiCore™ intervertebral disk[43] is also a metal on metal prosthesis with a ball and socket joint. This prevents dislocation of the superior end plate from the inferior end plate, and offers a rotational stop to prevent the facets from being overstressed.

Artificial disk implantation is still in its investigatory phase. Charité is the oldest device and has been implanted for several years. In retrospective long-term follow-up studies (four to five years) the success rates are high (70–80 percent).[44, 45] In a large randomized study ($n = 304$), they found the overall clinical success rate (defined as ≥ 25 percent improvement in Oswestry Disability Index score at 24 months, no device failure, no major complication, and no neurological deterioration) to be significantly higher in the Charité-treated group as compared with anterior lumbar interbody fusion group.[46] However, when the criteria mentioned above were analyzed separately, only the ODI scores were significantly higher. The Charité group recovered faster and reported lower pain scores in the first year, but the difference was not statistically significant after two years.[46] Neurological complications were not more common in the Charité group.[47] The study by Blumenthal has been criticized for comparing disk replacement to a kind of surgery that has been abandoned because it fails.[48] In a small RCT comparing ProDisc II to anterior fusion surgery, a greater improvement in ODI scores and motion was found, but no significant difference in pain scores.[49]

REFERENCES

1. Schwarzer AC, Aprill CN, Derby R *et al*. The prevalence and clinical features of internal disc disruption in patients with chronic low back pain. *Spine*. 1995; **20**: 1878–83.

2. Crock HV. Internal disc disruption. A challenge to disc prolapse fifty years on. *Spine*. 1986; **11**: 650–3.

3. Bogduk N. The lumbar disc and low back pain. *Neurosurgery Clinics of North America*. 1991; **2**: 791–806.

4. Barendse GA, van Den Berg SG, Kessels AH *et al*. Randomized controlled trial of percutaneous intradiscal radiofrequency thermocoagulation for chronic discogenic back pain: lack of effect from a 90-second 70 C lesion. *Spine*. 2001; **26**: 287–92.

5. Saal JS, Saal JA. Management of chronic discogenic low back pain with a thermal intradiscal catheter. A preliminary report. *Spine*. 2000; **25**: 382–8.

6. Saal JA, Saal JS. Intradiscal electrothermal treatment for chronic discogenic low back pain: a prospective outcome study with minimum 1-year follow-up. *Spine*. 2000; **25**: 2622–7.

7. Finch PM. The use of radiofrequency heat lesions in the treatment of lumbar discogenic pain. *Pain Practice*. 2002; **2**: 235–40.

8. Borggrefe M, Hindricks G, Haverkamp W, Breithardt G. Catheter ablation using radiofrequency energy. *Clinical Cardiology*. 1990; **13**: 127–31.

9. Goldberg SN, Gazelle GS, Dawson SL *et al*. Tissue ablation with radiofrequency: effect of probe size, gauge, duration, and temperature on lesion volume. *Academic Radiology*. 1995; **2**: 399–404.

10. Kleinstueck FS, Diederich CJ, Nau WH *et al*. Acute biomechanical and histological effects of intradiscal electrothermal therapy on human lumbar discs. *Spine*. 2001; **26**: 2198–207.

11. Houpt JC, Conner ES, McFarland EW. Experimental study of temperature distributions and thermal transport during radiofrequency current therapy of the intervertebral disc. *Spine*. 1996; **21**: 1808–12.

12. Wall MS, Deng XH, Torzilli PA *et al*. Thermal modification of collagen. *Journal of Shoulder and Elbow Surgery*. 1999; **8**: 339–44.

13. Holm S, Indahl A, Solomonow M. Sensorimotor control of the spine. *Journal of Electromyography and Kinesiology*. 2002; **12**: 219–34.

14. Lam KS, Carlin D, Mulholland RC. Lumbar disc high-intensity zone: the value and significance of provocative discography in the determination of the discogenic pain source. *European Spine Journal*. 2000; **9**: 36–41.

15. Saifuddin A, Braithwaite I, White J *et al*. The value of lumbar spine magnetic resonance imaging in the demonstration of anular tears. *Spine*. 1998; **23**: 453–7.

16. Derby R, Kim BJ, Lee SH *et al*. Comparison of discographic findings in asymptomatic subject discs and the negative discs of chronic LBP patients: can discography distinguish asymptomatic discs among morphologically abnormal discs? *Spine Journal*. 2005; **5**: 389–94.

17. Moneta GB, Videman T, Kaivanto K *et al*. Reported pain during lumbar discography as a function of anular ruptures and disc degeneration. A re-analysis of 833 discograms. *Spine*. 1994; **19**: 1968–74.

18. Vanharanta H, Sachs BL, Spivey MA *et al*. The relationship of pain provocation to lumbar-disk deterioration as seen by CT-discography. *Spine*. 1987; **12**: 295–8.

19. Sachs BL, Vanharanta H, Spivey MA *et al*. Dallas discogram description – a new classification of CT – discography in low-back disorders. *Spine*. 1987; **12**: 287–94.

* 20. Pauza KJ, Howell S, Dreyfuss P *et al*. A randomized, placebo-controlled trial of intradiscal electrothermal therapy for the treatment of discogenic low back pain. *Spine Journal*. 2004; **4**: 27–35.

21. Bogduk N. Discography guidelines. *The International Spine Intervention Society Newsletter*. 2003; **3**.

22. Sharps LS, Isaac Z. Percutaneous disc decompression using nucleoplasty(r). *Pain Physician*. 2002; **5**: 121–6.

23. Carragee EJ, Alamin TF, Miller J, Grafe M. Provocative discography in volunteer subjects with mild persistent low back pain. *Spine Journal*. 2002; **2**: 25–34.

24. Derby R, Lee SH, Kim BJ *et al*. Pressure-controlled lumbar discography in volunteers without low back symptoms. *Pain Medicine*. 2005; **6**: 213–21.

* 25. Carragee EJ, Alamin TF, Carragee JM. Low-pressure positive discography in subjects asymptomatic of significant low back pain illness. *Spine*. 2006; **31**: 505–09.

26. Karasek M, Bogduk N. Twelve-month follow-up of a controlled trial of intradiscal thermal anuloplasty for back pain due to internal disc disruption. *Spine*. 2000; **25**: 2601–7.

27. Derby R, Eek B, Chen Y *et al*. Intradiscal electrothermal annuloplasty (IDET): a novel approach for treating chronic discogenic back pain. *Neuromodulation*. 2000; **3**: 69–75.

28. Freeman BJ. IDET: a critical appraisal of the evidence. *European Spine Journal*. 2006; **15**: 448–57.

29. Freeman BJ, Fraser RD, Cain CM *et al*. A randomized, double-blind, controlled trial: intradiscal electrothermal therapy versus placebo for the treatment of chronic discogenic low back pain. *Spine*. 2005; **30**: 2369–77.

30. Erdine S, Yucel A, Celik M. Percutaneous annuloplasty in the treatment of discogenic pain: retrospective evaluation of one year follow-up. *Agri: The journal of the Turkish Society of Algology*. 2004; **16**: 41–7.

31. Finch PM, Price LM, Drummond PD. Radiofrequency heating of painful annular disruptions: one-year outcomes. *Journal of Spinal Disorders and Techniques*. 2005; **18**: 6–13.

32. Kapural L, Hayek S, Malak O *et al*. Intradiscal thermal annuloplasty versus intradiscal radiofrequency ablation for the treatment of discogenic pain: a prospective matched control trial. *Pain Medicine*. 2005; **6**: 425–31.

* 33. Pomerantz SR, Hirsch JA. Intradiscal therapies for discogenic pain. *Seminars in Musculoskeletal Radiology*. 2006; **10**: 125–35.

34. Watanabe I, Masaki R, Min N *et al*. Cooled-tip ablation results in increased radiofrequency power delivery and lesion size in the canine heart: importance of catheter-tip temperature monitoring for prevention of popping and impedance rise. *Journal of Interventional Cardiac Electrophysiology*. 2002; **6**: 9–16.

35. Cohen SP, Larkin T, Polly Jr DW. A giant herniated disc following intradiscal electrothermal therapy. *Journal of Spinal Disorders and Techniques*. 2002; **15**: 537–41.

36. Ackerman III WE. Cauda equina syndrome after intradiscal electrothermal therapy. *Regional Anesthesia and Pain Medicine*. 2002; **27**: 622.

37. Hsia AW, Isaac K, Katz JS. Cauda equina syndrome from intradiscal electrothermal therapy. *Neurology*. 2000; **55**: 320.

38. Wetzel FT. Cauda equina syndrome from intradiscal electrothermal therapy. *Neurology*. 2001; **56**: 1607.

39. Djurasovic M, Glassman SD, Dimar JR, Johnson JR. Vertebral osteonecrosis associated with the use of intradiscal electrothermal therapy: a case report. *Spine*. 2002; **27**: E325–8.

40. Cohen SP, Larkin T, Abdi S *et al*. Risk factors for failure and complications of intradiscal electrothermal therapy: a pilot study. *Spine*. 2003; **28**: 1142–7.

41. Urrútia G, Kovacs F, Nishishinya MB, Olabe J. Percutaneous thermocoagulation intradiscal techniques for discogenic low back pain. *Spine*. 2007; **32**: 1146–54.

42. Maurer P, Block JE, Squillante DPA-C. Intradiscal electrothermal therapy (IDET) provides effective symptom relief in patients with discogenic low back pain. *Journal of Spinal Disorders and Techniques*. 2008; **21**: 55–62.

∗ 43. Errico TJ. Why a mechanical disc? *Spine Journal*. 2004; **4**: 151S–7.

44. Cinotti G, David T, Postacchini F. Results of disc prosthesis after a minimum follow-up period of 2 years. *Spine*. 1996; **21**: 995–1000.

45. Lemaire JP, Skalli W, Lavaste F *et al.* Intervertebral disc prosthesis. Results and prospects for the year 2000. *Clinical Orthopaedics and Related Research*. 1997; **1**: 64–76.

∗ 46. Blumenthal S, McAfee PC, Guyer RD *et al.* A prospective, randomized, multicenter Food and Drug Administration investigational device exemptions study of lumbar total disc replacement with the CHARITE artificial disc versus lumbar fusion: part I: evaluation of clinical outcomes. *Spine*. 2005; **30**: 1565–75.

47. Geisler FH, Blumenthal SL, Guyer RD *et al.* Neurological complications of lumbar artificial disc replacement and comparison of clinical results with those related to lumbar arthrodesis in the literature: results of a multicenter, prospective, randomized investigational device exemption study of Charite intervertebral disc. Invited submission from the Joint Section Meeting on Disorders of the Spine and Peripheral Nerves, March 2004. *Journal of Neurosurgery. Spine*. 2004; **1**: 143–54.

48. Mirza SK. Point of view: Commentary on the research reports that led to Food and Drug Administration approval of an artificial disc. *Spine*. 2005; **30**: 1561–4.

49. Zigler JE. Clinical results with ProDisc: European experience and US investigation device exemption study. *Spine*. 2003; **28**: S163–6.

SECTION E

Pediatric techniques

38

Pain assessment in children

NANCY F BANDSTRA AND CHRISTINE T CHAMBERS

KEY LEARNING POINTS

- The assessment of pain in children can be a challenge.
- The best evidence exists for self-report and behavioral measures.
- Measures that are age-appropriate should be selected.

- Specialized measures are available for use with neonates and children with developmental disabilities, as well as for children experiencing chronic pain.
- Involving parents, and paying attention to cultural and ethnic factors, can improve pain assessment.

INTRODUCTION

Pain is a common experience for children and can present in the form of everyday bumps and bruises or can occur as a result of medical procedures, such as immunizations, and recurrent pains, such as headaches and stomachaches. Given the subjective nature of the pain experience and the communicative limitations often present when working with children, accurate pain assessment is one of the most difficult yet imperative challenges facing health professionals and researchers who work with children. Historically, children have been administered significantly less pain medication than is prescribed.[1] Difficulties assessing pain have frequently been cited as barriers to optimal pain management in children.[2] Unfortunately, despite the dramatic growth in knowledge about pain in children over the last 30 years, pediatric pain assessment and management continues to be substandard in many settings.[3]

The purpose of this chapter is to provide a review of commonly used measures for assessing pain in children and to summarize the research evidence in support of these various measures. The focus of this chapter will be primarily on acute pain; however, we will also provide a brief review of measures appropriate for use with pediatric patients experiencing chronic pain. We also highlight a number of special issues to consider when assessing pediatric pain, such as pain assessment among children with developmental disabilities, pain assessment in infants and neonates, the role of parents, and ethnic and cultural considerations.

ASSESSMENT OF ACUTE PAIN

Measurement of acute pain (rather than chronic pain) in children has received the most attention in the pediatric research literature by far. It is generally accepted that there are three primary approaches to assess acute pain in children:

1. self-report measures (i.e. what a child says or verbally indicates about their pain);
2. behavioral measures (i.e. the child's observed behavior in response to pain);
3. physiological measures (i.e. how the child's body reacts to pain).

A variety of measures designed to assess each of these three areas currently exists.[4] However, given that pain is a highly individualized and subjective event, a child's self-report (when available) is thought to be the most direct means of assessing pain experience and it has been suggested that it should be considered the gold standard for pain assessment.[5] For this reason, we begin our discussion with self-report measures and then progress to summarizing the literature on behavioral and physiological measures of pain.

Self-report measures

Self-report measures provide an opportunity for children to communicate (i.e. beyond simple verbalizations) their own pain to parents and/or health professionals. These measures typically require children to rate their pain intensity by using photographs/schematized faces, words, and/or numbers.[6] In most cases, self-reports are the most practical, quick, and cost-effective method of obtaining a pain assessment. Unfortunately, not all children are able to provide reliable and valid self-reports of pain, although there is no clear consensus regarding the age at which children can provide a self-report of pain. It is generally accepted that by the age of seven years, most children can provide an appropriate self-report using a pain measure,[7, 8, 9, 10] and mixed evidence exists that some children as young as three years of age may also be capable of doing so.[6]

Some of the advantages and disadvantages associated with use of self-report measures of pain are shown in **Table 38.1**.

A recent systematic review assessed the psychometric properties of the various self-report pain intensity measures available for use in children and adolescents. For a detailed discussion of the psychometric properties of each recommended self-report scale, see Ref. 11. Of the 34 self-report pain measures identified for consideration in this review, six measures were determined to have well-established evidence of reliability and validity. The measures recommended were the following:

- Faces Pain Scale (FPS);[12]
- Faces Pain Scale-Revised (FPS-R);[13]
- Wong-Baker FACES Pain Rating Scale;[14]
- Oucher;[15]
- Visual analog scale (VAS);
- Pieces of Hurt Tool (also known as the Poker Chip Tool).[16]

Each of these measures is summarized below. Of the six measures described in the review by Stinson and colleagues,[11] no single measure demonstrated sufficient reliability and validity for children across the age/developmental span. In addition, each measure displayed varying levels of preference by children as well as varying rates of failure, suggesting some children's inability to accurately use these measures. For these reasons, at the conclusion of each measure description below, an age-based recommendation for its use is provided.[11]

FACES SCALES

Faces scales give children the opportunity to rate their pain using a series of ranked faces. Some of these self-report measures provide schematized pictures of faces (e.g. FPS, FPS-R, Wong-Baker FACES Pain Rating Scale) and others provide real photographs of children (e.g. the Oucher). Both types have shown sufficient reliability and validity, but have varying degrees of interpretability and feasibility for clinicians, as well as acceptability by children.[11]

The FPS and FPS-R illustrate gender-neutral faces representing expressions ranging from "no pain" to "most pain possible." The child is asked to point to the face that corresponds to the level of pain he/she is experiencing. The original FPS depicts seven faces.[12] A revised version of this scale, the FPS-R,[13] uses six faces and is generally scored from 0 to 10 (see **Figure 38.1**) to facilitate

Table 38.1 The advantages and disadvantages associated with use of self-report measures of pain.

Advantages	Disadvantages
Most children above the age of seven can reliably report their own pain	Not appropriate for use in nonverbal/preverbal children
Self-report is typically the most valid and reliable measure of a child's pain	May be inappropriate for neurologically impaired children
	Some children may be too distressed to accurately self-report
Measures generally require little training to learn or time to conduct	May elicit exaggerated (or minimized) reports depending on a variety of factors (e.g. social, situational influences)

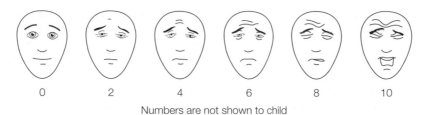

Numbers are not shown to child

Figure 38.1 Faces Pain Scale-Revised. Instructions to the child are: "These faces show how much something can hurt. This face (point to left-most face) shows no pain (or hurt). The faces show more and more pain (point to each from left to right) up to this one (point to right-most face) – it shows very much pain. Point to the face that shows how much you hurt (right now)." Do not use words like "happy" or "sad." This scale is intended to measure how children feel inside, not how their face looks. Numbers are not shown to children; they are shown here only for reference. The instructions for administration are currently available in over 32 languages from www.painsourcebook.ca. Reproduced from Hicks CL, von Baeyer CL, Spafford PA *et al*. The Faces Pain Scale – Revised: toward a common metric in pediatric pain measurement. *Pain*. 2001; **93**: 173–83. Scale adapted from: Bieri D, Reeve RA, Champion G *et al*. The Faces Pain Scale for the self-assessment of the severity of pain experienced by children: development, initial validation and preliminary investigation for ratio scale properties. *Pain*. 1990; **41**: 139–50. Used with permission from the International Association for the Study of Pain [IASP]®.

comparison with other self-report and observational scales using the same 0–10 scoring metric. Ratings of three out of seven or more on the FPS signifies clinically meaningful pain[17] and both scales have shown evidence of responsivity following pharmacological intervention.[18, 19] In fact, a change of one face over time is generally considered a clinically significant change.[20] Both the FPS and FPS-R are appropriate for the assessment of procedural, postoperative, and disease-related pain in children.[11] In addition, administration instructions for the FPS-R have been translated into over 32 languages and are available from www.painsourcebook.ca.

The Wong-Baker FACES Pain Rating Scale is composed of six hand-drawn faces.[14] The faces range from smiling (representing "no hurt") to crying (representing "hurts worst"). The scale itself is scored from 0 to 5 (see **Figure 38.2**). The measure has established adequate responsivity to procedural[21, 22, 23, 24, 25] and postoperative pain.[26] Although often preferred by children relative to other assessment measures[14, 22, 27, 28] the Wong-Baker FACES Pain Rating Scale's use of smiling/crying anchors has been identified as problematic. Scales that begin with neutral faces (such as the FPS-R) are considered a more valid measure of pain intensity because scales with tears or smiles are generally more tied to an emotional component[29] and may be more likely to confound more general negative emotions and distress with pain intensity.[30]

While the FPS, FPS-R, and the Wong-Baker FACES Pain Rating Scale all rely on schematized faces, the Oucher[15] uses real photographs of children to measure pain intensity. The Oucher provides a measurement using not only a scale of six faces (scored from 0 to 5), but also a corresponding 0–100-mm vertical rating scale (scored from 0 to 100; see **Figure 38.3**). The Oucher can detect changes from pre- to postoperation and following pharmacological interventions.[31, 32, 33, 34] Because the Oucher consists of both a numerical rating scale and a photograph scale, it may only be appropriate for older children who can comprehend these types of serial tasks.[35] As is discussed below under the section entitled Cultural and ethnic considerations, the Oucher has also been validated using photographs of African-American and Hispanic children.[36]

Stinson and colleagues[11] recommend using the FPS-R as the measure of choice for school-aged (i.e. 4- to 12-year-old) children. The FPS-R should be used with caution in the lower end of this age range as children below the age of seven years may have difficulties using such measures reliably.[11]

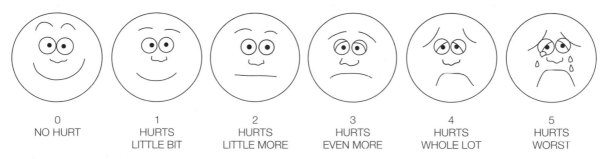

Figure 38.2 Wong-Baker FACES Scale. Point to each face using the words to describe the pain intensity. Ask the child to choose face that best describes their own pain and record the appropriate number. Reprinted from Hockenberry MJ, Wilson D, Winkelstein ML. *Wong's Essentials of Pediatric Nursing*, 7th edn. St. Louis: Mosby, 2005, p. 1259. Used with permission. Copyright, Mosby.

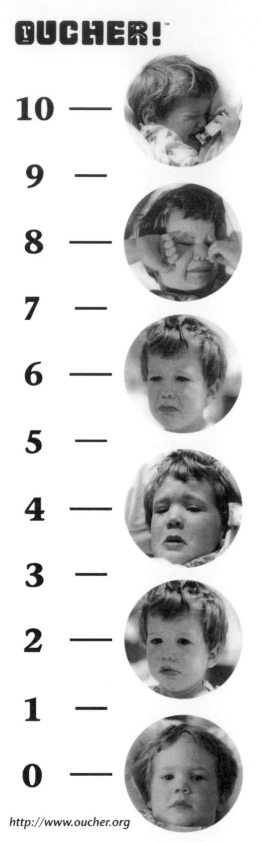

OUCHER!™

http://www.oucher.org

Figure 38.3 The Oucher self-report pain scale. Reprinted from Beyer JE, Denyes MJ, Villaruel AM. The creation, validation, and continuing development of the Oucher: a measure of pain intensity in children. *Journal of Pediatric Nursing.* 1992; **7**: 335–46. Used with permission from Judith E. Beyer.

VISUAL ANALOG SCALES

The VAS is generally a 10-cm vertical or horizontal line with ends representing the extreme levels of pain intensity (e.g. "no pain" and "worst pain," see **Figure 38.4**). Children are asked to make a mark or point to their own level of pain. Scores typically range from 0 to 100 mm (depending on the scale's length) and changes of 10 to 13 mm are usually considered clinically meaningful.[37, 38] Varying versions of the VAS have been used to assess procedural, postoperative, and disease-related pain. Furthermore, the VAS has shown responsivity to change following surgery,[39] as well as pharmacological interventions.[31, 39, 40] However, mixed results have indicated that the strength of these findings may be contingent upon a child's age, level of comprehension, and type of pain.[32, 41, 42] The VAS should be used cautiously with children between the ages of 8 and 12 years, but is recommended for use with children >12 years. Using the FPS-R as a secondary assessment tool in these younger children may be helpful.

PIECES OF HURT TOOL (ALSO KNOWN AS THE POKER CHIP TOOL)

Although faces scales and VASs are appropriate for use in older children, the ability of children under the age of seven years to use these measures varies. A self-report measure often used with younger children is the Pieces of Hurt Tool.[16] This simple measure consists of four poker chips described as representing different amounts of hurt (e.g. from "a little hurt" to "the most hurt you could ever have"; instructions are available at: www.painresearch.utah.edu/cancerpain/attachb7.html). The child is asked to choose "how many pieces of hurt" he/she is currently experiencing and the tool is scored from 0 to 4. The Pieces of Hurt Tool has shown evidence of responsivity from pre- to postsurgery[32] and pre- to postanalgesia.[33] The Pieces of Hurt Tool is recommended as the measure to use with preschool-aged children in acute and postoperative pain settings. However, it is advised that this tool be used in conjunction with behavioral measures[11] since self-report ratings in young children may be affected by external, non-pain-related variables (e.g. cognitive, emotional, situational factors).[43]

Behavioral measures

Behavioral measures are designed to assess pain and distress by observing a child's response to pain (e.g. vocalizations, facial expressions, behavior). Although self-report measures are often considered the gold standard in pediatric pain assessment, health professionals working with neonates, toddlers, and noncommunicative children are unable to utilize this type of assessment tool. When children are unable to voice their own levels of discomfort, health professionals must look to behavioral

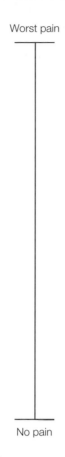

Worst pain

No pain

Figure 38.4 Visual analog scale.

measures as their primary source of pain measurement.[44] Unlike self-report measures, which tend to be applicable across acute pain settings, observational pain scales are often designed for and validated in distinct pain settings.

The advantages and disadvantages of behavioral pain measures are shown in **Table 38.2**.

A recent systematic review assessed the psychometric properties of the various observational/behavioral pain intensity measures available for use in children and adolescents.[44] Of the 20 behavioral pain measures included in the evaluation, six measures were determined to have well-established evidence of reliability and validity.[44] These measures include two scales recommended for procedural and postoperative pain assessment in hospital, an additional scale recommended for postoperative pain assessment at home, one measure specifically for critical care, and finally, two scales specifically designed to assess the important corresponding constructs of pain-related distress and fear:

- Face, Legs, Arms, Cry, Consolability (FLACC);[45]
- Children's Hospital of Eastern Ontario Pain Scale (CHEOPS);[46]
- Parents' Postoperative Pain Measure (PPPM);[47]
- COMFORT Scale;[48]
- Procedure Behavior Check List (PBCL);[49]
- Procedure Behavioral Rating Scale-Revised (PBRS-R).[50]

Table 38.2 The advantages and disadvantages of behavioral pain measures.

Advantages	Disadvantages
Able to assess pain in preverbal/ nonverbal children	May be time-consuming to conduct and score
Yield detailed information on a number of behavioral domains	May require training to administer
Unobtrusive	No behavior does not equal no pain

Each of these measures is discussed below in detail. It should be noted that, in addition to these broad-band behavioral measures, measures of facial expression alone (e.g. Neonatal Facial Coding System,[51] Child Facial Coding System[52]) have been used frequently in research but may have limited feasibility for use in clinical practice.

PROCEDURAL PAIN

Two well-established behavioral measures (FLACC and CHEOPS) are recommended for pain associated with medical procedures.[44] The FLACC is designed to assess the behavioral reaction to pain in children one year of age and above.[45] As the name implies, raters assess each of the five categories (face, legs, arms, cry and the child's consolability). Each category is scored from 0 to 2 representing a gradual increase of distressed behavior (see Table 38.3). Advantages of the FLACC include quick administration and easy interpretation.[44]

Similarly, the CHEOPS has raters report on six different categories (crying, facial expression, verbal expression, torso position, touch, and leg position)[46] and has been used to measure pain in children across the age range.[44] Unlike the FLACC, the behavioral categories on the CHEOPS are scored from 0 to 3 to allow for differential rating of each included behavior (see **Table 38.4**). Total scores from four to six points represent no pain. Like the FLACC, the CHEOPS has substantial evidence of reliability and validity. Unlike the FLACC, the CHEOPS requires more time to complete and has a less-recognized metric with scores ranging from 0 to 13 (versus 10 in the FLACC). However, a distinct advantage of the CHEOPS is that it does not require raters to try to comfort the distressed child after the procedure (as is done to assess the "consolability" category in the FLACC). Used to assess procedural pain, both the FLACC and the CHEOPS are also appropriate pain assessment tools postoperatively.

POSTOPERATIVE PAIN

Although used with procedural pain quite often, the FLACC was originally validated as a postoperative pain

Table 38.3 FLACC scale.

Item	Score		
	0	**1**	**2**
Face	No particular expression or smile	Occasional grimace or frown, withdrawn, disinterested	Frequent to constant quivering chin, clenched jaw
Legs	Normal position or relaxed	Uneasy, restless, tense	Kicking or legs drawn up
Activity	Lying quietly, normal position, moves easily	Squirming, shifting back and forth, tense	Arched, rigid or jerking
Cry	No cry (awake or asleep)	Moans or whimpers; occasional complaint	Crying steadily, screams or sobs, frequent complaints
Consolability	Content, relaxed	Reassured by occasional touching, hugging or being talked to, distractible	Difficult to console or comfort

Reproduced with permission from Merkel SI, Voepel-Lewis T, Shayevitz JR, Malviya S. The FLACC: a behavioral scale for scoring postoperative pain in young children. *Pediatric Nursing.* 1997; **23**: 293–7. © 2002, The Regents of the University of Michigan.

Table 38.4 Children's Hospital of Eastern Ontario Pain Scale (CHEOPS) items.

Item	Behavior	Score	Definition
Cry	No cry	1	Child is not crying
	Moaning	2	Child is moaning or quietly vocalizing, silent cry
	Crying	2	Child is crying but the cry is gentle or whimpering
	Scream	3	Child is in a full-lunged cry; sobbing; may be scored with complaint or without complaint
Facial	Composed	1	Neutral facial expression
	Grimace	2	Score only if definite negative facial expression
	Smiling	0	Score only if definite positive facial expression
Child verbal	None	1	Child is not talking
	Other complaints	1	Child complains but not about pain, e.g. "I want to see my mommy," or "I am thirsty"
	Pain complaints	2	Child complains about pain
	Both complaints	2	Child complains about pain and about other things, e.g. "It hurts; I want mommy"
	Positive	0	Child makes any positive statement or talks about other things without complaint
Torso	Neutral	1	Body (not limbs) is at rest; torso is inactive
	Shifting	2	Body is in motion in a shifting or serpentine fashion
	Tense	2	Body is arched or rigid
	Shivering	2	Body is shuddering or shaking involuntarily
	Upright	2	Child is in vertical or upright positions
	Restrained	2	Body is restrained
Touch	Not touching	1	Child is not touching or grabbing at wound
	Reach	2	Child is reaching for but not touching wound
	Touch	2	Child is gently touching wound or wound area
	Grab	2	Child is grabbing vigorously at wound
	Restrained	2	Child's arms are restrained
Legs	Neutral	1	Legs may be in any position but are relaxed; includes gentle swimming or serpentine-like movements
	Squirming/kicking	2	Definitive uneasy or restless movements in the legs and/or striking out with foot or feet
	Drawn up/tensed	2	Legs tensed and/or pulled up tightly to body and kept there
	Standing	2	Standing, crouching, or kneeling
	Restrained	2	Child's legs are being held down

Reproduced from McGrath PJ, Johnson G, Goodman JT *et al.* CHEOPS: A behavioral scale for rating postoperative pain in children. In: Fields HL, Dubner R, Cervero F (eds). *Advances in pain research and therapy.* New York: Raven Press, 1985: 395–402.

measure.[45] The extensive reliability and validity data supporting the FLACC makes it the first choice for postoperative assessment while in hospital.[44] Generally, postoperative pain tends to last over a longer period of time than the pain associated with medical procedures, making the category of "consolability" a more meaningful measure of pain assessment.

Following surgery, children are sent home and parents are given the duty of supplying the care needed during postsurgical recovery. Chambers and colleagues[47] developed an assessment measure called the Parents' Postoperative Pain Measure to assist parents in assessing the pain of their children once discharged from hospital care. The PPPM is comprised of 15 items, each describing a behavior typically exhibited by a child postsurgery (see Table 38.5). Parents are asked to rate their child's current behavior as compared to his/her normal behavior. Use of the PPPM is relatively quick and easy, resulting in a low level of burden for parents. Originally validated with children between the ages of 2 and 12 years,[47] the PPPM has been used to measure pain in children as young as one year of age.[44]

Postoperative pain measures (with the exception of the PPPM) have primarily been validated in the period shortly after surgery. These types of scales become unreliable for assessing the long-term pain that often follows surgery since many of the behaviors described may habituate over time.[53] For this reason, care should be taken when using these types of measures to assess pain over a long period of time.

Table 38.5 Parent's Postoperative Pain Measure items.

Items
Whine or complain more than usual?
Cry more easily than usual?
Play less than usual?
Not do the things s/he normally does?
Act more worried than usual?
Act more quiet than usual?
Have less energy than usual?
Refuse to eat?
Eat less than usual?
Hold the sore part of his/her body?
Try not to bump the sore part of his/her body?
Groan or moan more than usual?
Look more flushed than usual?
Want to be close to you more than usual?
Take medication when s/he normally refuses?

Items are scored "Yes" or "No." Items scored as "Yes" are summed for a total score out of 15. A score of at least 6 out of 15 signifies clinically significant pain.
Reprinted by permission from Chambers CT, Reid GJ, McGrath PJ, Finley GA. Development and preliminary validation of a postoperative pain measure for parents. *Pain.* 1996; **68**: 307–13.

CRITICAL/INTENSIVE CARE

Only one assessment tool has been validated for use in situations of critical care or when children are on ventilator support. Designed for children across the age spectrum (from newborns to 17 years), the COMFORT Scale[48] takes into account the restricted physical motion and limited behavioral reaction of children in critical care. The scale assesses alertness, calmness/agitation, respiration, physical movement, blood pressure change, heart rate change, muscle tone, and facial tension (each category scored 1 to 5; see **Table 38.6**).

ASSESSMENT OF PAIN-RELATED FEAR AND DISTRESS

When children are approached with a painful procedure, they rarely experience just pain. Often the corresponding emotions of fear and anxiety are present. This is especially true for children who have undergone multiple procedures due to chronic illness (e.g. cancer) or severe injury (e.g. burn). Acute pain over a long period of time may lead to the development of significant levels of anxiety and fear. In fact, research with survivors of childhood cancer has indicated a high likelihood of posttraumatic stress symptoms,[54] as well as the possible development of posttraumatic stress disorder (PTSD).[55]

Two scales designed to measure distress and pain-related fear are the Procedure Behavior Check List[49] and the Procedure Behavioral Rating Scale-Revised.[50] These measures include a series of behavioral items that relate to fear and distress rather than pain. They are often included in studies of painful procedures and can provide helpful information regarding a child's distress level in addition to the information available about pain via other measures. Both the PBCL and the PBRS-R were originally designed or have been subsequently used to assess distress and pain-related fear in children across the age range.[44]

Physiological measures

Physiological measures provide a quantification of how a child's body reacts to pain. Although it would be desirable to have a direct way of measuring the body's response to pain, in the same way that a thermometer provides a direct measure of body temperature, given the subjective and complex nature of the pain experience, it should not be surprising that, to date, no such measure has been identified. The most commonly used physiological measures are heart rate, vagal tone, respiratory rate, blood pressure, oxygen saturation, transcutaneous oxygen, palmar sweating, intracranial pressure, and stress response and all have shown at least some validity as pain measures in some instances.[56] The advantages and disadvantages of physiological measures of pain are shown in **Table 38.7**.

There is insufficient evidence to recommend physiological measures as a primary approach for pain

Table 38.6 COMFORT Scale items.

Indicator	Score	Behavior	Definition
Alertness	1	Deeply asleep	The state of least responsiveness to the environment. The patient's eyes are closed, breathing is deep and regular, and the patient shows minimal responses to changes in the environment
	2	Lightly asleep	The patient has their eyes closed throughout most of the observation period, but still responds somewhat to the environment as evidenced by slight movements, facial movements, unsuccessful attempts at eye openings, etc.
	3	Drowsy	The patient closes their eyes frequently or makes labored attempts to open eyes and is less responsive to the environment
	4	Alert and awake	The patient is responsive and interactive with the environment, but without an exaggerated response to the environment. The patient's eyes remain open most of the time or open readily in response to ambient stimuli
	5	Hyper-alert	The patient is hyper-vigilant, may be wide-eyed, attends rapidly to subtle changes in the environmental stimuli and has exaggerated responses to environmental stimuli
Calmness/ agitation	1	Calm	The patient appears serene and tranquil. There is no evidence of apprehension or emotional distress
	2	Slightly anxious	The patient is not completely calm. The patient shows slight apprehension and emotional distress
	3	Anxious	The patient appears somewhat apprehensive and emotionally distressed but remains in control
	4	Very anxious	The patient appears very apprehensive. Emotional distress is apparent but the patient remains somewhat in control
	5	Panicky	The patient's total demeanor conveys immediate and severe emotional distress with loss of behavioral control
Respiratory response	1	No coughing or no spontaneous respiration	Only ventilator generated breaths are apparent. No respiratory movement is apparent between ventilator breaths. No oral movement or chest wall movement occurs, except as created by the ventilator
	2	Spontaneous respiration	The patient breathes at a regular, normal respiratory rate in synchrony with the ventilator. No oral movement or chest wall movement occurs which is contrary to the ventilator movement
	3	Occasional cough/resists ventilator	The patient has occasional oral or chest wall movement contrary to the ventilator pattern. The patient may occasionally breathe out of synchrony with the ventilator
	4	Actively breathes against ventilator	The patient has frequent oral or chest wall movement contrary to the ventilator pattern, coughs regularly, or frequently breathes out of synchrony with the ventilator
	5	Fights ventilator – coughs/ chokes/gags	The patient actively makes oral or chest wall movement contrary to the ventilator pattern, coughs and/or gags in a manner which may interfere with ventilation
Physical movement	1	None	The patient shows complete absence of independent movement
	2	Occasional, slight movements	The patient shows three or fewer small amplitude movements of the fingers or feet, or very small head movement
	3	Frequent, slight movement	The patient shows more than three small amplitude movements of the fingers or feet, or very small head movements
	4	Vigorous movements of extremities only	The patient shows movements of greater amplitude, speed or vigor of hands, arms or legs. The head may move slightly. Movement is vigorous enough to potentially disrupt cannulas
	5	Vigorous movements of extremities, torso and head	The patient shows movements of greater amplitude, speed or vigor of the head and torso, such as head thrashing, back arching, or neck arching. Extremities may also move. Movement is vigorous enough to potentially disrupt placement of an endotracheal tube

(Continued over)

Table 38.6 COMFORT Scale items (continued).

Indicator	Score	Behavior	Definition
Blood pressure	1		Blood pressure below baseline
	2		Blood pressure consistently at baseline
	3		Infrequent elevations of 15% or more (1–3 during observation period)
	4		Frequent elevations of 15% or more (more than 3 during observation period)
	5		Sustained elevation greater than or equal to 15%
Heart rate	1		Heart rate below baseline
	2		Heart rate consistently at baseline
	3		Infrequent elevations of 15% or more (1–3 during observation period)
	4		Frequent elevations of 15% or more (more than 3 during observation period)
	5		Sustained elevation greater than or equal to 15%
Muscle tone	1	Relaxed/None	Muscle tone is absent. There is no resistance to movement
	2	Reduced muscle tone	The patient shows less resistance to movement than normal, but muscle tone is not totally absent
	3	Normal muscle tone	Resistance to movement is normal
	4	Increased tone/flexionof fingers/toes	The patient shows resistance to movement that is clearly greater than normal, but the joint is not rigid
	5	Extreme rigidity/flexion of fingers/toes	Muscle rigidity is the patient's predominant state throughout the observation period. This may be observed even without manipulating an extremity
Facial tension	1	Relaxed	The patient shows no facial muscle tone, with absence of normal mouth and eye closing. The mouth may look slack and the patient may drool
	2	Normal tone	The patient shows no facial muscle tension with mouth and eyes closing appropriately
	3	Some tension	This does not include sustained tension of muscle groups such as the brow, forehead, or mouth
	4	Full facial tension	The patient shows notable, sustained tension of facial muscle groups including the brow, forehead, mouth, chin, or cheeks
	5	Hyper-alert	The patient demonstrates facial grimacing with an expression that conveys an impression of crying, discomfort, and distress. This generally includes extreme furrowing of brow and forehead and contortion of the mouth

Total scores can range between 8 and 40. A score of 17–26 generally indicates adequate sedation and pain control. Reproduced from Ambuel B, Hamlett KW, Marx CM, Blumer JL. Assessing distress in pediatric intensive care environments: the COMFORT scale. *Journal of Pediatric Psychology*. 1992; **17**: 95–109, by permission of the Society of Pediatric Psychology, Division 54 of the American Psychological Association.

Table 38.7 The advantages and disadvantages of physiological measures of pain.

Advantages	Disadvantages
Objective	Habituate over time to long-lasting pain
	Are not specific to pain and measure other states (e.g. distress, anxiety)
	Rarely correlated with other self-report and behavioral measures of pain

assessment in children at this time, although they may be helpful to include as part of a broader pain assessment battery for some populations and context (e.g. neonates in the intensive care unit).

ASSESSMENT OF CHRONIC PAIN

In contrast to the considerable research conducted in the area of acute pain assessment in children, significantly less attention has been devoted to measures of chronic pain in children and adolescents. Often, many of the self-report measures summarized above will be used to provide an assessment of chronic pain (e.g. VAS or FPS-R can be used to have children rate the pain from their most recent headache). Because of its complex nature, chronic pain assessment often also encompasses measurement of domains known to be related to pain, such as physical (e.g. interference with daily activities, sleep) and psychological variables (e.g. depression, anxiety). Some of the most common measures used in pediatric chronic pain assessment include the Functional Disability Inventory (FDI),[57] the Pain Coping Questionnaire (PCQ),[58] and the Pain Catastrophizing Scale for Children (PCS-C).[59] A review of measures commonly used in the assessment of adolescent chronic pain by Eccleston and colleagues[60] revealed that of a total of 43 different measures that had been cited as part of an assessment battery, only 12 of these measures actually had been validated for use with adolescents with chronic pain. This review also revealed considerable diversity in measures applied for chronic pain assessment across studies, making it difficult to interpret results and compare across studies.

A better approach to this more piecemeal assessment method is the use of comprehensive questionnaires designed to document pain intensity, as well as other pain-related variables, such as the affective qualities associated with the pain or pain-related interference. In the past, the most commonly used multidimensional questionnaire for assessing childhood chronic pain is the Varni/Thompson Pediatric Pain Questionnaire (PPQ)[61] which provides separate forms for children, parents, and clinicians. The measure was modelled after the most widely used adult pain instrument, the McGill Pain Questionnaire (MPQ)[62] and assesses pain intensity, location, and the sensory, evaluative and affective qualities of the pain experience. The measure has been validated primarily for use with children with arthritis[63] and sickle cell disease,[64] although it is frequently used with children experiencing a variety of painful conditions.

More recently, a comprehensive measure of the impact of adolescent chronic pain has been developed by Eccleston and colleagues.[65] The Bath Adolescent Pain Questionnaire (BAPQ) is a 61-item measure used to assess functioning in seven domains: social functioning, physical functioning, depression, general anxiety, pain specific anxiety, family functioning, and development. Although the items on this measure are similar to those included on separate, individual measures of these various areas, this measure has the advantage of being integrated and validated on samples of adolescents with chronic pain. The BAPQ shows promise as a tool that could be useful in research, as well as in clinical practice. Greater consistency in the applications of measures to chronic pain assessment would represent a significant advance for the field.

ASSESSMENT OF PAIN IN CHILDREN WITH DEVELOPMENTAL DISABILITIES

An area that has received considerable attention and shown rapid growth in the last ten years is the assessment of pain in children with developmental disabilities.[66] For many years, it was believed that individuals with developmental disabilities were incapable of experiencing and/or expressing pain. It is now generally accepted that this belief was false and unfounded and, in fact, these children may be particularly vulnerable to both acute and chronic forms of pain as they frequently have comorbid painful medical conditions and are more likely to require surgeries and other painful medical procedures than children without disabilities.[67]

In terms of pain assessment, measures validated for use with children without disabilities have sometimes been helpful (e.g. FLACC), but fortunately several measures have been developed and validated specifically for use in assessing pain in children with developmental disabilities.[68] The most commonly used and cited measure is the Non-Communicating Children's Pain Checklist (NCCPC).[69] Two current versions of the NCCPC are available; one to assess general pain (NCCPC-R; see **Table 38.8**)[70] and another to assess postoperative pain.[71] The measure assesses the presence of a series of behavioral indicators of pain (e.g. moaning, changes in sleep, facial expression). Two similar measures are also available: the Échelle Douleur Enfant San Salvadour (DESS)[72] and the Pediatric Pain Profile (PPP),[73] although these measures are not as strongly supported in the literature as the NCCPC. The availability of these validated measurement tools for children with developmental disabilities has drawn attention to the importance of pain in this population whose suffering was often previously ignored. Unfortunately, the majority of work that has been conducted to validate these measures has included samples of children with many different forms of disability. However, a child with autism may express pain in a very different way than a child with Down syndrome. Additional focus on variation in pain expression and pain assessment as a function of the nature of the disability present should help to further improve pain assessment for these children.

ASSESSMENT OF PAIN IN NEONATES AND INFANTS

In the 25 years since the recognition that neonates and infants feel pain, there has been tremendous growth in the area of pain assessment among this population. For obvious reasons, pain assessment in this age group is one of the more challenging tasks faced by health professionals working with children. In the past, the challenge was that there were no reliable or valid pain measures that could be used with neonates and infants. Now the clinician has the opposite dilemma; a systematic review conducted by Duhn and Medves[74] revealed that there are now over

Table 38.8 The Non-Communicating Children Pain Checklist-Revised items.

Subscale	Item
Vocal subscale	Moaning, whining, whimpering (fairly soft)
	Crying (moderately loud)
	Screaming/yelling (very loud)
	A specific sound or word for pain (for example, a word, cry, or type of laugh)
Eating/sleeping subscale	Eating less, not interested in food
	Increase in sleep
	Decrease in sleep
Social subscale	Not co-operating, cranky, irritable, unhappy
	Less interaction with others, withdrawn
	Seeking comfort or physical closeness
	Being difficult to distract, not able to satisfy or pacify
Facial subscale	A furrowed brow
	A change in eyes, including squinching of eyes, eyes opened wide; eyes frowning
	Turning down of mouth, not smiling
	Lips puckering up, tight, pouting, or quivering
	Clenching or grinding teeth, chewing or thrusting tongue out
Activity subscale	Not moving, less active, quiet
	Jumping around, agitated, fidgety
Body/limb subscale	Floppy
	Stiff, spastic, tense, rigid
	Gesturing to or touching part of the body that hurt
	Protecting, favoring, or guarding part of the body that hurts
	Flinching or moving the body part away, being sensitive to touch
	Moving the body in specific way to show pain (e.g. head back, arms down, curls up, etc.)
Physiological signs subscale	Shivering
	Change in color, pallor
	Sweating, perspiring
	Tears
	Sharp intake of breath, gasping
	Breath holding

Each item is scored as how often it was observed (not at all, just a little, fairly often, very often) during a two-hour period. The Eating/sleeping subscale is scored for the entire day (not just a two-hour period).
Reprinted with permission from Breau LM, McGrath PJ, Camfield CS, Finley GA. Psychometric properties of the non-communicating children's pain checklist–revised. *Pain.* 2002; **99**: 349–57.

three dozen measures available for assessing pain in infants, all with varying degrees of psychometric support. Sadly, despite this proliferation of measures, there is still no consensus on what the best measure is for assessing pain in this age group.[75]

There are two main approaches to assessing pain in neonates and infants, including unidimensional and multidimensional measures.[75] Unidimensional measures are those that include either only one indicator (e.g. cry) or several similar indicators (e.g. different facial actions). Probably the most commonly used and well-recognized unidimensional measure of pain is the Neonatal Facial Coding System (NFCS).[51] The NFCS codes nine different facial movements (e.g. brow bulge, taut tongue) to yield an overall facial activity score which has been found to be reflective of pain. Multidimensional measures of pain provide an assessment based on more than one indicator or domain; for example, including different behavioral items (e.g. facial action, cry) or coming up with a composite assessment based on multiple domains (e.g. a combination of behavioral and physiological parameters). One of the most widely used multidimensional measures of neonatal pain is the Premature Infant Pain Profile (PIPP).[76] The PIPP provides a composite score based on three behavioral (facial actions: brown bulge, eye squeeze, and nasolabial furrow), two physiologic (heart rate and oxygen saturation), and two contextual (gestational age and behavioral state) factors.

As with pain assessment in older children, the specific measure selected for use depends on a variety of factors, including the type of pain to be assessed, the age and characteristics of the infant (e.g. preterm versus term), and the setting in which the pain is to be assessed. An excellent review of pain assessment and management in infants and neonates is available in the new volume by Anand *et al.*[77]

THE ROLE OF THE PARENT IN PAIN ASSESSMENT

This chapter has focused primarily on providing an overview of pain measures that rely on direct input from or observation of the child. It is important to note that parents play a critical role in pain assessment. Parents are the experts on their child and some pain measurement tools (e.g. PPPM, NCCPC) explicitly acknowledge the parent as an important resource about departures from normal behavior that may signify pain. Whenever possible, parents should be asked to provide ratings of their children's pain (which can often be done using the same measure the child is using to facilitate comparisons). It is interesting to note, however, that parents (as well as health professionals) often underestimate children's pain when adult ratings are directly compared to children's ratings using the same measures.[78] It is unclear what might explain the tendency for parents and other adults to underestimate children's pain, but it is important for clinicians to take into account the likelihood that parental pain ratings may represent an underestimation of the child's actual pain experience.

CULTURAL AND ETHNIC CONSIDERATIONS

The majority of the measures included within this chapter were developed and validated primarily with English-speaking populations. Caution must be used when assessing children whose first language is something other than English. Concepts developed for a measure within one culture may not readily translate into another language.[79] The simple translation of materials is often not accurate and should not be used without proper validation. Therefore, if available, pain assessment measures should only be used if validated in the translated form. The Oucher is one example of a pain measure that has been validated in both African-American and Hispanic children.[33] The FPS-R has been translated into over 32 different languages, with validation studies in several languages currently under way.[80] Cultural notions of pain and pain expression are also an important aspect of the pain experience and should not be overlooked in pain assessment.

CONCLUSIONS

This chapter provides a summary of pain assessment measures available for use with children and draws attention to a number of important clinical issues that relate to pain assessment. There are a variety of self-report and behavioral measures for assessment of acute pain in children that are well supported in the research literature. Physiological measures of pain have not demonstrated sufficient specificity to pain to be recommended for clinical use. Measures are also available for assessment of pediatric chronic pain in children and for children with developmental disabilities. The clinician working with children in pain is urged to consider the important role of the parent in pain assessment, as well as the influence of cultural and ethnic factors of pain experience and measurement. Unfortunately, despite the myriad of pain assessment tools available for use with children, including special populations of children such as those with developmental disabilities or the very young, pain remains a variable that often goes underrecognized and undertreated. Pain is generally given a low priority in hospitals and the lack of education about pain among health professionals may contribute to needless pain and suffering in children that would otherwise be assessed and subsequently managed more appropriately. While children in pain would certainly benefit from the development of new and improved pain measures, it is critical for research attention to now be directed towards exploring creative and interactive methods for increasing the likelihood that existing measures are actually adopted for routine use in clinical care.[81, 82]

Pain assessment should be assessed at regular intervals, like vital signs, and recorded in patients' clinical charts. Selecting pain measures for use with children that are evidence-based and strongly supported in the research literature will help lead to improved care and decrease suffering.

ACKNOWLEDGMENTS

NF Bandstra is supported by a doctoral award from the Nova Scotia Health Research Foundation (NSHRF) and an honorary Killam Predoctoral Scholarship. She is a trainee member of Pain in Child Health (PICH), a Strategic Training Initiative in Health Research of the Canadian Institutes for Health Research (CIHR). CT Chambers is supported by a Canada Research Chair. The authors are grateful to Marie-Claude Grégoire and Kelly Hayton for their assistance with the preparation of this chapter.

REFERENCES

1. Mather L, Mackie J. The incidence of postoperative pain in children. *Pain*. 1983; **15**: 271–82.
2. Craig KD, Lilley CM, Gilbert CA. Social barriers to optimal pain management in infants and children. *Clinical Journal of Pain*. 1996; **12**: 232–42.
3. Scott-Findlay S, Estabrooks CA. Knowledge translation and pain management. In: Finley GA, McGrath PJ, Chambers CT (eds). *Bringing pain relief to children: treatment approaches*. Totowa, NJ: Humana Press, 2006: 199–228.

4. Finley GA, McGrath PJ (eds). *Measurement of pain in infants and children*. Seattle, WA: IASP Press, 1998.

5. Merskey H, Bogduk N (eds). *Classification of chronic pain: descriptions of chronic pain syndromes and definitions of pain terms*, 2nd edn. Seattle, WA: IASP Press, 1994.

6. Champion GD, Goodenough B, von Baeyer CL, Thomas W. Measurement of pain by self-report. In: Finley GA, McGrath PJ (eds). *Measurement of pain in infants and children*. Seattle, WA: IASP Press, 1998: 123–60.

7. McGrath PJ. There is more to pain measurement in children than "ouch". *Canadian Psychology*. 1996; **37**: 63–75.

8. Shields BJ, Palermo TM, Powers JD *et al*. Predictors of a child's ability to use a visual analogue scale. *Child: Care, Health and Development*. 2003; **29**: 281–90.

9. Shields BJ, Cohen DM, Harbeck-Weber C *et al*. Pediatric pain measurement using a visual analogue scale: a comparison of two teaching methods. *Clinical Pediatrics*. 2003; **42**: 227–34.

10. Stanford EA, Chambers CT, Craig KD. The role of developmental factors in predicting young children's use of a self-report scale for pain. *Pain*. 2006; **120**: 16–23.

* 11. Stinson JN, Kavanagh T, Yamada J *et al*. Systematic review of the psychometric properties, interpretability and feasibility of self-report pain intensity measures for use in clinical trials in children and adolescents. *Pain*. 2006; **125**: 143–57.

* 12. Bieri D, Reeve RA, Champion GD *et al*. The Faces Pain Scale for the self-assessment of the severity of pain experienced by children: development, initial validation, and preliminary investigation for ratio scale properties. *Pain*. 1990; **41**: 139–50.

* 13. Hicks CL, von Baeyer CL, Spafford PA *et al*. The Faces Pain Scale-Revised: toward a common metric in pediatric pain measurement. *Pain*. 2001; **93**: 173–83.

* 14. Wong DL, Baker CM. Pain in children: comparison of assessment scales. *Pediatric Nursing*. 1988; **14**: 9–17.

* 15. Beyer JE, Denyes MJ, Villaruel AM. The creation, validation, and continuing development of the Oucher: a measure of pain intensity in children. *Journal of Pediatric Nursing*. 1992; **7**: 335–46.

* 16. Hester NK. The preoperational child's reaction to immunization. *Nursing Research*. 1979; **28**: 250–5.

17. Gauthier JC, Finley GA, McGrath PJ. Children's self-report of postoperative pain intensity and treatment threshold: determining the adequacy of medication. *Clinical Journal of Pain*. 1998; **14**: 116–20.

18. Migdal M, Chudzynska-Pomianowska E, Vause E *et al*. Rapid, needle-free delivery of lidocaine for reducing the pain of venipuncture among pediatric subjects. *Pediatrics*. 2005; **115**: e393–8.

19. Taddio A, Soin HK, Schuh S *et al*. Liposomal lidocaine to improve procedural success rates and reduce procedural pain among children: a randomized controlled trial. *Canadian Medical Association Journal*. 2005; **172**: 1691–5.

20. Bulloch B, Tenenbein M. Validation of 2 pain scales for use in the pediatric emergency department. *Pediatrics*. 2002; **110**: e33.

21. Gharaibeh M, Abu-Saad H. Cultural validation of pediatric pain assessment tools: Jordanian perspective. *Journal of Transcultural Nursing*. 2002; **13**: 12–18.

22. Keck JF, Gerkensmeyer JE, Joyce BA, Schade JG. Reliability and validity of the Faces and Word Descriptor Scales to measure procedural pain. *Journal of Pediatric Nursing*. 1996; **11**: 368–74.

23. Kendall JM, Reeves BC, Latter VS. Nasal Diamorphine Trial Group. Multicentre randomised controlled trial of nasal diamorphine for analgesia in children and teenagers with clinical fractures. *British Medical Journal*. 2001; **322**: 261–5.

24. Robert R, Brack A, Blakeney P *et al*. A double-blind study of the analgesic efficacy of oral transmucosal fentanyl citrate and oral morphine in pediatric patients undergoing burn dressing change and tubbing. *Journal of Burn Care and Rehabilitation*. 2003; **24**: 351–5.

25. Stein PR. Indices of pain intensity: construct validity among preschoolers. *Pediatric Nursing*. 1995; **21**: 119–23.

26. Robertson J. Pediatric pain assessment: validation of a multidimensional tool. *Pediatric Nursing*. 1993; **19**: 209–13.

27. Chambers CT, Hardial J, Craig KD *et al*. Faces scales for the measurement of postoperative pain intensity in children following minor surgery. *Clinical Journal of Pain*. 2005; **21**: 277–85.

28. West N, Oakes L, Hinds PS *et al*. Measuring pain in pediatric oncology ICU patients. *Journal of Pediatric Oncology Nursing*. 1994; **11**: 64–8.

29. Chambers CT, Craig KD. An intrusive impact of anchors in children's faces pain scales. *Pain*. 1998; **78**: 27–37.

30. Chambers CT, Giesbrecht K, Craig KD *et al*. A comparison of faces scales for the measurement of pediatric pain: children's and parents' ratings. *Pain*. 1999; **83**: 25–35.

31. Aradine CR, Beyer JE, Tompkins JM. Children's pain perception before and after analgesia: a study of instrument construct validity and related issues. *Journal of Pediatric Nursing*. 1988; **3**: 11–23.

32. Beyer J, Aradine C. Patterns of pediatric pain intensity: a methodological investigation of a self-report scale. *Clinical Journal of Pain*. 1987; **3**: 130–41.

33. Beyer JE, Knott CB. Construct validity estimation for the African-American and Hispanic versions of the Oucher Scale. *Journal of Pediatric Nursing*. 1998; **13**: 20–31.

34. Ramritu P. Use of Oucher Numeric and Word Graphic Scale in children aged 9–14 years with post operative pain. *Journal of Clinical Nursing*. 2000; **9**: 763–72.

35. Beyer J, Aradine C. The convergent and discriminant validity of a self-report measure of pain intensity for children. *Children's Health Care*. 1988; **16**: 274–82.

36. Villarruel AM, Denyes MJ. Pain assessment in children: theoretical and empirical validity. *Advances in Nursing Science*. 1991; **14**: 32–41.

37. Gallagher EJ, Liebman M, Bijur PE. Prospective validation of clinically important changes in pain severity measured on a visual analog scale. *Annals of Emergency Medicine.* 2001; **38**: 633–8.

38. Powell CV, Kelly AM, Williams A. Determining the minimum clinically significant difference in visual analog pain score for children. *Annals of Emergency Medicine.* 2001; **37**: 28–31.

39. Tyler DC, Tu A, Douthit J, Chapman CR. Toward validation of pain measurement tools for children: a pilot study. *Pain.* 1993; **52**: 301–09.

40. Abu-Saad H, Holzemer WL. Measuring children's self-assessment of pain. *Issues in Comprehensive Pediatric Nursing.* 1981; **5**: 337–49.

41. Beales JG, Keen JH, Holt PJ. The child's perception of the disease and the experience of pain in juvenile chronic arthritis. *Journal of Rheumatology.* 1983; **10**: 61–5.

42. Goodenough B, Addicoat L, Champion GD *et al.* Pain in 4- to 6-year-old children receiving intramuscular injections: a comparison of the Faces Pain Scale with other self-report and behavioral measures. *Clinical Journal of Pain.* 1997; **13**: 60–73.

43. Chambers CT, Johnston C. Developmental differences in children's use of rating scales. *Journal of Pediatric Psychology.* 2002; **27**: 27–36.

∗ 44. von Baeyer CL, Spagrud LJ. Systematic review of observational (behavioral) measures of pain for children and adolescents aged 3 to 18 years. *Pain.* 2007; **127**: 140–50.

∗ 45. Merkel SI, Voepel-Lewis T, Shayevitz JR, Malviya S. The FLACC: a behavioral scale for scoring postoperative pain in young children. *Pediatric Nursing.* 1997; **23**: 293–7.

∗ 46. McGrath PJ, Johnson G, Goodman JT *et al.* CHEOPS: A behavioral scale for rating postoperative pain in children. In: Fields HL, Dubner R, Cervero F (eds). *Advances in pain research and therapy.* New York: Raven Press, 1985: 395–402.

∗ 47. Chambers CT, Reid GJ, McGrath PJ, Finley GA. Development and preliminary validation of a postoperative pain measure for parents. *Pain.* 1996; **68**: 307–13.

∗ 48. Ambuel B, Hamlett KW, Marx CM, Blumer JL. Assessing distress in pediatric intensive care environments: the COMFORT scale. *Journal of Pediatric Psychology.* 1992; **17**: 95–109.

∗ 49. LeBaron S, Zeltzer L. Assessment of acute pain and anxiety in children and adolescents by self-reports, observer reports, and a behavior checklist. *Journal of Consulting and Clinical Psychology.* 1984; **52**: 729–38.

∗ 50. Katz ER, Kellerman J, Siegel SE. Behavioral distress in children with cancer undergoing medical procedures: developmental considerations. *Journal of Consulting and Clinical Psychology.* 1980; **48**: 356–65.

51. Grunau RV, Craig KD. Pain expression in neonates: facial action and cry. *Pain.* 1987; **28**: 395–410.

52. Chambers CT, Cassidy KL, McGrath PJ *et al. Child Facial Coding System revised manual.* Halifax, NS: Dalhousie University, 1996.

53. Beyer JE, McGrath PJ, Berde CB. Discordance between self-report and behavioral pain measures in children aged 3–7 years after surgery. *Journal of Pain and Symptom Management.* 1990; **5**: 350–6.

54. Stuber ML, Kazak AE, Meeske K, Barakat L. Is posttraumatic stress a viable model for understanding responses to childhood cancer? *Child and Adolescent Psychiatric Clinics of North America.* 1998; **7**: 169–82.

55. American Psychiatric Association. *Diagnostic and statistical manual of mental disorders,* 4th edn. Washington, DC: American Psychiatric Association Press, 1994.

56. Sweet SD, McGrath PJ. Physiological measures of pain. In: Finley GA, McGrath PJ (eds). *Measurement of pain in infants and children.* Seattle: IASP Press, 1998: 59–81.

57. Claar RL, Walker LS. Functional assessment of pediatric pain patients: psychometric properties of the Functional Disability Inventory. *Pain.* 2006; **121**: 77–84.

58. Reid GJ, Gilbert CA, McGrath PJ. The Pain Coping Questionnaire: preliminary validation. *Pain.* 1998; **76**: 83–96.

59. Crombez G, Bijttebier P, Eccleston C *et al.* The child version of the Pain Catastrophizing Scale (PCS-C): a preliminary validation. *Pain.* 2003; **104**: 639–46.

60. Eccleston C, Jordan AL, Crombez G. The impact of chronic pain on adolescents: a review of previously used measures. *Journal of Pediatric Psychology.* 2006; **31**: 684–97.

∗ 61. Varni JW, Thompson KL, Hanson V. The Varni/Thompson Pediatric Pain Questionnaire. I. Chronic musculoskeletal pain in juvenile rheumatoid arthritis. *Pain.* 1987; **28**: 27–38.

∗ 62. Melzack R. The McGill Pain Questionnaire: major properties and scoring methods. *Pain.* 1975; **1**: 277–99.

63. Thompson KL, Varni JW, Hanson V. Comprehensive assessment of pain in juvenile rheumatoid arthritis: an empirical model. *Journal of Pediatric Psychology.* 1987; **12**: 241–55.

64. Walco GA, Dampier CD. Pain in children and adolescents with sickle cell disease: a descriptive study. *Journal of Pediatric Psychology.* 1990; **15**: 643–58.

65. Eccleston C, Jordan A, McCracken LM *et al.* The Bath Adolescent Pain Questionnaire (BAPQ): development and preliminary psychometric evaluation of an instrument to assess the impact of chronic pain on adolescents. *Pain.* 2005; **118**: 263–70.

66. Oberlander TF, Symons FJ (eds), *Pain in children and adults with developmental disabilities.* Baltimore: Paul H Brookes, 2006.

67. Bottos S, Chambers CT. The epidemiology of pain in developmental disabilities. In: Oberlander TF, Symons FJ (eds). *Pain in children and adults with developmental disabilities.* Baltimore: Paul H Brookes, 2006: 67–87.

68. Breau LM, McGrath PJ, Zabalia M. Assessing pediatric pain and developmental disabilities. In: Oberlander TF, Symons FJ (eds). *Pain in children and adults with developmental disabilities.* Baltimore: Paul H Brookes, 2006: 149–72.

∗ 69. Breau LM, Camfield C, McGrath PJ *et al*. Measuring pain accurately in children with cognitive impairments: refinement of a caregiver scale. *Journal of Pediatrics.* 2001; **138**: 721–7.

∗ 70. Breau LM, McGrath PJ, Camfield CS, Finley GA. Psychometric properties of the Non-Communicating Children's Pain Checklist-Revised. *Pain.* 2002; **99**: 349–57.

∗ 71. Breau LM, Finley GA, McGrath PJ, Camfield CS. Validation of the Non-Communicating Children's Pain Checklist-Postoperative version. *Anesthesiology.* 2002; **96**: 528–35.

∗ 72. Collignon P, Giusiano B. Validation of a pain evaluation scale for patients with severe cerebral palsy. *European Journal of Pain.* 2001; **5**: 433–42.

∗ 73. Hunt A, Goldman A, Seers K *et al*. Clinical validation of the Paediatric Pain Profile. *Developmental Medicine and Child Neurology.* 2004; **46**: 9–18.

74. Duhn LJ, Medves JM. A systematic integrative review of infant pain assessment tools: beyond the basics. *Advances in Neonatal Care.* 2004; **4**: 126–40.

75. Stevens BJ, Pillai Riddell RR, Oberlander TE, Gibbins S. Assessment of pain in neonates and infants. In: Anand KJS, Stevens BJ, McGrath PJ (eds). *Pain in neonates and infants*, 3rd edn. Edinburgh: Elsevier, 2007: 67–90.

76. Stevens B, Johnston C, Petryshen P, Taddio A. Premature Infant Pain Profile: development and initial validation. *Clinical Journal of Pain.* 1996; **12**: 13–22.

77. Anand KJS, Stevens BJ, McGrath PJ (eds). *Pain in neonates and infants*, 3rd edn. Philadelphia: Elsevier, 2007.

78. Chambers CT, Reid GJ, Craig KD *et al*. Agreement between child and parent reports of pain. *Clinical Journal of Pain.* 1998; **14**: 336–42.

79. Chang AM, Chau JP, Holroyd E. Translation of questionnaires and issues of equivalence. *Journal of Advanced Nursing.* 1999; **29**: 316–22.

80. von Baeyer CL. The Faces Pain Scale-Revised. Pediatric pain sourcebook of protocols, policies, and pamphlets. Last updated August 2007, cited February 2008. Available from: http://painsourcebook.ca/docs/pps92.html

81. Franck LS, Allen A, Oulton K. Making pain assessment more accessible to children and parents: can greater involvement improve the quality of care? *Clinical Journal of Pain.* 2007; **23**: 331–8.

82. Simons J, MacDonald LM. Changing practice: implementing validated paediatric pain assessment tools. *Journal of Child Health Care.* 2006; **10**: 160–76.

39

Procedures for pediatric pain management

RICHARD F HOWARD

KEY LEARNING POINTS

- Analgesic pharmacology during infancy and childhood is increasingly well understood, and consequently effective and safe analgesic protocols can be developed for the management of acute pain in children of all ages.
- Pain should be assessed using a valid, developmentally appropriate method and assessments should be repeated

at frequent intervals in order to evaluate the effectiveness of analgesia.

- Guidelines are available relating to many aspects of pain management in children, including acute postoperative and procedural pain in children. They should be consulted and implemented.

GENERAL CONSIDERATIONS

In recent years, there have been many advances in the range and complexity of techniques available for pain management in infants and children.[1, 2] Considerable experience has been gained in the safe and effective use of potent analgesia at all ages, even in the youngest infant. Children's pain management has been revolutionized in the last few years by a better understanding of the factors that contribute to safe and effective pain control. The use of developmentally appropriate pain assessment (see Chapter 38, Pain assessment in children), an appreciation of the need for suitable physiological monitoring with close supervision by trained pediatric staff, the benefits of pediatric pain management teams (see Chapter 50, Organization of pediatric pain services) and the widespread use of pain management protocols are all important considerations.

Multimodal analgesia, i.e. the use of a number of complementary pharmacological and nonpharmacological

approaches in conjunction with each other, underpins the management of pain in children. The value of effective pain assessment cannot be overstated, but assessments must be repeated at frequent intervals, and indications of pain lead to appropriate remedial action which should be outlined in a clear and effective management plan (**Table 39.1**).

This chapter outlines the practical details of pharmacological pain management, including protocols for techniques, such as patient-controlled analgesia (PCA) and nurse-controlled analgesia (NCA), and technical descriptions of physical interventions, such as epidural analgesia and other local anesthetic techniques. Psychological pain management strategies have an increasingly important place, particularly in the management of painful procedures. These are discussed in Chapter 40, Mind/body skills for children in pain, and Chapter 16, Psychological interventions for acute pediatric pain in the *Acute Pain* volume of this series.

Professionals involved in the routine medical care of children are expected to have an understanding of the

Table 39.1 Pain score–pain management action plan.

Pain score			
P 0	No pain[a]	Reassess frequently	
P 1–3	Mild pain[a]	Review analgesia	
		NCA	Give bolus ten minutes before activity
		PCA	Encourage bolus ten minutes before activity
		Epidural	Assess level
P 4–7	Moderate pain[a]	Give analgesia	
		NCA	Give bolus
		PCA	Encourage bolus
		Epidural	Assess level, increase rate
P 8–10	Severe pain[a]	Give analgesia – review regimen	
		NCA	Give bolus, assess, and repeat
		PCA	Review usage; consider background infusion
		Epidural	Assess level, increase rate

[a] Ensure supplementary analgesia is given (paracetamol+an NSAID if appropriate).
NCA, nurse-controlled analgesia; NSAID, nonsteroidal anti-inflammatory drugs; PCA, patient-controlled analgesia.

principles of contemporary pain management and to be aware of current good practice. Although when compared with adults there is less high quality research evidence in children to guide practice, a number of examples of evidence-based guidelines on aspects of pediatric pain management are now available, they should be consulted and their recommendations implemented when designing analgesic protocols.[3, 4, 5]

Routes of administration for analgesics

The route of administration of analgesia is an important consideration in children and one that can profoundly influence its effectiveness. The palatability of oral formulations and the acceptability of any other route must be taken into account to ensure compliance when planning regimens. For example, the use of intramuscular analgesics has been cited as a major cause of undermedication in children. Many of them would rather endure even quite severe pain than be subjected to a distressing and in itself painful intramuscular analgesic injection. Nurses are also reluctant to administer such unpleasant treatments to unwilling children and therefore analgesia is unlikely to be given.[6]

Whenever possible, protocols and prescriptions for analgesia to be administered on demand should allow for several choices of route for maximum flexibility, e.g. paracetamol (acetaminophen) can be given orally, rectally, or intravenously.

ORAL

When it is available, the oral route is always preferred over other methods. Children will usually accept oral analgesia,

but they may have strong preferences regarding the consistency or flavor of medication. In general, liquids are preferred over tablets or capsules, and in addition they are often mixed with small amounts of a favorite drink. Liquid formulations also have the advantage that they are homogeneous and can be more easily and accurately diluted and divided into smaller doses for young patients.

RECTAL

Rectal administration of analgesics has become very popular, especially for paracetamol and the nonsteroidal anti-inflammatory drugs (NSAIDs). Easy administration and slow absorption kinetics are convenient and allow plasma levels to be maintained with relatively infrequent dosing. Drawbacks are that rectal absorption can be erratic and unpredictable for some drugs, leading to uncertainty about the correct dose and redosing interval, and that some children or their families perceive it to be unpleasant or unacceptable.[7] The rectal pharmacokinetics of paracetamol have been particularly well investigated in infants and children. Higher initial doses are required to reliably achieve adequate plasma levels, and the maintenance dose and dosing interval depend on clearance of the drug, which is age-dependent.[8, 9]

SUBLINGUAL, BUCCAL, AND INTRANASAL

Although these routes are not frequently used in children, they are popular for some analgesics, notably the opioids. Rapid absorption, lack of hepatic "first-pass effect" leading to relative increases in efficacy and potency and improvements in compliance are possible advantages. Intranasal diamorphine, fentanyl, and sufentanil have been used for procedural pain, sublingual and buccal oxycodone for postoperative pain, and buccal or "oral transmucosal" fentanyl for premedication or procedural pain.[10, 11, 12, 13]

INTRAVENOUS, SUBCUTANEOUS, AND INTRAMUSCULAR

Potent analgesia is frequently given by the intravenous route due to its convenience, rapid onset, and predictable bioavailability. Subcutaneous administration is also useful, particularly when venous access is limited. The intramuscular route for analgesia should generally be avoided in children, but it may have a limited place in the anesthetized or heavily sedated child as a predictable and convenient short-term solution.

NEURAXIAL

Local anesthetics, opioids, ketamine, and clonidine are frequently given neuraxially, particularly by the epidural route. Advantages are that relatively widespread analgesia is possible with low doses and few systemic side effects. Many analgesics have synergistic effects when given neuraxially. Catheters can be placed in the epidural space so that analgesic solutions can be infused for several days if necessary.

INHALATIONAL

Nitrous oxide has analgesic properties and can be inhaled at concentrations of 50–70 percent for pain relief during medical procedures, such as dressing changes, bone marrow aspiration, removal of sutures, or lumbar puncture. The use of nitrous oxide is discussed in Chapter 27, Acute pain management in children in the *Acute Pain* volume of this series.

SYSTEMIC ANALGESIA FOR MILD TO MODERATE PAIN

Mild and moderate acute and long-term pain is usually satisfactorily managed with oral analgesia. Paracetamol and the NSAIDs are the mainstay of postoperative pain management following minor procedures, after sprains and minor acute injuries, and for many types of long-term pain, including chronic headache, some musculoskeletal pain, and joint pain. They are frequently used concurrently as part of a multimodal analgesic technique, and for moderate pain not controlled by this combination, the addition of a low potency opioid such as codeine or tramadol is usually beneficial. **Table 39.1** lists analgesics and doses commonly used for mild/moderate pain in

pediatric practice, the pharmacology of these analgesics is discussed in Chapter 3, Clinical pharmacology: opioids; Chapter 4, Clinical pharmacology: traditional NSAIDs and selective COX-2 inhibitors; Chapter 5, Clinical pharmacology: paracetamol and compound analgesics; and Chapter 27, Acute pain management in children in the *Acute Pain* volume of this series.

Paracetamol

This is a low potency analgesic when used alone, but is much more effective in combination with NSAIDs and/or opioids. Paracetamol is the first-line mild analgesic in children, it is also used as an antipyretic. As with most analgesics, the pharmacokinetics of paracetamol are developmentally regulated, the principal adverse effect is hepatotoxicity in overdose. Single doses less than 150 mg/kg are not generally associated with toxicity, the use of maximum doses for more than five days is not generally recommended without close medical supervision.[14][III] The dose of paracetamol depends on both age and route of administration (**Table 39.2**).

Nonsteroidal anti-inflammatory drugs

Although there may be some interindividual differences in the response to NSAIDs, and their potential to cause adverse effects, these drugs are largely used interchangeably for acute pain indications. The choice of NSAID depends on availability and convenience; some drugs are easily obtainable in child-friendly formulations and presentations. NSAIDs are not currently used for analgesia in the neonatal period, they are used under direct medical supervision in infants of one to three months of age. After six months of age, they appear to have a similar side-effect profile to that in older children and adults. Ibuprofen is the most investigated and therefore first-choice NSAID in the very young, where its safety profile is comparable to that of paracetamol.[15][II] Caution is advised when using this group of drugs in the presence of asthma, renal impairment, bleeding tendency, and peptic ulceration, although risks appear to be small for short-term use, especially for ibuprofen.[16][II] Cross-sensitivity with aspirin-induced asthma can occur, but NSAIDs do not appear to affect respiratory function in other ashmatics.[17] Their use after surgery where there is a high risk of postoperative bleeding, e.g. tonsillectomy, is controversial and is discussed in Chapter 27, Acute pain management in children in the *Acute Pain* volume of this series.

Codeine

Codeine is a low potency opioid, the efficacy of which depends on its metabolism to morphine by the

Table 39.2 Analgesics for mild to moderate pain in infants and children.

Drug	Class of analgesic	Route of administration	Doses
Paracetamol	Antipyretic-analgesic	Oral/rectal[a]	15–20 mg/kg qid
			90 mg/kg/day maximum
			60 mg/kg/day term neonate
			30–45 mg/kg/day preterm
		Intravenous[b]	10–15 mg/kg qid
			40 mg/kg/day term neonate
			60 mg/kg/day, <50 kg body weight
			4 g daily, >50 kg body weight
		Intravenous[b]	Propacetamol 180 mg/kg/day
Ibuprofen	NSAID	Oral	20 mg/kg/day, <6 months
			30 mg/kg/day >6 months (maximum 2.4 g/day)
Diclofenac	NSAID	Oral	1 mg/kg tid (3 mg/kg/day)
		Rectal	1 mg/kg tid (3 mg/kg/day)
Ketorolac	NSAID	Oral	0.5–1 mg/kg qid (max 10 mg/dose)
		Intravenous	0.5 mg/kg qid (maximum 10 mg/dose)
Codeine	Opioid	Oral	1 mg/kg qid
		Rectal	1 mg/kg qid
		Intravenous	Not recommended
Tramadol	Opioid/monoaminergic	Oral	1–2 mg/kg qid
		Intravenous	1 mg/kg qid

NSAID, nonsteroidal anti-inflammatory drugs; qid, four times a day; tid, three times a day.
[a]See also **Table 27.5**, Chapter 27, Acute pain management in children in the *Acute Pain* volume of this series.
[b]See also **Table 27.6**, Chapter 27, Acute pain management in children in the *Acute Pain* volume of this series.

cytochrome P450 enzyme CYP2D6. The activity of the enzyme is genetically and developmentally regulated, which complicates its use in that it is not possible to predict whether individual patients will benefit from the drug.[18] Nevertheless, there is evidence that variability in the response to codeine is less when it is combined with other analgesics, such as paracetamol.[19][I] Codeine has an excellent safety record in children and can be used if reliable methods of pain assessment are also employed.

Tramadol

Tramadol is a moderate potency analgesic, usually classified as an opioid, but with both opioid and nonopioid modes of action.[20] It has become popular in pediatric practice, mainly in Europe, because opioid side effects may be less prominent.[21][II], [22][II] The opioid effects of tramadol are mediated through direct but weak μ-agonist activity, and more potent (× 2–300) μ-agonist effects by an active metabolite O-desmethyltramadol. Tramadol also appears to act through serotonergic and noradrenergic mechanisms.[20] As the active metabolite of tramadol is produced by the cytochrome P450 enzyme CYP2D6 (see above under Codeine), unanswered questions arise regarding the effects of genetic polymorphisms and development on the efficacy of tramadol.[23] Nevertheless, tramadol has been used widely in children, including in the neonate. Tramadol pharmacokinetics have been investigated; clearance is reduced in the neonatal period but reaches 44 percent of the mature value by one month and is similar to adults by one year.[24]

ANALGESIA FOR MODERATE TO SEVERE PAIN

Moderate to severe self-limiting pain is usually treated with analgesic combinations that include a potent opioid such as morphine. Multimodal analgesia with paracetamol and NSAIDs may also be supplemented with novel analgesics, such as ketamine or clonidine, that are included especially when pain proves to be difficult to treat or if opioid side effects are troublesome. Localized pain, particularly postoperative pain, can often be managed with single shot or continuous local anesthesia (LA) in combination with systemic analgesics.

Opioids

Opioids have been used extensively for many years in the management of pain in infants and children. Morphine is the most tried and tested and therefore the best understood and commonly prescribed, especially for neonates and young children. Other opioids have also become popular in some countries for specific indications, or because of convenient formulations; for example, the use of oral oxycodone, transcutaneous fentanyl, neuraxial hydromorphone, and intranasal diamorphine have all been described.

Because the interindividual variation in response to opioids is great, they are usually titrated to initial effect, with subsequent doses and dose intervals determined by response and a knowledge of developmental pharmacokinetics. The initial doses for different routes of administration of the most frequently prescribed opioids for children are given in **Table 39.3**. The principal initial side effects include sedation, respiratory depression, nausea and vomiting, and itching. These effects should be monitored and treated accordingly, see below under Side effects of opioid analgesia and **Table 39.4**. In longer-term use, constipation, tolerance, and physical dependence are also a feature of opioid therapy, especially if infused over more than four or five days, and therefore opioids should not be rapidly withdrawn if they have been used for more than a few days at high doses. For acute pain indications, most of these unwanted effects can easily be managed, but they are more problematic when opioids are used for weeks or months. The use of opioids in the treatment of cancer pain in children is discussed in Chapter 25, Pediatric cancer pain in the *Cancer Pain* volume of this series.

MORPHINE

Morphine is by far the most extensively investigated opioid in children and it can be used safely, provided developmentally appropriate dosage regimens and suitable monitoring for adverse effects such as respiratory depression are implemented. Morphine is inexpensive

Table 39.4 Suggested monitoring for children receiving parenteral opioids.

Parameter	Method
Analgesia	Validated pain score
Sedation	Sedation scale[a]
Respiration	Respiratory rate, pulse oximetry (in air)
Cardiovascular	Heart rate/blood pressure
Nausea and vomiting	Nausea scale

[a]For example, University of Michigan Sedation Score.[25]

and versatile, it is reliably absorbed orally with a bioavailability of 0.5 compared to parenteral routes, it can be given i.v., i.m., and s.c., and it is effective in the epidural space and intrathecally.

Parenteral morphine is required postoperatively after major surgery and for severe pain when intestinal function is likely to be disturbed. Morphine can be given by intermittent dosing, continuous infusion, or using a demand-led system such as PCA or NCA. Onset of analgesia is rapid after i.v. injection and therefore the initial dosage (**Table 39.3**) can be titrated to effect by repeating the dose at five- to ten-minute intervals until analgesia is achieved.

The developmental pharmacokinetics of morphine have been well investigated, clearance is reduced in the neonate rising to 80 percent of values similar to older children and adults by six months of age.[26, 27] Clinically,

Table 39.3 Initial doses and routes for opioids in children.

Drug	Routes of administration	Initial and maintenance dose
Morphine	Oral	0.1 mg/kg (<1 month)
		0.2 mg/kg (>1 month)
	Intravenous	0.02–0.05 mg/kg (<1 month)
		0.05–0.1 mg/kg (>1 month)
	Subcutaneous	0.05 mg/kg
	Epidural	0.02–0.05 mg/kg
Oxycodone	Oral	0.2 mg/kg
Hydrocodone	Oral	0.2 mg/kg
Methadone	Oral	0.2 mg/kg
	Intravenous	0.1–0.2 mg/kg
Fentanyl	OTFC[a]	See relevant product information
	Transdermal	Available as 12, 25, and 50 µg/hour patches (see relevant product information)
	Intravenous	0.0005 mg/kg
	Epidural	0.001 mg/kg
Hydromorphone	Oral	0.06 mg/kg
	Intravenous	0.005–0.015 mg/kg
	Subcutaneous	0.005–0.015 mg/kg
	Epidural	0.001–0.003 mg/kg

[a]OTFC, oral transmucosal fentanyl citrate.

infusion rates for children greater than one month of age are adjusted within the initial range of 10–30 µg/kg per hour (0.01–0.03 mg/kg per hour). Infusion rates are reduced for neonates (or dose intervals are increased) and titrated according to response within the starting range of 2–12 µg/kg per hour (0.002–0.012 mg/kg per hour). Suggested regimens for intravenous infusion of morphine in neonates and older children are given in **Table 39.5**.

PATIENT-CONTROLLED ANALGESIA

Popular in adult practice (see Chapter 11, Patient-controlled analgesia in the *Acute Pain* volume of this series), PCA has similar advantages and indications in children. It is generally considered suitable for those aged six years and above, provided they are able to understand the concept and physically able to operate the handset, there have been reports of successful use of PCA in children as young as four years of age. In practice, children are likely to need special help in the form of pre-use education, frequent reeducation during use, encouragement, and reminders, if the technique is to work well. It is important to emphasize that the safety of PCA depends on self-administration and therefore only the patient should operate the handset. In children younger than 12 years, a small continuous (background) infusion is often used, a typical PCA regimen is given in **Table 39.6**.

NURSE-CONTROLLED ANALGESIA

The lack of flexibility of a simple morphine infusion can be improved by allowing fixed-volume extra doses of analgesia to be given by nursing staff using a PCA-type programmable infusion pump. Extra doses can be given according to assessed analgesic requirements, before movement, or before painful care such as physiotherapy. Typical nurse-controlled analgesia uses a continuous infusion rate of 10–20 µg/kg per hour (0.01–0.02 mg/kg per hour) and extra doses of the same amount every 15–20 minutes (**Table 39.6**).[28] Advantages of NCA are flexibility to treat rapidly changing analgesic requirements, accuracy, and convenience. NCA is suitable for children who are too young or unable to use PCA, or in situations where frequent painful procedures are carried out. NCA can also be used in the neonatal period, in which case the continuous infusion is reduced or omitted until opioid requirements are established: a recommended regimen is shown in **Table 39.6**.

FENTANYL

Fentanyl is an extremely potent rapidly acting opioid with a terminal half-life of about 30 minutes. An advantage of fentanyl is that it may have less effect on the pulmonary vasculature than morphine and is therefore used in the presence of, or in patients who are at risk of, pulmonary

Table 39.5 Intravenous morphine infusion for neonates and children age >1 month.

	Preparation	Concentration	Initial dose	Infusion rate
Morphine infusion (neonate)	Morphine sulfate 1 mg/ kg in 50 mL solution	20 µg/kg/mL (0.02 mg/kg/mL)	0.5–2.5 mL (0.01–0.05 mg/kg)	0.1–0.6 mL/hour (0.002–0.012 mg/kg/hour)
Morphine infusion (age >1 month)	Morphine sulfate 1 mg/ kg in 50 mL solution	20 µg/kg/mL (0.02 mg/kg/mL)	1.0–5.0 mL (0.02–0.1 mg/kg)	0.5–1.5 mL/hour (0.01–0.03 mg/kg/hour)

Table 39.6 Suggested morphine NCA and PCA protocols for neonates, infants, and children.

	Preparation	Concentration	Initial dose	Programming		
				Background infusion	NCA/PCA dose	Lockout interval (minutes)
NCA for neonatal use	Morphine sulfate 1 mg/kg in 50 mL solution	0.02 mg/kg/mL	0.5–2.5 mL (0.01–0.05 mg/ kg)	0–0.5 mL (0–0.01 mg/kg/ hour)	NCA 0.5–1.0 mL (0.01–0.02 mg/ kg)	20–30
NCA for infants and children >1 month	Morphine sulfate 1 mg/kg in 50 mL solution	0.02 mg/kg/mL	2.5–5.0 mL (0.05–0.1 mg/ kg)	0.5–1.0 mL/hour (0.01–0.02 mg/ kg/hour)	NCA 0.5–1.0 mL (0.01–0.02 mg/ kg)	15–20
PCA	Morphine sulfate 1 mg/kg in 50 mL solution	0.02 mg/kg/mL	2.5–5 mL (0.05–0.1 mg/ kg)	0–0.2 mL/hour (0–0.004 mg/ kg/hour)	PCA 0.5–1.0 mL (0.01–0.02 mg/ kg/hour)	5

NCA, nurse-controlled analgesia; PCA, patient-controlled analgesia.

hypertension. Owing to its high lipid solubility, fentanyl is used in a number of novel analgesic delivery systems, including oral-transmucosal and transdermal, which have been used for procedural pain and cancer pain, respectively. A disposable iontophoretic transdermal fentanyl PCA device has been developed recently which may be suitable for teenagers and older children, but which has not been investigated in this age group.[29]

OXYCODONE AND HYDROCODONE

These are semi-synthetic opioids with moderately high efficacy that are used frequently in proprietary analgesics in combination with paracetamol and NSAIDs. They are better absorbed orally, but may have little other advantage in comparison with morphine. Oral oxycodone and controlled-release oral oxycodone are popular in the management of cancer pain.[30]

HYDROMORPHONE AND METHADONE

Hydromorphone is a morphine derivative with a relatively long duration of action. Like morphine, it is considered a hydrophilic opioid but has a greater water solubility allowing a smaller volume/dose. It is also popular for epidural use because it appears to have an advantageous efficacy/side-effect profile in comparison with morphine and the more lipid soluble fentanyl.[31, 32][II]

Methadone is a long-acting opioid with N-methyl-D-aspartate (NMDA) antagonist properties. Although it is often regarded as an "old" opioid because it has been available for many years, there is renewed interest in its use as an analgesic for neuropathic pain and in order to reduce opioid tolerance. Methadone has traditionally been used in the management of opioid withdrawal and in addiction states because of its long duration of action.

SIDE EFFECTS OF OPIOID ANALGESIA

The adverse effects of opioid analgesics are largely predictable and dose related. Naloxone, the opioid antagonist, may selectively reverse side effects when infused in low doses with little obvious effect on analgesia.[33][II] Opioid partial agonists are sometimes used to treat opioid side effects, but they have been little investigated in children.

Nausea and vomiting

Nausea and vomiting due to opioids can sometimes be treated by adjustments to dosing regimens, e.g. reducing the rate of delivery of PCA and NCA bolus doses, more commonly antiemetic drugs are required. The use of antiemetics in children for PONV has been reviewed recently, and consensus guidelines developed.[34][II] Children deemed to be at risk should be given prophylaxis

with either dexamethasone or a 5HT antagonist, such as ondansetron. Treatment can be with either of these first-line antiemetics or, if they are not effective, combination with a second-line drug, such as prochlorperazine or cyclizine, should be used.[34][II]

Respiratory depression

Clinically significant depression of respiration due to therapeutic use of opioids for pain is a rare event, provided recommended doses are used. Certain groups may be more at risk such as patients with sleep apnea syndromes or other types of airway compromise.[35] Neonates have traditionally been considered to be more sensitive to opioid-induced respiratory depression, but this did not appear to be true when depression of the carbon dioxide response curve by morphine at different ages was measured.[36] Age-related differences in pharmacokinetics are probably responsible for the relative increase in respiratory effects for a given dose seen clinically in young patients. Nevertheless, neonates and infants at risk for apnea due to age or following general anesthesia, who are also receiving opioids, should be treated as high risk.

There is no agreement on minimum standards of monitoring for children receiving parenteral opioids. Most authorities recommend that the level of sedation is monitored in addition to respiratory rate because somnolence is a more sensitive measure of depression of respiration (**Table 39.4**). Patients who are at risk will obviously need more intensive observation; continuous pulse oximetry may be helpful, but it is an insensitive measure of respiratory depression if patients are receiving supplementary oxygen.

Ketamine

Ketamine, a phencyclidine derivative and NMDA antagonist, is a dissociative general anesthetic agent with analgesic properties in subanesthetic doses. The principal analgesic uses of ketamine in pediatrics are for postoperative pain as a neuraxial analgesic, or less commonly as a supplement to intravenous opioids. It is also used for the management of procedural pain. Ketamine is a racemic mixture and the S-isomer has approximately twice the analgesic potency of its racemate with a better side-effect profile and is probably preferred when available.[37] If ketamine is used as a neuraxial analgesic, the solution must of course be preservative-free. The developmental neurotoxic safety of ketamine itself is not conclusively established, and as it is not licensed for use by this route in adults or children it has not undergone the usual rigorous testing required; nevertheless, there are no reports of such toxicity after many years of clinical use. The authors of a systematic review concluded that more investigation should be undertaken before epidural ketamine can be recommended, others have argued that S-ketamine in particular has been shown to be safe.[37, 38]

POSTOPERATIVE ANALGESIA: CAUDAL KETAMINE

There are numerous descriptive studies of the use of caudal epidural ketamine, with or without LA. Ketamine at a dose of 0.25–0.5 mg/kg prolongs the effect of caudal LA following a range of subumbilical surgery, such as orchidopexy, hypospadias, or inguinal hernia repair.[4, 38][I]

Studies in adults have shown that postoperative, intravenous ketamine may have opioid-sparing effects and reduce opioid-related side effects,[39][I], [40][I] In children, this remains to be proven, but nevertheless low-dose ketamine is used to supplement i.v. opioids when pain is refractory or difficult to manage, a typical regimen is 10–50 μg/kg per hour (**Table 39.7**).

PROCEDURAL PAIN

Ketamine 1–2 mg/kg i.v. is used in emergency departments, oncology units, burns units, and elsewhere for the management of painful procedures, such as dressing changes, simple fracture reduction, lumbar puncture, and bone marrow biopsy. The use of ketamine in this way by physicians not trained in anesthesia is controversial, but provided certain criteria are fulfilled it is regarded as safe by some practitioners.[41, 42, 43]

Clonidine

The α2 adrenergic agonist clonidine is used fairly extensively for caudal epidural analgesia with or without LA at a dose of 1–2 μg/kg, where, like ketamine, it appears to prolong analgesia.[38][I], [44] Clonidine shows a marked developmental effect in regard to its sedative properties, and severe respiratory depression has been reported in neonates.[45, 46] Clonidine neurotoxicity has been more extensively investigated than that of ketamine, but again as it is not licensed for neuraxial analgesia in children there is some debate concerning its use.[38, 44]

LOCAL ANESTHETIC PROCEDURES

Local anesthetic blocks are an extremely important part of pediatric pain management, particularly for acute postoperative and procedural pain. Enthusiasm for regional anesthesia in children originates from the realization in the early 1980s that the residual effects of anesthesia and the adverse consequences of opioids could be minimized by the use of LA. The prevalence of day surgery in pediatrics and the relative simplicity of many LA blocks in children that are appropriate for the most common operations has meant that they have become part of standard care.

General considerations

Children dislike needles and will not usually cooperate with uncomfortable or prolonged procedures, consequently, with few exceptions local anesthetic blocks are performed under general anesthesia. This is in direct contrast to practice in adults where it has been argued that neurological damage due to direct needle trauma can be avoided if the patient reports paresthesia during placement of a block. There is a consensus of opinion that block placement under general anesthesia is the preferred option in children, and evidence of its safety has been provided by a number of outcome studies.[47, 48, 49]

In recent years, there has been interest in the use of ultrasound to aid accurate placement of LA, and positioning of catheters for LA infusion, in both peripheral and epidural blocks.[50] The technique has been extended to children and descriptions of the successful use of ultrasound for ilio-inguinal, umbilical, and epidural block have been published in the last few years.[51, 52, 53] Although special skills and equipment are needed, possible advantages are faster and more accurate placement, higher success rates, reduced dose of LA needed, and lower incidence of complications.[51, 53, 54]

PERIPHERAL NERVE BLOCKS

Penile block

Indications

This block is used for intra- and early postoperative analgesia for circumcision, meatoplasty, and distal hypospadias. For circumcision, penile block is comparable to caudal block with low rates of complications.[55][I] In neonates shortly after birth, circumcision is sometimes performed without general anesthesia; penile block is more effective than either subcutaneous ring block or topical local anesthesia in this circumstance, but the

Table 39.7 Doses of clonidine and ketamine.

Drug		Dose		
		Oral	Intravenous	Epidural (caudal)
Clonidine	a₂-adrenergic agonist	0.001–0.002 mg/kg	0.001–0.002 mg/kg	0.001–0.002 mg/kg ± local anesthetic
Ketamine	NMDA receptor antagonist	0.5–1 mg/kg	0.1 mg/kg	0.25–0.5 mg/kg ± local anesthetic

NMDA, *N*-methyl-D-aspartate.

authors of a systematic review noted that none of these entirely eliminated the pain response during the procedure.[56][I]

Anatomy

The two dorsal nerves of the penis supply its distal two-thirds. They arise as terminal branches of the pudendal nerves and can be blocked as they emerge from under the pubic bone in the subpubic space at the base of the penis. The nerves then run close to the dorsal penile arteries and veins on the corpora cavernosa of the penis. The subpubic space is covered anteriorly by the skin and the superficial and deep layers of fascia of the anterior abdominal wall. It is divided into two compartments (each containing a nerve and vessels) by the suspensory ligament of the penis.

Method

Injections are made lateral to the symphisis pubis on both sides at the base of the penis. After antisepsis, a short-bevel 22-gauge regional block needle is inserted posteriorly through the two fascial layers which can be felt as separate slight reductions in resistance about 0.5 cm or more from the skin. After gentle aspiration, 0.1 mL/kg of local anesthetic solution is injected on either side.

Local anesthetic solutions

Only plain (no vasoconstrictor) solutions of local anesthetic should be used. 0.5 percent bupivacaine, levobupivacaine, or ropivacaine are suitable.

Complications

Hematoma due to puncture of vessels or corpora cavernosa is possible. Compression due to large hematoma may cause edema or swelling of the penis.

Ilio-inguinal/iliohypogastric block

Indications

This block is indicated for abdominal surgery below the level of the umbilicus, particularly inguinal hernia repair.[4] [I] Ultrasound-guided block may have the advantage of increasing reliability and reducing the required dose of LA.[57][III] Extension of the block by including the genital branch of the genitofemoral nerve with a second injection may improve the quality of analgesia, but a difference could only be detected during intraoperative cord traction in one study.[58][II]

Anatomy

The ilio-inguinal and iliohypogastric nerves supply the inguinal region, they arise from the lumbar plexus, and lie conveniently close together medial to the anterior–superior iliac spine (ASIS). These nerves and a third, the genital branch of the genitofemoral nerve, also supply the skin of the scrotum on that side. The ilio-inguinal and iliohypogastric nerves lie beneath the external oblique

aponeurosis, between the internal oblique and transversus abdominis muscles.

Method

A short-bevel 22-gauge regional block needle is inserted one fingers' breadth medial to the ASIS, the infant or child's index finger provides an age-appropriate measure. The needle is advanced until a change in resistance, sometimes described as a "click" or "pop," is felt as it passes through the external oblique aponeurosis. The position can be confirmed by observing the needle supported by the fascia moving with respiration when it is released. After gentle aspiration, a volume of 0.2–0.5 mL/kg of the local anesthetic is injected. The genital branch of the genitofemoral nerve can be blocked by injecting 0.1–0.2 mL/kg close to the pubic tubercle on that side.

Local anesthetic solution

Bupivacaine or levobupicaine 0.25 percent, or ropivacaine 0.2 percent up to a maximum dose of 2–2.5 mg/kg (1 mL/kg).

Complications

Unwanted motor block of the femoral nerve can occur producing leg weakness.[59]

Fascia iliaca compartment block

Indications

The femoral, obturator, and lateral cutaneous nerves of the thigh can be blocked together by injecting local anesthetic into the confined space of the fascia iliaca compartment in which they lie. The block is used for superficial surgery of the anterolateral thigh, fracture of the femur, and femoral osteotomy.[60] A catheter may be inserted to provide continuous postoperative analgesia.[61]

Anatomy

The nerves arise from the lumbar plexus and run beneath the inguinal ligament deep to the fascia iliaca which is itself continuous with the deep layers of the ligament. In the thigh, the fascia iliaca lies beneath the fascia lata and forms the roof of the compartment. Inferior to the inguinal ligament, the fascia iliaca forms the roof of a space known as the "lacuna musculorum", which is continuous with the fascia iliaca compartment above. Local anesthetic injected into the lacuna musculorum spreads to block the nerves as they pass through the compartment.

Method

A short-bevel 22-gauge regional block needle is inserted 0.5 cm below the inguinal ligament, two-thirds of the distance laterally from the pubic tubercle. The needle is advanced at an angle of 60° to the skin in a cephalad direction using a saline-filled syringe to detect loss of resistance, which is detected twice as the needle tip penetrates the fascia lata and the fascia iliaca. After gentle aspiration, the local anesthetic solution is injected.

Local anesthetic solution

Bupivacaine or levobupivacaine 0.25 percent 0.5 mL/kg, or a similar volume of ropivacaine 0.2 percent 0.7 mL/kg has been recommended for children under 20 kg.

Infraorbital nerve block

Indications

The nerve supplies the skin and mucous membrane of the upper lip and lower eyelid and the skin between. It has been particularly advocated for cleft lip repair and is also suitable for surgery of the supplied area of the face and to the maxillary incisors, canine, and premolar teeth, it is superior to peri-incisional wound infiltration with LA.[62][II]

Anatomy

The infraorbital nerve, which runs in the infraorbital canal, emerges through the infraorbital foramen of the maxilla which is palpable below the midpoint of the infraorbital margin. The foramen is located approximately halfway between this point and the angle of the mouth and medial (at least 0.75 cm) to the base of the nasal ala.

Method

The nerve is blocked either percutaneously or intraorally through the labial sulcus. The intraoral technique utilizes the dentition as a landmark and is therefore more suitable for the older child.

- **Percutaneous technique:** the needle is introduced perpendicular to and through the skin at the site of the infraorbital foramen. It is advanced until bony resistance is established and then slightly withdrawn and the local anesthetic injected.
- **Intraoral technique:** The midpoint of the infraorbital ridge is palpated externally with the index finger. The infraorbital foramen is then identified as a bony depression just below this point with the fingertip. Using the thumb of the same hand, the upper lip is retracted and the needle advanced through the labial sulcus opposite the first premolar or first primary molar. Infiltration of local anesthetic below the palpating index finger will be felt as a slight swelling at that point.
- **Local anesthetic solution:** 0.5–0.75 mL of bupivacaine, levobupivacaine, or ropivacaine 0.5 percent with epinephrine is injected.

Brachial plexus blocks

Indications

Brachial plexus blocks are indicated for upper limb surgery of the hand and forearm. The nerve supply to the upper limb is provided by the brachial plexus formed from the nerve roots of the fifth cervical (C5) to first thoracic (T1) spinal nerves with variable contributions from C4 and T2. The nerves of the plexus pass through the neck and below the mid-point of the clavicle into the axilla. Many methods of blocking the plexus have been described using the axilliary, supraclavicular, and infraclavicular approaches, and they are described in specialist texts on the subject. The axillary approach, described here, is the best studied and is considered to be safer, and hence the method of choice where analgesia to forearm and hand are required.[63] Continuous block using a catheter is possible and the infraclavicular approach is sometimes favored for this, as it is easier to fix the catheter to the less mobile skin of the chest. Ultrasound-guided infraclavicular approaches are likely to be safer than blind techniques and may be faster and more reliable than nerve stimulator-guided placement.[64][II] Supraclavicular brachial plexus block has been little used in children, except in expert hands, due to the need to inject in close proximity to the pleura and vital structures of the neck; nevertheless, case series have demonstrated its feasibility.[65]

Axillary approach: anatomy

The three composite cords of the brachial plexus are closely related to the axillary artery in the axilla. The nerves and artery are ensheathed in fascia forming a number of compartments which are discontinuous with those above the clavicle, limiting spread of the local anesthetic solution.

Method

In the supine position, the arm is abducted to 90° with the elbow flexed. The axillary artery is palpated with the index finger high in the axilla and overlying the humerus against which it can be compressed. The finger is moved along the artery to the mid-point of the axilla and the regional block needle (attached to a short extension tube) is inserted just above this point towards the artery until it enters the fascial sheath, identifiable by a sudden reduction in resistance. The location is confirmed by observing pulsations of the unsupported needle and failure to aspirate blood before injection. A catheter can also be located in this position to allow reinjection or infusion of local anesthetic. If the artery is unintentionally entered, it should be transfixed and two injections made one on either side, followed by compression of the vessel to avoid hematoma formation.

Local anesthetic solution with 0.5 mL/kg of 0.25 percent bupivacaine or levobupivacaine, or 0.2 percent ropivacaine is followed by further injections or an infusion not exceeding the maximum recommended doses of local anesthetic.

Intercostal and paravertebral nerve block

Cutaneous segmental sensory innervation in the thorax and upper abdomen is supplied by consecutive intercostal nerves that can be individually blocked by one or more injections, or more commonly by the use of catheters in various sites in order to provide more extensive and continuous analgesia. These techniques are used for rib fracture, post-thoracotomy pain, or localized pain of the chest wall.

Intercostal block

Classical approaches to the intercostal space have been used successfully in children; the mid-axillary line approach is the most commonly chosen. The child lies in the lateral position with the arm extended to above the head and the mid-axillary line identified. The lower edge of the rib corresponding to the nerve is marked in the mid-axillary line and using a short-bevel 22- or 25-gauge needle advanced at right angles to the skin until it strikes the lower edge of the rib. The needle bevel cephalad is slightly withdrawn and then advanced until it passes immediately below the lower edge of the rib and a slight loss of resistance is felt. 0.05–0.1 mL/kg of LA with vasoconstrictor is injected into each intercostal space (maximum 2 mL per space).

Catheter techniques

- **Subcostal.** A catheter placed in one or more intercostal spaces allows infusion of local anesthesia.
- **Paravertebral block.** Local anesthesia in the paravertebral space, which exists between T1 and T12 where it is obliterated by the psoas muscle, allows unilateral multiple spinal segments to be blocked by a single injection. Catheters in the paravertebral space allow infusion of local anesthetic and extended analgesia which may be comparable to epidural blockade.

Anatomy

As in the adult, the paravertebral space in children is a potential space communicating from T1 to T12 lateral to the thoracic vertebral bodies. Dorsally, the space is limited by the transverse process of the vertebra and the costotransverse ligament, anterolaterally by the parietal pleura. The space contains the intercostal nerve and thoracic sympathetic chain, as well as the intercostal vesels.

Method

In the lateral decubitus position, a Tuohy needle is inserted about 1 cm lateral to the vertebral spinous process and advanced perpendicularly until contact is made with the transverse process. The needle is withdrawn slightly and then "walked" along the transverse process either above or below where it is advanced close to the bone. The paravertebral space is detected by loss of resistance on piercing the costotransverse ligament and injection made and a catheter inserted. For thoracotomy, puncture should be at T5/6 and for abdominal surgery (unilateral incision), at T9/10. A catheter can also be placed directly in the paravertebral region during thoracic surgery.

Local anesthetic solution using bupivacaine 0.25 percent, 0.5 mL/kg is followed by infusion of 0.2 mg/kg per hour.

CENTRAL NERVE BLOCKS

Epidural analgesia

Neuraxial spread of solution in the epidural space allows relatively extensive analgesia for a given dose of analgesic. The toxicity of LA means that dose limits must be strictly observed and so neuraxial analgesia has distinct advantages, especially in the very young. The duration of action of epidural LA is relatively extended in comparison with peripheral nerve block and intrathecal block, but does not exceed four hours even with the longest acting drugs. Catheters can easily be placed into the epidural space and considerable experience has been gained of prolonged epidural analgesia by infusion of local anesthetic. The duration of action of single-shot caudal or lumbar epidurals can be extended by drugs with an additive neuraxial effect, e.g. opioids, clonidine, or ketamine.

Caudal approach: indications

Caudal analgesia is effective for surgery below the umbilicus including abdominal, perineal, and lower limb procedures. Caudal analgesia is particularly strongly indicated for circumcision, hypospadias surgery, orchidopexy, and inguinal hernia repair.[4][II]

Anatomy

Ossification of the five sacral vertebral segments begins with the two lowest at the age of about 18 years and is complete by the end of the second decade. The sacral hiatus is a defect in the fifth verebra and it is covered by ligaments, subcutaneous fat, and skin. The size of the hiatus decreases with maturity and may become ossified in the adult. The sacral canal contains the distal (caudal) epidural space, cauda equina, dura extending to S3 at birth and S2 in childhood. Identification of the sacral hiatus is usually easy in infancy and childhood. It is palpable as a soft depression between the sacral cornua of S5. It is also located at the apex of an equilateral triangle whose base is between the posterior iliac spines. An alternative approach, with the child in the lateral position, is to find the hiatus at the midline intersection of a line drawn perpendicularly from the greater trochanter of the femur when the leg is flexed at the hip.

Method

Once the hiatus is located, under aseptic conditions, a needle is inserted through the skin in the midline at an angle of 45° aiming cranially. There is a sudden change in resistance as the needle passes through the relatively dense membrane and into the space. Intravascular or intradural location of the needle are excluded by gentle aspiration on the needle and by removing the syringe from the needle for 30 seconds or longer. An intravascular canula (22 gauge) can also be used, which is gently advanced over the needle for 2 or 3 cm once the space is entered.

The extent of local anesthetic block depends on the volume of solution injected (see Table 27.7 in Chapter 27, Acute pain management in children in the *Acute Pain* volume of this series). Other analgesics used alone or in combination with caudal local anesthetic include clonidine 1–2 µg/kg, ketamine 0.5 mg/kg, and opioids, e.g. morphine 20–50 µg/kg in preservative-free solutions.

Alternatively, a catheter can also be advanced into the caudal space and for some considerable distance higher, if it is desired to reach lumbar or thoracic epidural segments. The relatively short and straight spine of neonates and infants allows the catheter to be reliably sited at the required level. Catheter location can be confirmed by radiography using a small amount of radiographic contrast if required. Special catheters have been devised which will allow their location to be confirmed either by electrical stimulation, electrocardiogram (ECG) guidance or ultrasound.[66, 67, 68]

Lumbar and thoracic epidural analgesia

Indications

Epidural analgesia is effective for major surgery of the thorax, abdomen, spine, and lower limbs. It is particularly indicated in patients with potential respiratory compromise or where muscle spasm is likely to be a problem postoperatively.

Anatomy

The principal surface landmarks and technique of epidural analgesia are similar at all ages except that vertebral column is less curved and intersegmental distances are much less in early life. In the neonate, the pelvis is relatively flat and therefore a line drawn vertically between the anterior superior iliac crests in the lateral position crosses the border of L5/S1 in the neonate and the vertebral body of L5 in young children. Lack of sacral ossification also means that it is possible to access the epidural space through the sacral intervertebral spaces. The supraspinous ligament and the ligamentum flavuum are much softer and less readily identifiable in childhood and they are incapable of supporting the weight of a standard Tuohy epidural needle, which must therefore be supported at all times during the procedure of catheter insertion.

Technique

In children, general anesthesia is a prerequisite with full cardiorespiratory monitoring. An 18-gauge Tuohy epidural needle is suitable for all ages and shorter versions of the needle are available for children less than 10 kg (one year of age). Nineteen-gauge needles are also available and preferred by some practitioners for very small infants and neonates, but the fine 23-gauge epidural catheter which must be used with this needle is prone to technical problems. It is not necessary to fluid preload children less than six years old, but blood pressure and heart rate should be monitored throughout.

Identification of the epidural space

A technique of loss of resistance (LORT) to continuous pressure on a "low friction" syringe filled with saline is preferred by most practitioners, but many modifications have been described.[47, 69, 70] Air is not recommended to detect loss of resistance in children due to the risk of venous air embolus, unblocked dermatomes due to air pockets in the epidural space, and a possible association with neurological damage. Dural tap or accidental penetration of the dura has been reported in children, but the incidence is very low if the above technique is used to locate the space.[28] The use of an epidural test dose is controversial; epinephrine-containing solutions may detect intravascular injection, but high rates of false-positive and false-negative tests have been reported. Previous estimation of the depth of the epidural space may be helpful and a number of formulae have been suggested; however, interindividual variation is common. In the neonate, the lumbar epidural space is between 0.4 and 1.5 cm from the skin, depending on approach. Under six months of age, there is little correlation between depth, age, and weight. In older infants and children between six months and ten years, 1 mm/kg is a good approximation, or depth (cm) $= 1 + 0.15 \times$ age (years), and depth (cm) $= 0.8 + 0.05 \times$ weight (kg), respectively.[71, 72]

Epidural catheters

An epidural catheter, if indicated, is placed through the needle. A standard 21-gauge catheter is preferred, and a minimum length of 4 cm is normally left in the space as this reduces the chances of dislodgment of the catheter due to movement.[73] The catheter should be fixed at the skin using a clear plastic dressing such that the entry site can easily be inspected later, it is usually also taped to the child's back as far as the shoulder. Minor technical complications are common, particularly occlusion and kinking of fine catheters; disconnection and dislodgment also occur more frequently in pediatric practice. The use of larger catheters where possible, experience and improved fixation technique should reduce these to a minimum. Retrograde leakage of the infusate back to the insertion site also occurs, but does not usually reduce efficacy. The infection rate of epidural catheters is low, even when located below the nappy line. Slight redness at the insertion site is common, inflammation with redness and swelling or visible pus is an indication for removal of the catheter, skin swab culture, and appropriate antibiotic therapy if indicated.[74]

Epidural drugs and infusions

Drugs, doses, and infusion rates for epidural analgesia are given in **Table 39.8**. An initial dose of local anesthetic,

Table 39.8 Typical drugs, doses, and infusion rates for epidural analgesia.

Drug	Initial dose	Infusion	Rate
Levobupivacaine-morphine	Levobupivacaine 0.25% 0.5–0.75 mL/kg	Levobupivacaine 0.125% with preservative-free morphine 0.001%	0.1–0.4 mL/hour[a]
Levobupivacaine-fentanyl	Levobupivacaine 0.25% 0.5–0.75 mL/kg	Levobupivacaine 0.125% with fentanyl 1–2 µg/mL	0.1–0.4 mL/hour[a]
Ropivacaine	Ropivacaine 0.2% 0.5–0.75 mL/kg	Ropivacaine 0.2%	0.1–0.4 mL/hour[a]

[a] Maximum rate 0.2 mL/hour in neonates.

with or without opioid, is followed by a continuous infusion of the solution. For intraoperative use, concentrated local anesthetic solutions, e.g. levobupivacaine 0.25 percent, are usually required initially to establish a sensory-motor block; for postoperative or other acute pain, analgesia can be provided by more dilute solutions. Augmentation of analgesia using opioids is common; morphine, hydromorphone, and fentanyl are all popular.

Patient-controlled epidural analgesia (PCEA) is used in some centers. Epidural solutions are similar to those described previously. A small continuous "background" infusion of 0.2 mL/kg per hour together with demand doses of 1–3 mL with a lockout of 15–30 minutes has been suggested.[75]

Complications

Accidental intravascular injection, unwanted motor block, and toxicity due to accidental overdose or cumulation of LA after prolonged infusion can all occur. Meticulous technique, monitoring, and frequent review of infusion rates should minimize these problems.

Inadequate analgesia may be due to a poorly located catheter or inadequate spread of local anesthetic; tachyphylaxis also occurs. Relocation of the catheter by judicious withdrawal of a short (1 cm) length, increasing the volume or strength of the analgesic infusion, or the addition of adjunctive neuraxial analgesics may help.

Epidural local anesthetic–opioid combinations are popular, but improvements in analgesia are obtained at the expense of the introduction of opioid-related complications. Sedation, respiratory depression, and itching can be treated with small doses of naloxone; nausea and vomiting is managed with antiemetics.

Retention of urine is a bothersome complication of epidural analgesia that occurs more frequently when opioids are used, when thoracic dermatomes are blocked, and in older children. Prophylactic urinary catheterization is indicated for high-risk groups, otherwise urine output is monitored.

Long-term neurological complications following epidural analgesia are very rare, occurring at an estimated maximum rate of 1:10,000, which is comparable to that in adults.[49, 76]

Monitoring during epidural analgesia

Staff caring for patients with continuous epidural analgesia should receive appropriate training, be aware of the potential complications and competent to manage them. In addition to cardiorespiratory monitoring, assessment of pain, and sedation, a regular estimation of the dermatomal height of sensory block and presence and degree of motor block should be undertaken. The insertion site of the catheter should also be inspected at least daily for signs of infection or dislodgment. Cardiorespiratory monitoring is usually continued for 24 hours after cessation of the epidural if opioids have been infused as delayed respiratory depression has been reported.[77]

REFERENCES

* 1. Howard R. Current status of pain management in children. *Journal of the American Medical Association.* 2003; **290**: 2464–9.

* 2. Lonnqvist P, Morton N. Postoperative analgesia in infants and children. *British Journal of Anaesthesia.* 2005; **95**: 59–68.

* 3. Royal College of Nursing. *Clinical guidelines for the recognition and assessment of acute pain in children.* London: Royal College of Nursing, 1999.

* 4. Good Practice in Postoperative and Procedural Pain Management. *Pediatric Anesthesia.* 2008; (in press).

* 5. Australian and New Zealand College of Anaesthetists. *Acute pain management: scientific evidence*, 2nd edn. Melbourne: Australian and New Zealand College of Anaesthetists, 2005. Available from: www.nhmrc.gov.au/publications.

6. Schechter N, Allen D, Hanson K. Status of pediatric pain control: a comparison of hospital analgesic usage in children and adults. *Pediatrics.* 1986; **77**: 11–15.

7. Seth N, Llewellyn N, Howard R. Parental opinions regarding the route of administration of analgesic medication in children. *Paediatric Anaesthesia.* 2000; **10**: 537–44.

8. Anderson B, Woolard G, Holford N. Pharmacokinetics of rectal paracetamol after major surgery in children. *Paediatric Anaesthesia.* 1995; **5**: 237–42.

9. Anderson B, Woollard G, Holford N. A model for size and age changes in the pharmacokinetics of paracetamol in neonates, infants and children. *British Journal of Clinical Pharmacology.* 2000; **50**: 125–34.

10. Kendall J, Reeves B, Latter V. Multicentre randomised controlled trial of nasal diamorphine for analgesia in children and teenagers with clinical fractures. *British Medical Journal (Clinical research ed.).* 2001; **322**: 261–5.

11. Galinkin JL, Fazi LM, Cuy RM *et al.* Use of intranasal fentanyl in children undergoing myringotomy and tube placement during halothane and sevoflurane anesthesia. *Anesthesiology.* 2000; **93**: 1378–83.

12. Kokki H, Rasanen I, Lasalmi M *et al.* Comparison of oxycodone pharmacokinetics after buccal and sublingual administration in children. *Clinical Pharmacokinetics.* 2006; **45**: 745–54.

13. Binstock W, Rubin R, Bachman C *et al.* The effect of premedication with OTFC, with or without ondansetron, on postoperative agitation, and nausea and vomiting in pediatric ambulatory patients. *Paediatric Anaesthesia.* 2004; **14**: 759–67.

14. Howell T. Paracetamol-induced fulminant hepatic failure in a child after 5 days of therapeutic doses. *Paediatric Anaesthesia.* 2000; **10**: 344–5.

15. Lesko S, Mitchell A. The safety of acetaminophen and ibuprofen among children younger than two years old. *Pediatrics.* 1999; **104**: e39.

*16. Lesko S, Mitchell A. An assessment of the safety of pediatric ibuprofen. A practitioner-based randomized clinical trial. *Journal of the American Medical Association.* 1995; **273**: 929–33.

17. Short J, Barr C, Palmer C *et al.* Use of diclofenac in children with asthma. *Anaesthesia.* 2000; **55**: 334–7.

18. Williams D, Hatch D, Howard R. Codeine phosphate in paediatric medicine. *British Journal of Anaesthesia.* 2001; **86**: 421–7.

19. Moore A, Collins S, Carroll D, McQuay H. Paracetamol with and without codeine in acute pain: a quantitative systematic review. *Pain.* 1997; **70**: 193–201.

*20. Bozkurt P. Use of tramadol in children. *Paediatric Anaesthesia.* 2005; **15**: 1041–7.

21. Engelhardt T, Steel E, Johnston G, Veitch D. Tramadol for pain relief in children undergoing tonsillectomy: a comparison with morphine. *Paediatric Anaesthesia.* 2003; **13**: 249–52.

22. Ozalevli M, Unlugenc H, Tuncer U *et al.* Comparison of morphine and tramadol by patient-controlled analgesia for postoperative analgesia after tonsillectomy in children. *Paediatric Anaesthesia.* 2005; **15**: 979–84.

23. Allegaert K, Van den Anker J, Verbesselt R *et al.* O-demethylation of tramadol in the first months of life. *European Journal of Clinical Pharmacology.* 2005; **61**: 837–42.

24. Allegaert K, Anderson B, Verbesselt R *et al.* Tramadol disposition in the very young: an attempt to assess in vivo cytochrome P-450 2D6 activity. *British Journal of Anaesthesia.* 2005; **95**: 231–9.

25. Malviya S, Voepel-Lewis T, Tait A *et al.* Depth of sedation in children undergoing computed tomography: validity and reliability of the University of Michigan Sedation Scale (UMSS). *British Journal of Anaesthesia.* 2002; **88**: 241–5.

26. Bouwmeester N, Anderson B, Tibboel D, Holford N. Developmental pharmacokinetics of morphine and its metabolites in neonates, infants and young children. *British Journal of Anaesthesia.* 2004; **92**: 208–17.

*27. Kart T, Christrup L, Rasmussen M. Recommended use of morphine in neonates, infants and children based on a literature review: Part 1. Pharmacokinetics. *Paediatric Anaesthesia.* 1997; **7**: 5–11.

*28. Lloyd-Thomas A, Howard R. A pain service for children. *Paediatric Anaesthesia.* 1994; **4**: 3–15.

29. Chelly J. An iontophoretic, fentanyl HCl patient-controlled transdermal system for acute postoperative pain management. *Expert Opinion on Pharmacotherapy.* 2005; **6**: 1205–14.

*30. Kalso E. Oxycodone. *Journal of Pain and Symptom Management.* 2005; **29**: S47–56.

31. Sucato DJ, Duey-Holtz A, Elerson E, Safavi F. Postoperative analgesia following surgical correction for adolescent idiopathic scoliosis: a comparison of continuous epidural analgesia and patient-controlled analgesia. *Spine.* 2005; **30**: 211–17.

32. O'Hara Jr JF, Cywinski JB, Tetzlaff JE *et al.* The effect of epidural vs intravenous analgesia for posterior spinal fusion surgery. *Paediatric Anaesthesia.* 2004; **14**: 1009–15.

33. Maxwell L, Kaufmann S, Bitzer S *et al.* The effects of a small-dose naloxone infusion on opioid-induced side effects and analgesia in children and adolescents treated with intravenous patient controlled analgesia: a double-blind, prospective, randomized, controlled study. *Anesthesia and Analgesia.* 2005; **100**: 953–8.

*34. Gan TJ, Meyer T, Apfel CC *et al.* Consensus guidelines for managing postoperative nausea and vomiting. *Anesthesia and Analgesia.* 2003; **97**: 62–71.

35. Strauss S, Lynn A, Bratton S, Nespeca M. Ventilatory response to CO_2 in children with obstructive sleep apnea from adenotonsillar hypertrophy. *Anesthesia and Analgesia.* 1999; **89**: 328–32.

36. Lynn A, Nespeca M, Opheim K, Slattery J. Respiratory effects of intravenous morphine infusions in neonates, infants, and children after cardiac surgery. *Anesthesia and Analgesia.* 1993; **77**: 695–701.

*37. Koinig H, Marhofer P. S(+)-ketamine in paediatric anaesthesia. *Paediatric Anaesthesia.* 2003; **13**: 185–7.

*38. Ansermino M, Basu R, Vandebeek C, Montgomery C. Nonopioid additives to local anaesthetics for caudal blockade in children: a systematic review. *Paediatric Anaesthesia.* 2003; **13**: 561–73.

39. Elia N, Tramer M. Ketamine and postoperative pain – a quantitative systematic review of randomised trials. *Pain.* 2005; **113**: 61–70.

40. Subramaniam K, Subramaniam B, Steinbrook R. Ketamine as adjuvant analgesic to opioids: a quantitative and qualitative systematic review. *Anesthesia and Analgesia.* 2004; **99**: 482–95.

41. Morton NS. Ketamine is not a safe, effective, and appropriate technique for emergency department paediatric procedural sedation. *Emergency Medicine Journal*. 2004; **21**: 272–3.

42. Howes MC. Ketamine for paediatric sedation/analgesia in the emergency department. *Emergency Medicine Journal*. 2004; **21**: 275–80.

∗ 43. Migita RT, Klein EJ, Garrison MM. Sedation and analgesia for pediatric fracture reduction in the emergency department: a systematic review. *Archives of Pediatrics and Adolescent Medicine*. 2006; **160**: 46–51.

44. Ecoffey C. Pediatric regional anesthesia – update. *Current Opinion in Anaesthesiology*. 2007; **20**: 232–5.

45. Galante D. Preoperative apnea in a preterm infant after caudal block with ropivacaine and clonidine. *Paediatric Anaesthesia*. 2005; **15**: 708–09.

46. Hansen T, Henneberg S. Caudal clonidine in neonates and small infants and respiratory depression. *Paediatric Anaesthesia*. 2004; **14**: 529–30.

∗ 47. Dalens B. Some current controversies in paediatric regional anaesthesia. *Current Opinion in Anaesthesiology*. 2006; **19**: 301–8.

48. Giaufre E, Dalens B, Gombert A. Epidemiology and morbidity of regional anesthesia in children: a one-year prospective survey of the French-Language Society of Pediatric Anesthesiologists. *Anesthesia and Analgesia*. 1996; **83**: 904–12.

∗ 49. Llewellyn N, Moriarty A. The national pediatric epidural audit. *Paediatric Anaesthesia*. 2007; **17**: 520–33.

50. Grau T. Ultrasonography in the current practice of regional anaesthesia. *Best Practice and Research. Clinical Anaesthesiology*. 2005; **19**: 175–200.

51. Willschke H, Marhofer P, Bosenberg A et al. Ultrasonography for ilioinguinal/iliohypogastric nerve blocks in children. *British Journal of Anaesthesia*. 2005; **95**: 226–30.

52. de Jose Maria B, Gotzens V, Mabrok M. Ultrasound-guided umbilical nerve block in children: a brief description of a new approach. *Paediatric Anaesthesia*. 2007; **17**: 44–50.

53. Willschke H, Marhofer P, Bosenberg A et al. Epidural catheter placement in children: comparing a novel approach using ultrasound guidance and a standard loss-of-resistance technique. *British Journal of Anaesthesia*. 2006; **97**: 200–07.

54. Marhofer P, Bosenberg A, Sitzwohl C et al. Pilot study of neuraxial imaging by ultrasound in infants and children. *Paediatric Anaesthesia*. 2005; **15**: 671–6.

55. Allan CY, Jacqueline PA, Shubhda JH. Caudal epidural block versus other methods of postoperative pain relief for circumcision in boys. *Cochrane Database of Systematic Reviews*. 2003; **CD003005**.

∗ 56. Brady-Fryer B, Wiebe N, Lander JA. Pain relief for neonatal circumcision. *Cochrane Database of Systematic Reviews*. 2004; **CD004217**.

57. Willschke H, Bosenberg A, Marhofer P et al. Ultrasonographic-guided ilioinguinal/iliohypogastric nerve block in pediatric anesthesia: what is the optimal volume? *Anesthesia and Analgesia*. 2006; **102**: 1680–4.

58. Sasaoka N, Kawaguchi M, Yoshitani K et al. Evaluation of genitofemoral nerve block, in addition to ilioinguinal and iliohypogastric nerve block, during inguinal hernia repair in children. *British Journal of Anaesthesia*. 2005; **94**: 243–6.

59. Roy-Shapira A, Amoury R, Ashcraft K et al. Transient quadriceps paresis following local inguinal block for postoperative pain control. *Journal of Pediatric Surgery*. 1985; **20**: 554–5.

60. Dalens B, Vanneuville G, Tanguy A. Comparison of the fascia iliaca compartment block with the 3-in-1 block in children. *Anesthesia and Analgesia*. 1989; **69**: 705–13.

61. Ivani G, Tonetti F. Postoperative analgesia in infants and children: new developments. *Minerva Anestesiologica*. 2004; **70**: 399–403.

62. Prabhu K, Wig J, Grewal S. Bilateral infraorbital nerve block is superior to peri-incisional infiltration for analgesia after repair of cleft lip. *Scandinavian Journal of Plastic and Reconstructive Surgery and Hand Surgery*. 1999; **33**: 83–7.

63. Thornton KL, Sacks MD, Hall R, Bingham R. Comparison of 0.2% ropivacaine and 0.25% bupivacaine for axillary brachial plexus blocks in paediatric hand surgery. *Paediatric Anaesthesia*. 2003; **13**: 409–12.

64. Marhofer P, Sitzwohl C, Greher M, Kapral S. Ultrasound guidance for infraclavicular brachial plexus anaesthesia in children. *Anaesthesia*. 2004; **59**: 642–6.

65. Pande R, Pande M, Bhadani U et al. Supraclavicular brachial plexus block as a sole anaesthetic technique in children: an analysis of 200 cases. *Anaesthesia*. 2000; **55**: 798–802.

66. Rapp H, Folger A, Grau T. Ultrasound-guided epidural catheter insertion in children. *Anesthesia and Analgesia*. 2005; **101**: 333–9.

67. Tsui B, Seal R, Koller J. Thoracic epidural catheter placement via the caudal approach in infants by using electrocardiographic guidance. *Anesthesia and Analgesia*. 2002; **95**: 326–30.

68. Goobie S, Montgomery C, Basu R et al. Confirmation of direct epidural catheter placement using nerve stimulation in pediatric anesthesia. *Anesthesia and Analgesia*. 2003; **97**: 984–8.

69. Tsui B, Wagner A, Cunningham K et al. Can continuous low current electrical stimulation distinguish insulated needle position in the epidural and intrathecal spaces in pediatric patients? *Paediatric Anaesthesia*. 2005; **15**: 959–63.

70. Williams D, Howard R. Epidural analgesia in children. A survey of current opinions and practices amongst UK paediatric anaesthetists. *Paediatric Anaesthesia*. 2003; **13**: 769–76.

71. Hasan M, Howard R, Lloyd-Thomas A. Depth of epidural space in children. *Anaesthesia*. 1994; **49**: 1085–7.

72. Bosenberg A, Gouws E. Skin-epidural distance in children. *Anaesthesia*. 1995; **50**: 895–7.

73. Sage F, Lloyd Thomas A, Howard R. Paediatric lumbar epidurals: a comparison of 21-G and 23-G catheters in patients weighing less than 10 kg. *Paediatric Anaesthesia*. 2000; **10**: 279–82.

74. Seth N, Macqueen S, Howard R. Clinical signs of infection during continuous postoperative epidural analgesia in children: the value of catheter tip culture. *Paediatric Anaesthesia*. 2004; **14**: 996–1000.

75. Birmingham P, Wheeler M, Suresh S *et al*. Patient-controlled epidural analgesia in children: can they do it? *Anesthesia and Analgesia*. 2003; **96**: 686–91.

76. Auroy Y, Narchi P, Messiah A *et al*. Serious complications related to regional anesthesia: results of a prospective survey in France. *Anesthesiology*. 1997; **87**: 479–86.

77. Krane E. Delayed respiratory depression in a child after caudal epidural morphine. *Anesthesia and Analgesia*. 1988; **67**: 79–82.

40

Mind/body skills for children in pain

TIMOTHY CULBERT, STEFAN FRIEDRICHSDORF, AND LEORA KUTTNER

KEY LEARNING POINTS

- Pain represents a complex mind/body process and therefore effective treatment approaches must address both physiological and psychological aspects of the pain experience.
- Mind/body treatments such as hypnosis and biofeedback represent time and cost-effective strategies for treating pediatric pain (acute and chronic).

- Mind/body techniques offer a way to teach children and adolescents about self-regulation abilities.
- Appropriate training in mind/body techniques for healthcare professionals working with children is important and readily available through a number of professional organizations.

INTRODUCTION

The pain experience is inherently psychophysiologic in nature. It always includes both a biologic, objective component – the actual tissue damage, inflammation, or insult – and an affective, cognitive, subjective component – the experience of discomfort, suffering, and the attribution of the sensation as painful and unpleasant. Self-regulation techniques, such as hypnosis and biofeedback, represent integrative approaches that directly address this essential mind–body unity.[1]

Hypnosis, biofeedback, and related self-regulation approaches have come to the forefront as evidence-based, practical, and potent therapeutic strategies[2, 3, 4] for children and adolescents with a variety of acute, recurrent, and chronic pain problems (**Boxes 40.1** and **40.2**). In addition, because these strategies tap into children's innate developmental drives for mastery, fantasy, and curiosity, they serve as ideal vehicles for teaching children

to actively help themselves through pain and associated anxiety symptoms.[5]

This chapter covers some key pediatric concerns in the pain research literature and provides in-depth clinical applications with illustrative case examples of hypnosis and biofeedback as prototype mind/body strategies for children and adolescents to manage acute and chronic pain. The chapter includes a discussion of the theoretical rationale and commonalities of mind/body techniques in therapeutic practice, the limitations for their use, and closes with information about certification and training.

Definitions

Self-regulation (or mind/body) skills are defined as psychophysiological strategies that use focused attention and self-directed practice to train a person to identify and control unwanted symptoms by modifying undesirable

Box 40.1 Examples of pain-related conditions for which mind/body approaches are helpful

- Acute pain
- Burns
- Cancer
- Chronic/recurrent pain
- Complex regional pain syndrome type I and II (formerly: Reflex sympathetic dystrophy)
- Gastrointestinal problems (severe constipation, encopresis, functional abdominal pain, Irritable bowel syndrome)
- Headache: migraine, tension type, or mixed
- Human immunodeficiency virus (HIV)/ acquired immune deficiency syndrome (AIDS)-associated pain
- Juvenile rheumatoid arthritis
- Myofascial pain
- Neuromuscular disorders
- Orthopedic conditions
- Pain related to chronic medical conditions (cancer, cystic fibrosis, diabetes)
- Raynaud's syndrome
- Sickle cell anemia
- Somatization/somatoform disorders

Box 40.2 Examples of painful medical procedures for which mind/body approaches are helpful

- Bone marrow aspiration
- Biopsies
- Dental procedures
- Dressing changes
- Finger prick
- Gynecological examination
- Intramuscular drug application (obsolete for analgesia!)
- Lumbar puncture
- Port-a-Cath needle access
- Subcutaneous drug application
- Trauma management
- Preoperative/perioperative interventions
- Procedural pain
- Surgical/orthopedic procedures
- Sutures
- Throat culture
- Venipuncture/intravenous placement

physiologic responses, behaviors, and thought patterns so that a desired level of health and wellness may be achieved. Applied psychophysiology is the area of study that examines links between behavioral/emotional/cognitive phenomena and physiologic response patterns.[6] Ongoing research suggests that mind/body techniques elicit responses via the psychoneuroendoimmunologic axis.[7]

A number of mind/body methods fall into this area (**Table 40.1**). The term mind/body techniques (or skills) has become widely accepted as a way to describe this broad domain of strategies using a variety of techniques to facilitate the mind's capacity to affect bodily function and symptoms. These techniques are seen as increasingly important in the management of acute and chronic pain and can be integrated with pharmacologic strategies effectively.[8, 9, 10]

Developmental issues

Traditionally, young children have been regarded as too young to understand their physiological processes and too immature to cooperate and learn how to modify them. The concept that young children can regulate their pain sensation and perception may seem radical, but it is well within a preschooler's ability.[11] Adapted to each stage of development from the age of three to the teenage years, self-regulation methods such as bubble blowing, regulated breathing, relaxation techniques, imagery, hypnosis, and biofeedback methods (using videogame-style computer software), can be taught to children in pain or who are anticipating pain and distress.

It is essential to correctly gauge each child's emotional and cognitive age so that age-appropriate language is used, level of understanding is determined, and the therapeutic partnership is productive (not confusing or boring).[12] Chronological age is not always an accurate measure, as anxiety and pain tend to make a child regress in areas of social, emotional, and behavioral functioning. Consequently, the clinician must be creative and sensitive, and must observe the child closely during the introduction to select the best-suited self-regulation method and then adjust the direction and coaching to the changes in the child.[12] This becomes more challenging when the techniques are used to modify pain perception during medical procedures. Under these conditions, the clinician must coordinate with the team and pace the child to maximize self-coping during the more painful part of the procedure.

With developmentally appropriate language, adequate support, and trust, children of all ages can learn coping and self-regulation skills to reduce pain and anxiety for surgery, invasive medical procedures, chronic diseases, and recurring painful conditions.[2, 3, 5, 13, 14, 15, 16] Whatever the child's age, when successfully integrated by the child as a way of dealing with pain and discomfort, these

Table 40.1 Some examples of mind/body strategies.

Strategy	Description
Hypnosis (mental imagery)	An altered state of awareness usually, but not always, involving relaxation during which participants experience heightened suggestibility
Biofeedback	The use of electronic or electromechanical equipment to measure and then feedback information about physiologic processes which can then be modulated by the individual in desirable directions
Breath control training	Teaching paced, diaphragmatic breathing technique for relaxation purposes
Progressive muscle relaxation	Sequenced tensing and relaxing of various muscle groups in the body for the purpose of enhanced body awareness and relaxation
Self-monitoring	Using symptom dairies, visual analog scales and related tools to keep track of one's physiological and psychological events and changes over time
Positive self-talk	A component of cognitive-behavioral therapy, involves teaching the awareness of negative, inaccurate, and unhelpful thought patterns and cultivation of positive, helpful internal thoughts
Meditation	Defined as the intentional self-regulation of attention with a systematic mental focus on particular aspects of inner or outer experience
Autogenics	Repetitive, systematic, hypnotic-like self-suggestions about the body becoming warm, heavy, and relaxed

methods have long-term benefits[15] and can be used throughout the person's life for other incidental or accidental pain, well beyond the original reason for the pain management referral. When well established in the child's repertoire, these active, self-directed coping skills can also play a crucial part in easing the approach to death, as part of the palliative therapeutic regimen. Self-regulation training provides children with the opportunity to experience mastery and control, even when external obstacles seem insurmountable.

Integrative approaches to pediatric pain management

The term "integrative" refers to the blending of all relevant therapeutic interventions – conventional and complementary-biological and psychological – to fit each patient's needs and preferences for effective pain and symptom management. State of the art pain management in the twenty-first century demands that pharmacological management is no longer the sole approach to the management of a child's pain and suffering.[4, 10, 16] Physical and psychological responses to acute pain during childhood are interrelated and may affect short-term health directly as well as influencing the development of chronic pain later in life.

A comprehensive, holistic approach to manage a child's pain requires combining the most appropriate pharmacological intervention with a variety of other options including physical methods (such as cuddle/hug from family, massage, transcutaneous electric nerve stimulation (TENS), comfort positioning, heat, cold, etc.), mind/body techniques (such as biofeedback, hypnosis, abdominal breathing, distraction) as well as modalities such as acupressure/acupuncture, music therapy, and aromatherapy as deemed most appropriate for the

individual child. In most cases, utilizing behavioral techniques for management of acute pain and distress does not add significant time and in certain situations can actually decrease the time required for an uncomfortable procedure.[8] A recent study by Zeltzer et al.[9] supported an integrative approach for children with a variety of chronic pain conditions, which combined hypnosis and acupuncture. Children receiving six weeks of weekly sessions with the combined approach were noted to experience less pain and functional impairment and >90 percent of the pediatric subjects involved (ages 6–18 years), found this treatment combination acceptable.

Anxiety, fear, and pain

Even in the best of situations, because of the intrinsically disturbing nature of experiencing pain, children may become sensitized and develop specific fears or more generalized anxiety about medical procedures and interventions perceived to cause pain.[16, 17, 18] Successful pain management almost always includes interventions for the anticipatory anxiety component of pain. There is a reciprocal relationship for most individuals between pain and anxiety-interventions whereby less anxiety may dramatically decrease pain and vice versa. Therefore, completion of a thorough pain history, reviewing previous pain experiences, family and cultural pain attitudes, and comfort preferences, is important. Mind/body therapies can be utilized to address both the anxiety and the pain experience simultaneously.

One helpful and important way to promote comfort and reduce distress for children experiencing pain is to appropriately recognize and support parental involvement. A recent review of the literature on the role of parental presence in the context of children's medical procedures by Piira et al.[19] underscores this theme. The authors point out that although overall findings are mixed, it is appropriate for care providers to provide parents with the opportunity to be present during their child's painful procedure. Clinical experience suggests that when trained and provided with a defined, clear role in these situations, parents can be an invaluable resource in supporting their child in these challenging encounters.

Benefits of mind/body skills training

Clinical experience suggests that there are substantial advantages for children and adolescents who learn and practice mind/body skills. Their active participation in the therapeutic process leads to greater maturity and independence in managing their pain symptoms, enhanced self-confidence, reduced disabling effects of recurring or long-term pain, and increased ability to participate in normal daily activities. There is consistent clinical evidence that children learn these methods more rapidly than do adults, and generally children are more adept than adults in using hypnotherapy for control of pain. Children are also more proficient at physiologic control, as described by Attanasio et al.[20] and confirmed by others. Thus, children are excellent candidates for self-regulation training.

More has been written about the use of mind/body methods with adults than with children and adolescents. However, over the last 20 years, there has been a notable increase in the demand for training in the clinical application of pediatric mind/body methods within children's hospitals worldwide by pediatric healthcare professionals, including nurses, psychologists, pediatricians, anesthesiologists, and child life specialists. In the last ten years, the number of attendees and requests for mind/body training workshops by professional organizations, such as the Society for Developmental and Behavioral Pediatrics, the American Clinical Hypnosis Society, Professional Pain Societies and the Association for Applied Psychophysiology and Biofeedback, and Biofeedback Foundation of Europe, has notably increased. The practical benefits and ease of implementation of self-regulatory methods within pediatric settings is making them acceptable and more commonly practiced in North America, Australia, and western Europe. Parents are increasingly interested in mind–body, nondrug approaches for their children.

CLINICAL APPLICATIONS OF MIND/BODY TECHNIQUES

This section proceeds with definitions, case examples, and descriptions of treatment approaches for foundational mind/body strategies – progressive muscle relaxation, diaphragmatic breathing, hypnosis, and biofeedback. The section also defines and describes the phenomenon of hypnoanalgesia.

Basic relaxation skills

MUSCLE RELAXATION TECHNIQUES

General muscle relaxation is a pleasant experience for children aged five to six years and older as a step in the self-regulation training of physiologic pain processes.[21] With younger children, relaxation generally happens automatically. As a general rule, they do not yet have the degree of kinesthetic awareness to control and release specific muscle groups without an active biofeedback signal. Of course, there are individual differences, and if physical tension is a concern for a child younger than six, the "Raggedy Ann" doll game is developmentally appropriate to teach relaxation without the child having to lie down and close their eyes.

Demonstrating with a floppy doll how each of her limbs flops and her body bends and hangs down comfortably, the preschool child is encouraged to imitate the doll with floppy arms and legs and finally to hang loosely over the arm of the clinician "like a floppy, happy Raggedy Ann." Parents and the child are then instructed to practice being a floppy Raggedy Ann before the feared procedure, or when the child gets pain, so that it does not hurt as much and the pain can drain away.

Muscle tightness and muscle group asymmetries can cause and/or contribute to a variety of pain conditions. Muscle relaxation helps children to become more aware of their bodies in helpful ways, and to refocus and relax. Alternating sequentially through the body between tightening and relaxing different muscle groups, children are taught discrimination and control of areas of muscle tension. After completion of several rounds of squeezing and letting go, many older children and teenagers are able to discharge excessive nervous and muscle tension, improving their level of comfort.

An alternative and less demanding relaxation technique is to cover the older child with a blanket and invite him or her to "Close your eyes and let the relaxation begin to seep into your body." Starting at the child's toes, move slowly up the body and describe each part of the body becoming "heavier, warmer, and more relaxed." Over a five- to seven-minute period, slowly guide the child's attention to the growing comfort and release that is occurring in their body, particularly in and around the areas of pain or ache. Making an audio recording of this enables the child to regularly practice relaxation, increasing the ability to release muscle tension, pain, and discomfort. This method is particularly helpful for bedridden children who are compromised by disease, surgery, treatments such as during bone marrow transplantation, or who are in end-of-life care.

DIAPHRAGMATIC BREATHING

Regulated and rhythmic diaphragmatic breathing is an easy first step to teach the beginnings of self-regulation[11, 13, 22] and yields immediate results in "being boss of your own body." Little preparation is required, and as such it is useful in first encounters with a fearful child in an acute or procedural pain situation. To start, the child is instructed to "exhale" rather than the conventional request to "inhale." Releasing breath allows a frightened child to "let go" tension and then breathe in more deeply. Emphasizing "Blow out slowly!" interrupts mounting anxiety and enables the child or teenager to gain a modicum of self-control.

Physiologically, acute pain and acute anxiety are manifested as a shift into sympathetic arousal, and are seen behaviorally in the child's shallow rapid breathing, sometimes hyperventilation, increased muscular tension, attentional vigilance, and often whimpering or tears. The instruction to "Breathe out the pain – blow it far away!" interrupts the mounting fight or flight response. Maintained over three to five exhalations, with encouragement to slow these exhalations down, physiological markers change. The child's breathing shifts from quick and shallow chest breathing to deeper diaphragmatic breathing, which is more relaxing. We typically recommend asking children to breathe in through the nose and then out through the mouth, slowly and effortlessly. Children report feeling more in control and less overwhelmed by the pain, anxiety, or panic as they control their breathing. This physiological shift can be achieved and stable within five minutes and hence is ideal for blood draws and intravenous (i.v.) injections. Breathing at a rate of five to seven breaths per minute for most people seems to promote an optimal state of autonomic nervous system (ANS) balance.

One interactive, child-friendly way to teach relaxation breathing is by using props such as pinwheels and bubbles.[13] With children ten years and under, blowing bubbles is a more child-centered way of placing the child in charge of the process, maintaining the breathing, and diverting attention away from the pain onto the task of creating, tracking, and counting the bubbles. This technique has surprised us with its usefulness, particularly for immunizations and other minor painful pediatric procedures. Furthermore, bubble blowing and regulated deep breathing establishes the concept of self-regulation and the awareness of how to modify body responses. It has been effective with toddlers and preschoolers in acute pain, for anticipatory anxiety prior to a procedure, or during invasive medical procedures.

Hypnosis

DEFINITIONS AND BACKGROUND

Hypnosis involves cultivation of an altered state of awareness, leading to heightened suggestibility, that allows for changes in a child's perception and experience of pain without complete conscious effort.[2] It is an internal imaginative process that differs from other techniques such as distraction, which focuses the child's attention on external objects. Hypnosis uses the child's imagination as the agent of change. The clinician enters the child's world, using the child's frame of reference and language to create an alternate experience, then addresses the pain through suggestions for altering sensations and increasing comfort. As such, the therapeutic process of hypnosis is in step with the apparent involuntary nature and manifestation of pain. The stages of hypnosis are shown in **Table 40.2**.

The therapeutic use of hypnosis for pain is clinically highly valued. It has been said that there is no other psychological tool so efficacious in creating comfort out of discomfort yet with none of the adverse side effects associated with medical treatments of similar efficacy.

The goal of using hypnosis during pain is to:

- eliminate fear and passive coping by increasing the child's understanding of pain signals;
- reduce the intensity of the pain and/or create distance from the pain, altering its distressing impact;
- retrain the nervous system to alter the experience of pain and its role in a child's functioning.

A hypnotic trance state is an altered state of consciousness in which perception, memory, emotions, and sensation can be therapeutically changed. To ease a child's pain, a trance is created during which the following occur:

- the child's attention is intensified and narrowed during hypnotic inductions and imaginative involvements to create an alternate or competitive experience;

Table 40.2 The stages of hypnosis.

Stages of hypnosis	
Induction	Initiating the experience of hypnosis typically by practicing a procedure or activity that narrows and focuses attention, evokes curiosity and/or that facilitates relaxation
Deepening	Intensification of the trance experience utilizing various strategies such as imagery, sensory awareness, relaxation
Therapeutic suggestion	Suggestions – direct, indirect, metaphorical – about creating desired therapeutic change
Re-alerting	The client returns to their usual state of awareness
De-briefing	Discussion of the experience, planning for the ongoing practice of self-hypnosis and arranging follow-up

- suggestions for positive change that are immediate or posthypnotic are provided;
- the pain sensations are positively reframed to have a signal value, directing the child to the area where pain perception can then be modulated;
- time distortion may be experienced for long-term benefit and to reduce fatigue.

HYPNOANALGESIA

The term hypnoanalgesia refers to the facilitation of decreased pain sensation within the hypnotic state. Much of the evidence for the effectiveness of the use of hypnoanalgesia has been derived from studies in acute care settings,[2, 17, 18, 23, 24, 25, 26] as well as treatments for procedural pain in oncology treatments[27, 28] addressing the pain and distress associated with lumbar punctures and bone marrow aspirations for children with leukemias or other medical procedures. A number of studies highlight the usefulness of hypnosis for acute procedural pain and associated distress, as detailed below.

- Goldie,[18] in one of the earliest controlled studies with hypnosis, used hypnoanesthesia in the emergency room during surgery for patients aged three to seven years. When hypnosis was used, Goldie noted a significant reduction in the percentage of patients needing pharmacotherapeutic analgesia or anesthesia for suturing and the reduction of fractures.
- Over the intervening years, there have been a number of studies on the use of hypnosis as an adjunct to pediatric anesthesia in order to decrease the use of preoperative medication, to enable greater ease during anesthetic induction, to reduce the amount of anesthesia and requirements for analgesics postoperatively, and to increase postoperative comfort.[23, 24]
- In a prospective, controlled, randomized trial comparing hypnoanalgesia with propanolol and placebo, Olness et al.[29] found that the use of hypnosis was significantly more effective in reducing the frequency of headaches than either propranolol or placebo, which did not differ from each other.
- Butler et al.[8] utilized hypnosis training for a group of children undergoing voiding cystourethrogram (VCUG) radiographic procedures and who had previously experienced distress with that procedure. After brief training in a hypnotic exercise, the child was then coached during the VCUG procedure itself by a trained therapist. Compared to a control group who received standard behavioral approaches, the hypnosis intervention group displayed less distress as rated by both parents and medical staff, were more compliant with the procedure, and on average required 14 minutes less time to complete the VCUG.

- Liossi et al.[26] demonstrated that children undergoing lumbar puncture (LP) experienced less anticipatory anxiety and procedure-related pain when hypnosis was combined with topical EMLA as an intervention than when children were given only the topical EMLA alone or when the EMLA was combined with attention from a therapist.
- Calipel et al.[23] compared midazolam and hypnosis as a preoperative intervention for children aged two to eleven years and found that children in the hypnosis group experienced less anxiety during the mask induction phase of anesthesia as well as demonstrating less behavioral difficulty at days one and seven postoperatively.
- Studies also suggest the efficacy of mental imagery for functional recurrent abdominal pain.[30, 31]

Various techniques, metaphors, and therapeutic suggestions can be utilized to facilitate the child's modulation of pain experience. Hypnoanalgesia promotes dissociation from the pain, such as the "pain switch" technique or the "magic glove."[13, 14, 15]

In the pain switch technique, the child is told how the brain receives and interprets nerve signals from all parts of the body:

> Right now the nerves in your body are sending a lot of pain information about your e.g. broken wrist. Your brain instantly understands these nerve signals, and sends messages back to the body, that keeps you aware of the pain. Now, I'm going to teach you how to focus your attention on the switches in your brain that control those incoming pain signals so that you can turn them down. As you do that your body will receive weaker pain messages and therefore feel less pain. The more you practice this the better you'll get at turning the pain switches down more quickly. And you'll feel less pain and be in more control.

During hypnotic induction, the child moves into a trance and is instructed to focus on the switch inside their brain that goes to the painful body part. This is the deepening process of the hypnotic trance. With each deep exhalation during diaphragmatic deep breathing, the child is guided to turn down the pain switch as much as possible until comfort is experienced, or until a satisfactory plateau in the pain perception is achieved. The child is encouraged through posthypnotic suggestion to maintain that decreased pain level, and with each subsequent practice to achieve greater levels of comfort and pain relief. The child is then brought out of the trance state.

The criterion for success is that the child feels a significant difference between the pain levels during and after the hypnotic trance. It is important to emphasize that the goal of the "pain switch" is not to remove all pain, which is often an unrealistic goal, but to decrease the perceived pain and to increase the child's mastery over this pain as well as improving daily functional activities. Obviously, this method has particular value for children with recurring or chronic pain conditions.

In an emergency – a startling environment for most – children often spontaneously move into a hypnotic trance with narrowed absorption and attention to the pain.[17] In this situation, relaxation is not required; rather, a spontaneous active–alert trance often occurs. The child in this altered state of awareness is highly suggestible. The clinician's task is to recognize and use this spontaneously altered state of consciousness to diminish pain perception and distress, and to promote rapid healing.

A simple and highly effective hypnotic intervention for trauma pain is to talk calmly and directly, defining with the child precisely *where the pain is* and *where the pain is not*. Defining where it is not is as important as knowing the areas of pain. It draws the child's attention to the limits of the pain. This enables the clinician to provide suggestions for reducing the area affected by the pain and for increasing the spread of comfort from the nonaffected areas. This intervention works synergistically with any needed analgesics, increasing the efficacy of both.

The therapeutic work is to sustain the child's absorption so that they no longer feel overwhelmed. Panic and anxiety are reduced by providing limits to the pain sensation, which was feared to be endless.

Case example: hypnoanalgesia

Jonathan, a 14-year-old, traumatically amputated the top joints of two fingers on his right hand during a woodworking class. After plastic surgery to reshape tips for these fingers, he was discharged with paracetamol (acetaminophen) with codeine to control his pain. He was referred for hypnosis by his family physician. Jonathan was in shock that his hand was forever altered and experienced throbbing pain in the top of his digits, which he rated six out of ten. In the first session, he was trained to use the pain switch and was able to reduce the pain to three out of ten. He was also given posthypnotic suggestions for seeing his hand as normal and being able to use it naturally with comfort and growing ease.

An audio tape was made of the hypnotic process so that he could practice it as often as he needed during the subsequent days. His progress was rapid, and on the second session five days later he reported pain levels of three and the ability to get the pain down to one using the hypnotic tape. His hand was continuing to heal well and he was feeling less self-conscious about displaying it. The third session was a follow-up two weeks later – Jonathan reported that "the nightmare was over." His new finger tips were somewhat sensitive, but no longer painful, and he was getting accustomed to using them again. He planned to return to his passion of drumming.

Case commentary

With the traumatic nature of this injury, the therapeutic concern was that Jonathan could develop phantom digit pain. Since the trauma, shock, and pain were addressed simultaneously, he did not develop this distressing phenomenon. In acute situations, only a few hypnotic interventions are needed as part of the pain therapy to improve the course of recovery.

HYPNOSIS WITH PRESCHOOL CHILDREN

Since hypnosis with preschool-age children is so different from that with the school-age child and adolescent, it is not strictly accurate to refer to the experience as true hypnosis. A better term for the preschooler's trance is protohypnosis or imaginative involvement.[2] The different manifestations with the younger child are that:

- closing eyes is invariably associated with going to sleep – something that most alert or anxious preschoolers will not willingly do, particularly when in pain in an unfamiliar environment;
- their grasp of their world shifts fluidly between the world of fantasy and reality. This is the age of imaginary playmates and the spontaneous playing out of fears or concerns;
- younger children do not easily settle and become still. They are usually unfamiliar with the concept of relaxing and so instructions "to relax" may be meaningless;
- their active imagination is often physically expressed through movement. Their hypnotic trance thus occurs with eyes open, and sometimes wriggling and moving.

Children under six years old consequently require an informal, activity-based method during which they are free to move around. Props such as puppets, teddy-bears, bubbles, music, or a favorite story can also be helpful in promoting and maintaining the child's trance. It is important to be highly flexible, engaging, and informal, and to speak in a manner that absorbs attention and not the quiet soothing tone used with adults.

Despite these differences, children as young as three years have been found capable of significantly altering their sensations and relieving pain during painful medical procedures.[11] These effects occur rapidly, and young children can create partial anesthesia or sensation alteration within a few minutes. Sometimes, during hypnosis, the child's gaze often becomes more fixed – a sign of greater absorption.

Inviting a very young child to enter a hypnotic trance to cope with pain requires a creative fit between the type of pain and the child's frame of reference.

Case example: preschool child and i.v. pain

Logan, a bright five year old, complained about her weekly i.v. vincristine treatments in which she gets cranky, unhappy, and sometimes weepy. The diphenhydramine she was given only took some of the edge off, so her oncologist suggested using hypnosis "to help the time go quicker and for her to feel easier about these treatments." Here are some excerpts from the audiotape made with Logan for her to use during i.v. chemotherapy.

Logan was invited to breathe out and travel inside to her favorite place. Nodding her head when she was there, she began reexploring her "Make-a-Wish" trip to a Carribean resort. She was invited to see its Pegasus horses at the entrance, the aquarium with sharks, manta-rays, and other surprising underwater creatures. "There is so much to see and wonder at, that your whole body can now begin to feel easy, comfortable, while you have fun at the same time. Yes with enough time to have fun, time just goes so quickly… So that when you're ready you can get your bathers on and immediately go down the water slide, feeling the whoosh so fast, yet feeling so safe… and before you know it your chemo would be over and you can go home, happy and satisfied that you did well."

Case commentary

Time distortion is an inherent potential in the hypnotic experience. For a child like Logan, who finds chemo distressing, being able to "leave" the treatment by traveling into her imagination to a favorite experience, enables a negative situation to be transformed into a more pleasant alternative. Adding suggestions for "time going quicker" or being surprised "how soon it is time to go home," is a simple but highly effective suggestion to help taxing situations become more tolerable.

HYPNOSIS WITH SCHOOL-AGE CHILDREN AND ADOLESCENTS

Fit the trance to the nature of the child's pain, their interests, and their beliefs. Gather this information from the child or adolescent, parent, or nurse and incorporate it within the trance experience to increase absorption and improve outcome.

Useful questions to ask are:

- Where would you rather be than here?
- What helped you best when you were in pain before?
- What did you do or think that best helped the pain to go away?
- Where are your favorite places/what are your favorite things to do?

Use this information to weave a relevant and absorbing trance for the child.

- The peak of children's hypnotizability is from 8 to 12 years.[2]
- Most children six years or older are able to sit or lie still, attend, respond to verbal direction, and easily move into a hypnotic trance. They can close their eyes and follow the process of relaxing and releasing muscle tension around the painful site.

- Adolescents' trances more closely resemble those of adults: they will often need longer trances for therapeutic benefit; they take longer to relax and shift away from present reality and longer to return back.
- After their hypnotic trances, children often report their own spontaneous elaborations that reveal the degree to which the child made the trance his own relevant experience. These can be included in future hypnotic sessions.

Case example: school-aged child with headaches

Michael, a somewhat obsessive ten year old, suffered for three years with frequent tension migraine headaches. When asked the questions above, he answered that he would rather be snorkeling in Hawaii. He felt best when he was away from his sister (significantly, he mishcard the second question) and he did not have anything that helped the pain go away, which is a common reply from children with a long history of chronic or recurring pain.

Using a favorite induction method, Michael moved rapidly into trance and confirmed that he was snorkeling in Hawaii. He was able to identify the fish that swam by, the underwater sea life forms he encountered, and continued to provide minute details of this inner experience as it unfolded. He was encouraged to let the seawater wash his headache pain out of his forehead and temples, and to note that the further he went into the coral reef the better and better his head felt. Four minutes into the experience, he reported no headache remaining. With a posthypnotic suggestion that with each practice the pain would drain away faster and he would remain headache free for longer and longer periods, he was invited to return to the room.

Case commentary

The need for control in this intense, somewhat obsessive, boy made it appropriate that he take the lead in developing his trance experience. The more he invested himself in this experience, the more effective it would be. His lead would also ensure a quicker relief from pain. Michael required only one session as follow-up. He remained in charge of his now infrequent headaches and at follow-up proudly confirmed that they were "not a hassle" anymore.

Biofeedback

DEFINITIONS AND BACKGROUND

Biofeedback refers to the use of electronic or electromechanical equipment to measure and then feedback information about physiologic functions.[32] The child or adolescent uses this physiologic information to improve body awareness and gain control of the selected physiologic response in the desired direction. Feedback is provided in a variety of auditory, visual, and even multimedia "game" formats that the patient finds most appealing and understandable. **Figure 40.1** shows two game presentation formats for feedback delivery.

Biofeedback is an ideal self-regulation skill for many children and adolescents because of its immediacy.

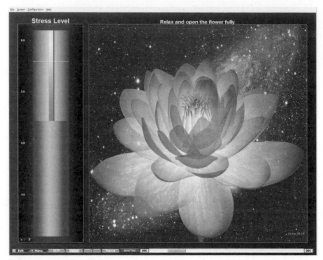

(a)

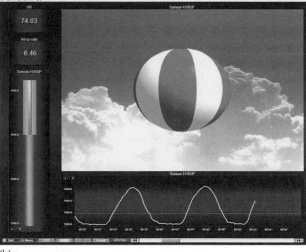

(b)

Figure 40.1 Examples of biofeedback technology from BioTrace software for the NeXus Biofeedback System: (a) The flower animation displayed here is controlled by the child's sweat gland activity (called electrodermal response) which is directly related to "stress level" or sympathetic nervous activity. The child is "rewarded" with the action of the flower opening up, as they are able to relax and reduce sweat gland activity by lowering arousal. (b) The balloon animation displayed here is linked to a device measuring the movement of the child's abdomen in response to breathing. As the child breathes in and the abdomen expands, the balloon increases in size. As the child exhales and the abdomen decreases in size, the balloon deflates. This sequence is useful in teaching "diaphragmatic" breathing as a relaxation technique. Screenshots provided by Stens Corporation (www.stens-biofeedback.com).

Patients quickly and convincingly see the evidence of physiologic control and also dramatically see the evidence for mind–body connections. We have found that children delight in seeing profound, rapid changes in heart rate, breathing, muscle tension, and other physiologic parameters achieved simply by imagining different situations (active versus passive activities) or by thinking of different emotional states (fear versus happiness). With improved somatic awareness and mastery in physiologic control, children can truly see that "a change in thinking causes a change in your body's response." Armed with this confidence, children can take charge of pain-related symptoms in a variety of ways.[5]

Early in the biofeedback experience, it is useful to complete a psychophysiologic stress profile on each child. This identifies the unique pattern of ANS reactivity (an individual's ANS "fingerprint") to different types of stressful stimuli and their ability to recover from such stress. During this procedure, the child is attached to various sensors (temperature, electromyogram (EMG), electrodermal activity (EDA), heart rate (photoplethmysography, PPG), and breathing) and a two-minute baseline is recorded of one relaxation condition with eyes open followed by one with eyes closed. The child is then led through a set of different standardized stressors (such as: cognitive stressor –doing a rapid series of age-appropriate math calculations; physical stressor – controlled painful stimulus such as placing an extremity in an ice-water bath). After each stressor the subject then once again relaxes in eyes-open and eyes-closed conditions to allow for "recovery." The recording is then reviewed and the pattern from arousal to relaxation examined.

The profile can be reviewed with the child as a dramatic example of mind–body connections and as evidence for their ability to recover from stressors. Information about preferred response modality helps to determine which modality to train in subsequent sessions. For example, some children will be sensitive temperature responders with rapid and large changes across each condition in the profile, whereas for others the heart rate or sweat gland activity (EDA) responds more dramatically.

Biofeedback adds precision to the self-regulation skills training experience for both the child in pain and the clinician.

- Biofeedback therapy is designed to enhance each child's sense of mastery and control, promoting a shift from a more external to a more internal "locus of control."
- In certain pain-related conditions, such as headache and Raynaud syndrome, mastering physiologic change in specific ways to specific thresholds, for example increasing peripheral temperature to greater than 92°F, is very helpful in reducing headaches.[32]
- For chronic and recurring pain, physiological control training via biofeedback builds confidence and often

allows the tapering of pain medication. The child develops more trust in the internal healing ability and pain coping strategies, and becomes less reliant on the external help of medication.

- It is highly beneficial in teaching children to control excessive sympathetic nervous system activity, to relax tight muscles, and to change dysfunctional breathing patterns, all of which can commonly be associated with the anxiety component of the pain experience.
- Because of its game-like quality, biofeedback is a user-friendly strategy that is culturally syntonic with today's high-technology youth. It provides immediate, concrete reinforcement with rapid attainment of skill.

Studies have shown that children are excellent at physiologic control of a variety of physiologic functions and are usually better than adults.[20] Biofeedback is currently being used in inpatient and outpatient medical settings and in school-based and community mental health centers. Biofeedback modalities that are most commonly utilized are described in **Table 40.3**.

TEACHING BIOFEEDBACK TO CHILDREN

Biofeedback training with pediatric patients can proceed in an organized fashion while considering the following aspects of training.

- Schedule:
  - Most children can be taught and coached in biofeedback techniques within six to eight 40-minute biofeedback sessions, spaced one to two weeks apart.
  - In the first biofeedback session, the coached children develop an increase in body awareness and physiological control, which is immediately and strongly reinforcing.
  - The first three or four sessions are scheduled approximately one week apart and subsequent sessions are spaced at two-week intervals.
- Practice:
  - The practicing of these self-regulation and relaxation skills at home, at school, and in other relevant settings is emphasized for achieving succesful results.
  - Some patients do best with scheduling daily practice sessions at home in an organized routine, for example a minimum of two five-minute practice sessions at home per day. Other patients do best with situation-specific practice, for example "prior to your math test, breath deeply and relax your muscles."
  - Brief (30 seconds to two minutes) and frequent relaxation minibreaks are also helpful for children with persistent pain complaints.

Table 40.3 Biofeedback modalities and abbreviations and explanations.

Modality	Abbreviation	Explanation
Peripheral temperature (thermography)	TMP	Measures finger temperature, which serves as an indirect measurement of ANS balance; the more stress activity (reflecting increased sympathetic arousal), the less peripheral blood flow, the lower the finger temperature. Relaxation improves peripheral vasodilation and increases finger temperature
Breathing (pneumography)	PNG	Measures abdominal or thoracic movement during respiration utilizing a "stretch" sensor
Exhaled carbon dioxide level (capnography)	CAP	Measures exhaled carbon dioxide. During hyperventilation persons drop CO_2 below the normal range of 38–42 torr
Heart rate (photoplethmysography)	PPG	Measures heart rate via finger pulse
Heart rate variability	HRV	Measures heart rate and related parameters and then utilizes mathematical calculations to look at the balance of the ANS as reflected in heart rate acceleration and deceleration effects. Likely affected by emotional state as well as breathing pattern and rate
Muscle tension (electromyography)	EMG	Measures muscle electrical activity
Skin conductance/ electrodermal activity	EDA	Measures sweat gland activity on the hands by measuring relative skin surface electrical conductance or resistance (which is a function of the number of sweat glands open or closed). Sweat gland activity is sensitive to sympathetic nervous system changes
EEG biofeedback or neurofeedback	EEG	Measures the amount of delta, theta, alpha, and beta waves in various geographic locations on the brain using scalp surface electrodes

– Children are asked to keep a daily log or symptom diary that details practice progress and describes symptoms using a VAS rating system for symptom severity.

– Eventually, a number of cues can be developed with the patient that serve as helpful reminders to use their chosen pain control technique.

Parental involvement

In the first one or two sessions, parents are invited to observe in order to get a general sense of the process, what the practice expectations are, and their role in coaching their child at home. After that, children are usually invited to participate alone with the clinician, so that they give their full attention. This emphasizes their responsibility, choice, and sense of partnership in participating in the therapeutic process.

Physiologic modality

A variety of physiologic modalities may be explored to determine what would be the most responsive to ameliorate the pain symptom. For certain patients, the modality to be trained, for example, temperature, muscle tension, or breathing, is determined by their particular pain symptom. For others, the physiologic modality that is most "hotly" reactive is identified and then trained. There is some debate within the biofeedback field about whether training the specific modality is more important or whether the general process issues are more important. For certain problems where specific etiologic mechanisms can be identified, training to that parameter is indicated.

- Migraine headaches have a vascular reactivity component. Training peripheral finger temperature to increase to levels above 92–95°F on a regular basis decreases migraine frequency and severity. The mechanism includes autonomic nervous system balance changes that may then affect vascular reactivity patterns and/or neurologic irritability.[33]
- Chronic tension headaches display tight and/or asymmetric muscle groups on EMG evaluation in the neck, face, and shoulders. Training in muscle relaxation and symmetry can decrease symptoms.[33]
- Complex regional pain syndrome (CRPS) may involve sympathetic nervous system (SNS) dysregulation in the affected limb and blod flow changes. EDA training to decrease excess SNS activity and peripheral temperature work to enhance blood flow can be helpful. As SNS arousal decreases, blood flow often improves and pain intensity may decrease.
- Raynaud's disorder involves decreased blood flow to the hands and feet, causing pain particularly in cold weather. Peripheral temperature biofeedback training restores normal blood flow ability and ameliorates these symptoms.
- Functional gastrointestinal problems such as irritable bowel syndrome (IBS) and recurrent abdominal pain are often exacerbated with stress activity. Training children in heart rate variability (HRV) biofeedback, peripheral temperature, EDA, or breath control with PNG can be useful in reestablishing ANS balance and decreasing symptoms.[34]

Beyond its value in providing information to the pediatric patient about their body, biofeedback equipment provides physiologic data that are helpful for therapy. Some clinicians routinely monitor physiologic changes during sessions, but do not initially disclose the information. Watching SNS activity and changes when talking about sensitive or uncomfortable topics gives helpful data in determining which themes, topics, and life experiences affect the patient and which are particularly distressing or stimulating. This is particularly helpful with complex pain or somatization disorders in which the physiologic monitoring helps to identify possible emotional and other triggers that, at a minimum, may be exacerbating the child's pain.

Physiologic monitoring can also evaluate progress with other self-regulatory strategies, such as relaxation training or response to certain types of thematic material or mental imagery. These data can be reviewed at a later time in order to facilitate understanding certain response patterns to pain or to reinforce progress or the possibilities for change.[32]

Techniques

In each biofeedback training session, thought is given to select the visual screen displays and auditory feedback options that optimally engage and appropriately challenge each child. Additional therapeutic techniques are used within any one session and across subsequent sessions.

- Mental imagery is commonly employed to provide the opportunity for imaginary or "*in vivo*" rehearsal, to enhance physiologic change, and to deepen the relaxation experience.
- Reframing the problem in manageable terms and with an emphasis on daily function, rather than the limitations created by the symptom.
- A positive self-talk repertoire is developed collaboratively to encourage self-efficacy. As with hypnosis, adjustments to language should reflect each child's developmental level, individual interests, and perspectives.

Case example: biofeedback for headaches

Fifteen-year-old Jenni was referred for chronic daily headaches, which began eight months earlier when school started. Previously, she had experienced only occasional minor headaches. The headaches she reported had continued, unabated, every day since the beginning of the school year. Rated on a VAS to be a "7," Jenni described them as bitemporal and somewhat diffuse and as occurring each day from the time she awoke until midday. In addition, approximately once every two weeks, she would have a more severe, pounding headache associated with nausea which she would have to "sleep off." These were likely migraine headaches. She was missing school more often and her mother was concerned. Ibuprofen and propranolol had not been helpful, and Jenni did not want to try other medications. Jenni liked school, was a good student, and had a close group of friends. She thought stress played some role in the exacerbation of her headaches, which had become a topic of frequent discussion at home.

At the first session, a psychophysiologic stress profile was completed and Jenni saw with interest that even with a mild cognitive stressor (she was asked to do some challenging math problems) her SNS reacted briskly with a decrease in peripheral temperature, increases in heart rate and EDA, and changes in breathing. She recovered to baseline quickly after stress, and this was pointed out as a healthy sign. She learned a basic progressive muscle relaxation and mental imagery exercise and how to track her headaches in a symptom diary.

One week later, at the second session, she brought her calendar and her ratings had not changed much. Diaphragmatic breathing and self-hypnosis on themes of control, healthy functioning, and decreased pain were explored and developed. Jenni was encouraged to reframe her thoughts about headaches and the control they were exerting over her life and, instead, focus on the things she enjoyed doing and could do.

At the third session, Jenni noted she had begun to experience a drop in her daily pain ratings from an unchanging "7" on her VAS to an occasional "4–6 range" rating on some days. She reported that she forgot about headaches altogether while doing her self-hypnosis practice. She had had one probable migraine event that week and had missed one day of school. Her mother also commented that Jenni seemed to be talking less about her headaches at home. At this session, the link between peripheral (finger) temperature and headaches was explored with Jenni. Her baseline finger temperature (nondominant hand, index finger) was 78°F. With direct visual feedback using a colorful pyramid display, Jenni was able to increase finger temperature to 90°F after eight minutes of relaxation. Specific images about warmth and blood flow were explored as another way to facilitate the finger-warming phenomena. Jenni was given temperature bands for home training and instructed in their use, so she could see the same benefits and success with her home practice.

By the fourth session, Jenni was doing much better and had experienced several headache-free days and no migraine episodes. With home training combining breathing, self-hypnosis, and muscle relaxation, she was consistently achieving finger temperatures of 90–92°F. At long-term follow-up a few months later, she had only rare headaches and was utilizing her self-management skills in both preventative and abortive modes for headache

control. She felt confident about her pain control skill, and no longer felt the need to use medication.

Case commentary

The literature supporting biofeedback and relaxation skills training as effective for relieving juvenile migraine and tension-type headaches is quite robust. Randomized, controlled trials and meta-analyses have described the long- and short-term benefits of self-regulation training as being superior to pharmacotherapy.[29, 33] Bifrontal EMG and peripheral temperature training are particularly successful, although the mechanisms by which they effect therapeutic change are not completely understood.

Children and adolescents with chronic, mixed headaches, such as in Jenni's case, can be the most refractory to any treatments. Self-regulation training coupled with effective education about mind–body links and stress management are key ingredients for success. In our experience, the majority of children who suffer from migraine can taper or eliminate medication use, whether it be abortive or preventative medication, after self-regulation training. Decreased reliance on medication and increased self-efficacy are the keys to a successful outcome for this complex pain problem.

Case example: biofeedback for needle phobia

Abbi, a 12-year-old girl, was referred for self-regulation training to control severe needle phobia. She needed immunizations within a few weeks to go on a family overseas trip, and the referring pediatrician had been unsuccessful in gaining Abbi's cooperation for these vaccinations. She screamed and cried uncontrollably at the doctor's office and her parents and professional staff were at a loss to know how to help her.

Abbi recalled only one other experience, a few years prior, when she had venipuncture, which required many attempts to get the sample. She recalls feeling out of control as people held her down. Since that time, she has had a strong fear of needles. Despite those fears, she expressed the desire to help herself.

During the first session, Abbi was taught basic EMG biofeedback and breath control, emphasizing mastery themes. Abbi enjoyed this and did well. During the next session, she was trained in EDA biofeedback as an easy way for her to track her own nervous system's anxiety responses to needles. Over that and the two subsequent sessions, Abbi focused on controlling her SNS response with graduated exposure to elements of the vaccination experience. She learned to control her breathing, heart rate, and SNS activity, as reflected in her maintenance of low EDA readings. She particularly liked a biofeedback screen called "kaleidoscope," in which she erased a complex design of colorful lines and shapes as she decreased her EDA to the desired threshold level.

A vaccination visit plan was then discussed and role-played using actual equipment, but stopped short of giving the injection. She practiced by playing the nurse and giving a "pretend" vaccination to her favorite stuffed animal. Mental imagery was added to her practice regimen, including the idea of imagining herself getting the vaccination, maintaining good control, and noticing how proud she felt. The following week in the biofeedback room, with her EDA sensor attached and running, Abbi demonstrated her self-regulation skill by keeping her EDA at desired levels, staying in control, and receiving her vaccination with minimal distress. She was very proud of her accomplishment.

Case commentary

Needle phobia is a common problem in a variety of settings for children of all ages. Many children report afterwards that the anticipatory anxiety and emotional distress is often worse than the actual "shot" itself. Direct desensitization with the monitoring of a relevant physiologic modality such as EDA, breathing, or heart rate offers an excellent opportunity to reinforce the desired behavioral change. The engaging nature of visual feedback and the ability to set concrete "goals" are helpful for many young children to reinforce their sense of control. Imagery (self-hypnosis) can add a sense of positive expectation for success. Finally, the use of these techniques can heighten curiosity and provide attentional shifts, thus enhancing the focus on something other than the injection pain.

Additionally, it may be helpful to keep in mind how to prevent "needle phobia." We know that children of all ages are overwhelmed by the experience of a painful procedure in a hospital environment and especially by the loss of control. All efforts should be made by the medical team, especially during the first pain painful procedure (as this experience will influence all future events), to empower the child to regain control. Helpful approaches include:

- offering choices to the child as to where to place an EMLA patch;
- choices of where to perform the procedure (such as parent's lap, while standing, sitting, lying, etc.);
- unless in a life-threatening event, children should not be held down for a painful procedure;
- painful procedure should not be performed in a child's hospital bed, as this should be a "safe place;"
- designating a mind/body skills "coach" to facilitate the use of coping, relaxation, and distraction techniques (one healthcare professional or family member has to be solely present for the child's comfort engaging him or her);
- refocus of the patient immediately after the painful event (offer little present out of "treasure box") with praise and commendation on how well the child has done;
- practicing and using bubble blowing or diaphragmatic exhalation to reduce anxiety and increase coping.

DESIGNING SUCCESSFUL MIND/BODY TREATMENT STRATEGIES

A sequential model for mind/body skills training

Children often understand the idea that in pain situations they are in many ways experiencing a mind/body system that is "out of balance." In clinical biofeedback and other types of mind/body skills training, it is helpful to follow a hierarchical structure of tasks from an initial phase where the individual is taught to discriminate (or discern) the difference between a "balanced" and "out of balance" mind/body system to the next step of developing control (where they learn to rebalance the mind/body system in specific ways) and then finally to generalize this skill application to the their everyday life – home, school, sports or wherever.

In the *discern* phase of training, children are taught about mind–body links and physiologic control and are assisted in learning to discriminate differences between states of relaxation (low SNS arousal) and tension/anxiety (high SNS arousal), negative and positive thoughts/feelings, and notice any associated phenomena. They are also coached to carefully and completely tune into inner bodily events and sensations. For example, for the child with muscle tension as part of their pain symptom complex, early recognition of tension in specific muscle groups (such as trapezia or neck muscles) is important in the discern phase. "How does your muscle feel; how fast is your heart beating? Notice your breathing – is it fast or slow? Are you breathing in your chest or shoulders or down in your belly?" Following this the child is asked what these symptoms and body sensations mean or symbolize. Increasing self-awareness of the range of internal messages associated with the pain prepares the child for appropriate and therapeutic responses to those messages.

An efficient and enjoyable way to train an initial sense of body awareness is by discrimination training with surface EMG. Children can quickly learn to identify even low levels of tension and/or muscle asymmetry with biofeedback and then correct this problem. Eventually, they can do this without the presence of immediate visual or auditory feedback. They develop acute awareness of the target symptom or sensation and then can act preemptively to control it. One of the distinct benefits of biofeedback training is the enhanced capacity for "somatic awareness."

It is important to note that, for children, baseline values for individual physiologic modalities may vary somewhat. Baseline values across sessions can also vary, particularly for EDA and peripheral temperature.

In the control phase of training, patients are coached to master specific skills and to achieve certain trends or threshold goals in training a specific physiologic function.

- The child might be helped to consistently maintain a bifrontal EMG reading below 3 mV, an EDA below

5 µmho with directed relaxation, or a finger temperature of 93–95°F. All of these would be common goals and would reflect a desirable level of lowered SNS activity.

- With diaphragmatic breathing, children master the ability to relax chest and thoracic musculature, achieve good abdominal movement (measured by PNG), breathe at a slow pace, and maintain an inhalation time of two to three seconds with an exhalation time of five to six seconds.
- With favorite place imagery, a child can be coached to develop a general sense of comfort and relaxation.

We begin with a home practice recommendation of five minutes twice a day to foster comfort, confidence, and experience with these techniques. Note that for children it is not necessary to achieve rigidly defined predetermined goals for any given physiologic change. General trends in physiologic change (warmer hands, less muscle tension) are indicative of a desired shift to a more balanced state of mind and body and are more important than absolute magnitude of change. In this training phase, many children find that specific mental imagery enhances the rapidity with which they can regulate their level of change for a given modality; for example, imagining warmth- and relaxation-related experiences to facilitate their own peripheral temperature change.

The generalize phase is often the most challenging part of biofeedback training as the patient begins to apply the learned skills successfully in the appropriate real-life situation or environment without the machine or the clinician. Most children enjoy quick success in the discern and control sessions, and within three to five sessions most are achieving the desired physiologic control goals in the biweekly office-based sessions.

For transfer of skills to take place:

- Triggers and cues are identified with the patient that will alert them to apply their self-management skills. Early pain signals that were previously ignored now cue the child to engage in the selected helpful strategies.
- Parents and teachers are encouraged to help cue in ways that are agreed upon with the child.
- Role playing specific situations with the patient to elicit emotional arousal and/or imaginal rehearsal techniques can prepare them for the real-life stimulus.
- Usually, one or two long-term follow-up sessions or refresher sessions are set up two to four months from the initial sessions to check on long-term progress and to offer any support and adjustments needed to the plan.
- Clients can be sent home with portable hand-held biofeedback trainers so that daily biofeedback practice can occur between office visits.

Integrating mind/body therapies

Mind/body skills can be used to facilitate the therapeutic relationship and have many positive attributes.

- Biofeedback is a comfortable, nonthreatening, and quite playful way to begin the pain management process, build rapport, and elicit a sense of curiosity while concretely demonstrating bidirectional mind–body influences.
- Relaxation enhances emotional comfort and willingness to communicate.
- Biofeedback is similar to that of induction techniques used in hypnosis and hypnotherapy. Watching the visual feedback and listening to a monotonous auditory-guiding feedback tone tends to narrow attention and increase awareness of internal body events and sensations, which open the door to further discussion of these phenomena.
- States of deep relaxation enhance access to unconscious material and facilitate fantasy and imagery. With the development of an alternative state of awareness during biofeedback training, the child may be more open to therapeutic suggestion for pain and distress reduction.

Self-hypnosis can be a very useful addition in the later stages of biofeedback training. Adding "age progression," in which the child sees himself in the future as healthy, functional, and pain free, brings that possibility closer and sets a positive expectation for symptom control in a finite time span.

- It may be that most mind/body techniques including hypnosis and biofeedback training are pathways to the same end point – a state of heightened suggestibility and lowered ANS arousal where patients can make choices about pain perception, control, and change.
- Diaphragmatic breathing, relaxation methods, biofeedback, and hypnosis are commonly integrated in the therapeutic process of relieving a child's pain. In fact, for most pediatric patients, biofeedback training leads to an altered state of awareness with narrowed, highly focused attention, facilitation of a state of comfort and relaxation, and facilitation of a sense of control – just like that described in hypnosis.
- Some children and adolescents enjoy the added visual and sensory feedback elements and find that they accelerate their somatic awareness and subsequent pain modulation ability. Others move quickly beyond the need for external feedback cues and cultivate the "internal" imagery experience in mastering their pain symptoms.
- Simply training a child to change a physiologic modality such as heart rate or breathing does not

necessarily result in immediate pain reduction. However, by integrating this body control training with somatic awareness, therapeutic suggestions, and new ways of understanding self-control, many children experience benefits.

- Children and adolescents are highly active participants in therapy and are offered several approaches or options depending on their interests, developmental level, and coping style. Our role is as a "coach." The ultimate responsibility for success rests with the patient. Nevertheless, skilled guidance, rapport, honesty, and a true sense of partnership are key ingredients in this undertaking to control pain.

Mind/body therapies: mechanism of therapeutic change

Thoughts and emotions can directly influence physiologic response systems and processes, such as blood flow, muscle tension, release of hormones, neuropeptides, inflammatory mediators, and other immune system changes, all of which play a role in the production of pain. In addition to spinal control mechanisms of nociceptive transmission, descending pathways that originate in the cortex and thalamus can play a significant role in modulating each person's pain perception and experience. The gate control theory of pain suggests that thoughts, beliefs, and emotions may affect how much pain you feel from any given physical sensation.[35] The ability to plan and actively modulate pain perception via connecting pathways from the central nervous system (CNS) gives rise to consideration of a number of therapeutic interventions that may work centrally to "close the gates" via these descending CNS influences.[36]

Melzack[37] postulates an essential interplay between central and peripheral nervous systems with regard to the pain experience and pain experience pathways that are partly innate and partly learned. Calling this neural network "the neuromatrix," the likely basis for one's physical wiring, he proposes that it plays a role in pain and somatic awareness. Being somewhat malleable, it acquires its individual reaction patterns or its "neurosignature" through repeated activation. Perhaps self-regulatory strategies modify these pain reaction pathways both consciously and unconsciously to reconfigure an individual's response tendency.

We do not fully understand the hypnotic process, but it is agreed that, as a state of altered consciousness, hypnosis is different both from the normal waking state and from the different stages of sleep. Hypnosis resembles various meditative states, with its narrowly focused attention, primary process thinking, and ego-receptivity.[2] Some have postulated that hypnosis decreases anxiety rather than affecting the pain sensation itself. Hypnosis does decrease anxiety and thereby increases pain tolerance, but this is not the predominant mechanism of action for hypnoanalgesia and hypnoanesthesia. Recent studies also support that individuals undergoing certain hypnotic experiences demonstrate significant changes in regional cerebral bloodflow as evidenced by function MRI techniques.[38] The neurobiological impact of imagery is also being explored. One study in 2005 by Raij et al.[39] demonstrated that individuals who experienced hypnosis-induced pain show evidence for activation of the brain's cerebral pain circuitry similar to that which occurs in response to pain of organic origin (laser irritation of skin). Studies also suggest that within the hypnotic state, ANS balance as reflected in heart rate variability patterns is modulated mostly by decreasing sympathetic nervous system activity but may reflect increased parasympathetic activity as well.[40, 41]

With the discovery of endorphins, there was speculation that the key to the mechanism of action of hypnoanalgesia had been found. The hypothesis that hypnosis is the natural way of releasing endorphins has not yet been supported by research.[42] Hypnotic analgesia for experimental pain was not reversed by the administration of naloxone hydrochloride. Furthermore, in contrast to the elevated endorphin levels in patients experiencing acupuncture,[43] patients experiencing hypnotic analgesia showed no increase in endorphin levels.[42] Current findings in this intriguing area of inquiry may have methodological pitfalls, particularly problems in measurement. Melzack and Wall's gate control theory of pain provides one rationale for the effectiveness of hypnosis in the control of pain.[35] The theory is far from a full explanation of hypnotic action.

Research suggests that successful self-regulation strategies operate on multiple levels with multifactorial mechanisms of therapeutic change.[44] A variety of potential mediators in pain control, both specific and nonspecific, may play a role.

Potential specific mechanisms of pain control with mind/body strategies may include:

- decreased sympathetic nervous system activity: there is evidence that SNS activity up-modulates pain conduction;[45]
- specific physiologic changes that are condition specific: such as muscle relaxation and symmetry training in tension headache; reduction in excessive SNS activity in irritable bowel syndrome; reduction in inflammatory mediators secondary to specific therapeutic suggestion for burns;
- downregulation of pain activity through the descending inhibitory pathway;
- unidentified neuroelectrical/neurochemical/ neurometabolic/somatic changes.

Potential nonspecific mechanisms of pain control with mind/body strategies include:

- the shift from an external to a more internal locus of control enhances sense of self-efficacy in the control of pain;

- positive expectancy, also called placebo factor, "faith factor," and hopefulness;
- the active partnership and rapport with the clinician;
- cognitive reframing of the pain, which occurs particularly in many mind/body techniques, does not necessarily change pain intensity but shifts its relevance, quality, attention, and secondary gain factors allowing for enhanced functioning.

Limitations of mind/body therapies

Biofeedback and hypnosis are not panaceas, and care must be taken to understand their indications, contra-indications, and limitations.[2]

- Biofeedback training and hypnosis are usually not suitable for children who are psychotic or severely depressed, and should be undertaken with extreme caution in children with posttraumatic stress disorder (PTSD) and other severe emotional problems.
- In certain cases, the scientific literature supports the use of a specific biofeedback modality for a specific disorder. Seek supervision and case consultation when in doubt.[3]
- Only use biofeedback training with children who present with pain complaints/diagnoses that are well within one's scope of training and expertise.
- Be honest with parents and with patients about the expected length of therapy and reasonable expectations for hypnosis and the biofeedback training process.
- Mind/body skills should not be pursued in place of necessary, life-saving conventional treatments and treatment approaches should be appropriately prioritized after discussion with all relevant parties.[46]

In a 1987 study, Olness and Libbey[47] found that 20 percent of children referred for self-regulation training (primarily hypnosis) had a previously undiagnosed biologic etiology for their condition. This study underscores that all children presenting with pain symptoms require thorough medical and neurologic evaluation to rule out organic conditions that may contribute to the presenting symptom. For example, children with headaches and abdominal pain need specific medical and neurologic evaluation to rule out tumor, infectious, and metabolic problems that may cause recurrent pain.

Concurrent use of psychotropic, anti-inflammatory or analgesic medication is not a contraindication to self-hypnosis, biofeedback or other relaxation training, but needs to be carefully managed on a case-by-case basis. Certain psychotropic agents will change ANS responsivity and so may affect baseline biofeedback measurements and the child's ability to modulate certain modalities, such as peripheral temperature, heart rate, and skin conductance. Some children can reduce or even eliminate the need for certain medications when mind/body skills training is successful (e.g. decrease or eliminate analgesic use in juvenile migraine). This must be carefully coordinated with the prescribing physician.

TRAINING AND CERTIFICATION

Formal training is recommended for those interested in applying this powerful group of techniques. Training in hypnosis occurs through the Society for Developmental and Behavioral Pediatrics Workshops (www.sdbp.org) and The American Society for Clinical Hypnosis (www.asch.org). Certification in hypnosis is available through the American Society for Clinical Hypnosis and also through the American Boards of Clinical Hypnosis. Training in biofeedback is available by contacting the Association for Applied Psychophysiology and Biofeedback (www.aapb.org) or the Biofeedback Foundation of Europe (www.bfe.org). Professional certification is available through the Biofeedback Certification Institute of America (www.bcia.org). Certification in either field includes both course work and clinical supervision, as well as written and practical exams.

CONCLUSION

Every human has the capacity to examine, appreciate, and regulate our inner experience and reactions to pain. Mind/body strategies, such as hypnosis and biofeedback, uniquely and directly cultivate these internal abilities to modulate and reduce pain phenomena. Within the last decade, self-regulation strategies have moved to the forefront of evidence-based, practical approaches for clinical pediatric pain management. The strategies continue to be supported by empirical research and by practical application and success in clinical settings. These uniquely valuable tools for managing pain in children and adolescents are: (1) biofeedback, with its "hi-tech" appeal; (2) hypnosis, which uses innate imaginative abilities; (3) diaphragmatic breathing, a fundamental physiological index of distress and pain; and (4) other relaxation approaches (meditation, yoga, autogenics), all of which offer training to counteract the tension and preoccupation of pain.

Pain drains a child's energy and reduces their ability to cope. The experience of pain is demonstrated to have potential long-term, negative effects on children and adolescents. However, the practice of self-regulation techniques appears to mitigate much of the negative impact of pain on children and their functioning. These methods facilitate competency and a sense of mastery over nociception, anxiety, and distress, and also enable children to take a more active part in and responsibility for treatment and recovery.

Individuals who actively engage in some form of self-regulation appear to have an improved quality of life.[48]

Children who master self-regulation skills acquire special "life skills" that can be utilized in future experiences of pain and stress. Early training in self-regulation skills, self-hypnosis, or biofeedback may also be an important disease-prevention tool in pediatrics due to growing evidence that effective management of pain and associated emotional distress improves long-term prognosis.

The most commonly raised objection from medical and nursing staff to the use of self-regulatory strategies is "I don't have time." This assumes that self-regulation training is lengthy and removed from medical treatment. It need not be. Over the last 25 years, we have learned a great deal about how rapidly patients in pain respond to hypnosis, and how shock and anxiety increase a person's receptivity to suggestion. Teaching children about mind–body connections does not necessarily require expensive computerized biofeedback equipment. Imagination and creative thinking combined with a thermometer in the clinic room, a pulse oximeter in the emergency room, or a scale in the triage room – these can all be used as "biofeedback" devices to help patients to understand their bodies and begin to develop self-control, confidence, and relief from pain. What is required by the practitioner is the ability to engage with children creatively, flexibly, with passion, and a sense of humor. Mind/body strategies and related nondrug approaches should be integrated with appropriate pharmacologic interventions in all settings where pediatric pain is managed and it is certain that they will continue to serve as powerful, front-line tools for children of all ages.

REFERENCES

* 1. Astin J. Mind-Body Therapies for the management of pain. *Clinical Journal of Pain.* 2004; **20**: 27–32.
* 2. Olness K, Kohen DP. *Hypnosis and hypnotherapy with children*, 3rd edn. New York: Guilford Press, 1996.
* 3. Culbert T, Banez G. Pediatric Applications of biofeedback other than headache. In: Schwartz M, Andrasik F (eds). *Biofeedback: a practitioners guide*, 3rd edn. New York: Guilford Press, 2003.
* 4. Tsao J, Zeltzer L. Complementary and alternative medicine approaches for pediatric pain: a review of the state-of-the-science. *Evidence-based Complementary and Alternative Medicine.* 2005; **2**: 149–59.
  5. Sussman D, Culbert T. Pediatric self-regulation. In: Levine MD, Crocker AC, Carey WB (eds). *Developmental–behavioral pediatrics*, 3rd edn. Philadelphia: WB Saunders, 1999.
  6. Astin J, Shapiro S, Eisenberg D, Forys K. Mind-body medicine: state of the science, implications for practice. *Journal of the American Board of Family Medicine.* 2003; **16**: 131–47.
  7. Cohen S, Herbert T. Health psychology: psychological factors and physical disease from the perspective of human psychoneuroimmunology. *Annual Review of Psychology.* 1996; **47**: 113–42.
  8. Butler LD, Symons BK, Henderson SL *et al.* Hypnosis reduces distress and duration of an invasive medical procedure for children. *Pediatrics.* 2005; **115**: e77–85.
  9. Zeltzer LK, Tsao JC, Stelling C *et al.* A phase I study on the feasibility and acceptability of an acupuncture/hypnosis Intervention for chronic pediatric pain. *Journal of Pain and Symptom Management.* 2002; **24**: 437–46.
  10. World Health Organization (WHO) Guidelines. *Cancer pain relief and palliative care in children.* Geneva: World Health Organization, 1998: 24–8.
* 11. Kuttner L. *A child in pain, how to help, what to do.* Vancouver: Hartley and Marks, 1996. Available from: www.bookstore.cw.bc.ca
  12. Gerik S. Pain management in children: developmental considerations and mind-body therapies. *Southern Medical Journal.* 2005; **98**: 295–302.
  13. Sugarman L. *Imaginative medicine: hypnosis is pediatric practice.* Video documentary (70 min), 1997. Available from: www.laurencesugarman.com.
  14. Kuttner L. *No fears, no tears, children with cancer coping with pain.* Video documentary (27 min), Boston, MA, USA: Fanlight Productions, 1985. Available from: www.fanlight.com.
  15. Kuttner L. *No fears, no tears – 13 years later.* Video documentary on the long-term impact of children's pain control, Boston, MA, USA: Fanlight Productions, 1998. Available from: www.fanlight.com.
* 16. Blount R, Piira T, Cohen L, Cheng P. Pediatric procedural pain. *Behavior Modification.* 2006; **30**: 24–49.
  17. Kohen D. Application of relaxation mental imagery in pediatric emergencies. *International Journal of Clinical and Experimental Hypnosis.* 1986; **34**: 283–94.
  18. Goldie C. Hypnosis in the casualty department. *British Medical Journal.* 1956; **2**: 1340–2.
  19. Piira T, Sugiura T, Champion GD *et al.* The role of parental presence in the context of children's medical procedures: a systematic review. *Child: Care, Health and Development.* 2005; **31**: 233–43.
  20. Attanasio V, Andrasik F, Burke E *et al.* Clinical issues in utilizing biofeedback with children. *Clinical Biofeedback and Health.* 1985; **8**: 134–41.
  21. Culbert T. Biofeedback with children and adolescents. In: Schaefer C (ed.). *Innovative psychotherapy techniques in child and adolescent therapy*, 2nd edn. New York: John Wiley & Sons, 1999.
  22. Kajander R, Peper E. Teaching diaphragmatic breathing to children. *Biofeedback.* 1998; **26**: 14–17.
  23. Calipel S, Lucas-Polomeni MM, Wodey E, Ecoffey C. Premedication in children: hypnosis versus midazolam. *Pediatric Anaesthesia.* 2005; **15**: 275–81.
  24. Lambert S. The effects of hypnosisguided imagery on the postoperative course of children. *Journal of Developmental and Behavioral Pediatrics.* 1996; **17**: 307–10.

25. Lassetter J. The effectiveness of complementary therapies on the pain experience of hospitalized children. *Journal of Holistic Nursing.* 2006; **24**: 196–208.

26. Liossi C, White P, Hatira P. Randomized clinical trial of local anesthetic versus a combination of local anesthetic with self-hypnosis in the management of pediatric procedure-related pain. *Health Psychology.* 2006; **25**: 307–15.

27. Liossi C, Hatira P. Clinical hypnosis in the alleviation of procedure related pain in pediatric oncology patients. *International Journal of Clinical and Experimental Hypnosis.* 2003; **51**: 4–28.

28. Richardson J, Smith J, McCall G, Pilkington K. Hypnosis for procedure related pain and distress in pediatric cancer patients: a systematic review of effectiveness and methodology related to hypnosis interventions. *Journal of Pain and Symptom Management.* 2006; **31**: 7084.

29. Olness K, MacDonald J, Uden D. Comparison of self-hypnosis and propranolol in the treatment of juvenile classic migraine. *Pediatrics.* 1987; **79**: 593–7.

30. Anbar R. Self hypnosis for the treatment of functional abdominal pain in childhood. *Clinical Pediatrics.* 2001; **40**: 447–51.

31. Weydert JA, Shapiro DE, Acra SA *et al.* Evaluation of guided imagery as treatment for recurrent abdominal pain in children: A randomized controlled trial. *BMC Pediatrics.* 2006; **6**: 29.

* 32. Culbert T, Reamcy J, Kohen D. Cyberphysiologic strategies for children: the clinical hypnosis, biofeedback interface. *International Journal of Clinical and Experimental Hypnosis.* 1994; **442**: 97–117.

33. Andrasik F, Schwartz M. Behavioral assessment and treatment of pediatric headache. *Behavior Modification.* 2006; **30**: 93–113.

34. Humphreys P, Gevirtz R. Treatment of recurrent abdominal pain: components analysis of four treatment protocols. *Journal of Pediatric Gastroenterology and Nutrition.* 2000; **31**: 47–51.

35. Melzack R. From the gate to the neuromatrix. *Pain.* 1999; (Suppl. 6): S121–6.

36. Holyrod J. Hypnosis treatment of clinical pain: understanding why hypnosis is useful. *International Journal of Clinical and Experimental Hypnosis.* 1996; **44**: 33–51.

37. Melzack R. Phantom limb pains and the concept of the neuromatrix. *Trends in Neurosciences.* 1990; **13**: 88–92.

38. Raz A, Fan J, Posner M. Hypnotic suggestion reduces conflict in the human brain. *Mental Health Nursing.* 2005; **102**: 9978–83.

39. Raij TT, Numminen J, Närvänen S *et al.* Brain correlates of subjective reality of physically and psychologically induced pain. *Proceedings of the National Academy of Sciences of the United States of America.* 2005; **102**: 2147–51.

40. DeBenedittis G, Cigada M, Bianchi A *et al.* Autonomic changes during hypnosis: a heart rate variability power spectrum analysis as a marker of sympatho-vagal balance. *International Journal of Clinical and Experimental Hypnosis.* 1994; **42**: 140–52.

41. Hippel C, Hole G, Kaschka W. Autonomic profile under hypnosis as assessed by heart rate variability and spectral analysis. *Pharmacopsychiatry.* 2001; **34**: 111–13.

42. Moret V, Forster A, Laverrière *et al.* Mechanism of analgesia induced by hypnosis and acupuncture: is there a difference? *Pain.* 1991; **45**: 135–40.

43. Pintov S, Lahat E, Alstein M *et al.* Acupuncture and the opiod system: implications in the management of migraine. *Pediatric Neurology.* 1997; **17**: 129–33.

44. Jensen MP, McArthur KD, Barber J *et al.* Satisfaction with and beneficial side effects of hypnotic analgesia. *International Journal of Clinical and Experimental Hypnosis.* 2006; **54**: 432–47.

45. Baron R, Levine JD, Fields HL. Causalgia and reflex sympathetic dystrophy: does the sympathetic nervous system contribute to the generation of pain? *Muscle and Nerve.* 1999; **22**: 678–95.

46. Cohen M, Kemper K. Complementary therapies in pediatrics: a legal perspective. *Pediatrics.* 2005; **115**: 774–80.

47. Olness K, Libbey P. Unrecognized biologic basis for behavioral symptoms in children referred for hypnotherapy. *American Journal of Clinical Hypnosis.* 1987; **30**: 1–8.

48. Bakal D. *Minding the body: clinical uses of somatic awareness.* New York: The Guilford Press, 1999.

PART III

CLINICAL TRIALS

41

Placebo and nocebo

LUANA COLLOCA, DAMIEN G FINNISS, AND FABRIZIO BENEDETTI

KEY LEARNING POINTS

- A placebo is a treatment with no specific therapeutic action and the placebo effect is the outcome following its administration.
- The placebo effect is a psychobiological phenomenon and must not be confounded with other phenomena, such as spontaneous remission.
- The effects following the administration of a placebo are due to the psychosocial context around the therapy.
- A positive psychosocial context may induce a placebo effect whereas a negative context may lead to a nocebo effect.

- There is not a single placebo effect but many, in different systems and diseases and with different mechanisms.
- The placebo analgesic effect is mediated by the endogenous opioid systems in some circumstances.
- The nocebo hyperalgesic effect is mediated by anxiety-induced activation of cholecystokininergic systems.
- If an analgesic treatment is administered covertly, its effects are smaller than when given overtly.

INTRODUCTION

Over the past two decades the placebo effect has shifted from being a nuisance in clinical research to a promising model of an emerging neuroscience of mind–brain–body interactions. In fact, the interest in and the success of placebo research resides in its multifaceted meaning, which involves key issues in modern science – from neurobiology to philosophy, from ethics to social psychology, and from clinical trials design to medical practice.[1] Thus, the placebo effect, which has long been neglected by the neuroscience community, is today considered a real and detectable biological phenomenon, and the question of whether placebos work has been reframed as to how they work. The purpose of this chapter is to introduce the reader to the nature and extent of the placebo phenomenon and to present the interesting implications of the new evidence that arises from recent research in this field. The relatively extensive overview and reference base will permit a more detailed exploration of specific topics, issues, and questions. Overall, this chapter presents what we know today about the neural mechanisms underlying the placebo effect, as well as the clinical and ethical implications in routine medical practice and in clinical trials.

Placebo is the Latin word for "I shall please" and although it would seem that there are some anomalies in both the origin and the translations of the word placebo, the term "placebo" entered the medical lexicon to indicate sham treatments and inert substances (such as sugar pills and saline solutions) that physicians give deliberately to please or placate anxious patients.[2, 3, 4]

Physicians have perhaps always been conscious of the fact that patients get better after taking inert drugs.[5, 6, 7] However, it is clear that the history of placebos is not the history of the placebo effects. In fact, the history of placebos concerns their use in clinical trials for the validation of new treatments, whereas the history of placebo effects pertains to the studies on the psychosocial therapeutic effect following the administration of inert medical treatments.

Brody[8] emphasized the role of symbolic meaning, defining the placebo effect as a change in the body, or the body-mind unit, that occurs as a result of the symbolic significance which one attributes to an event or object in the healing environment. This definition is embedded in the notion that symbols induce expectations of an outcome, thus emphasizing the crucial role of meaning[9, 10] and expectation.[11] In other words, the therapeutic context has a meaning that induces expectations which, in turn, shape experience and behavior, as emphasized by Kirsch.[11, 12, 13] According to Moerman,[9, 10] the term placebo effect deflects our attention from what is really important (the meaning and the meaning-induced expectations), and aims it at what is not (the inert pills and, in general, the inert medical treatments).

The concept of the placebo effect as a context effect has been stressed by several authors.[14, 15] The context is made up of words, attitudes, provider's behavior, and medical devices, or in other words what Balint[16] called the whole atmosphere around the treatment. It has often been pointed out that the term "context effect" and "placebo effect" could be used, at least in part, interchangeably[14, 15] in order to overcome the negative connotations associated with the term placebo and to highlight the therapeutic nature of the healthcare context. The weight of context in facilitating cognitive and emotional modulation of a therapeutic outcome definitively emerges from different therapeutic outcomes after an open or hidden administration of the same drug. The main finding is that when the patient is completely unaware that a treatment is being given, the treatment is less effective than when it is given overtly according to routine medical practice.[17] Therefore, under such conditions, the placebo effect can be defined as the difference between open and hidden administration of the treatment, even though no placebo is given. The result of this subtraction represents the placebo component of a treatment. According to the context and to context-induced expectations, placebos may produce either positive or negative outcomes. To distinguish the pleasing from the noxious effects of placebo, several authors introduced and elaborated the term nocebo.[18, 19, 20, 21] The term *nocebo* ("I shall harm") was specifically chosen to denote the counterpart of the term *placebo*. If the meaning of the context is reversed in the opposite direction, a nocebo effect can be obtained. However, Kennedy[18] and Kissel and Barrucand[19] differentiate nocebo from placebo only in terms of negative or positive outcomes, not in terms of expectations.[20, 21, 22]

In spite of all these definitions, the term placebo/ nocebo effect often remains a source of confusion and of dangerous misconception. "Placebos are inert and don't cause anything" asserts Moerman.[9] As an anthropologist, he suggests the use of the formulation "meaning response" rather than "placebo response." The meaning response is defined as the physiological or psychological effects of meaning on the treatment or illness. Conceptualizing the issue in terms of meaning may be important from an evolutionary perspective.[23]

ATTEMPTS TO QUANTIFY THE PLACEBO EFFECT

Over the years, many researchers have turned to clinical trials literature to learn more about the placebo effect. We will be presenting the most representative. The first attempt to quantify the therapeutic effect of placebos was by Henry K Beecher in 1955,[24] who published "The powerful placebo," a paper reviewing 15 controlled trials involving 1802 patients. Defining positive outcomes as "percent satisfactorily relieved by placebo," Beecher reported effect sizes ranging from 26 to 58 percent with an average of 35 percent. The notion that approximately one-third of patients respond to placebo has since permeated medical text and teachings, even though Henry K Beecher did not report that number. This early work has been criticized on methodological grounds.[7, 25, 26]

However, despite some methodological limitations, Beecher's view represents a seminal demonstration of the placebo effect in medical practice.[24] In the 1950s, he suspected that some surgical treatments may also lead to a placebo effect. At the time, mammary artery ligation was provided for patients suffering from angina pectoris. In 1959, Cobb and co-workers[27] tested this procedure using a double-blind design. Surgeons were shown a randomization card after skin incision, telling them whether to proceed with surgery or to close the wound (sham procedure). Patients and outcomes observers were blinded as to the allocation of the real or the sham procedure. Patients in both groups improved dramatically, with trends favoring skin incision. After further similar results,[28] Beecher[29] concluded that a placebo effect is also demonstrable for surgery.

Opposite claims about the placebo effect are made by Hróbjartsson and Gøtzsche.[30] These authors conducted a systematic review of clinical trials in which patients were randomly assigned to either placebo or no treatment. Today, this review remains a source of intense debate. The goal was to study the clinical effect of placebos discerning whether patients randomized to placebo under blind conditions have better outcomes than those randomized to no treatment. One hundred and thirty trials were identified and 40 different clinical outcomes investigated by selecting binary (e.g. the proportion of alcohol abusers and nonalcohol abusers) and continuous (e.g. the amount of alcohol consumed) outcomes. They considered the effect of three types of placebos: pharmacological (e.g. a pill), physical (e.g. a manipulation), and psychological (e.g. conversation). They calculated the pooled relative risk for binary outcomes and the pooled standardized mean differences for continuous outcomes, where pooled relative risk was defined as the ratio of the number of patients with an unwanted outcome to the total number of patients in the placebo group, divided by the same ratio in the untreated group. The standardized mean difference was defined as the difference between the mean values for unwanted outcomes in the placebo and untreated groups divided by the pooled standard deviation. A negative value indicated a beneficial effect of placebo both for binary and continuous outcomes. The findings of Hróbjartsson and Gøtzsche's review did not detect a significant effect of placebo, as compared with no treatment, in pooled data from trials with subjective or objective binary or continuous objective outcomes. However, they found a significant difference between placebo and no treatment in trials with subjective outcomes and in trials involving the treatment of pain. There was also some evidence that placebos had greater effect in small trials with continuous outcomes than in large trials, with an inverse relation between trial size and placebo size. Furthermore, in an update of their first review, Hróbjartsson and Gøtzsche argued further that when a large effect of a placebo intervention is not present, small effects on continuous outcomes, for example in pain, could not be clearly distinguished from biases.[31] Thus, the observed significant effect of placebo on subjective outcomes may have been due to biased reports of subjects rather than to true placebo effects.

However, it is important to note that they used very broad inclusion criteria and failed to recognize that placebos are not expected to work uniformly across diseases or disorders.[32, 33, 34, 35, 36, 37, 38, 39, 40, 41, 42, 43, 44, 45, 46] Aggregating without regard to the heterogeneity of disorders does not allow us to discern whether a placebo effect really exists. In fact, different sizes of placebo effects might occur among different disorders that do not have the same mechanism of action. Another problematic aspect of the Hróbjartsson and Gøtzsche's meta-analysis is the fact that in this analysis, it is impossible to consider many critical factors involved in placebo responses, such as the consideration of the patient's and physician's expectations, the healing context, and the many cues and factors that can influence the efficacy of an intervention.[1, 9, 14, 15, 22, 47]

In another study aimed at investigating the placebo effect in analgesic studies only, Vase et al.[48] conducted one meta-analysis that included 23 of the 29 clinical trials from the meta-analysis by Hróbjartsson and Gøetzsche[30] and another meta-analysis of 14 studies that investigated placebo analgesic mechanisms. Although this study has been criticized by Hróbjartsson and Gøtzsche,[49] Vase et al.[48] found that the magnitudes of the placebo analgesic effects were higher in studies that investigated placebo analgesic mechanisms compared with clinical trials where the placebo was used only as a control condition. Vase et al.[48] suggest that this difference might be due to the different placebo instructions and suggestions given in the clinical trial setting compared to the experimental setting. In fact, clinical trial investigators typically avoid giving oral suggestions of analgesia in favor of neutral instructions, whereas investigators of the placebo effect typically emphasize the analgesic suggestions.

The literature is full of other studies indicating that beliefs and expectations can play a relevant role in human health. For example, it has long been known that placebo injections are more powerful than placebo pills,[50, 51] placebos taken four times a day are more powerful than placebos taken twice a day,[3] red and yellow tables make better stimulants, while blue or green tablets better tranquilizers,[52] and sham devices (validated sham acupuncture needle) have greater effects than placebo pill on self-reported pain and severity of symptoms.[53]

In general, these meta-analyses are worthy of consideration because they present the scenario for two different ways of investigating the placebo effect: on the one hand the randomized clinical trial (RCT), and on the other, the clinical/experimental setting specifically designed to investigate the placebo effect.

HOW TO DETECT REAL PLACEBO RESPONSES

The term "placebo effect" is often used interchangeably with the term "placebo response." However, the term "placebo effect" refers to any average improvement in the condition of a group of subjects that has received a placebo manipulation. Conversely, the term "placebo response" refers to the change in an individual caused by a placebo manipulation. In order to detect a real placebo response, it is important to consider some confounding factors in addition to the appropriateness of the experimental design. In fact, the investigation of the placebo effect is full of drawbacks and pitfalls because for a placebo response to be demonstrated several other phenomena must be ruled out.[1, 54, 55, 56] These phenomena are natural history, regression to the mean, false-positive errors, and co-interventions (**Figure 41.1**).

For example, many pathological conditions show spontaneous variation and fluctuation of symptoms over time that is known as natural history.[57, 58] Relapses and remissions can occur in the absence of any treatment manipulation. If a subject takes a placebo just before his/her discomfort starts decreasing, he/she may believe that the placebo is effective, although that decrease would have occurred anyway. Clearly, this is not a placebo effect but a spontaneous remission that leads to a misinterpretation

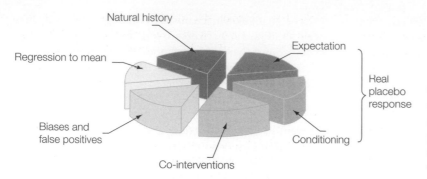

Figure 41.1 Confounding factors which must be ruled out in order to demonstrate real placebo responses (expectation and/or conditioning). The percentages of each factor does not necessarily reflect reality, as there are no studies providing this information.

of the cause–effect relationship. To demonstrate a placebo effect one must show a difference between the natural history and the placebo intervention. Another example is related to regression to the mean. This refers to the phenomenon where a variable will tend to move closer to the center of the distribution from initial to later measurements. This is a mathematical property of all measurements subject to random error. Subsequent measurements tend to be lower, because of the regression to the mean, even if no biologically or psychologically mediated placebo effects are present.[59] If individuals tend to receive their initial clinical assessment when their pain is near its greatest intensity, then their pain level is likely to be lower when they return for a second pain assessment. In this case also, the improvement cannot be attributed to any intervention they might have undergone. Regression to the mean often appears together with placebo effects in clinical trials, and the only reliable way to see what proportion of an observed improvement might actually be attributable to the placebo manipulation is again to compare a group receiving a placebo to a group receiving no treatment. A further source of confusion is represented by a particular type of error made by the patient and/or physician, a false-positive error. This is known as signal detection theory (SDT) and was described by Allan and Siegel[60] as a possible mechanism of placebo effects. The ambiguity of a symptom may lead to biases following verbal suggestion of benefit. In other words, a patient can report that a substance makes him or her feel better, detecting by mistake a symptomatic relief – this is termed false-positive errors. False-positive errors are common in medical decision-making, both by physicians who diagnose a patient's symptom and by patients who report symptom severity.

Thus, in clinical practice and uncontrolled trials, the reported success rate may be due to one or more of the described phenomena – natural history, regression to the mean, and subject biases. The success rate may also be due to unidentified co-interventions, producing parallel effects on the observed benefit, and to the effect of being under study (Hawthorne effect).

The literature is full of examples where investigators have failed to account for these artifacts. This point is definitely clarified by Ernst and Resch[61] who suggested a distinction between the perceived and the true placebo

effect. The former is the response observed in the placebo group of a randomized controlled trial. The true placebo effect equals this response minus the confounding effects described above. Thus, the perceived placebo effect is equal to the true placebo effect only if no effects are observed in the untreated control group when compared with the placebo group.

WHAT PARADIGM TO STUDY THE PLACEBO EFFECT

Together with the exclusion of the above-mentioned confounding factors, it is crucial to select an appropriate paradigm when we want to investigate the placebo phenomenon.

The use of placebo and untreated groups in clinical trials is not aimed at identifying the true placebo effect.[61, 62, 63] Trialists, clinicians, and drug companies are mainly interested in seeing whether the active drug is more effective than the placebo, and they are not interested in the placebo effect itself. Fortunately, clinical trials are not the only methodology available and are not the best model for investigating the placebo effect. Most of our knowledge of the placebo effect comes from the laboratory setting where the experiments are designed to shed light on its neurobiological aspects. Studying the placebo effect in the laboratory setting gives us the opportunity to control psychological and physiological variables, and to rule out possible confounding factors for the placebo effect. For example, in the laboratory setting it is possible to conduct trials using three randomly selected, equally matched groups: (1) the natural history (NH) group or untreated group, which receives no treatment of any kind; (2) the placebo group, which receives an inert treatment that simulates the active one; (3) the active treatment, which receives the real treatment. The comparison between the placebo and the natural history group allows us to detect and measure the placebo effect. Regression to the mean can be ruled out by using, for example, experimental pain. False-positive errors and scaling biases can be eliminated through the evaluation of objective physiological parameters (e.g. hormones, autonomic responses).

Although most clinical trials use the placebo-controlled design, other experimental paradigms have been devised, including the balanced placebo design, the double-blind versus deceptive design, and the open-hidden paradigm (**Figure 41.2**). A brief overview of the characteristics of these paradigms follows.

The balanced placebo design, formulated by Ross and co-workers,[64] refers to a methodology for studying many aspects of human behavior and drug effects, orthogonally manipulating instructions (told drug versus told placebo) and drug administered (received drug versus received

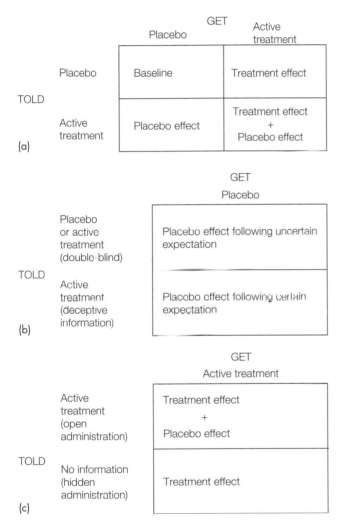

Figure 41.2 Paradigms to study a placebo response. (a) Balanced placebo design. The table shows the different combinations of what the patients receive and what they are told, allowing investigators to identify the modulation of drug action by verbal suggestions. (b) Double-blind versus deceptive design. Placebos are administered to patients by changing the information about the treatment. In fact, double-blind design provides uncertain expectations whereas the deceptive design provides certain expectations. (c) Open-hidden administration of an active treatment. It consists in the administration of the active treatment while the patient is either aware or unaware that a medical therapy is being given.

placebo) (**Figure 41.2a**). It has been used in many conditions, such as alcohol research,[65, 66] smoking,[67] amphetamine effects,[68] and psychiatric disorders.[69, 70] This design is particularly interesting for the investigation of placebo effects because it indicates that verbally induced expectations can modulate the therapeutic outcome, both in the placebo group and in the active treatment group. For example, Flaten et al.[71] showed that carisoprodol, a centrally acting muscle relaxant resulted in different outcomes, either relaxant or stimulant, depending on the combination of verbal suggestion and drug administration (including the placebo) and Keltner et al.[72] confirmed that different activation patterns are produced in the brain following different combinations of suggestions. The balanced placebo design produces information that cannot be derived from conventional clinical trials. For example, it provides a baseline against which drug and placebo effects can be measured, and provides a direct assessment of the drug effect with the placebo component removed. The problem with the balanced placebo design is that it entails deception (**Table 41.1**).

The second example is the double-blind versus deceptive design (**Figure 41.2b**). This design compares the therapeutic outcomes of a double-blind administration of an active drug with a deceptive one. Although outside the clinical setting, Kirsch and Weixel[73] showed that different verbal suggestions produce different outcomes. In one group, they administered regular coffee or decaffeinated coffee according to the usual double-blind design, and the subjects received the information that either the active or decaffeinated substance was being administered. In the second group, decaffeinated coffee was deceptively presented as real coffee. The authors found that the placebo responses were higher following the deceptive administration than the double-blind paradigm, concluding that uncertainty induces less expectation and, in turn, smaller placebo effect.

Similar findings arise from a study by Pollo and co-workers.[74] Thoracotomized patients were treated with buprenorphine on request for three consecutive days, together with a basal intravenous infusion of saline solution. However, the verbal instructions that were given to the patients were changed in three different groups of patients. The first group was told nothing

Table 41.1 Manipulation of expectations through different experimental designs. Use of a placebo (+) or not (−) is reported along with the use of deception.

	Placebo administration	Deception
Balanced placebo design	+	+
Double blind/deceptive design	+/+	−/+
Open-hidden design	−	−

about any analgesic effect (natural history). The second group was told that the basal infusion was either a powerful painkiller or a placebo (classic double-blind administration). The third group was told that the basal infusion was a potent painkiller (deceptive administration). The analgesic effect of the saline basal infusion was measured by recording the doses of buprenorphine requested over the three-day treatment. It was found that buprenorphine requests decreased in the double-blind group by 20.8 percent compared with natural history, and the reduction in the deceptive administration group was even greater, reaching 33.8 percent. These results indicate that little differences in verbal instructions ("It can be either a placebo or a painkiller and therefore we are not certain that the pain will subside" versus "It is a potent painkiller, and therefore we expect the pain will subside soon") produce different placebo analgesic effects, which in turn trigger a dramatic change of behavior leading to a significant reduction in opioid intake.

Recently, the open-hidden paradigm has become an interesting way to isolate the placebo effect as a context effect. Also termed "overt-covert design," the name refers to the modality of administration of a treatment: doctor-initiated versus machine-initiated therapy. The former is the classical situation of routine medical practice whereby an active treatment is administered to the patient, who is conscious that a medical therapy is being carried out. In this case, the therapeutic outcome is represented by the sum of the specific effects of the treatment itself and the placebo effect. The latter (machine-initiated) consists of the administration of the active treatment while the patient is completely unaware that it is being given (**Figure 41.2c**). It is possible to perform this hidden administration of a drug by means of a computer-controlled infusion pump that is pre-programmed to deliver the drug at the established time. The crucial point here is that the patient does not know when the infusion starts and ends, but he/she knows that a drug will be given.[17] Therefore, in this case there is full informed consent without any deception (**Table 41.1**).

Despite its obvious appeal, the open-hidden paradigm has been studied in only a few situations. In studies of analgesia, Levine et al.[75] and Levine and Gordon[76] found that in postoperative pain following the extraction of the third molar, a hidden injection of morphine (6–8 mg) provided the same effect as the injection of saline solution administered in full view of the patient. To obtain an effectiveness greater than the placebo, the hidden morphine dose needed to be increased to 12 mg. Recently, a careful analysis of the differences between open and hidden injections has been performed where the effects of four widely used painkillers (buprenorphine, tramadol, ketorolac, and metamizol), administered in either open or hidden manner, were investigated.[77] In all cases, a hidden injection was less effective than an open one. These results have been further extended to conditions other than pain, such as anxiety and Parkinson's disease.[17, 78, 79] What

these studies tell us is that the knowledge about a treatment and the expectation of clinical benefit affects the therapeutic outcome. The importance of this point has been recently demonstrated in a clinical condition, Alzheimer's disease (AD). The cognitive impairment that occurs in this pathological condition is a natural model to assess the difference between the open (expected) and hidden (unexpected) treatments, as the disruption of expectation/placebo-related analgesic mechanisms may eliminate the weight of the psychosocial component. Benedetti et al.[80] applied a local anesthetic, either overtly or covertly, to the skin of AD patients to reduce burning pain after venipuncture. They correlated the placebo component with both cognitive status and functional connectivity among different brain regions. They found that AD patients with reduced Frontal Assessment Battery scores showed a reduced placebo component of the analgesic treatment. The disruption of the placebo component occurred when reduced connectivity of the prefrontal lobes with the rest of the brain was present. Remarkably, the loss of these placebo-related mechanisms reduced treatment efficacy, such that a dose increase was necessary to produce adequate analgesia.

The findings from studies using the open-hidden paradigm underscores the active role of cognition in the overall therapeutic outcome and highlights the interesting possibilities for both clinicians and scientists. The open-hidden paradigm, where applicable, gives us the chance to study the placebo effect without the administration of any placebo, overcoming certain ethical constraints. This design has some similarities with the balanced placebo design without recourse to deception.[81, 82] Therefore, by isolating the psychosocial component of the context from the medical treatment itself, it is possible to shed light on the interaction between biopsychosocial and pharmacological processes.

Finally, conditioning protocols represent a good way to elicit a placebo response. Apart from expectation theories which are based on the assumption that a placebo produces an effect because the recipient expects it,[12, 13] classical conditioning may be another mechanism that generates placebo responses. However, expectation and conditioning theories do not necessarily contrast each other, and may represent two sides of the same coin.[83] In fact, placebo responses seem to be mediated by expectation and cognitive factors when conscious functions, such as pain and motor performance are involved, whilst they appear to be mediated by conditioning when unconscious functions, such as hormone secretion, come into play.[79]

NEUROCHEMISTRY OF PLACEBO/NOCEBO EFFECTS

Studies conducted in the laboratory setting have been able to minimize many of the problems encountered in the clinical trial setting and have provided important and reliable evidence about the nature of the placebo effect. Pain has been the main area of study of the placebo effect and comprises the largest body of research examining the placebo response. If we want to critically look at current knowledge about placebo effects, we must begin with a review of the literature on placebo analgesia.

Starting in the 1970s, placebo analgesia received considerable support in its legitimacy by way of two distinct but converging lines of research that demonstrated a physiological pathway for the placebo effect. Levine et al.[84] and Grevert et al.[85] showed that placebo analgesia is antagonized by the opioid antagonist, naloxone, thus suggesting that it is mediated by endogenous opioids. These findings have been confirmed and extended by other studies.[76, 86, 87, 88] First, Fields and Levine[57] hypothesized that placebo analgesia may be mediated by nonopioid mechanisms as well.[57, 89] The involvement of opioids depends on the procedure used to induce the placebo analgesic response.[90] In fact, by using the experimental ischemic arm pain model, it was found that if the placebo response is induced by means of strong expectation cues, it can be blocked by naloxone, whereas if the expectation cues are reduced, it proves to be naloxone-insensitive. In addition, if the placebo response is obtained after previous exposure to opioid drugs, it is naloxone-reversible. Conversely, if the placebo response is obtained after prior exposure to nonopioid drugs, it is naloxone-insensitive. All these data clearly suggest that

opioid and nonopioid mechanisms come into play in different circumstances. There is also evidence of somatotopic organization of placebo analgesia. Specific placebo analgesic responses can be obtained in different parts of the body[91, 92] and these responses are naloxone-reversible.[87]

Placebo-activated endogenous opioids have also been found to affect the respiratory centers and to induce respiratory depression.[88, 93] The cardiovascular system has also been found to be influenced by endogenous opioids during placebo analgesia,[94] thus indicating that placebo-induced release of opioids affects different systems and apparatuses (**Figure 41.3**).

In a second line of research, the cholecystokinin (CCK) antagonist, proglumide, has been found to enhance the placebo analgesic effect,[86, 95] thus suggesting that CCK has an inhibitory role in placebo-induced analgesia.

In addition, an extension of the action of CCK as an anti-analgesia system comes from work on nocebo hyperalgesia.[96, 97, 98] By using experimental ischemic arm pain in healthy volunteers, it was found that verbally induced nocebo suggestions produced hyperalgesia and hyperactivity of the hypothalamic–pituitary–adrenal (HPA) axis, as assessed by means of adrenocorticotropic hormone and cortisol plasma concentrations. The administration of the CCK antagonist proglumide blocked nocebo hyperalgesia completely, but had no effect on HPA hyperactivity, suggesting a specific involvement

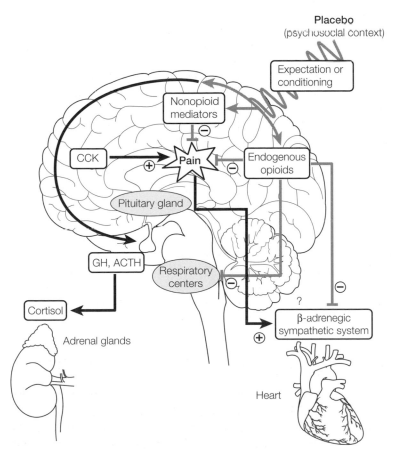

Figure 41.3 Cascade of biochemical events that may take place in the brain after placebo administration. Placebo administration along with verbal suggestions of analgesia (psychosocial context) may reduce pain through opioid and/or nonopioid mechanisms. Placebos have also been found to affect the respiratory centers, the cardiovascular system, and serotonin (5HT)-dependent hormone secretion. Redrawn by permission from Colloca L, Benedetti F. Placebos and painkillers: is mind as real as matter? *Nature Reviews. Neuroscience.* 2005; **6**: 545–52.

of CCK in the hyperalgesic but not in the anxiety component of the nocebo effect. These findings are in line with the study by Andre et al.[99] who demonstrated that the CCK-B receptor antagonist, CI-988, prevents anxiety-induced hyperalgesia in rodents. Thus, placebo suggestions activate endogenous opioids, whereas nocebo suggestions activate CCK, which confirms the anti-nociceptive action of opioids versus the pro-nociceptive action of CCK.

NEUROANATOMY OF PLACEBO/NOCEBO EFFECTS

Although the pharmacological approach with agonist and antagonist drugs has produced important information on the biochemical events triggered by context-induced expectations, pharmacological analysis does not allow identification of specific brain regions. Recently, functional imaging techniques, such as functional magnetic resonance imaging (fMRI), positron emission tomography (PET), and electroencephalography (EEG) have provided the opportunity to also define the neuroanatomical bases of placebo analgesia.[100]

The first imaging study of placebo analgesia showed that a subset of brain regions are similarly affected by either a placebo or a μ-opioid agonist. In fact, by using PET, it was found that the very same regions in the brain are affected by both a placebo and the opioid agonist remifentanil, thus indicating a related mechanism in placebo-induced (psychological effect) and opioid-induced analgesia (pharmacodynamic effect).[101] In particular, the administration of a placebo induced the activation of the rostral anterior cingulate cortex (rACC), the orbitofrontal cortex (OrbF), and the anterior insula (aINS), and there was a significant covariation in activity between rACC and the lower pons/medulla, and a subsignificant covariation between rACC and the periacqueductal gray (PAG), therefore suggesting that a descending rACC/PAG/pons/medulla pain-modulating circuit is involved in placebo analgesia, as previously suggested by other authors.[102, 103]

An opioid neuronal network in the cerebral cortex and the brain stem has been described as a descending pain-modulating pathway that connects, either directly or indirectly, the cerebral cortex to the brain stem.[92, 102, 104] In particular, ACC and OrbF project to PAG which, in turn, modulates the activity of the rostral ventromedial medulla (RVM). The ACC and PAG, together with some other nuclei in the brain stem (e.g. the parabrachial nuclei), are rich with opioid receptors. Therefore, this pain-modulating circuit appears to be the same, which is activated in placebo analgesia. The activation of μ-opioid receptors is implicated in a number of functions and the current hypothesis is that they work through a descending pattern of activation that is identifiable in the rACC-PAG-pons-medulla circuit.[103] The μ-opioid receptors are

heavily distributed involving cortical and subcortical regions such as the thalamus, the ACC, the nucleus accumbens, the amygdala, and the PAG.[105, 106]

Recently, Zubieta et al.[107] have confirmed the role of μ-opioid receptors in placebo analgesia. By using PET imaging and carbon-11-carfentanil, which binds selectively to the μ-opioid receptor, it was shown that the placebo analgesic response involved μ-opioid transmission. The pain stimulus was associated with a significant activation of endogenous opioid in the dorsal ACC, medial prefrontal cortex (mPFC), right INS, ventral basal ganglia (nucleus accumbens extending to ventral pallidum), medial thalamus (mTh), right amygdala, temporal cortex, and PAG. Placebo administration increased μ-opioid transmission in the left dorsolateral PFC, rACC, ipsilateral nucleus accumbens, and aINS.

Further studies performed with functional magnetic resonance imaging analyzed the brain regions involved in placebo analgesia. These studies revealed that the activity of pain regions, particularly the thalamus, aINS and caudal rACC, was reduced by a placebo treatment, thus indicating that placebos reduce nociceptive transmission along the pain pathways.[108, 109, 110, 111] In addition, during the anticipation phase of the placebo analgesic response, an activation of the dorsolateral prefrontal cortex (DLPFC), OrbF, rostral medial and anterior PFC, superior parietal cortex (SPC), and PAG was found, suggesting the activation of a cognitive-evaluative network just before the placebo response.[109] The increased activity of the PAG also suggests the activation of endogenous opioids in the anticipatory phase of the placebo response.[109, 112]

Cognitive factors, such as anticipation and expectation, have also been found to affect the pain matrix when a pain increase is expected.[113, 114, 115, 116, 117] For example, fMRI activation is significantly reduced when a high-intensity noxious stimulus is anticipated and accompanied by a low-intensity visual cue,[72] whereas expectation of painful stimulus enhances brain responses to a nonpainful stimulus.[118, 119] The hypothesis is that top-down mechanisms could inhibit pain signals at the level of the spinal cord.[103] This idea is supported by a recent study showing that expectancy induces a reduction of secondary hyperalgesia, which is known to involve spinal mechanisms.[120] Constantly, ACC is reported to be involved in placebo analgesia, suggesting its activation in response to a homeostatic imbalance requiring motivation for protective behavior.

These experimental approaches are important in better defining the neuroanatomy of placebo effect and further understanding the neuroscience of placebo phenomena.

PLACEBO EFFECTS IN CONDITIONS OTHER THAN PAIN

The release of endogenous substances following a placebo procedure is a phenomenon which is not confined to the field of pain, but it is also present in motor disorders, such as Parkinson's disease, depression, endocrine and immune systems, and addiction.[121]

It has been shown that parkinsonian patients respond to placebos quite well.[122, 123] A first study used PET in order to assess the release of endogenous dopamine. This study showed that placebo-induced expectation of motor improvement activates endogenous dopamine in the striatum of parkinsonian patients.[124] Interestingly, it was also shown that a placebo manipulation affects the firing pattern of neurons of the subthalamic nucleus and this is correlated to clinical improvement and subjective report of well-being.[125]

Depression is another condition that has been investigated, although several ethical constraints limit our understanding of the action of placebos in depressed patients. In fact, although both electrical and metabolic changes in the brain have been described, adequate controls are still lacking. Placebos have been found to induce EEG changes in the prefrontal cortex of patients with major depression, particularly in the right hemisphere[126, 127] and changes in brain glucose metabolism, as assessed by PET, in subcortical areas, including the brain stem and hippocampus, and cortical regions, such as the posterior ACC, the DLPFC, the premotor cortex, the dorsal ACC, and the inferior parietal posterior INS.[128]

The immune system has also been found to be affected by placebos.[129] In 1896, MacKenzie showed that some people who are allergic to flowers developed an allergic reaction when presented with something that superficially looks like a flower, but contains no pollen (a placebo flower).[130] Ader and colleagues widely demonstrated that a conditioned (placebo) enhancement of antibody production is possible using an antigen as an unconditioned stimulus of the immune system.[131, 132, 133, 134, 135] Recently, these findings have been confirmed in humans. In fact, repeated associations between cyclosporin A (unconditioned stimulus) and a flavored drink (conditioned stimulus) induced conditioned immunosuppression, where the flavored drink (the placebo) alone produced a suppression of the immune functions, as assessed by means of interleukin-2 (IL-2) and interferon-gamma (IFN-γ) mRNA expression, *in vitro* release of IL-2 and IFN-γ, as well as lymphocyte proliferation.[136] In this case, the placebo response can be interpreted as a genuine conditioned response.

Robust evidence also corroborates the presence of conditioning-mediated placebo effects in the endocrine system. By using the analgesic drug sumatriptan, a serotonin agonist of the 5-$HT_{1B/1D}$ receptors that stimulates growth hormone (GH) and inhibits cortisol secretion, it was shown that a conditioning procedure is capable of producing hormonal placebo responses (**Figure 41.3**). In fact, if a placebo is given after repeated administrations of sumatriptan, a placebo GH increase and a placebo cortisol decrease can be found. In contrast, verbally induced expectations of increase/decrease of GH and cortisol do not have any effect on the secretion of these hormones, suggesting a pivotal role of conditioning.[78, 79]

Recently, the effect of methylphenidate on brain glucose metabolism has been analyzed in two different conditions in both cocaine abusers and nondrug abusers: (1) when they expected to receive the drug; and (2) when they expected to receive a placebo. In the former case, the effect was approximately 50 percent greater than in the latter, thus indicating that expectation enhanced the pharmacological effect of the drug.[137, 138]

All these studies need to be considered when placebo analgesia is studied, as they support the integration of the understanding of placebo mechanisms in pain and analgesia with other illnesses. This is fundamental and necessary to identify similarities and differences that may help to better understand of the many facets of the placebo effect.

CLINICAL IMPLICATIONS

Many of the studies discussed in this chapter raise implications for both clinical practice and clinical trial design. Interestingly, there has been far less investigation into the nocebo response, even though the clinical implications may carry the same degree of importance as those of placebo mechanisms. As the study of placebo and nocebo mechanisms advances, it is hoped that more is learned about how to identify and exploit these mechanisms to improve both clinical practice and patient's quality of life, and to develop new clinical trial designs.

The open-hidden paradigm has been discussed as an interesting paradigm for studying placebo effects.[139] Overall, at least three important clinical and methodological implications derive from this paradigm.[17] First, the lesser effectiveness of hidden treatments indicates the crucial role of the patient–provider interaction. Second, by using the hidden paradigm, the efficacy of some treatments can be assessed without the need for placebo administration, thus overcoming the ethical problem of placebo administration and deception. Third, the hidden paradigm can change the conception of how clinical trials must be viewed and conducted. In fact, it is possible to isolate the specific action of a treatment (such as the pharmacological properties of a drug) from the overall effect of the treatment (the specific action plus the context-driven placebo mechanisms). One important implication of this paradigm is that it can demonstrate that even though a drug may show strong analgesic efficacy in a normal RCT design, it may in fact have little or no specific analgesic properties. This was demonstrated in a study by Benedetti and coworkers,[95] whereby the CCK antagonist proglumide was tested in both a standard RCT design and a hidden fashion. When administered in full view of the patient, proglumide was shown to be an effective analgesic. However, when the patients did not know they were receiving the drug, it had no effect on pain, demonstrating that the drug had no specific analgesic properties (**Figure 41.4**). The action of the CCK antagonist proglumide consists in the potentiation of top-down placebo mechanisms and it does not act directly on pain pathways. This valuable information would not be obtained using a standard RCT design and therefore the open-hidden paradigm may represent an excellent alternative for studying certain treatments. It also underscores the power of the expectation component of an active treatment on the overall effectiveness of the treatment. In other words, proglumide induces a reduction of pain if, and only if, associated with a placebo procedure. Today we know that proglumide is not a painkiller, but it acts on placebo-activated opioid mechanisms.

We have no *a priori* knowledge of which substances act on pain pathways and which on expectation mechanisms, and indeed virtually all drugs may interfere with the top-down mechanisms. In the same way as the Heisenberg uncertainty principle of physics states that a dynamical disturbance is necessarily induced on a system by a measurement, in clinical trials a dynamical disturbance may be induced on the brain by virtually any kind of drug. Thus, this uncertainty cannot be solved with the standard clinical trial design.[1] The only way to partially solve this problem is to make the expectation pathways, so to speak, silent.

The power of patient's perception or expectations is also highlighted by some of the previously mentioned studies,

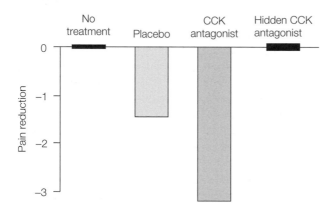

Figure 41.4 How the open-hidden paradigm is changing our conception of clinical trials. A clinical trial with three arms (No treatment, Placebo, CCK antagonist) shows that placebo is better than no treatment and proglumide (CCK-antagonist) is better than placebo in relieving pain. According to classical clinical trial methodology, this leads to the erroneous belief that the CCK-antagonist acts specifically on pain pathways as a painkiller. This interpretation is wrong, as demonstrated by the total ineffectiveness of the same CCK-antagonist when it is given covertly, with the patient completely unaware that a drug is being administered (Hidden CCK antagonist). Since the drug has analgesic effects only in association with a placebo procedure, its action is not specifically directed to the pain pathways, but rather to the expectation pathways, enhancing the placebo analgesic response (data from Benedetti *et al.*[95]).

whereby the manipulation of expectations were able to improve the efficacy of a stimulant drug[137, 138] and result in reduced drug intake in postoperative pain.[74] This is also underscored by some recent clinical trials whereby the patient's perceived assignment to either a placebo or active treatment better predicted the outcome to human fetal mesencephalic transplantation (a treatment for Parkinson's disease)[140] and acupuncture[141, 142, 143] than did the actual allocation. These studies clearly demonstrate that those patients who experienced placebo responses show better therapeutic outcomes and request fewer drugs than those who are not under the effect of expectations.

Whether one wishes to look at placebo responses in the light of meaning or context effects, it is clear that the psychosocial context surrounding a given treatment can play a significant role in the outcome of the treatment by the activation of placebo and nocebo mechanisms. At the center of this is the clinician, the patient, and the overall treatment environment, and at this stage much more research is needed to identify how changes in these factors can potentiate placebo mechanisms and improve therapy.

At the same time, an ethical debate aimed at avoiding the misuse of placebos in clinical trials, surgery, and medical practice is necessary.[1, 54, 55, 144]

The Declaration of Helsinki maintains that it is unethical to assign patients to receive a placebo when effective treatment exists.[145] However, the note of clarification on paragraph 29 of the WMA Declaration of Helsinki reads:

> …a placebo-controlled trial may be ethically acceptable, even if proven therapy is available, under the following circumstances:
>
> - where for compelling and scientifically sound methodological reasons its use is necessary to determine the efficacy or safety of a prophylactic, diagnostic or therapeutic method; or
> - where a prophylactic, diagnostic or therapeutic method is being investigated for a minor condition and the patients who receive placebo will not be subject to any additional risk of serious or irreversible harm;
> - all other provisions of the Declaration of Helsinki must be adhered to, especially the need for appropriate ethical and scientific review.[146]

Significant and controversial criticism has been made in relation to the document. In general, the arguments that are advocated for or against the use of the placebo in clinical studies can be summarized as follows. Placebo defenders sometimes use the utilitarian argument whereby exposing subjects to placebo treatment is justified by the knowledge gained for future patients, whereas placebo opponents reply that ethical obligations to the single individual take precedence over science and society. Placebo defenders also affirm that the approval of the Institutional Review Board and the patient's informed consent are sufficient, whereas placebo opponents contend that most informed consent forms are incomprehensible, thus making the patient unable to judge the experimental situations. Another point raised by many placebo defenders deals with the use of placebos for symptomatic treatments and not for curative therapies. Placebo opponents argue that there is no justification even for minor discomfort.

An emergent view among researchers and ethicists argues that not only is the use of sham surgery ethical, but that it should also be mandatory when conducting trials to evaluate the effectiveness of surgical procedures.[147] There are, however, some opponents to placebo surgery who emphasize the role of evidence-based medicine.[148]

As far as medical practice is concerned, a positive therapist–patient interaction does not require an ethical discussion and is, indeed, an essential ingredient of any therapy. Yet, deception remains a critical issue. On the one hand, it is considered to damage the medical profession, contributing to the erosion of confidence and trust in medical staff and caregivers.[149, 150] On the other hand, it may be justified by the concept of paternalism, in which the physician's purpose is not actually to deceive but to cure.[151, 152]

What is clear now is that when looking at a given therapy, one needs to not only look at the active properties of the intervention but also at the context in which it is given and the particularly powerful role the clinician's words on the patient's brain.[153] It is hoped that future research will further identify placebo mechanisms and ways of accessing and harnessing these mechanisms in the clinical setting for the benefit of the patient.

ACKNOWLEDGMENTS

This work was supported by grants from Regione Piemonte and San Paolo IMI.

REFERENCES

* 1. Colloca L, Benedetti F. Placebos and painkillers: is mind as real as matter? *Nature Reviews Neuroscience.* 2005; **6**: 545–52.
2. Brown WA. The placebo effect. *Scientific American.* 1998; **278**: 90–5.
3. de Craen AJ, Kaptchuk TJ, Tijssen JG, Kleijnen J. Placebos and placebo effects in medicine: historical overview. *Journal of the Royal Society of Medicine.* 1999; **92**: 511–15.
4. Wall PD. The placebo and the placebo response. In: Wall PD, Melzack R (eds). *The textbook of pain.* New York: Churchill Livingstone, 1999: 1419–30.
5. Brown WA, Johnson MF, Chen MG. Clinical features of depressed patients who do and do not improve with placebo. *Psychiatry Research.* 1992; **41**: 203–14.
6. Turner JA, Deyo RA, Loeser JD et al. The importance of placebo effects in pain treatment and research. *Journal of the American Medical Association.* 1994; **271**: 1609–14.
7. Wall PD. The placebo effect: an unpopular topic. *Pain.* 1992; **51**: 1–3.
8. Brody H. *The placebo response.* New York: Harper Collins, 2000.
9. Moerman DE, Jonas WB. Deconstructing the placebo effect and finding the meaning response. *Annals of Internal Medicine.* 2002; **136**: 471–6.
* 10. Moerman DE (ed.). *Meaning, medicine and the placebo effect.* Cambridge: University Press, 2002.
11. Kirsch I (ed.). *How expectancies shape experience.* Washington, DC: American Psychological Association, 1999.
12. Kirsch I. Response expectancy as determinant of experience and behaviour. *American Psychologist.* 1985; **40**: 1189–202.
13. Kirsch I (ed.). *Changing expectations: A key to effective psychotherapy.* Pacific Grove, CA: Brooks/Cole, 1990.
* 14. Di Blasi Z, Harkness E, Ernst E et al. Influence of context effects on health outcomes: a systematic review. *Lancet.* 2001; **357**: 757–62.
15. Benedetti F. How the doctor's words affect the patient's brain. *Evaluation and the Health Professions.* 2002; **25**: 369–86.
16. Balint M. The doctor, his patient, and the illness. *Lancet.* 1955; **1**: 683–8.
* 17. Colloca L, Lopiano L, Lanotte M, Benedetti F. Overt versus covert treatment for pain, anxiety, and Parkinson's disease. *Lancet Neurology.* 2004; **3**: 679–84.
18. Kennedy WP. The nocebo reaction. *Medicina Experimentalis. International Journal of Experimental Medicine.* 1961; **95**: 203–05.
19. Kissel P, Barrucand D (eds). *Placebos et effect placebo en medicine.* Paris: Masson, 1964.
20. Hahn RA. A sociocultural model of illness and healing. In: White L, Tursky B, Schwartz GE (eds). *Placebo: theory, research, and mechanisms.* New York: Guilford, 1985: 167–95.
21. Hahn RA. The nocebo phenomenon: concept, evidence, and implications for public health. *Preventive Medicine.* 1997; **26**: 607–11.
22. Moerman DE. Doctors and patients: the role of clinicians in the placebo effect. *Advances in Mind–Body Medicine.* 2003; **19**: 14–22.
23. Humphrey N (ed.). Great expectations: the evolutionary psychology of faith healing and the placebo response. In: *The mind made flesh: essays from frontiers of psychology and evolution.* Oxford: Oxford University Press, 2002: 255–85.
24. Beecher HK. The powerful placebo. *Journal of the American Medical Association.* 1955; **159**: 1602–06.

25. Kienle GS, Kiene H. Placebo effect and placebo concept: a critical methodological and conceptual analysis of reports on the magnitude of the placebo effect. *Alternative Therapies in Health and Medicine.* 1996; **2**: 39–54.

26. Kienle GS, Kiene H. The powerful placebo effect: fact or fiction? *Journal of Clinical Epidemiology.* 1997; **50**: 1311–8.

27. Cobb LA, Thomas GI, Dillar DH *et al.* An evaluation of internal-mammary-artery ligation by a double-blind technique. *New England Journal of Medicine.* 1959; **269**: 115–8.

28. Dimond EG, Kittle CF, Crockett JE. Comparison of internal mammary artery ligation and sham operation for angina pectoris. *American Journal of Cardiology.* 1960; **5**: 483–6.

29. Beecher HK. Surgery as placebo. A quantitative study of bias. *Journal of the American Medical Association.* 1961; **176**: 1102–07.

30. Hróbjartsson A, Gøtzsche PC. Is the placebo powerless? An analysis of clinical trials comparing placebo with no treatment. *New England Journal of Medicine.* 2001; **344**: 1594–602.

31. Hróbjartsson A, Gøtzsche PC. Is the placebo powerless? Update of a systematic review with 52 new randomized trials comparing placebo with no treatment. *Journal of Internal Medicine.* 2004; **256**: 91–100.

32. Shapiro AK, Shapiro E. The placebo: is it much ado about nothing. In: Harrington A (ed.). *The placebo effect – an interdisciplinary exploration.* Harvard: University Press, 1997: 12–36.

33. Ader R. Much ado about nothing. *Advances in Mind–Body Medicine.* 2001; **17**: 293–5.

34. Brody H, Weismantel D. A challenge to core beliefs. *Advances in Mind–Body Medicine.* 2001; **17**: 296–8.

35. DiNubile MJ. Is the placebo powerless? *New England Journal of Medicine.* 2001; **345**: 1278.

36. Einarson TE, Helmes M, Stolk P. Is the placebo powerless? *New England Journal of Medicine.* 2001; **345**: 1277.

37. Greene PJ, Wayne PM, Kerr CE *et al.* The powerful placebo: doubting the doubters. *Advances in Mind–Body Medicine.* 2001; **17**: 298–307.

38. Kaptchuk TJ. Is the placebo powerless? *New England Journal of Medicine.* 2001; **345**: 1277.

39. Kirsch I, Scoboria A. Apples, oranges, and placebos: heterogeneity in a meta-analysis of placebo effects. *Advances in Mind–Body Medicine.* 2001; **17**: 307–09.

40. Kupers R. Is the placebo powerless? *New England Journal of Medicine.* 2001; **345**: 1278.

41. Lilford RJ, Braunholtz DA. Is the placebo powerful? *New England Journal of Medicine.* 2001; **345**: 1277–8.

42. Miller FG. Is the placebo powerless? *New England Journal of Medicine.* 2001; **345**: 1277.

43. Papakostas YG, Daras MD. Placebos, placebo effect, and the response to the healing situation: the evolution of a concept. *Epilepsia.* 2001; **42**: 1614–25.

44. Shrier I. Is the placebo powerless? *New England Journal of Medicine.* 2001; **345**: 1278.

45. Spiegel D, Kraemer H, Carlson RW. Is the placebo powerless? *New England Journal of Medicine.* 2002; **345**: 1276.

46. Wickramasekera I. The placebo efficacy study: problems with the definition of the placebo and the mechanisms of placebo efficacy. *Advances in Mind–Body Medicine.* 2001; **17**: 309–12; discussion 312–8.

∗ 47. Benedetti F, Mayberg HS, Wager TD *et al.* Neurobiological mechanisms of the placebo effect. *Journal of Neuroscience.* 2005; **25**: 10390–402.

48. Vase L, Riley 3rd JL, Price DD. A comparison of placebo effects in clinical analgesic trials versus studies of placebo analgesia. *Pain.* 2002; **99**: 443–52.

49. Hróbjartsson A, Gøtzsche PC. Unsubstantiated claims of large effects of placebo on pain. Serious errors in meta-analysis of placebo analgesia mechanism studies. *Journal of Clinical Epidemiology.* 2006; **59**: 336–8.

50. de Craen AJ, Tijsssen JG, de Gans J, Kleijnen J. Placebo effect in the acute treatment of migraine: subcutaneous placebos are better than oral placebos. *Journal of Neurology.* 2000; **247**: 183–8.

51. Moerman DE. The meaning response and the ethics of avoiding placebos. *Evaluation and the Health Professions.* 2002; **25**: 399–409.

52. de Craen AJ, Roos PJ, Leonard de Vries A, Kleijnen J. Effect of colour of drugs: systematic review of perceived effect of drugs and of their effectiveness. *British Medical Journal.* 1996; **313**: 1624–6.

53. Kaptchuk T, Stason WB, Davis RB *et al.* Sham device v inert pill: randomized controlled trial of two placebo treatments. *British Medical Journal.* 2006; **332**: 391–7.

54. Benedetti F, Colloca L. Placebo-induced analgesia: methodology, neurobiology, clinical use, and ethics. *Review in Analgesia.* 2004; **7**: 129–43.

55. Colloca L, Benedetti F. The placebo in clinical studies and in medical practice. In: Price DD, Bushnell C (eds). *Psychological methods of pain control: basic science and clinical perspectives.* Seattle, WA: IASP Press, 2004: 187–205.

56. Pollo A, Benedetti F. Toward understanding the biological mechanisms of placebo analgesia. In: Price DD, Bushnell C (eds). *Psychological methods of pain control: basic science and clinical perspectives.* Seattle, WA: IASP Press, 2004: 171–86.

57. Fields HL, Levine JD. Placebo analgesia – a role for endorphins. *Trends in Neurosciences.* 1984; **7**: 271–3.

∗ 58. Hoffman GA, Harrington A, Fields HL. Pain and the placebo: what we have learned. *Perspectives in Biology and Medicine.* 2005; **48**: 248–65.

59. Davis CE. Regression to the mean or placebo effect? In: Guess HA, Kleinman A, Kusek JW, Engel LW (eds). *The science of the placebo: toward an interdisciplinary research agenda.* London: BMJ Books, 2002: 158–66.

60. Allan LG, Siegel S. A signal detection theory analysis of the placebo effect. *Evaluation and the Health Professions.* 2002; **25**: 410–20.

61. Ernst E, Resch KL. Concept of true and perceived placebo effects. *British Medical Journal.* 1995; **311**: 551–3.

62. Lewis JA, Jonsson B, Kreutz G *et al.* Placebo-controlled trials and the Declaration of Helsinki. *Lancet.* 2002; **359**: 1337–40.

63. Michels KB, Rothman KJ. Update on unethical use of placebos in randomised trials. *Bioethics.* 2003; **17**: 188–204.

64. Ross S, Krugman AD, Lyerly SB, Clyde DJ. Drugs and placebos: a model design. *Psychological Reports.* 1962; **10**: 383–92.

65. Marlatt GA, Demming B, Reid JB. Loss of control drinking in alcoholics: An experimental analogue. *Journal of Abnormal Psychology.* 1973; **81**: 223–41.

66. Epps J, Monk C, Savage S, Marlatt GA. Improving credibility of instruction in the balanced placebo design: a misattribution manipulation. *Addictive Behaviours.* 1998; **23**: 426–35.

67. Sutton SR. Great expectations: some suggestions for applying the balanced placebo design to nicotine and smoking. *British Journal of Addiction.* 1991; **86**: 659–62.

68. Mitchell SH, Laurent CL, de Wit H. Interaction of expectancy and the pharmacological effects of d-amphetamine: subjective effects and self-administration. *Psychopharmacology.* 1996; **125**: 371–8.

69. Rohsenow DJ, Bachorowski J. Effects of alcohol and expectancies on verbal aggression in men and women. *Journal of Abnormal Psychology.* 1984; **93**: 418–32.

70. Wilson GT, Niaura RS, Adler JL. Alcohol: selective attention and sexual arousal in men. *Journal of Studies on Alcohol.* 1985; **46**: 107–15.

71. Flaten MA, Simonsen T, Olsen H. Drug-related information generates placebo and nocebo responses that modify the drug response. *Psychosomatic Medicine.* 1999; **61**: 250–5.

72. Keltner JR, Furst A, Fan C *et al.* Isolating the modulatory effect of expectation on pain transmission: a functional magnetic resonance imaging study. *Journal of Neuroscience.* 2006; **26**: 4437–43.

73. Kirsch I, Weixel LJ. Double-blind versus deceptive administration of a placebo. *Behavioral Neuroscience.* 1988; **102**: 319–23.

74. Pollo A, Amanzio M, Arslanian A *et al.* Response expectancies in placebo analgesia and their clinical relevance. *Pain.* 2001; **93**: 77–84.

75. Levine JD, Gordon NC, Smith R, Fields HL. Analgesic responses to morphine and placebo in individuals with postoperative pain. *Pain.* 1981; **10**: 379–89.

76. Levine JD, Gordon NC. Influence of the method of drug administration on analgesic response. *Nature.* 1984; **312**: 755–6.

77. Amanzio M, Pollo A, Maggi G, Benedetti F. Response variability to analgesics: a role for non-specific activation of endogenous opioids. *Pain.* 2001; **90**: 205–15.

78. Benedetti F, Maggi G, Lopiano L *et al.* Open versus hidden medical treatments: the patient's knowledge about a therapy affects the therapy outcome. Prevention and treatment. 2003. Available online: http://journals.apa.org/prevention/volume6/toc-jun-03.html.

79. Benedetti F, Pollo A, Lopiano L *et al.* Conscious expectation and unconscious conditioning in analgesic, motor and hormonal placebo/nocebo responses. *Journal of Neuroscience.* 2003; **23**: 4315–23.

80. Benedetti B, Arduino C, Costa S *et al.* Loss of expectation-related mechanisms in Alzheimer's disease makes analgesic therapies less effective. *Pain.* 2006; **121**: 133–44.

81. Bootzin R. Studying the context in which treatments are delivered: observations on "open versus hidden medical treatments". Prevention and treatment. 2003. Available online: http://journals.apa.org/prevention/volume6/toc-jun-03.html.

82. Kirsch I. Hidden administration as ethical alternatives to the balanced placebo design. Prevention and treatment. 2003. Available online: http://journals.apa.org/prevention/volume6/toc-jun-03.html.

83. Stewart-Williams S, Podd J. The placebo effect: dissolving the expectancy versus conditioning debate. *Psychological Bulletin.* 2004; **130**: 324–40.

84. Levine JD, Gordon NC, Fields HL. The mechanism of placebo analgesia. *Lancet.* 1978; **23**: 654–7.

85. Grevert P, Albert LH, Goldstein A. Partial antagonism of placebo analgesia by naloxone. *Pain.* 1983; **16**: 129–43.

86. Benedetti F. The opposite effects of the opiate antagonist naloxone and the cholecystokinin antagonist proglumide on placebo analgesia. *Pain.* 1996; **64**: 535–43.

87. Benedetti F, Arduino C, Amanzio M. Somatotopic activation of opioid systems by target-directed expectations of analgesia. *Journal of Neuroscience.* 1999; **19**: 3639–48.

88. Benedetti F, Amanzio M, Baldi S *et al.* Inducing placebo respiratory depressant responses in humans via opioid receptors. *European Journal of Neuroscience.* 1999; **11**: 625–31.

89. Gracely RH, Dubner R, Deeter WD, Wolskee PJ. Clinicians' expectations influence placebo analgesia. *Lancet.* 1985; **1**: 43.

90. Amanzio M, Benedetti F. Neuropharmacological dissection of placebo analgesia: expectation-activated opioid systems versus conditioning-activated specific sub-systems. *Journal of Neuroscience.* 1999; **19**: 484–94.

91. Montgomery GH, Kirsch I. Mechanisms of placebo pain reduction: An empirical investigation. *Psychological Science.* 1996; **7**: 174–5.

92. Price DD. Placebo Analgesia. In: Price DD (ed.). *Psychological mechanisms of pain and analgesia.* Progress in Pain Research and Management, 15. Seattle: IASP Press, 1999: 155–81.

93. Benedetti F, Amanzio M, Baldi S *et al.* The specific effects of prior opioid exposure on placebo analgesia and placebo respiratory depression. *Pain.* 1998; **75**: 313–19.

94. Pollo A, Vighetti S, Rainero I, Benedetti F. Placebo analgesia and the heart. *Pain.* 2003; **102**: 125–33.

95. Benedetti F, Amanzio M, Maggi G. Potentiation of placebo analgesia by proglumide. *Lancet*. 1995; **346**: 1231.

96. Benedetti F, Amanzio M, Casadio C *et al*. Blockade of nocebo hyperalgesia by the cholecystokinin antagonist proglumide. *Pain*. 1997; **71**: 135–40.

97. Benedetti F, Amanzio M. The neurobiology of placebo analgesia: from endogenous opioids to cholecystokinin. *Progress in Neurobiology*. 1997; **52**: 109–25.

* 98. Benedetti F, Amanzio M, Vighetti A, Asteggiano G. The biochemical and neuroendocrine bases of the hyperalgesic nocebo effect. *Journal of Neuroscience*. 2006; **26**: 12014–22.

99. Andre J, Zeau B, Pohl M *et al*. Involvement of cholecystokininergic systems in anxiety-induced hyperalgesia in male rats: behavioral and biochemical studies. *Journal of Neuroscience*. 2005; **25**: 7896–904.

100. Tracey I. The neural matrix of pain processing and placebo analgesia: evidence from functional imaging. *Headache Currents*. 2005; **2**: 123–6 (available online at www.blackwell-synergy.com/toc/hec/2/6).

*101. Petrovic P, Kalso E, Petersson KM, Ingvar M. Placebo and opioid analgesia – imaging a shared neuronal network. *Science*. 2002; **295**: 1737–40.

102. Fields HL, Price DD. Towards a neurobiology of placebo analgesia. In: Harrington A (ed.). *The placebo effect: an interdisciplinary exploration*. Cambridge: Harvard University Press, 1997: 93–116.

103. Fields HL. State-dependent opioid control of pain. *Nature Reviews. Neuroscience*. 2004; **5**: 565–75.

104. Fields HL, Basbaum AI. Central nervous system mechanism of pain modulation. In: Wall PD, Melzack R (eds). *Textbook of pain*. New York: Churchill Livingstone, 1994: 243–57.

105. Willoch F, Tolle TR, Wester HJ *et al*. Central pain after pontine infarction is associated with changes in opioid receptor binding: a PET study with 11 C-diprenorphine. *AJNR American Journal of Neuroradiology*. 1999; **20**: 686–90.

106. Willoch F, Schindler F, Wester HJ *et al*. Central poststroke pain and reduced opioid receptor binding within pain processing circuitries: a [11C]diprenorphine PET study. *Pain*. 2004; **108**: 213–20.

*107. Zubieta JK, Bueller JA, Jackson LR *et al*. Placebo effects mediated by endogenous opioid activity on μ-opioid receptors. *Journal of Neuroscience*. 2005; **25**: 7754–62.

108. Lieberman MD, Jarcho JM, Berman S *et al*. The neural correlates of placebo effects: a disruption account. *Neuroimage*. 2004; **22**: 447–55.

*109. Wager TD, Rilling JK, Smith EE *et al*. Placebo-induced changes in FMRI in the anticipation and experience of pain. *Science*. 2004; **303**: 1162–7.

110. Kong J, Gollub RL, Rosman IS *et al*. Brain activity with expectancy-enhanced placebo analgesia as measured by functional magnetic resonance imaging. *Journal of Neuroscience*. 2006; **26**: 381–8.

111. Price DD, Craggs J, Nicholas Verne G *et al*. Placebo analgesia is accompanied by large reductions in pain-related brain activity in irritable bowel syndrome patients. *Pain*. 2007; **127**: 63–72.

112. Wager TD. Expectations and anxiety as mediators of placebo effects in pain. *Pain*. 2005; **115**: 225–6.

113. Buchel C, Morris J, Dolan RJ, Friston KJ. Brain systems mediating aversive conditioning: an event-related fMRI study. *Neuron*. 1998; **20**: 947–57.

114. Chua P, Krams M, Toni I *et al*. A functional anatomy of anticipatory anxiety. *Neuroimage*. 1999; **9**: 563–71.

115. Hsieh JC, Stone-Elander S, Ingvar M. Anticipatory coping of pain expressed in the human anterior cingulate cortex: a positron emission tomography study. *Neuroscience Letters*. 1999; **262**: 61–4.

116. Ploghaus A, Tracey I, Gati JS *et al*. Dissociating pain from its anticipation in the human brain. *Science*. 1999; **284**: 1979–81.

117. Porro CA, Baraldi P, Pagnoni G *et al*. Does anticipation of pain affect cortical nociceptive systems? *Journal of Neuroscience*. 2002; **22**: 3206–14.

118. Sawamoto N, Honda M, Okada T *et al*. Expectation of pain enhances responses to nonpainful somatosensory stimulation in the anterior cingulated cortex and parietal operculum/posterior insula: an event-related functional magnetic resonance imaging study. *Journal of Neuroscience*. 2000; **20**: 7438–45.

119. Koyama T, McHaffie JG, Laurienti PJ, Coghill RC. The subjective experience of pain: where expectations became reality. *Proceedings of the National Academy of Sciences of the United States of America*. 2005; **102**: 12950–5.

120. Matre D, Casey KL, Knardahl S. Placebo-induced changes in spinal cord pain processing. *Journal of Neuroscience*. 2006; **26**: 559–63.

121. Colloca L, Lopiano L, Benedetti F, Lanotte M. The placebo response in conditions other than pain. *Seminars in Pain Medicine*. 2005; **3**: 43–7 (available online at www.blackwell-synergy.com/toc/hec/2/6).

122. Shetty N, Friedman JH, Kieburtz K *et al*. The placebo response in Parkinson's disease. *Clinical Neuropharmacology*. 1999; **22**: 207–12.

123. Goetz CG, Leurgans S, Raman R, Stebbins GT. Objective changes in motor function during placebo treatment in Parkinson's disease. *Neurology*. 2000; **54**: 710–14.

*124. de la Fuente-Fernandez R, Ruth TJ, Sossi V *et al*. Expectation and dopamine release: mechanism of the placebo effect in Parkinson's disease. *Science*. 2001; **293**: 1164–6.

*125. Benedetti F, Colloca L, Torre E *et al*. Placebo-responsive Parkinson patients show decreased activity in single neurons of subthalamic nucleus. *Nature Neuroscience*. 2004; **7**: 587–8.

126. Leuchter AF, Cook IA, Witte EA *et al*. Changes in brain function of depressed subjects during treatment with placebo. *American Journal of Psychiatry*. 2002; **159**: 122–9.

127. Leuchter AF, Morgan M, Cook IA *et al*. Pretreatment neurophysiological and clinical characteristics of placebo

responders in treatment trials for major depression. *Psychopharmacology.* 2004; **177**: 15–22.

128. Mayberg HS, Silva JA, Brannan SK *et al.* The functional neuroanatomy of the placebo effect. *American Journal of Psychiatry.* 2002; **159**: 728–37.

*129. Pacheco-Lopez G, Engler H, Niemi MB, Schedlowski M. Expectations and associations that heal: Immunomodulatory placebo effects and its neurobiology. *Brain, Behavior, and Immunity.* 2006; **20**: 430–46.

130. MacKenzie JN. The production of the so-called 'rose-cold' by means of an artificial rose. *American Journal of the Medical Sciences.* 1896; **91**: 45–45.

131. Ader R, Cohen N. Behaviourally conditioned immunosuppression and murine systemic lupus erythematosus. *Science.* 1982; **215**: 1534–6.

132. Ader R, Cohen N. The influence of conditioning on immune responses. In: Ader R, Felten DL, Cohen N (eds). *PsychoNeuroImmunology.* San Diego: Academic Press, 1991: 611–46.

133. Ader R, Cohen N. Psychoneuroimmunology: Conditioning and Stress. *Annual Review of Psychology.* 1993; **44**: 53–85.

134. Olness K, Ader R. Conditioning as an adjunct in the pharmacotherapy of lupus erythematosus. *Journal of Developmental and Behavioral Pediatrics.* 1992; **13**: 124–5.

135. Giang DW, Goodman AD, Schiffer RB *et al.* Conditioning of cyclophosphamide-induced leucopenia in humans. *Journal of Neuropsychiatry and Clinical Neurosciences.* 1996; **8**: 194–201.

136. Goebel MU, Trebst AE, Steiner J *et al.* Behavioral conditioning of immunosuppression is possible in humans. *FASEB Journal.* 2002; **16**: 1869–73.

137. Volkow ND, Wang GJ, Ma Y *et al.* Expectation enhances the regional brain metabolic and the reinforcing effects of stimulants in cocaine abusers. *Journal of Neuroscience.* 2003; **23**: 11461–8.

138. Volkow ND, Wang GJ, Ma Y *et al.* Effects of expectation on the brain metabolic responses to methylphenidate and to its placebo in non-drug abusing subjects. *Neuroimage.* 2006; **32**: 1782–92.

139. Finniss DG, Benedetti F. Mechanisms of the placebo response and their impact on clinical trials and clinical practice. *Pain.* 2005; **114**: 3–6.

140. McRae C, Cherin E, Yamazaki TG *et al.* Effects of perceived treatment on quality of life and medical outcomes in a double-blind placebo surgery trial. *Archives of General Psychiatry.* 2004; **61**: 412–20.

141. Bausell RB, Lao L, Bergman S *et al.* Is acupuncture analgesia an expectancy effect? Preliminary evidence based upon participants' perceived assignments in two placebo controlled trials. *Evaluation and the Health Professions.* 2005; **28**: 9–26.

*142. Linde K, Witt CM, Streng A *et al.* The impact of patient expectations on outcomes in four randomized controlled trials of acupuncture in patients with chronic pain. *Pain.* 2007; **128**: 193–4.

143. Benedetti F. What do you expect from this treatment? Changing our mind about clinical trials. *Pain.* 2007; **128**: 264–71.

*144. Price DD. New facts and improved ethical guidelines for placebo analgesia. *Journal of Pain.* 2005; **6**: 213–4.

145. World Medical Association. Declaration of Helsinki. Amended by 52nd WMA General Assembly, Edinburgh, Scotland. *Journal of the American Medical Association.* 2000; **284**: 3043–5.

146. World Medical Association. *Declaration of Helsinki.* Note of clarification on Paragraph 29. Washington. 2002; Last updated September 10, 2004; cited December 2007. Available from: www.wma.net/e/policy/ b3.htm#paragraphe29.

147. Horng S, Miller FG. Is placebo surgery unethical? *New England Journal of Medicine.* 2002; **347**: 137–9.

148. Polgar S, Ng J. Ethics, methodology and the use of placebo controls in surgical trials. *Brain Research Bulletin.* 2005; **67**: 290–7.

149. Bok S. The ethics of giving placebos. *Scientific American.* 1974; **231**: 17–23.

150. Bok S. Ethical issues in use of placebo in medical practise and clinical trials. In: Guess HA, Kleinman A, Kusek JW, Engel LW (eds). *The science of the placebo: toward an interdisciplinary research agenda.* London: BMJ Books, 2002: 63–73.

151. Rawlinson MC. Truth-telling and paternalism in the clinic: philosophical reflection on the use of placebo in medical practice. In: White L, Tursky B, Scwartz GE (eds). *Placebo: theory, research, and mechanisms.* New York: Guilford Press, 1985: 403–16.

152. Lichtenberg P, Heresco-Levy U, Nitzan U. The ethics of the placebo in clinical practice. *Journal of Medical Ethics.* 2004; **30**: 551–4.

153. Benedetti F, Lanotte M, Lopiano L, Colloco L. When words are painful: unraveling the mechanisms of the nocebo effect. *Neuroscience.* 2007; **147**: 260–71.

42

Clinical trials: acute and chronic pain

AUDUN STUBHAUG AND HARALD BREIVIK

KEY LEARNING POINTS

- A clinical trial is a a prospective comparison of outcomes in patients assigned to test or control treatment(s). If possible, assignment should be by randomization, and all participants and observers should be blinded for intervention type.
- The purpose of the study must be clearly defined, meaningful, and aimed at increasing our knowledge and improving patient care.
- One primary efficacy variable should be chosen.
- Document assay sensitivity (i.e. that the study is able to find a true difference between groups) to make interpretation of outcome data possible.
- Knowledge of the placebo response (i.e. context-sensitive treatment effect) is essential in studies of pain.
- Placebo control is not unethical, but rescue pain relief must be available for all patients taking part in pain studies.

- Parallel studies are more easily analyzed and interpreted, but require larger numbers of patients than crossover studies.
- Evoked pain (e.g. pain during deep breathing and coughing after a thoracotomy) may be a more sensitive and important measure of treatment outcome than pain at rest.
- Besides measurement of pain, physical functioning, emotional functioning, participant ratings of global improvement and satisfaction with treatment, and side effects are important outcomes in pain studies.
- Report outcomes that can be used in meta-analyses (e.g. number of patients with 30 and 50 percent reduction in pain intensity).
- The trial should be registered in an open-access register, and the results published according to the CONSORT guidelines.

INTRODUCTION

A clinical trial is a planned experiment designed to assess the efficacy of a treatment by comparing the outcomes in a group of patients treated with a test treatment with those observed in a similar control group of patients (**Box 42.1**). The patients should normally be assigned to one of the groups by a randomization procedure, and enrolled and followed prospectively over the same time period. Thus, studies using historical controls do not qualify as clinical trials. Even if most published clinical trials assess drug treatment, effects of other kinds of interventions can, and should, be tested in the same way, e.g. surgical procedures, physical therapy, nursing procedures, and patient information. This chapter will specifically address trial methodology in assessment of analgesic drugs, but most issues are relevant for other interventions as well.

Box 42.1 An overview of the randomized controlled clinical trial (RCT)

1. Define the purpose of the study. Perform a thorough literature search. State specific hypotheses.
2. Define clearly main outcome(s), classification variables, and confounding variables.
3. Design the study. Controls. Placebo? Blinding. Calculate sample size.
4. Apply for approval from ethical committee and drug regulatory authorities (where applicable).
5. Use an adequate randomization method and maintain allocation concealment.
6. Register the trial in an open-access trial register before you start.
7. Conduct the trial. Make sure there is no unmasking of patient or observer blinding.
8. Analyze the results. Use descriptive statistics, test the hypotheses, and estimate treatment effect size.
9. Draw conclusions with care. Be careful with *a posteriori* hypotheses.
10. Publish the results in sufficient detail to permit an informed judgment of the validity of your conclusions.

EXPLANATORY AND PRAGMATIC ATTITUDES

Explanatory studies seek to find a causal relationship that has general validity outside the particular clinical situation studied – a biological principle.[1] A strict study design may be necessary to obtain a precise answer to a specific question.

Pragmatic studies, on the other hand, seek to find the best way to treat patients in specific clinical situations.[1] Results of a pragmatic study are not necessarily valid for other populations or circumstances than those studied.

Often clinical trials have elements of both these orientations. It is important to be aware of the differences. Much too often, general conclusions are drawn from pragmatic studies, or limitations of the study are not sufficiently emphasized and understood. **Table 42.1** summarizes typical differences between explanatory and pragmatic studies.

WHAT IS THE PURPOSE OF THE STUDY?

A preliminary research question needs a thorough literature search before you define clearly the specific purpose of the study. How will the proposed research advance our knowledge and potentially lead to improved patient care? Check the World Health Organization (WHO) web portal for ongoing clinical trials in your field (www.who.int/trialsearch).

DEFINE A PRIMARY EFFICACY VARIABLE

If many efficacy variables are measured and tested statistically, a problem arises. Even if there is no true difference between two treatments, the probability (p) of finding a statistically significant difference at the 0.05 level if ten different independent variables are tested is

---

Table 42.1 Important differences between explanatory and pragmatic.

Design issue	Explanatory	Pragmatic
Main question	General biological principle, e.g. can presurgical treatment prevent postoperative hypersensitivity?	What is the best treatment in clinical practice? For example, paracetamol with or without NSAID
Patient selection	Selective	Inclusive
Treatments	Specific actions (e.g. selective receptor agonists/antagonists)	Clinical favorites, including combinations
Controls	Placebo	Other active medication
Dose	High, often fixed	Titrate as in clinic
Treatment conditions	Optimal	Corresponding to clinical practice
Outcomes	Biologically meaningful	Clinically relevant
Analysis	Per protocol	Intention to treat

NSAID, nonsteroidal anti-inflammatory drug.

$1 - 0.95^{10} = 0.40$ (i.e. 40 percent). To avoid this problem, a primary efficacy variable should be chosen before the start of the study. This primary efficacy variable should be the basis for the sample size determination. Ideally, the primary efficacy variable should be a biologically or clinically meaningful outcome. However, sometimes a surrogate end point must be used. A surrogate end point can be defined as an observed variable that relates in some way to the variable of primary interest. Outcomes used in studies in pain relief are discussed in more detail below under More about outcomes in trials of pain treatment.

STUDY DESIGN

The randomized, double-blind, placebo-controlled trial has become the gold standard in investigation of new analgesics. In general, inadequately controlled clinical trials yield larger estimates of treatment effects than adequately controlled trials.[2] Thus, proper randomization and blinding are essential. It is also of crucial importance that the study is designed so that it is capable of finding a real difference. The study must have assay sensitivity.

ASSAY SENSITIVITY

Demonstration of assay sensitivity means that a study is documented to be able to show a significant difference between a standard analgesic and placebo, between two active drugs known to have different effects, or between two different doses of an active drug. One classical pitfall continues to appear frequently in published studies. A comparison of two active drugs finds no difference, and the authors conclude erroneously that the two drugs are equally effective (see below under Equivalence trials).

Assay sensitivity can be divided into upside sensitivity (the ability to discriminate between two active drugs) and downside sensitivity (the ability of a study to discriminate between an active drug and placebo). The score of placebo and standard active drug in a pain model decides upside and downside sensitivity in that pain model. In general, it is difficult to have both high upside sensitivity and high downside sensitivity in the same trial.[3]

CHOICE OF TREATMENTS AND CONTROLS

The number of treatment groups necessary depends on the aim of the study. The aim could be to demonstrate:

- superiority;
- equivalence;
- the relative potency;
- additive effect;
- synergy.

Superiority studies

A typical example is a critical trial of a new analgesic. As a minimum, the new drug is compared with placebo, and the aim is to show superiority over placebo. To help in interpretation, at least a third group should be added, using a standard analgesic drug in order to document assay sensitivity of the trial (**Figure 42.1**). For a complete discussion of design and interpretation of superiority studies, see the interactive textbook chapter by Max.[4]

Equivalence trials

The aim of an equivalence study is to show that one active drug (e.g. a new cyclooxygenase-2 (COX-2)-specific inhibitor) has equal efficacy to a standard drug (e.g. a nonselective COX inhibitor). The problem with this kind of study is that very large numbers of subjects are needed to prove that there is no clinically significant difference. If the two drugs are truly equivalent and give 75 percent overall treatment success, and we want to prove that the two treatments do not differ with more than 10 percent success rate, we will need 232 patients in each group to find this with 80 percent confidence ($p \leq 0.05$).

Underlying the interpretation of any equivalence trial is the assumption that the standard therapy is effective under the experimental conditions of the study. This is not necessarily true and is a threat to the validity of such trials. Assay sensitivity is not proven unless a third group is added, either placebo, two doses of the active comparator, or two active drugs with known efficacy difference.

Another problem is to know what a clinically important difference is under the specific conditions of the trial. A third group receiving placebo could both serve as a yardstick in judgment of what difference is clinically significant and prove presence of assay sensitivity.[5, 6, 7]

Relative potency

To find the relative potency, i.e. the relative size of a standard drug necessary to produce an effect equivalent to a test drug unit, at least four groups are needed. With two groups of standard and test drugs, there must be parallel dose response and overlap in effect size to correctly calculate relative potency. Several doses of each drug would be preferable. Relative potency may vary depending on whether peak analgesia or total analgesia over a time period is used for analysis if the drugs have different kinetics.[8]

During recent years, some studies have aimed at deciding relative potency by use of the patient-controlled

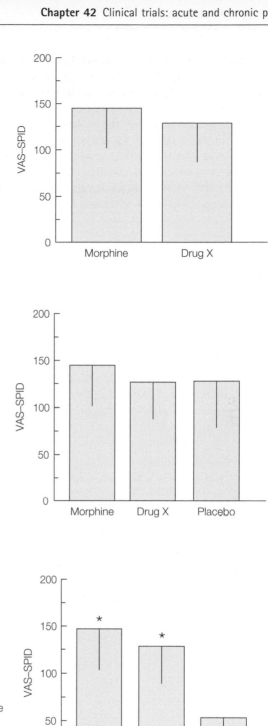

Figure 42.1 The pain intensity (left) and the corresponding summed pain intensity differences (SPID; right) are based on observed pain intensity (visual analog scale, VAS). Pain intensity difference (PID) is the pain intensity at drug intake minus the pain intensity at a given later time point. SPID is the area under the curve multiplied by the trapezoid rule (see **Figure 42.3**). *Significantly different from placebo. Panels (a), (b), and (c) show three different results. (a) No difference between drug X and the standard active drug. Possible interpretations: 1, the drugs are equally effective; 2, study methods are insensitive. (b) Study methods are insensitive to the analgesic effect of the standard analgesic. Assay sensitivity is not demonstrated. No conclusions can be drawn. (c) Assay sensitivity is demonstrated – the study can detect the analgesic effect of the standard active. Drug X is superior to placebo. Upside sensitivity is not tested. Reproduced with permission from Stubhaug A, Breivik H. Post-operative analgesic trials: some important issues. In: Breivik H (ed.). *Post-operative pain management. Baillière's Clinical Anaesthesiology: International Practice and Research 9*. London: Baillière Tindall, 1995: 555–84.[3]

analgesia (PCA) technique. This technique relies on a number of assumptions. The principle of PCA is that each patient will be able to titrate his plasma concentration and effect–organ concentration to constantly lie around the MEAC (minimum effective analgesic concentration). By comparing drug consumption, one should, in theory, be able to calculate relative potencies of different drugs.

Objections to the validity of PCA comparisons are, however, numerous. The pharmacokinetic profiles of the drugs being compared should be similar. If the duration of analgesia differs, the relative potency calculated is influenced by the duration of the study period. The PCA drug (e.g. morphine) may relieve one component of the pain experience (e.g. acute nociceptive pain), but not another pain component (e.g. acute neuropathic pain). Especially in such situations, the severity of pain is not the only factor that determines whether or not the patient will push the dose-demand button. Patients may choose not to push the demand button because they have the impression that the drug gives rise to side effects, such as unpleasant cognitive dysfunction, sedation, and nausea, and a patient may prefer some pain to these side effects. Thus, both analgesic profile and side effect profile of the drugs being compared should also be similar when the PCA technique is used to explore relative potency between analgesic drugs. In addition, groups of patients receiving the same drug in different bolus sizes should be included as a test of assay sensitivity of the method.[9, 10]

Additive effects

To document the additive effects of treatments is of interest when two drugs examined represent different classes of drugs (different mechanisms of action) with different side effect profiles. A typical design would then have four groups: placebo, each of the drugs separately, and a fourth group with the combination of both drugs. Ideally, it should also have groups with high doses of the single drugs. This would ideally prove that the combination of smaller doses of both drugs is beneficial compared with a higher dose of either single drug owing to fewer side effects or to a limiting ceiling effect of analgesia of the single drugs.

Synergy

To distinguish between additive and synergistic combinations requires more advanced designs and statistical expertise. Several doses of each drug and the combination are needed.[11] A graphical presentation as an isobologram is easily interpreted (**Figure 42.2**). If the combination (with confidence limits) lies below the line of additivity, synergy has been proven.

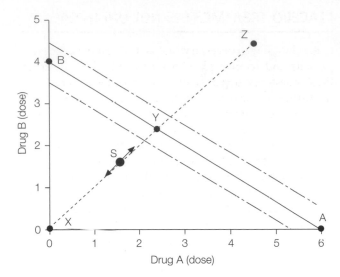

Figure 42.2 Isobologram showing doses of drugs A and B that have been calculated to give, for example, a 50 percent reduction in pain intensity (points A and B are calculated by regression from groups receiving escalating doses of A and B as single drugs). With simple additive effect, the doses of a combination of A and B necessary to give a 50 percent reduction in pain lie along the line A–B (shown with the confidence interval as dashed lines). Several groups receiving escalating doses of the combination in a defined dose relation (in this case 1:1) have been tested. Line X–Z indicates the possible mixtures of this combination. The doses necessary to give 50 percent pain relief are calculated by regression. Point Y represents a simple additive effect; points along the line X–Y show synergism; points along line Y–Z show antagonism. If the calculated dose of the combination lies along X–Y and confidence limits do not cross the confidence limits for line A–B, the synergism has been proven, as indicated by point S (arrows represent the confidence interval for S).

WHY IS KNOWLEDGE OF THE PLACEBO RESPONSE ESSENTIAL IN STUDIES OF PAIN?

There is a huge variation between subjects that undergo similar procedures.[12, 13, 14] Even if we only include patients with a certain pain intensity magnitude, one major problem in trials of pain relief is that we do not know how large the spontaneous reduction of pain without any treatment at all would be.[13, 14] For ethical reasons, we are unable to measure it. A placebo group receiving placebo treatment and an adequate rescue drug when needed is the closest we can get. The placebo response, measured as the reduction of pain after placebo treatment, is of course also part of the active drug response. Thus, knowledge of the placebo response in a study helps with interpreting the active drug response. It is shown that there are huge differences in the placebo response between studies.[15] This makes use of historical data on placebo response worthless. This must be kept in mind when evaluating trials that have included only active drugs.

PLACEBO TREATMENT IS NOT UNETHICAL

Is the clinical trial necessary, and is it ethical to randomize patients and to give placebo treatment? The answer to these questions depends on what we know about the treatments in question. In medical practice, potentially harmful treatments are often given without any documentation of effect. The major ethical question is to evaluate the balance between the importance of the objective of the study and the inherent risk to the participating subject. The degree of risk and discomfort must be favorably balanced by the probability of benefit to the patient or to patients in general. Participation in a clinical trial may have several advantages for the patient. However, even a modest additional discomfort or risk would be unethical if the study were designed in a way to preclude useful conclusions, or if the results for some reason are withheld from publication. Thus, proper study design, including placebo when relevant and publication of the results, are important ethical imperatives.[16]

Placebo treatment is never inactive, without effects, or equivalent to no treatment. The context of the administration of a treatment always influences the outcome. Unless the context-sensitive treatment effects ("placebo effects") are controlled, these may confound the outcome measures of a trial. This is especially true when measures of outcome rely on a subjective experience such as pain. Even proxy outcome measures of pain trials, such as functions, can be strongly influenced by context factors. For an in-depth discussion of these aspects of clinical trials, see Chapter 41, Placebo and nocebo.

METHOD OF RANDOMIZATION AND ALLOCATION CONCEALMENT

As previously mentioned, randomization is crucial. Randomization is an insurance against imbalance between treatment groups with respect to important, but often unknown, confounding factors. Variables that are known to affect results can be controlled for by stratified randomization (e.g. sex, age, diagnosis).[14, 17] The method is to produce a separate block randomization list for each subgroup (stratum).[17]

The exact method used for production of the treatment allocation list should be chosen carefully (e.g. envelope method, computer generation, use of lists of random numbers, randomization in blocks, etc.).[17, 18, 19] Proper randomization minimizes systematic allocation bias, but with small sample sizes randomization does not prevent random imbalance. In small clinical trials, stratified randomization is not effective and minimization is the accepted method of ensuring balance between groups for several known prognostic factors.[20] Minimization should be done by an independent person who allocates the next participant in a trial to the treatment that best minimizes imbalance between treatment groups across multiple predefined prognostic factors. A random element should normally be included in the process, and use of specially designed software like Minim (www-users.york.ac.uk/~mb55/guide/minim.htm) is recommended.[20]

After proper randomization, adequate allocation concealment must be continued. Proper allocation concealment prevents those who admit participants to the trial from knowing the upcoming assignments.[21, 22] Thus, quasi-randomization, such as allocating to active or placebo on alternating weeks, or allocation by day of birth, is not acceptable.

Both open access and commercial programs and websites offer help with randomization. A directory of randomization services has been made available by Martin Bland (www-users.york.ac.uk/~mb55/guide/randsery.htm).

INCLUSION OF PATIENTS: INCLUSION BASED ON PAIN MECHANISMS? ENRICHED ENROLLMENT

A careful selection and description of the population under study is important. The protocol must define clearly the inclusion criteria and the exclusion criteria. The CONSORT statement also requires that the settings and locations where the data were collected are reported.[23, 24] This makes extrapolation of results to other settings and populations easier.

Normally, a baseline pain above a certain level will increase the sensitivity of the trial. If patients with a low baseline pain are included, the potential treatment effect may be small compared with random fluctuations in pain intensity.

There is now a trend toward a mechanism-based pain diagnosis and treatment. Inclusion criteria based on an understanding of the pain mechanism should be considered in clinical pain trials.[25] As an example, zoster patients with severe allodynia may respond differently to a treatment compared with zoster patients insensitive to peripheral stimulation. In chronic pain trials, a screening period before a patient is randomized to treatment is usually necessary. This is important to document that pain intensity and other variables are relatively stable.

Sometimes, an enriched enrollment procedure is indicated to exclude nonresponders that make the study insensitive. Enriched enrollment means that only subjects who respond to the test treatment or a similar treatment, enter the study. If, for example, a new oral N-methyl-D-aspartate (NMDA) receptor antagonist is to be tested against neuropathic pain but is expected to help only a small subgroup of patients that are difficult to define on the basis of clinical judgment, it may be acceptable to include only patients who respond to an intravenous infusion of a known NMDA receptor antagonist like ketamine. Such an enriched enrollment strategy is meant to increase sensitivity and to reduce the risk of type II error (see below under Statistical issues), but it may easily introduce bias and problems with the interpretation of the results. If the patients use the test treatment in an open enrichment phase, they will more easily detect the active treatment in the blinded study phase (see below under Blinding and unblinding: active placebo). In patients on stable use of analgesics, a "flare of pain" if the drug is stopped will indicate that the patient is sensitive for that class of drug, and this flare can be an inclusion criterium and thus guide the enriched enrollment. However, abrupt opioid withdrawal may aggravate chronic pain even if long-term opioid treatment had minimal analgesic effect.

BLINDING AND UNBLINDING: ACTIVE PLACEBO

Blinding of treatment is especially important when subjective responses are measured. A double-blind procedure means that neither the patient nor the observer can identify the assigned treatment. A randomized, double-blind technique is a gold standard that should be used whenever possible. It is important to be aware that the possibility of unblinding of patient and observer is a serious threat to the validity of the study. The risk of unblinding increases with the duration of the study, and especially with crossover designs. After several weeks on an active drug, both patients and investigators often correctly guess the treatment allocation. Active placebo aims to mimic typical side effects of active drugs, such as sedation and dry mouth, without having any direct pharmacodynamic effect on pain. Drugs such as benzatropine and benzodiazepines have been used to reduce the risk of unblinding.[26, 27]

When the patient knows that he may receive placebo treatment and he guesses, correctly or incorrectly, from the onset of significant pain relief or side effects, that he received an active treatment, the pain relieving effect of the active drug, or of placebo will be increased, and vice versa.[28, 29]

The CONSORT statement (item 11b) proposes that the success of blinding is reported.[23, 24] However, very few studies do this.[30] One good example from the pain field is a study by Gilron et al.[31] The study reports not only the patient's guesses, but also the basis for the guess (absence or presence of analgesia or side effects). Such information may be very helpful in interpretation of results.

PARALLEL OR CROSSOVER STUDIES?

This is often an important question. A parallel design is never wrong, but will often require a much higher number of patients to answer the question than a crossover design. Parallel studies are preferred by regulatory agencies for pivotal trials of new drugs. Single centers may

be forced to use a crossover design to be able to include a sufficient number of patients to answer the research question. Whereas a parallel study is easy to analyze, the crossover design has several possible pitfalls.

The most serious problem with crossover designs is the interaction between treatments (carryover effects). This means that the effects of a treatment persist into the subsequent period. A period effect means a systematic difference between periods, irrespective of the treatment. Other problems with the crossover design include an increased length of study with more variation in pain, loss of data as a result of more dropouts than in parallel studies, and an increased risk of unblinding.

Parallel studies are by far the most common in postoperative analgesic trials: each patient is allocated to receive only one of the treatments tested. Parallel studies are the most straightforward, are easy to analyze, and are preferred by the majority of clinical trialists.[32] If the study population of a parallel trial is very heterogeneous, the problems that are likely to arise include variability of results, overlap between groups, and a low test power; no difference between drugs can be demonstrated even if a true difference exists. If the treatment effect is clinically meaningful, but nevertheless is small compared with interindividual variance, statistical power can be increased considerably by use of a crossover design.

With crossover trials it is important to remember that period effects and carryover effects exist, having both pharmacological and psychological reasons. To reduce the influence of these effects, a balanced design is necessary. Patients are randomized to predefined sequences (**Tables 42.2, 42.3,** and **42.4**). Carryover effects and period effects can also be calculated and accounted for in the efficacy analysis. However, both design and analysis of such studies are much more complicated than in parallel studies, and should be avoided if statistical expertise is not available. For a thorough discussion of crossover designs, see Jones and Kenward.[33]

MORE ABOUT OUTCOMES IN TRIALS OF PAIN TREATMENT

What is a meaningful end point?

Self-report measures are considered the gold standard in pain studies because they reflect the subjective nature of pain. Pain intensity is naturally often chosen as the primary outcome in studies of analgesics. From experimental studies there is substantial evidence that patients' assessment of pain intensity is a valid measure of experienced pain.[34] Often only the sensory dimension of pain (pain intensity) is measured, but the overall burden of suffering may depend on other aspects than the intensity of pain, e.g. affective, emotional aspects and interference with activities and sleep.

Table 42.2 Typical two-treatment crossover design.

Sequence	Treatment	
	Period 1	Period 2
1	A	B
2	B	A

Table 42.3 A three-group, complete crossover design.

Sequence	Treatment		
	Period 1	Period 2	Period 3
1	A	C	B
2	B	A	C
3	C	B	A
4	A	B	C
5	B	C	A
6	C	A	B

Table 42.4 Four-group complete crossover as a reduced, balanced, Latin square design.

Sequence	Treatment			
	Period 1	Period 2	Period 3	Period 4
1	A	D	B	C
2	B	A	C	D
3	C	B	D	A
4	D	C	A	B

This Latin square ensures that: (1) each subject has all treatments; (2) each treatment occurs with equal frequency in each period; and (3) that each treatment pair (e.g. A followed by D) occurs with equal frequency.

It is a good idea to ask what the patients think is an important outcome. In a qualitative study in chronic pain patients on opioid treatment, the patients chose the most meaningful end points to be (in descending order of importance): decreased pain, decreased frequency of scheduled doses, decreased opioid dose, decreased constipation, decreased drowsiness, improved sleep, improved activity of living, and improved concentration.[35] This demonstrates that simply assessing pain intensity may be an oversimplification of the measurement of effects of an analgesic drug. Similarly, important outcomes in acute pain include the ability to mobilize, to take deep breaths, and the absence of distressing side effects such as nausea, sedation, and cognitive dysfunction. A group called IMMPACT (Initiative on Methods, Measurement and Pain Assessment in Clinical Trials) has reviewed this area carefully and proposed core outcomes for studies in chronic pain.[36]

Pain intensity, pain unpleasantness, pain quality, and pain relief

Pain intensity is most commonly evaluated by an 11-point numerical rating scale (NRS) (0–10; 0 = no pain, 10 = worst pain imaginable), by a visual analog scale (VAS) (100-mm scale anchored at the two ends by the descriptors "no pain" and "worst pain imaginable"), or a four- to five-point categorical verbal rating scale (VRS) (e.g. 0 = no pain, 1 = weak pain, 2 = moderate pain, 3 = severe pain). Both the VAS and the 11-point NRS are proven to discriminate better than the four-point VRS in acute and chronic pain.[37] The 11-point NRS is often the preferred scale because of its simplicity and ease of use for most patients. Assessment of pain affect or unpleasantness is supported by the evidence that the affective component of pain can be distinguished from the sensory component (pain intensity) and may be differentially responsive to treatments.[38] Further description of pain qualities can be sampled with the Short-Form McGill Pain Questionnaire (SF-MPQ),[39] which assesses 15 specific sensory and affective pain descriptors and provides a total score and sensory and affective subscale scores. Pain relief can be calculated from pain intensity differences, but can also be assessed directly with similar instruments as pain intensity. For a thorough discussion on pain measurement, see Chapter 2, Practical methods for pain intensity measurements and Chapter 3, Selecting and applying pain measures.

Evoked pain

Instead of simply assessing "pain at rest," additional information can be achieved by using several types of stimuli to evoke pain. Mechanical (**Table 42.5**), thermal, and electrical stimuli can be used to measure pain thresholds and to assess responses to suprathreshold stimuli. Likewise, a standardized body movement can be a clinically meaningful stimulus (e.g. coughing, walking, and moving the arms after breast surgery).

In a postoperative study, a low dose of ketamine was shown to block the development of static hyperalgesia (measured with von Frey filaments) around a nephrectomy incision, although it had only a minor effect on pain at rest.[40] Correspondingly, in a dental postoperative model, Gilron and colleagues[41] found that an AMPA/kainate glutamate receptor antagonist (LY 293558) had only a minimal effect on resting pain, but had a robust effect on pain evoked by mouth opening. This demonstrates that simply testing new drugs for their effect on pain intensity at rest may falsely lead to the conclusion that they are without efficacy.

In trials on chronic pain patients, use of thermal, mechanical, and electrical stimuli have produced interesting new information about disease mechanisms and treatment effects.[42, 43, 44]

Table 42.5 Evoked mechanical pain: nature of stimuli and proposed research tools.

Nature of mechanical stimulus	Research tool
Static	
Punctate	Von Frey filaments
Blunt	Pressure algometer
Dynamic	
Spatial distribution	Artist's brush
	Cotton wool swab
	Toothbrush
Temporal distribution	Repetitive von Frey filament stimulation, e.g. 2 Hz

Repeated measurements: create a summary measure such as SPID or TOTPAR

Pain intensity and pain relief are usually measured repeatedly in studies on acute pain. Very often, there are different time intervals between the measurements. In such cases, it is a good idea to create a summary measure for a study-relevant time period and use this as the main efficacy variable.[45] Summed pain intensity difference (SPID) (**Figure 42.3**) is an example of one such summary measure. Note that it is not simply a sum of measurements, but an area under the curve (AUC) that takes time intervals between measurements into account. Correspondingly, TOTPAR is the AUC for pain relief (categorical scale) multiplied by time data. Also, in chronic pain trials, adequate use of baseline and repeated outcome measurement in the analysis may increase the statistical power.[46]

Consumption of rescue analgesia and remediation time

In many studies, in both acute and chronic pain, patients are offered a rescue drug when needed. This is necessary for ethical reasons. In such cases, group differences after the primary intervention will be divided into two outcomes: pain and rescue drug consumptions. As shown in **Figure 42.4**, this may reduce the sensitivity of each of the two outcomes, but can be compensated for by increasing the number of patients included.[40] The PCA consumption as the single main outcome has weaknesses that have been discussed above (see above under Relative potency). A composite score that takes into account both pain intensity and consumption of rescue analgesic can be a useful tool in analyzing data from such studies, but has not been used much.[47, 48]

In trials where a single dose is given, the time when a rescue drug is needed and the subsequent response to the rescue drug should be recorded. This remediation time is

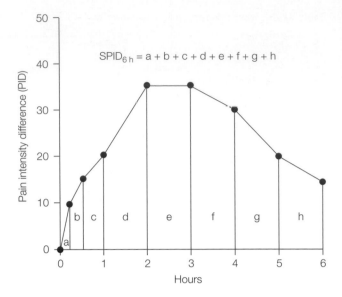

Figure 42.3 Graphical display of individual pain intensity differences in a study of acute pain. Pain intensity difference (PID) is pain intensity at drug intake minus pain intensity at a given time point. SPID is the total (summed) area under the PID curve, each subarea calculated by the trapezoid rule. In this case, pain intensity is measured after 15 minutes, 30 minutes, 1 hour, 2 hours, 3 hours, 4 hours, 5 hours, and 6 hours. SPID corresponds to the areas $a+b+c+d+e+f+g+h$.

a useful summary score, and the response to a standard rescue drug gives important additional information.[3]

Onset of analgesia

There is no generally accepted definition of how the onset of analgesia should be assessed clinically in acute pain. Onset can be described in terms of both the probability of obtaining onset and, for patients who obtain onset, the distribution of time to onset. One relatively new method is the use of patient-operated stopwatches. The watches are started when the trial drug has been administered. The patient is instructed to stop one watch the moment a defined clinically significant amount of pain relief is first experienced, e.g. when the first perception of pain relief is present or when meaningful pain relief is first experienced.[49] For many patients, the first perception of pain relief is not followed by a lasting meaningful pain relief. Time to meaningful pain relief seems more robust against placebo onset than time to first perception of pain relief. Onset can also be derived from the pain relief readings at prefixed time points. A common estimate of onset is the midpoint of the time interval between the first interview at which the patient reported onset and the preceding interview. This derived onset variable is a calculated value, not a measured one, and is often unable to discriminate between active drugs and placebo, even if the active drugs are superior in other efficacy measures.

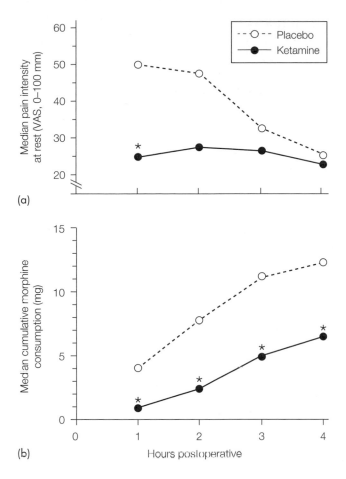

(a)

(b)

Hours postoperative

Figure 42.4 Difference in pain intensity and morphine consumption (patient-controlled analgesia, PCA) for the first four postoperative hours between a group receiving a low dose of ketamine and placebo. Note that an initial difference in pain intensity at one hour leads to a higher opioid consumption in the group with more pain. This leads to reduced pain, but never a full compensation. The initial group difference in pain intensity is divided between the two variables of pain intensity and opioid consumption. After four hours, no group difference is present (data not shown). Reproduced with permission from Stubhaug A, Breivik H, Eide PK et al. Mapping of punctuate hyperalgesia surrounding a surgical incision demonstrates that ketamine is a powerful suppressor of central sensitization to pain following surgery. *Acta Anaesthesiologica Scandinavica.* 1997; **41**: 1124–32.[40]

Regardless of method, it will be difficult to calculate one single value to characterize onset: for example, how should one correct for patients who do not experience onset before they receive rescue drug? Laska *et al.*[49] have proposed a clinically useful way to express relief and onset characteristics of a drug using a set of percentiles. A hypothetical example could read as follows, "For patients whose pain is similar to that experienced by patients examined in this study, it may be expected that 80 percent will experience an effect from the drug. Of those who have an effect, 25 percent will feel that they are obtaining meaningful relief by ten minutes or sooner, 50 percent by

20 minutes or sooner, 75 percent by 40 minutes or sooner, and almost all who obtain an effect will have obtained it by 60 minutes."

Similar to measurement of onset, the patient can be asked to stop a second watch when the clinically significant pain relief is no longer felt (offset).

Pain interference with daily life (physical and emotional functioning). Health-related quality of life

IMMPACT recommendations include assessment of pain interference with physical functioning and emotional functioning.[37] A disease-specific measure is recommended if a well-accepted one exists, as for example WOMAC for osteoarthritis pain.[50] One simple general inventory for measuring physical functioning is the Brief Pain Inventory (BPI). The patient scores how the pain interferes with general activity, mood, walking ability, work, relations with other people, sleep, and enjoyment of life.[51] Proposed inventories for emotional functioning are the Beck Depression Inventory[52] and the Profile of Mood States (POMS).[53] Further developments of such instruments are under way, and the use of item response theory will allow individual questions depending on known patients characteristics and previous answers.[54]

Generic measures of health-related quality of life (QoL) like the SF-36[55] allow comparison with other disorders. It is an impressive finding that patients suffering from chronic nonmalignant pain have as low health-related QoL as patients in the terminal phase of cancer.[56] Clearly, clinical trials on chronic pain should assess QoL in addition to more traditional pain assessment.[36]

Side effects

In many clinical settings, the side effects are as important as the treatment effect. The quality of reporting varies a great deal.[57] Studies using only open-ended question like, "Have you experienced any side effects?" in general report fewer side effects than studies using more structured interviews. Specific questions regarding important side effects with assessment of intensity, duration, and interference give valuable information.

Global assessment

A global question, such as "What is your overall satisfaction with the treatment?" is an important question at the end of the study because it gives the patient an opportunity to evaluate the positive effects (analgesia, better sleep, etc.), the negative drug effects (side effects), and the comfort and feasibility of the method employed. A patient with total analgesia but unacceptable side effects may choose to give a low score on the global assessment.

Global assessment scales should have options for both improvement and worsening. One such scale is the Patients Global Impression of Change (PGIC) which is suitable for chronic pain trials. The participants rate their response during a trial with the options "very much improved," "much improved," "minimally improved," "no change," "minimally worse," "much worse," and "very much worse."[3, 36]

What is a clinically important change in pain outcomes?

Two studies by Farrar et al.[58, 59] concluded that an approximate reduction of 30 percent in pain intensity corresponds well with the patient's experience of clinically meaningful pain relief. Thus, if pain intensity is the main outcome, it seems reasonable to design a study that is large enough to be able to detect a 30 percent reduction in pain intensity. This topic has been carefully reviewed and benchmark values for several core outcomes have been proposed.[60]

Outcomes that can easily be extracted for use in a meta–analysis (responder analysis)

With the increased focus on systematic reviews, there has been a call for standardization of outcomes and reporting in trials in pain relief to make it easier to compare and reproduce research results.

For use in systematic reviews, quantitative data have been dichotomized into success or failure before data from several studies are combined. Until now, the fraction of patients achieving > 50 percent of the maximum possible pain relief has most frequently been extracted from acute pain trials, and the fraction achieving an estimation of 50 percent pain relief has been extracted from studies in chronic pain.[61] A significant change in the mean may be the result of both a moderate change in many patients and a major change in a small number of patients. Therefore, extraction of data should ideally be based on individual data of a standard dichotomous or dichotomizable outcome. Number of patients with > 30 percent reduction and 50 percent reduction in pain intensity is suggested by IMMPACT in a recent concensus report.[36, 62]

LONG-TERM TRIALS: ASSESSMENT OF QUALITY OF LIFE

There is a considerable lack of long-term trials in chronic pain. Most trials last only a few weeks at the most. One reason is that it is ethically difficult to keep patients on placebo for long periods. A solution is a second open-label phase after the initial blinded trial. Longer-term trials are necessary to assess whether treatment effects are lasting and, most importantly, to assess the impact of treatment on a patient's global situation, taking into account side effects and measures of quality of life.

STATISTICAL ISSUES

It is beyond the scope of this chapter to cover statistical issues in any detail. Statistical planning before the start of the study is very important: if you think you will need help with the statistics, this is the time to seek it.

One critical aspect in the planning of a clinical study is to estimate the sample size required. The number of subjects necessary to obtain a certain power depends upon the magnitude of the difference that is considered interesting to detect and the variance of the variable under study in the population. It follows that knowledge about the variation is critical. Sample size calculations based on pilot results are generally more reliable than results based on results in the literature. The purpose of the sample size determination is to avoid both false-positive (type I error), with choice of a sufficiently low α (usually 0.05), and false-negative (type II error) results (**Table 42.6**). If the sample is too small, it will be impossible to show that even large differences are due to anything other than chance. The sample size is normally set so that if the chosen difference exists, then it is more than 80 percent chance (80 percent power, i.e $\beta = 0.20$) that a statistically significant result will be obtained.

How do we treat drop outs? Intention–to–treat versus per–protocol analysis

Randomization and blinding is not sufficient to secure an unbiased comparison between treatments. In addition,

Table 42.6 Cells A–D show four possible results of a clinical trial; small sample sizes increase the risk of the results shown in cells B and C.

		Objective truth	
		Difference between treatments	No difference between treatments
Conclusion of the clinical trial	Difference between treatments	A: Correct conclusion of the clinical trial (true-positive)	C: Incorrect conclusion (false-positive); type I error
	No difference between treatments	B: Incorrect conclusion (false-negative); type II error	D: Correct conclusion of the clinical trial (true-negative)

missing data should be ignorable. This is seldom the case in pain studies.

In acute pain, single-dose trials, it is common that patients leave the study when they receive rescue medication (in accordance with the protocol). Usually, they are assigned the baseline pain intensity or the last real observation immediately before rescue for the rest of the trial (last observation carried forward (LOCF)). This introduces potential bias.[3, 63] At the end of the trial, the proportion of real assessments may be small.

Pain intensity at withdrawal will tend to be higher for those who leave the study early versus those who leave the study late. A drug with early onset and moderate effect may score better than a drug with late onset good effect due to the effect of observations carried forward after rescue.[3]

In long-term trials, patients do not normally leave the study even if they use rescue drug. However, they may stop using the drug under study, e.g. due to lack of effect or to side effects. Should such patients be excluded from the efficacy analysis?

A per-protocol (PP) analysis compares outcomes only in those patients who are sufficiently compliant with the protocol. This means that both the intervention and the assessments are undertaken according to a minimum defined in the protocol. A per-protocol analysis gives an estimate of the so-called **method-effectiveness**, which is often of interest to clinicians as long as proper information is given about all patients entering the study.[64]

However, all postrandomization exclusions may inflate the risk of type I error (finding a difference when a true difference does not exist). An intention to treat (ITT) analysis is based on the initial treatment intent (the randomization), not on the treatment eventually received by the patient. The reasons why the patient did not receive the treatment as randomized are ignored. The ITT analysis estimates the **use-effectiveness**. A true ITT analysis requires complete follow up, including main outcomes and side effects, regardless of compliance with the intervention. This is not always possible, and authors often define the ITT population less strictly, e.g. all patients with usable outcome assessment. Both ITT and PP analysis give information of interest.[65] In many studies, both analyses should be presented with a strict definition of the populations.[24] If the PP analysis and the ITT analysis differ, the reasons for this must be further investigated. A simple example of ITT and PP analysis in a study with many drop outs is presented in **Table 42.7**.

In crossover studies, drop outs create additional problems. Paired analysis can only be undertaken with patients who have outcomes from all periods. This makes true ITT analysis impossible for efficacy evaluation. In addition, drop outs may invalidate a balanced design. A complete description of the patient flow and reasons for postrandomization exclusions must be given.[23, 24]

REGISTER YOUR TRIAL

Publication bias means that studies finding a difference between treatments are more likely to be published than negative ones. Not to report study results is increasingly seen as scientific and ethical misconduct, and the pressure to register trials to reduce underreporting is growing.[66] Prospective registration of all trials in an open access register is the solution. This gives transparency regarding ongoing trials, their planned study size, chosen primary outcome, and several other key items. Several registers exist today.

The ISRCTN register (http://isrctn.org) and the NIH-based register (http://clinicaltrials.gov) are the largest with >2000 and >1000 pain studies registered, respectively. In 2007, the WHO opened a web search portal for clinical trials from several primary registers (www.who.int/ictrp/en).

PUBLISH YOUR TRIAL

The revised CONSORT statement presents a checklist of 22 items that should be properly reported and a flow diagram to show the passage of patients through a randomized controlled trial.[23, 24] A template and updated guidelines are available from the CONSORT website (www.consort-statement.org). There is no reason not to use these guidelines when applicable.

According to the revised Helsinki Declaration, all results should be published.[16] For studies not fully published in peer-reviewed journals, there is at present no formal consensus on standards for the minimum of results reporting. It is expected that guidelines for results reporting will be established as part of the WHO clinical trial registry platform. In the near future, study approval might be given only on the condition that the trial is registered and that main results will be reported in an open register.

Table 42.7 A simple example of a study where intention-to-treat- and per-protocol analysis lead to different conclusions.

	New	Old	Analysis	Interpretation
Randomized subjects	100	100	Intention-to-treat:	
Responders	50	50	50 responders/100 versus 50 responders/100	New = Old
Received intervention	60	90	Per-protocol:	New, better than Old
Responders	45	45	45 responders/60 versus 45 responders/90	

CONCLUSIONS

A clinical trial is a comparison of outcomes in patients randomized to test or control treatment(s). If possible, all participants should be blinded for the intervention type(s). An explanatory trial seeks to explore a general biological principle by finding a causal relationship that has general validity outside the particular clinical situation studied, whereas a pragmatic trial seeks to find the best treatment for a particular condition or group of people. The purpose of the study must be clearly defined, meaningful, and aimed at increasing our knowledge. It is important to choose one primary efficacy variable. In order to make interpretation of outcome data possible, one should document upside assay sensitivity (i.e. an active control treatment is effective) and downside assay sensitivity (unspecific ("placebo") control is less effective). Knowledge of the placebo response (i.e. context-sensitive treatment effect) is essential in studies of pain. Placebo control is not unethical, but rescue pain relief must be available for all patients taking part in pain studies. Undertaking a study that gives results that cannot be interpreted is unethical.

True randomization of patients to the interventions being studied and allocation concealment reduces bias. Blinding of participants and observers to test treatment(s) also reduces bias; unblinding (e.g. because of effects or side effects) may increase or decrease active treatment effects.

Parallel studies are more easily analyzed and interpreted, but require larger numbers of patients than crossover studies.

About 30 percent reduction in pain intensity is considered meaningful by patients.

Evoked pain (e.g. pain during deep breathing and coughing after a thoracotomy) is often a more sensitive and important measure of treatment outcome than pain at rest. Other patient-reported outcomes like pain interference with physical and emotional functioning should be assessed in addition to pain intensity. Report outcomes that can be used in meta-analyses (e.g. proportion of patients with more than 30 percent pain relief). Seek statistical help while planning the trial. Register your trial in an open access register. Publish your trial results. Follow the CONSORT guidelines for reporting a randomized controlled trial.

REFERENCES

1. Schwartz D, Lellouch J. Explanatory and pragmatic attitudes in therapeutical trials. *Journal of Chronic Diseases.* 1967; **20**: 637–48.

* 2. Schulz KF, Chalmers I, Hayes RJ, Altman DG. Empirical evidence of bias. Dimensions of methodological quality associated with estimates of treatment effects in controlled trials. *Journal of the American Medical Association.* 1995; **273**: 408–12.

* 3. Stubhaug A, Breivik H. Post-operative analgesic trials: some important issues. In: Breivik H (ed.). *Post-operative pain management. Baillière's Clinical Anaesthesiology: International Practice and Research 9.* London: Baillière Tindall, 1995: 555–84.

* 4. Max MB. The design of clinical trials of pain treatment. In: Max MB, Lynn J. editors. *Symptom research. Methods and opportunities. An interactive textbook.* Last updated October 2003, cited February 2008. Available from: http://symptomresearch.nih.gov/chapter_1/index.htm.

5. Tramer MR, Reynolds DJ, Moore RA, McQuay HJ. When placebo controlled trials are essential and equivalence trials are inadequate. *British Medical Journal.* 1998; **317**: 875–80.

6. Landow L. Current issues in clinical trial design: superiority versus equivalency studies. *Anesthesiology.* 2000; **92**: 1814–20.

7. Stubhaug A. Comparison of tramadol with morphine for post-operative pain following abdominal surgery. *European Journal of Anaesthesiology.* 1996; **13**: 416–17.

8. Beaver WT, Wallenstein SL, Houde RW, Rogers A. A clinical comparison of the effects of oral and intramuscular administration of analgesics: pentazocine and phenazocine. *Clinical Pharmacology and Therapeutics.* 1968; **9**: 582–97.

9. Owen H, Plummer JL, Armstrong I *et al.* Variables of patient-controlled analgesia. 1. Bolus size. *Anaesthesia.* 1989; **1**: 7–10.

* 10. Max MB. Divergent traditions in analgesic clinical trials. *Clinical Pharmacology and Therapeutics.* 1994; **56**: 237–41.

11. Tallarida RJ, Stone DJ, Raffa RB. Efficient designs for studying synergistic drug combinations. *Life Sciences.* 1997; **61**: 417–25.

12. Parkhouse J, Lambrechts W, Simpson BRJ. The incidence of postoperative pain. *British Journal of Anaesthesia.* 1961; **33**: 345–53.

13. McQuay HJ, Bullingham RE, Moore RA *et al.* Some patients don't need analgesics after surgery. *Journal of the Royal Society of Medicine.* 1982; **75**: 705–08.

14. Rosseland LA, Stubhaug A. Gender is a confounding factor in pain trials: Women report more pain than men after arthroscopic surgery. *Pain.* 2004; **112**: 248–53.

* 15. Turner JA, Deyo RA, Loeser JD *et al.* The importance of placebo effects in pain treatment and research. *Journal of the American Medical Association.* 1994; **271**: 1609–14.

* 16. World Medical Association Declaration of Helsinki: ethical principles for medical research involving human. *Journal of the American Medical Association.* 2000; **284**: 3043–45.

* 17. Altman DG, Bland JM. How to randomise. *British Medical Journal (Clinical research ed.).* 1999; **319**: 703–04.

* 18. Meinert CL. *Clinical trials. Design, conduct and analysis.* New York: Oxford University Press, 1986.

* 19. Pocock SJ. *Clinical trials. A practical approach.* New York: John Wiley & Sons, 1983.

20. Altman DG, Bland JM. Treatment allocation by minimisation. *British Medical Journal (Clinical research ed.).* 2005; **330**: 843.

21. Schulz KF. Randomised trials, human nature, and reporting guidelines. *Lancet.* 1996; **348**: 596–8.

* 22. Pildal J, Hrobjartsson A, Jorgensen K *et al.* Impact of allocation concealment on conclusions drawn from meta-analyses of randomized trials. *International Journal of Epidemiology.* 2007; **36**: 847–57.

* 23. Moher D, Schulz KF, Altman DG. The CONSORT statement: revised recommendations for improving the quality of reports of parallel-group randomised trials. *Lancet.* 2001; **357**: 1191–4.

* 24. Altman DG, Schulz KF, Moher D *et al.* CONSORT GROUP (Consolidated Standards of Reporting Trials). The revised CONSORT statement for reporting randomized trials: explanation and elaboration. *Annals of Internal Medicine.* 2001; **134**: 663–94.

* 25. Woolf CJ, Max MB. Mechanism-based pain diagnosis: issues for analgesic drug development. *Anesthesiology.* 2001; **95**: 241–9.

26. Watson CP, Moulin D, Watt-Watson J *et al.* Controlled-release oxycodone relieves neuropathic pain: a randomized controlled trial in painful diabetic neuropathy. *Pain.* 2003; **105**: 71–78.

27. Khoromi S, Cui L, Nackers L, Max MB. Morphine, nortriptyline and their combination vs. placebo in patients with chronic lumbar root pain. *Pain.* 2007; **130**: 66–75.

28. Max MB, Schafer SC, Culnane M *et al.* Association of pain relief with drug side effects in postherpetic neuralgia: a single-dose study of clonidine, codeine, ibuprofen, and placebo. *Clinical Pharmacology and Therapeutics.* 1988; **43**: 363–71.

29. Romundstad L, Breivik H, Niemi G *et al.* Methylprednisolone intravenously 1 day after surgery has sustained analgesic and opioid-sparing effectys. *Acta Anaesthesiologica Scandinavica.* 2004; **48**: 1223–31.

30. Hróbjartsson A, Forfang E, Haahr MT *et al.* Blinded trials taken to the test: an analysis of randomized clinical trials that report tests for the success of blinding. *International Journal of Epidemiology.* 2007; **36**: 654–63.

31. Gilron I, Orr E, Tu D *et al.* A placebo-controlled randomized clinical trial of perioperative administration of gabapentin, rofecoxib and their combination for spontaneous and movement-evoked pain after abdominal hysterectomy. *Pain.* 2005; **113**: 191–200.

32. Sriwatanakul K, Lasagna L, Cox C. Evaluation of current clinical trial methodology in analgesimetry based on experts' opinions and analysis of several analgesic studies. *Clinical Pharmacology and Therapeutics.* 1983; **34**: 277–83.

33. Jones B, Kenward MG. *Design and analysis of cross-over trials.* London: Chapman and Hall, 1989.

34. Nielsen CS, Stubhaug A, Price DD *et al.* Individual differences in pain sensitivity: Genetic and environmental contributions. *Pain.* 2008; **136**: 21–9.

35. Casarett D, Karlawish J, Sankar P *et al.* Designing pain research from the patients perspective: what trial end points are important to patients with chronic pain? *Pain Medicine.* 2001; **2**: 309–16.

* 36. Dworkin RH, Turk DC, Farrar JT *et al.* Core outcome measures for chronic pain clinical trials: IMMPACT recommendations. *Pain.* 2005; **113**: 9–19.

37. Breivik EK, Bjornsson GA, Skovlund E. A comparison of pain rating scales by sampling from clinical trial data. *Clinical Journal of Pain.* 2000; **16**: 22–8.

38. Price DD, Harkins SW, Baker C. Sensory-affective relationships among different types of clinical and experimental pain. *Pain.* 1987; **28**: 297–307.

39. Melzack R. The short-form McGill Pain Questionnaire. *Pain.* 1987; **30**: 191–7.

40. Stubhaug A, Breivik H, Eide PK *et al.* Mapping of punctuate hyperalgesia surrounding a surgical incision demonstrates that ketamine is a powerful suppressor of central sensitization to pain following surgery. *Acta Anaesthesiologica Scandinavica.* 1997; **41**: 1124–32.

41. Gilron I, Max MB, Lee G *et al.* Effects of the AMPA/kainate antagonist LY293558 on spontaneous and evoked postoperative pain. *Clinical Pharmacology and Therapeutics.* 2000; **68**: 320–7.

42. Attal N, Brasseur L, Parker F *et al.* Effects of gabapentin on the different components of peripheral and central neuropathic pain syndromes: a pilot study. *European Neurology.* 1998; **40**: 191–200.

43. Sjolund KF, Belfrage M, Karlsten R *et al.* Systemic adenosine infusion reduces the area of tactile allodynia in neuropathic pain following peripheral nerve injury: a multi-centre, placebo-controlled study. *European Journal of Pain.* 2001; **5**: 199–207.

44. Jørum E, Warncke T, Stubhaug A. Cold allodynia and hyperalgesia in neuropathic pain: the effect of N-methyl-D-aspartate (NMDA) receptor antagonist ketamine; a double blind, cross-over comparison with alfentanil and placebo. *Pain.* 2003; **101**: 229–35.

* 45. Matthews JN, Altman DG, Campbell MJ, Royston P. Analysis of serial measurements in medical research. *British Medical Journal (Clinical research ed.).* 1990; **300**: 230–5.

46. Vickers AJ, Altman DJ. Statistics notes: Analysing controlled trials with baseline and follow up measurements. *British Medical Journal (Clinical research ed.).* 2001; **323**: 1123–4.

47. Silverman DG, O'Connor TZ, Brull SJ. Integrated assessment of pain scores and rescue morphine use during studies of analgesic efficacy. *Anesthesia and Analgesia.* 1993; **77**: 168–70.

48. Romundstad L, Breivik H, Roald H *et al.* Methylprednisolone reduces pain, emesis, and fatigue after breast augmentation surgery: a single-dose, randomized, parallel-group study with methylprednisolone

125 mg, parecoxib 40 mg, and placebo. *Anesthesia and Analgesia.* 2006; **102**: 418–25.

49. Laska EM, Siegel C, Sunshine A. Onset and duration: measurement and analysis. *Clinical Pharmacology and Therapeutics.* 1991; **49**: 1–5.

50. Bellamy N, Buchanan WW, Goldsmith CH *et al.* Validation study of WOMAC: a health status instrument for measuring clinically important patient relevant outcomes to antirheumatic drug therapy in patients with osteoarthritis of the hip or knee. *Journal of Rheumatology.* 1988; **15**: 1833–40.

51. Cleeland CS, Ryan KM. Pain assessment: global use of the Brief Pain Inventory. *Annals of the Academy of Medicine of Singapore.* 1994; **23**: 129–38.

52. Beck AT, Ward CH, Mendelson M *et al.* An inventory for measuring depression. *Archives of General Psychiatry.* 1961; **4**: 561–71.

53. McNair DM, Lorr M, Droppleman LF. *Profile of mood states.* San Diego, CA: Educational and Industrial Testing Service, 1971.

54. Turk DC, Dworkin RH, Burke LB *et al.* Developing patient-reported outcome measures for pain clinical trials: IMMPACT recommendations. *Pain.* 2006; **125**: 208–15.

55. Ware JE, Sherbourne CD. The MOS 36-item short-form health survey (SF-36). I. Conceptual framework and item selection. *Medical Care.* 1992; **30**: 473–83.

56. Fredheim O, Kaasa S, Fayers P *et al.* Chronic non-malignant pain patients report as poor health related quality of life as palliative cancer patients. *Acta Anaesthesiologica Scandinavica.* 2008; **52**: 143–8.

57. Edwards JE, McQuay HJ, Moore RA, Collins SL. Reporting of adverse effects in clinical trials should be improved: lessons from acute postoperative pain. *Journal of Pain and Symptom Management.* 1999; **18**: 427–37.

58. Farrar JT, Portenoy RK, Berlin JA *et al.* Defining the clinically important difference in pain outcome measures. *Pain.* 2000; **88**: 287–94.

59. Farrar JT, Young Jr JP, LaMoreaux L *et al.* Clinical importance of changes in chronic pain intensity measured on an 11-point numerical pain rating scale. *Pain.* 2001; **94**: 149–58.

∗ 60. Dworkin RH, Turk DC, Wyrwich KW *et al.* Interpreting the clinical importance of treatment outcomes in chronic pain clinical trials: IMMPACT recommendations. *Journal of Pain.* 2008; **9**: 105–21.

∗ 61. McQuay H, Moore A. *An evidence-based resource for pain relief.* Oxford: Oxford University Press, 1998.

62. Farrar JT, Dworkin RH, Max MB. Use of the cumulative proportion of responders analysis graph to present pain data over a range of cut-off points: making clinical trial data more understandable. *Journal of Pain and Symptom Management.* 2006; **31**: 369–77.

63. Thaler HT, Friedlander-Klar H, Cirrincione C *et al.* A statistical approach to measuring analgesic response. In: Bond MR, Charlton J, Woolf C (eds). *Proceedings of the VIth World Congress on Pain.* Amsterdam: Elsevier, 1991: 539–42.

64. Sheiner LB, Rubin DB. Intention-to-treat analysis and the goals of clinical trials. *Clinical Pharmacology and Therapeutics.* 1995; **57**: 6–15.

65. Lachin JM. Statistical considerations in the intent-to-treat principle. *Controlled Clinical Trials.* 2000; **21**: 167–89.

66. De Angelis C, Drazen JM, Frizelle FA *et al.* Clinical trial registration: a statement from the International Committee of Medical Journal Editors. *Annals of Internal Medicine.* 2004; **141**: 477–8.

43

Clinical trials: dental pain

ELSE K BREIVIK HALS

KEY LEARNING POINTS

- The dental pain model = patients in postoperative pain (first 12 hours) after surgical removal of mandibular third molars.
- The patient population is young and healthy patients largely unencumbered by concurrent disease and thus concomitant medication.
- Oral analgesics are best tested using this model.

- Thorough planning of protocol and keeping to the protocol.
- Adherence to randomized controlled trials.
- Good clinical trial practice, i.e. approval from ethical committee and Medicinus Agency.
- The primary outcome measure should be the direct assessment of change in pain intensity.

INTRODUCTION

Surgical removal of mandibular impacted or incompletely erupted third molars in ambulatory patients is a common procedure, both in general dental practice and in oral surgery practice (**Figure 43.1**). The operative procedure results in hyperalgesia two to four hours later, with cardinal signs of inflammation (rubor, calor, tumor, dolor, functio laesa) involving the alveolar bone, surrounding mucosa, and masticatory organs. The study of pain and pain relief after this type of surgery is often referred to as "the dental pain model." The postoperative pain experienced varies from mild to severe following dissipation of the local anesthetic block, reaching its peak within the first six hours. Following this initial period, acute pain abates and the patient requires less analgesic medication.[1] Although the duration of pain and discomfort may last for more than four postoperative days, it is usually transient and is limited to one to three postoperative days.[2] Other sequelae, such as trismus with reduced mouth opening and facial swelling, may also appear gradually, peaking at between 48 and 72 hours.[3][II] The majority of these patients are healthy young adults (18–30 years old) without former experience of oral disability or consuming medication, which could influence pain assessment or interact with the analgesic under study.

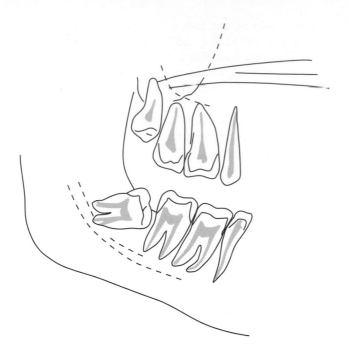

Figure 43.1 Surgical removal of impacted third molars is a useful setting for acute postoperative pain trials. The impacted third molar in the lower jaw requires surgical removal, a procedure that will be associated with postoperative pain of moderate to severe intensity in approximately 50 percent of patients.

This chapter will predominantly address trials for the relief of postoperative pain after third molar surgery and only briefly discuss other acute dental pains that have been employed for the evaluation of analgesics.

Using the dental pain model, Lökken and coworkers[4] [II] published the first study on acute pain and inflammation following third molar removal in 1975, and in the subsequent decade they published several clinical studies which examined the efficacy of oral analgesics using this model.[5] A crossover design was originally used in patients who required bilateral surgical removal of third molars, with each patient undergoing unilateral surgery on two separate occasions and receiving alternate interventions on each. However, this crossover design has lost some of its popularity because of the limited number of test drug groups possible in this design (see Improving and documenting assay sensitivity) and because of a potential carryover effect when each patient acts as his or her own control. The parallel group design is now more common, in which each patient undergoes one operation and receives a single treatment only. The parallel design also enables more than two test drugs to be examined, and carryover effects are absent because each subject participates only once. A drawback of the parallel design, however, is a greater variation in assessments between patients than in the assessments from each patient on two separate occasions using the crossover design. The dental pain model has been extensively used in the evaluation of

the pain-relieving effects of nonsteroidal anti-inflammatory drugs (NSAIDs), paracetamol (acetaminophen), opioids, local anesthetics, and combinations of these given before, during, or after surgery.[1] Not only traditional and new analgesic and anti-inflammatory drugs, but also antibiotics, corticosteroids, homeopathic treatment, low-energy-level laser, and complementary healing have been evaluated using the dental pain model.[1, 6][II], [7][II], [8, 9][II], [10, 11][II]

ADVANTAGES OF THE DENTAL PAIN MODEL

The dental pain model is generally considered to be sensitive in documenting whether the analgesic effectiveness of "mild" analgesics is superior to that of placebo,[12][II] as well as in discriminating between analgesic drugs of differing analgesic potencies.[13] In fact, McQuay and Moore[14] recommend the removal of lower third molars as their model of choice for an explanatory trial of an oral analgesic in the latest *Textbook of Pain*. In most oral maxillofacial surgical units, there is an abundance of otherwise healthy young adult patients undergoing third molar surgery, of whom approximately half will require analgesia. Most patients are willing to participate and, being young adults, will understand instructions and comply with protocol requirements when well informed by the investigator. The surgical procedure is usually elective and postoperative pain is confined to one area of the body. The large number of patients undergoing third molar surgery at oral maxillofacial surgical units means that an adequate supply of patients can be found within a reasonable time frame for trial execution. Thus, the readily available patients, the relative simplicity of the procedure, and the immediate pain experienced create an ideal setting for analgesic trials.[15][II]

LIMITATIONS OF THE DENTAL PAIN MODEL

The natural course of postoperative pain following third molar surgery is fairly short. Time to peak pain intensity after removal of impacted wisdom teeth is approximately six hours after surgery.[16][I] Therefore, trials can only be of limited duration, ideally taking place within the first 6–11 postoperative hours. Variation in baseline pain after third molar surgery is large,[17][II] with only 40–60 percent of patients reporting moderate to severe pain.[18][II], [19][II], [20][II] The dental pain model has been recommended only for single-dose studies owing to this variability among patients.[21] Only 20–40 percent of patients undergoing unilateral mandibular third molar surgery have been reported to experience pain and discomfort during the first three postoperative days,[22][I] whereas 37–75 percent of patients undergoing surgical removal of all four third molars experience pain and discomfort during the first three postoperative days.[23][I] Owing to this variation of pain intensity during the first postoperative days, repeated dose analgesic trials lasting more than 11 hours may thus not have sufficient assay sensitivity for differences to be detected between analgesic test drugs.

Surgical removal of third molars is usually performed on outpatients under local anesthesia, but occasionally general anesthesia is employed. Recovery from general anesthesia is often complicated by side effects which may hinder pain intensity evaluations. The postoperative facilities at the oral maxillofacial surgical units may also be insufficient for pain assessment.

THE PROTOCOL AND GOOD CLINICAL TRIAL PRACTICE

The study of subjective experience such as pain is notoriously subject to bias. Meticulous protocol design and subsequent close adherence to it and monitoring improves the quality of the trial. Analgesic trials using the dental pain model should adhere to the general rules of good clinical trial practice,[24] which demand not only high ethical and scientific standards but also meticulous conduct, recording, terminating, and reporting of trials according to preestablished criteria in the study protocols. Inadequate methodological standards correlate with bias in estimation of treatment effect, and blind assessments of analgesics produce significantly lower and more consistent measurements than open assessments.[25] Analgesic trials therefore require strict adherence to the principles of randomized controlled trials (RCTs).[25, 26]

The essence of good clinical trial design and execution is to:

- define a clear purpose and hypothesis;
- describe the effect variables and how they will be measured;
- describe any known confounding variables and control for them by exclusion criteria or by stratified randomization;
- justify study design: parallel groups or crossover; single dose or multiple repeated doses of test drug. Control group(s): standard active, one or more doses, and placebo;
- calculate sample size to achieve sufficient statistical power. If necessary, perform pilot study to be able to estimate variation and sample size;
- receive ethical committee approval and Medicinus Agency approval prior to starting the trial;
- sign patient insurance if needed according to hospital policy;
- randomize using accepted methodology;
- mask test drugs and secure blinding of patients and observer;
- receive oral and written informed patient consent;

- guide, inform, and support patients to ensure protocol compliance and to ensure that there is no unblinding of patients nor of observers;
- ensure blinding of patients and observers throughout the study period and beyond evaluation of effect variables measured in each patient (= double blind);
- analyze data using descriptive statistics and test statistics. Estimate treatment effects with confidence intervals;
- make conclusions based on findings and statistical analysis;
- record details of dropouts, missing data, rescue treatment;
- publish the study according to the CONSORT statement, allowing the reader to evaluate the validity of your findings.[26]

PATIENT INFORMATION, CONSENT, AND MONITORING

The principles of the Declaration of Helsinki should be adhered to when asking eligible patients to participate in analgesic trials. Thus, patients should be informed of the basis for conducting the trial, the stage of test drug development, the expected test drug efficacy, and the expected side effects of active control groups and placebo when included. Patients should be informed that they do not have to give a reason for not participating in the trial and that their consent to participate or refuse will not affect the standard of clinical care that they will receive. Written informed consent must be obtained prior to surgical procedure.

Our experience is that the majority of patients do not decline when asked to participate, and, if they do, the usual reason is the inconvenience of staying in the clinic for baseline pain assessments and instructions. This refusal is less often the case if they have been informed of trial procedures at an earlier visit. In trials in which placebo is included, however, more patients are reluctant to participate, despite the availability of rescue medication.

OPERATIVE PROCEDURES

To reduce variability in pain due to surgical trauma, the surgical technique should be strictly standardized and the operation preferably performed by a single surgeon.[27][II] Surgical removal of mandibular impacted third molars is usually performed under local anesthesia using, for example, lidocaine (lignocaine) 20 mg/mL and epinephrine (adrenaline) 12.5 µg/mL (Xylocain–Adrenaline, AstraZeneca, Sweden) block of the nervus alveolaris inferior and infiltration of nervus bukkalis. This technique allows evaluation of baseline pain approximately three hours later.[28][II] A 3- to 4-cm soft-tissue incision is performed and the mucoperiosteum reflected to visualize the tooth. Cortical alveolar bone is then removed by burr under saline irrigation and the impacted tooth is sectioned and elevated. Finally, the mucoperiosteal flap is repositioned with sutures and an inlay of a 2×1 cm gauze drain saturated with 3 percent chlortetracycline ointment (Terramycin-Polymyxin B, Pfizer, USA) is left in the wound opening. No other antibiotics, sedatives, or other drugs are administered to the patients eligible for trial participation. The procedure should be performed in the morning, so that assessments are taken during the afternoon and early evening for all patients.

PATIENT UNDERSTANDING OF INSTRUCTIONS AND COMPLIANCE WITH PROTOCOL

To adequately measure the baseline pain intensity of trial participants, patients should remain in the clinic until full recovery from the local anesthetic block is clearly evident. One investigator has the responsibility for patient surveillance. Patients are instructed to rate their present pain intensity half-hourly after surgery or extraction on a visual analog scale (VAS), or a numerical rating scale (NRS). A categorical verbal rating scale has been demonstrated to be a less sensitive measure of pain intensity and is no longer used in our department.[29][II], [30][II] After dissipation of the effects of the local anesthetic, patients who do not report a pain intensity of more than 50 mm on a 100-mm VAS are excluded and discharged from the clinic with routine postoperative instructions; routine analgesics are prescribed. The duration of the conduction block (inferior alveolar nerve block) with lidocaine 20 mg/mL with epinephrine 12.5 μg/mL is, on average, 85 minutes for the dental pulp and 190 minutes for the oral soft tissue.[28] In our studies, patients did not experience moderate to severe pain until 3–3.5 hours after injection of local anesthesia.[20][II], [29][II]

Patients who do report a pain intensity equal to or greater than 50 mm on a 100-mm VAS are randomized, given the test drug, and asked to remain for a further 30 minutes in order to rate pain relief on a five-point verbal pain relief scale (PAR). Patients then record the remaining pain intensity assessments after they have left the clinic. By now, the observer will have an impression of the patient's ability to understand instructions and use the VAS and the PAR.

Since most of the pain diaries will be attended to after the patients have left the clinic, the patients must be contactable by the investigator or monitor to ensure the quality of the trial data. Contacting participants by telephone in the afternoon increases patient compliance, reminds patients of their obligations as trial participants, and serves as an extra service for the patient if they have questions regarding their postoperative course, assessments in their home diary, or rescue drug intake. Overall ratings of drug efficacy and side effects are performed at the end of the observation period as a global score on a VAS or a categorical scale. The home diary is returned on the seventh postoperative day when sutures and chlortetracycline gauze are removed.

Inclusion criteria for trial participants prior to drug administration

- Indications for surgical removal of third molars are present[31] (**Box 43.1**).
- Either sex, between 18 and 40 years old.
- No history of chronic pain.
- Asymptomatic mandibular third molar on the day of operation (no symptomatic pericoronitis or pulpitis).
- Baseline pain intensity (i.e. pain at drug intake) of predetermined magnitude (see Baseline pain intensity as a confounding factor).

Exclusion criteria for trial participants prior to drug administration

- Concomitant medication (except oral contraceptives).
- Any form of systemic steroid treatment during the last month.
- Known hypersensitivity to the test drugs.
- Bronchial asthma or gastrointestinal ulcerative disease (if test drug is an NSAID).
- Inflammatory gastrointestinal disease (Crohn's disease or ulcerative colitis).
- Hepatic or renal disease.
- Pregnant or lactating women.
- Anxiety related to dental treatment.
- Alcohol consumption one day or less preoperatively.
- Deviation from surgical procedure as specified in the protocol.
- No pain or inadequate pain intensity level after offset of local anesthesia (baseline pain).
- When motivation and compliance with protocol is questionable.

Box 43.1 Report of a workshop on the management of patients with third molar teeth.[31] Indications for third molar removal according to The National Institute of Health (NIH), USA

- One or more episodes of pericoronitis.
- Unrestorable caries in the third molar tooth.
- Distal caries in the adjacent tooth.
- Periodontal disease (resulting in bone destruction).
- Evidence of follicular enlargement.
- Resorption of the third molar or adjacent tooth.

IMPROVING AND DOCUMENTING ASSAY SENSITIVITY

The objectives of comparative analgesic trials are to demonstrate that the effectiveness of one treatment is significantly better than another, or that a new drug is superior to placebo and at least as effective as a "standard" analgesic. Interpretation problems arise when no difference is revealed between the treatments in a trial that does not embody placebo or standard analgesic comparators.[32] As a result, it cannot be ascertained whether the outcome for the test drug indicates that it is equally effective or whether the assay sensitivity is inadequate. Study error could occur, for example, due to patient distress in the clinical setting to respond normally to medication or to understand properly the pain questionnaires/pain diaries. The procedure or the information from the clinical investigator could be insufficient, or contain confounding factors, or data could vary merely because of random variation. Selection of adequate control groups (standard analgesics in two doses, or placebo, or both) is therefore essential to verify and document that the study methodology can distinguish between degrees of analgesic effectiveness. Testing the analgesic drug against a placebo control will detect whether it is an analgesic. Testing the analgesic drug against a standard analgesic control, for example paracetamol, can indicate how much of the pain relief is caused by placebo effects.[32]

The importance of documenting assay sensitivity was well illustrated in another dental test model for the evaluation of oral analgesics: acute apical periodontitis or acute apical abscess causes moderate to severe odontalgia. The dental treatment is usually pulpectomy and analgesics are usually prescribed for the management of postoperative pain. In patients with moderate to severe baseline pain, pulpectomy combined with placebo medication resulted in a 50 percent reduction in pain during the first 24 hours.[33][II] This means that most of these patients receive pain relief from the dental treatment alone. Analgesic trials performed on endodontic emergency patients must therefore also have test drug comparators that enable assay sensitivity to be controlled. Assay sensitivity was documented, for example by Doroschak and coworkers,[33][II] through the superior analgesic effect of the combination of flurbiprofen plus tramadol compared with placebo on endodontic pain.

BASELINE PAIN INTENSITY AS A CONFOUNDING FACTOR

Adequate and homogeneous baseline pain intensity is an important factor in determining the outcome of a trial of analgesic drugs.[34] Even in standardized forms of surgery, such as the surgical removal of impacted third molars, patients vary tremendously in their reported discomfort.[17][II] Mild pain may be sufficient in a trial

where the aim is to document that a weak analgesic drug is superior to placebo.[17][II] However, patients who enter the study suffering from severe pain have a greater potential for pain relief, as measured by the decrease in pain intensity, than patients who enter the study with a lower pain intensity. Thus, in trials designed to document whether two or more analgesic drugs are significantly different from each other, at least moderate to strong pain intensity is required.[20][II], [34][II]

It is well documented that postoperative pain intensity after third molar surgery increases with the extent of the surgical intervention.[2, 35][I], [36][I] This was confirmed in a trial of 293 patients who were stratified into groups according to the extent of trauma of third molar removal: extraction of one upper third molar, surgical removal of one mandibular impacted third molar, or surgical removal of two ipsilateral impacted third molars.[17][II] Although baseline pain intensity was related to the extent of surgical trauma, the variation in pain intensity experienced by patients with similar degrees of surgical trauma was large (**Figure 43.2**). The duration and degree of surgical trauma are thus only partly responsible for the postoperative pain intensity. Two factors which seem to considerably confound the pain intensity are: psychological status and the degree of tissue trauma (i.e. skill of operator), despite difficulty in extraction. In a follow-up study in which patients were screened for their baseline

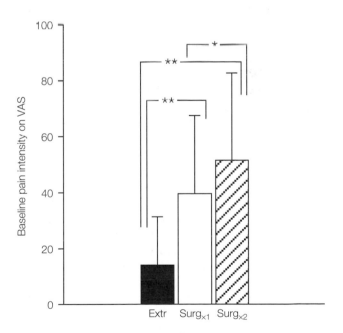

Figure 43.2 Mean (standard deviation) baseline pain intensity in the three clinical groups following third molar removal. Extr, extraction of one fully erupted maxillary third molar ($n = 100$); Surg $_{\times 1}$, surgical removal of one impacted mandibular third molar ($n = 95$); Surg $_{\times 2}$, surgical removal of two ipsilateral impacted third molars ($n = 98$); VAS (0–100 mm). $^{*}p < 0.05$; $^{**}p < 0.01$ (Kruskal–Wallis). (Modified from Breivik and Bjornsson.[17])

pain before leaving the clinic, one in two patients did not reach a postoperative pain intensity of 50 mm or above on a 100-mm VAS after local anesthetic offset.[20][II] In a follow-up study, 46 of 166 patients (38 percent) experienced less pain intensity than 50 mm on a 100-mm VAS after surgical removal of impacted third molars.[29][II]

Similarly, Desjardins[37][II] reported that a substantial proportion (30–50 percent) of patients undergoing extraction of erupted third molars did not develop postoperative pain. Patients undergoing more extensive procedures involving mucoperiostal flaps and removal of alveolar bone (e.g. periodontal surgery or surgical removal of impacted third molars) less frequently had no or little postoperative pain (10–20 percent).[38][II] Hansson et al.[18][II] found that 14 of 100 patients did not report any pain at all and 40 patients (40 percent) did not use any analgesics during the 70-hour observation period following surgical removal of third molars. Nörholt[19][II] stated that 34 percent of patients after surgical removal of third molar(s) reported no pain or only mild pain. Therefore, in the dental pain model, pain intensity varies substantially irrespective of the extent of surgery, and a predetermined intensity of baseline pain should be met before patients are finally included in the trial.[39, 40]

Despite efforts to include only patients with a certain degree of pain intensity, there might be upper outliers of baseline pain that need adjusting for. Adjusting for baseline pain intensity as a covariant should thus be part of the statistical analysis of the outcome data.

DOWNSIDE ASSAY SENSITIVITY

It is vital that the study is designed so that a clinically meaningful and statistically significant difference between placebo and the active drug can be measured, particularly for the study of analgesics of modest efficacy. This is called downside assay sensitivity, which can be quantified by the inclusion of a standard analgesic and placebo arm in the protocol.[21] An example of this is a single-dose study designed to compare a novel analgesic (FS 205-397) with aspirin 650 mg as a standard and with placebo following oral surgery. As the standard analgesic (aspirin) was associated with significantly better pain relief than placebo, it was possible to conclude that the study design was of sufficient downside sensitivity.[41][II]

UPSIDE ASSAY SENSITIVITY

When a new drug is compared with a standard active analgesic drug only (without a placebo control group), the study must document upside assay sensitivity.[21] This means that the study must be capable of illustrating clinically meaningful and statistically significant differences between two standard analgesic drugs of differing efficacy, or between two doses of a known standard analgesic drug.[23, 32] An example of this is a single-dose study designed to compare diflunisal with paracetamol with or without codeine following oral surgery in which paracetamol with codeine afforded significantly more pain relief than paracetamol alone.[42][II] Consequently, sound conclusions can be drawn from the analysis of efficacy data of diflunisal in that the study design demonstrated sufficient upside sensitivity.

PLACEBO CONTROL?

Although the inclusion of a placebo arm in dental pain trials is desirable, its omission can be occasionally justified, for example when the use of a placebo group is ethically difficult (e.g. evaluation in children) or when placebo has previously been compared with an active standard analgesic comparator. Instead, a second dose level of the standard analgesic will ensure that meaningful interpretation of the analgesic assay data is possible.[32]

An inert placebo arm or an active comparator is mandatory in RCTs to demonstrate the efficacy of a test drug,[32] and withholding an active treatment is unlikely to result in serious harm in short-term analgesic trials. Nevertheless, the Declaration of Helsinki states that "every patient should be assured of the best proven, diagnostic and therapeutic method"; therefore, efforts should be made to limit the number of trials which include placebo controls. However, placebo control is necessary when one needs to establish whether the test drug is an active analgesic in the study population. Inclusion of a placebo arm is also required when there is reason to doubt whether a dental pain model has satisfactory downside assay sensitivity. This was not the case in a dental pain study designed to investigate whether the efficacy of two standard analgesics (paracetamol 1 g and paracetamol 1 g plus codeine 60 mg) differed. A placebo arm was not included as the downside assay sensitivity had previously been established in an identical dental pain study, and therefore the use of placebo might be considered unethical.[20][II] Adequate upside assay sensitivity was documented in another study by including two standard analgesics arms (paracetamol 1 g and paracetamol 1 g plus codeine 60 mg), the results demonstrating that paracetamol plus codeine was superior to paracetamol alone for pain relief (**Figure 43.3**).[29][II]

RESCUE ANALGESIC DRUG

Whenever a placebo treatment or a test drug of uncertain analgesic efficacy is included in a clinical trial, the provision of rescue analgesia is mandatory.[32] In practice, this means that such analgesic trials must ensure that a rescue analgesic of proven efficacy is available to all patients included in the study. This can be accomplished by giving all participants rescue medication in sealed envelopes

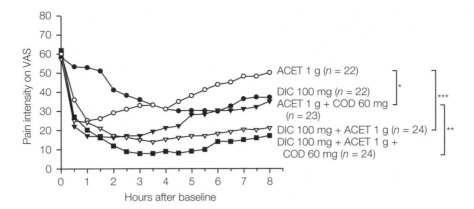

Figure 43.3 Comparison of mean pain intensity ratings on a 100-mm VAS when various analgesic combinations are taken after surgical removal of third molars. In a randomized, double-blind study, 120 patients with moderate to strong pain after surgery received in a single oral dose combinations of diclofenac (DIC; enteric coated tablets), acetaminophen (ACET), and codeine (COD). Diclofenac plus acetaminophen with or without codeine was superior to diclofenac alone or acetaminophen alone (***$p < 0.01$). Diclofenac plus acetaminophen plus codeine was superior to acetaminophen plus codeine (**$p = 0.01$). Adequate upside assay sensitivity was documented as acetaminophen plus codeine was superior to acetaminophen alone (*$p < 0.05$) (GLM). (Modified from Breivik et al.[29])

with written instructions, or prescriptions of a standard rescue analgesic, or both.

CONCLUSIONS

Pain following surgical removal of wisdom teeth is a simple tool for assessing the efficacy of analgesics. However, there are many pitfalls in performing clinical trials on outpatients. The dental pain model needs thorough planning and rigid control during execution in order to provide valid and reproducible results. One needs to adhere to ethical guidelines, randomized controlled trials, establish baseline pain intensity and assay sensitivity, as well as patient compliance. It is time consuming and rewarding to carry through a dental pain study. The outcome should be reliable if guidelines are followed.

PRACTICAL TIPS

- The visual analog scale should be printed, not copied, to avoid distortion of size when copying the sheet.
- The direct assessment of change in pain intensity in patients reporting similar baseline pain intensity should be the primary outcome measure in an analgesic trial on acute postoperative pain.
- Recovery rooms for trial participants and patients being screened for trial participation should be separate from the other patients at the clinic.
- A simple screening procedure at the end of the studies, such as asking the participants what test drug they thought they had been given, will document that a double-blind procedure was not

inadvertently unblinded during the trial, e.g. by side effects or other cues.[43][II], [44][II]

The postsurgical dental pain model used for analgesic efficacy evaluation has many advantages, such as pain confined to one area of the body and young and healthy patients largely unencumbered by concurrent disease and thus concomitant medication. The potential study population is large, and therefore studies of sufficient power can be conducted. Limitations of the dental pain model are the relatively transient duration of pain and the large interindividual variation in pain experienced following the oral surgical procedure. However, adherence to the principles of protocol design, meticulous planning, protocol compliance, and trial execution will result in reliable data when using this pain model.

REFERENCES

* 1. Seymour RA, Walton JG. Pain control after third molar surgery. *International Journal of Oral Surgery*. 1984; **13**: 457–85.
2. Szmyd L, Shannon IL, Mohnac AM. Control of postoperative sequela in impacted third molar surgery. *Journal of Oral Therapeutics and Pharmacology*. 1965; **21**: 491–6.
3. Troullos E, Hargreaves KM, Butler DP, Dionne RA. Comparison of nonsteroidal anti-inflammatory drugs, ibuprofen and flurbiprofen, with methylprednisolone and placebo. *Journal of Oral and Maxillofacial Surgery*. 1990; **48**: 945–52.
* 4. Løkken P, Olsen I, Norman-Pedersen K. Bilateral surgical removal of impacted lower third molar teeth as a model for drug evaluation: a test with ibuprofen. *European Journal of Clinical Pharmacology*. 1975; **8**: 209–16.

5. Lökken P, Skjelbred P. Aspirin or paracetamol? *Lancet*. 1981; **2**: 1346–7.

6. Baxendale BR, Vater M, Lavery KM. Dexamethasone reduces pain and swelling following extraction of third molar teeth. *Anaesthesia*. 1993; **48**: 961–4.

7. Fernando S, Hill CM, Walker R. A randomised double blind comparative study of low level laser therapy following surgical extraction of lower third molar teeth. *British Journal of Oral and Maxillofacial Surgery*. 1993; **31**: 170–2.

∗ 8. Meechan JG, Seymour RA. The use of third molar surgery in clinical pharmacology. *British Journal of Oral and Maxillofacial Surgery*. 1993; **31**: 360–5.

9. Wirth DP, Brenlan DR, Levine RJ, Rodriguez CM. The effect of complementary healing therapy on postoperative pain after surgical removal of impacted third molar teeth. *Complementary Therapies in Medicine*. 1993; **1**: 133–8.

∗ 10. Urquhart E. Analgesic agents and strategies in the dental pain model. *Journal of Dental Research*. 1994; **22**: 336–41.

11. Lökken P, Straumsheim PA, Tveiten D, Skjelbred P. Effects of homeopathy on pain and other events after acute trauma: placebo controlled trial with bilateral oral surgery. *British Medical Journal*. 1995; **310**: 1439–42.

∗ 12. Cooper SA. Models for clinical assessment of oral analgesics. *Journal of the American Medical Association*. 1983; **75**: 24–9.

∗ 13. Forbes JA. Oral surgery. In: Max M, Portenoy R (eds). *Advances in pain research and therapy*, vol. 18. New York: Raven Press, 1991: 347–74.

14. McQuay HJ, Moore A. Methods of therapeutic trials. In: Wall, Melzack (eds). *Textbook of pain*, 5th edn. London: Elsevier Churchill Livingstone, 2006: 415–26.

∗ 15. Cooper SA, Beaver WT. A model to evaluate mild analgesics in oral surgery. *Clinical Pharmacology and Therapeutics*. 1976; **20**: 241–50.

16. Fisher SE, Frame JW, Rout PGJ. Factors affecting the onset and the severity of pain following the surgical removal of unilateral impacted mandibular third molar teeth. *British Dental Journal*. 1988; **164**: 351–4.

17. Breivik EK, Björnsson GA. Variation in surgical trauma and baseline pain intensity: effects on assay sensitivity of an analgesic trial. *European Journal of Oral Sciences*. 1998; **106**: 844–52.

18. Hansson P, Ekblom A, Thomsson M, Fjellner B. Pain development and consumption of analgesics after oral surgery in relation to personality characteristics. *Pain*. 1989; **37**: 271–7.

∗ 19. Nörholt SE. Treatment of acute pain following removal of mandibular third molars. *International Journal of Oral and Maxillofacial Surgery*. 1998; **27**: 1–41.

20. Breivik EK, Haanæs HR, Barkvoll P. Upside assay sensitivity in a dental pain model. *European Journal of Pain*. 1998; **2**: 179–86.

∗ 21. Cooper SA. Single dose analgesic studies: the upside and downside of assay sensitivity. In: Max M, Portenoy R,

Laska E (eds). *Advances in pain research and therapy*, vol. 18. New York: Raven Press, 1991: 117–23.

22. Berge TI, Bøe OE. Predictor evaluation of postoperative morbidity after surgical removal of mandibular third molars. *Acta Odontologica Scandinavica*. 1994; **52**: 1–8.

23. Shugars DA, Benson K, White RP et al. Developing a measure of patient perceptions of short-term outcomes of third molar surgery. *Journal of Oral and Maxillofacial Surgery*. 1996; **54**: 1402–08.

∗ 24. Meinert CL. *Good clinical trial practice*. Nordic Guidelines, Uppsala: Nordic Council of Medicine, 1989.

25. Jadad RA, Moore RA, Carroll D et al. Assessing the quality of reports of randomized clinical trials: is blinding necessary? *Controlled Clinical Trials*. 1996; **17**: 1–12.

∗ 26. Moher D, Schultz KF, Altman DG. The CONSORT statement: revised recommendations for improving the quality of reports of parallel-group randomised trials. *Lancet*. 2001; **357**: 1191–4.

27. Bjørnsson GA, Bjørnland T, Skoglund LA. Reproducibility of postoperative courses after surgical removal of symmetrically impacted wisdom teeth. *Methods and Findings in Experimental and Clinical Pharmacology*. 1995; **17**: 345–56.

28. Yagiela JA. Local anesthetics. In: Dionne RA, Phero JC (eds). *Management of pain and anxiety in dental practice*. Amsterdam: Elsevier Science, 1993: 109–34.

29. Breivik EK, Barkvoll P, Skovlund E. Combining diclofenac with paracetamol or paracetamol–codeine after oral surgery: a randomised, double blind, single oral dose study. *Clinical Pharmacology and Therapeutics*. 1999; **66**: 625–35.

30. Breivik EK, Björnsson GA, Skovlund E. A comparison of pain rating scales by sampling from clinical trial data. *Clinical Journal of Pain*. 2000; **16**: 22–8.

31. Anonymous. Report of a workshop on the management of patients with third molar teeth. *Journal of Oral and Maxillofacial Surgery*. 1994; **52**: 1102–12.

∗ 32. Max MB, Laska EM. Single-dose analgesic combinations. In: Max M, Portenoy R (eds). *Advances in pain research and therapy*, vol. 18. New York: Raven Press, 1991: 55–95.

33. Doroschak AM, Bowles WR, Hargreaves KM. Evaluation of the combination of Flurbiprofen and Tramadol for management of endodontic pain. *Journal of Endodontics*. 1999; **25**: 660–3.

∗ 34. Lasagna L. The psychophysics of clinical pain. *Lancet*. 1962; **2**: 572–5.

35. Houmes RJ, Voets MA, Verkaaik A et al. Efficacy and safety of tramadol versus morphine for moderate and severe postoperative pain with special regard to respiratory depression. *Anesthesia and Analgeia*. 1992; **74**: 510–14.

36. Oikarinen K. Postoperative pain after mandibular third molar surgery. *Acta Odontologica Scandinavica*. 1991; **49**: 7–13.

37. Desjardins PJ. Analgesic efficacy of piroxicam in postoperative pain. *Journal of the American Medical Association*. 1988; **84**: 35–41.

38. Jorkjend L, Skoglund L. Effect of non-eugenol- and eugenol-containing periodontal dressing on the incidence and severity of pain after periodontal soft tissue surgery. *Journal of Clinical Periodontology.* 1990; **17**: 341–4.

39. Sriwatanakul K, Lasagna L, Cox C. Evaluation of current clinical trial design methodology in analgesimetry based on experts' opinions and analysis of several studies. *Clinical Pharmacology and Therapeutics.* 1983; **34**: 277–83.

40. Breivik EK. Analgesic trials in oral surgery. Methodological aspects of the dental pain model with special emphasis on assay sensitivity and effects of combining paracetamol with codeine and/or diclofenac. Doctoral thesis. Oslo, Norway, University of Oslo, 1999.

41. Mehlisch DR, Sterling WR, Mazza FA, Singer JM. A single-dose study of the efficacy and safety of FS 205-397 (250 mg or 500 mg) versus aspirin and placebo in the treatment of postsurgery dental pain. *Journal of Clinical Pharmacology.* 1990; **30**: 815–23.

42. Forbes JA, Beaver WT, White EH *et al.* Diflunisal. A new oral analgesic with an unusually long duration of action. *Journal of the American Medical Association.* 1982; **248**: 2139–42.

43. Hughes JR, Krahn D. Blindness and the validity of the double-blind procedure. *Journal of Clinical Psychopharmacology.* 1985; **5**: 138–42.

44. Carroll KM, Rounsville BJ, Nich C. Blind man's bluff: effectiveness and significance of psychotherapy and pharmacotherapy blinding procedures in a clinical trial. *Journal of Consulting and Clinical Psychology.* 1994; **62**: 276–80.

44

Clinical trials: cancer pain

ULF E KONGSGAARD AND MADS U WERNER

KEY LEARNING POINTS

- Epidemiolological surveys have demonstrated that a large proportion of cancer patients suffers from significant pain.
- High quality trials in cancer pain patients are needed to improve treatment strategies and techniques.
- Cancer pain comprises a group of heterogeneous disorders characterized by fluctuations in pain intensity and variable responses to treatment.
- Extrapolated data from experimental chronic pain models or animal research are not always representative of clinical cancer pain.
- Research in analgesics have mainly focused on postoperative pain with few studies on cancer patients.

- Extrapolation from acute pain to chronic cancer pain is not always possible.
- Reliable prediction and identification of patients at risk for unrelieved pain is important.
- Many studies have failed to recognize a clinical perspective of cancer patients, particularly in respect of a potentially terminal disease.
- We need to develop multimodal research methodology, validated instruments, and assessment tools that more clearly define these dimensions.
- Uniformity of design and reporting of trials furthermore requires an interdisciplinary and multiprofessional collaboration.

INTRODUCTION

Cancer is a common cause of death in our society, and pain caused by cancer or cancer therapy occurs frequently. A number of epidemiological surveys have demonstrated that approximately 25 percent of patients with localized disease report pain, and that the prevalence of pain can be as high as 90 percent in patients with advanced cancer.[1, 2] A number of patients with metastatic disease suffer from

significant pain long before the terminal stage of their cancer. Studies have indicated that effective pain control can be achieved in up to 88 percent of patients with cancer-related pain,[3] however, many patients still do not receive adequate pain management.[2, 3] Unrelieved pain impairs functional status, compromises quality of life, and may interfere with anticancer treatment.

Patients with advanced cancer often present complex patterns of symptoms, of which pain is the most prevalent.

Furthermore, patients regularly present with extremely heterogeneous pain profiles, particularly during unstable disease.[2] In the past, the study of pain and pain management in this population has often been ignored. Pain treatment has mostly been empirical, incomplete, and often resulted in unnecessary suffering for many patients.

Pain in the cancer patient may be caused by:

- cancer growth or spread *per se*;
- diagnostic or therapeutic procedures;
- paraneoplastic syndromes;
- disability or immobilization due to the disease or therapy;
- conditions unrelated to cancer.

The multidimensionality in the pain experience is evident from the description of cancer pain as "a mosaic composed of acute pain, chronic pain, tumor-specific pain, and treatment-related pain cemented together by ongoing psychological, social, and existential responses of distress and suffering."[4] The temporal aspects of pain may influence the strategy and the aggressiveness of the therapy. The pathophysiological substrate for pain and the clinical characteristics of cancer pain and its response to analgesic treatment have not been firmly established.[5]

ANALGESIC REQUIREMENTS

An important factor complicating the study of pain in cancer patients is the remarkable variability in dose–response patterns to most analgesics. Confusion in the terms of analgesic efficacy and responsiveness has contributed to the controversy of opioids in pain conditions. The term "efficacy" only addresses analgesia, but does not consider the occurrence of side effects. Effective pain treatment considers a favorable balance between pain relief and undesirable side effects. Portenoy *et al.*[6] have introduced the term "responsiveness" to characterize the degree of analgesia achieved at a dose associated with tolerable and manageable side effects. This implies individual dose titration aiming at a balance between pain relief and side effects, leading to satisfactory analgesia with a minimum of tolerable side effects. This emphasizes the analgesic response as a relative phenomenon that accounts for interindividual variability and the occurrence of dose-dependent side effects.

The development of tolerance is another factor to consider regarding opioid responsiveness. Tolerance is a complex phenomenon, which has led to some controversy regarding its relevance in the clinical management of cancer pain. Prolonged administration of an opioid may lead not only to adaptation, but during certain conditions also to hyperalgesic responses.[7] Dose escalation, without any signs of disease progression or complication, is used as a clinical indicator of tolerance development. Surveys using this criterion indicate that the rate and extent of

tolerance differ dramatically among cancer patients.[8] It seems, however, that the most common reason for dose escalation in patients with cancer pain is disease progression. Even if tolerance does not appear to be of major clinical significance in most patients, it should be considered a confounding factor in the assessment of analgesic requirements in clinical trials.

Variability in responsiveness may also be associated with pharmacokinetic factors. Renal impairment may prolong the duration of analgesia but also enhance opioid toxicity, due to the accumulation of active metabolites dependent upon renal excretion. Recent data indicate that pharmacogenetic variability may be responsible for individual differences in the analgesic efficacy of morphine.[9, 10, 11] Other factors also have to be considered, such as patient age, drug interactions, cognitive abilities, fear, anxiety, and mood disorders.

Elements of variability in analgesic requirements

- Biopsychosocial and existential factors.
- Factors related to the cancer and its treatment.
- Pain type (nociceptive/neuropathic).
- Tolerance development.
- Pharmacogenetics.
- Pharmacokinetics (drug interactions/drug elimination).

PAIN FLUCTUATION

Patients with chronic cancer-related pain usually experience fluctuations in pain intensity. When these episodes of increased pain intensity are clinically significant and interrupt a background pain that is otherwise well-controlled and tolerated, they are commonly described as episodes of breakthrough pain. Breakthrough pain is extremely heterogeneous,[12] and may vary in etiology, pathophysiology, frequency, temporal pattern, severity, quality, and impact.[13, 14] At present, there is no unanimous definition of breakthrough pain, however, breakthrough pain is often defined as a transient increase in pain to greater than moderate intensity, which occurs on a baseline pain of moderate intensity or less. For practical purposes, it can be divided into:

1. incident pain (predictable pain precipitated by mobilization or physiological activity);
2. spontaneous pain (stimulus-independent episodic flares of pain); and
3. end-of-dose failure (inadequate duration of a sustained release preparation).

The paucity of data may relate to the difficulties in defining and measuring subtypes of pain. The methodological challenge in studying a highly variable subjective experience that may or may not occur during any planned assessment period is evident. From a methodological perspective it is also often difficult to interpret pain intensity ratings after the administration of a rescue analgesic drug.

Baseline drift (natural fluctuations of symptoms not associated with the intervention) is important in respect to both symptoms and the pharmacological actions from analgesics.[15] This should include assessments of pain intensity at several specific time points of the day and preferably during standardized conditions. Studies are needed to clarify the true effectiveness of the conventional therapeutic approaches to breakthrough pain, for example by comparing escalation of the baseline dose with optimal use of rescue dose as alternative interventions for breakthrough pain. Additional studies that evaluate the dose and timing of the rescue medication are needed.[12]

Temporal aspects of pain

- Background pain.
- Recurrent pain.
- Pain fluctuations.
- Breakthrough pain:
    - incident pain;
    - spontaneous pain;
    - end-of-dose failure.

PAIN ASSESSMENT IN CANCER PAIN TRIALS

Pain is a subjective experience and as such is influenced by a number of variables that are difficult to control, both in the clinical situation and in the context of a controlled trial.[5] A comprehensive assessment of the patient with cancer pain is of course mandatory in any study of pain epidemiology or treatment outcomes, but may also have important clinical implications in evaluating disease progression, complications, and in the planning of adjuvant oncological therapy.

A number of experimental studies, in animal models of bone metastases[16] and perineural tumor invasion,[17] indicate that the pathophysiological changes induced by cancer may differ from changes seen in conventional nociceptive, inflammatory, or neuropathic injury models. The peripheral and central inflammatory responses to cancer may contain cancer-specific components that may require specific pharmacological treatment modalities.[18] Although animal experiments are obviously important for increased understanding of pain mechanisms and analgesia, extrapolation of data from animals to humans experiencing cancer pain should be exercised with caution.

In an analysis of discomfort in the cancer patient, it is important to distinguish between the terms nociception,

pain, and suffering. Nociception is defined as activity in the nervous system following tissue damage. Pain is the conscious perception of acute or chronic nociception, including sensory-discriminative, affective-emotional, and cognitive-evaluative processes. Suffering may be defined as a perceived threat to the integrity of the personality. Suffering in the cancer patient affects quality of life (**Figure 44.1**). Although pain has an important influence on suffering, other factors such as anxiety, depression, vulnerability, catastrophizing behavior, dependence, physical immobility, and social isolation also affect quality of life.[19, 20, 21, 22] Depression, anxiety, and sleep disturbances are particularly common in the cancer patient population and it would therefore seem prudent to consider these variables when designing cancer pain trials.[5]

There are numerous ways to categorize the types of pain that occur in cancer patients. These include definitions based on the pathophysiological mechanisms of pain, its temporal aspects, its intensity, the cancer type, and the specific pain syndromes that occur with different cancer types. It is important to acknowledge the wide disagreement on the best outcome measures for pain clinical trials.[23] In a systematic evidence report on management of cancer pain, including 218 relevant trials, 125 distinctly different pain outcomes were assessed.[4]

Tools for pain assessment can be divided into two main categories: intensity scales and questionnaires intended to capture the multidimensionality of cancer pain. The intensity scales most commonly used are the visual analog scales (VAS), numerical rating scales (NRS), and verbal categorical rating scales (VRS).[24] In acute pain, NRS and VAS scales may demonstrate higher sensitivity in detecting differences in outcomes of pain intensity than VRS.[25] However, generally, most of the intensity scales seem to be equally effective in pain rating.[26] Generally, pain intensity ratings (from baseline to postmedication assessment point) are correlated with changes in pain relief rating, but significant differences may still exist and

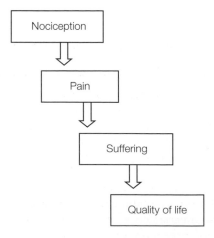

Figure 44.1 The pain experience: steps in the production and perception of pain.

therefore it has been recommended to use both pain intensity and pain relief scales in analgesic trials.

We cannot rely on pain intensity or pain relief measures alone to evaluate treatment efficacy, and therefore a series of currently validated assessment instruments are available for the multidimensional evaluation of cancer pain. Furthermore, there are scenarios when self-reports of pain will be difficult, for instance in the cognitively impaired or in the elderly, and alternatives, such as observation of behavior or assessment of physiological variables, will have to be considered.

Validated assessment instruments for multidimensional evaluation of cancer pain

- McGill Pain Questionnaire.[27]
- Brief Pain Inventory.[28]
- Memorial Pain Assessment Card.[29]

In general, four criteria are important in choosing a measure appropriate for clinical trials as well as for clinical practice.[30]

1. **Validity** (accuracy). An accurate method should give values near the true value or the reference value.
2. **Reliability** (precision). A precise method should give the same value if applied repeatedly under circumstances in which the underlying characteristics are believed to be unchanged, i.e. if staff changes, it is important that the measurement does not.
3. **Responsiveness**. Clinically important changes should be detectable.
4. **Appropriateness**. Patients, families, and staff should feel comfortable using the measure in this setting, should not be burdened by it, and should find it clinically useful as well as intuitively meaningful.

POLYPHARMACY AS A PROBLEM FOR CANCER PAIN TRIALS

A large number of cancer pain patients will eventually, in addition to the trial drug, be treated with other analgesics and adjuvant analgesics (also called co-analgesics) – other drugs to control distressing symptoms as well as drugs to combat the disease itself. This practice of polypharmacy may confound the interpretation of clinical trials. A study of 676 patients with advanced cancer found widespread use of adjuvant drugs for symptom control; the adjuvants most frequently used were major tranquilizers, sedatives, anxiolytics, antidepressants, anticonvulsants, and antiemetics.[31] The concomitant use of this heterogeneous group of drugs may affect the pharmacokinetics and

pharmacodynamics of analgesics. The true influence of these drugs on opioid effects, however, may be difficult to determine. Besides drug interactions, the side effects of adjuvant drugs may confound the side effects, such as sedation and confusion, of the trial medications.

Improvement in pain treatment is likely to require drug combinations, however, few analgesic combinations have been studied, particularly in a chronic setting with multiple dosing.

Drug interactions (therapeutic effects as well as side effects)

- Additive effects.
- Synergistic (supra-additive) effects.
- Antagonistic effects.

Randomized controlled clinical trials of dose titration are required in order to establish the efficacy and safety margins of a new analgesic drug. When comparing efficacy or when changing from one opioid agonist to another, equianalgesic conversion tables are generally being used. However, there is still a lack of consensus on standard conversion procedures for these drugs. The recommended oral equianalgesic dose conversion ratio between hydromorphone and morphine is in one standard textbook 1:4[32] and in another 1:7.5[33] and following subcutaneous administration 1:4 and 1:7.5, respectively. Oxycodone versus morphine equianalgesic dose ratios varies in textbooks between 1:1[34] to 1:1.5–2[33] after oral administration and 1:1[32] to 1:1.5[34] after subcutaneous administration. Another example is the equianalgesic dose ratio of methadone that increases in a dose-dependent manner with higher morphine requirements. Morphine equivalence of single dose (for acute pain) of methadone is very different from repeated doses (due to the pharmacokinetics of methadone). This is different from other opioid agonists in which the equianalgesic ratio appears to be independent of the opioid exposure. These findings suggest that there is only partial cross-tolerance between opioid agonists.[35]

Ethical reasons dictate a ready availability of rescue medication at all times for breakthrough pain. The potential limitations of the use of an additional dose of rescue medication as an outcome measure also have to be considered. Clearly, factors other than pain intensity may play a role in the patient's decision to take a rescue dose.[23] The use of rescue medication is affected by both patient and perhaps, even by healthcare provider beliefs.[36] Despite the complex issues involved in the interpretation of rescue medication usage in clinical trials, however, patients in a placebo group can be expected to administer more of a rescue treatment than patients allocated to an efficacious investigation treatment. Together with pain intensity ratings, the requirement of rescue medication may provide an important measure of the efficacy of the treatment being evaluated.[36] In trials where rescue analgesics are given early to a significant proportion of study patients, the numbers of "true" pain observations after test drugs decline rapidly, therefore, a composite score based on actual pain observations (both before and after rescue) and rescue analgesic consumption during a defined time period can be useful.[37, 38]

Administration of several opioid agonists simultaneously could influence the interpretation of analgesic requirements and drug-induced toxicity. Authors have reported significant improvement, or even complete disappearance of opioid side effects, with both opioid rotation and dose reduction.[39] In a systematic review[40] comprising 53 reports, all but one concluded that opioid switching was a useful clinical strategy for improving pain control and/or reducing opioid-related side effects. However, in contrast, the conclusion of the review was that the evidence to support the practice of opioid switching was largely anecdotal or based on observational and uncontrolled studies.

FUNDAMENTALS OF CLINICAL TRIALS IN CANCER PAIN

Some trial results are so unequivocal that a comparison group does not seem to be needed. Successful results of this magnitude, however, are rare. Given the wide spectrum of the natural history of cancer in general and cancer pain in particular, and even the variability of an individual patient's response to any intervention, the need for a defined control or comparison group is obvious. However, conducting controlled clinical trials in the palliative cancer pain setting is a particular challenge. It is difficult to recruit patients and to conduct trials successfully due to the serious nature of the disease and the likelihood of symptom progression.[5]

Several research projects designed to investigate clinical cancer pain syndromes are based on conclusions from research with healthy subjects experiencing experimental pain. Furthermore, clinical studies on drugs for cancer pain are frequently investigating patients in an early stage of cancer. These studies often contain several exclusion criteria, selecting patients without any confounding factors, and the results from these studies are then extrapolated to the terminally ill cancer pain population.[41]

ISSUES OF STUDY DESIGN IN CANCER PAIN TRIALS

Historical control study designs

The simplest approach to evaluate a new treatment is to compare a single group of patients given the new treatment with a group previously treated with an alternative regimen. The argument for using a historical control design is that all new participants can receive the new intervention, which facilitates and accelerates recruitment. Historical control studies have undoubtedly contributed to medical knowledge, but there are important limitations since historical controls are particularly vulnerable to bias due to changes in study conditions over time.[42] Sacks *et al.*[43] compared trials of the same treatments in which randomized or historical controls were used and found a consistent tendency for historically controlled trials to yield more optimistic results than prospective, randomized trials. The historical control study may, despite its limitations, still have a place in scientific investigations as a rapid, relatively inexpensive method of obtaining initial feedback regarding a new therapy. In addition to its hypothesis-generating potential, the use of historical controls can be justified in controlled situations of relatively rare conditions, such as in evaluating treatments for refractory pain symptoms in advanced cancer. In such situations, blinding is usually not possible and randomization may not always be justifiable. For instance, in a clinical trial of an invasive therapy for pain management, it may be unethical to allocate patients to an invasive placebo group.

The only justification for investigating invasive procedures, especially the ones that are irreversible (i.e. midline myelotomy, anterolateral cordotomy), is a reasonable expectation of a high benefit–harm ratio. Unfortunately, there are few animal models that can serve as templates for the requirement of "reasonable expectation" of therapeutic effective pain treatment. To justify the higher risks and costs of invasive interventions, direct comparisons with noninvasive therapies are needed. Even when direct comparisons are not feasible, the goal should be to retain all the methodological features of a well-conducted trial other than the randomization.[44]

Sequential trials

A sequential trial depends at any stage on the results so far obtained. Since patients are started on treatment serially and not simultaneously, it is possible to assess the response to treatment as it becomes available in sequential order. This conveys an ethical advantage, with the possibility of terminating the trial quickly when one intervention is an important new advance. The trials are not defined for a fixed period, but the study terminates when one treatment shows a clear superiority or it is highly unlikely that any important difference will be seen. Group sequential trials call for an early discontinuation if one treatment is clearly superior or carries unacceptable adverse events. Thus, a sequential trial is most appropriate when the response is obvious soon after treatment is started. Repeated measurements are by their own nature multidimensional (a patient has multiple pain evaluations in time) and, for this reason, summary measures analysis should be preferred.[45, 46, 47] The summary of multidimensional data is itself part of the analysis, and results can be reported in a clinically significant way, provided the choice of the outcome measure is clinically relevant.[23, 48]

Multivariate sequential procedures (observation and analysis of more than one statistical variable at a time), in which several experimental treatments are compared with a common control, have also been considered.[49] Methodology has been developed for the construction of sequential stopping rules when the first interim analysis involves selection of the most promising experimental treatment. These trials may prove time-efficient and helpful as a guide to determine the variance of the measurements and design of the final trial protocol.

Randomized controlled trials

The randomized controlled trial (RCT) has become the ideal standard for clinical investigations and provides the essential background for evidence-based medicine. Nevertheless, a randomized placebo-controlled trial should only be used when there is genuine doubt about the efficacy of the treatments and when adequate precautions have been taken to secure that patients allocated to the placebo group do not experience a clinically significant reduction in quality of care.

ADVANTAGES OF THE RANDOMIZED DESIGN

- Removes potential bias in the allocation of participants.
- Tends to produce comparable groups.
- Facilitates blinding.
- Validity of statistical tests of significance is guaranteed.

Investigators should carefully weigh the advantages and disadvantages of crossover versus parallel study designs to ensure validity without compromising effectiveness. Although certain situations will provide preferences, both designs can at times be employed, as illustrated by Deschamps et al.[50] and Parris et al.,[51] who conducted trials comparing immediate release analgesics with sustained release analgesics.

Parallel study designs

The standard parallel study design is the most commonly used and has the advantage of simplicity in that a single treatment or a combination of treatments is given to each group and a fixed number of patients are involved (**Figure 44.2**). Parallel designs are less dependent on assumption about disease progression and they are more appropriate than crossover designs when the patient's condition may change over time. Parallel designs should also be favored when there is a possibility of significant carryover effects. Furthermore, parallel study designs are advantageous when baseline homogeneity between treatment groups is present, or when precautions such as stratification or various techniques of adaptive randomization (e.g. block randomization) have been considered. In cancer patients, this last condition may be difficult to accomplish; moreover, a large number of patients may be needed to obtain the desired statistical power. In general, parallel group trials allow for longer follow-up with regular assessment of outcomes. Even if the duration of a parallel study is longer compared to a crossover study, the dropout rate may be smaller.[52] In a parallel-group trial, precision may be increased when the within-subject variance is lower than that of the between-subject variance and baseline measurements are employed to provide within-subject data.

WHEN TO CONSIDER THE STANDARD PARALLEL STUDY DESIGN

- Long duration of treatment.
- There is a likelihood of significant carryover effects.
- A number of treatments are to be compared.
- Patient recruitment is facilitated compared with the crossover design.

Crossover study designs

Crossover designs are used to increase the sensitivity of a study by using each patient as his or her own control (**Figure 44.3**).

This increases validity and reduces the required sample size compared with a parallel study design. A crossover design requires a chronic and stable condition that reverts to its original state with discontinuation of the treatment. This is far from the scenario in long-term studies of

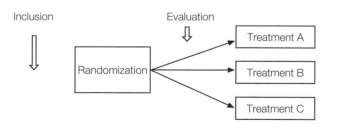

Evaluation

Figure 44.2 Standard parallel designs to assess the effects of three treatments (A, B, and C).

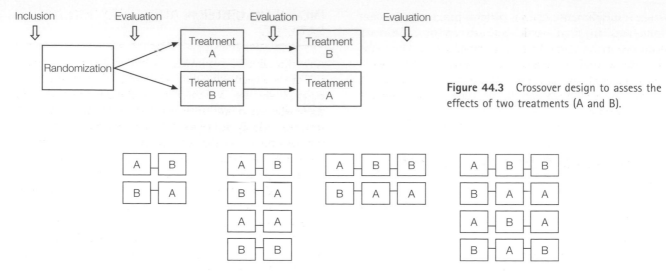

Figure 44.3 Crossover design to assess the effects of two treatments (A and B).

Figure 44.4 Examples of different crossover designs used to compare two treatments (A and B). The three more complex designs on the right are more able to distinguish treatment from carryover effects.

patients with advanced cancer, who in most cases will experience disease progression and deterioration of physical function. Therefore, crossover designs are preferred in studies of relatively short duration in order to reduce the number of withdrawals. Crossover trial designs are recommended when the therapeutic effects of the drug cease soon after it is discontinued during the washout period. A difference between treatments may either be the result of a carryover effect of one treatment into the next period, or of a general time effect – a so-called order effect. During the washout period it is obviously required that the design allows patients to receive adequate rescue medication.

WHEN TO CONSIDER THE CROSSOVER TRIAL

- Carryover effects are limited.
- Within-subject variation is restricted.
- An order effect is absent or can be balanced out.
- An extension of the treatment period does not alter the difference between the treatment effects.
- Prolongation of the trial will not result in a large increase in dropouts.
- Difficulties in obtaining baseline measurements.

Addition of other treatment sequences or a third treatment period offer possible unbiased estimates of treatment effects even in the presence of various types of carryover effects (**Figure 44.4**).

Enriched enrollment study designs

A variant of the crossover design, the enriched enrollment design, may be useful in studying treatments to which only a restricted number of patients respond.[53] Patients

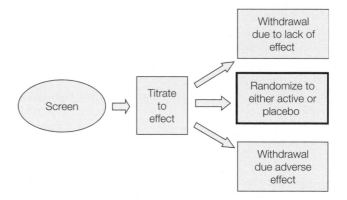

Figure 44.5 Enriched enrollment randomized withdrawal design.

initially undergo a therapeutic selection trial from which only the responders are enrolled in the subsequent study trial. However, these designs are open to criticism that prior exposure to the treatment may jeopardize the double-blind procedures and may result in spurious positive results (**Figure 44.5**).[54]

Cluster-randomized trials

Cluster-randomized trials represent an important experimental design that may supplement ordinary randomized clinical trials.[55] These are trials in which individuals are randomized in groups (i.e. the groups are randomized, not the individuals). Reasons for performing cluster randomized trials vary. Sometimes the intervention can only be administered to the group, sometimes the motivation is to avoid contamination (all participants in the trial are affected by the intervention, even if it is only given directly to some of them); sometimes the design is simply more convenient or economical. Cluster-randomized trials are particularly relevant in evaluations of interventions at the level of a clinic, a hospital, a district, or a region. Sample sizes have to be greatly increased, and an adequate number of clusters are essential as well. One should rigorously guard against selection bias.

SELECTION AND STRATIFICATION OF PATIENTS WITH CANCER PAIN

The final study protocol must include a detailed specification of patient eligibility and patient selection criteria. It is important to focus on patient groups considered most likely to benefit from the new intervention. In most cases, patients are selected from a study population defined by the eligibility criteria and investigators therefore face the problem of extrapolating conclusions from the trial to the study population, and to the general population with the disease.

The large variability in cancer pain patients necessitates implementation of strategies that may reduce heterogeneity in treatment groups in clinical trials. One strategy is to select patients with specific characteristics, such as type and stage of tumor, pain syndrome, pain category, or functional status. This would increase the validity of the study, but at the expense of a reduction in the number of potentially available study participants and that findings may only be relevant for a selected cohort of patients. While stratification may provide an improved balance between treatment groups, it also increases the complexity of the trial and the need for a larger sample size and in most cases tends to reduce the number of degrees of freedom. Moreover, extended subset analyses increase the risk of spurious results produced by chance effects alone (type I error).

An alternative approach to reduce stratification to a manageable size would be to categorize patients into a confined number of strata on the basis of a configuration of variables. A standardized staging system of cancer pain that could be used for such purposes, similar to those developed to classify various malignancies, is needed. Bruera et al.[56] have assessed the accuracy of a staging system for cancer pain which included the assessment of pain, previous opioid dose, cognitive function, psychological distress, opioid tolerance, and past history of alcohol or drug abuse.

Whether patients receiving oncological concomitant management with radiotherapy, chemotherapy, or immunomodulating therapy should be excluded from drug trials of cancer pain depends on the trial design. In studies of long duration, inclusion of these patients could be a confounding factor. In short-term studies this presents a lesser problem, however, acute analgesic effects or side effects of the oncological therapies have to be considered.

INCLUSION CRITERIA AND ACCRETION OF PATIENTS

Any clinical trial requires a precise definition of which patients are eligible for the inclusion. Studies often include patients who are in a more stable clinical condition than those who could potentially benefit from the new treatment regimens. Ideally, strategies should be designed to include a sample population that corresponds to patients clinically most likely to benefit from the intervention. This is not, however, always possible with cancer patients. Many trials of controlled release opioid preparation have included patients with stable low-intensity pain requiring a moderate dose of opioid. In the systematic review by Bell et al.[5] including 34 studies, almost half of the studies recruited patients in treatment with weak opioids (WHO ladder step 2). The results from these studies may not always be relevant or applicable to patient groups with severe pain, who require much higher opioid doses and who frequently require a parenteral route of administration.

Participation in a specific drug trial excludes the patient from taking part in any other parallel investigational drug trial. In larger university centers this may limit the potential number of patients available for a particular cancer pain study.

Significant organ dysfunction is a major exclusion criteria in most trials of analgesics. Thus, many patients who initially qualify for inclusion may have a borderline renal or hepatic dysfunction that may increase during the study and thus have to be withdrawn from the trial. This might limit the relevance of the results obtained when applied to patients with advanced cancer. To make the results of trials more generalizable, it may be necessary to extend the range of acceptable biochemical indices for organ function for patient inclusion into these trials. However, decisions regarding the level of clinical dysfunction at which patients are still eligible for participation in clinical trials rely on the clinical judgment of researchers and represent a source of bias.[55]

Rigorous patient selection may exclude a large proportion of terminal cancer patients with partially impaired cognitive function or affective disorders. Depression is common in cancer patients and its severity may increase as the disease progresses.[57] There is also a correlation between pain intensity and psychomotor impairment, as well as a relationship between pain intensity and fatigue and vigor.

Problems with inclusion criteria and accretion of patients

- Unstable pain.
- Impaired cognitive function.
- Depression.
- Organ dysfunction.
- Impaired drug distribution and elimination.
- Participation in other trials.

SIZE AND DURATION OF STUDY

A trial has to be large enough to detect clinically important differences between treatments. Strict inclusion criteria are important but they should not be so restrictive that enrollment becomes almost impossible and the findings only applicable to a small subset of the population. Large multicenter trials may be preferable and provide larger groups of study patients, although this may lead to inflation in inclusion criteria and violation of protocol adherence due to the increased number of investigators.

In standard textbooks on medical statistics it is seen that in binary outcome studies three variables are used in a priori calculations of sample size: the minimal, relevant difference, the significance level (α) and the power of the study $(1-\beta)$. The significance level indicates the probability of a type I error, i.e. that a significant outcome is expected to occur by chance alone with no true difference in treatment efficacy. Thus, with a significance level of 0.05 a significant outcome is expected to occur by chance alone in one of twenty trials. The power of the study indicates the probability of a type II error, i.e. that a false negative outcome is expected to occur by chance alone. Thus, with a power of 0.9 ($\beta = 0.1$) a negative outcome is expected to occur by chance alone in one of ten trials with a significant, positive outcome. Obviously, studies of cancer pain must be large enough to control for factors likely to confound results.[52]

Factors influencing the number of subjects required in a study

- Study design.
- The objectives defined for the trial.
- The number of primary endpoint measurements.
- The variance of the end-point measurements.
- The use of summated measures.
- Significance level (the statistical power of the study).

Researchers must also consider how many potentially eligible patients can be included in the trial within a reasonable time frame. The achievable accrual rate of patients is often less than half what is estimated.

Factors causing a decreased accrual rate

- Investigators may be overenthusiastic in their prediction of patient recruitment.
- Some patients will not be eligible for the trial.
- Some eligible patients may not wish to participate in the trial.
- Some patients may not be evaluable.

The absence of a critical mass of qualified researchers and of a central institution able to coordinate trials in this area are important constraints for patient accrual.[58] Another dimension is the selected nature of patients who may agree to take part in such studies. Consent rates of only 8–14 percent in eligible patients may be likely.[59]

The duration of intervention may be fixed for all patients or depend on the therapeutic progress of each patient. The former is easier to interpret but sometimes fails to incorporate sufficient flexibility to tailor the therapy to each patient's best interest. Short, fixed periods of therapy are often satisfactory for phase II trials of short-term efficacy. However, for trials of more long-term effects, the duration of therapy may require a more complex definition that incorporates plans for dealing with side effects, dose modification, and patient withdrawal. Treatment periods should be long enough to ascertain that the patient has reached maximal target response.

FACTORS DIFFICULT TO CONTROL IN CANCER PAIN TRIALS

Cancer pain comprises a group of heterogeneous disorders characterized by variable responses to treatment. Few of the experimental conditions used in chronic pain models or animal research are representative of the patient with cancer and pain. Therefore, a number of factors difficult to control can influence clinical trials in cancer pain patients.

The incidence of side effects

Accurate data concerning the incidence of side effects are difficult to obtain in cancer patients owing to ongoing oncological therapies. There is, in any case, little agreement about what constitutes acceptable versus unacceptable side effects. Ultimately, the patient must be regarded as the final authority on when a side effect is sufficiently disagreeable. There is a paucity of sensitive tools to accurately characterize these effects, and their apparent incidence and seriousness will naturally differ with changes in the methods used to characterize them.

Two dimensions need to be considered when evaluating the severity of side effects: intensity and duration. Deschamps et al.[50] employed an index that took into account both the intensity and duration of side effects to assess toxicity. In addition to the descriptive statistics provided, this index had the advantage of allowing comparison of the relative importance of each side effect. Side effects may indicate whether that drug has reached its site of action. However, common opioid effects such as nausea and constipation may indicate peripheral (gastrointestinal) opioid receptor effects, not CNS effects.[60]

Accumulation of opioids and their metabolites may result in excitatory toxicities such as myoclonus, seizures, hyperalgesia, and hyperactive delirium/hallucinations. A number of psychoactive drugs, including midazolam, phenobarbital, and baclofen, have been tried for the management of opioid-induced neurotoxicity. These drugs, however, are more likely to increase sedation and lead to impairment of cognitive functions. The route of administration of opioids, either systemically or spinal, may also influence the dose at which side effects would appear.

Patient compliance

The design of the study should remain sufficiently straightforward to be adhered to without causing confusion or inconvenience for the participants. All clinical studies have problems with noncompliance, but in analgesic studies in advanced cancer these problems seem even more complex and challenging.

Assuming that adequate and reliable pain assessment scales have been included in the study, the temporal procedure for data collection may not be sensitive enough to detect fluctuations in pain that may occur throughout the day. Some patients may report more pain in the morning than during the rest of the day or vice versa.[15, 52] Cancer patients often express reservations about opioid use due to fear of addiction, sedation, and impairment of cognitive functions. Myths regarding addiction and the stigmata of using controlled substances still affect patients' perceptions and may compromise participation in clinical trials. In addition, patients may fail to comply because they are concerned that using opioids too early will endanger pain relief when they have more pain, or because they fear that initiation of an opioid treatment signals that death is near. A number of patients may also underreport the severity of pain and the lack of adequate pain relief because of a variety of reasons, such as not wanting to acknowledge disease progression, not wanting to divert the physician's attention from treatment of the disease, and not wanting to tell the physician that pain treatments are unsuccessful. Weiss *et al.*[61] showed that a large proportion of patients with pain chose to tolerate pain instead of increasing pain therapy.

Patient withdrawals

Poor participant adherence may be a significant problem in long-term studies. Cognitive impairment and progressively limited physical mobility may interfere with data acquisition during clinical trials. Ideally, patient enrollment in clinical trials should be restricted in later stages of their disease. However, prediction of life expectancy in patients with cancer is notoriously inaccurate.[32] Many patients entering clinical trials are likely to

deteriorate in their physical or cognitive abilities or die during the trial. In a study by Kongsgaard and Poulain[62] evaluating the efficacy and safety of transdermal delivery of fentanyl in chronic cancer pain, 138 patients were recruited and entered the dose-titration phase. Owing to disease progression and inadequate symptom control, only 72 patients completed the double-blind study. Even studies of short duration may experience significant patient withdrawal: in a placebo-controlled drug trial in cancer patients, 90 percent of the placebo group withdrew in the first day.[63] Loss to follow-up is one of the significant reasons for exclusions after randomization. At times, participants lost to follow-up could still be included in the analysis if outcome information could be obtained from another source. Such opportunities, however, seldom arise. In any case, exclusions, withdrawals, and losses to follow-up should always be reported in clinical studies.[64]

Supplementary treatment

Psychological interventions to reduce anxiety, depression, and pain have been shown to mitigate symptoms and improve quality of life for cancer patients.[65] Significant contributions of supplementary treatment of this type may influence the nature of the study, introduce bias, and interfere with the correct interpretation of results in clinical trials. Nevertheless, confining such ancillary initiatives as well as other treatment measures, for example palliative radiation therapy and chemotherapy, in cancer patients already participating in a study would be unethical, irrespective of ideal requirements of clinical trials.

ETHICAL ISSUES

Ethical conduct, which should be a self-evident element of any clinical trial, means treating the patient with the intervention believed to be the best for the patient. However, the reason that a clinical trial is being considered at all is that there is uncertainty about the potential benefits of a new treatment. The inclusion of untreated controls does not obviate treatment effects and introduces bias because there is no blinding. How should informed consent be performed? Are the ethical aspects of randomization discussed? Are placebo controls necessary, possible, ethical, and interpretable?

Individual versus collective ethics

Volunteer studies can present obvious ethical and experimental constraints. Direct comparison between therapies does not always offer patients a sufficiently similar experience upon which to make assessments or to draw firm conclusions.[44] Thus, provisions of adequate, yet ethical controls are often impossible. Individual ethics mean that each patient should be offered the treatment which is thought to be most beneficial to control the symptoms. Collective ethics are concerned with achieving medical progress as efficiently as possible so that all patients may subsequently benefit from superior therapy. Most people feel instinctively that we should pay exclusive attention to individual ethics. Individual ethics invariably are compromised to some extent since otherwise patients would be exposed to improvised therapy based on clinical opinion, circumstantial and insubstantial evidence.[5] Each clinical trial requires a balance between individual ethics and collective ethics. Society as a whole, as well as guidelines and laws on medical ethics, have perhaps not fully appreciated the reality of clinical trials, yet.

Placebo treatment

Placebos in medical practice are given with the expectation that patients will benefit from nonspecific effects, so efforts are made to maximize these effects. Placebo-controlled studies seem only to be of relevance in studies with continuous subjective outcomes, such as management of pain, emesis, and dyspnea.[66] However, it cannot be excluded that placebo effects may exist in disorders such as irritable bowel syndrome or idiopathic constipation.

In clinical trials, placebo effects should be balanced between groups to allow the specific effect to show. However, a placebo cannot be employed if there is definite evidence that withholding standard treatment would be detrimental to the patient. Although it would be unethical to withhold an active analgesic for a prolonged period, administration may be delayed for a short interval, for example in postoperative pain, when the patient has immediate access to rescue medication, either via nurse-administration or a patient-controlled device for delivery of rescue analgesic. If pain relief is not achieved at the end of that period, a more potent rescue treatment must be given. Thus, arguments for using a placebo in this situation can be justified provided that the patient has given an informed consent and rescue medication is available whenever the patient requests it.

Placebo-controlled efficacy trials of oral opioids for cancer pain are lacking. Bell et al.[5] recommend use of a placebo control in selected trials with low-intensity pain. However, such trials will have low assay sensitivity and the risk of not being able to demonstrate clinical efficacy is another major ethical problem.

Some argue that the use of placebo should be avoided in trials, wherever a relevant reference drug is available. The reference drug should have a recognized evidence-base for use in cancer pain, its efficacy should have been well documented and it should be a clinically relevant comparator drug. In trials of opioids, or in trials of neuropathic pain, the comparator drugs could be morphine and gabapentin, respectively. Use of comparators with a higher analgesic efficacy than placebo will lead to fewer unintended episodes of breakthrough pain in the trial. Data from "head-to-head," active comparator-controlled trials, are probably more meaningful for clinical management of pain, but unfortunately they may require very large-scale studies, unless noninferiority or equivalence trials designs are used.

Generally, chronic administration of a placebo cannot be justified in pain that normally responds to established therapy. In these situations, the only feasible way to conduct placebo-controlled trials may be to give both placebo and active treatment groups access to a standard rescue analgesic at the expense of a more complex interpretation of analgesic requirements and drug-induced toxicity, as outlined earlier. In such studies, requirement of rescue analgesic becomes another important outcome measure. This type of efficacy study should have a limited duration and therefore does not pose any ethical problem different from the clinical scenario of management of breakthrough pain.

If the use of placebo group is not justifiable, an alternative approach is to use a second dose level of the standard analgesic. It could furthermore be argued that the ethics of using a placebo control should be compared to the potential ethical dilemma of exposing seriously ill patients to trials which do not produce reliable results due to lack of power, sensitivity, or other methodological problems.

Patient information and consent

The common trial design requires informed consent from the patient prior to randomization, but Zelen[67] has suggested that randomization can precede informed consent so that only those allocated to the new treatment are asked to participate. Even if this strategy does increase recruitment, the approach is impossible in double-blind or single-blind trials and there will always be a risk of introduction of a systematic bias. Cognitive aspects of "informed consent" is another facet of the problem. A number of studies have demonstrated that subjects rarely have an adequate understanding of consent forms[68, 69] and often do not even understand the meaning or implication of the randomization procedure.[70] Patients in a late palliative stage are especially vulnerable, and balancing the roles of a researcher and a clinician are frequently experienced as difficult.[71] Patients suffering from a terminal illness or refractory symptoms may pay little attention to the informed consent process if they perceive enrollment in a clinical research protocol as their last hope for effective treatment. Patients as well as physicians tend to overestimate the potential benefit they will receive from enrollment, which can blur the line between enrollment in research and receiving medical treatment.

Despite increasing international collaboration, cross-cultural knowledge, and competence, there are internationally widely divergent attitudes towards informed consent for every patient entering a clinical trial.[72] In multicenter trials, this could influence results in spite of detailed criteria and adequate protocol adherence.

When designing a clinical protocol, attention should be paid to the guidelines set out in the revised CONSORT statement in the manuscript. These guidelines also provide useful advice during manuscript preparation, particularly in regard to the inclusion of a flow diagram.[64]

CONCLUSION

Cancer pain remains a problem in spite of immense efforts aimed at improving treatment through education campaigns, guidelines, treatment algorithms, and growing research. Why have we not succeeded? Perhaps we need to assess the pertinent question: Is pain in cancer patients different from that in patients with a noncancer diagnosis? Of course there are some specific pathophysiologic changes in cancer patients that could explain some of the differences, such as patients with gradual compression of nerves from tumors, chemotherapeutic agent-induced neuropathy, or specific cytokine release from bone metastases. However, more important is probably the multidimensionality in the pain experience characterized by fluctuations in pain intensity and variable responses to treatment, along with the challenge of disease progression and existential suffering. This means that extrapolated data from acute pain, chronic pain, or animal research are not always representative of clinical cancer pain. Thus, we need to develop multimodal research methodology, validated instruments, and assessment tools that are tailored to address cancer patients, particularly in respect of a potentially terminal disease.

REFERENCES

1. Jacox A, Carr DB, Payne R. New clinical-practice guidelines for the management of pain in patients with cancer. *New England Journal of Medicine*. 1994; **330**: 651–5.
2. Bruera E, Kim HN. Cancer pain. *Journal of the American Medical Association*. 2003; **290**: 2476–9.
3. Zech DF, Grond S, Lynch J et al. Validation of World Health Organization Guidelines for cancer pain relief: a 10-year prospective study. *Pain*. 1995; **63**: 65–76.
∗ 4. Carr DB, Goudas LC, Balk EM et al. Evidence report on the treatment of pain in cancer patients. *Journal of the National Cancer Institute Monographs*. 2004; **32**: 23–31.
∗ 5. Bell RF, Wisloff T, Eccleston C, Kalso E. Controlled clinical trials in cancer pain. How controlled should they be? A qualitative systematic review. *British Journal of Cancer*. 2006; **94**: 1559–67.
6. Portenoy RK, Foley KM, Inturrisi CE. The nature of opioid responsiveness and its implications for neuropathic pain: new hypotheses derived from studies of opioid infusions. *Pain*. 1990; **43**: 273–86.
7. Chang G, Chen L, Mao J. Opioid tolerance and hyperalgesia. *Medical Clinics of North America*. 2007; **91**: 199–211.
8. Portenoy RK. Tolerance to opioid analgesics: clinical aspects. *Cancer Surveys*. 1994; **21**: 49–65.
∗ 9. Klepstad P, Dale O, Skorpen F et al. Genetic variability and clinical efficacy of morphine. *Acta Anaesthesiologica Scandinavica*. 2005; **49**: 902–08.
10. Stamer UM, Bayerer B, Stuber F. Genetics and variability in opioid response. *European Journal of Pain*. 2005; **9**: 101–04.
∗ 11. Somogyi AA, Barratt DT, Coller JK. Pharmacogenetics of opioids. *Clinical Pharmacology and Therapeutics*. 2007; **81**: 429–44.
∗ 12. Portenoy RK, Payne D, Jacobsen P. Breakthrough pain: characteristics and impact in patients with cancer pain. *Pain*. 1999; **81**: 129–34.
∗ 13. Svendsen KB, Andersen S, Arnason S et al. Breakthrough pain in malignant and non-malignant diseases: a review of prevalence, characteristics and mechanisms. *European Journal of Pain*. 2005; **9**: 195–206.
∗ 14. Caraceni A, Martini C, Zecca E et al. Breakthrough pain characteristics and syndromes in patients with cancer pain. An international survey *Palliative Medicine*. 2004; **18**: 177–83.
15. Odrcich M, Bailey JM, Cahill CM, Gilron I. Chronobiological characteristics of painful diabetic neuropathy and postherpetic neuralgia: Diurnal pain variation and effects of analgesic therapy. *Pain*. 2006; **120**: 207–12.
16. Donovan-Rodriguez T, Dickenson AH, Urch CE. Superficial dorsal horn neuronal responses and the emergence of behavioural hyperalgesia in a rat model of cancer-induced bone pain. *Neuroscience Letters*. 2004; **360**: 29–32.
17. Shimoyama M, Tatsuoka H, Ohtori S et al. Change of dorsal horn neurochemistry in a mouse model of neuropathic cancer pain. *Pain*. 2005; **114**: 221–30.
18. Donovan-Rodriguez T, Dickenson AH, Urch CE. Gabapentin normalizes spinal neuronal responses that correlate with behavior in a rat model of cancer-induced bone pain. *Anesthesiology*. 2005; **102**: 132–40.
19. Wasan AD, Davar G, Jamison R. The association between negative affect and opioid analgesia in patients with discogenic low back pain. *Pain*. 2005; **117**: 450–61.
∗ 20. Zaza C, Baine N. Cancer pain and psychosocial factors: a critical review of the literature. *Journal of Pain and Symptom Management*. 2002; **24**: 526–42.
21. Sullivan MJ, Thorn B, Haythornthwaite JA et al. Theoretical perspectives on the relation between catastrophizing and pain. *Clinical Journal of Pain*. 2001; **17**: 52–64.
22. Keefe FJ, Abernethy AP, Campbell C. Psychological approaches to understanding and treating disease-related pain. *Annual Review of Psychology*. 2005; **56**: 601–30.

∗ 23. Farrar JT, Portenoy RK, Berlin JA et al. Defining the clinically important difference in pain outcome measures. *Pain*. 2000; **88**: 287–94.

∗ 24. Melzack R, Katz J. Pain assessment in adult patients. In: McMahon SB, Koltzenburg M (eds). *Wall and Melzack's textbook of pain*, 5th edn. Philadelphia: Elsevier Churchill Livingstone, 2006: 291–304.

25. Breivik EK, Bjornsson GA, Skovlund E. A comparison of pain rating scales by sampling from clinical trial data. *Clinical Journal of Pain*. 2000; **16**: 22–8.

26. Jensen MP, Chen C, Brugger AM. Postsurgical pain outcome assessment. *Pain*. 2002; **99**: 101–09.

27. Melzack R. The McGill Pain Questionnaire: major properties and scoring methods. *Pain*. 1975; **1**: 277–99.

28. Daut RL, Cleeland CS, Flanery RC. Development of the Wisconsin Brief Pain Questionnaire to assess pain in cancer and other diseases. *Pain*. 1983; **17**: 197–210.

29. Fishman B, Pasternak S, Wallenstein SL et al. The Memorial Pain Assessment Card. A valid instrument for the evaluation of cancer pain. *Cancer*. 1987; **60**: 1151–8.

30. Ramsay M, Winget C, Higginson I. Review: measures to determine the outcome of community services for people with dementia. *Age and Ageing*. 1995; **24**: 73–83.

31. Walsh TD. Adjuvant analgesic therapy in cancer pain. In: Foley KM, Bonica JJ, Ventafridda V (eds). *Advances in pain research and therapy*. New York, NY: Raven Press, 1990: 155–69.

32. Hanks G, Cherny NI, Fallon M. Opioid analgesic therapy. In: Doyle D, Hanks G, Cherny N, Calman K (eds). *Oxford textbook of palliative medicine*, 3rd edn. Oxford: Oxford University Press, 2004: 316–41.

33. Twycross RG. Opioids. In: Wall PD, Melzack R (eds). *Textbook of pain*, 4th edn. New York: Churchill Livingstone, 1999: 1187–214.

∗ 34. Ripamonti C. Pharmacology of opioid analgesia: clinical principles. Cancer pain. In: Bruera ED, Portenoy RK (eds). *Assessment and management*. Cambridge: Cambridge University Press, 2003: 124–49.

35. Bruera E, Pereira J, Watanabe S et al. Opioid rotation in patients with cancer pain. A retrospective comparison of dose ratios between methadone, hydromorphone, and morphine. *Cancer*. 1996; **78**: 852–7.

∗ 36. Dworkin RH, Turk DC, Farrar JT. Core outcome measures for chronic pain clinical trials: IMMPACT recommendations. *Pain*. 2005; **113**: 9–19.

37. Silverman DG, O'Connor TZ, Brull SJ. Integrated assessment of pain scores and rescue morphine use during studies of analgesic efficacy. *Anesthesia and Analgesia*. 1993; **77**: 168–70.

38. Romundstad L, Breivik H, Roald H et al. Methylprednisolone reduces pain, emesis, and fatigue after breast augmentation surgery: a single-dose, randomized, parallel-group study with methylprednisolone 125 mg, parecoxib 40 mg, and placebo. *Anesthesia and Analgesia*. 2006; **102**: 418–25.

39. de Stoutz ND, Bruera E, Suarez-Almazor M. Opioid rotation for toxicity reduction in terminal cancer patients. *Journal of Pain and Symptom Management*. 1995; **10**: 378–84.

40. Quigley C. Opioid switching to improve pain relief and drug tolerability. *Cochrane Database of Systematic Reviews*. 2004; **CD004847**.

41. Kaasa S, De Connoy F. Palliative care research. *European Journal of Cancer*. 2001; **37**: S153–9.

42. Grimes DA, Schulz KF. Bias and causal associations in observational research. *Lancet*. 2002; **359**: 248–52.

43. Sacks H, Chalmers TC, Smith Jr H. Randomized versus historical controls for clinical trials. *American Journal of Medicine*. 1982; **72**: 233–40.

44. Clark PI, Leaverton PE. Scientific and ethical issues in the use of placebo controls in clinical trials. *Annual Review of Public Health*. 1994; **15**: 19–38.

45. Matthews JN, Altman DG, Campbell MJ, Royston P. Analysis of serial measurements in medical research [see comments]. *British Medical Journal*. 1990; **300**: 230–5.

∗ 46. Senn S, Stevens L, Chaturvedi N. Repeated measures in clinical trials: simple strategies for analysis using summary measures. *Statistics in Medicine*. 2000; **19**: 861–77.

∗ 47. Caraceni A, Brunelli C, Martini C et al. Cancer pain assessment in clinical trials. A review of the literature (1999–2002). *Journal of Pain and Symptom Management*. 2005; **29**: 507–19.

48. Farrar JT, Young Jr JP, LaMoreaux L et al. Clinical importance of changes in chronic pain intensity measured on an 11-point numerical pain rating scale. *Pain*. 2001; **94**: 149–58.

49. Vincent E, Todd S, Whitehead J. A sequential procedure for comparing two experimental treatments with a control. *Journal of Biopharmaceutical Statistics*. 2002; **12**: 249–65.

50. Deschamps M, Band PR, Hislop TG et al. The evaluation of analgesic effects in cancer patients as exemplified by a double-blind, crossover study of immediate-release versus controlled-release morphine. *Journal of Pain and Symptom Management*. 1992; **7**: 384–92.

51. Parris WC, Johnson Jr BW, Croghan MK et al. The use of controlled-release oxycodone for the treatment of chronic cancer pain: a randomized, double-blind study. *Journal of Pain and Symptom Management*. 1998; **16**: 205–11.

52. Kerr IG. Clinical trials to study pain in patients with advanced cancer: practical difficulties. *Anticancer Drugs*. 1995; **6**: 18–28.

53. Byas-Smith MG, Max MB, Muir J, Kingman A. Transdermal clonidine compared to placebo in painful diabetic neuropathy using a two-stage 'enriched enrollment' design. *Pain*. 1995; **60**: 267–74.

54. Leber PD, Davis CS. Threats to the validity of clinical trials employing enrichment strategies for sample selection. *Controlled Clinical Trials*. 1998; **19**: 178–87.

55. Portenoy RK. Cancer pain general design issues. In: Max M, Portenoy R, Laska R (eds). *Advances in pain research and therapy*. New York: Raven Press, 1991: 233–66.

56. Bruera E, Schoeller T, Wenk R *et al.* A prospective multicenter assessment of the Edmonton staging system for cancer pain. *Journal of Pain and Symptom Management.* 1995; **10**: 348–55.

57. Spiegel D, Sands S, Koopman C. Pain and depression in patients with cancer. *Cancer.* 1994; **74**: 2570–8.

58. MacDonald N, Bruera E. Clinical trials in cancer pain research. In: Foley KM, Bonica JJ, Ventafridda V (eds). *Advances in pain research and therapy.* New York: Raven Press, 1990: 443–9.

59. Stambaugh JE. Commentary: issues for chronic pain models with specific emphasis on the chronic cancer pain model. In: Max M, Portenoy R, Laska R (eds). *Advances in pain research and therapy.* New York: Raven Press, 1991: 287–9.

60. Kurz A, Sessler DI. Opioid-induced bowel dysfunction: pathophysiology and potential new therapies. *Drugs.* 2003; **63**: 649–71.

61. Weiss SC, Emanuel LL, Fairclough DL, Emanuel EJ. Understanding the experience of pain in terminally ill patients. *Lancet.* 2001; **357**: 1311–15.

62. Kongsgaard UE, Poulain P. Transdermal fentanyl for pain control in adults with chronic cancer pain. *European Journal of Pain.* 1998; **2**: 53–62.

63. Stambaugh Jr JE, Drew J. The combination of ibuprofen and oxycodone/acetaminophen in the management of chronic cancer pain. *Clinical Pharmacology and Therapeutics.* 1988; **44**: 665–9.

∗ 64. Moher D, Schulz KF, Altman DG. The CONSORT statement: revised recommendations for improving the quality of reports of parallel-group randomized trials. *Annals of Internal Medicine.* 2001; **134**: 657–62.

65. Syrjala KL, Donaldson GW, Davis MW *et al.* Relaxation and imagery and cognitive-behavioral training reduce pain during cancer treatment: a controlled clinical trial. *Pain.* 1995; **63**: 189–98.

∗ 66. Hrobjartsson A, Gotzsche PC. Is the placebo powerless? An analysis of clinical trials comparing placebo with no treatment. *New England Journal of Medicine.* 2001; **344**: 1594–602.

67. Zelen M. A new design for randomized clinical trials. *New England Journal of Medicine.* 1979; **300**: 1242–5.

68. Lavelle-Jones C, Byrne DJ, Rice P, Cuschieri A. Factors affecting quality of informed consent. *British Medical Journal.* 1993; **306**: 885–90.

69. Joffe S, Cook EF, Cleary PD *et al.* Quality of informed consent in cancer clinical trials: a cross-sectional survey. *Lancet.* 2001; **358**: 1772–7.

70. Snowdon C, Garcia J, Elbourne D. Making sense of randomization; responses of parents of critically ill babies to random allocation of treatment in a clinical trial. *Social Science and Medicine.* 1997; **45**: 1337–55.

71. Casarett DJ, Karlawish JH. Are special ethical guidelines needed for palliative care research? *Journal of Pain and Symptom Management.* 2000; **20**: 130–9.

∗ 72. Rivera R, Borasky D, Rice R *et al.* Informed consent: an international researchers' perspective. *American Journal of Public Health.* 2007; **97**: 25–30.

45

Clinical trials: neuropathic pain

ANDREW SC RICE

KEY LEARNING POINTS

- The "gold standard" tool for assessing therapeutic interventions in neuropathic pain is the double-blind randomized controlled trial (RCT).
- The most conventional design of RCT is a parallel group study, but crossover designs can be justified in certain circumstances, for example rare clinical conditions or expensive interventions.
- Postherpetic neuralgia and painful diabetic neuropathy are the conditions most frequently examined in neuropathic pain RCTs to date.

- Most RCTs to date have used placebo as a comparator. However, as the evidence base of established therapies becomes stronger, it will be increasingly difficult to justify the use of placebo in neuropathic pain RCTs and equivalence or superiority trials will be required.
- Careful phenotyping of subjects prior to randomization, for example of sensory phenotype by quantitative sensory testing, may enable subgroups of responders to be identified.

INTRODUCTION

A clinical trial is a prospective experiment conducted to test the effects of a medical intervention in human subjects and is the key methodological tool for establishing an evidence base. In the context of neuropathic pain, most interventions being tested will be pharmacological and thus the effects examined will be efficacy, tolerability, and adverse events.

The current evidence base for neuropathic pain therapies increasingly comprises data from phase II or III drug development trials (**Table 45.1**). Consequently, placebo-controlled trials are popular and few published trials have directly examined drug equivalence or synergy, a notable

exception being a recent combination study of gabapentin and morphine in painful diabetic neuropathy and postherpetic neuralgia.[3] Today's climate of increased regulation, for example the burden imposed by European Union Clinical Trials Directive[4, 5] (www.medicines.mhra.gov.uk/ourwork/licensingmeds/types/clintrialdir.htm), considered in the light of a relatively poor track record of major nonindustrial funding for academic neuropathic pain clinical trials, predicates that in the foreseeable future we can expect few major trials to be conducted without commercial sponsorship. However, there are several important areas in which there is little incentive for industry sponsored trials, notably head to head comparisons of drugs and drug combination studies,[6] and

Table 45.1 Phases of drug development studies.[1, 2]

Phase	
I	The earliest studies carried out in humans. Small number of healthy volunteers (<20) to investigate the clinical pharmacology of a drug (pharmacodynamics, pharmacokinetics) and its toxicity of drug in humans
II	First studies in patients, often for proof of concept in order to provide early efficacy data required for a decision as to whether to commit to phase III studies. Usually to determine optimal dose and regimen and to further investigate safety
	Can be divided into phase IIa and phase IIb. Often involve 200–300 patients. Not necessarily randomized or placebo controlled
III	Large trials to determine efficacy and safety. For a particular indication. Usually performed for the purposes of providing data to support a submission to regulatory authorities. Randomized and controlled, usually placebo controlled. Depending on indication, 100–3000 patients.
IV	After registration of a product with a regulatory authority. Usually performed for marketing purposes or as part of postmarketing surveillance.

therefore calls for academic collaborations have been made to address this shortcoming.[7] Therefore, this chapter will focus on the design requirements of trials which are performed primarily for regulatory purposes.

Although trials of preventative strategies have been performed in the context of neuropathic pain (e.g. vaccines for postherpetic neuralgia[8]), most trials examine pain relief in the context of established neuropathic pain. The latter scenario will be the focus of this chapter.

The European Medicines Agency has adopted a guideline for clinical trials of neuropathic pain therapies.[9] Additionally, all clinical trials must be conducted in accordance with Good Clinical Practice (GCP) Guidelines[10, 11] (www.ich.org), shown in **Box 45.1**.

ETHICS

All medical research in humans, including clinical trials, must protect subjects against harm. The World Medical Association's (WMA) Declaration of Helsinki states the principles governing this requirement and it is reexamined and updated on a regular basis, the latest version at the time of writing being dated October 9, 2004 (www.wma.net/e/policy/b3.htm).

The International Association for the Study of Pain has produced ethical guidelines, specifically geared to the conduct of pain research in humans (www.iasp-pain.org/ethics-h.html).[12] These are shown in **Box 45.2**.

A discussion of the complex ethical matters relating to clinical research is not within the scope of this chapter, other than to state that it is mandatory that the protocol of a trial be examined by a legitimate ethical review committee and that the approval of that committee is granted before commencing the trial.

The provision of rescue medication should be considered.[9] The choice of rescue medication should be evidence-based for each individual disease. In the specific context of a chronic neuropathic pain study, the protocol should probably state that once a subject has taken rescue medication, then they should be withdrawn for lack of efficacy and the data up to the point of withdrawal analyzed on an intent to treat basis.

HYPOTHESIS AND QUESTION

As dictated by "scientific method," the conventional starting point for a clinical trial is the statement of a hypothesis (e.g. "Gabapentin is superior to placebo in alleviating the continuous pain of postherpetic neuralgia"). This statement will naturally lead to a definition of a set of questions which will need to be answered in a trial, in order to test the hypothesis.

TRIAL DESIGN

The exact design of a clinical trial will be dictated by the hypothesis to be tested. Most neuropathic pain studies reported to date sought to demonstrate superiority of a test drug over placebo. However, there is now an argument that a position has been reached whereby there are sufficient evidence-based therapies for neuropathic pain and therefore it may no longer be ethical to unnecessarily expose subjects to placebo in neuropathic pain studies (see Controls). Furthermore, there is also a necessity to directly compare the existing and novel therapies in equivalence/superiority studies and to directly examine the additive or synergistic effects of a combination of treatments in clinical trials, although there is little incentive for industry to fund such studies.

Bias elimination

A major factor in the design of a trial is the elimination of bias, which can be defined as any systematic deviation from the truth. Bias is a potentially confounding factor in any clinical trial and possible sources of bias must be identified at the design stage, and tools employed to reduce or eliminate the effect of these. Many types of bias can be identified (Table 8 in Earl-Slater[1]), but perhaps the most relevant to neuropathic pain trials are:

Box 45.1 Principles of GCP in clinical trials

1. Clinical trials should be conducted in accordance with the ethical principles that have their origin in the Declaration of Helsinki, and that are consistent with GCP and the applicable regulatory requirement(s).
2. Before a trial is initiated, foreseeable risks and inconveniences should be weighed against the anticipated benefit for the individual trial subject and society. A trial should be initiated and continued only if the anticipated benefits justify the risks.
3. The rights, safety, and well-being of the trial subjects are the most important considerations and should prevail over interests of science and society.
4. The available nonclinical and clinical information on an investigational product should be adequate to support the proposed clinical trial.
5. Clinical trials should be scientifically sound, and described in a clear, detailed protocol.
6. A trial should be conducted in compliance with the protocol that has received prior institutional review board (IRB)/independent ethics committee (IEC) approval/favorable opinion.
7. The medical care given to, and medical decisions made on behalf of, subjects should always be the responsibility of a qualified physician or, when appropriate, of a qualified dentist.
8. Each individual involved in conducting a trial should be qualified by education, training, and experience to perform his or her respective task(s).
9. Freely given informed consent should be obtained from every subject prior to clinical trial participation.
10. All clinical trial information should be recorded, handled, and stored in a way that allows its accurate reporting, interpretation, and verification.
11. The confidentiality of records that could identify subjects should be protected, respecting the privacy and confidentiality rules in accordance with the applicable regulatory requirement(s).
12. Investigational products should be manufactured, handled, and stored in accordance with applicable good manufacturing practice (GMP). They should be used in accordance with the approved protocol.
13. Systems with procedures that assure the quality of every aspect of the trial should be implemented.

Reproduced with permission from Ref. 11, www.ich.org

- Selection bias occurs when the subjects participating in the trial are not a representative sample of the disease population to be examined. There are several methods for overcoming this difficulty, for example by recruiting a strict series of consecutive patients presenting to a clinic. Particular care must be exercised to eliminate cultural, gender, geographic, social class, and ethnic bias in multicenter studies by careful selection of centers and balancing of recruitment between centers. Enriched sample (selecting patients who have responded (or excluding those who have not) to the test or similar treatment before) may overestimate the effect of a test drug.
- Allocation bias occurs when the manner in which subjects are allocated to the arms of the trial is distorted; it can be eliminated by the use of randomization when allocating subjects to study arms. Lack of randomization can overestimate treatment effect by approximately 40 percent.[13] Indeed, the presence or lack of randomization can even yield contradictory results when the same intervention is tested.[14] Randomization can be simple or restricted (e.g. stratification by age or sensory testing findings). Block randomization maintains the balance of subjects allocated to each arm at all time points during the execution of the trial.

- Subject bias occurs when the subjects in a trial are aware of the treatment which they are receiving. This can occur unintentionally, for example if particular side effects reveal the nature of a treatment to a subject. For example, in an acute pain trial, it was revealed that a subject who guessed correctly that they received an active analgesic reported a more pronounced pain-relieving effect, compared with a subject who received the same active analgesic but who guessed that they received placebo.[15] The inclusion of tools to detect possible unblinding of the subject should be considered in the trial design.
- Observer bias occurs when the researcher taking measurements, collecting, and/or analyzing data is aware of the treatment which a subject is receiving.
- Subject and observer bias can be reduced by "blinding" subjects or observers to the nature of treatments. When this is applied to both parties a trial is described as "double blind." Failure to use a double-blind technique will increase treatment effect by approximately 17 percent.[13, 16]
- Analysis bias results from inappropriate handling of data from subjects who withdraw from a trial. Analysis of data on an "intent to treat" basis (analysis which includes all data from all subjects actually randomized and who received at least one

---

Box 45.2 International Association for the Study of Pain Ethical Guidelines for Pain Research in Humans

1. The health, safety, and dignity of human subjects have the highest priority in pain research. The investigator is personally responsible for the conduct of research and its effects on the experimental subject at all times, even though the patients have given their consent to participate.
2. Before starting any study of human subjects, the proposed experimental protocol must be reviewed and approved by an independent committee on human research. The functions of the committee are as follows:
    a. to ensure that participants are not coerced or harmed;
    b. to evaluate the potential for undesirable physical or psychological effects occurring during the research;
    c. to decide whether the proposed research should be the subject of regular review;
    d. the committee should be appropriately constituted and normally should include scientists, health care practitioners, and lay members;
    e. the scientific merit of the proposal and the research methods proposed should normally be the subject of independent evaluation by an appropriately constituted peer review committee. The scientific review process normally should take place before the consideration of ethical matters.
3. Potential participants should be informed fully about the goals, procedures, and risks of the study before giving their consent.
4. Healthy subjects and patients must be able to decline, or to terminate, participation at any stage without risk or penalty whatsoever.
5. Written consent must be obtained to indicate that the subject understands the nature and purpose of the proposed study, has had the opportunity to ask questions and agrees to participate on a voluntary basis. Where possible, informed consent should be endorsed by an independent signatory.
6. There is a duty to protect those who may be incapable of giving fully informed and voluntary consent. These include children, the elderly, the mentally handicapped, prisoners, and those very ill with other disease. Such persons should not be used for medical research unless they are essential for the goals of the proposed research. In such cases, consent must be obtained, also from those who have legal responsibility for their welfare.
7. In any pain research, stimuli should never exceed a subject's tolerance limit and subjects should be able to escape or terminate a painful stimulus at will. The minimal intensity of noxious stimulus necessary to achieve the goals of the study should be established and not exceeded.
8. In all circumstances, including studies that employ placebo and sham treatment methods, an effective, accepted method of pain relief must be provided on request of the patient or subject. The availability of alternative pain relief should be made clear in the consent form and the instruction before the study begins.

Reproduced from (www.iasp-pain.org/ethics)[12] with permission from the International Association for the Study of Pain.

---

dose of the test or comparator treatment) will reduce bias related to withdrawals, including those withdrawals due to treatment effects (e.g. lack of efficacy or adverse events).

- Reporting bias relates from incomplete or selective reporting of data. Advance registration of clinical trial protocol should help to eliminate this.[17]

Therefore, the "gold standard" tool for the assessment of a therapy for efficacy and safety is the randomized double-blind controlled trial.

Parallel group or crossover?

Most trials performed for regulatory purposes use parallel group designs (each subject allocated only to a single treatment), although the comparatively large sample which has to be recruited to achieve statistical power using such designs is something of a disadvantage. Superficially, crossover designs (subject allocated to two or more treatments at different times) might appear to have an advantage over a parallel group approach, in that a smaller sample is required to achieve power (see **Figure 45.1**). Crossover studies also have an advantage that each subject acts as their own control. However, crossover designs have several disadvantages and in practice are employed less frequently than before and are generally not preferred by most regulatory authorities. There are several reasons of this which include the following.

- Carryover effect. This occurs when the effect of a treatment in one arm of the study complicates the next phase. This is usually eliminated by the

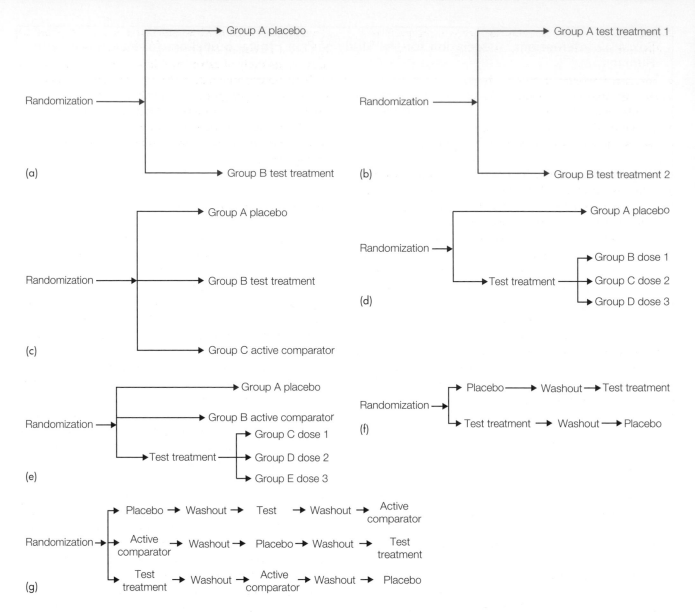

Figure 45.1 Schematic examples of various parallel group and crossover trial designs: (a) simple parallel group with placebo control; (b) parallel group equivalence trial; (c) parallel group with placebo and active comparator; (d) parallel group placebo control, multiple dose; (e) parallel group placebo control, active comparator, multiple dose; (f) placebo controlled simple crossover; (g) three-way crossover.

inclusion of washout periods, but the exact requirements of a washout period can be difficult to determine for drugs which have variable, unpredictable, or prolonged elimination characteristics, such as cannabinoids. Furthermore, a washout period can expose subjects to a period of no treatment, even a rebound increase of pain (for example, after a period with an opioid), which might be considered unethical.

- Unintentional unblinding of subjects in one arm, for example by side effects, thus revealing the nature of a treatment in another arm.
- Period (or order) effect: A time-dependent variation in the nature of a disease or symptom between the treatment periods could complicate a crossover

design. For example, a subject could report a different baseline pain intensity for each treatment phase. Pain intensity can vary across time for any number of reasons and some diseases associated with neuropathic pain can be progressive (e.g. cancer pain, multiple sclerosis, or painful diabetic neuropathy).
- Complicated statistical analysis.

Crossover designs might be acceptable in certain circumstance, such as for a rare disease when a sufficient number of subjects is unlikely to be recruited for a parallel group study or when a very expensive therapy is to be tested.

Despite the greater numbers of subjects which need to be recruited to parallel group studies, the advantages of such a design dictate that this has become the preferred option for most investigators.[7] Advantages include:[1]

- consistent baseline for each subject;
- lack of carryover or period effects;
- simpler statistical analysis;
- can be used to determine causality;
- each subject receives only one intervention.

Neither conventional parallel group nor crossover designs are efficient at elucidating adverse effect frequency and therefore drug safety, this is mainly because the observations are limited to the relatively short duration treatment period in a trial. This period is obviously much shorter than the usual period of clinical therapy and therefore adverse effects which take time to become apparent may not be detected in conventional trials, for example the long-term risks of mental illness associated with cannabinoid therapy cannot be detected in the short-term trials which have been conducted to date.[18] Furthermore, the sample size for most trials (see below under Sample size) is calculated on the basis of analgesic efficacy and therefore infrequently occurring adverse effects (or those restricted to subsets of patients) are unlikely to be detected.

Sample size

The sample size for a trial needs to be not only sufficiently large to ensure that false-negative results are not obtained by chance, but also, conversely, small enough to be efficient and to expose the minimum number of subjects to risk. In a classic review of 383 trials published in major journals, 275 reported "negative" results, but only 16 percent of these "negative" trials had recruited a sufficient sample size to detect a 25 percent relative difference between groups.[19] Underpowered studies also tend to overestimate treatment effects by approximately 30 percent.[20, 21]

For any given trial the calculation of the sample size required to achieve sufficient statistical power will be based on a number of assumptions peculiar to that trial (see Ref. 22 for an explanation of power calculations and worked examples). However, an impression of approximate sample sizes required for placebo-controlled parallel group neuropathic pain studies can be gained by examining published trials. For example, in a three arm parallel group study of gabapentin in postherpetic neuralgia, a sample size of 118 subjects randomized per arm was predicted to yield 90 percent power on the assumption of efficacy being indicated by a 1.0 cm (estimated standard deviation 2.35) change on a 10 cm numeric rating scale (NRS) pain intensity scale.[23] Similarly, a two arm study of gabapentin in postherpetic neuralgia which assumed a definition of efficacy of a 1.5 point change on an 11 point NRS pain intensity scale (estimated standard

deviation 3.4) required 80 subjects per arm in order to achieve a power of 80 percent.[24] Finally, a two arm parallel group study of gabapentin in a population of painful diabetic neuropathy patients predicted that a sample size of 75 subjects per group was required to yield 90 percent power to detect a difference between gabapentin and placebo in being associated with a "moderate" improvement measured using a seven-point global impression of change scale.[25]

Inclusion/exclusion criteria

The precise inclusion/exclusion criteria must be clearly stated in the trial protocol. The precise nature of these will be dictated by the needs of the individual trial, but an idea of "generic" criteria can be formed by consulting previous key studies.[23, 24, 25, 26, 27, 28, 29] Nevertheless, some special factors do need to be considered as described below.

Traditionally, neuropathic pain studies recruit from specific populations on the basis of underlying disease (e.g. postherpetic neuralgia, painful diabetic neuropathy, HIV-related neuropathy, etc.), but it has been hypothesized that the classification of neuropathic pain for treatment purposes should rather be based upon the pain mechanism(s) operating in individual patients.[30] However, the validation of practical, sensitive, specific, and reliable methods for detecting pain mechanism(s) operating in individual neuropathic pain patients is probably many years away and therefore clinical trial recruitment can be expected to be disease-based for the foreseeable future. Nevertheless, it is certainly advisable to record patterns of symptoms, clinical signs, and other features, such as psychological state, in individual subjects at recruitment. Similarly, although costly, it is certainly possible to phenotype neuropathic pain patients on the basis of findings from formal quantitative sensory testing, perhaps into broad "hyposensory" and "hypersensory" groups.[31] This may be important in conditions such as postherpetic neuralgia and traumatic neuropathy where distinct subpopulations exist.[32] This information could be used in *post hoc* analyses to indentify subsets of "drug-responders" whose "analgesic signals" may be otherwise obscured within the "noise" of the overall trial populations. Dissemination, collation, and examination of such stratified data, especially when combined with data relating to pain relief associated with different drugs with discreet mechanisms of action, could yield important information about neuropathic pain mechanisms.

In designing a trial protocol, decisions have to be made regarding the concurrent use of other therapies in clinical trials. The simple choice is whether to continue existing medications which may have efficacy in the condition being studied or to stop them. If the choice is to cease therapy with certain drugs then there must be a sufficient washout period in the screening phase before the trial begins. If concurrent drugs are allowed, then these must only be permitted at a stable dose throughout the study.[9] Provided the inclusion criteria contain the safeguard of a predetermined threshold of baseline pain intensity (see below), then concurrent medications should not present too much of a problem, although pharmacological interactions with trial medications must be considered, as the existing therapies are self-evidently not completely effective. The information about concurrent drugs must be recorded so that analysis of the data can be stratified by groups/doses of concurrent drugs.

Enriched enrolment into a trial, for example by including or excluding subjects who have or have not responded to a certain drug in the past, can present problems with interpretation. Active enriched enrolment policies are to be discouraged as they can distort the evidence base. If such an approach is to be used then it must be fully justified and transparently reported. However, there are practical issues here since the probability of recruiting sufficient treatment-naive subjects with an established neuropathic pain condition is low. For instance, in trials of gabapentin in a sample of post-herpetic neuralgia patients, most subjects had previously tried two to three different drugs for their pain and approximately 70 percent had tried an anticonvulsant and 80 percent had tried amitriptyline.[23]

It is conventional to exclude subjects with insufficient severe pain intensity at the baseline screening phase, for example less than 4 on an 11-point scale.[9, 23, 24, 26, 29, 33, 34]

The population from which subjects are to be recruited also needs to be carefully considered. Most trials recruit from secondary or tertiary care pain medicine clinics. However, it could be argued that this population, almost by definition, represents the extreme of neuropathic pain patients who are likely to be resistant to conventional analgesic drugs, be taking multiple medications, display high levels of comorbidity and have high pain intensity scores. It may be more appropriate to recruit from a primary care base to obtain a study population more reflective of the main population of the particular disease under study. One way of achieving this is by advertising-based recruitment, but this approach has its own risks, particularly of introducing selection bias.[33]

Models

Most neuropathic pain studies attempt to study pain within the context of a single disease, although the veracity of extrapolating efficacy from one neuropathic pain condition to another is questionable.[35] Some trials have been reported which examined a mixture of neuropathic conditions, but these have been difficult to interpret.[26]

Postherpetic neuralgia is a frequent choice as a disease model for neuropathic pain, and is certainly one with which regulatory authorities are familiar.[36] Advantages of postherpetic neuralgia include that it is relatively easy to define and diagnose, once established it runs a relatively stable course, and it is not complicated by an underlying disease process. However, the fact that it occurs predominantly in elderly subjects (e.g. median 75 years[23]) can complicate studies, particularly from the adverse events perspective.

Painful diabetic neuropathy has also been studied in large trials.[37] However, this model does suffer from the complicating factors of an underlying disease process which may be progressive, variable blood glucose concentrations potentially influencing pain intensity and concurrent illness complicating drug elimination. There is also a possibility of a trial effect associated with the entry of a diabetic subject into a study, which may encourage better self-control of blood glucose concentration, which could in turn theoretically increase the magnitude of the placebo response.

There are other potential trial models, which so far have not been very popular,[37] but certainly have some attractive features. For example, HIV and certain drug-related neuropathies (e.g. nucleoside reverse transcriptase inhibitors, taxols, statins, and vinca alkaloids) are associated with the development of small fiber axonal neuropathies which may be painful and therefore amenable to study. Traumatic neuropathies are another under-studied group, but perhaps the heterogeneity of peripheral nerve injuries which may result in neuropathic pain makes it difficult to recruit a sufficiently homogenous population to study.

The choice of models also raises the question of whether a study in a single disease entity can be extrapolated to reflect evidence of effectiveness in a broader range of neuropathic pain conditions. This is a difficult question to answer and certainly there are groups of medications (e.g. tricyclic antidepressants, gabapentin, and related drugs) for which evidence of efficacy exists across a broad range of indications.[37] Conversely, whilst tricyclic antidepressants are efficacious, for example in postherpetic neuralgia[36] and other conditions,[37] they do not appear to be associated with efficacy in HIV-related neuropathies.[37]

A further problem with studying single disease models is that the overall result may obscure subpopulations in whom an intervention is actually more or less effective than in the overall study population. Confounding factors such as different pain mechanisms or sensory phenotype operating in different subjects drawn from the same disease population, or genetic or environmental variations in drug pharmacodynamics or kinetics, might not be exposed unless detailed phenotyping of subjects and *post hoc* analyses were employed for all potential confounding factors, which is clearly impossible since they are not all known. For example, in an equivalence study in postherpetic neuralgia subjects whilst efficacy was demonstrated for both tricyclic antidepressants and opioids, there was no correlation between opioid and tricyclic antidepressant responsiveness, implying that distinct subpopulations in the sample were sensitive to opioids or tricyclic antidepressants.[27] This finding is perhaps not altogether surprising when one considers that these drugs have distinct mechanisms of action. One way around this problem might be to screen subjects for their responsiveness to certain drugs or their sensory phenotype prior to randomization and perform an analysis with this variable.

Controls

The major purpose of control groups is to permit discrimination between observed effects which are caused by the test treatment and those related to other factors. The factors governing choice of controls have been considered in detail by the European Medicines Agency,[38] which has identified five broad types of control.

1. Placebo: The placebo should be identical in all aspects to the test treatment, other than that it does not contain the active drug. Not only does placebo control permit examination of the efficacy of the test therapy, but it can also determine the relationship of the test treatment to adverse events. Furthermore, since there are many placebo-controlled trials in the evidence base for neuropathic pain, placebo control can, to a certain extent, also be used as a measure of internal assay sensitive of the study design. Because there is generally a greater measurable difference in efficacy between placebo and efficacious test medications, as opposed to between different test medications, the use of placebo permits an efficient study as fewer subjects will have to be randomized to achieve sufficient statistical power, than, for example, in a superiority study. Whilst placebo controls might be regarded as the "gold standard" control, the use of placebo does present some special problems. For example:
   a. Inadvertent unblinding. The test drug might be associated with particular efficacy or side effects which reveal the nature of the treatment to subjects. This is a particular problem with crossover studies. This could be overcome by using an "active placebo" which has a similar side-effect profile as the test drug, but no superiority in terms of efficacy than placebo for the primary outcome measure. The inclusion of two or more placebos (double dummy) may also mitigate this problem if an active placebo is not available.
   b. There are ethical concerns in exposing patients to the harm of unrelieved pain in a neuropathic pain trial, but it should also be emphasized that placebo does not equate to no

treatment since most large studies reveal a significant efficacy associated with placebo. However, it is questionable whether the use of placebo can be justified when there are now established therapies for a particular medical condition. The position of the World Medical Association on this subject is clear (see **Box 45.3**), although some regulatory authorities appear not to wholly concur with this view. Therefore, justification for the use of placebo for neuropathic pain trials is a difficult judgment which is continually changing as the evidence base for neuropathic pain therapies expands. This complicated and contentious issue is without the remit of this chapter and is discussed in detail elsewhere.[39]

2. Active treatment comparator. This is useful when placebo is considered unethical. Additionally, comparison of the test drug to another is a useful

---

Box 45.3 Extracts from the World Medical Association 2000 revision of the Declaration of Helsinki regarding the position on the use of placebo in clinical trials

In paragraph 29: "The benefits, risks, burdens, and effectiveness of a new method should be tested against those of the best current prophylactic, diagnostic, and therapeutic methods. This does not exclude the use of placebo, or no treatment, in studies where no proven prophylactic, diagnostic, or therapeutic method exists".

Subsequent reconsideration of this issue has led to the following clarification: "The WMA hereby reaffirms its position that extreme care must be taken in making use of a placebo-controlled trial and that in general this methodology should only be used in the absence of existing proven therapy. However, a placebo-controlled trial may be ethically acceptable, even if proven therapy is available, under the following circumstances: a. Where for compelling and scientifically sound methodological reasons its use is necessary to determine the efficacy or safety of a prophylactic, diagnostic or therapeutic method; or b. Where a prophylactic, diagnostic or therapeutic method is being investigated for a minor condition and the subjects who receive placebo will not be subject to any additional risk of serious or irreversible complication".

internal measure of assay sensitivity (the property of trial design which defines the ability to distinguish between treatments of differing efficacy). If the active control has been extensively studied to provide an evidence base of known effectiveness, then an active control study will be an equivalence (or superiority/inferiority) trial. However, equivalence studies generally require much larger numbers of subjects to be randomized in order to achieve statistical power than placebo-controlled studies, since the difference between two efficacious treatments will generally be expected to be less than that between placebo and a test therapy. A problem with active controls arises when the active has not been externally validated, if both treatments are shown to be equivalent is this because neither or both treatments were effective? In this case the inclusion of a placebo control is necessary for correct interpretation of the results.

3. Comparisons of multiple doses of the test treatment under investigation. This has the advantage of yielding dose/response data. When used alone, this type of control suffers from not being able to estimate the placebo effect and having no internal assay sensitivity, but when combined with placebo as zero dose, and perhaps an active control, it becomes a more attractive option. An important issue is determining how the final dose for each group is reached, especially as some treatments may require dose titration to minimize adverse effects. Forced titration of final dose determined at randomization is the optimal approach, but some studies may allow "patient satisfaction" to determine the final dose, although this has the disadvantage of effectively removing randomization.

4. No treatment. As no-treatment controls cannot be blinded, the risk of introducing subject bias dictates that this is not an appropriate strategy for neuropathic pain studies. There are also ethical concerns with this design, especially for pain studies.

5. External controls not studied concurrently with investigated treatment, for example retrospective controls, are not generally employed in neuropathic pain trials, because several forms of bias are inherent in this design.

It is possible to include multiple controls (e.g. placebo, active, and multiple dose) in a single multi-arm study combining the advantages of each type of control. This approach is attractive, but has the disadvantages of expense and requiring the recruitment of a large number of subjects. The European regulators advise three arm (placebo–test drug-active comparator) for phase II/III studies, when an established active comparator exists.[9]

Outcome measures

Recommendations have been published by the IMMPACT group on core outcome measures for use in chronic pain trials[40] (see **Table 45.2**). Whilst these are a welcome and useful tool in design of trials, they should not be regarded

Table 45.2 IMMPACT recommendations.[40]

Recommendations	
Recommended core outcome measure for clinical trials of chronic pain treatment efficacy and effectiveness	
Pain	11-point (0–10) numerical rating scale of pain intensity
	Usage of rescue analgesics
	Categorical rating of pain intensity (none, mild, moderate, severe) in circumstances in which numerical ratings may be problematic
Physical functioning (either one of two measures)	Multidimensional Pain Inventory Interference Scale
	Brief Pain Inventory interference items
Emotional functioning (at least one of two measures)	Beck Depression Inventory
	Profile of mood states
Participant ratings of global improvement and satisfaction with treatment	Patient Global Impression of Change
Symptoms and adverse events	Passive capture of spontaneously reported adverse events and symptoms and use of open-ended prompts
Participant disposition	Detailed information regarding participant recruitment and progress through the trial, including all information specified in the CONSORT guidelines

Reprinted from *Pain*, 113, Dworkin RH, Turk DC, Farrar JT *et al*. Core outcome measures for chronic pain clinical trials: IMMPACT recommendations, 9–19, © (2005), with permission from the International Association for the Study of Pain.

as being totally proscriptive and, as McQuay pointed out in an accompanying editorial, they must be widely debated before being generally accepted.[5, 41] In this editorial it was also emphasized that whilst few would disagree with the broad domains identified by the IMMPACT group (pain; physical functioning; emotional functioning; participant ratings of global improvement and satisfaction with treatment; symptoms and adverse events; participant disposition), more evidence and debate is required to inform recommendations of exactly which tools should be preferred to make measurements within those domains. The following discussion is based on the IMMPACT recommendations, with the proviso that these are under debate.

PRIMARY OUTCOME MEASURE

There is a general consensus amongst published trials in neuropathic pain, and IMMPACT, that the primary outcome measure in neuropathic pain studies should be a form of self-reported pain intensity measurement (see also Chapter 14, Outcome measurement in chronic pain in the *Chronic Pain* volume of this series). An 11 point (0–10) NRS is a reasonable first choice,[9] but the choice of particular scale and collection method (e.g. paper diary versus electronic diary versus telephone reporting) is a more difficult decision for which we do not really have sufficient evidence at the current time. Categorical scales can be used in situations where the use of an NRS is difficult and they are often employed as secondary measures.

However, pain intensity measures are of limited value for measuring anything other than ongoing pain. Many patients suffering from neuropathic pain also suffer from episodic evoked and paroxysmal pain, and in some conditions almost exclusively so (e.g. trigeminal neuralgia). In these situations, it is important to include an event rate measure. It is conceivable that some medications may influence evoked or paroxysmal pain more than ongoing pain, so it is important to record and analyze the data accordingly.

There are difficulties in determining the optimal method for expressing derived data from an NRS. One approach is a simple predetermined degree of change in an NRS. However, for data analysis this is probably inappropriate, the problem being that a simple change does not take into account baseline pain values. A common approach is therefore to take a percentage change in baseline pain. Nevertheless, a difficulty emerges when one attempts to set a certain percentage change in baseline pain intensity as a cut-off for the purposes of defining treatment responders. On one level, the precise cut-off level is not of major relevance since the same measure will be applied to both control and test groups and it could be set high (e.g. 90 percent) or low (e.g. 10 percent) and whilst the numbers of responders will be small or large, respectively, the proportion of responders may not vary too much between the different definitions. However, a

consistent definition of responder across trials where similar measurement tools are used is useful for comparison and evidence accumulation purposes. Fifty percentage change is widely used in meta-analyses,[36, 37, 42] partly because of the ease of data extraction, whereas 30 percent has been shown to equate to certain measures of patient satisfaction in a database of chronic pain trials.[43] It is probably appropriate that, at least for the time being, data derived from both definitions of responder rate are reported in publications of neuropathic pain trials.[9]

SECONDARY OUTCOME MEASURES

An important feature of a neuropathic pain is the quantification of the impact of treatment upon "nonpain" features which often accompany neuropathic pain. A full discussion of these is without the realm of this chapter and the IMMPACT recommendations can be accepted for the time being[40] (**Table 45.2**) (see also Chapter 14, Outcome measurement in chronic pain in the *Chronic Pain* volume of this series). However, some additional measures which might be considered, for example a qualitative measure of pain quality and influence on affect such as the well-validated and widely used short form McGill Questionnaire.[9, 44] A specific measure of sleep interference (although it is included in the brief pain inventory) and global quality of life measure such as the SF-36 health survey (or one of its shortened versions) might be also considered. Secondary outcome measures, especially those associated with quality of life, physical, and emotional functioning, may also provide a measure of the impact of side effects associated with a novel therapy.

A point arises when the interpretation of secondary outcome data is considered in the context of the primary outcome, pain intensity. A positive change in an association with an improvement in pain intensity might be regarded as being causally related. However, it is possible to envisage other scenarios; for instance, an efficacious therapy with unacceptably severe or frequent adverse events might have a negative impact on secondary measures in the face of a positive change or unchanged in pain intensity. Alternatively, a subject may choose to function to a certain level of pain intensity, in this case an effective therapy may not have much impact on measure pain intensity, but secondary measures might improve.

In designing a trial, consideration must be given to the temporal aspects of data collection, especially in the context of drug administration and symptom patterns peculiar to the disease model.[9]

Duration

For short-term proof of efficacy studies of a parallel group design it is probably sufficient to continue the treatment phase for six to eight weeks, although for most of the major pregabalin and gabapentin studies, the treatment effect was apparent by one to two weeks of treatment and slight variations were more likely to be related to variations in dose escalation.[23, 24, 25, 26, 27, 28, 29] European regulators advise a minimum of 12 weeks of study after a stable dose of the test drug has been reached.[9] However, a more open question is how long one needs to continue a study in order to demonstrate if any apparent efficacy will be sustained in the long term, for example if tolerance is an issue with a new drug? To investigate this scenario, the European regulators recommend consideration of a 6–12-month open label extension study.[9]

The duration of study required to properly reflect the adverse events profile of a novel therapy is a more difficult judgment. Frequent adverse events which appear soon after commencing therapy are likely to be detected in six- to eight-week studies powered to detect efficacy; however, longer periods of study may be required to detect adverse events which only appear after longer-term treatment. The need to detect late adverse events has to be weighed against the undesirability of exposing subjects to placebo for long periods; a widely adopted solution is to extend placebo-controlled studies with a longer (often one year) open label study to monitor adverse events, including extension of the placebo group. However, as events surrounding the identification of the cardiovascular risks associated with cyclooxgenase (COX)-2 inhibitors imply, this strategy may not be sufficient to detect significant adverse events which have a long latency or occur only in distinct subgroups of the population.[45] These can only be detected by closely monitoring large populations for prolonged periods of time. Safety assessment of new drugs over long periods in large populations is usually undertaken as a "postmarketing surveillance" exercise, usually reliant on voluntary reporting. This is probably insufficiently rigorous for the current era and it could be argued that regulatory authorities should perhaps grant provisional registration for a new drug based on conventional phase III studies, for a prolonged period when enforced monitoring of safety is a requirement.

MONITORING

Trials in progress should be monitored to protect subjects being unnecessarily exposed to risk and the monitoring tools must be clearly stated in the protocol. Of the various scenarios which might be identified during the course of a clinical trial, the most important are:

- **Futility**: It may become evident during the course of a clinical trial that, for example, the test medication is not superior to placebo. The trial is then deemed futile and should be stopped.
- **Harm**: Trials should be monitored to serious and frequent unexpected adverse events and stopped if unreasonable harm to subjects is a possibility.

- **Scientific misconduct**: Trials should be externally and independently monitored to verify the quality and veracity of data being obtained and to actively seek inconsistencies which may indicate scientific misconduct on the part of an investigator.

The responsibility for monitoring these scenarios is usually discharged by a data and ethics monitoring committee which is completely independent of the investigators and the institutions conducting the study (www.mrc.ac.uk/pdf-ctg.pdf).[10] This committee monitors the data from the trial on a continuous ongoing basis and has the responsibility to recommend premature termination of the study. As the data monitoring committee is independent it should have procedures in place to ensure investigator blinding is not compromised.

TERMINATION

A design feature that might be employed as an additional measure of assay sensitivity might be to allow a period of no treatment at the termination of a trial, during which it would be expected that baseline pain intensities be reachieved, assuming that the disease baseline has not shifted during the course of the trial.

An important ethical question arises at the end of a trial of a novel therapy, if the trial demonstrates that the test therapy is effective. Is it permissible to offer a subject an effective therapy in the context of a clinical trial and then not to offer that subject the opportunity to continue with that therapy after the trial? This is a difficult question, especially in the context of trials performed for drug regulatory purposes, because the medication in question may not have received regulatory approval at the termination of the study. The World Medical Association has considered this point (**Box 45.4**) and the responsibility inherent in its position might, for example, be discharged by conducting a long-term open label study of the test medication, which follows on from the main trial and into which subjects are invited. Such a study could have the primary intention of collecting long-term safety data.

DISSEMINATION

Dissemination is a key phase of any clinical trial and the method of proposed dissemination must be stated in the trial protocol. All trials of neuropathic pain therapies contribute to the clinical evidence base from which clinical decisions are made. Therefore, it is imperative that all data, including "negative" data are in the public domain, preferably in the form of a peer-reviewed paper. In order to understand and interpret clinical trials sufficient information must be given to a reader and the trial must be reported in a transparent fashion. The Consolidated Standard of Reporting Trials (CONSORT) were published

Box 45.4 The position of the World Medical Association Declaration of Helsinki on access to treatment after a trial has been completed

"At the conclusion of the study, every subject entered into the study should be assured of access to the best proven prophylactic, diagnostic and therapeutic methods identified by the study."

This position was later clarified by the statement: "It is necessary during the study planning process to identify post-trial access by study participants to prophylactic, diagnostic and therapeutic procedures identified as beneficial in the study or access to other appropriate care. Post-trial access arrangements or other care must be described in the study protocol so the ethical review committee may consider such arrangements during its review".

Reproduced with permission from (www.wma.net/e/policy/pdf/17c.pdf. (Accessed December 20, 2006); and www.wma.net/e/policy/b3.htm (Accessed December 20, 2006)). Copyright 2007, World Medical Association. All Rights Reserved.

in 1996 (revised 2001) and have been adopted by most major journals.[46] There are few good reasons not to publish trials in accordance with the CONSORT recommendations. CONSORT provides a check list for authors and editors and flow chart (**Figure 45.2**) which should be included in the published report of a trial (www.consort-statement.org).

Duplicate and selective publication of trial results are not in the interests of compiling an accurate evidence base for neuropathic pain therapies. Covert duplicate publication of clinical trial data overestimates a treatment effect, for example a meta-analysis of trials of ondansetron for postoperative emesis found that duplicate publication of data was associated with a 23 percent overestimation of efficacy.[47] Selective publication, particularly of adverse events, is unhelpful, as emphasized by the arguments surrounding the risks associated with, for example COX-2 inhibitors and paroxetine.[45, 48] It is therefore important that all the raw data, including those for adverse events, are available for public scrutiny and analysis and there have been outline agreements which move towards this position.[49] A safeguard against this practice is the registration of clinical trials and their protocols prior to commencement, indeed this is now a requirement for publication in major journals.[17, 50, 51]

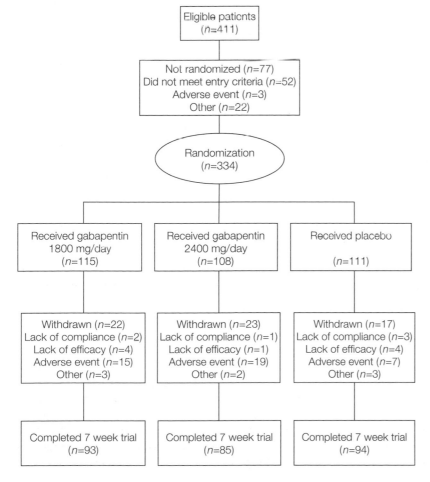

Figure 45.2 Example of a CONSORT flow diagram from a trial of gabapentin in postherpetic neuralgia. Redrawn from *Pain*, **94**, Rice ASC, Maton S, Gabapentin in postherpetic neuralgia; a randomised, double-blind, controlled study, 215–24, © (2001), with permission from the International Association for the Study of Pain.

APPENDIX: USEFUL INTERNET-BASED RESOURCES

- Bandolier (well-respected evidence-based healthcare site with many useful resources for practitioners and investigators. Also links to the Oxford Pain Internet Site for evidence based views on pain medicine) www.jr2.ox.ac.uk/bandolier
- World Medical Association (Declaration of Helsinki) www.wma.net
- European Medicines Agency (European Regulatory Authority, useful guidelines on neuropathic pain trials) www.emea.eu.int
- Medicines and Healthcare Products Regulatory Agency (United Kingdom Regulatory Authority) www.mhra.gov.uk
- Food and Drug Administration (United States Regulatory Authority) www.fda.gov
- International Association for the Study of Pain (ethical guidelines for the study of pain in humans) www.iasp-pain.org
- Medical Research Council (United Kingdom Funding Agency – Source of useful information and guidelines, including Good Clinical Practice guidelines) www.mrc.ac.uk
- International Conference on Harmonization of Technical Requirements for Registration of Pharmaceuticals for Human Use (international body aiming to achieve harmonization in drug registration processes in Europe, Japan, and the United States) www.ich.org.

REFERENCES

1. Earl-Slater A. *The handbook of clinical trials and other research*, 1st edn. Abingdon: Radcliffe Medical Press, 2002.
2. Day S. *Dictionary for clinical trials*, 1st edn. Chichester: John Wiley & Sons, 1999.
3. Gilron I, Bailey JM, Tu D *et al.* Morphine, gabapentin, or their combination for neuropathic pain. *New England Journal of Medicine*. 2005; **352**: 1324–34.
4. European Parliament. Directive 2001/20/EC of the European Parliament and of the Council of 2001. *Official Journal of the European Communities*. L121/34. 2001: 4th April.
5. Woods K. Implementing the European clinical trials directive. *British Medical Journal*. 2004; **328**: 240–1.
6. Black DR, Sang CN. Advances and limitations in the evaluation of analgesic combination therapy. *Neurology*. 2005; **65**: S3–6.
7. Max MB. Afterword: Five steps to increase the payoff of chronic pain trials. *Neurology*. 2005; **65**: S74–7.
8. Oxman MN, Levin MJ, Johnson GR *et al.* A vaccine to prevent herpes zoster and postherpetic neuralgia in older adults. *New England Journal of Medicine*. 2005; **352**: 2271–84.
* 9. Committee for Medicinal Products for Human Use. Guideline on clinical investigation of medicinal products intended for use in the treatment of neuropathic pain. London: European Medicines Agency; 2004. Report No.: CHMP/EWP/252/03.
* 10. Medical Research Council. *MRC guidelines for good clinical practice in clinical trials*. MRC Clinical Trials Series. London: Medical Research Council, 1998.
* 11. International Conference on Harmonisation of Technical Requirements for Registration of Pharmaceuticals for Human Use. Guideline for Good Clinical Practice, 1996.
* 12. Charlton E. Ethical guidelines for pain research in humans. Committee on Ethical Issues of the International Association for the Study of Pain. *Pain*. 1995; **63**: 277–8.
13. Schulz KF, Chalmers I, Hayes RJ, Altman DG. Empirical evidence of bias. Dimensions of methodological quality associated with estimates of treatment effects in controlled trials. *Journal of the American Medical Association*. 1995; **273**: 408–12.
* 14. Carroll D, Tramer M, McQuay H *et al.* Randomization is important in studies with pain outcomes: systematic review of transcutaneous electrical nerve stimulation in acute postoperative pain. *British Journal of Anaesthesia*. 1996; **77**: 798–803.
15. Romundstad L, Breivik H, Niemi G *et al.* Methylprednisolone intravenously 1 day after surgery has sustained analgesic and opioid-sparing effects. *Acta Anaesthesiologica Scandinavica*. 2004; **48**: 1223–31.
16. Ernst E, White AR. Acupuncture for back pain: a meta-analysis of randomized controlled trials. *Archives of Internal Medicine*. 1998; **158**: 2235–41.
17. Abbasi K. Compulsory registration of clinical trials. *British Medical Journal*. 2004; **329**: 637–8.
18. Rice ASC, Lever IJ, Zarnegar R. Cannabinoids and analgesia, with special reference to neuropathic pain. In: McQuay HJ, Kalso E, Moore RA (eds). *Systematic reviews and meta-analyses in pain*. Seattle: IASP Press, 2007: 233–46.
* 19. Moher D, Dulberg CS, Wells GA. Statistical power, sample size, and their reporting in randomized controlled trials. *Journal of the American Medical Association*. 1994; **272**: 122–4.
20. Moore RA, Tramer M, Carroll D *et al.* A quantitative systematic review of topically applied non-steriodal anti-inflammatory drugs. *British Medical Journal*. 1998; **316**: 333–8.
21. Moore RA, Gavaghan D, Tramer MR *et al.* Size is everything – large amounts of information are needed to overcome random effects in estimating direction and magnitude of treatment effects. *Pain*. 1998; **78**: 209–16.
22. Cohen J. A power primer. *Psychological Bulletin*. 1992; **112**: 155–9.
23. Rice ASC, Maton S. Post Herpetic Neuralgia Study Group. Gabapentin in postherpetic neuralgia; a randomised, double-blind, controlled study. *Pain*. 2001; **94**: 215–24.

24. Rowbotham MC, Harden N, Stacey B *et al.* Gabapentin for treatment of postherpetic neuralgia. *Journal of the American Medical Association.* 1998; **280**: 1837–43.

25. Backonja M, Beydoun A, Edwards KR *et al.* Gabapentin for the symptomatic treatment of painful neuroapthy in patients with diabetes mellitus. *Journal of the American Medical Association.* 1998; **280**: 1831–6.

26. Serpell MG. Neuropathic Pain Study Group. Gabapentin in neuropathic pain syndromes: a randomised, double-blind, placebo-controlled trial. *Pain.* 2002; **99**: 557–66.

27. Raja SN, Haythornwaite J, Pappagallo M *et al.* Opioids versus antidepressants in postherpetic neuralgia. *Neurology.* 2002; **59**: 1015–21.

28. Sabatowski R, Galvez R, Cherry DA *et al.* Pregabalin reduces pain and improves sleep and mood disturbances in patients with post-herpetic neuralgia: results of a randomised, placebo-controlled clinical trial. *Pain.* 2004; **109**: 26–35.

29. Dworkin RH, Corbin AE, Young Jr JP *et al.* Pregabalin for the treatment of postherpetic neuralgia: A randomized, placebo-controlled trial. *Neurology.* 2003; **60**: 1274–83.

* 30. Woolf CJ. Dissecting out mechanisms responsible for peripheral neuropathic pain: Implications for diagnosis and therapy. *Life Sciences.* 2004; **74**: 2605–10.

* 31. Rolke R, Magerl W, Campbell KA *et al.* Quantitative sensory testing: a comprehensive protocol for clinical trials. *European Journal of Pain.* 2006; **10**: 77–88.

* 32. Fields HL, Rowbotham MC, Baron R. Postherpetic neuralgia: irritable nociceptors and deafferentation *Neurobiology of Disease.* 1998; **5**: 209–27.

* 33. Dworkin RH, Katz J, Gitlin MJ. Placebo response in clinical trials of depression and its implications for research on chronic neuropathic pain. *Neurology.* 2005; **65**: S7–19.

34. Sabatowski R, Galvez R, Cherry DA *et al.* Pregabalin reduces pain and improves sleep and mood disturbances in patients with post-herpetic neuralgia: results of a randomised, placebo-controlled clinical trial. *Pain.* 2004; **109**: 26–35.

* 35. Rowbotham MC. Mechanisms of neuropathic pain and their implications for the design of clinical trials. *Neurology.* 2005; **65**: S66–73.

* 36. Hempenstall K, Nurmikko TJ, Johnson RW *et al.* Analgesic therapy in postherpetic neuralgia: a quantitative systematic review. *Public Library of Science - Medicine.* 2005; **2**: 628–44.

* 37. Finnerup NB, Otto M, McQuay HJ *et al.* Algorithm for neuropathic pain treatment: an evidence based proposal. *Pain.* 2005; **118**: 289–305.

* 38. European Agency for the Evaluation of Medicinal Products. Choice of control group in clinical trials. London: European Agency for the Evaluation of Medicinal Products; 2000. Report No.: CPMP/ICH/364/96.

* 39. Nagasako EM, Kalauokalani DA. Ethical aspects of placebo groups in pain trials: Lessons from psychiatry. *Neurology.* 2005; **65**: S59–65.

* 40. Dworkin RH, Turk DC, Farrar JT *et al.* Core outcome measures for chronic pain clinical trials: IMMPACT recommendations. *Pain.* 2005; **113**: 9–19.

41. McQuay H. Consensus on outcome measures for chronic pain trials. *Pain.* 2005; **113**: 1–2.

42. McQuay HJ, Moore RA. *An evidence-based resource for pain relief,* 1st edn. Oxford: Oxford University Press, 1998.

43. Farrar JT, Young JP, LaMoreaux L *et al.* Clinical importance of changes in chronic pain intensity measured on an 11-point numerical pain rating scale. *Pain.* 2001; **94**: 149–58.

44. Melzack R. The short-form McGill Pain Questionnaire. *Pain.* 1987; **30**: 191–7.

45. Anonymous. Taking stock of coxibs. *Drugs and Therapeutics Bulletin.* 2005; **43**: 1–6.

* 46. Moher D, Schulz F, Altman G, Lepage L. The CONSORT statement: revised recommendations for improving the quality of reports of parallel-group randomised trials. *Lancet.* 2001; **357**: 1191–4.

47. Tramer MR, Reynolds DJ, Moore RA, McQuay HJ. Impact of covert duplicate publication on meta-analysis: a case study. *British Medical Journal.* 1997; **315**: 635–40.

48. Dyer O. GlaxoSmithKline faces US lawsuit over concealment of trial results. *British Medical Journal.* 2004; **328**: 1395.

49. Mayor S. Drug companies agree to make clinical trial results public. *British Medical Journal.* 2005; **330**: 109.

* 50. De Angelis CD, Drazen JM, Frizelle FA *et al.* Is this clinical trial fully registered? A statement from the International Committee of Medical Journal Editors. *Lancet.* 2005; **365**: 1827–9.

* 51. De Angelis C, Drazen JM, Frizelle FA *et al.* Clinical trial registration: a statement from the International Committee of Medical Journal Editors. *Lancet.* 2004; **364**: 911–12.

46

Techniques of systematic reviews and meta-analysis in pain research

LESLEY A SMITH

KEY LEARNING POINTS

- Systematic reviews may resolve uncertainty where individual studies are inconclusive or disagree.
- Explicit methods limit bias and improve reliability and accuracy of conclusions.
- Meta-analysis increases power to detect differences between interventions and enhances precision of treatment effects.

- There are different statistical models for performing meta-analysis, but no one correct method.
- Sensitivity analyses should be conducted to assess impact of different methods, inclusion criteria and assumptions. Exploration of variability between study results is essential.

INTRODUCTION

What we call scientific knowledge today is a body of statements of varying degrees of certainty. Some of them are most unsure; some of them are nearly sure; but none is absolutely certain.

How you get to know is what I want to know.

Richard Feynman[1]

Healthcare professionals have ever increasing amounts of information to digest merely to keep up with new research findings. Individual trials often give conflicting results, and it can be almost impossible to assimilate and assess all of the available information on a particular topic. Systematic reviews aim to overcome some of the difficulties by bringing together all the available evidence relevant to a particular research question, and provide clear statements about the effects of healthcare interventions and, where possible, how different interventions compare. A systematic review can be defined as a review that has been prepared using a systematic approach to minimize biases, and the approach is recorded in a methods section.[2] The key features of a systematic review are outlined in **Box 46.1**. They differ from traditional literature reviews in which one or more of these key characteristics are absent.[3]

Systematic reviews provide strong evidence to underpin evidence-based policy and practice decisions. With the generation of clinical guidelines and recommendations for healthcare practice increasingly based on systematic reviews, there is a need for healthcare professionals to understand the strengths and weaknesses of such reviews. It is important to appraise a review to understand how the conclusions have been reached, in order to successfully incorporate their findings into the decision-making process.

The aim of this chapter is to introduce the reader to the basic principals of the systematic review process, focusing on reviews to evaluate the effectiveness of an intervention. It provides an overview of the main procedures involved. Each step is illustrated using a worked example and additional sources where more detailed guidance can be found is given. The steps involved in conducting a review include:

- formulating a clear research question;
- searching for all available evidence;
- selection and appraisal of studies;
- summarizing and combining results from relevant studies;
- and interpretation of review findings.

Box 46.1 Key features of a systematic review

- Clearly defined research question.
- Inclusion and exclusion criteria defined a priori.
- Comprehensive and rigorous searches for potentially relevant studies.
- Methods used to appraise and abstract information from individual studies predefined, explicitly reported, and conducted in duplicate to minimize errors.
- Methods used to synthesis data predefined and explicitly reported and variability between studies explored.
- Presentation of raw data rather than just a summary.
- May include a meta-analysis, but not a requirement.

It is easy to underestimate the time and resources required to complete a review. Each stage requires much painstaking work, and a review is likely to take months to complete rather than weeks.

FRAMING THE QUESTION

The first step of a systematic review involves clearly defining the research question. The methods adopted for conducting the review are guided by the questions the review poses. Questions may be broad such as "Are parenteral opioids effective and safe for labor pain?" or more specific such as "Does celecoxib have greater gastrointestinal tolerability than other nonsteroidal anti-inflammatory drugs (NSAID)?"

In formulating the question, it is useful to think about elements of the question in terms of population, intervention(s) or exposure(s), comparison group(s), and outcome(s) (PICO).

- Population – who is the population or patient group that will be studied?
- Intervention or exposure – which dose, route, duration, formulation, one drug or all drugs in a class of drugs?
- Comparison group(s) – which comparison groups, for example other drugs, placebo, waiting list control, no treatment control, sham treatment, or any comparison?
- Outcomes – which outcomes, all or prespecified specific outcomes, quality of life, mortality, etc?

Table 46.1 illustrates PICO for the two examples given above.

Based on choices made for PICO, the reviewer can then decide which study designs are the most appropriate for the review. The gold standard for any review must be one that includes the highest quality evidence available to answer the question. What constitutes good evidence? The best evidence to evaluate treatment effectiveness comes from large, well-designed and executed

Table 46.1 Formulating the review question.

		Celecoxib	Parenteral opioids
1	Which study designs?	Randomized controlled trials	Randomized controlled trials
2	Which participants?	Adults with OA or RA	Women in labor
3	Which intervention(s)?	Celecoxib at licensed therapeutic doses	Parenteral opioids given as mono- or co-therapy
4	Which comparison groups?	NSAID or placebo	Any including: epidural, cervical block, placebo, or another opioid or nonopioid drug
5	Which outcomes?	Pain, mobility, gastrointestinal safety	Pain relief, maternal and neonatal outcomes efficacy, and safety outcomes

randomized controlled trials (RCT). Inadequate randomization procedures, lack of blinding, and exclusion of participants from final analyses may risk overestimation of treatment effects.[4, 5, 6] For example, RCTs where allocation was not concealed adequately from trial investigators led to overestimation of treatment effects by approximately 30 percent.[6] This is further illustrated in a systematic review of transcutaneous electrical nerve stimulation (TENS) for postoperative pain, in which the RCTs overwhelmingly showed no significant difference between TENS and sham TENS for pain relief, whereas the nonrandomized trials showed a significant benefit with TENS.[5] Although there are clinical questions which cannot be answered efficiently by RCTs, for example evaluation of rare adverse events, systematic reviews of nonrandomized studies may generate misleading results. This chapter, therefore, concentrates on systematic reviews of randomized trials.

Once the question has been formulated, it is advisable to develop a protocol outlining the methods to be used to identify, select, appraise, and combine the results of relevant studies. The aim of the protocol is to reduce the number of decisions that may be based on what is found reported in existing studies which could potentially introduce bias.

FINDING THE EVIDENCE

Having framed the review question, it is important to look for all relevant studies. A review can only be considered as systematic when it includes a thorough search of all the available evidence.

The steps involved in generating a list of potentially relevant studies include identification of appropriate search terms, selection of relevant databases, and retrieval of citations from the searches.

A good starting point is to develop a search based on the key concepts that apply to the question using PICO. A list of terms that describes each search concept comprehensively is generated. These should be both free text vocabulary, for example the author's terminology in the title and abstract, and controlled vocabulary such as thesaurus terms. When listing free text terms, think about all synonyms (operation OR surgery), alternate spelling variants (paediatric OR pediatric), abbreviations (nonsteroidal anti-inflammatory drug OR NSAID) and pleural or singular variants (NSAID OR NSAIDS). Do not rely on one term to find all articles on a subject.

Once a comprehensive list of terms has been generated, these can be combined with the Boolean operators AND and OR. Firstly, free text and controlled vocabulary terms for each individual concept can be combined with the OR operator, then two or more concepts are combined with the AND operator. The number of concepts that are combined will determine the number of articles subsequently retrieved. There are two main approaches to constructing an efficient search strategy.

The aim of a highly sensitive search is to identify as many references as possible in order to minimize the possibility of missing potentially relevant studies. With this approach, there is a higher risk of identifying and retrieving studies that do not meet the inclusion criteria, but there is less likelihood of missing studies. A highly sensitive search for studies evaluating acupuncture for treatment of chronic back pain might include terms for the population of interest (chronic back pain) combined with terms for intervention of interest (acupuncture).

In contrast, the aim of a highly precise search is to target the studies more specifically. A precise search for studies would involve combining several concepts such as: population (chronic back pain) AND intervention (acupuncture) AND outcome (quality of life) AND study design (RCT). By requiring citations to have at least one term in each concept, it will generate fewer hits and a greater proportion of them will be relevant. The more concepts that are added, the more precise the search becomes. The risk of this approach is that some studies may be missed, something to consider if there is a paucity of studies in the area being reviewed.

In practice, a balance somewhere between the two is recommended. Examples of search strategies are shown in **Box 46.2**.

There are many electronic databases available for searching, and each has information on the subject area and journals covered on its own website (**Table 46.2**). The choice of which and how many to search depends on the review question and the clinical area – CENTRAL is particularly recommended for searches of RCTs. There is a degree of overlap between databases, but searches across many decreases the likelihood of missing potentially relevant studies.

Inevitably, initial searches will miss potentially relevant studies, and additional strategies must be employed. Studies identified by initial searches should be retrieved and reference lists scanned for articles not originally identified. Also, it is advisable to conduct a citation search, using Science Citation Index for example, to identify articles that have cited identified relevant studies, and which may be subsequent studies. Writing to experts in the field of study and clinical trial registries can also yield otherwise unavailable data. However, it may be difficult to locate and obtain all studies, published and unpublished, therefore, the reviewer must be aware of the influence of potential publication bias on the findings and overall conclusions. It is important to collate all of the studies found from the different sources in one central database and to document all aspects of the search strategy as part of the systematic review.

> ## Box 46.2 Sensitive search strategy for identifying reports of randomized controlled trials in MEDLINE (OVID version)
>
> Celecoxib for osteoarthritis and rheumatoid arthritis
> (cyclooxygenase 2 inhibitors.MeSH OR celecoxib.tw OR celebrex.tw OR SC-58635.tw)
> *and*
> (osteoarthritis.MeSH OR osteoarthritis.tw or osteoarthrosis.tw or osteoarthritic.tw OR "degenerative joint disease".tw OR Arthritis, Rheumatoid.MeSH OR rheumatoid adj arthrit*.tw OR arthritis.tw)
> *and*
> highly sensitive search strategy from Cochrane Handbook 4.2.6 September 2006 appendix 5.b
> (randomized controlled trial [pt] OR controlled clinical trial [pt] OR randomized controlled trials [mh] OR random allocation [mh] OR double-blind method [mh] OR single-blind method [mh] OR clinical trial [pt] OR clinical trials [mh] OR ("clinical trial" [tw]) OR ((singl* [tw] OR doubl* [tw] OR trebl* [tw] OR tripl* [tw]) AND (mask* [tw] OR blind* [tw])) OR (placebos [mh] OR placebo* [tw] OR random* [tw] OR research design [mh:noexp]) NOT (animals [mh] NOT humans [mh])
>
> MeSH and mh denote Medical subject heading field, tw denotes text word.
> *denotes wildcard.

APPRAISING THE EVIDENCE

Assessing for eligibility

The aim of eligibility assessment is to avoid bias in the study selection process. Eligibility criteria are based on which studies definitely answer the question(s) posed by the review, and should be determined at the protocol stage. Potentially relevant citations are selected from the searches, and articles obtained, these are then screened for eligibility in duplicate by two independent assessors. The choice of whether to assess the reports blind or open is down to the resources available as it is very time-consuming. Blind assessment (not knowing the author, journal, year of publication, etc.) has not been demonstrated to be worth the effort, but may be advisable for controversial reviews.

Assessing for likelihood of bias

Quality assessment plays an important role in interpretation of the study findings, and helps determine the strength of evidence on which to base recommendations for practice. The principle of quality assessment is to assess each study for the likelihood of bias using an explicit and standardized procedure. The elements assessed will depend on generic factors related to the study design, and specific factors related to the review topic. Components important to assess are susceptibility to selection bias and confounding, measurement bias, and attrition bias. For example, in the systematic review of effectiveness and tolerability of celecoxib we assessed the following potential sources of bias:

- method of generation of the random allocation;
- concealment of allocation at randomization;
- blinding of trial participants and investigators;
- completeness of treatment and follow-up;
- methods used to compensate for missing outcome data.

Further details of how these were appraised are given in **Box 46.3**.

Numerous checklists and quality assessment scales have been developed, many of which assign an overall score to each study in order to differentiate between studies of variable quality. One such scale commonly used is the Jadad scale.[7] However, assignment of a quality score is problematic, and no longer recommended due to the assessment and subsequent score being highly dependent on the scale used, with discordant results produced by different scales.[8] As with eligibility assessment, it is important for the quality assessment to be conducted independently in duplicate with discrepancies resolved through discussion or consultation with another reviewer.

Incorporating the outcome of quality assessment in the systematic review makes intuitive sense. One approach is to exclude studies unless they meet a predetermined quality threshold, for example only double-blind studies included. Alternatively, a more inclusive approach may be preferable where studies are included regardless of blinding status, and the impact of the presence or absence of adequate blinding on the overall review findings is assessed through sensitivity analyses. The latter approach avoids excluding potentially informative data. Regardless, the possible influence of variable quality on study findings should always be investigated. A systematic review of the effectiveness of acupuncture compared with placebo acupuncture for relief of back and neck pain was conducted by Ernst and White.[9] Nine RCTs comparing acupuncture with a control group were pooled in a meta-analysis and showed that there was 39 percent increased risk of pain reduction with acupuncture compared with control RR 1.39 (95 percent CI: 1.16, 1.67). The authors concluded that acupuncture was effective and failed to investigate the potential impact of bias on the results. Pooling of the four RCTs considered to be of higher quality, i.e. less likely to be biased due to blinding of outcome assessment, produces a smaller benefit which is not statistically significant 1.17 (95 percent CI: 0.91, 1.51),

Table 46.2 Electronic bibliographic databases.

Database	Available from	Details
MEDLINE	Freely available via PubMed at www.ncbi.nlm.gov/PubMed	The major bibliographic database for biomedical literature, US focus
EMBASE	www.embase.com	Pharmacology and biomedicine, European focus
CENTRAL (Cochrane Central Register Controlled Trials)	Freely available for many users via: www3.interscience.wiley.com/cgi-bin/mrwhome/106568753/HOME	Clinical trials from bibliographic databases (notably MEDLINE and EMBASE), and other published and unpublished sources
CINAHL (Cumulative Index to Nursing and Allied Health Literature)	www.cinahl.com/prodsvcs/prodsvcs.htm	Literature on all aspects of nursing and allied health disciplines
PsycINFO	www.apa.org/psycinfo/	World's serial literature on psychology and related disciplines
AMED (Allied and Complementary Medicine)	www.bl.uk/collections/health/amed.html	Literature covering complementary medicine, occupational therapy, physiotherapy, occupational therapy, speech and language therapy, and palliative care
LILACS (Latin American and Caribbean Health Sciences Literature)	http://bases.bireme.br/cgi-bin/wxislind.exe/iah/online/?IsisScript=iah/iah.xis&base=LILACS&lang=i	Covers literature related to the health sciences published in Latin America and the Caribbean, and is published by WHO Regional Offices. Contains articles and documents such as: theses, books, conference proceedings, scientific reports, and governmental publications
ASSIA (Applied Social Science Index and Abstracts)	www.csa.com/factsheets/assia-set-c.php	Database covering health, social services, psychology, sociology, economics, politics, race relations, and education
SIGLE (System for Information on Grey Literature)	http://stneasy.fiz-karlsruhe.de	European nonconventional literature covering pure and applied natural sciences, for example, dissertations, conference proceedings, and reports
Science Citation Index	http://scientific.thomson.com/products/sci/	May be used to identify other relevant citations on a related topic by identifying records citing a relevant author or authors
National Research Register	www.nrr.nhs.uk/	
MetaRegister of Current Controlled Trials	http://controlled-trials.com	
US National Cancer Institute register of ongoing RCTs:	www.cancer.gov/clinicaltrials	
Information on other research registers from:	www.york.ac.uk/inst/crd/htadbase.htm#3	

however, for the five lower quality studies which were not blind, the pooled RR was higher 1.70 (1.30, 2.22) and statistically significant. This indicates that a pooled average effect, without taking quality into account, may be misleading and overestimate the true effect. The studies were variable in terms of acupuncture regimens, outcome assessment, and control group and perhaps more importantly the likelihood of bias was high in the majority of the studies precluding performing a meta-analysis on these studies.[10] Juni and colleagues[8] provide a useful outline of the pros and cons of the various ways of incorporating study quality into meta-analysis.

Data extraction

Data extraction involves recording relevant information from each study. Decisions about what information to extract should be decided before extraction, ideally at the protocol stage, and usually includes details such as

Box 46.3 Quality assessment components

The method of generation of treatment allocation rated as:

- Adequate if sequences were unpredictable. Acceptable methods are: computer generated random numbers, table of random numbers, coin toss, card shuffle, throwing dice, drawing lots or envelopes, or any other method guaranteeing the principle of unpredictable group assignment.
- Inadequate if sequences were predictable. Inadequate methods are use of patient numbers, birth date, alternate allocation, or some other systematic method.
- Unclear if insufficient information given.

Concealment of allocation at randomization rated as:

- Adequate if trial investigators were unaware of treatment allocation of each participant before they entered the trial. Acceptable methods are: list kept at a central office or pharmacy, serially numbered opaque envelopes, identical treatments in serially numbered pots, or any other method that guarantees concealment.
- Inadequate if the next assignment can be predicted. Inadequate methods are: open allocation schedule, nontamperproof envelopes, and all procedures based on inadequate generation of allocation sequences.
- Unclear if insufficient information given.

The blinding of trial participants and investigators and how it was achieved. The success of the blinding procedure also assessed if reported in the original studies.

To assess completeness of follow-up, the following information is assessed.

- Information on the type of analysis conducted: intention-to-treat or observed case analysis.
- Whether participants were analyzed in the groups to which they were randomized.
- The proportion of people who were excluded from the analysis in each treatment group with reasons why.
- The proportion of withdrawals and drop-outs in each treatment group with reasons why.
- Methods used to compensate for missing data.

study design, population, intervention or exposure, comparison group(s), outcome measures, and results. Ideally, data extraction should be performed independently by at least two reviewers to improve reliability. As with eligibility and quality assessment, disagreements should be resolved by consensus or arbitration. Where agreement cannot be reached, the potential influence of any uncertainty should be investigated through sensitivity analysis. It is common for more than one publication of the same data to occur. These may be in the form of serial publications where each represents different outcomes or lengths of follow-up, or may actually report duplicate data. Studies reporting positive results are more likely to be reported in duplicate; therefore, care should be taken to avoid inclusion of duplicate data. For example, in a review of an antiemetic agent, Tramer and colleagues[11] found 17 percent of the RCTs were published more than once. It is advisable and can be fruitful to contact authors of the original study reports to obtain additional information if it has not been reported fully in the article.

SUMMARIZING THE EVIDENCE

The aim of data synthesis is to gather and summarize the results of the included studies in order to provide an estimate of average effectiveness, investigate if the effect varies between studies, and investigate possible sources of the differences.

This may be achieved through a narrative synthesis with or without the addition of formal statistical techniques (meta-analysis). There are situations where it may be inadvisable to combine studies in a meta-analysis, particularly if disparate methodologies, populations, interventions, or outcomes have been used, as with the acupuncture review.[10] Or it may simply be impossible if insufficient data are reported.[12] A meta-analysis is by no means essential in order to make a review "systematic." Although a quantitative synthesis has the advantage of producing an overall estimate of the treatment effect, a clear and comprehensive summary of the studies relevant to a particular question is also of value. Presentation of study characteristics and results in a summary table in a clear consistent format will aid interpretation and facilitate reaching clear and constructive conclusions.[10, 12]

In a meta-analysis, data from similar studies are pooled to estimate a weighted average effect in which more weight is given to studies contributing more information (larger sample sizes and more precise estimates of treatment effects) than studies contributing less information. It is important to note that studies are not pooled as if data came from one large study, but involves a two-step process where the between group difference is calculated for each study first, then these are pooled to estimate the average effect.

A criticism sometimes levelled at systematic reviews is that lumping together information from different trials gives unreliable results. It is legitimate to combine information as long as thoughtful consideration is given to the choice of which studies to pool. For example, for the review of celecoxib for treatment of osteoarthritis (OA) and rheumatoid arthritis (RA), separate meta-analyses were undertaken for each comparison and outcome. Studies comparing celecoxib with placebo were pooled separately from comparisons with another active agent (NSAIDs). Additionally, studies on participants with OA that evaluated pain using the Western Ontario and MacMaster universities (WOMAC) index were pooled separately from studies on participants with RA that evaluated pain using the American College of Rheumatology (ACR-20) responder index.[13]

If factors vary across trials, then it may be more appropriate to carry out subgroup analyses, for example of different drug doses or different patient groups, or to consider a qualitative review. For example, a review of epidural corticosteroids for sciatica[14] carried out subgroup analyses based on the time at which pain relief was measured: short-term (1–60 days following epidural) and long-term (12–52 weeks) pain relief.

The choice of which summary statistic to use is dependent on the type of data to be analyzed, and the expected and observed variation in results between studies. The types of data most frequently encountered for systematic reviews are as follows:

- Binary or dichotomous where a participant may be in one of two states such as in pain or pain-free. Binary data are summarized using either relative measures of effect: risk ratios (RR) or odds ratios (OR) which describes the effect in one group relative to another group, or absolute measures of effect: risk differences (RD) which describes the difference in event rate between the intervention and control groups. The number needed to treat (NNT) describes the number of people that must receive a treatment in order to prevent one extra person having the outcome that would have had they received placebo. It is calculated from the RD and though often used to summarize results from individual RCTs, it cannot be combined in a meta-analysis.
- Continuous data such as blood pressure or measurement using an assessment scale which is usually summarized using means. Comparison between mean values in an intervention and a control group generates a difference in means (MD). A standardized mean difference (SMD) may be calculated if studies have evaluated an outcome using different scales such as pain measured using different measurement scales. This is a standardized value with-out any units, and is often referred to as an effect size.
- Time-to-event data which give the time to the occurrence of an event such as death, and are usually summarized as a hazard ratio (HR). The HR describes the reduction in risk on treatment compared with control over the entire follow-up period.

- Other outcome data that may be encountered include counts which are events that can happen to a person more than once, such as the number of migraine episodes that occur a month. These may be analyzed as continuous data when the frequency of the event is common, or when the outcome is rare, analyzed as rates. A rate describes the frequency of the event in a stated period of time in all participants in a treatment group, for example eight migraine episodes occurred in 120 person-years of follow-up, and therefore, the rate is 0.067 per person-year. The rate ratio compares the rate in one group divided by the other group.
- Pain may be assessed using short ordinal measurement scales which categorize pain such as none, mild, moderate, or severe. A score may be assigned to the categories and longer scales treated as continuous data. Sometimes these scales are dichotomized and then treated as binary data. For example, in RCTs evaluating treatments for migraine, headache relief is defined as headache pain reduced from moderate or severe to mild or none according to a four-point categorical scale.[15]

See the Cochrane Handbook Section 8.6.1 (freely downloadable from www.cochrane.org/resources/handbook/index.htm) for a thorough discussion of choice of summary statistics and methods of meta-analysis.[16]

Random versus fixed effects

Statistical methods of combining results utilize a fixed effects or random effects model. The fixed effect model assumes that each study is estimating the same underlying treatment effect, i.e. it is fixed across studies. The assumption is there is no statistical heterogeneity, and that any differences between study results are only due to chance. Studies pooled using a fixed effects model calculate the variance of the pooled effect based on the inverse of the sum of the weights of each study. The assumption of the random effects model is that each study is estimating a different effect, but one which follows a distribution, such as a normal distribution. Thus variation between study effects is random. The random effects model adds variance to the pooled effect in proportion to the variability of the results of the individual studies, generating wider confidence intervals around the pooled effect than for the fixed effect model. For this reason it produces a more conservative estimate of effect.

Heterogeneity

Heterogeneity between studies may arise due to differences in methodology and differences in clinical characteristics which can be minimized by making careful pooling decisions. Statistical heterogeneity refers to differences between study effects greater than would be expected due to chance. Statistical testing for heterogeneity should be performed routinely, but commonly used statistical tests lack power so that while a positive test for heterogeneity suggests that trials were not similar, a negative test does not provide complete reassurance that there is no heterogeneity.[17] For this reason, a p-value higher than the usual value of 0.05 is recommended ($p<0.1$). More recently, a test that quantifies the amount of heterogeneity present is recommended: I^2. This value describes the proportion of variability across studies due to true differences rather than random error.[18]

Investigating heterogeneity

If heterogeneity is detected, meta-analysis may not be advisable, particularly if heterogeneity is excessive ($I^2 > 75$ percent). If a meta-analysis is conducted, a random effects model may be used instead of a fixed effects model to account for the heterogeneity, but it is not a substitute for investigation of possible sources. Ideally, exploratory analyses should be preplanned, limited to as few as possible and based on sound scientific and empirical considerations.

One such exploratory analysis is sensitivity analysis, which evaluates how robust the findings of the meta analysis are to decisions made about pooling studies. For example, findings and interpretation of the efficacy and tolerability of celecoxib did not change when the unpublished studies were removed from the main analysis.[13] The overall findings are strengthened if results are similar, whether or not questionable studies are included.

Another type of exploratory analysis is subgroup analysis. Subgroups may be generated by either grouping subsets of participants; for example, the benefit of celecoxib in participants not taking aspirin seemed greater (73 percent reduction in ulcer incidence, 52 to 84 percent), than in participants taking aspirin (51 percent reduction, 14 to 72 percent) (**Figure 46.1**).[13] Alternatively, by grouping subsets of studies whereby different studies would be in each subgroup as shown with the previous example for epidural corticosteroids for sciatica.[14]

Lastly, meta-regression is a technique to investigate potential differences in effect according to a particular characteristic or to investigate heterogeneity. Its use is limited by the requirement for at least ten studies to make meaningful investigations, frequently unavailable in any single meta-analysis. Nonetheless, it sometimes yields interesting findings. A meta-regression analysis by Derry and Loke[19] showed no significant relationship between risk of gastrointestinal hemorrhage and daily aspirin dose. The relative reduction in the incidence of gastrointestinal hemorrhage was 1.5 percent per 100 mg reduction of dose, but this was not significant ($p = 0.3$).[19]

In practice, many of these exploratory analyses have many pitfalls, and cautious interpretation of their findings is advised as they may generate spurious relationships. They may, however, generate useful hypotheses.

	Celecoxib	NSAID
No prophylactic aspirin use		
Study 071(D)	11/129	28/274
Study 071(I)	12/129	66/235
Zhao 1999(N)	14/260	29/116
Simon 1999(N)	20/383	36/128
Study 062(N)	11/182	75/186

RR = 0.27 (0.16 to 0.48)
Heterogeneity: Q=17.79, p=0.001

Prophylactic aspirin use		
Study 071(D)	1/18	8/32
Study 071(I)	1/18	12/41
Zhao 1999(N)	6/45	5/30
Simon 1999(N)	3/40	0/9
Study 062(N)	7/29	12/28

RR = 0.49 (0.28 to 0.86)
Heterogeneity: Q=3.12, p=0.54

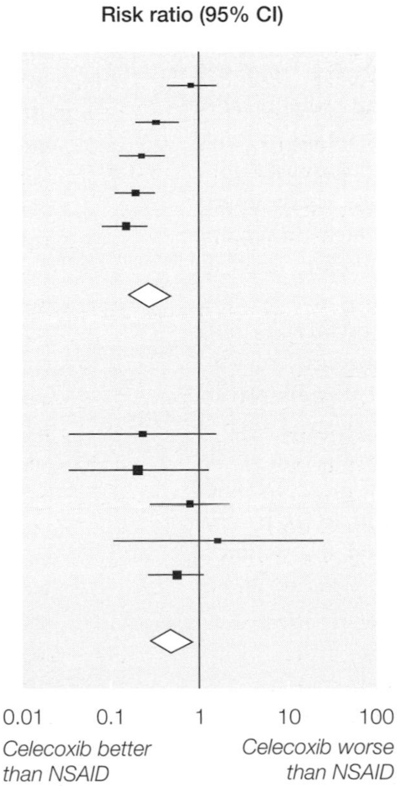

Figure 46.1 Forest plot showing impact of prophylactic aspirin on incidence of ulcers in randomized trials of celecoxib versus NSAIDs. D, diclofenac 75 mg twice daily; I, ibuprofen 800 mg thrice daily; N, naproxen 500 mg twice daily.

Publication bias

Publication bias occurs when the chance of publication of a study is related to the significance of its results: a study is more likely to be published if it shows significant effects. Evidence for this comes from a meta-analysis of four groups of research projects approved by ethics committees or institutional review boards in the USA, UK, and Australia which found that the odds of publication was 2.4 times greater if the results were statistically significant.[20]

Additionally, studies are more likely to be published sooner,[21] in English language journals,[22] be cited more frequently,[23, 24] and published in multiple publications[11] if they demonstrate significant effects. More recently, outcome reporting bias has also been identified as an additional source of publication bias.[25, 26, 27] A retrospective review of publications of RCTs identified the odds of reporting a significant outcome was approximately twice that of nonstatistically significant outcomes.[27]

All of the above biases are more likely to affect small studies rather than large. Larger studies require a greater investment of time and money and are therefore more likely to be published even when results are not significant. A commonly used method for exploring publication bias is the "funnel plot." A funnel plot is a scatter plot of individual study effects plotted according to the precision of the estimate. In the absence of bias, studies will be evenly scattered forming a symmetrical inverted funnel shape. Smaller studies with less precise estimates appear more widely scattered at the bottom, and larger studies with more precise estimates appear towards the top. If small studies remain unpublished because they fail to show significant effects, an asymmetrical plot will result. Asymmetrical plots may also be due to clinical or methodological heterogeneity. Inferences are also limited by having sufficient studies to create a meaningful plot. Formal statistical tests are available to test if asymmetry is likely to be due to chance, but they lack power and often give inconsistent results and therefore are not recommended.

Publication bias and poor reporting quality are both serious threats to the validity of systematic reviews. Reviewers should make every effort to identify all relevant studies, published or unpublished. Trial registries such as those shown in **Table 46.2** will aid identification in the future. Adherence to recommendations of the CONSORT statement for improving the reporting of RCTs by trial authors should improve the assessment and abstraction of reliable data from relevant studies by interested reviewers.

CONCLUSION

In summary, this chapter aims to provide a framework for carrying out a review, taking into account the most important methodological issues. A good review pays careful attention to susceptibility to bias, reports on outcomes which are meaningful to healthcare professionals, consumers, and researchers, and expresses results in a clear and useful way.

ACKNOWLEDGMENTS

Henry McQuay, Andrew Moore, Eija Kalso, Geoff Gourlay, and Anna Oldman provided many useful suggestions and ideas in writing the first edition of this chapter.

REFERENCES

1. Feynman RP. *The meaning of it all*. London: Penguin Books, 1999: 27.
2. Chalmers I, Altman D (eds). *Systematic reviews*. London: BMJ Publishing Group, 1994.
3. Mulrow CD. The medical review article: state of the science. *Annals of Internal Medicine*. 1987; **106**: 485–8.
* 4. Schulz KF, Chalmers I, Hayes RJ, Altman DG. Empirical evidence of bias: dimensions of methodological quality associated with estimates of treatment effects in controlled trials. *Journal of the American Medical Association*. 1995; **273**: 408–12.
* 5. Carroll D, Tramer M, McQuay H *et al.* Randomization is important in studies with pain outcomes: systematic review of transcutaneous electrical nerve stimulation in acute postoperative pain. *British Journal of Anaesthesia*. 1996; **77**: 798–803.
* 6. Juni P, Altman DG, Egger M. Systematic reviews in health care: Assessing the quality of controlled clinical trials. *British Medical Journal*. 2001; **323**: 42–6.
* 7. Jadad AR, Moore RA, Carroll D *et al.* Assessing the quality of reports of randomized clinical trials: is blinding necessary? *Controlled Clinical Trials*. 1996; **17**: 1–12.
* 8. Juni P, Witschi A, Bloch R, Egger M. The hazards of scoring the quality of clinical trials for meta-analysis. *Journal of the American Medical Association*. 1999; **282**: 1054–60.
9. Ernst E, White AR. Acupuncture for back pain: a meta-analysis of randomized controlled trials. *Archives of Internal Medicine*. 1998; **158**: 2235–41.
10. Smith LA, Oldman AD, McQuay HJ, Moore RA. Teasing apart quality and validity in systematic reviews: an example from acupuncture trials in chronic neck and back pain. *Pain*. 2000; **86**: 119–32.
11. Tramer MR, Reynolds DJ, Moore RA, McQuay HJ. Impact of covert duplicate publication on meta-analysis: a case study. *British Medical Journal*. 1997; **315**: 635–40.
12. Bricker L, Lavender T. Parenteral opioids for labor pain relief: a systematic review. *American Journal of Obstetrics and Gynecology*. 2002; **186**: S94–109.

13. Deeks JJ, Smith LA, Bradley MD. Efficacy, tolerability, and upper gastrointestinal safety of celecoxib for treatment of osteoarthritis and rheumatoid arthritis: systematic review of randomised controlled trials. *British Medical Journal.* 2002; **325**: 619.

14. Watts RW, Silagy CA. A meta-analysis on the efficacy of epidural corticosteroids in the treatment of sciatica. *Anaesthesia and Intensive Care.* 1995; **23**: 564–9.

15. Oldman AD, Smith LA, McQuay HJ, Moore RA. Pharmacological treatments for acute migraine: quantitative systematic review. *Pain.* 2002; **97**: 247–57.

∗ 16. Higgins JPT, Green S (eds). *Cochrane handbook for systematic reviews of interventions 4.2.5*, 2005 [updated May 2005] Available from: http://www.cochrane.org/resources/handbook/hbook.htm.

17. Gavaghan DJ, Moore RA, McQuay HJ. An evaluation of homogeneity tests in meta-analyses in pain using simulations of individual patient data. *Pain.* 2000; **85**: 415–24.

∗ 18. Higgins JP, Thompson SG, Deeks JJ, Altman DG. Measuring inconsistency in meta-analyses. *British Medical Journal.* 2003; **327**: 557–60.

19. Derry S, Loke YK. Risk of gastrointestinal haemorrhage with long term use of aspirin: meta-analysis. *British Medical Journal.* 2000; **321**: 1183–7.

∗ 20. Dickersin K. How important is publication bias? A synthesis of available data. *AIDS Education and Prevention.* 1997; **9**: 15–21.

21. Ioannidis JP. Effect of the statistical significance of results on the time to completion and publication of randomized efficacy trials. *Journal of the American Medical Association.* 1998; **279**: 281–6.

22. Egger M, Zellweger-Zahner T, Schneider M *et al.* Language bias in randomised controlled trials published in English and German. *Lancet.* 1997; **350**: 326–9.

23. Gotzsche PC. Reference bias in reports of drug trials. *British Medical Journal (Clinical Research ed.).* 1987; **295**: 654–6.

24. Ravnskov U. Cholesterol lowering trials in coronary heart disease: frequency of citation and outcome. *British Medical Journal.* 1992; **305**: 15–19.

∗ 25. Chan AW, Hrobjartsson A, Haahr MT *et al.* Empirical evidence for selective reporting of outcomes in randomized trials: comparison of protocols to published articles. *Journal of the American Medical Association.* 2004; **291**: 2457–65.

26. Chan AW, Krleza-Jeric K, Schmid I, Altman DG. Outcome reporting bias in randomized trials funded by the Canadian Institutes of Health Research. *Canadian Medical Association Journal.* 2004; **171**: 735–40.

27. Chan AW, Altman DG. Identifying outcome reporting bias in randomised trials on PubMed: review of publications and survey of authors. *British Medical Journal.* 2005; **330**: 753.

PART IV

ORGANIZATION OF MULTIDISCIPLINARY PAIN MANAGEMENT TEAMS

47

Organization and role of acute pain services

DAVID COUNSELL, PAMELA E MACINTYRE, AND HARALD BREIVIK

KEY LEARNING POINTS

- Postoperative and other acute pain continue to be poorly managed, causing unnecessary suffering and increasing risk of complications after surgery and injury.
- The institution of acute pain services (APS) leads to improved pain relief and reduces treatment-related side effects.
- There are many models of APS; the superiority of one over another has not been shown and local circumstances may determine which will function best.
- Staff education, a key role of an APS, is a prerequisite for better pain assessment, improved prescribing practices, and better acute pain relief.

- Improved acute pain management results more from the APS educational activities and appropriate organizational delivery of pain relief than from the techniques themselves.
- When attention is given to education, patient assessment, documentation, and provision of appropriate guidelines and policies, even basic "low-tech" techniques of pain relief are more effective.
- Close liaison with all personnel involved in the care of the patient is required for successful management of acute pain. This goal is reached by an ongoing educational program delivered by a well-staffed and well-trained APS.

INTRODUCTION

Objectives in acute pain management can be summarized in four broad categories. These may help to determine the requirements for analgesic management in terms of the technique and service structure required for delivery of effective acute pain relief.

Humanitarian

The need to prevent or reduce unnecessary pain and suffering is clearly important.[1, 2, 3] It would seem an obvious intention, but the evidence from *Pain after surgery*[4] suggests that before this report the prevailing attitude was that pain, often severe pain, was to be expected after surgery and that medical and nursing staff were ill-equipped to deal with it.

Avoidance of the pathophysiological consequences of untreated severe pain

It is now realized that pain may have significant adverse physiological and psychological effects and that many of the well-recognized complications of surgery are precipitated or aggravated by poorly treated acute pain.[5]

In high risk patients, i.e. those having major thoracic or abdominal surgery or with significant medical comorbidities, the need for effective analgesia becomes paramount in attempts to reduce perioperative morbidity. Especially important is the ability to achieve "dynamic analgesia," i.e. to reduce pain provoked by movement, e.g. with coughing and deep breathing early in the postoperative period.

Reducing the risk of chronic pain

Some common operations may lead to chronic pain syndromes.[6, 7, 8] Increased understanding of nociception and pain impulse processing in the central nervous system has raised hopes that better acute pain management may lead to a reduction in the incidence of severe chronic postoperative pain.[9, 10] For more information on the prevalence of chronic pain after surgery and evidence for its prevention see Chapter 31, Preventing chronic pain after surgery, in the *Acute Pain* volume of this series, and Chapter 30, Chronic pain after surgery, in the *Chronic Pain* volume of this series.

Preservation of vital organ functions and fast-track recovery

This is of particular importance in accelerated recovery (fast-track surgery) programs where early mobilization and nutrition are primary objectives that cannot be achieved unless acute pain is well managed.[11, 12, 13, 14, 15]

It could be argued that all these objectives are universal in pain management and indeed that is so. What perhaps distinguishes acute pain management from chronic pain management is the urgency with which effective analgesia is required, particularly if patients are at risk of pain-related adverse events.

The World Health Organization (WHO) analgesic ladder is a well-known tool for managing pain relief that is often applied inappropriately in the acute pain setting with simple analgesics being prescribed as first line resulting in undertreatment of pain. That said, the ladder is useful in the treatment of acute pain, providing one realizes the need to descend rather than ascend the ladder beginning with strong opioids or invasive analgesic techniques and reducing to simple analgesics as the acute response to injury subsides.

Increasing recognition of inadequate acute pain management

Despite these objectives, studies over the last few decades have consistently shown that acute pain management is often still suboptimal, with up to two-thirds of surgical and medical patients experiencing moderate to severe pain during their hospital stay.[16, 17, 18, 19, 20, 21, 22]

The consequences have been increasing use of more sophisticated methods of pain relief in general hospital wards and in ambulatory settings, the development of acute pain services (APS), and guidelines and reports relevant to acute pain management. Some of these guidelines and reports are listed below.

- The Royal College of Surgeons and College of Anaesthetists: *Working party report on pain after surgery*, 1990.[4]
- Faculty of Anaesthetists and Royal Australasian College of Surgeons: *Statement on acute pain management*, 1991.[23]
- International Association for the Study of Pain (IASP) *Task Force on Acute Pain: Management of acute pain: a practical guide*, 1992.[24]
- US Department of Health and Human Services, Agency for Health Care Policy and Research (AHCPR), Clinical Practice Guideline. *Acute pain management: operative or medical procedures and trauma*, 1992.[25]
- American Society of Anesthesiologists (ASA): *Practice guidelines for acute pain management in the perioperative setting*, 1995.[26]
- College of Paediatrics and Child Health Working Party Report: *Prevention and control of pain in children*, 1997.[27]
- Association of Anaesthetists of Great Britain and Ireland: *The anaesthesia team*, 1998.[28]
- UK Audit Commission Report: *Anaesthesia under examination*, 1998.[29]
- Europain: *Minimum standards for the management of postoperative pain*, 1998.[30]
- National Health and Medical Research Council (Australia) Working Party Report: *Acute pain management: scientific evidence*, 1999.[31]
- Veterans Health Administration and Department of Defense in the USA: *Clinical practice guidelines for the management of postoperative pain*.[32] An updated copy of these guidelines can be found at www.oqp.med.va.gov/cpg/PAIN/PAIN_GOL.htm
- Joint publication by several UK professional bodies: *Good practice in the management of continuous epidural analgesia in the hospital setting*, 2004.[33]
- American Society of Anesthesiologists (ASA): *Practice guidelines for acute pain management in the perioperative setting: an updated report by the American Society of Anesthesiologists Task Force on Acute Pain Management*.[34]
- Australian and New Zealand College of Anaesthetists and Faculty of Pain Medicine: *Acute pain management: scientific evidence*, 2nd edn, 2005.[35]
- Australian and New Zealand College of Anaesthetists and Faculty of Pain Medicine: *Guidelines on acute pain management*, 2007.[36]
- British Pain Society publication: *Pain and substance misuse: improving the patient experience*, 2007.[37]
- PROSPECT: *Procedure-specific postoperative pain management*.[38]

The report of the Royal College of Surgeons and College of Anaesthetists[4] stated that an APS "should be introduced in all major hospitals performing surgery in the UK" and later recommendations from the Faculty of Anaesthetists,[23] AHCPR,[25] and American Society of Anesthesiologists[26] agreed that all major acute care centers should have an APS.

In part as a result of the earlier reports and guidelines, as well as increasing awareness of the need to treat acute pain and the potential benefits of providing good-quality analgesia, the proportion of hospitals with APS has risen, as has recognition of the need for an APS. Although the model of APS may vary (see below under Organization of acute pain services), in the UK[39] and Canada[40] around 90 percent of hospitals now have an APS. However, the definition of what constitutes an APS can vary from institution to institution. In a postal survey of APS in hospitals in the UK (81 percent response rate), 86 percent provided a weekday service with a reduced service at other times; only 5 percent provided 24-hour service, seven days a week.[41]

THE DEVELOPMENT AND GROWTH OF ACUTE PAIN SERVICES

Advanced pain relief techniques, such as patient-controlled analgesia (PCA) and epidural analgesia, had been used for the management of acute pain for some years before the advent of APS. However, their use in a general ward setting did not become widespread until after APS had been established.

While the idea for an anesthesiologist-led analgesia team to supervise acute pain relief and take responsibility for education, was mooted as early as 1976,[42] the development of these teams did not start until a decade later. The landmark publication by Ready et al. in 1988,[43] which described the beginning of their APS in the USA and the first 18 months' experience, heralded the start of the rapid development and growth of organized APS. Starting within a short time after this and then increasing rapidly over the next 20 years, other countries including Australia,[44, 45] the UK,[46, 47, 48] New Zealand,[49] Germany,[50, 51] Canada,[52] Ireland,[53] Spain,[54] Israel,[55, 56] Belgium,[57, 58] Italy,[59] Norway and Switzerland,[60] Sweden,[61] Denmark,[62] Poland,[63] Saudi Arabia,[64] Hong Kong,[65, 66] Malaysia,[67, 68] Singapore,[69, 70] and Thailand[71] followed suit.

The changing role of the acute pain service

The APS started by Ready et al.[43] over 20 years ago aimed primarily to manage acute postoperative pain using one of the more "high-tech" methods of pain relief, such as PCA and epidural analgesia. Changes over time have seen APS play a major role in also improving the effectiveness of more conventional "low-tech" methods of pain relief, so that more patients in a hospital will benefit.[72, 73]

The concept of the APS, as a postoperative pain management service, has also changed over that period, both in the way that these services are run and in the range of services they provide.

In the early days, the focus followed the excellent recommendations in *Pain after surgery*[4] summarized below:

- responsibility for the day-to-day management of acute pain after surgery;
- organization of services so that the level of care and monitoring is appropriate for both the clinical condition of the patient and the technique involved;
- provision of in-service training for medical and nursing staff involved in the management of postoperative pain;
- establishment of programs for the diagnosis and management of the complications and hazards of particular forms of treatment;
- audit of the beneficial and detrimental outcomes of existing methods of treatment and evaluation of new techniques;
- clinical research into the relief of acute pain.

In recent years, APS have found themselves being called upon to provide assistance in other areas of the hospital where pain management is problematic, away from the primary remit of managing postoperative pain. In many hospitals, input from APS has facilitated improvements in pain management for daycase surgery,[74, 75] in emergency medicine departments,[76, 77, 78] and pediatric wards,[79, 80, 81] and also pioneered techniques to manage procedural pain in many situations.[82, 83, 84, 85, 86, 87] In addition to these roles, APS have come under increasing pressure to assume a role in improving pain management on medical wards, where poor pain relief remains a major concern.[17, 88]

Other developments in the understanding of pain have demonstrated that acute pain and chronic pain are not separate entities, but part of a pain continuum, and that neuropathic pain is often a factor in the acute pain setting. This requires APS teams to recognize and implement early treatment using drugs and techniques more traditionally associated with chronic pain therapies.[7, 89]

Acute pain services are also called upon to deal with increasingly more complex pain management issues, such as acute on chronic pain, acute pain after spinal cord injury, and other major trauma, and acute medical pain (e.g. acute herpes zoster, sickle cell crisis, pain associated with HIV/AIDS, cardiac pain) and increasingly more complex patient groups (e.g. opioid-tolerant patients, patients with a substance abuse disorder, the elderly, and patients with obstructive sleep apnea).[35, 72] In view of the wider demands on modern APS, and the increased knowledge required by individuals previously seen as acute pain practitioners, it might be that the term "inpatient pain service" is now a more appropriate title than acute pain service.

Finally, members of some APS teams are becoming more involved in perioperative medicine[15] and outreach critical care services,[90, 91] as well as accelerated postoperative recovery programs following major surgery. These fast-track programs rely heavily upon the provision of effective analgesia and present new challenges in providing pain relief that facilitates early mobilization and early oral intake.[11, 15, 92]

Models of APS organization

There has been some debate as to the best form of APS and there is, as yet, no consensus about the best model or even agreed definitions of what might constitute an APS. Therefore, the structure of APS varies widely, depending on local patients' profiles, local traditions, and responsibilities for care of surgical and medical patients. For the purposes of training in multidisciplinary pain medicine, the Faculty of Pain Medicine in Australia states that an APS must have at least one specialist anesthesiologist session (a session is a half day) and one nursing session allocated each weekday, as well as 24-hour availability of a specialist anesthesiologist for consultation.[93] For training in anesthesia, both the Royal College of Anaesthetists in the UK and the Australian and New Zealand College of Anaesthetists require all institutions with anesthesia trainees to have an APS. Similar requirements exist in Norway and the other Nordic countries. In Australia, 91 percent of training hospitals have an APS run by the Department of Anaesthesia, with daily input from medical staff (Australian and New Zealand College of Anaesthetists, personal communication). A recent survey of training hospitals in the in the UK showed that while 90 percent of hospitals reported having an APS, dedicated medical staff sessions did not exist in 37 percent, were limited to one to two sessions per week in 49 percent, and in only 4 percent were there five or more sessions.[39]

Currently, APS structures vary from nurse-based/ anesthesiologist-led, without daily participation by an anesthesiologist[55, 73] to anesthesiologist-based/nurse-supported – anesthesiology leadership being common because the knowledge required and techniques used are similar to those used in anesthesia.[43, 44, 49] All rely on APS nurses and, regardless of the model chosen, an organized team approach is essential.

The nurse-based, anesthesiologist-supervised model described by Rawal[73] seeks to involve all nurses in the provision of better analgesia, regardless of technique used. It proposes that improved education and regular monitoring of pain and pain relief ("making pain visible") will lead to better analgesia for all patients. The anesthesiologist-led model of Ready et al.[43] has been criticized as

being costly because only a small proportion of patients receive its benefits.[94] That is, it forgets the many patients whose pain will be treated using one of the more conventional analgesic regimens (e.g. intermittent intramuscular or oral opioids), prescribed by junior medical staff. However, this need not and should not be the case (see below under Selection of analgesic regimens).

Werner et al.[95] performed a systematic review of articles relating to APS. Of the 73 articles they reviewed which discussed organizational aspects, the APS was physician-based (usually anesthesiologist) in 56 (77 percent) and 17 (23 percent) were nurse-based. There was no evidence to suggest that either model is superior.

Unfortunately, some anesthesiologist-based APS have tended to concentrate on the high-tech approaches to pain relief, placing less emphasis on improving simple methods of pain relief throughout their hospital. This approach benefits only a small proportion of patients. This need not be the case, if, as with the nurse-based service, the anesthesiologist-based APS assists in the development of better protocols for all analgesic regimens used throughout the hospital.[72, 96]

Story et al.[90] reported on the results of a combined physician-based critical care outreach and APS team comprising both anesthesiologists and nursing staff. They conducted a prospective, before-and-after trial of standard acute pain management followed by a period when high-risk postoperative patients were reviewed for the first three days after their return to a general ward by a combined APS and medical emergency team they called IMPACT (Inpatient Management of acute Pain and Advice on Clinical Treatment). They showed that an APS providing critical care outreach may improve postoperative outcome: the incidence of serious adverse events decreased from 23 events per 100 patients to 16 events per 100 patients and the 30-day mortality decreased from 9 to 3 percent ($p = 0.004$).[90]

In the UK and Nordic countries, APS appear to have developed following two basic models often determined by the priorities of the physician originally directing the service. Setting up an APS was undertaken in many hospitals by clinicians already involved in chronic pain work. Under these circumstances, provision of acute pain management is under the umbrella of a comprehensive pain service with the same nurses and doctors providing input into both acute and chronic pain management.

In contrast, other services were initiated by clinicians with an interest in improving perioperative care, seeing pain as a crucial element in patient management during this critical period. Such services have frequently developed as distinct APS separate from the chronic pain service (CPS) resources and personnel and often with links into perioperative care initiatives, such as outreach critical care services,[97] which in the UK have developed using a nurse practitioner model similar to that of many UK APS.[91] Advocates of this latter model suggest that acute and chronic pain management services do not sit comfortably together arguing that acute pain work is largely inpatient-based, while chronic pain work is largely in outpatients and that the urgency required in acute pain work is at odds with the long review times for most chronic pain therapies.

However the APS is organized, cooperation between acute and chronic sectors is crucial if appropriate management of complex patients is to be facilitated, as these patients frequently require input from practitioners with chronic pain knowledge during the inpatient phase of their treatment and subsequent follow up as an out-patient. It is also important to keep clear business objectives for both arms of the service as the requirements of each are often very different, and to ensure that staff appointed to APS duties are not assimilated into running CPS to the detriment of the APS (and vice versa). Clear thinking, even to the point of submitting separate business plans, helps to clarify the requirements of both services and presents an opportunity to clarify the resource requirements and objectives of the two services.

Regardless of the model chosen, the philosophy with which to approach acute pain work is that of "working to put the acute pain team out of business" by striving, through education and training, to disseminate the work of the team down to ward level. To some degree, this philosophy has been successful with concepts such as multimodal analgesia now being widely understood and with PCA and epidural analgesia being largely managed at ward level by ward staff. That said, it is unlikely that APS will ever be unemployed due to the ever-increasing demands brought on by the increasing number of complex challenges (see above under The changing role of the acute pain service).

Initiating an acute pain service

Initiating and developing an APS is a major undertaking which requires the support of medical and nursing staff and hospital managers. Also needed are all of the factors covered below under Resources required which looks at organization of an APS – education, appropriate selection of analgesic regimens, provision of standardized protocols and guidelines, and audit and quality improvement programs.

The management of this change can be difficult. For further information on change management using the establishment of APS as an example, see Chapter 48, Acute pain services and organizational change.

RESOURCES REQUIRED

At an institutional level, a key factor limiting the effectiveness of acute pain management is a lack of resources. Such resources include adequate staffing (medical and nursing) both within- and after-hours, the time and personnel required for education of staff and patients, the time and personnel required for assessment and appropriate monitoring of patients, and the provision of appropriate drugs and equipment.

It is also recognized that once established, an APS may rapidly have requests to expand the service, for example into daycase surgery,[74, 75] emergency medicine departments,[76, 77, 78] pediatric wards,[79, 80, 81] procedural settings,[82, 83, 84, 85, 86, 87] and medical wards.[17, 88]

The director of the APS has to ensure that the work being undertaken by the service does not exceed available resources. It is, of course, desirable to run an APS that is inclusive and able to deal with all aspects of pain management in the inpatient population, but this must be tempered with common sense regarding priorities when resources are limited – as they inevitably are. Patients in severe acute pain in the early postoperative period must continue to take precedence as this situation may lead on to increased postoperative morbidity and possibly even mortality. These patients may require urgent intervention 24 hours, seven days per week.

As the service expands its role, it is essential to identify and highlight the increased resource requirements of these developments well in advance so as not to undermine existing service provision. Service expansion is inevitable and indeed desirable, facilitating improvements in pain management in many sectors of the hospital, but resources must be forthcoming. In order to ensure success in developing resources, it is vital that the surgical and medical staff, as well as the hospital administration, understand and support the APS.

Benefits of an acute pain service

POSTOPERATIVE PATIENT OUTCOME

Randomized controlled trials looking at the benefits or otherwise of APS have not been undertaken. However, there are data from studies of lower methodological quality that have attempted to compare pain relief and other patient outcomes in patients under the care of an APS with those patients who are not.

Although firm conclusions about the benefits of APS are difficult to make because of the heterogeneity of APS models, recent reviews have suggested that implementation of APS programs is associated with significant improvements in pain relief and reduction in the incidence of side effects after surgery.[34, 95, 98]

In the systematic review by Werner et al.,[95] 48 studies containing outcome data were identified. Twenty-five were prospective studies and of these, five were controlled trials (including one using historical controls) and ten analyzed outcome before and after provision of a formal APS. Twenty-three of the studies included in the review used retrospective data. The outcome variables most frequently reported were pain ratings, treatment-related side effects, and adverse events; less often the studies reported on postoperative complications, cost, and length of hospital stay. In summary, the authors concluded that implementation of an APS is associated with a significant decrease in patients' postoperative pain ratings and that the incidence of nausea and vomiting may be reduced, but that evidence for other benefits is weak.

As Werner et al.[95] note in their paper, "segmenting the effects of an APS from the effects of the increased awareness of postoperative pain and/or improvements in postoperative pain techniques by multimodal pain-relieving techniques and improvements in surgical technique (minimal invasive surgery) is difficult." Outcome, such as postoperative morbidity and hospital stay, are dependent on many other factors in addition to good pain relief, including programs for postoperative care and rehabilitation, orders for mobilization and oral nutrition, and defined discharge criteria.

It could be argued that an APS "represents an instrument to improve pain relief"[95] and to assist in postoperative rehabilitation and fast-track surgery programs. It could also be argued that any improvement in pain is due to the analgesic technique used, the general increase in awareness of the importance of good pain management, the use and increasing availability of improved treatment regimens, and knowledge about and use of better treatment strategies for analgesia-related side effects, rather than the presence of the APS. However, widespread use of some more sophisticated techniques (e.g. epidural analgesia) in most institutions is only possible because of supervision by an APS.

There are some individual studies that show better outcome when use of a specific analgesic technique is supervised by an APS. For example, when a comparison was made between PCA managed by an APS or primary ward doctor, the incidence of postoperative nausea and urinary retention was less in APS-supervised patients, despite an increase in opioid consumption.[99] Similarly, the incidence of epidural-related hypotension decreased after the introduction of an APS[45, 100] and pain relief with PCA[45, 100] and epidural analgesia[45] improved. Input from an APS can also significantly improve the effectiveness of more traditional opioid analgesic administration.[48, 101]

Other individual studies showing marked improvements in pain relief with fewer side effects after the inception of an APS are those by Salomaki et al.[102] and a survey of 23 hospitals in the US, 49 percent of which had anesthesiologist-based APS.[103]

Improved patient outcomes in terms of decreased morbidity and mortality may also be seen if high-risk postoperative patients are regularly reviewed by a combined APS-critical care outreach team – see above under Models of APS organization.[90]

REDUCTION OF PERSISTENT PAIN

A number of studies have shown association between the intensity of acute pain (both postoperative and acute pain

from medical conditions) and the development of persistent pain.[10, 104, 105, 106, 107, 108, 109] There is no evidence that treatment of acute pain, *per se*, will reduce the risk of persistent pain.[110] There is, however, some evidence that more aggressive acute pain relief with epidural analgesia started before surgery and continued after surgery under the supervision of an APS may reduce the incidence of persistent pain after thoracotomy[106, 111] and severe phantom pain after leg amputation,[112] although not the incidence of phantom pain overall.[113] Amitriptyline given in the early stages of acute herpes zoster may reduce the risk of chronic postherpetic neuralgia.[114] Members of an APS team may also be more likely to recognize the onset of early neuropathic pain associated with surgery, trauma, or medical disease, and institute appropriate treatment with antihyperalgesic drugs and techniques.[110]

ECONOMIC CONSIDERATIONS

Increasingly, healthcare decision-makers are using economic analyses to help allocate limited healthcare resources effectively. Unfortunately, as yet there are no good data about the cost-effectiveness of APS or the relative cost-effectiveness of the different models of APS, despite the rapid increase and widespread availability of APS in many countries (see above under The development and growth of acute pain services).

A recent review of economic evaluations[115] concluded that there was a lack of high-quality economic studies to support the cost-effectiveness and cost-benefits of APS, that the cost of APS for surgical patients from direct and indirect effects (improved pain management from education in patients not receiving APS) varied from US$2.28 to US$5.08 per patient per day, and that there were insufficient data to identify which APS model (anesthesiologist-based/nursing-supported or nurse-based/anesthesiologist-supervised) was more cost-effective. This cost is similar to that estimated more than a decade before by Breivik[116] – US$2–4 per patient per day for a nurse-based/anesthesiologist-supported APS.

Individual studies have, however, suggested that an APS may be cost-effective. In one of these,[51] a prospective evaluation of the cost-effectiveness of an APS-supervised multimodal epidural PCA program, an overall cost-saving was seen because of a shorter stay in the high-dependency wards, even though a greater degree of supervision was needed for the patient-controlled epidural analgesia (PCEA)-treated patients. The other study[58] looked at cost-effectiveness before and after the introduction of an APS; pain ratings and the incidence of postoperative complications (after some surgery) related to inadequate acute pain relief decreased, but there was no difference in duration of hospital stay and postoperative mortality rate. There was an increase in the cost per patient of 19 Euro per day.[58] While this is not an insignificant amount, it is a direct cost;

cost per patient per day would be less if indirect effects of an APS on all patients were taken into account.[116]

ORGANIZATION OF ACUTE PAIN SERVICES

Education

One of the reasons for past and current deficiencies in the management of acute pain is inadequate education of medical, nursing and allied health staff and students, patients and their families and friends. Inadequate knowledge, misconceptions, and the persistence of some of the myths that surround pain management continue to result in barriers that prevent optimal analgesia in many patients. Better education of all groups is needed, if more sophisticated methods of pain relief (such as patient-controlled and epidural analgesia) are to be managed safely and effectively and if better results are to be gained from conventional methods of pain relief.

PATIENTS

While the evidence for any benefit from preoperative patient education is varied and conflicting in terms of decreases in anxiety, analgesic use, and perceptions of pain intensity,[35, 117] it is only appropriate that patients who are cared for by the APS be given information about the pain relief methods that are available and the choices that they have. In order to make the decision on whether to consent to a treatment, they need the following information:

- likely benefits and the probabilities of success;
- risks and side effects;
- how their pain relief and its treatment (including any side effects or complications that may occur) will be monitored and assessed;
- a reminder that they can change their mind or have a second opinion;
- where applicable, details of costs or charges that have to be met.

Patients should know why effective analgesia is important for their recovery, as well as their comfort and the benefits of physiotherapy and early mobilization should be explained. Information should be given to each patient and tailored to the needs of that patient. It can be presented in a number of ways including verbally, in booklet form, on a video/CD, or made available on the Internet. Examples of the latter include:

- Australian and New Zealand College of Anaesthetists, Faculty of Pain Medicine:
  - Managing acute pain: a guide for patients (available from: www.anzca.edu.au/resources/ books-and-publications);

- Royal College of Anaesthetists:
  - Epidurals for pain relief after surgery (available from: www.rcoa.ac.uk/docs/eprs.pdf);
  - Nerve damage associated with a spinal or epidural injection (available from: www.rcoa.ac.uk/docs/ nerve-spinal.pdf).

The accuracy of some information available to patients remains limited, particularly in terms of risks associated with techniques, such as epidural analgesia. Past studies in this area, concentrating largely on epidural abscess formation,[118, 119, 120] suggested a complication rate between 1:800 and 1:10,000. However, more recent evidence from the UK,[121] and Australia[122] suggests an incidence of major complications (epidural abscess and hematoma) as high as 1:1030[122] to 1:660,[121] although not all patients suffered permanent neurological damage. Similar findings were reported from Sweden.[123] Clearly, this is one major task of an APS: to secure a robust monitoring regimen, to be able to discover early symptoms of impending major complications, and then treating them before irreparable damage can occur.[60, 124] The Third National Audit Project (NAP III) being undertaken by the Royal College of Anaesthetists is studying the complication rates associated with anesthetic and pain management neuraxial procedures. It is expected to report on its findings in late 2008.

When needed, patients should be given information at the time of discharge about ongoing pain relief at home, as well as, in the case of patients who have had epidural analgesia, the need to report back to the APS should they develop signs and symptoms that could suggest the onset of an epidural abscess. An example of a letter given to patients at the time of discharge is shown in **Box 47.1**.

NURSING AND MEDICAL STAFF

Ward nurses and medical staff play a key role in ensuring that analgesia, whether simple or sophisticated, is safely and effectively managed. It is known that improvements in the awareness and assessment of pain,[48, 94, 101] as well as improved postoperative pain relief and prescribing practices can result from staff education and the introduction of medical and nursing guidelines.[48, 101] Education and accreditation programs are therefore essential.

All medical and nursing personnel should be aware of the detrimental effects that unrelieved pain can have on patient well-being and outcome after trauma and surgery and understand the physiological and psychological benefits of good pain relief. They should have a good understanding of the techniques being used, potential problems including drug interactions, and the recognition and treatment of complications and side effects. They should also understand issues arising from the treatment of pain in cognitively impaired patients and in patients from different cultures.

Box 47.1 Example of letter given to patients after epidural analgesia

Postepidural infusion/injection patient instruction leaflet/discharge instructions

Serious complications from epidural analgesia are rare (1 in 10,000). Because the epidural space is close to the spinal cord a collection of pus, or a blood clot can cause pressure on the spinal cord. In the unlikely event that there is pressure on the spinal cord, it is crucial to diagnose and treat it as quickly as possible; this must be done by expert hospital doctors to prevent delays in treatment and long lasting damage. This leaflet tells you what to look for and what action to take if you think that you have a problem.

Assessment before the removal of epidural catheter

At the end of treatment with your epidural infusion, the team of doctors and nurses caring for you will examine you to ensure that you don't have any residual numbness or weakness of legs from the action of the drugs in your epidural infusion. They will ask to you move your legs and examine you to make sure that the sensation in your legs is as it was before the operation. It is important to remember that some operations can cause altered sensation in the legs, therefore any changes experienced may be as a result of the surgery and not the epidural. If you do have altered sensation when the epidural is removed, the attending team can discuss this with you.

If you experience any of the listed signs and symptoms (see list below) as a new problem, after your epidural infusion has been stopped as an inpatient ask the nurse in charge of the ward to contact the pain team or on call anaesthetist immediately.

If you have been discharged, it is important that you contact the on-call anaesthetist at the hospital immediately. After speaking to the on-call anaesthetist, they will arrange to see you in the Accident and Emergency department in order to examine you.

Signs and symptoms

- Redness, pus, tenderness, or pain at the epidural wound site;
- Feeling generally unwell, despite the fact that all seems to be well with the surgical wound;
- High temperature, neck stiffness;
- Numbness and or weakness in your legs/inability to weight bear;
- Difficulty passing water/incontinence of faeces.

Reproduced with permission of Wrexham Maelor Hospital, North East Wales NHS Trust. © North East Wales HNS Trust, UK.

Many APS require some form of certification or accreditation before nurses can assume responsibility for a patient using one of the more advanced methods of pain relief, such as PCA and epidural analgesia. Education and accreditation programs often consist of verbal and written information (e.g. lectures or workshops and booklets), written assessment (e.g. multiple choice questionnaires), and a practical assessment (e.g. demonstration of ability to program machines, administer epidural bolus doses).[72, 94] Reaccreditation every one to two years will help ensure that knowledge and practices are regularly updated. Formal education programs need to be supplemented with informal one-on-one bedside teaching in the ward.

Anesthesiologists and trainees involved with the APS must receive training and be made familiar with local guidelines. Teaching should be offered to medical students and doctors in training. It is important that surgeons and physicians at all grades of seniority are also offered continuing medical education in acute pain.

Selection of analgesic regimens

SELECTION OF ANALGESIC TECHNIQUE

The selection of analgesic techniques to be used by an APS is based on:

- availability of drugs, equipment, and expertise;
- risks and benefits of the drugs and techniques;
- operative procedure and associated risk factors, particularly size and location of primary incision;
- patient factors, particularly medical comorbidity.

The decision to offer a particular method of analgesia should be based on current knowledge of the benefits and limitations of the methods available, patient case mix, cultural differences, and staffing levels and training. In the first instance at least, it may be best to introduce just a small range of standard analgesic techniques, so that staff become knowledgable about and confident in their use.

A detailed discussion of analgesic techniques, including risks and benefits, is outside the scope of this chapter, but the range of methods that could be used by an APS includes:

- simple multimodal analgesia including paracetamol (acetaminophen), nonselective NSAIDs and COX-2-selective inhibitors in selected patients – see Chapter 4, Clinical pharmacology: traditional NSAIDs and selective COX-2 inhibitors, and Chapter 5, Clinical pharmacology: paracetamol and compound analgesics, in the *Acute Pain* volume of this series;
- optimized intermittent intravenous, intramuscular, subcutaneous, and oral opioid analgesia – see Chapter 3, Clinical pharmacology: opioids, in the *Acute Pain* volume of this series;
- patient-controlled i.v. opioid analgesia – see Chapter 11, Patient-controlled analgesia, in the *Acute Pain* volume of this series, and Chapter 24, Intravenous and subcutaneous patient-controlled analgesia;
- epidural analgesia, including patient-controlled epidural analgesia – see Chapter 13, Epidural and spinal analgesia, in the *Acute Pain* volume of this series, and Chapter 26, Epidural analgesia for acute pain after surgery and during labor, including patient-controlled epidural analgesia;
- single-dose intrathecal opioid analgesia – see Chapter 13, Epidural and spinal analgesia, in the *Acute Pain* volume of this series;
- continuous or intermittent regional blockade (other than epidural analgesia) – see Chapter 12, Continuous peripheral neural blockade for acute pain, in the *Acute Pain* volume of this series and Chapter 23, Peripheral nerve blocks: practical aspects;
- premixed nitrous oxide and oxygen (Entonox);
- treatments for neuropathic pain (including ketamine, antidepressants, anticonvulsants, and membrane stabilizers) – see Chapter 6, Clinical pharmacology: other adjuvants, in the *Acute Pain* volume of this series, and Chapter 12, Antiepileptics, antidepressants, and local anesthetic drugs;
- novel analgesic delivery systems, e.g. transdermal, iontophoretic transdermal, intranasal – see Chapter 10, Routes of administration, in the *Acute Pain* volume of this series, and Chapter 25, Alternative opioid patient-controlled analgesia delivery systems – transcutaneous, nasal, and others;
- nonpharmacological therapies, such as cognitive-behavioral approaches, hypnosis, relaxation exercises, and physical methods, such as transcutaneous electrical nerve stimulation (TENS), acupuncture, and massage – see Chapter 14, Transcutaneous electrical nerve stimulation (TENS) and acupuncture for acute pain; Chapter 16, Psychological interventions for acute pediatric pain; Chapter 15, Psychological therapies – adults, in the *Acute Pain* volume of this series; Chapter 17, Transcutaneous electrical nerve stimulation; and Chapter 18, Acupuncture.

While many APS still regard the care of patients receiving PCA, epidural analgesia including PCEA, single-dose spinal opioid analgesia, and continuous regional techniques as the bulk of their clinical work, it is inevitable that the use of more complex therapies in more complex patients will increase as the concept of a comprehensive, multidisciplinary inpatient pain service matures.

A number of factors will influence the appropriateness of a particular method of analgesia relating to the patient and to the planned surgical procedure. Although analgesic requirements vary from patient to patient, certain operative procedures are usually more painful than others. Thoracic and upper abdominal wounds tend to be the most painful. The anticipated severity and duration of pain will influence the choice of postoperative analgesia.

Patient factors are also very important and it is necessary therefore to take a careful history. The patient's underlying cardiovascular and respiratory status may influence the choice of analgesia. Certain analgesics may be inappropriate because of potential interactions with concomitant drug therapy or renal, hepatic, or endocrine disease. It is also important to ascertain the patient's past experience and expectations of pain relief and their preoperative use of opioids, alcohol, and other drugs, such as cannabis, cocaine, amphetamines, and benzodiazepines. Poor understanding or limited motor skills may limit the use of patient-controlled techniques. While making these assessments, it is possible to make some informal judgments of the patient's personality and coping style, which also help determine the most appropriate method of analgesia.

SELECTION OF EQUIPMENT AND DRUGS

The APS will require infusion pumps for the provision of PCA, epidural analgesia, continuous regional blockade, and the administration of drugs, such as ketamine. If continuous infusions are to be used, it may also be safer to use pumps where the rate of infusion can be capped (i.e. rate-limited), so that inadvertent high infusion rates cannot be delivered. Pumps used for epidural infusions and PCEA must have a high pressure tolerance to facilitate delivery of a bolus dose through the high resistance epidural filters and catheter without activation of the high pressure alarm.

The pumps used for PCA and for PCEA need to be portable and robust, easy to program, and lockable to prevent tampering with the program or reservoir. These lockable pumps may also be used to deliver continuous infusions of other drugs where diversion of that drug may be a risk (e.g. ketamine). The patient's PCA control button needs to be large enough to be easy to use and should have a retaining strap for less dexterous patients. In some circumstances, an alternative to a hand-held patient demand button may be needed (see Chapter 11,

Patient-controlled analgesia in the *Acute Pain* volume of this series). New developments in PCA technology may make cumbersome PCA pumps unnecessary for some patients, being replaced by adhesive iontophoretic PCA systems using transdermal fentanyl.[125, 126]

Although individualization of treatment is important, it is suggested that a limited number of drugs and drug regimens for pain relief is agreed within the hospital. The potential for error existing in a system where each anesthesiologist prescribes their own recipe for PCA, epidural analgesia, or single-dose intrathecal opioids is immense. Increasing evidence about optimal regimens of, for example, epidural analgesia[127] reduces the need for a wide variety of epidural analgesic combinations. Limiting the available regimens allows the hospital pharmacy to provide PCA syringes and infusion bags for epidural analgesia, allows the ward staff to become familiar with those techniques and their problems, and facilitates evaluation by the APS. Where possible, use of prefilled syringes or other drug reservoirs will minimize the risk of prescription errors and bacteriological contamination (see Chapter 26, Epidural analgesia for acute pain after surgery and during labor, including patient-controlled epidural analgesia).

Standardization of protocols and guidelines

Standard orders and guidelines are commonly used for the more advanced methods of pain relief such as PCA and epidural analgesia (see Chapter 11, Patient-controlled analgesia and Chapter 13, Epidural and spinal analgesia, in the *Acute Pain* volume of this series). However, standardization may also help to make traditional methods of pain relief, such as intermittent i.v. or i.m. opioid analgesia, safer and more effective.[48, 101, 124]

Consideration should therefore be given to standardizing a number of aspects of all acute pain management regimens, regardless of drug or technique used and regardless of whether the analgesia is considered simple or advanced.[72] These include:

- prescribing and documentation, for example:
  - drugs used (analgesic and nonanalgesic, e.g. for the treatment of nausea and vomiting);
  - drug doses and drug concentrations;
  - the use (if any) of concurrent anticoagulant and antiplatelet drugs and the timing of removal of epidural catheters in patients receiving such drugs;
  - nondrug treatment (e.g. supplemental oxygen).
- assessment of pain and the response to inadequate analgesia;
- monitoring for adverse effects and the response to and treatment of side effects.

As with all guidelines, the aim is to try and improve the quality of clinical decision-making and eliminate inappropriate/reduce unnecessary variations in clinical practice, not to dictate practice.

STANDARDIZED PRESCRIBING AND DOCUMENTATION

If the drugs and analgesic techniques can be agreed upon, charts can be preprinted with the standard regimen (some centers may use adhesive labels with preprinted drug concentrations), thus avoiding transcription errors. Similarly, guidance on alterations of doses, prohibition of other opioids or sedatives, use of supplemental oxygen, monitoring requirements, management of inadequate analgesia, recognition and treatment of side effects, and who to call if there are problems, can all be included in standardized orders. Examples of preprinted PCA and epidural analgesia standardized orders, which incorporate a bedside flow chart, are shown in **Figures 47.1** and **47.2**.

Standardized prescribing guidelines should not be limited to techniques such as PCA and epidural analgesia. An APS can help devise evidence-based guidelines for all analgesic regimens, advanced or simple, used for acute pain management.[72] See examples of APS-initiated guidelines for intermittent subcutaneous and oral opioid in **Figures 47.3** and **47.4**.

STANDARDIZED ASSESSMENT OF PAIN

The International Association for the Study of Pain defines pain as, "an unpleasant sensory and emotional experience associated with actual or potential tissue damage or described in terms of such damage."[128] In other words, pain is a subjective, highly individual experience. Therefore, whenever possible, its assessment should be by the person experiencing the pain.

Correlations between observer and patient assessment of pain are usually low or moderate, even using specifically trained nursing staff with rationally derived rating scales.[129] Nurses consistently and significantly rate patients' pain lower than do the patients themselves.[130] However, patients think that nurses do know how much pain they are experiencing and this further impedes communication and treatment.

The assessment of pain (as the fifth vital sign) is therefore an essential component of acute pain management and should be a routine part of clinical practice, incorporated into standard nursing assessments and recorded in conjunction with assessments of respiration, blood pressure, pulse, and temperature measurements.

In the acute pain setting, unidimensional measures of pain intensity are most commonly used, such as the Visual Analog Scale, Verbal Numerical Rating Scale, and Categorical Rating Scale (using words to describe the pain). Each of these methods is reasonably reliable as long as any end points and adjectives employed are carefully selected and standardized. While often used to compare levels of pain between patients, these methods of scoring pain are probably of most use as measures of change in the level of pain within each patient and the effectiveness of treatment of that pain. The use of pain scores and other methods of acute pain assessment are outlined in Chapter 2, Practical methods for pain intensity measurements and Chapter 8, Assessment, measurement, and history, in the *Acute Pain* volume of this series.

It can be very difficult to get a meaningful and totally subjective assessment of pain if the patient is acutely ill, disorientated, is cognitively impaired, or if there are language barriers to communication. Other methods of pain assessment will then be needed (see Chapter 8, Assessment, measurement, and history, in the *Acute Pain* volume of this series).

Whatever scale is used, it is important to assess pain intensity on movement as well as at rest, thus assessing dynamic analgesia. Assessing pain only at rest can easily give a false impression of comfort. It is important that patients are able to deep breathe and cough in the early postoperative period, to mobilize when required, and to participate in other rehabilitation activities. Pain relief can only be counted as fully effective if it allows the patient to perform these activities; if they cannot, then recovery will be impaired. Therefore an assessment of the functional impact of pain is useful.

One way of assessing and documenting this has been suggested – the Functional Activity Scale (FAS).[131] The possible scores are A, B, or C and the activity assessed is determined on an individual patient basis – for example, coughing may be an appropriate target after upper abdominal surgery, but joint mobility and ability to comply with physiotherapy an appropriate target after knee or hip replacement surgery.

Using this simple categorical score:

A = no limitation (there is no limitation of activity due to pain);
B = mild limitation (the patient is able to undertake the activity, but experiences moderate to severe pain);
C = significant limitation (the patient is unable to complete the activity due to pain).

It is also important to ensure that there is an adequate and timely response to inadequate analgesia or functional impairment. If patients are to gain maximum benefit from any techniques, then attention to detail is paramount as is the 24-hour availability of staff (medical and nursing), so that inadequate pain relief can be managed quickly.

STANDARDIZED MONITORING

Patients with acute pain must be assessed at frequent intervals in order to optimize analgesia and detect or manage side effects or complications at an early stage. Therefore, as well as regular assessments of pain, patients should also be observed for the onset of side effects and complications related to the analgesic technique in use.

Such assessments need to be done using clearly described and standardized criteria and tools. However, there will be little benefit from this unless these assessments are coupled with clearly defined trigger levels for intervention, and strategies need to be in place to manage deviation from expected values. Therefore, requirements for monitoring and documentation should be accompanied by guidelines for the recognition and treatment of adverse effects and complications. As well as orders for the treatment of common side effects, such as nausea and vomiting, itching and hypotension, there should be very clear guidelines that enable early recognition and treatment of respiratory depression and early recognition and notification of motor and sensory deficit or increasing back pain associated with epidural analgesia.

Respiratory depression

Fear of respiratory depression has limited the rational use of opioid analgesia by any route for many years. However, the incidence of respiratory depression after PCA and epidural analgesia is no higher than that seen with conventional as-needed intramuscular analgesia.[35]

There remains significant confusion about the best method of monitoring for respiratory depression. Measurement of arterial pCO_2 levels is the most sensitive and accurate, but not possible in most patients, particularly on a regular basis. Therefore, reliance must be placed on clinical measures.

It is well known that respiratory rate is an unreliable guide to respiratory depression and hypoxemia;[35, 132] indeed, respiratory depression can coexist with a normal respiratory rate,[72] but that increasing sedation almost inevitably precedes significant respiratory depression. The patient's level of sedation should therefore be assessed on a regular basis. One common sedation scoring system used is that in **Table 47.1**. Note that it indicates that patients should be roused to assess their level of sedation. If this is not done, the early onset of respiratory depression can be missed, sometimes with fatal results.[133] If a sedation score of 2 or more is reported, a reduction in

Table 47.1 Sedation scores.

Score	Description
0	Wide awake
1	Easy to rouse[a]
2	Constantly drowsy, easy to rouse but unable to stay awake (e.g. falls asleep during conversation); early respiratory depression
3	Severe; somnolent, difficult to rouse; severe respiratory depression

[a]Some centers also add a "1S," which indicates asleep, but easy to rouse.

ROYAL ADELAIDE HOSPITAL
ACUTE PAIN SERVICE
PATIENT-CONTROLLED ANALGESIA (PCA)
Standard Orders

PATIENT LABEL

Unit Record No.: _____

Surname: _____

Given Names: _____

Date of Birth: _____ Sex: _____

PCA PROGRAM ORDERS:

1. **DRUG:** ....
    * = order in mg or microgram as appropriate

    Place appropriate drug label here

2. **CONCENTRATION:***...................................../mL

3. **BOLUS DOSE:***
    Dose:

    ....   ** = sign and date any changes

    .... **

    If pain not controlled:

    Bolus dose may increase to ....

    Bolus dose may increase to .... **

4. **CONTINUOUS (BACKGROUND) INFUSION:***

    .... /hr (.................... mL/hr)

    .... /hr (.................... mL/hr) **

5. **LOADING DOSE:**   0 (zero)

6. **DOSE DURATION:**   "stat"

7. **LOCKOUT:**   5 minutes

ROUTE (if other than IV): ....

GENERAL ORDERS:

1. Oxygen at *2 to 4 L/min via nasal specs or 6 to 8 L/min via mask* while orders are in effect.

2. No systemic opioids or sedatives to be given except as ordered by the APS.

3. Naloxone to be immediately available.

4. One-way anti-reflux valve to be used in IV line and an anti-syphon valve must be in-line between patient and syringe at all times.

5. *Monitoring requirements:* see overleaf.

6. Record current total dose per syringe in mg or microgram as appropriate. Reset total dose to zero when syringe changed.

7. Cease PCA if the patient becomes confused.

8. For inadequate analgesia or other problems related to the analgesia, contact the rostered APS anaesthetist.

TREATMENT OF SIDE EFFECTS:

RESPIRATORY DEPRESSION (EXCESSIVE SEDATION):

1. If sedation score = 2, reduce size of the bolus dose by half and cease any background infusion.

2. If sedation score = 3 (irrespective of respiratory rate) OR sedation score = 2 and respiratory rate 6/min, give 100 microgram NALOXONE IV stat. Repeat 2 minutely PRN up to a total of 400 microgram. Cease PCA and call the APS anaesthetist.

3. If sedation score 2 revert to hourly sedation scores until sedation score < 2 for at least 2 hours.

NAUSEA AND VOMITING:

1. Give METOCLOPRAMIDE 10mg IV 4 hourly PRN.

2. If ineffective after 15 minutes, add TROPISETRON 2 mg IV daily PRN.

3. If still ineffective after another 15 minutes, add DROPERIDOL 500 microgram IV 4 hourly PRN (250 microgram if > 70 years).

SIGNATURE OF ANAESTHETIST: .... Date: ....

(Print name ....)

Cease above orders:

Signature of anaesthetist: .... Date: .... Time: ....

APS-PATIENT CONTROLLED ANALGESIA   **MR 98.2**

(a)

Figure 47.1 Example of preprinted (a) standard orders (continued over). Reproduced with permission of the Royal Adelaide Hospital, South Australia.

opioid dose is mandated, regardless of the patient's pain score.[72] If the patient is uncomfortable, alternative and less sedating forms of pain relief need to be added to the analgesic regimen.

The importance of increasing sedation as a clinical sign of early respiratory depression was highlighted by Vila *et al.*[134] In an attempt to improve pain relief in a cancer setting they introduced a numerical pain treatment

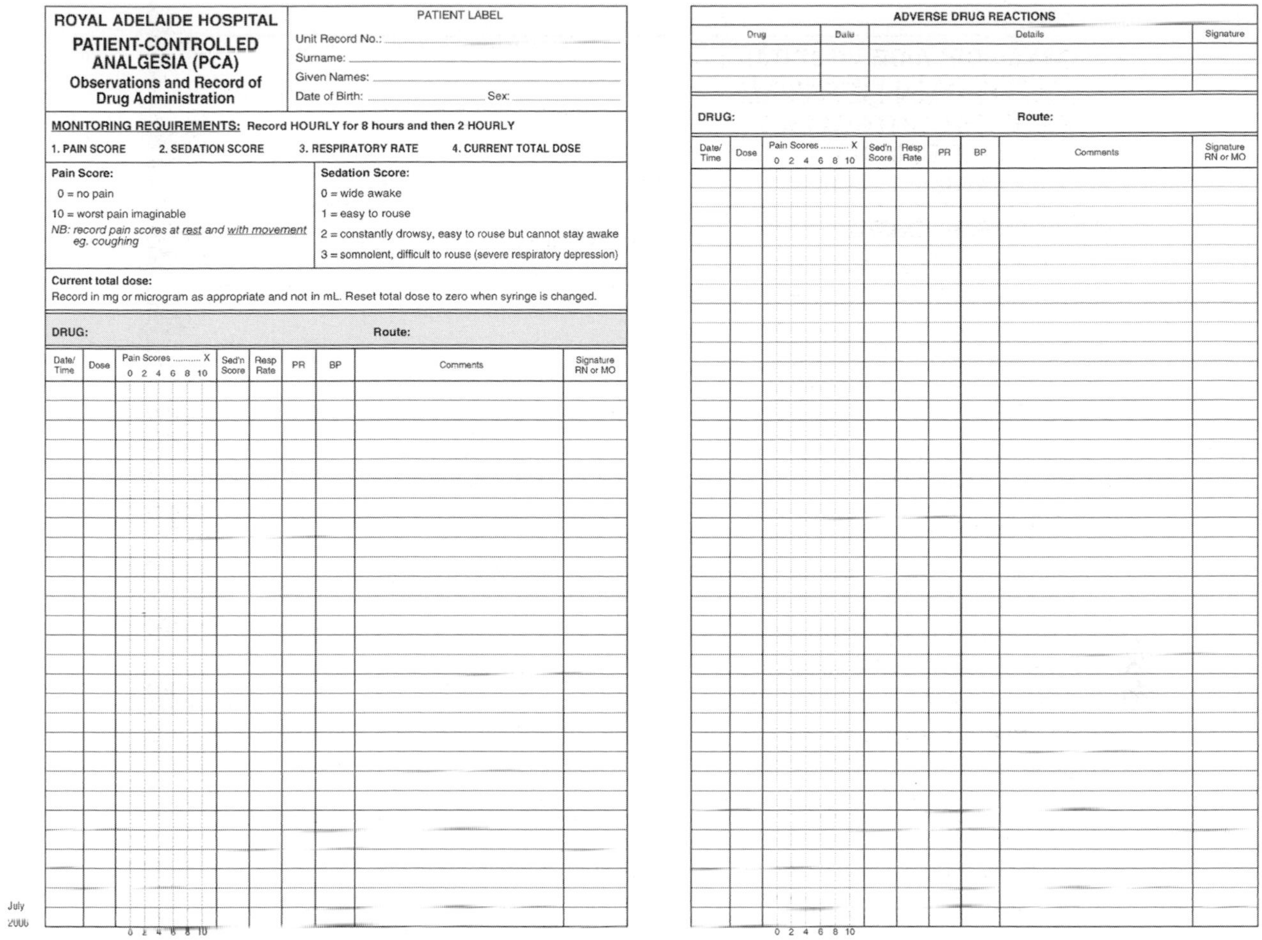

ROYAL ADELAIDE HOSPITAL

PATIENT-CONTROLLED ANALGESIA (PCA)
Observations and Record of Drug Administration

PATIENT LABEL

Unit Record No.: _____
Surname: _____
Given Names: _____
Date of Birth: _____ Sex: _____

MONITORING REQUIREMENTS: Record HOURLY for 8 hours and then 2 HOURLY

1. PAIN SCORE 2. SEDATION SCORE 3. RESPIRATORY RATE 4. CURRENT TOTAL DOSE

Pain Score:
0 = no pain
10 = worst pain imaginable
NB: record pain scores at rest and with movement eg. coughing

Sedation Score:
0 = wide awake
1 = easy to rouse
2 = constantly drowsy, easy to rouse but cannot stay awake
3 = somnolent, difficult to rouse (severe respiratory depression)

Current total dose:
Record in mg or microgram as appropriate and not in mL. Reset total dose to zero when syringe is changed.

DRUG: _____ **Route:** _____

Date/Time	Dose	Pain Scores .... X 0 2 4 6 8 10	Sed'n Score	Resp Rate	PR	BP	Comments	Signature RN or MO

July 2006

0 2 4 6 8 10

(b)

ADVERSE DRUG REACTIONS			
Drug	Date	Details	Signature

DRUG: _____ **Route:** _____

Date/Time	Dose	Pain Scores .... X 0 2 4 6 8 10	Sed'n Score	Resp Rate	PR	BP	Comments	Signature RN or MO

0 2 4 6 8 10

Figure 47.1 (b) Example of preprinted flow sheet for patient-controlled analgesia (continued).

algorithm in which opioids were given to patients in order to achieve satisfactory pain scores. A review of this intervention showed a two-fold increase in the risk of respiratory depression. Importantly, the authors noted that respiratory depression was usually not accompanied by a decrease in respiratory rate. Of the 29 patients who developed respiratory depression (either before or after the introduction of the algorithm), only three had a respiratory rates of <12 breaths per minute, but 27 had a decrease in their level of consciousness. As well as confirming that increasing sedation is a more reliable way of detecting opioid-induced respiratory depression, this study highlighted the risk of titrating opioid (or other pharmacological therapies) solely to achieve a desirable pain score without appropriate patient monitoring.

Oxygen saturation (as measured by pulse oximetry) is often used as an easy and noninvasive measure of blood oxygen levels. However, care must be taken in the interpretation of any readings. If the patient is receiving supplemental oxygen, the added oxygen may mask deterioration in respiratory function (i.e. "normal" oxygen saturation levels may still be seen).

Hypotension

The reported incidence of hypotension associated with epidural analgesia varies widely[135] and depends on the dose of local anesthetic used and the criteria used to define hypotension. It can be minimized if appropriate dose regimens are used.[72, 124]

However, patients may become hypotensive in the hours following major surgery for many reasons. Unfortunately, if the patient is receiving epidural analgesia, the first response of the ward staff may be discontinuation of the epidural infusion, when the underlying cause is usually hypovolemia.[136] As a result, inadequate analgesia may be added to the patient's existing problems. In order to prevent this happening, a program of education should be introduced to all staff to help them differentiate between common causes of hypotension – for example, bleeding and relative hypovolemia in the presence of an epidural block.

ROYAL ADELAIDE HOSPITAL
ACUTE PAIN SERVICE
EPIDURAL/INTRATHECAL/ REGIONAL ANALGESIA
Standard Orders

PATIENT LABEL

Unit Record No.: _____

Surname: _____

Given Names: _____

Date of Birth: _____ Sex: _____

ANALGESIA ORDERS: *(sign and date any changes)*

1. **DRUG:** ....

Place appropriate drug label here

2. **CONCENTRATION:** ....

3. **BOLUS DOSE:**

   .... to .... mL 2 hourly PRN

4. **INFUSION RATE:** ** = sign and date any changes

   .... to .... mL/hr

   .... to .... mL/hr**

ROUTE: ....

GENERAL ORDERS:

1. Oxygen at *2 to 4 L/min via nasal specs or 6 to 8 L/min via mask* while orders are in effect.

2. No systemic opioids or sedatives to be given except as ordered by the APS.

3. No anticoagulant or antiplatelet medications to be given (other than heparin for prevention of DVTs) before consulting with the APS.

4. Naloxone to be immediately available.

5. An anti-syphon valve must be in-line between patient and syringe at all times.

6. Maintain IV access while orders are in effect.

7. *Monitoring requirements:* see overleaf.

8. Record current total volume per syringe in mL and reset to zero when syringe changed.

9. For inadequate analgesia or other problems related to the analgesia, contact the rostered APS anaesthetist.

INTRATHECAL MORPHINE DETAILS (as needed)

Dose .... microgram

Time given ....

TREATMENT OF SIDE EFFECTS:

RESPIRATORY DEPRESSION (EXCESSIVE SEDATION):

1. If sedation score = 2, reduce rate of infusion by one quarter to one third.

2. If sedation score = 3 (irrespective of respiratory rate) OR sedation score = 2 and respiratory rate ≤ 6/min, give 100 microgram NALOXONE IV stat. Repeat 2 minutely PRN up to a total of 400 microgram. Cease infusion and call the APS anaesthetist.

3. If sedation score ≥ 2 revert to hourly sedation scores until sedation score < 2 for at least 2 hours.

NAUSEA AND VOMITING:

1. Give METOCLOPRAMIDE 10mg IV 4 hourly PRN.

2. If ineffective after 15 minutes, add TROPISETRON 2 mg IV daily PRN.

3. If still ineffective after another 15 minutes, add DROPERIDOL 500 microgram IV 4 hourly PRN (250 microgram if > 70 years).

SEVERE ITCHING:

Give 100 microgram NALOXONE IV stat. Repeat 10 minutely PRN up to a total of 400 microgram.

SIGNATURE OF ANAESTHETIST: .... Date: ....

(Print name ....)

Cease infusion: Date: .... Time: .... **Remove analgesia catheter:** Date: .... Time: ....

Give next dose of heparin at: Date: .... Time: ....

Signature of Anaesthetist: ....

Catheter removed and complete: Signature of RN: .... Date: .... Time: ....

APS-EPIDURAL/INTRATHECAL/REGIONAL ANALGESIA   MR 98.0

(a)

Figure 47.2 Example of preprinted (a) standard orders (continued over). Reproduced with permission of the Royal Adelaide Hospital, South Australia.

Recent studies have suggested a benefit from moderate fluid restriction during and after some major surgical procedures.[137, 138, 139] After colorectal surgery, Brandstrup *et al.*[138] found that a restricted regimen aimed at maintaining perioperative body weight resulted in significant decreases in cardiorespiratory and tissue healing complications. Similarly, Holte *et al.*[139] reported an improvement in pulmonary function – although it was

ROYAL ADELAIDE HOSPITAL

EPIDURAL/INTRATHECAL/ REGIONAL ANALGESIA
Observations and Record of Drug Administration

PATIENT LABEL

Unit Record No.: _____

Surname: _____

Given Names: _____

Date of Birth: _____ Sex: _____

MONITORING REQUIREMENTS: Record Items 1 to 6 EACH HOUR for 8 hours and then 2 HOURLY

1. PAIN SCORE
2. SEDATION SCORE
3. RESPIRATORY RATE
4. BP AND HEART RATE
5. MOVEMENT AND SENSATION
6. CURRENT TOTAL DOSE
7. EPIDURAL INSERTION SITE: Once per shift, record any inflammation, tenderness, swelling or leakage at the epidural insertion site; reinforce dressing if needed – do not remove and replace.

After administration of a bolus dose:
Record Items 1 to 5 every 5 minutes for 20 minutes.

After removal of an epidural catheter:
Record movement and sensation every 4 HOURS for 24 HOURS.

Pain Score:	Sedation Score:
0 = no pain	0 = wide awake
10 = worst pain imaginable	1 = easy to rouse
NB: record pain scores at rest and with movement eg. coughing	2 = constantly drowsy, easy to rouse but cannot stay awake
	3 = somnolent, difficult to rouse (severe respiratory depression)

Current total dose:
Record in mL. Reset total dose to zero when syringe is changed.

Movement and Sensation:
- Ask the patient if they have any numbness/weakness. Unless injured, get the patient to flex their hips and knees (ie, draw their knees up to their chest).
- IF ALL IS NORMAL, record M✓ S✓ in the M/S column: otherwise document and call the APS immediately.

DRUG: _____ **Route:** _____

Date/ Time	Dose	Pain Scores .... X 0 2 4 6 8 10	Sed'n Score	Resp Rate	PR	BP	M/S	Comments	Signature RN or MO

0 2 4 6 8 10

July 2006

(b)

ADVERSE DRUG REACTIONS

Drug	Date	Details	Signature

DRUG: _____ **Route:** _____

Date/ Time	Dose	Pain Scores .... X 0 2 4 6 8 10	Sed'n Score	Resp Rate	PR	BP	M/S	Comments	Signature RN or MO

0 2 4 6 8 10

Figure 47.2 (b) Example of preprinted flow sheet for patient-controlled analgesia (continued).

only transient (differences in forced vital capacity (FVC) and forced expiratory volume (FEV) were significant at six hours after surgery only); there was an increase in the concentrations of cardiovascularly active stress response hormones (renin, aldosterone, and angiotensin) and no differences in the rate of overall recovery.

Adherence to restrictive regimens could further complicate the provision of epidural analgesia and may increase the need for vasoconstrictor use, which may not always be to the patient's benefit. The perioperative period is extremely complex and the studies regarding fluid restriction to date seldom make allowance for conflicting issues such as the quality of analgesia, which might also influence outcome; thus the case for such regimens is not yet proven.[140] That said, Holte et al.[139] expressed some concern about the trend to more anastomosis leakages in the patients on restrictive regimens, so their suggestion that individualized goal-directed fluid administration strategies (which could take into account the use of epidural analgesia) may be the sensible way forward.

Motor and sensory blockade and block height

A major concern about the use of epidural analgesia is the risk of spinal cord compression and paraplegia from an epidural hematoma or abscess. Although the risk is low (see above under Organization of acute pain services), early detection is the key to avoiding permanent neurological loss. Early diagnosis and, if indicated, immediate surgical decompression, will increase the likelihood of good neurological recovery.[141] Ideally, this will occur within eight hours of the onset of neurological symptoms, but even then the degree of residual damage is determined by the degree of compression and a complete recovery is not assured.

It is therefore important to use epidural regimens (drug doses and infusion rates) that minimize (ideally avoid) motor and sensory deficit (see Chapter 26, Epidural analgesia for acute pain after surgery and during labor, including patient-controlled epidural analgesia). As well as maximizing the chance of the development of an abscess or hematoma being diagnosed at an early stage, it

Royal Adelaide Hospital Guidelines
RAH Drug Committee
Revised May 2007
Planned Review Date June 2008

DOSAGE GUIDELINES
FOR INTERMITTENT SUBCUTANEOUS OPIOID ADMINISTRATION
For Acute Pain Management

• Subcutaneous, rather than intramuscular, administration is recommended
• For intermittent administration of intravenous opioids refer to appropriate RAH guidelines

- Recommended opioid doses are based on average analgesic requirements of opioid-naïve patients following moderate to major surgery
- Avoid co-administration of sedatives with opioids where possible
- Avoid co-administration of other opioids - ensure 1 hour has elapsed since the last dose when changing to a different immediate-release opioid.
- Consideration should be given to dosage amendment in differing clinical situations.
- Dose requirements of opioids for analgesia for patients on long term opioid therapy may be higher.
- The best clinical predictor of opioid dose is patient age[1]

[1] Macintyre PE, Jarvis DA. Age is the best predictor of postoperative morphine requirements. Pain 64(2): 357-64 1996

Please direct any queries to:
• Acute Pain Service OR
• Medicines Information Centre Pharmacy Department Phone 25546

Table : Initial Opioid Orders		
Age (Years)	MORPHINE Dose range (mg)	OXYCODONE Dose range (mg)
< 15	*	*
15 - 39	7.5 - 12.5	7.5 - 12.5
40 - 59	5 - 10	5 - 10
60 - 69	2.5 - 7.5	2.5 - 7.5
70 - 85	2.5 - 5	2.5 - 5
>85	2 - 3	2 - 3

* Contact WCH Drug Information Centre or WCH Department of Anaesthesia for advice on opioid doses for children <15 years

- Order recommended dose of opioid 2 hourly prn.
- Suggest start in middle of dose range.
- Upper limit of dose range can be increased if analgesia is inadequate, and if sedation score is less than 2 and respiratory rate greater than 8/min.
- Oxycodone is the preferred second-line opioid.
  Note that the equianalgesic dose (same analgesic efficacy) for SC oxycodone is equal to that of SC morphine but is half the oral oxycodone dose. That is 10 mg SC oxycodone = 10 mg SC morphine = 20 mg oral oxycodone (see RAH guidelines for oral oxycodone administration)

MONITORING OF THERAPY IS ESSENTIAL

For monitoring requirements, refer to RAH Guidelines for Intermittent Subcutaneous Opioid Administration

(a)

Figure 47.3 Example of guidelines for intermittent subcutaneous opioids administration (continued over). Reproduced with permission of the Royal Adelaide Hospital, South Australia.

will also help maximize the patient's ability to move and walk (both proprioception and muscle strength will be preserved) and reduce the risk of hypotension. Note that a patient with an epidural abscess may not be febrile.[35]

Also importantly, patients must be reminded (and ideally given written information prior to discharge – see example in **Box 47.1**) that they should contact the APS urgently should they develop increasing (new) back pain or motor or sensory loss after they have left hospital. Signs and symptoms of epidural abscesses may not develop until some time after discharge.[122]

Neurological deterioration in any patient with, or having recently had, an epidural catheter in place should prompt urgent radiological investigation to exclude treatable cord compression. If a patient with epidural analgesia develops motor or significant sensory block of one or both limbs, it is important to exclude the presence of epidural hematoma or abscess, or inadvertent subarachnoid infusion, by switching off the infusion and reassessing the patient regularly over the next one to three

hours for signs of resolution of the blockade. Failure of the block to resolve should prompt early investigation by magnetic resonance (MR) (preferably) or computed tomography (CT) scan.

It is therefore essential that sensory and motor function should be tested informally (by inquiring if the patient has any numbness and asking them to flex their hip: movement at ankle or toes only is not sufficient[72] or formally (using a recognized scale such as that suggested by Bromage[142]) on a regular basis. Testing should be performed both during the time of epidural analgesia and for a period after removal of the epidural catheter. One should be aware that epidural hematoma and abscess may occur subsequent to the removal of the catheter or even several days later.

Regular monitoring of the level of block during epidural analgesia has been common practice in many hospitals with a block level above T4 mandating reductions in epidural infusion rates. However, in modern practice with epidural catheters sited at the upper dermatome for abdominal and

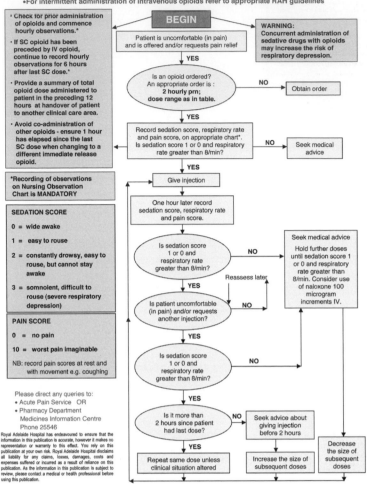

Figure 47.3 Example of guidelines for intermittent subcutaneous opioids administration. Reproduced with permission of the Royal Adelaide Hospital, South Australia (continued).

(b)

thoracic surgery, block levels above T4 are common and should not be cause for concern in the absence of motor loss or significant hypotension or bradycardia. Experience in cardiac surgery, with blocks routinely sited at T4, have demonstrated that respiratory function is maintained even in the presence of demonstrable loss of power and paresthesia in the upper limbs leading to monitoring systems based on arm power in different myotomes.[143] This should not be necessary in noncardiac surgery, but suggests that monitoring for arm symptoms is adequate in everyday practice, rather than assessing the formal level of block which becomes increasingly unreliable the weaker the local anesthetic used. In some centers, routine observations of bilateral upper and lower sensory level for cold (ice-cube in a glove) is done by nurses on the ward, in order to assist in the earlier detection of a dislodged epidural catheter (see Chapter 26, Epidural analgesia for acute pain after surgery and during labor, including patient-controlled epidural analgesia).[124]

Back pain

Patients should also be asked if they have any back pain as increasing (and new) back pain may be the first sign of an epidural hematoma or abscess following epidural analgesia.[35]

Audit and quality improvement

The delivery of an APS is a high-volume activity and patient safety is paramount. Errors occur and may have serious implications, but understanding the causes of errors are an important way of preventing repeat occurrences. Critical analysis of errors can be used to initiate changes in patient care, equipment, and organization of the APS.[144] Efforts to improve pain management therefore involve much more than just improving pain assessment and documentation, and an APS should include the use of evidence-based treatment regimens,

RAH Drug Committee
Revised August 2006
Planned Review Date August 2007

Royal Adelaide Hospital Guidelines
DOSAGE GUIDELINES FOR INTERMITTENT IMMEDIATE-RELEASE ORAL OXYCODONE ADMINISTRATION
For Acute Pain Management

- Recommended opioid doses are based on average analgesic requirements of opioid-naïve patients following moderate to major surgery
- Avoid co-administration of sedatives with opioids where possible
- Avoid co-administration of other opioids (eg morphine, hydromorphone, Panadeine Forte) – ensure 1 hour has elapsed since the last dose when changing to a different immediate-release opioid.
- Consideration should be given to dosage amendment in differing clinical situations.
- Dose requirements of opioids for analgesia for patients on long term opioid therapy may be higher.
- The best clinical predictor of opioid dose is patient age[1]
- Slow-release oxycodone (Oxycontin) is not recommended for management of acute pain. At the RAH, patients can only be commenced on Oxycontin by the Pain Management, Palliative Care or Cancer Services

[1] Macintyre PE, Jarvis DA. Age is the best predictor of postoperative morphine requirements. Pain 64(2): 357-64 1996

Table : Initial Immediate-release Oral Oxycodone Orders

Age (Years)	Oxycodone Dose range (mg)
< 15	*
15 - 39	15 - 25
40 - 59	10 – 20
60 - 69	5 – 15
70 - 85	5 – 10
> 85	2.5 - 5

Please direct any queries to:
- Acute Pain Service OR
- Medicines Information Centre Pharmacy Department Phone 25546

* Contact WCH Drug Information Centre or WCH Department of Anaesthesia for advice on opioid doses for children <15 years

- Order recommended dose of oxycodone 2 hourly prn.
- Suggest start in middle of dose range.
- Upper limit of dose range can be increased if analgesia is inadequate, and if sedation score is less than 2 and respiratory rate greater than 8/min.

Use of Oxycodone as a discharge medication
- Oxycodone is not recommended for routine prescription on discharge
- If it is to be prescribed, both the patient and the patient's general practitioner should be informed that it is recommended that it be used only for a maximum of a week after discharge and in decreasing daily doses. Re-prescription is not recommended. If the patient's pain persists they should be reviewed.

MONITORING OF THERAPY IS ESSENTIAL
For monitoring requirements, refer to RAH Guidelines for Intermittent Oral Oxycodone Administration

Royal Adelaide Hospital has endeavoured to ensure that the information in this publication is accurate, however it makes no representation or warranty to this effect. You rely on this publication at your own risk. Royal Adelaide Hospital disclaims all liability for any claims, losses, damages, costs and expenses suffered or incurred as a result of reliance on this publication. As the information in this publication is subject to review, please contact a medical or health professional before using this publication

(a)

Figure 47.4 Example of guidelines for intermittent oral oxycodone (continued over). Reproduced with permission of the Royal Adelaide Hospital, South Australia.

pain management quality improvement (QI) measures, and increased patient involvement.[145]

Traditionally, three aspects of an APS can be audited:

1. **Outcome** – patient satisfaction, analgesic efficacy, side effects (e.g. emesis, pruritus), critical incidents, length of hospital stay, complications, mobilization, bowel and bladder function;
2. **Structure** – staff, equipment;
3. **Process** – patients (e.g. number, origin, age, surgical procedure), techniques (e.g. type, duration, drug, failure rate), service (e.g. response times, missed follow up), documentation (e.g. pain, side effects).

Recommended quality indicators and suggested measures for acute pain management have been published by the American Pain Society[145] and the Royal College of Anaesthetists.[146]

The key to effective QI is the cycle whereby audit information is collected, analyzed, and reviewed; changes are then agreed and standards set; the changes are implemented; and after a period of time the cycle repeated. Institutional barriers to this labor-intensive QI approach must be addressed in order for this process to be effective. Such barriers include lack of administrative support and resources for data collection, analysis, and review of changes needed; a reliance on written information rather than face-to-face information and education sessions with staff in order to facilitate implementation of change; and resistance to change (see Chapter 48, Acute pain services and organizational change).[145] Gordon et al.[145] also highlight the critical role of physician leadership in QI programs and change, rather than just physician involvement, and that an interdisciplinary team approach is essential to change as an individual person or discipline acting alone often fails to achieve the desired outcomes.

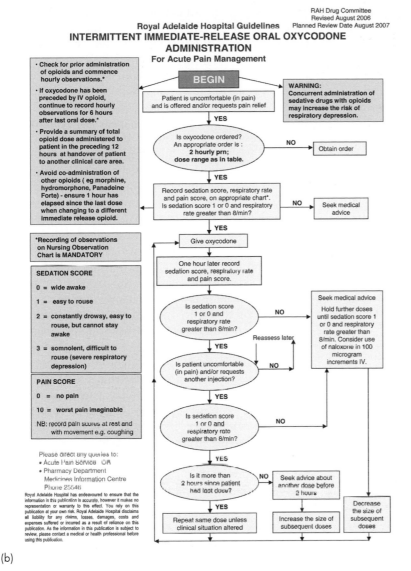

Figure 47.4 Example of guidelines for intermittent oral oxycodone. Reproduced with permission of the Royal Adelaide Hospital, South Australia (continued).

Regular audit of the activity and outcomes of an APS will allow appropriate review and adjustment of management protocols and continuing staff education. However, this requires a reliable method of data collection.

In recent years, the use of personal digital assistants (PDA) on APS rounds has become increasingly common.[147, 148, 149, 150] Chan et al.[148] compared a PDA-based data management system with their previous paper system, looking at factors such as ease of use, the time taken to conduct the APS round, and the amount of paper saved. While they found no difference in user satisfaction, there was a significant saving in paper and man-hours with the PDA system. Lee et al.[147] also reported that a PDA system resulted in much faster data management.

It is very difficult to maintain interest in reporting and to achieve any degree of completeness over long periods of time. Reporting procedures need to be available, simple, confidential, involve feedback, and result in effective changes. An enthusiastic and vigilant coordinator is essential.

Communication and collaboration

Within each institution there must be clearly defined lines of communication and accountability for acute pain management.[145] Communication between the acute pain team and the varied departments accommodating patients is vitally important and can be facilitated by the designation of nurse unit teachers or link nurses. These can be involved in regular meetings with the APS and be responsible for the two-way dissemination of information between the APS and their clinical areas. The members of the APS team should also meet regularly to review problems and progress and to revise management strategies as needed. Surgeons and physicians responsible for other clinical areas and administrative, medical, and nursing managers need to be kept abreast of the APS developments through meetings and reports.

In addition, and in view of the complexity (medical comorbidities and/or pain issues) of patients often seen by an APS and the likelihood of shared care of a patient, members of the APS team will need to communicate and collaborate with members of other medical and nursing services. This may include, but is not limited to, chronic pain clinics, palliative care services, and drug and alcoholic services.

Arrangements for cover out of normal hours should be detailed in the APS documentation and all staff made aware of these. Different disciplines may be responsible for different aspects of the service and lines of communication and continuity of care need to be clearly delineated. This is also true for the relationship with and responsibility for any chronic pain inpatients and for other shared patients. Therapy commenced during the inpatient phase of treatment is often aimed at dealing with the immediate problem to facilitate discharge; mechanisms to ensure appropriate follow up of these patients is essential.

CONCLUSIONS

Acute pain services are essential to the organization of care for patients who have acute pain following surgery, trauma, or medical conditions. Their introduction has led to improved pain relief as a result of a multidisciplinary approach to education, training, and assessment and the safe introduction of more effective methods of analgesia.

The role of an APS has changed significantly since the first APS was implemented. APS teams now commonly manage more complex pain problems and acute pain in increasingly more complex patients. APS can also play a significant role in admission planning by taking an active part in preoperative assessment – not just in terms of patient education and explanations about acute pain management, but also in identifying those patients who have high predictors for the risk of developing persistent postsurgical pain or with more complex comorbidities such as opioid tolerance, substance abuse disorders, or chronic pain.

Although the early emphasis on acute pain management alone was essential, experience over the last 20 years has resulted in an increased awareness of two features of treating this particular (acute pain) patient population that would be improved by integration with other clinicians and other clinical services.

The first is that treatment of pain *per se* will not necessarily improve surgical outcome and that analgesia should not be considered in isolation but as a component of a multimodal clinical pathways approach to perioperative care to facilitate rehabilitation and recovery.[2]

Second, separation of APS teams from existing CPS may result in a simplistic approach to pain relief, emphasizing the treatment of the nociceptive element of postoperative pain. This may result in the underdiagnosis and undertreatment of neuropathic pain occurring in the early postinjury period, with the subsequent development of chronic pain states and referral to CPS. In addition, this artificial distinction between the two types of services may lead to suboptimal management of patients presenting at the interface of acute and chronic pain management.

One possibility in the future is that pain services are defined as inpatient and outpatient, rather than APS and CPS to ensure appropriate resources for both arms of the service whilst recognizing that pain has few, if any, artificial boundaries and that a comprehensive approach to pain is required in both circumstances. Whatever nomenclature is used, services must be structured to allow flow between inpatient and outpatient services and the training of medical and nursing staff must reflect the wider range of skills and knowledge required by inpatient clinicians beyond the traditional need to manage only acute pain.

In addition to the need to ensure the development of a comprehensive integrated pain service, one must not forget the needs of perioperative patients and the need to integrate pain management strategies with other overlapping issues, such as postoperative nausea and vomiting, thromboprophylaxis, fluid and electrolyte management, control of blood pressure, sepsis, and hypoxemia and other respiratory complications. The importance of the expertise gained by the members of APS and their role in perioperative medicine, as part of a fast-track team, and in the development of critical care outreach teams is to be encouraged.

ACKNOWLEDGMENTS

This chapter is updated and expanded from Wheatley RG and Madej TH. Organization of an acute pain service. In: Rowbotham DJ and Macintyre PE (eds). *Clinical Pain Management: Acute Pain*, 1st edn. London: Hodder Arnold, 2003.

REFERENCES

1. Cousins MJ, Brennan F, Carr DB. Pain relief: a universal human right. *Pain.* 2004; **112**: 1–4.
2. Werner MU. The acute pain service: present and future role. *Current Anaesthesia and Critical Care.* 2007; **18**: 125–9.
3. Rawal N. Organization, function, and implementation of acute pain service. *Anesthesiology Clinics of North America.* 2005; **23**: 211–25.
* 4. Royal College of Surgeons and College of Anaesthetists. *Working party report on pain after surgery.* London: Royal College of Surgeons and College of Anaesthetists, 1990.

5. Duncan FM, Counsell DJ. Pain relief in the high risk patient. In: McConachie I (ed.). *Anaesthesia in the high risk patient.* Cambridge: Cambridge University Press, 2001: 51–64.

6. Perkins FM, Kehlet H. Chronic pain as an outcome of surgery. A review of predictive factors. *Anesthesiology.* 2000; **93**: 1123–33.

7. Kehlet H, Jensen TS, Woolf CJ. Persistent postsurgical pain: risk factors and prevention. *Lancet.* 2006; **367**: 1618–25.

8. Macrae WA. Chronic pain after surgery. *British Journal of Anaesthesia.* 2001; **87**: 88–98.

9. Katz WA, Rothenberg R. Section 3: The nature of pain: pathophysiology. *Journal of Clinical Rheumatology.* 2005; **11**: S11–15.

10. Poleshuck EL, Katz J, Andrus CH *et al.* Risk factors for chronic pain following breast cancer surgery: a prospective study. *Journal of Pain.* 2006; **7**: 626–34.

11. Kehlet H. Future perspectives and research initiatives in fast-track surgery. *Langenbeck's Archives of Surgery.* 2006; **391**: 495–8.

12. Kehlet H. Fast-track colonic surgery: status and perspectives. *Recent Results in Cancer Research.* 2005; **165**: 8–13.

13. Breivik H. The future role of the anaesthesiologist in pain management. *Acta Anaesthesiologica Scandinavica.* 2005; **49**: 922–6.

14. Kehlet H, Wilmore DW. Fast-track surgery. *British Journal of Surgery.* 2005; **92**: 3–4.

15. White PF, Kehlet H, Neal JM *et al.* The role of the anesthesiologist in fast-track surgery: from multimodal analgesia to perioperative medical care. *Anesthesia and Analgesia.* 2007; **104**: 1380–96.

16. Apfelbaum JL, Chen C, Mehta SS, Gan TJ. Postoperative pain experience: results from a national survey suggest postoperative pain continues to be undermanaged. *Anesthesia and Analgesia.* 2003; **97**: 534–40.

17. Dix P, Sandhar B, Murdoch J, MacIntyre PA. Pain on medical wards in a district general hospital. *British Journal of Anaesthesia.* 2004; **92**: 235–7.

∗ 18. Dolin SJ, Cashman JN, Bland JM. Effectiveness of acute postoperative pain management: I. Evidence from published data. *British Journal of Anaesthesia.* 2002; **89**: 409–23.

19. Warfield CA, Kahn CH. Acute pain management. Programs in U.S. hospitals and experiences and attitudes among U.S. adults. *Anesthesiology.* 1995; **83**: 1090–4.

20. Rocchi A, Chung F, Forte L. Canadian survey of postsurgical pain and pain medication experiences. *Canadian Journal of Anaesthesia.* 2002; **49**: 1053–6.

21. Yates P, Dewar A, Edwards H *et al.* The prevalence and perception of pain amongst hospital in-patients. *Journal of Clinical Nursing.* 1998; **7**: 521–30.

22. Oden R. Acute postoperative pain: Incidence, severity, and the etiology of inadequate treatment. *Anesthesiology Clinics of North America.* 1989; **7**: 1–5.

23. Faculty of Anaesthetists and Royal Australasian College of Surgeons. *Statement on acute pain management.* Melbourne: Faculty of Anaesthetists and Royal Australasian College of Surgeons, 1991.

24. Ready LB, Edwards WT. *Taskforce on Acute Pain. Management of acute pain; a practical guide.* Seattle: IASP Publications, 1992.

25. Carr DB, Jacox AK, Chapman CR *et al. Acute pain management: operative or medical procedures and trauma, clinical practice guideline.* Rockville, MD: Agency for Health Care Policy and Research PHS, US Department of Health and Human Services, 1992.

26. American Society of Anesthesiologists. Practice guidelines for acute pain management in the perioperative setting. A report by the American Society of Anesthesiologists Task Force on Pain Management, Acute Pain Section. *Anesthesiology.* 1995; **82**: 1071–81.

27. College of Paediatrics and Child Health Working Party. *Prevention and control of pain in children.* London: BMJ Publishing, 1997.

28. Association of Anaesthetists of Great Britain and Ireland. *The anaesthesia team.* London: Association of Anaesthetists of Great Britain and Ireland, 1998.

∗ 29. Audit Commission. *Anaesthesia under examination.* London: Audit Commission, 1997.

30. Europain. *Minimum standards for the management of postoperative pain.* Goring on Thames: Pegasus Healthcare International, 1998.

31. National Health and Medical Research Council of Australia. *Acute pain management: scientific evidence.* Canberra: National Health and Medical Research Council of Australia, 1999.

∗ 32. Department of Veterans Affairs. *Clinical practice guidelines for the management of postoperative pain.* Last updated October 2001, cited February 2008. Available from: www.oqp.med.va.gov/cpg/PAIN/PAIN_base.htm.

33. The Royal College of Anaesthetists, the Royal College of Nursing, the Association of Anaesthetists of Great Britain and Ireland, the British Pain Society and the European Society of Regional Anaesthesia and Pain Therapy joint publication. *Good practice in the management of continuous epidural analgesia in the hospital setting.* Last updated November 2004, cited February 2008. Available from: www.rcoa.ac.uk/docs/Epid-Analg.pdf.

∗ 34. American Society of Anesthesiologists. Practice guidelines for acute pain management in the perioperative setting: an updated report by the American Society of Anesthesiologists Task Force on Acute Pain Management. *Anesthesiology.* 2004; **100**: 1573–81.

∗ 35. Australian and New Zealand College of Anaesthetists and Faculty of Pain Medicine. *Acute pain management: scientific evidence,* 2nd edn. Melbourne: Australian and New Zealand College of Anaesthetists. Last updated December 2007, cited February 2008. Available from: www.anzca.edu.au/resources/books-and-publications/acutepain_update.pdf.

36. Australian and New Zealand College of Anaesthetists and Faculty of Pain Medicine. *Guidelines on acute pain management.* Last updated February 2007, cited February 2008. Available from: www.anzca.edu.au/resources/professional-documents/professional-standards/ps41.html.

37. British Pain Society. *Pain and substance misuse: improving the patient experience 2007.* Last updated April 2007, cited February 2008. Available from: www.britishpainsociety.org/pub_professional.htm#misuse.

∗ 38. PROSPECT. *Procedure specfic postoperative pain management.* Cited February 2008. Available from: www.postoppain.org.

39. Nagi H. Acute pain services in the United Kingdom. *Acute Pain.* 2004; **5**: 89–107.

40. Goldstein DH, VanDenKerkhof EG, Blaine WC. Acute pain management services have progressed, albeit insufficiently in Canadian academic hospitals. *Canadian Journal of Anaesthesia.* 2004; **51**: 231–5.

41. Powell AE, Davies HT, Bannister J, Macrae WA. Rhetoric and reality on acute pain services in the UK: a national postal questionnaire survey. *British Journal of Anaesthesia.* 2004; **92**: 689–93.

42. Editorial (Anonymous). *Anaesthesia and Intensive Care.* 1976; **4**: 95.

∗ 43. Ready LB, Oden R, Chadwick HS *et al.* Development of an anesthesiology-based postoperative pain management service. *Anesthesiology.* 1988; **68**: 100–06.

44. Macintyre PE, Runciman WB, Webb RK. An acute pain service in an Australian teaching hospital: the first year. *Medical Journal of Australia.* 1990; **153**: 417–21.

45. Sartain JB, Barry JJ. The impact of an acute pain service on postoperative pain management. *Anaesthesia and Intensive Care.* 1999; **27**: 375–80.

46. Wheatley RG, Madej TH, Jackson IJ, Hunter D. The first year's experience of an acute pain service. *British Journal of Anaesthesia.* 1991; **67**: 353–9.

47. Cartwright PD, Helfinger RG, Howell JJ, Siepmann KK. Introducing an acute pain service. *Anaesthesia.* 1991; **46**: 188–91.

48. Gould TH, Crosby DL, Harmer M *et al.* Policy for controlling pain after surgery: effect of sequential changes in management. *BMJ.* 1992; **305**: 1187–93.

49. Schug SA, Haridas RP. Development and organizational structure of an acute pain service in a major teaching hospital. *Australia and New Zealand Journal of Surgery.* 1993; **63**: 8–13.

50. Maier C, Kibbel K, Mercker S, Wulf H. [Postoperative pain therapy at general nursing stations. An analysis of eight year's experience at an anesthesiological acute pain service]. *Anaesthesist.* 1994; **43**: 385–97.

51. Brodner G, Mertes N, Buerkle H *et al.* Acute pain management: analysis, implications and consequences after prospective experience with 6349 surgical patients. *European Journal of Anaesthesiology.* 2000; **17**: 566–75.

52. Zimmermann DL, Stewart J. Postoperative pain management and acute pain service activity in Canada. *Canadian Journal of Anaesthesia.* 1993; **40**: 568–75.

53. Hu P, Owens T, Harmon D. A survey of acute pain services in teaching hospitals in the Republic of Ireland. *Irish Journal of Medical Science.* 2007; **176**: 225–8.

54. Blanco J, Blanco E, Rodriguez G *et al.* One year's experience with an acute pain service in a Spanish University Clinic hospital. *European Journal of Anaesthesiology.* 1994; **11**: 417–21.

55. Shapiro A, Zohar E, Kantor M *et al.* Establishing a nurse-based, anesthesiologist-supervised inpatient acute pain service: experience of 4,617 patients. *Journal of Clinical Anesthesia.* 2004; **16**: 415–20.

56. Barak M, Poppa E, Tansky A, Drenger B. The activity of an acute pain service in a teaching hospital: five years' experience. *Acute Pain.* 2006; **8**: 155–9.

57. Bardiau FM, Braeckman MM, Seidel L *et al.* Effectiveness of an acute pain service inception in a general hospital. *Journal of Clinical Anesthesia.* 1999; **11**: 583–9.

58. Stadler M, Schlander M, Braeckman M *et al.* A cost-utility and cost-effectiveness analysis of an acute pain service. *Journal of Clinical Anesthesia.* 2004; **16**: 159–67.

59. Moizo E, Berti M, Marchetti C *et al.* Acute Pain Service and multimodal therapy for postsurgical pain control: evaluation of protocol efficacy. *Minerva Anestesiologica.* 2004; **70**: 779–87.

60. Breivik H, Hogstrom H, Niemi G *et al.* Safe and effective postoperative pain relief: introduction and continuous quality improvement of comprehensive postoperative pain management programmes. In: Breivik H (ed.). *Postoperative pain management. Baillière's Clinical Anaesthesiology: International Practice and Research.* London: Baillière Tindall, 1995; **9**: 423–60.

61. Rawal N, Berggren L. Organization of acute pain services: a low-cost model. *Pain.* 1994; **57**: 117–23.

62. Bredahl C, Dahl BL, Toft P. [Acute pain service. Organization and results]. *Ugeskrift for Laeger.* 1998; **160**: 6070–4.

63. Kubler A, Zolnowska A, Zielinski S *et al.* [Organization of services for treatment of postoperative pain – 3-year experience]. *Przeglad Lekarski.* 1998; **55**: 325–7.

64. Anwari JS, Ahmed F, Mustafa T. An audit of acute pain service in Central, Saudi Arabia. *Saudi Medical Journal.* 2005; **26**: 298–305.

65. Tsui SL, Irwin MG, Wong CM *et al.* An audit of the safety of an acute pain service. *Anaesthesia.* 1997; **52**: 1042–7.

66. Hung CT, Lau LL, Chan CK *et al.* Acute pain services in Hong Kong: facilities, volume, and quality. *Hong Kong Medical Journal.* 2002; **8**: 196–201.

67. Vijayan R, Delilkan AE. First year's experience with an acute pain service – University Hospital Kuala Lumpur. *Medical Journal of Malaysia.* 1994; **49**: 385–400.

68. Neelima G, Chieng DC, Lim TA, Inbasegaran K. A review of the acute pain service in Hospital Kuala Lumpur. *Medical Journal of Malaysia*. 2003; **58**: 167–79.

69. Shah MK. Acute pain service, Kandang Kerbau Hospital, 1995 – a first year's experience. *Singapore Medical Journal*. 1997; **38**: 375–8.

70. Wong LT, Koh LH, Kaur K, Boey SK. A two-year experience of an acute pain service in Singapore. *Singapore Medical Journal*. 1997; **38**: 209–13.

71. Yimyaem PR, Kritsasaprakornkit W, Thienthong S *et al.* Postoperative pain management by an acute pain service in a university hospital in Thailand. *Acute Pain*. 2006; **8**: 161–7.

72. Macintyre PE, Schug SA. *Acute pain management: a practical guide*, 3rd edn. London: Saunders, 2007.

73. Rawal N. Organization of acute pain services – a low-cost model. *Acta Anaesthesiologica Scandinavica Supplement*. 1997; **111**: 188–90.

74. Rawal N. Postoperative pain treatment for ambulatory surgery. *Best Practice and Research. Clinical Anaesthesiology*. 2007; **21**: 129–48.

75. Shang AB, Gan TJ. Optimising postoperative pain management in the ambulatory patient. *Drugs*. 2003; **63**: 855–67.

76. Grant PS. Analgesia delivery in the ED. *American Journal of Emergency Medicine*. 2006; **24**: 806–9.

77. Sandhu S, Driscoll P, Nancarrow J, McHugh D. Analgesia in the accident and emergency department: do SHOs have the knowledge to provide optimal analgesia? *Journal of Accident and Emergency Medicine*. 1998; **15**: 147–50.

78. Goodacre SW, Roden RK. A protocol to improve analgesia use in the accident and emergency department. *Journal of Accident and Emergency Medicine*. 1996; **13**: 177–9.

79. McArthur E, Cunliffe M. Pain assessment and documentation – making a difference. *Journal of Child Health Care*. 1998; **2**: 164–9.

80. Golianu B, Krane EJ, Galloway KS, Yaster M. Pediatric acute pain management. *Pediatric Clinics of North America*. 2000; **47**: 559–87.

81. Walker SM. Acute pain management in pediatric patients. *International Anesthesiology Clinics*. 1997; **35**: 105–30.

82. Harvey AJ, Morton NS. Management of procedural pain in children. *Archives of Disease in Childhood. Education and Practice Edition*. 2007; **92**: ep20–6.

83. Summer GJ, Puntillo KA, Miaskowski C *et al.* Burn injury pain: the continuing challenge. *Journal of Pain*. 2007; **8**: 533–48.

84. Summer GJ, Puntillo KA. Management of surgical and procedural pain in a critical care setting. *Critical Care Nursing Clinics of North America*. 2001; **13**: 233–42.

85. Heafield RH. The management of procedural pain. *Professional Nurse*. 1999; **15**: 127–9.

86. Gallagher G, Rae CP, Kinsella J. Treatment of pain in severe burns. *American Journal of Clinical Dermatology*. 2000; **1**: 329–35.

87. Murat I, Gall O, Tourniaire B. Procedural pain in children: evidence-based best practice and guidelines. *Regional Anesthesia and Pain Medicine*. 2003; **28**: 561–72.

88. Lauri S, Lepisto M, Kappeli S. Patients' needs in hospital: nurses' and patients' views. *Journal of Advanced Nursing*. 1997; **25**: 339–46.

89. Gilron I. Review article: the role of anticonvulsant drugs in postoperative pain management: a bench-to-bedside perspective. *Canadian Journal of Anaesthesia*. 2006; **53**: 562–71.

* 90. Story DA, Shelton AC, Poustie SJ *et al.* Effect of an anaesthesia department led critical care outreach and acute pain service on postoperative serious adverse events. *Anaesthesia*. 2006; **61**: 24–8.

91. Counsell DJ. The acute pain service: a model for outreach critical care. *Anaesthesia*. 2001; **56**: 925–6.

92. Kehlet H, Dahl JB. Anaesthesia, surgery, and challenges in postoperative recovery. *Lancet*. 2003; **362**: 1921–8.

93. Faculty of Pain Medicine, Australian and New Zealand College of Anaesthetists. *Guidelines for units offering training in multidisciplinary pain medicine*. Last updated October 2005, cited February 2008. Available from: www.anzca.edu.au/fpm/resources/professional-documents/pm2.

94. Karlsten R, Strom K, Gunningberg L. Improving assessment of postoperative pain in surgical wards by education and training. *Quality and Safety in Health Care*. 2005; **14**: 332–5.

* 95. Werner MU, Soholm L, Rotboll-Nielsen P, Kehlet H. Does an acute pain service improve postoperative outcome? *Anesthesia and Analgesia*. 2002; **95**: 1361–72.

96. Breivik H. How to implement an acute pain service. *Best Practice and Research. Clinical Anaesthesiology*. 2002; **16**: 527–47.

97. Department of Health. *Comprehensive critical care: a review of adult critical care services*. London: Department of Health, 2000.

98. McDonnell A, Nicholl J, Read SM. Acute pain teams and the management of postoperative pain: a systematic review and meta-analysis. *Journal of Advanced Nursing*. 2003; **41**: 261–73.

99. Stacey BR, Rudy TE, Nelhaus D. Management of patient-controlled analgesia: a comparison of primary surgeons and a dedicated pain service. *Anesthesia and Analgesia*. 1997; **85**: 130–4.

100. Coleman SA, Booker-Milburn J. Audit of postoperative pain control. Influence of a dedicated acute pain nurse. *Anaesthesia*. 1996; **51**: 1093–6.

101. Harmer M, Davies KA. The effect of education, assessment and a standardised prescription on postoperative pain management. The value of clinical audit in the establishment of acute pain services. *Anaesthesia*. 1998; **53**: 424–30.

102. Salomaki TE, Hokajarvi TM, Ranta P, Alahuhta S. Improving the quality of postoperative pain relief. *European Journal of Pain*. 2000; **4**: 367–72.

103. Miaskowski C, Crews J, Ready LB *et al.* Anesthesia-based pain services improve the quality of postoperative pain management. *Pain.* 1999; **80**: 23–9.

104. Tasmuth T, Blomqvist C, Kalso E. Chronic post-treatment symptoms in patients with breast cancer operated in different surgical units. *European Journal of Surgical Oncology.* 1999; **25**: 38–43.

105. Katz J, Jackson M, Kavanagh BP, Sandler AN. Acute pain after thoracic surgery predicts long-term post-thoracotomy pain. *Clinical Journal of Pain.* 1996; **12**: 50–5.

106. Senturk M, Ozcan PE, Talu GK *et al.* The effects of three different analgesia techniques on long-term postthoracotomy pain. *Anesthesia and Analgesia.* 2002; **94**: 11–15.

107. Caumo W, Schmidt AP, Schneider CN *et al.* Preoperative predictors of moderate to intense acute postoperative pain in patients undergoing abdominal surgery. *Acta Anaesthesiologica Scandinavica.* 2002; **46**: 1265–71.

108. Nikolajsen L, Ilkjaer S, Kroner K *et al.* The influence of preamputation pain on postamputation stump and phantom pain. *Pain.* 1997; **72**: 393–405.

109. Jung BF, Johnson RW, Griffin DR, Dworkin RH. Risk factors for postherpetic neuralgia in patients with herpes zoster. *Neurology.* 2004; **62**: 1545–51.

110. Stubhaug A, Breivik H. Prevention and treatment of hyperalgesia and persistent neuropathic pain after surgery. In: Breivik H, Shipley M (eds). *Pain – best practice and research compendium.* London: Elsevier, 2007: 281–6.

111. Obata H, Saito S, Fujita N *et al.* Epidural block with mepivacaine before surgery reduces long-term post-thoracotomy pain. *Canadian Journal of Anaesthesia.* 1999; **46**: 1127–32.

112. Gehling M, Tryba M. [Prophylaxis of phantom pain: is regional analgesia ineffective?]. *Schmerz.* 2003; **17**: 11–19.

113. Nikolajsen L, Ilkjaer S, Christensen JH *et al.* Randomised trial of epidural bupivacaine and morphine in prevention of stump and phantom pain in lower-limb amputation. *Lancet.* 1997; **350**: 1353–7.

114. Bowsher D. The effects of pre-emptive treatment of postherpetic neuralgia with amitriptyline: a randomized, double-blind, placebo-controlled trial. *Journal of Pain and Symptom Management.* 1997; **13**: 327–31.

115. Lee A, Chan S, Chen PP *et al.* Economic evaluations of acute pain service programs: a systematic review. *Clinical Journal of Pain.* 2007; **23**: 726–33.

116. Breivik H. Benefits, risks and economics of postoperative pain management programmes. In: Breivik H (ed.). *Postoperative pain management.* London: Baillière Tindall, 1995: 403–22.

117. Johansson K, Nuutila L, Virtanen H *et al.* Preoperative education for orthopaedic patients: systematic review. *Journal of Advanced Nursing.* 2005; **50**: 212–23.

118. Kindler CH, Seeberger MD, Staender SE. Epidural abscess complicating epidural anesthesia and analgesia. An analysis of the literature. *Acta Anaesthesiologica Scandinavica.* 1998; **42**: 614–20.

119. Hearn M. Epidural abscess complicating insertion of epidural catheters. *British Journal of Anaesthesia.* 2003; **90**: 706–07.

120. Wang LP, Hauerberg J, Schmidt JF. Incidence of spinal epidural abscess after epidural analgesia: a national 1-year survey. *Anesthesiology.* 1999; **91**: 1928–36.

121. Christie IW, McCabe S. Major complications of epidural analgesia after surgery: results of a six-year survey. *Anaesthesia.* 2007; **62**: 335–41.

122. Cameron CM, Scott DA, McDonald WM, Davies MJ. A review of neuraxial epidural morbidity: experience of more than 8,000 cases at a single teaching hospital. *Anesthesiology.* 2007; **106**: 997–1002.

123. Moen V, Dahlgren N, Irestedt L. Severe neurological complications after central neuraxial blockades in Sweden 1990–1999. *Anesthesiology.* 2004; **101**: 950–9.

124. Breivik H, Curatolo M, Niemi G *et al.* How to implement an acute postoperative pain service: an update. In: Breivik H, Shipley M (eds). *Pain – best practice and research compendium.* London: Elsevier, 2007: 255–70.

125. Grond S, Hall J, Spacek A *et al.* Iontophoretic transdermal system using fentanyl compared with patient-controlled intravenous analgesia using morphine for postoperative pain management. *British Journal of Anaesthesia.* 2007; **98**: 806–15.

126. Rawal N, Langford RM. Current practices for postoperative pain management in Europe and the potential role of the fentanyl HCl iontophoretic transdermal system. *European Journal of Anaesthesiology.* 2007; **24**: 299–308.

127. Curatolo M, Schnider TW, Petersen-Felix S *et al.* A direct search procedure to optimize combinations of epidural bupivacaine, fentanyl, and clonidine for postoperative analgesia. *Anesthesiology.* 2000; **92**: 325–37.

128. Merskey H. Pain terms: a list with definitions and notes on usage. Recommended by the Subcommittee on Taxonomy. *Pain.* 1979; **6**: 249–52.

129. Teske K, Daut RL, Cleeland CS. Relationships between nurses' observations and patients' self-reports of pain. *Pain.* 1983; **16**: 289–96.

130. Seers K. Perceptions of pain. *Nursing Times.* 1987; **83**: 37–9.

131. Scott DA, McDonald W. *Measuring pain management.* Melbourne: Victorian Quality Council, 2004.

132. Catley DM, Thornton C, Jordan C *et al.* Pronounced, episodic oxygen desaturation in the postoperative period: its association with ventilatory pattern and analgesic regimen. *Anesthesiology.* 1985; **63**: 20–8.

133. Peady C. Unauthorised access to the contents of a Graseby 3300 PCA pump. *Anaesthesia.* 2007; **62**: 98–9; discussion 9.

∗134. Vila Jr H, Smith RA, Augustyniak MJ *et al.* The efficacy and safety of pain management before and after implementation of hospital-wide pain management standards: is patient safety compromised by treatment based solely on numerical pain ratings? *Anesthesia and Analgesia.* 2005; **101**: 474–80.

135. Cashman JN, Dolin SJ. Respiratory and haemodynamic effects of acute postoperative pain management: evidence from published data. *British Journal of Anaesthesia.* 2004; **93**: 212–23.

136. Wheatley RG, Schug SA, Watson D. Safety and efficacy of postoperative epidural analgesia. *British Journal of Anaesthesia.* 2001; **87**: 47–61.

137. Neal JM, Wilcox RT, Allen HW, Low DE. Near-total esophagectomy: the influence of standardized multimodal management and intraoperative fluid restriction. *Regional Anesthesia and Pain Medicine.* 2003; **28**: 328–34.

138. Brandstrup B, Tonnesen H, Beier-Holgersen R *et al.* Effects of intravenous fluid restriction on postoperative complications: comparison of two perioperative fluid regimens: a randomized assessor-blinded multicenter trial. *Annals of Surgery.* 2003; **238**: 641–8.

139. Holte K, Foss NB, Andersen J *et al.* Liberal or restrictive fluid administration in fast-track colonic surgery: a randomized, double-blind study. *British Journal of Anaesthesia.* 2007; **99**: 500–08.

140. MacKay G, Fearon K, McConnachie A *et al.* Randomized clinical trial of the effect of postoperative intravenous fluid restriction on recovery after elective colorectal surgery. *British Journal of Surgery.* 2006; **93**: 1469–74.

141. Horlocker TT, Wedel DJ, Benzon H *et al.* Regional anesthesia in the anticoagulated patient: defining the risks (the second ASRA Consensus Conference on Neuraxial Anesthesia and Anticoagulation). *Regional Anesthesia and Pain Medicine.* 2003; **28**: 172–97.

142. Bromage P. *Epidural analgesia.* Philadelphia: WB Saunders, 1978.

143. Abd Elrazek E, Scott NB, Vohra A. An epidural scoring scale for arm movements (ESSAM) in patients receiving high thoracic epidural analgesia for coronary artery bypass grafting. *Anaesthesia.* 1999; **54**: 1104–09.

144. Chen PP, Ma M, Chan S, Oh TE. Incident reporting in acute pain management. *Anaesthesia.* 1998; **53**: 730–5.

145. Gordon DB, Dahl JL, Miaskowski C *et al.* American Pain Society recommendations for improving the quality of acute and cancer pain management: American Pain Society Quality of Care Task Force. *Archives of Internal Medicine.* 2005; **165**: 1574–80.

146. Royal College of Anaesthetists. *Raising the standard: a compendium of audit recipes.* Last updated 2006; cited February 2008. Available from: www.rcoa.ac.uk/index.asp?PageID=125.

147. Lee YL, Wu JL, Wu HS *et al.* The use of portable computer for information acquirement during anesthesiologist's ward round in acute pain service. *Acta Anaesthesiologica Taiwanica.* 2007; **45**: 79–87.

148. Chan SS, Chu CP, Cheng BC, Chen PP. Data management using the personal digital assistant in an acute pain service. *Anaesthesia and Intensive Care.* 2004; **32**: 81–6.

149. Goldstein DH, Wilson R, VanDenKerkof EG. Electronic monitoring in an acute pain management service. *Pain Medicine.* 2007; **8**: S94–100.

150. VanDenKerkhof EG, Goldstein DH, Lane J *et al.* Using a personal digital assistant enhances gathering of patient data on an acute pain management service: a pilot study: [L'utilisation d'un assistant numerique personnel facilite la cueillette de donnees d'un service de traitement de la douleur aigue: une etude pilote]. *Canadian Journal of Anaesthesia.* 2003; **50**: 368–75.

48

Acute pain services and organizational change

ALISON E POWELL, HUW TO DAVIES, JONATHAN BANNISTER, AND WILLIAM A MACRAE

KEY LEARNING POINTS

- Despite many reports and recommendations, acute pain services have struggled to embed lasting changes in routine postoperative pain management.
- The challenges that acute pain services face stem from three inter-related aspects of organizational change: the content, context, and process of change.

- Improving postoperative pain management will require difficult and controversial changes in attitudes, beliefs, and local practices.

INTRODUCTION

Recognition that postoperative pain management was inadequate in many hospitals in the UK National Health Service (NHS) led to the development of acute pain services (APSs) in the 1990s, with successive reports over the decade endorsing and developing the early recommendations.[1] Similar developments were also occurring outside the UK.[2, 3, 4, 5] However, despite the hard work of many committed individuals, successive studies[1, 6, 7, 8, 9] show that services have struggled to secure funding and recognition, and are sometimes unable to embed changes in postoperative pain management practice across their hospitals. This chapter is rooted in the experience of implementing acute pain services in the UK, but many of the problems described here are reflected in the experience of APSs in other countries.[10, 11]

The chapter examines why implementing acute pain services in the NHS has been so difficult and suggests

areas that need to be addressed in order to make further progress. It draws on research on NHS acute pain services and on broader research on organizational change in health care and other settings. The chapter will not deal with the mechanics of setting up and running an acute pain service as these issues have been comprehensively covered elsewhere[5, 12, 13] (see Chapter 51, Where does pain fit within healthcare delivery systems and organizations? and Chapter 47, Organization and role of acute pain services, and Chapter 17, Postoperative pain management following day surgery in the *Acute Pain* volume of this series). Instead, it will shed light on some of the underlying organizational factors that have undermined efforts to implement acute pain services and improve postoperative pain management.

The chapter will be structured in four parts. First we will briefly review the policy background to acute pain services in the UK NHS. We will then look at what studies of pain services show about the problems experienced in trying to implement these policies. The third part of the chapter considers APS implementation as an example of organizational change and uses insights from the organizational change literature to explore why implementation has been so challenging. Finally, we suggest areas that will need to be addressed in order to make further progress. While these conclusions will be rooted in a detailed examination of NHS services, it is our contention that the lessons drawn have wider applicability.

THE POLICY BACKGROUND TO NHS ACUTE PAIN SERVICES

Published evidence of under-treatment of postoperative pain goes back at least as far as the 1950s[14] but the problem was not formally acknowledged in the NHS until the publication in September 1990 of the *Report of the Working Party on Pain after Surgery*.[15] Commonly referred to as *Pain after Surgery*, the report is widely acknowledged as having provided the impetus for the development of acute pain services in the NHS.[16] *Pain after Surgery* lacked much detail on how the new acute pain services should be implemented but the report nevertheless formally made the explicit recommendation that "This service should be introduced in all major hospitals performing surgery in the UK".[15] This recommendation was then further endorsed by a series of documents published in the NHS in the following decade by a range of bodies, including government departments and professional organizations (**Table 48.1**).

Although these UK policy documents varied in the amount of detail they had, and there were few specific details about the practicalities of service provision (e.g. the number of nursing staff required per patient group), there was nevertheless a set of broad expectations about what acute pain services were intended to do in key areas.[17] For example, the acute pain service was to ensure that the following were in place: a hospital-wide strategy for acute pain management that would benefit all surgical patients; a standardized approach to the routine assessment of postoperative pain throughout the organization; appropriate written and verbal information for patients; and arrangements in place to ensure continuity of pain control after discharge.

Despite the flurry of reports in the decade following *Pain after Surgery*, implementing acute pain services was far from complete by 2000. The most striking change was in the number of hospitals with an acute pain service. When *Pain after Surgery* was published in 1990, only around 3 percent of NHS hospitals had an acute pain service.[18] By 1994, around 43 percent of hospitals had some form of acute pain service,[6, 18] and by 1997 there was an acute pain service in the overwhelming majority of trusts (88 percent).[8] However, although many hospitals had responded to the headline recommendation and set up an acute pain service (in name at least), these services were often struggling to implement the spirit and the letter of the more detailed practice changes around postoperative pain management.

IMPLEMENTATION PROBLEMS IN ACUTE PAIN SERVICES

Acute pain services typically faced problems in four related areas:

1. securing funding and recognition;
2. changing the attitudes of health professionals and managers towards pain management;
3. encouraging effective working between health professionals;
4. providing training to enable health professionals to deliver high quality pain management.

Table 48.1 Main UK reports making recommendations on acute pain services and postoperative pain management published between *Pain after Surgery* (1990) and 2000.

Published UK reports making recommendations on acute pain services and postoperative pain management	
1992	Protocol for Investment in Health Gain; Pain, Discomfort and Palliative Care	NHS Directorate, Welsh Office, Welsh Health Planning Forum
1994	Guidance for Purchasers on Pain Management Services	Royal College of Anaesthetists
1996	The Provision of Services for Acute Postoperative Pain in Scotland	Scottish Office, Department of Health
1997	Provision of Pain Services	Association of Anaesthetists/Pain Society
1997	Anaesthesia under Examination	Audit Commission
1997	A Guide to Pain Management	NHS Wales
1998	The Anaesthesia Team	Association of Anaesthetists
1999	Guidelines for the Provision of Anaesthetic Services – Guidance on Pain Management Services (update of 1994 document)	Royal College of Anaesthetists
2000	Services for Patients with Pain	Clinical Standards Advisory Group

These problems led to important gaps in services (**Box 48.1**): many acute pain services could only focus on the care of patients who were using specialized forms of analgesia; routine pain assessment was patchy; and there were problems providing cover out of hours and at weekends. Data from the most recent UK survey[31] show the extent to which these problems are ongoing (**Box 48.2**).

This faltering implementation of acute pain services took place against a background of much debate about the role, structure, and remit of such services. In the discussion sections of empirical papers, in editorials, in discussion pieces, and in the correspondence pages of professional journals, acute pain clinicians wrestled with such issues as the role of the acute pain service and the key components of the service;[18, 32, 33] the future development of acute pain services and their relationship with other acute services;[34, 35, 36, 37, 38, 39, 40] and whether acute pain services should exist as discrete services or whether pain management should be delivered through integrated pain services covering all types of pain.[41, 42] It is possible therefore that implementation was impeded at least in part by the lack of clarity and consensus about these issues, which created uncertainty and provided a "loophole" for funders and professionals who did not want to

---

Box 48.1 Introducing acute pain services to the UK: key problems

- Difficulties making documented pain assessment a routine part of care for all postoperative patients.
- Problems providing a service out of hours and at weekends.
- Difficulties in providing a service for all postoperative patients and not just patients using specialized forms of analgesia (e.g. PCA/epidural).
- Low level of formal involvement of other health professionals (e.g. pharmacists, physiotherapists).
- Low levels of robust local audit; lack of national standards against which local services could be developed and audited.
- Education programs hampered by service workloads and high turnover of some staff (e.g. junior doctors).
- Problems developing high quality guidelines and protocols.
- Lack of information for patients.
- Limited attention to arrangements for control of pain after discharge home.

Derived from Refs 6, 7, 8, 18, 19, 20, 21, 22, 23, 24, 25, 26, 27, 28, 29, 30.

Box 48.2 Improvements needed in postoperative pain management: main results from a UK survey[31]

Data were received on 325 hospitals out of 403 contacted (81 percent): 270 hospitals had an Acute Pain Service (83 percent); 55 did not (17 percent). The data below are from the 270 hospitals with an APS.

Availability of the pain service

- The majority of acute pain services (84 percent) were only available in full during daytime hours Monday to Friday.
- In the majority of hospitals (61 percent), the only provision for pain services out of hours was the on-call anesthetist.

Pain scoring

- Less than two-thirds of hospitals carried out pain scoring with all surgical inpatients.
- Less than two-thirds of hospitals carried out pain scoring as often as recommended (i.e. with other observations or more frequently).
- Only one in six hospitals continued pain scoring until discharge home.
- Pain scoring was no more established in day surgery units: one in six DSUs carried out no pain scoring at all; less than half carried out pain scoring as often as recommended, and only a third continued pain scoring until discharge home.

Management of postoperative nausea and vomiting

- Only half of hospitals had a protocol/established practice for postoperative nausea and vomiting (PONV) management for all patients.
- In a quarter of hospitals, PONV management was left to the individual doctor.

Pain control after discharge

- One in three hospitals provided day surgery patients with less than three days supply of analgesics.
- Only a third of hospitals advised day case patients about over the counter (OTC) analgesics; less than a quarter advised inpatients about them.
- Less than half of hospitals gave day case patients written information on pain control; less than a third of hospitals did so for inpatients.

introduce the full APS model or who wanted to delay implementation pending further developments.

Despite the many areas of contention, there was some agreement. In particular, it was agreed that improving postoperative pain management was not necessarily a question of developing new treatments and delivery techniques.[31] Many clinicians thought that improvements could be made through organizational approaches to make the best use of existing techniques and expertise.[31]

Taking this perspective and looking at improving postoperative pain management as an organizational problem, we are able to draw on the substantial organizational literature. This literature contains many insights into how organizations function, but is not always well known or applied in health care. The next section uses insights from part of this literature to explore APS implementation problems further.

APS IMPLEMENTATION: INSIGHTS FROM THE ORGANIZATIONAL CHANGE LITERATURE

Putting an innovation such as acute pain services into the NHS is an example of a generic challenge faced by all organizations, that of organizational change. The organizational change literature is vast and spread across a range of organizational disciplines: the literature covers behavioral, structural, and cultural approaches that each have their own disciplinary roots and change focus.[43, 44] In order to structure this part of the chapter, we will use one influential framework which has been used by a range of authors in looking at aspects of organizational change in health care and in other settings.[45, 46]

The processual-contextual perspective or content, context, and process (CCP) framework emphasizes the interplay of three overlapping key aspects: the nature of the change, the context in which it occurs and the process by which change unfolds[47] (**Box 48.3**). We will consider the implementation difficulties of acute pain services under these three headings of content, context, and process.

Content issues

The content part of the content, context, and process framework considers the nature and objectives of the proposed change.

Looking at APS implementation, it is clear that one of the reasons why acute pain services struggled was that the nature and objectives of the changes were problematic. This was not only because of the practice changes that they entailed (on which individual health professionals had differing views), but also because the scope of the changes and the implementation mechanisms were not well defined. As we have shown, services struggled with such fundamental issues as the size and structure of an

---

Box 48.3 The content, context, and process framework

The CCP framework is one way of illustrating important dimensions of organizational change. The terms can be broadly defined as follows:

- **Content** – This refers to the nature (e.g. radical or incremental) and objectives (e.g. to introduce new technology for a particular procedure or to change professional roles) of the organizational change.
- **Context: outer** – This refers to the national economic, political, and social context in which the organizational change is taking place and includes policies and events at national and regional level (e.g. devolution, initiatives to manage health service performance).
- **Context: inner** – This refers to the ongoing strategy, structure, culture, management, and political processes at local level (e.g. in the health care organization).
- **Process** – This refers to the actions, reactions, and interactions of the interested parties as they negotiate around the proposals for organizational change.

These dimensions are not separate or fixed: they overlap and interact with each other and they change over time (e.g. as local debates lead to modifications to initial service plans). Source: adapted from Pettigrew et al.[48]

---

acute pain service, the role of the specialist nurse, and the relationship between the service and related services (e.g. critical care outreach).

There is now a substantial body of research (see for example Greenhalgh et al.[49]) that provides evidence that certain attributes of an innovation like a new technology or a new way of delivering services make it more likely that the innovation will be successfully adopted. Key attributes are listed in **Box 48.4**.

The APS recommendations lacked many of these attributes. In particular, they lacked what many commentators suggest is the key requirement for successful organizational change, that of "relative advantage." Relative advantage means that all key players accept that the changes have clear unambiguous advantage (in terms of effectiveness or cost-effectiveness) over the status quo. The advantages of improving postoperative pain management were not accepted by all key players: as studies of acute pain services clearly show, many policy-makers and managers appeared to be indifferent to the role that good postoperative pain management might play in improving

---

Box 48.4 Key attributes of an innovation (e.g. an acute pain service) that make it more likely to be adopted

---

- **Relative advantage**: clear unambiguous advantage that is accepted by all key players.
- **Codifiability**: the knowledge required to use the innovation can be codified (as opposed to being tacit).
- **Trialability**: can be experimented with by intended users on a limited basis.
- **Observability**: the benefits are visible to intended adopters.
- **Reinvention**: the innovation can be adapted to suit the needs of the adopters.
- **Rigorous evaluation** against defined goals and milestones.

Sources: derived from Refs 48, 49, 50, 51, 52, 53.

---

postoperative outcomes, and even many clinicians seemed unconvinced.[17] Acute pain services struggled to persuade their colleagues about the benefits of good postoperative pain management *per se* and about the need to improve local services (see for example Mackrodt[25]).

Not only did the APS recommendations lack relative advantage, they also lacked other important attributes. For example, they did not have the attribute of "trialability," the potential to try them out on an experimental basis before full adoption.[49, 50, 51, 52, 53] Partial implementation was difficult because of the multiplicity of departments and professionals involved, and because success was largely dependent on such coordinated working. For example, although methods of pain assessment could be trialled on one ward, the effectiveness of this would be compromised if patients returned from theater without pain scores or with pain scores obtained under a different scoring system (e.g. 0 to 3 rather than 1 to 10).

Planned dissemination programs need to include rigorous evaluation and monitoring against defined goals and milestones.[51, 54, 55, 56] This was absent in the case of the APS recommendations: there was no national dissemination program or evaluation and although attempts have been made to agree a national data set,[57] there remains as yet no national audit program on acute pain management. In contrast, other service areas such as cancer surgery did have such defined goals.

The APS changes therefore lacked many of the desirable attributes. Furthermore, even the desirable attribute that they did have appeared to work against them. The APS changes did have the positive attribute of "reinvention" (i.e. the innovation can be adapted to suit local needs).[49, 50, 51] Certainly, the APS proposals were open to local adaptation. Several of the policy documents and

commentaries placed emphasis on the extent to which the recommendations could be modified and implemented according to local circumstances, and indeed one such commentary published a few years after *Pain after Surgery* specifically recommended the "low cost" APS model as an alternative to the full-scale model.[58] However, this very flexibility and adaptability in the absence of defined goals or even broad specifications meant that it was difficult to put a case to managers or commissioners for adequate resources to introduce or develop an acute pain service. The very adaptability of the APS recommendations to local circumstances appears to have led, in some hospitals, to an initial "lowest common denominator" approach from which it was difficult to recover later in the decade when national targets (focused on other service areas than pain) began to dominate hospital agendas.

Thus by the late 1990s, the majority of hospitals providing surgery could claim to have adopted the proposals in that, in name at least, they did have an acute pain service. However, this implementation of the "headline" recommendation concealed significant variations in the extent to which hospitals had been able to implement the detailed recommendations aimed at improving postoperative pain management.[1, 7, 8, 9]

In summary, the APS recommendations therefore lacked a range of important attributes that are conducive to innovation uptake. However, there are also other considerations. The organizational change literature emphasizes that it is not simply the attributes of the innovation that matter. It is the innovation–context interaction that determines whether and how an innovation will be taken up[59, 60, 61] and so the characteristics of the adopting organization are also critical. We will now consider some of the context issues that undermined APS implementation.

Context issues

"Context" in the content, context, and process framework refers to the national and local political, economic, and social contexts and encompasses specific local events (e.g. a merger affecting particular hospitals) and broader social processes (e.g. trends towards greater centralization in government).

In organizational change terms, the APS changes had two major difficulties in relation to context: firstly they were being introduced into the NHS, which is recognized (in common with other health services) to be a particularly challenging organizational context, and secondly they were introduced in a particularly turbulent phase of NHS history. In particular, they suffered from two features of this period: the large number of mergers and ongoing service reorganizations, and the strong emphasis on the performance management agenda. Although this section describes some of the features of the UK NHS context, acute pain services in other industrialized countries have also been introduced against a background of substantial health service change:[62, 63, 64, 65]

Health care reform has been one of the worldwide epidemics of the 1990s (p. 299)[64]

THE NHS AS A CHALLENGING ORGANIZATIONAL CONTEXT

The organizational change literature acknowledges that health services like the NHS represent a particularly challenging context for organizational change (**Box 48.5**). Processes in the NHS are affected by additional demands and constraints to those found in industry. For example, change in the NHS is affected by the need to provide a year-round public service. In addition, the care process involving any one NHS patient may be highly complex and involve a range of different individuals and departments, drawing on a range of clinical skills and organizational resources.[46] For example, a patient who is admitted for elective surgery will have some contact with, or input from, a range of professionals including anesthetists, surgeons, outpatient clinic nurses, ward nurses, theater staff, radiographers, phlebotomists, and pharmacists. The care process is complicated further when the patient has multiple health conditions that may require coordinated input from a wider range of specialists. Thus there is limited scope for improving elements of a process (such as postoperative pain management) in isolation from the whole (i.e. the patient's perioperative care).

APS IMPLEMENTATION TAKING PLACE AT A TURBULENT TIME

Acute pain service implementation has taken place against a backdrop of significant organizational turbulence in the

---

Box 48.5 Features of the NHS that make it a particularly challenging context for organizational change

- Complexity of care processes in a year-round service.
- Multiple organizations and stakeholders in a highly politicized environment.
- History of partially implemented mechanistic top-down approaches to change.
- Major influence of health professionals in mediating change.
- Continuing power struggles between managers and some health professionals.
- General lack of resources for change initiatives.

Derived from Refs 62, 66, 67, 68, 69, 70, 71, 72, 73.

NHS. Firstly, the 1980s, the decade prior to the introduction of acute pain services, was a period of accelerating change in the NHS[74] with substantial restructuring and the introduction of "general management" aimed at changing "not only the structure of the NHS, but also its ruling assumptions and much of the service culture."[48] Secondly, acute pain services were introduced in the 1990s, a period when the scale and pace of NHS change increased markedly.[75] There were marked shifts in policy direction, successive structural reorganizations, and a plethora of diverse and sometimes conflicting initiatives aimed at changing aspects of the service.[76, 77, 78] There are extensive and ongoing debates in the literature about these changes: their nature and scale (e.g. Robinson[76]); their potential deleterious effects (e.g. Iliffe and Munro,[79] Smith et al.,[80] Simoens and McMaster,[81] Walshe[82]); and about the relationship between continuity and change. However, there is strong agreement (e.g. Walshe,[82] Ferlie[83]) that the period has been one of rapid and highly turbulent change, particularly since 1997, and that there are few signs that the process is slowing down.

Thus the period from 1990 was one of radical, extensive, and often disordered organizational change in the NHS. It was therefore a highly challenging time to be introducing new services like the acute pain service and for achieving the objectives of addressing long-standing deficits in postoperative pain management.

Acute pain services were affected both by the "background" turbulence and also by specific aspects of the NHS changes. Organizational turbulence in the NHS has been widely acknowledged to have had a range of impacts on different aspects of the service, including health professionals readiness to engage with service change and with other initiatives. It is argued that the turmoil has prompted widespread "change fatigue," encouraging a "wait and see" attitude and leading to a reactive rather than proactive approach.[63, 69, 80, 84, 85, 86, 87] Such an approach may be characterized by organizational actors as "surviving" rather than developing, and is likely to have had a considerable influence on responses to national initiatives like the APS recommendations.

DELIVERING NEW SERVICES AMID MERGERS AND SERVICE REORGANIZATIONS

The APS recommendations required effective communication and team working across health professionals in perioperative care. These requirements did not therefore fit well with the existing directorate-based and hospital-based patterns of working, and APS implementation was often hampered by the communication difficulties within hospitals and across different hospitals within the same healthcare organization. These problems were exacerbated by the large number of mergers and service reorganizations.

There were 99 mergers of trusts (NHS healthcare organizations) between 1997 and 2002,[70] a process that forced staff in trusts that were used to working independently and in different ways from neighboring trusts to work together as colleagues.[67] It is known that the anticipated benefits of mergers are not always realized and that mergers may lead to unintended consequences.[88] Hospital mergers are acknowledged to be a particularly problematic type of merger and may result in a range of adverse consequences that have a negative effect on delivering and developing services.[70, 89, 90, 91, 92, 93] Indeed "Projects for 'integration' of services across sites were more often than not seen as 'disintegration' by the people involved in them" (p. 199).[91] Organizational changes including mergers and large-scale reorganization may thus have hindered APS implementation by reinforcing "silo-based" working (e.g. in directorates or single professions) and introducing new communication problems across large merged organizations that had previously worked separately.

DEVELOPING ACUTE PAIN SERVICES AT A TIME WHEN THE NATIONAL PERFORMANCE AGENDA WAS FOCUSED ON OTHER CLINICAL SERVICES

APS implementation was also hindered by the strong emphasis on the performance agenda. This led managers and health professionals to concentrate primarily on certain clinical services that were the subject of specific initiatives and performance management and meant that other services (such as pain management) received less attention.

Literature on NHS change makes clear that one of the adverse effects of performance management is that attention is skewed towards the service areas covered by the targets and that other services can be neglected[94, 95] although the full impact is unknown.[96] Organizational change literature suggests that it is more difficult to secure commitment to initiatives that appear to be unrewarded, especially when the necessary effort may take resources away from initiatives to which incentives or sanctions are attached.[97] Managers and clinical staff were concerned with the task of meeting externally imposed targets and other mandatory requirements in a resource-limited environment, and improving postoperative pain management was seen as neither relevant nor useful to this task.[97]

The concept of change taking place along the path of least resistance[98] suggests that had the APS recommendations fitted with other performance targets, there might have been less difficulty in implementation. However, the APS recommendations were not part of the performance agenda and in many ways conflicted with it. For example, time taken by anesthetists on pain management (e.g. on pain ward rounds) reduced time available for them to administer the anesthetics needed to "get through the waiting list," while time spent siting epidurals in theater lengthened the time needed per case and thus reduced the number of operations that could be carried out in one staffed theater session.

The literature on innovations suggests that political mandates (making the innovation compulsory) increase the motivation (but not the capacity) of an organization to adopt the innovation.[49] However, there were no political mandates attached to improving postoperative pain management. Paradoxically, "performance" in surgical care or "delivering the service" did not explicitly include good postoperative pain management. Nor did the statutory duty to monitor and improve "quality" imposed on NHS organizations through the 1990 NHS Act and later under clinical governance[99] explicitly include pain management. There was no national service plan on acute pain (as there was for other clinical areas, e.g. coronary heart disease),[78] no reference to pain in the criteria for awarding ratings to hospitals,[100] and no targeted funding.

Not only did the APS recommendations not feature in the main performance agenda targets, but the recommendations were also out of step with other drivers because they appeared to be so different. In an environment in which increasing emphasis was placed on performance targets and on measurement, there was much about pain management that appeared to be subjective, difficult to measure, and hard to evaluate.

To summarize, acute pain services were introduced in an unreceptive and even resistant context: health professionals and managers were preoccupied with multiple successive reorganizations and with a range of quality and performance initiatives that did not include postoperative pain. Against this background, the APS changes were further undermined by some of the responses and actions of health professionals in perioperative care. We will now consider these "process" aspects.

Process issues

Process factors in the content, context, and process framework are concerned with the "actions, reactions, and interactions" of interested parties in relation to the organizational change.[48] Such actions and reactions are of course related to the content and context of the change.

An important attribute of successful innovations identified in the literature is compatibility,[50] defined as the extent to which the proposed innovation is compatible with the values, norms, and perceived needs of intended adopters.[49] In fact, the APS changes were not always fully compatible with the values and norms of intended adopters and this therefore affected how they were received.

Firstly, the APS changes cut across views that were strongly held by many health professionals in perioperative care about the nature of postoperative pain and about responsibility for its management. Secondly, the APS changes entailed working effectively across the different professions in perioperative care, and so they challenged the long-established boundaries within and between professions that governed daily clinical practice.

CHALLENGE TO EXISTING VALUES AND NORMS

The APS changes therefore presented a profound challenge to many aspects of existing values and norms among health professionals in perioperative care (**Box 48.6**) and were met with varying degrees and types of resistance that hindered their implementation. For example, some doctors were unwilling to take advice from specialist pain nurses; many health professionals had doubts about the validity of patients' self-report of pain in pain scoring; and some were reluctant to take action based on patients' scores or advice from other professional groups.

Acute pain services were not unique in facing these challenges. The literature on organizational change in healthcare settings provides strong evidence that many healthcare innovations are resisted because (among other reasons) they disturb traditional divisions of labor between nursing and medical staff and challenge deeply-rooted aspects of professional identity (e.g. doctors' autonomy to prescribe as they wish).[47, 101, 102]

- Many evidence-based healthcare innovations involve disturbing a division of labor traditionally agreed across occupational groups (e.g. between nurses and doctors) and it can be very difficult to cross these boundaries.
- Such innovations also threaten professional autonomy and can result in turf-defending activities; there is therefore only limited scope for managerial control of the implementation process.
- Doctors' views of their own clinical world are shaped by a strong sense of their own autonomy to develop practice in accordance with their experience.
- The ability to respond *selectively* to peer influence is seen by many doctors as a marker of professional independence.

DIFFICULT INTER-PROFESSIONAL WORKING

Problems with inter-professional working (both within professions and between members of different professions) and the effects of these problems on providing care and changing practice are well documented (**Box 48.7**).

Box 48.6 Examples of ways in which the APS changes challenged existing values and norms

The changes:

- challenged long-standing and deeply-rooted beliefs about the meanings of pain (e.g. about the normality of a degree of postoperative pain);
- challenged long-standing beliefs about the side effects of analgesics (e.g. the belief that the risk of patient addiction was greater than the risks of untreated pain) and fears about the risks of adopting more "aggressive" pain management regimens;
- required health professionals to acknowledge that current practice was unsatisfactory;
- entailed actively seeking the patient's self-report of pain and accepting this as the basis for action by health professionals;
- challenged the belief that postoperative pain management could remain the "special interest" of a few individuals rather than being an integral part of all perioperative care;
- challenged existing notions of division of labor (e.g. between HDU nurses and ward nurses) and entailed working across professional boundaries in ways that went against established norms (e.g. nurses challenging the practice of doctors);
- activated individual health professionals' concerns about their own competence or that of colleagues in relation to more complex methods of analgesia (e.g. epidurals).

Box 48.7 Key themes from the literature on nursing and medical boundaries and inter-professional working

- Differing interpretation between nursing and medical professions of key concepts such as "collaboration";[103, 104, 105] "cooperation";[106] and what is central to "treating patients."[107]
- Divisions within individual professions into "camps."[108, 109, 110]
- Differences between professions in styles of learning, career patterns, models of working, regulatory mechanisms, etc.[109, 111]
- Inequality between medical and nursing professions.[112, 113]
- Issues of power (e.g. members of powerless groups belittling each other).[114, 115, 116]
- Skill substitution driven by the needs of the medical profession and not by the nursing profession.[117, 118]
- Bullying in nursing[119] and in perioperative care settings in particular.[120]
- Differences in culture between medical specialties.[121]
- The impact of medical dominance in decision-making around patient care.[104, 122]

The APS studies show many acute pain examples: anesthetists express frustration at working with surgical and anesthetic colleagues who have different views on the importance of postoperative pain management; acute pain specialist nurses struggle for recognition by medical staff; ward staff often do not carry out pain scoring and see pain management as the responsibility of the APS. This is reflected in a typical comment made in one recent survey:[17, 31]

> Difficulty in persuading our surgical colleagues about the importance of good pain management post op, and maverick prescribing of oral analgesia by them despite an agreed protocol causes some tensions – not always in the patient's best interest
>
> Anesthetist

A major factor undermining APS implementation was, therefore, the "bedrock" of traditional boundaries and professional norms that affected who could do or say what in relation to postoperative pain management, and influenced health professionals' responses to APS efforts to change practice. Although professional boundaries are acknowledged to present an ongoing and significant barrier to service change, strategies to overcome such barriers and to improve dysfunctional relationships are less well identified.[123, 124, 125, 126]

APS implementation was also undermined by an unintended consequence of introducing acute pain services: the tendency for some health professionals to "pass the buck" and to refer all postoperative pain problems to the acute pain service. It is well recognized in the organizational change literature (e.g. Armenakis and Bedeian,[45] Harris and Ogbonna,[127] Hammersley[128]) that unintended consequences will arise in all forms of planned organizational change, and that the range of effects of new policies or new practices will encompass intended and unintended, foreseen and unforeseen effects.[50, 128] While *Pain after Surgery* aimed to address the lack of "an identifiable individual or group with responsibility for the relief of acute pain,"[15] this designation of an identifiable individual and group may have had the unintended consequence of legitimizing[47] postoperative pain management as the "special interest" of a few health professionals.

In summary then, reactions to the APS changes were affected by the ways in which the changes challenged existing values and norms among health professionals in perioperative care. The changes conflicted with strongly held views about responsibility for postoperative pain management, and the requirement for effective interprofessional working did not fit well with long-established boundaries within and between professions. In addition, in some hospitals, the development of acute pain services had the unintended consequence of encouraging some health professionals to delegate all responsibility

for postoperative pain management to the acute pain service.

ADDRESSING THE IMPLEMENTATION CHALLENGES

Looking across the three categories of the "content, context, and process" framework of the dimensions of organizational change, the APS changes were hampered because they were:

- not universally accepted as necessary and not well defined in terms of the nature and objectives of the change (*content*);
- introduced in a turbulent environment in which attention was focused elsewhere and in which rapid local organizational changes were hindering effective communication (*context*);
- not always fully compatible with the deeply rooted norms, practices and beliefs of many health professionals (*process*).

It is therefore not surprising that the organizational change of implementing acute pain services has been so challenging and that many of the improvements that acute pain services have achieved in routine postoperative pain management have been patchy and hard to sustain. Much has been achieved however, and official reports and respondents in research studies rightly pay tribute to the commitment and hard work of members of acute pain services. Nevertheless, the insights from the organizational change literature suggest that there are key areas that need to be addressed if acute pain services are to make further progress in improving postoperative pain management for all patients (**Box 48.8**). These issues will be discussed under the three separate categories (content, context, and process) for convenience but we emphasize that they are closely interlinked in practice. We also emphasize that while they are discussed only briefly here, each of these challenges would require considerable ongoing effort for clinicians, policy-makers, and researchers in devising, testing, implementing, and evaluating policy and practice initiatives.

Content issues

We discussed earlier how acute pain service implementation lacked key attributes that are known to be conducive to successful organizational change. The most significant deficit was that of "relative advantage": the absence of clear agreement among the key people involved (managers, health professionals, policy-makers, and patients) about the need to improve postoperative pain management and about the benefits (e.g. in terms of effectiveness of pain management, cost-effectiveness of services, and use of resources) that the changes would bring.

> ## Box 48.8 Implementing acute pain services and improving postoperative pain management: key lessons from the organizational change literature
>
> - Achieving even relatively small changes in complex health service organizations is very challenging: there are many interacting organizational factors and hence no easy or permanent solutions.
> - Improving postoperative pain management will need health professionals, managers, and policy-makers to address a range of complex challenges.
> - Three key areas are:
>   - health professionals and managers need actively to agree about the need to improve postoperative pain management and about the benefits that improved services will bring;
>   - the wider health service context at national and local level (e.g. performance measurement, education, and training) needs to support and facilitate improvements in postoperative pain management;
>   - strategies are needed to reduce the impact of long-standing beliefs, attitudes, and fears among health professionals that impede good postoperative pain management.

A range of strategies is needed to secure active agreement about the importance of good postoperative pain management. These might include:

- addressing the current gaps in the research base;
- attending to the existing literature on "what works" in diffusing and sustaining innovations in health services (e.g. Greenhalgh et al.,[49] Dopson and Fitzgerald,[101] Grol et al.[129]);
- using insights from other fields (e.g. marketing) to "sell" postoperative pain management to skeptical policy-makers, managers, and health professionals.

Acute pain services have also struggled from the lack of clarity about the form and function of an acute pain service and its relationship to other services (e.g. critical care outreach), and this has led to much duplication of debates and "experiments" at local level, and to difficulties in making the case for adequate resources. Strategies to address these problems might include:

- devising clear national specifications for acute pain services (e.g. about appropriate staffing levels) that could be used for standard-setting, resource allocation, benchmarking, and evaluating progress;

- formal evaluation of the role of acute pain services in relation to other related services (e.g. critical care outreach).

Context issues

In addition to suffering (with other services) from what has been described as "the re-disorganisation of the NHS"[80] in the 1990s, acute pain service implementation has also been at odds with the performance management agenda on which much attention has been focused.

The organizational change literature argues strongly that for successful organizational change in health services, it is essential to have a multilevel approach with coherence between policy at the different levels (e.g. national, regional, and local).[62, 72, 130] In order to make further progress it will therefore be necessary to ensure that the wider NHS context at national and local level supports the contributions of individual health professionals and acute pain services in improving postoperative pain management.

This might include:

- reducing the number and frequency of mergers and service reorganizations and taking steps to ensure that the unintended adverse consequences are minimized;
- ensuring that good postoperative pain management is recognized and funded as an explicit part of providing surgery and is mandatory for securing training approval;
- introducing defined goals and milestones to evaluate improvements in postoperative pain management;
- recognizing the adverse impact that performance measurement is known to have on nontargeted services and ensuring that performance measurement systems support good clinical care across the whole service.

Clearly these are substantial policy changes that are not under the control of local acute pain services.

Process issues

Acute pain service implementation has been hampered by: attitudes towards postoperative pain management and its management; poor working relationships between some health professions and individuals; and by the tendency of some health professionals to hand over all responsibility for postoperative pain management to the acute pain service.

This means that the following need to be considered in order to make further progress:

- strategies to reduce the impact of the long-standing beliefs, attitudes, and fears that impede good postoperative pain management and that lie behind some of the reactions of health professionals to the changes;

- strategies to promote good working relationships between and across professions;
- understanding and addressing the unintended and dysfunctional consequences of specialist teams.

These are long-standing and generic problems that are not readily amenable to change, but acknowledging them is an essential starting point.

CONCLUDING REMARKS

Many of the problems we have described in this chapter are reflected in the experience of acute pain services outside the UK, including acute pain services in other European countries, in the US, in Australia, and in New Zealand.[131, 132, 133, 134, 135] Making further progress and addressing the areas that we have outlined above will be very challenging. First, with regard to the substantive nature of the values, beliefs, and attitudes informing postoperative pain management, the literature on pain management and acute pain services shows that attitudinal barriers in relation to pain and its management have been part of health services throughout the world for at least 50 years.[14, 136, 137, 138, 139] Second, the organizational change literature makes clear that achieving even relatively minor forms of incremental change is not straightforward (e.g. Dawson,[44] Rosenfeld and Wilson[140]), and the task is compounded when working in large and complex multilevel political organizations like health services. Third, changing attitudes, beliefs, and values that affect how health professionals work together (i.e. cultural change) is characterized as second order transformational change,[141, 142] the most radical, controversial, and demanding form of change in scale and scope:

> ... it is the 'intangible' components of [those] organizations that may yield the greatest threat to or facilitation of organizational change.[143]

It is also a major challenge because it is ongoing. Each acute pain service has constantly to adapt to changes in local circumstances (e.g. loss of key individuals, changes in local facilities, local networks forming and dissolving). Acute pain services as a whole also have to adapt. The effective management of postoperative pain in the future (whether through acute pain services, integrated pain services, or something quite different) will need to respond to future changes in the social and healthcare environments.[64, 144, 145] These may include regulatory changes (e.g. in relation to the availability of opiates and other drugs or to the practice of health professionals); changes in the organization of health services (e.g. increasing diversity of providers, changes in hospital organization and governance); changes in clinical care (e.g. new drugs, changing patterns of surgery); demographic changes (e.g. age distribution of population,

changes in levels of literacy); and advances in technology (e.g. new analgesic techniques, advances in information technology).

Although there is much about the future that is uncertain, it is clear that difficult and controversial cultural changes will be needed: widespread changes in attitudes and practices around postoperative pain and its management. Further structural and incremental change alone is unlikely to be sufficient to achieve the goal of effective pain management for all postoperative patients.

REFERENCES

1. McDonnell A, Nicholl J, Read SM. Acute Pain Teams in England: current provision and their role in postoperative pain management. *Journal of Clinical Nursing.* 2003; **12**: 387–93.
2. Clinton JJ. Acute pain management can be improved. *Journal of the American Medical Association.* 1992; **267**: 19.
3. McCaffery M, Pasero C. *Pain: Clinical manual,* 2nd edn. St Louis: Mosby, 1999.
4. NICS. *Institutional approaches to pain assessment and management.* Adelaide: National Institute of Clinical Studies, 2003.
5. Wheatley RG, Madej TH. Organization of an acute pain service. In: Rowbotham DJ, Macintyre PE (eds). *Clinical pain management: acute pain.* London: Arnold, 2003: 183–202.
6. Harmer M, Davies KA, Lunn JN. A survey of acute pain services in the United Kingdom. *British Medical Journal.* 1995; **311**: 360–1.
7. Audit Commission. *Anaesthesia under examination.* London: Audit Commission, 1997.
* 8. Clinical Standards Advisory Group. *Services for patients with pain.* London: Department of Health, 2000.
9. Nagi H. Acute pain services in the United Kingdom. *Acute Pain.* 2004; **5**: 89–107.
* 10. Rawal N, Allvin R, EuroPain Acute Pain Working Party. Acute pain services in Europe: a 17-nation survey of 105 hospitals. *European Journal of Anaesthesiology.* 1998; **15**: 354–63.
11. Rawal N. 10 years of acute pain services – achievements and challenges. *Regional Anesthesia and Pain Medicine.* 1999; **24**: 68–73.
* 12. Breivik H, Curatolo M, Neimi G *et al.* How to implement an acute postoperative pain service – an update. In: Breivik H, Shipley M (eds). *Pain: best practice and research compendium.* London: Elsevier, 2007: 255–86.
13. Australian and New Zealand College of Anaesthetists and Faculty of Pain Medicine. *Acute pain management: scientific evidence,* 2nd edn. Melbourne: Australian and New Zealand College of Anaesthetists and Faculty of Pain Medicine, 2005.
14. Wallace PGM, Norris W. The management of postoperative pain. *British Journal of Anaesthesia.* 1975; **47**: 113–20.

* 15. Royal College of Surgeons of England, College of Anaesthetists. *Report of the Working Party on Pain after Surgery*. London: Royal College of Surgeons/College of Anaesthetists, 1990, 1, 28.

16. Pediani RC. Organizing acute pain management. In: Carter B (ed.). *Perspectives on pain: mapping the territory*. London: Arnold, 1998: 153–70.

17. Powell AE. Examining the implementation of acute pain services in the UK National Health Service. Unpublished PhD thesis, University of St Andrews, 2006.

18. Windsor AM, Glynn CJ, Mason DG. National provision of acute pain services. *Anaesthesia*. 1996; **51**: 228–31.

19. Cartwright P, Helfinger RG, Howell JJ, Siepman KK. Introducing an acute pain service. *Anaesthesia*. 1991; **46**: 188–91.

20. Wheatley R, Madej TH, Jackson IJB, Hunter D. The first year's experience of an acute pain service. *British Journal of Anaesthesia*. 1991; **67**: 353–9.

21. Kestin IG, Baglin M. The effect of introducing an acute pain service into a district general hospital. *Anaesthesia Points West*. 1994; **27**: 24–34.

22. McLeod G, Davies HTO, Colvin JR. Shaping attitudes to postoperative pain relief: the role of the acute pain team. *Journal of Pain and Symptom Management*. 1995; **10**: 1–5.

23. Humphries CA, Counsell DJ, Pediani RC, Close SL. Audit of opioid prescribing: the effect of hospital guidelines. *Anaesthesia*. 1997; **52**: 745–9.

24. Davies HTO, McLeod G, Bannister J, Macrae WA. Obstacles in organization of service delivery reduce potential of epidural analgesia. *British Medical Journal*. 1999; **319**: 1499–500.

25. Mackrodt K. An evaluation of the effect of a pain management strategy within a district general hospital. Unpublished Masters thesis, Leicester University, 1999.

26. Tan TK, Brown I, Seow CS *et al*. Pre-registration house officers: What do they know about pain management? *Acute Pain*. 1999; **2**: 115–24.

27. O'Higgins F, Tuckey JP. Thoracic epidural anaesthesia and analgesia: United Kingdom practice. *Acta Anaesthesiologica Scandinavica*. 2000; **44**: 1087–92.

28. Harmer M. When is a standard not a standard? When it is a recommendation. *Anaesthesia*. 2001; **56**: 611–12.

29. McLeod G, Davies HTO, Munnoch N *et al*. Postoperative pain relief using thoracic epidural analgesia: Outstanding success and disappointing failures. *Anaesthesia*. 2001; **56**: 75–81.

30. Sanders MK, Michel MZM. Acute pain services – How effective are we? *Anaesthesia*. 2002; **57**: 927.

31. Powell AE, Davies HTO, Bannister J, Macrae WA. Rhetoric and reality on acute pain services in the NHS: a national postal questionnaire survey. *British Journal of Anaesthesia*. 2004; **92**: 689–93.

32. Black AM. Taking pains to take away pain. *British Medical Journal*. 1991; **302**: 1165–6.

* 33. McQuay H, Moore A, Justins D. Treating acute pain in hospital. *British Medical Journal*. 1997; **314**: 1531–5.

34. Boscoe MJ. Introducing the postoperative care team. *British Medical Journal*. 1997; **314**: 1346.

35. Goldhill DR. Introducing the postoperative care team. *British Medical Journal*. 1997; **314**: 389.

36. Rosen M. Such teams deserve a trial of efficacy and cost (correspondence). *British Medical Journal*. 1997; **314**: 1346.

37. Russell RCG. Royal College of Surgeons has training programme for surgical trainees. *British Medical Journal*. 1997; **314**: 1346.

38. Counsell DJ. The acute pain service: A model for outreach critical care. *Anaesthesia*. 2001; **56**: 925–6.

39. Counsell DJ. Outreach critical care services. *Anaesthesia*. 2002; **57**: 285–6.

40. Goldhill DR, McGinley A. Outreach critical care. *Anaesthesia*. 2002; **57**: 183.

41. Notcutt WG, Austin J. The acute pain team or the pain management service? *The Pain Clinic*. 1995; **8**: 167–74.

42. Mackrodt K. The role of an acute pain service. *British Journal of Perioperative Nursing*. 2001; **11**: 492–7.

43. Wilson DC. *A strategy of change: concepts and controversies in the management of change*. London: Routledge, 1992.

44. Dawson P. *Understanding organizational change*. London: Sage, 2003.

45. Armenakis AA, Bedeian AG. Organizational change: a review of theory and research in the 1990s (Yearly Review of Management). *Journal of Management*. 1999; **25**: 293–307.

46. Buchanan DA. *Occasional Paper 64: The lived experience of strategic change: a hospital case study*. Leicester: Leicester Business School, 2001.

47. Pettigrew AM. *The awakening giant: continuity and change in Imperial Chemical Industries*. Oxford: Basil Blackwell, 1985.

* 48. Pettigrew A, Ferlie E, McKee L. *Shaping strategic change*. London: Sage Publications, 1992: 267.

* 49. Greenhalgh T, Robert G, Bate P *et al*. *How to spread good ideas: a systematic review of the literature on diffusion, dissemination and sustainability of innovations in health service delivery and organization*. London: NCCSDO, 2004.

50. Rogers EM. *Diffusion of innovations*, 4th edn. New York: The Free Press, 1995.

51. Gustafson D, Sainfort F, Eichler M *et al*. Developing and testing a model to predict outcomes of organizational change. *Health Services Research*. 2003; **38**: 751–76.

52. Fleuren M, Wiefferink K, Paulussen T. Determinants of innovation within health care organizations: literature review and Delphi study. *International Journal for Quality in Health Care*. 2004; **16**: 107–23.

53. Grol R, Wensing M. Characteristics of successful innovations. In: Grol R, Wensing M, Eccles M (eds). *Improving patient care: The implementation of change in clinical practice*. Edinburgh: Elsevier, 2005: 60–9.

54. Blumenthal D, Kilo CM. A report card on continuous quality improvement. *The Milbank Quarterly*. 1998; **76**: 625–48.

∗ 55. Shortell SM, Bennett CL, Byck GR. Assessing the impact of continuous quality improvement on clinical practice: what it will take to accelerate progress. *The Milbank Quarterly.* 1998; **76**: 593–624.

56. Grol R, Wensing M. Effective implementation: a model. In: Grol R, Wensing M, Eccles M (eds). *Improving patient care: The implementation of change in clinical practice.* Edinburgh: Elsevier, 2005: 41–57.

57. Sutherland P, Michel M. Acute pain service audit: A national survey to agree an optimal data set. *Acute Pain.* 2000; **3**: 10–14.

58. Rawal N, Berggren L. Organization of acute pain services: a low-cost model. *Pain.* 1994; **57**: 117–23.

59. Ferlie E, Fitzgerald L, Wood M. Getting evidence into clinical practice: an organizational behaviour perspective. *Journal of Health Services Research and Policy.* 2000; **5**: 96–102.

60. Smith W. An explanation of theories that guide evidence-based interventions to improve quality. *Clinical Governance: An International Journal.* 2003; **8**: 247–54.

61. Hawe P, Shiell A, Riley T. Complex interventions: how "out of control" can a randomised control trial be? *British Medical Journal.* 2004; **328**: 1561–3.

∗ 62. Ferlie E, Shortell SM. Improving the quality of health care in the United Kingdom and the United States: a framework for change. *The Milbank Quarterly.* 2001; **79**: 281–315.

63. McKee M, Aiken L, Rafferty AM, Sochalski J. Organizational change and quality of health care: an evolving international agenda. *Quality in Health Care.* 1998; **7**: 37–41.

64. Klein R. Big bang health care reform – does it work? The case of Britain's 1991 National Health Service reforms. *Milbank Quarterly.* 1995; **73**: 299–337.

65. Degeling P, Zhang K, Coyle B *et al.* Clinicians and the governance of hospitals: A cross-cultural perspective on relations between profession and management. *Social Science and Medicine.* 2006; **63**: 757–75.

66. Mintzberg M. *The structuring of organizations.* Englewood Cliffs: Prentice-Hall, 1979.

67. Joss R, Kogan M. *Advancing quality: total quality management in the National Health Service.* Buckingham: Open University Press, 1995.

68. Koeck C. Time for organizational development in healthcare organizations. *British Medical Journal.* 1998; **317**: 1267–8.

69. Powell AE, Davies HTO. Business process re-engineering: lost hope or learning opportunity? *British Journal of Health Care Management.* 2001; **7**: 446–9.

70. Fulop N, Protopsaltis G, Hutchings A *et al.* Process and impact of mergers of NHS trusts: multicentre case study and management cost analysis. *British Medical Journal.* 2002; **325**: 246.

71. Davies HTO, Harrison S. Trends in doctor-manager relationships. *British Medical Journal.* 2003; **326**: 646–9.

∗ 72. Ham C, Kipping R, McLeod H. Redesigning work processes in health care: lessons from the National Health Service. *The Milbank Quarterly.* 2003; **81**: 415–39.

∗ 73. McNulty T. Redesigning public services: challenges of practice for policy. *British Journal of Management.* 2003; **14**: S31–45.

74. Ashburner L, Ferlie E, Fitzgerald L. Organizational transformation and top-down change: the case of the NHS. *British Journal of Management.* 1996; **7**: 1–16.

75. Young AP. Competing ideologies in health care: a personal perspective. *Nursing Ethics.* 1997; **4**: 191–200.

76. Robinson R. The impact of the NHS reforms 1991-1995: a review of research evidence. *Journal of Public Health Medicine.* 1996; **18**: 337–42.

77. Davies HTO, Nutley SM. Developing learning organizations in the new NHS. *British Medical Journal.* 2000; **320**: 998–1001.

78. Leatherman S, Sutherland K. *The quest for quality in the NHS: A mid-term evaluation of the quality agenda.* London: The Nuffield Trust, 2003.

79. Iliffe S, Munro J. New Labour and Britain's National Health Service: An overview of current reforms. *International Journal of Health Services.* 2000; **30**: 309–34.

80. Smith J, Walshe K, Hunter DJ. The 'redisorganization' of the NHS. *British Medical Journal.* 2001; **323**: 1262–3.

81. Simoens S, McMaster R. Institutional change and trust in the National Health Service: examining the impact of reform on the NHS value structure. In: Rushmer RK, Davies HTO, Tavakoli M, Malek M (eds). *Organization development in health care: strategic issues in health care management.* Aldershot: Ashgate, 2002: 150–64.

82. Walshe K. Health care under New Labour: rebuilding or dismantling the NHS? *British Journal of Health Care Management.* 2005; **11**: 73–6.

83. Ferlie E. Strategic change in UK health care: an overview of some recent research. Published from the Organizational Behaviour in Health Care Conference, Banff, Alberta, 2004.

84. Garside P. Organizational context for quality: lessons from the fields of organizational development and change management. *Quality in Health Care.* 1998; **7**: S8–15.

∗ 85. Leatherman S, Sutherland K. Evolving quality in the new NHS: policy, process and pragmatic considerations. *Quality in Health Care.* 1998; **7**: S54–61.

86. Cortvriend P. Change management of mergers: the impact on NHS staff and their psychological contracts. *Health Services Management Research.* 2004; **17**: 177–87.

∗ 87. Fitzgerald L, Lilley C, Ferlie E *et al. Managing change and role enactment in the professionalised organization.* London: NCCSDO, 2006.

88. Cartwright S, Schoenberg R. Thirty years of mergers and acquisitions research: recent advances and future opportunities. *British Journal of Management.* 2006; **17**: S1–5.

89. Denis J-L, Lamothe L, Langley A. The dynamics of collective leadership and strategic change in pluralistic organizations. *Academy of Management Journal.* 2001; **44**: 809–37.

90. Hutchings A, Allen P, Fulop N *et al.* The process and impact of trust mergers in the National Health Service: a financial

perspective. *Public Money and Management.* 2003; **23**: 103–12.

91. Langley A, Denis J-L, Lamothe L. Process research in healthcare: towards three-dimensional learning. *Policy and Politics.* 2003; **31**: 195–206.

∗ 92. Sheaff R, Schofield J, Mannion R et al. *Organizational factors and performance: a review of the literature.* London: NCCSDO, 2003.

93. Canadian Health Services Research Foundation. Bigger is always better when it comes to hospital mergers. *Journal of Health Services Research and Policy.* 2004; **9**: 59–60.

∗ 94. Fitzgerald L, Ferlie E, Wood M, Hawkins C. Interlocking interactions, the diffusion of innovations in health care. *Human Relations.* 2002; **55**: 1429–49.

95. Marshall MN. Public reporting of information on health care performance. In: Leatherman S, Sutherland K (eds). *The quest for quality in the NHS: A mid-term evaluation of the ten-year quality agenda.* London: The Nuffield Trust, 2003: 225–40.

96. Bevan G, Hood C. Have targets improved performance in the English NHS? *British Medical Journal.* 2006; **332**: 419–22.

97. Gollop R, Whitby E, Buchanan D, Ketley D. Influencing sceptical staff to become supporters of service improvement: a qualitative study of doctors' and managers' views. *Quality and Safety in Health Care.* 2004; **13**: 108–14.

98. Stickland F. *The dynamics of change.* London: Routledge, 1998.

99. Halligan A, Donaldson L. Implementing clinical governance: turning vision into reality. *British Medical Journal.* 2001; **322**: 1413–17.

100. Harris C. England introduces star system for hospital trusts. *British Medical Journal.* 2001; **323**: 709.

∗101. Dopson S, Fitzgerald L (eds). *Knowledge to action? Evidence-based health care in context.* Oxford: Oxford University Press, 2005.

102. Ferlie E. Conclusion: from evidence to actionable knowledge? In: Dopson S, Fitzgerald L (eds). *Knowledge to action? Evidence-based health care in context.* Oxford: Oxford University Press, 2005: 182–97.

103. Davies HTO, Nutley SM, Mannion R. Organizational culture and quality of health care. *Quality in Health Care.* 2000; **9**: 111–19.

104. Coombs MA. *Power and conflict between doctors and nurses: Breaking through the inner circle in clinical care.* London: Routledge, 2004.

105. Reeves S, Lewin S. Interprofessional collaboration in the hospital: strategies and meanings. *Journal of Health Services Research and Policy.* 2004; **9**: 218–25.

106. Krogstad U, Hofoss D, Hjortdahl P. Doctor and nurse perception of inter-professional co-operation in hospitals. *International Journal for Quality in Health Care.* 2004; **16**: 491–7.

107. Degeling P, Kennedy J, Hill M. Mediating the cultural boundaries between medicine, nursing and

management – the central challenge in hospital reform. *Health Services Management Research.* 2001; **14**: 36–48.

108. Davies C. *Gender and the professional predicament in nursing.* Buckingham: Open University Press, 1995.

109. Allen D. The nursing-medical boundary: a negotiated order? *Sociology of Health and Illness.* 1997; **19**: 498–520.

110. Tod A, Palfreyman S, Burke L. Evidence-based practice is a time of opportunity for nursing. *British Journal of Nursing.* 2004; **13**: 211–16.

111. Doyal L, Cameron A. Reshaping the NHS workforce. *British Medical Journal.* 2000; **320**: 1023–4.

112. Salvage J, Smith R. Doctors and nurses: doing it differently. *British Medical Journal.* 2000; **320**: 1019–20.

113. Faugier J, Woolnough H. Valuing 'voices from below'. *Journal of Nursing Management.* 2002; **10**: 315–20.

114. Brooks I. Managerialist professionalism: the destruction of a non-conforming subculture. *British Journal of Management.* 1999; **10**: 41–52.

115. Brown RB, Brooks I. Emotion at work: identifying the emotional climate of night nursing. *Journal of Management in Medicine.* 2002; **16**: 327–44.

116. Sieloff CL. Leadership behaviors that foster nursing group power. *Journal of Nursing Management.* 2004; **12**: 246–51.

117. Banham L, Connelly J. Skill mix, doctors and nurses: substitution or diversification? *Journal of Management in Medicine.* 2002; **16**: 259–70.

118. Stubbings L, Scott JM. NHS workforce issues: implications for future practice. *Journal of Health Organization and Management.* 2004; **18**: 179–94.

119. Lewis MA. Will the real bully please stand up. *Occupational Health.* 2004; **56**: 22–8.

120. Gilmour D, Hamlin L. Bullying and harassment in perioperative settings. *British Journal of Perioperative Nursing.* 2003; **13**: 79–85.

121. Willcocks SG. Clinician managers and cultural context: comparisons between secondary and primary care. *Health Services Management Research.* 2004; **17**: 36–46.

122. Varcoe C, Rodney P, McCormick J. Health care relationships in context: an analysis of three ethnographies. *Qualitative Health Research.* 2003; **13**: 957–73.

∗123. Zwarenstein M, Bryant W. Interventions to promote collaboration between nurses and doctors. *Cochrane Database of Systematic Reviews.* 1997; **CD000072**.

124. Rosenstein AH, O'Daniel M. Disruptive behavior and clinical outcomes: perceptions of nurses and physicians. *Nursing Management.* 2005; **36**: 18–29.

125. Bhattacharyya C, Reeves S, Garfinkel S, Zwarenstein M. Designing theoretically-informed implementation interventions: Fine in theory, but evidence of effectiveness in practice is needed. *Implementation Science.* 2006; **1**: 5.

126. ICEBeRG. Designing theoretically-informed implementation interventions. *Implementation Science.* 2006; **1**: 4.

127. Harris LC, Ogbonna E. The unintended consequences of culture interventions: a study of unexpected outcomes. *British Journal of Management.* 2002; **13**: 31–49.

128. Hammersley M. Is the evidence-based practice movement doing more good than harm? Reflections on Iain Chalmers' case for research-based policy making and practice. *Evidence and Policy.* 2005; **1**: 85–100.

*129. Grol R, Wensing M, Eccles M (eds). *Improving patient care: The implementation of change in clinical practice.* Edinburgh: Elsevier, 2005.

130. Grol R, Grimshaw J. From best evidence to best practice: effective implementation of change in patients' care. *Lancet.* 2003; **362**: 1225–30.

131. Wilder-Smith OHG, Mohrle JJ, Martin NC. Acute pain management after surgery or in the emergency room in Switzerland: a comparative survey of Swiss anaesthesiologists and surgeons. *European Journal of Pain.* 2002; **6**: 189–201.

132. Manias E, Bucknall T, Botti M. Nurses' strategies for managing pain in the postoperative setting. *Pain Management Nursing.* 2005; **6**: 18–29.

133. Carr DB, Reines HD, Schaffer JS *et al.* The impact of technology on the analgesic gap and quality of acute pain management. *Regional Anesthesia and Pain Medicine.* 2005; **3**: 286–91.

134. Rawal N, Langford RM. Current practices for postoperative pain management in Europe and the potential role of the fentanyl HCl iontophoretic transdermal system. *European Journal of Anaesthesiology.* 2007; **24**: 299–308.

135. Werner MU, Nielsen PR. The acute pain service: present and future role. *Current Anaesthesia and Critical Care.* 2007; **18**: 135–9.

136. Weis O, Sriwatanakul K, Alloza J *et al.* Attitudes of patients, housestaff, and nurses toward postoperative analgesic care. *Anesthesia and Analgesia.* 1983; **62**: 70–4.

137. Cartwright P. Pain control after surgery: a survey of current practice. *Annals of the Royal College of Surgeons of England.* 1985; **67**: 13–16.

138. Edwards WT. Optimizing opioid treatment of postoperative pain. *Journal of Pain and Symptom Management.* 1990; **5**: S24–36.

139. Green CR, Tait AR. Attitudes of healthcare professionals regarding different modalities used to manage acute postoperative pain. *Acute Pain.* 2002; **4**: 15–21.

140. Rosenfeld RH, Wilson DC. *Managing organizations: Text, readings and cases*, 2nd edn. Maidenhead: McGraw Hill, 1999.

141. Ackerman Anderson L, Anderson D. Awake at the wheel: moving beyond change management to conscious change leadership. *OD Practitioner.* 2001; **33**: 3.

*142. Iles V, Sutherland K. *Organizational change: A review for health care managers, professionals and researchers.* London: NCCSDO, 2001.

143. Osborne SP, Brown K. *Managing change and innovation in public service organizations.* Abingdon: Routledge, 2005: 75.

144. Slote Morris Z, Dawson S. Who's going to govern? The role of the state in the future of health and healthcare. In: Slote Morris Z, Rosenstrøm Chang L, Dawson S, Garside P (eds). *Policy futures for UK Health.* London: The Nuffield Trust, 2004: 65–79.

145. Slote Morris Z, Detmer D. Chapter 4: Where will technology take us? In: Slote Morris Z, Rosenstrøm Chang L, Dawson S, Garside P (eds). *Policy futures for UK Health.* London: The Nuffield Trust, 2004: 129–45.

49

Comprehensive pain rehabilitation programs: a North American reappraisal

PETER R WILSON

KEY LEARNING POINTS

- Comprehensive pain rehabilitation programs are effective when cost and outcomes are measured.
- Components of effective programs are difficult to define, but are included in published criteria.
- The Commission for the Accreditation of Rehabilitation Facilities (www.carf.org) has guidelines for the United States, Canada, and other countries.

- The Institute for Clinical Systems Improvement (Minneapolis, Minnesota, USA: www.icsi.org) has guidelines primarily for local consumption.
- Interventional pain management modalities are largely unstudied, unregulated, and have a paucity of cost–benefit analysis.

INTRODUCTION

The concept of pain as a malignant force is as old as humankind itself. An efferent control system in the pain system was postulated by Melzack and Wall[1] in their gate control theory of pain in 1965. This was one of the stimuli for an explosion of scientific interest in nociception and its neurophysiologic mechanisms. Unfortunately, there has not been a corresponding translation into clinical practice. There are few scientific studies that have demonstrated adequate management of any acute or chronic disease state. It is usually not possible to practice contemporary "evidence-based medicine" with respect to chronic pain

states because of lack of evidence and lack of political will.[2] Patient advocacy groups and private websites bemoan the parlous state of pain relief available to the general public. This dismal state of affairs was recognized by the United States Congress, which declared the "Decade of pain control and research," which began on 1 January 2001.[3]

The concept of pain as a biopsychosocial disease rather than a hard-wired function is relatively recent. John Bonica[4] formalized the idea of pain management as a multidisciplinary diagnostic and therapeutic endeavor in his seminal opus in 1953. This concept has been generally accepted since that time, and pain clinics and centers have been established with this model as the basis.[5]

The Bonica model of multidisciplinary pain management has come under increasing scrutiny from payers, patients, and regulators in the US. The following factors are among those that have changed in the 20–30 years of the development of the model.

- Increasing emphasis on evidence-based medical practice.[6]
- Increasing emphasis on cost–benefit considerations of a particular therapy.[7]
- Decreasing emphasis on return to work as a criterion.
- Increasing emphasis on quality of life and other psychosocial measures.
- Increasing emphasis on decreasing medical utilization as a long-term goal.
- Decreasing emphasis on the physician as "captain of the ship."
- Increasing recognition of the patient needing to be an informed participant in the process.
- Increasing recognition that medications (even opioids) have a place in chronic pain management.
- Recognition that medicolegal issues do not necessarily prohibit rehabilitation.

These factors have influenced the philosophy and practice in management of chronic pain, at least in the United States.

CHRONIC PAIN PROGRAMS

There was a proliferation of chronic pain programs in the early 1970s. The Bonica model was widely accepted, and programs were designed to include all the specialists deemed necessary to address the complex consequences of chronic pain[8] in a particular patient in a particular setting (**Box 49.1**). A history of the evolution and development of a noted pain clinic has been recorded by one of the most successful protagonists of the multidisciplinary model.[9] A typical multidisciplinary pain clinic evaluation could involve as many as a dozen medical and allied health specialists. A patient would be evaluated in turn by each of these clinicians independently from her/his point of view. The group (clinicians, patient, significant others) would then typically meet for at least an hour for each patient for the initial planning session to arrive at a consensus diagnosis and management plan. The plan would be implemented, often in the context of a multidisciplinary pain program. The *sine qua non* of the process was that there was no specific "curative" treatment for the underlying pathology, if any. Plans were typically developed to address the consequences of the chronic pain state. In the absence of evidence to the contrary (and there were very few data in the first three decades of chronic pain programs), each patient was admitted to the

---

Box 49.1 Signs and symptoms of the chronic pain state, leading to an overall reduction in quality of life

- Physical deconditioning:
  - reduction in muscle tone, strength, endurance;
  - reduction in aerobic capacity;
  - reduction in joint flexibility;
  - chronic sleep deprivation;
  - fear of additional injury.
- Psychological deconditioning:
  - depression;
  - anger;
  - anxiety;
  - irritability;
  - anhedonia;
  - guilt.
- Behavioral deconditioning:
  - development of abnormal illness behaviors;
  - loss of self-esteem;
  - irritability;
  - secondary gains.
- Inappropriate medication use.
- Work and vocational deconditioning:
  - loss of job, work status.
- Family issues:
  - loss of companionship;
  - loss of libido and potentia.
- Financial issues:
  - loss of salary;
  - medical expenses.
- Legal issues:
  - worker compensation issues;
  - social security disability issues;
  - personal injury issues.
- Inappropriate medical system utilization.

---

particular program, and standard protocols were used for all patients admitted. Such programs were financially viable at that time because of the prevailing "fee for service" payment mechanism. Under such a system, every interaction with the patient by every clinician was potentially reimbursable.

It was assumed that all patients would benefit from a general physical and psychological retraining program. Early clinical impressions of outcomes appeared to justify their use of this empiric model. Unfortunately, even now there are still too few data to justify this assumption in all varieties of pain services. Turk[10] critically examined the question of customizing treatment more than a decade ago without being able to arrive at definite conclusions regarding the optimal combination of modalities for a particular patient/client.

There was usually emphasis on return to work, and some programs used this as the major outcome measure and for economic justification. The number of patients returning to the same work was usually small.[11] "Return to work" is a difficult concept, as it has different meanings to different stakeholders. There are variables that might be out of control of the patient and program. For example, the patient might not have the skills required in the workforce, full-time work might not be possible or available, and the original job would often become unavailable.

There was also usually emphasis on "detoxification," with reduction or elimination of all medications. There seemed to be lower successful completion of rehabilitation in oxycodone users,[12] but with few initial data indicating sustained improvement in function. These initial pain rehabilitation programs were usually of three to four weeks duration, full-time, and in the inpatient setting. There was little emphasis on cost–benefit issues, as third-party payers seemed to accept the novelty of the treatments and their empirically attractive concepts. Even now there are few data available on tracking of subsequent health care utilization. Payers do not make these data available and the use of unprescribed alternative and complementary modalities are usually not included in such analyses. When such data are available, as discussed in the American Pain Society (APS) study, they are strongly supportive of the long-term savings obtained after a successful chronic pain rehabilitation program.

Turk revisited the subject in 2002.[13] He concluded that there were difficulties in interpreting results within and across studies. Variables might include:

- differences in inclusion and exclusion criteria for admission;
- comparability of treatments;
- definition of "chronic";
- comparability of drug doses and equianalgesic potency;
- differences between pain syndromes;
- definition of "success";
- societal differences.

Pain programs were not shown to eliminate pain, or even reduce the reported intensity, but there were sometimes statistically significant changes on more sophisticated instruments. Whether such changes are clinically significant is hotly debated.

These programs appeared so intuitively correct in their approach to the multifactorial problems that there was very little close scrutiny of them by the patients, providers, or payers. There were early outcome studies, of course, that appeared to justify the results.[14] With the advent of improved evaluation tools, a better understanding of the issues has been possible. However, even then, the outcome data have to be interpreted cautiously.[15]

Components of an "ideal" program are mentioned in detail below. It is not possible to discuss each in detail. They are listed because of their intuitive correctness, not necessarily because there is scientific evidence for their validity. Not every program addresses all areas of putative dysfunction. Review of this literature is difficult because the specific components of the subject program are rarely defined.[16, 17, 18]

PHYSICAL RECONDITIONING/REHABILITATION

Some chronic pain patients may find themselves in a vicious cycle of pain, inactivity, loss of physical condition, fear of musculoskeletal pain and reinjury with the performance of "usual" physical activity (kinesiophobia),[19] with consequent inhibition of physical activity, and accelerated deconditioning. These are difficult attitudes and behaviors[20] to change. The patient has to be reassured that physical activity is beneficial and not harmful: in the vernacular "use it or lose it; no pain, no gain." The rehabilitation program has to be planned to increase the loads gradually, with time-contingent and not symptom-contingent progress. The exercise program has to be emphasized so that the patient will maintain and increase the level of physical activity and function after discharge from the program. The separate components of muscle tone, strength, endurance, aerobic capacity, and joint function are likely to be of variable importance and may need different emphasis in the two groups. It is likely that baseline evaluations of these variables are essential for monitoring progress, as it is assumed that improvement in overall function will be related to improvement in these also. Few programs make appropriate before and after measurements of musculoskeletal or cardiovascular function.[21]

PSYCHOLOGICAL RECONDITIONING

Controversy surrounds the interactions between chronic pain and depression (addressed in Chapter 18, Chronic pain and depression in the *Chronic Pain* volume of this series). It is not clear whether there is a cause-and-effect relationship or whether both represent a common biochemical change, manifested in 5-hydroxytryptamine (5-HT)/norepinephrine (noradrenaline; NE)/dopamine (DA) depletion. Suffice it to say here that the use of relatively small doses of selective or nonselective 5-HT/NE reuptake blockers may produce a significant reduction in the perception and/or report of pain.[20]

Anger often accompanies chronic pain,[22] and it would be reasonable to address this aspect of psychological functioning, either individually or in a group setting. It must be remembered that there is often cause (in the patient's mind) for the anger – hostile work environment, unsympathetic employer, incompetent physician, the adversarial legal system, an apparently unfeeling spouse. Creative and constructive avenues to express and reduce this anger have to be identified. There is good evidence that childhood or current physical or sexual abuse is associated with an increased incidence of chronic pain and increased utilization of medical resources.[23, 24, 25] Anhedonia is often related to the pain and depression, and may be expected to improve with effective treatment of the depression, pain, and insomnia. Loss of libido in any pain patient and decreased potentia (in males) may be related to the pain or depression, or to opioid analgesics, and may also be expected to resolve as the syndrome is successfully treated.[26] There may be no specific treatment, but urological evaluation may be necessary.

BEHAVIORAL ADJUSTMENT

Chronic pain states contribute to the development of abnormal illness behaviors.[27] These include any unproductive behavior with respect to that person's health. There are significant other adjustment disorders in chronic pain states.[28] Cognitive/behavioral therapies are therefore based on the assumption that maladaptive attitudes and behaviors are learned, and can therefore be modified by new learning experiences.[29]

Turner and Keefe[30] have reviewed the history and theoretical basis of cognitive-behavioral therapy (CBT) in chronic pain management. They also reviewed evidence of efficacy and found that the evidence was not yet good, and that firm conclusions were difficult to justify. More recent studies have been much more encouraging.[2, 31]

There have been reports of specific symptom control with CBT, for example insomnia,[32] back pain,[33] and musculoskeletal pain.[34]

MEDICATION ISSUES

Attitudes to the use of scheduled medications in chronic illness of nonmalignant origin have been negative, if the medications do not produce satisfactory functional improvement. Chronic pain is becoming accepted as a disorder of the neuromatrix with defined structural, chemical, and functional changes, and not a voluntary defect of personality. There has been a corresponding change in the attitudes of the various regulators, assisted in part by statements from the American Academy of Pain Medicine, American Pain Society, and other professional organizations. Similar changes are beginning to occur elsewhere.[35] As noted by Long,[9] pain clinics originally intended to "detoxify" all patients by elimination of "all narcotics, sedative-hypnotics, or other potentially harmful drugs." However, it was recognized even then that anxiety and depression might need to be treated pharmacologically.[36, 37, 38]

With the increasing use and acceptance of opioids for the long-term alleviation of nonmalignant pain has come the increasing recognition of the interaction of chronic pain behaviors and substance abuse/addiction[39] (see also Chapter 46, Pain management and substance misuse in the *Chronic Pain* volume of this series). The consensus panel of the American Academy of Pain Medicine and the American Pain Society introduced the concept of "pseudoaddiction" to define the state of drug-seeking that accompanies untreated or undertreated pain.[40] The American Society of Addiction Medicine has also promulgated position statements regarding the rights and responsibilities of physicians who use opioids for the treatment of pain.[41] Portenoy[42] had previously defined the rights and responsibilities of patients who are candidates for long-term opioid therapy, leading to the development of "opioid contracts."[43] These various incentives have led to regulatory changes that make well-documented and medically defensible prescribing of opioids less onerous.[44] Various states have enacted intractable pain legislation to reduce the onus on appropriate prescribers. It must be recognized that particular care must be taken to establish the veracity of the patient, as there are certain patients who will not report medication and substance use accurately.[45] It is becoming clear that the treatment of acute or chronic pain and addiction in the same patient have to be considered as separate but interrelated exercises.[46]

Addicted patients must not be denied appropriate acute pain management, even though it will probably include opioids.[47] The situation is more complex when an addicted patient also has complaints of chronic pain.[48]

Hooten and his colleagues showed that under certain situations in carefully selected patients opioid withdrawal could be accompanied by favorable outcomes.[49] Patients with symptomatically severe and disabling pain while taking maintenance opioid therapy experienced significant improvement in physical and emotional functioning after the pain rehabilitation program that incorporated opioid withdrawal. There was undoubtedly selection bias, as patients knew that opioid withdrawal was a major component in the program. The subjects were predominantly female, highly educated, and compliant. They were highly motivated, but had not improved with other interventions. Long-term follow-up is not yet available.

WORK ISSUES

Return to work is a difficult concept to measure. A recent review evaluated 4124 papers and only found ten of sufficient quality to include in the study.[50] This found that there was strong evidence that work disability duration was significantly reduced by work accommodation offers and contact between healthcare provider and workplace. In the adversarial system in the United

States, the healthcare provider is usually prohibited from direct contact with the employer. There was moderate evidence that a return to work coordinator was helpful. In the United States, this is usually the qualified rehabilitation counselor (QRC), employed by the insurance company.[51]

One implication of many studies is that there will be return to the same work without restrictions at the same reimbursement. There are other return to work scenarios: same work with restriction, different work with lower reimbursement, full-time and part-time options. Durability of the return is of critical importance. A three-year follow-up study from one pain clinic indicated that only about one-third of participants maintained their original improvement.[52] About half of a cohort of patients treated more than a decade previously reported gainful employment, although 68 percent reported significant pain.[53] In another study, actual return to work and long-term outcome appears to be determined largely by pain variables.[54]

FAMILY ISSUES

As discussed above, family issues are important factors in both the maintenance and rehabilitation of abnormal illness behaviors.[55] The spouse or other caregiver has to be taught that the patient has to become more self-sufficient. Children and adolescents have to be taught healthy behaviors, to prevent pain-related disability.[56, 57]

FINANCIAL ISSUES

There is no doubt that chronic pain imposes both direct and indirect financial burdens on patients and families.[58] These costs may include:

- decreased income;
- increased insurance premiums;
- physicians' fees;
- hospital fees;
- medical supplies;
- prescription and over-the-counter medications;
- emergency room and urgent care visits;
- travel and accommodation for physician and hospital visits;
- unreimbursed expenses;
- alternative and complementary therapy costs;
- legal expenses.

These are a source of hardship and stress,[59] and may be difficult or impossible to deal with. For example, even though a patient is theoretically protected by the Americans with Disabilities Act (ADA), it is most unlikely that a worker who has had back surgery will ever be employed in the blue-collar sector again. Although it is illegal to consider health issues in employment, other reasons not to hire a person are usually found.

MEDICAL UTILIZATION

Economic evaluation of chronic pain intervention costs is difficult.[59] However, durable reduction in medical utilization is an important outcome of a chronic pain rehabilitation program. It indicates that there has been a measurable change in the patient's abnormal illness behavior. This change has direct benefits to the patient, medical providers, and payers. There are indirect benefits to the patient's self-esteem and independence.[60] Unfortunately, such data are regarded as proprietary by the payers, and are not available for publication in the United States.

COMPREHENSIVE PAIN REHABILITATION ACCREDITATION

It has been very difficult to define on evidence the optimal model for a comprehensive pain rehabilitation program in the light of these various considerations. In the absence of evidence-based outcome data, the default standards are those derived from expert consensus. The Commission on Accreditation of Rehabilitation Facilities (CARF; www.carf.org) is a nongovernmental not-for-profit organization that has accredited general rehabilitation programs in the United States for the last 35 years. It is an organization composed of representatives of the rehabilitation community and other stakeholders in the rehabilitation process. These include representatives of relevant medical societies and allied health organizations, the insurance industry, the hospital industry, patient/public advocacy groups, and public members.

Accreditation criteria are developed and administered by CARF by a complex process involving expert committees and input from active programs in the community. National advisory committees (NACs) of experts involve providers, payers, persons served, and accreditation specialists from CARF. The final consensus product ("standards manual") is updated as required. NACs are convened at least every third year for each major section. Consensus is achieved where there are inadequate scientific/outcome data.

CARF interdisciplinary pain rehabilitation programs

The CARF definition (Section 3.C, 2007) states:

An interdisciplinary pain rehabilitation program provides outcomes-focused, coordinated, goal-oriented interdisciplinary team services to measure and improve the functioning of persons with pain and encourage their appropriate use of health care systems and services. The program can benefit persons who have limitations that interfere with their physical, psychological, social, and/or vocational functioning. Information about the scope of the services and the outcomes achieved is shared by the program with stakeholders.

The interdisciplinary team is determined by the needs of the person served, and, at a minimum, includes personnel with the competencies necessary to evaluate and facilitate the achievement of predicted/desired outcomes in the following dimensions:

- functional;
- medical;
- physical;
- psychological;
- social;
- vocational.

The team therefore should include:

- the person served;
- the pain team physician;
- the pain team psychologist;
- dependent on the assessed needs of the person served, individuals from, but not limited to, those listed below who will assist in the accomplishment of functional, physical, psychological, social, and vocational goals:
  - biofeedback therapist;
  - case manager;
  - exercise physiologist;
  - nurse practitioner;
  - occupational therapist;
  - pharmacist;
  - physical therapist;
  - physician assistant;
  - psychiatrist;
  - registered nurse;
  - social worker;
  - therapeutic recreation specialist;
  - vocational specialist;
- other stakeholders, as appropriate.

CARF is aware that data are currently not available to provide guidelines regarding team size.[7] Until recently, the pain team was defined as a minimum of five in number. This was clearly more expensive than the present recommendation as there were no data indicating that five were more effective or cost-effective than the current three. The person served and two specialists are, by definition, the minimum needed to provide an interdisciplinary function.

The increasingly important issues of clinical effectiveness and cost-effectiveness were addressed by Turk.[13] He reviewed representative published studies that evaluated the clinical effectiveness of pharmacological treatments, conservative (standard) care, surgery, spinal cord stimulators, implantable drug delivery systems, and pain rehabilitation programs.

One estimate suggested the cost of lost productivity alone might be of the order of US$60 billion per year.[61] Direct costs are also difficult to estimate, but it is thought that both prescription medications and over-the-counter medications cost several times this amount. Stanos and Houle[5] have suggested the current costs are in the US$70–120 billion range.

Comprehensive pain rehabilitation programs account for a relatively small proportion of the total US pain treatment costs. It is not possible to obtain accurate numbers, either of programs or of patients treated. For example, the United States CARF lists 79 CARF-accredited programs in 2007; 52 of these are in the state of Texas, 6 in Washington State, and the remainder in 16 other states. There is an unknown number of pain rehabilitation programs that are not accredited by CARF, for example, at the Mayo Clinic.

It is also difficult to estimate the number of modality-based "interventional practices" in the United States. Current estimates are that there may be some 7000 interventional practitioners in the USA (MA Huntoon, personal communication, 2007). The website of the American Society of Interventional Pain Physicians reports more than 3200 active physician members who provide "interventional" pain management in the form of injections, nerve blocks, radiofrequency neural ablations, implantation of spinal pumps and stimulators, and other invasive procedures (www.asipp.org). The International Spinal Intervention Society (which began as the International Spinal Injection Society) currently has active members in the United States providing interventional pain management (www.spinalinjection.com). The American Society of Regional Anesthesia and Pain Medicine has several thousand members, many of whom are interventionists (www.asra.com). However, it is evident that there are far more of these facilities than CARF-accredited ones in the US. This may be a reflection on reimbursement policies rather than the practice of evidence-based pain medicine and thorough cost-benefit analysis.

Dr Dennis Turk, then president of the American Pain Society, convened a Task Force on Comprehensive Pain Rehabilitation, chaired by Dr Robert Gatchell. The charge was to develop a report of published results that support the clinical and cost-effectiveness of comprehensive pain programs. The report appeared in the *Journal of Pain*.[62] The authors confronted the difficulties of estimating direct and indirect costs of chronic pain. They reported a crisis in much of the developed world (United States, The Netherlands, New Zealand,

Australia, Denmark, Canada, Spain, and Italy). It is very difficult to estimate direct and indirect costs of chronic pain to Americans, but it is suggested that it may be more than US$150 billion per year. Healthcare expenditures themselves may make up only 10 percent of the costs of chronic pain in the United States, the authors concluded. It is even difficult to estimate medication costs. Scheduled analgesic medications (primarily opioids) have more than 150 million prescriptions written each year, and this number is rapidly increasing, according to the Drug Enforcement Administration (www.usdoj.gov).

The concept of treatment "success" was discussed, as defined by the various stakeholders in the patient's illness: the individual with the chronic pain, healthcare providers, insurers, attorneys, and "society", which ultimately pays for much of the cost. The only treatment models that could be defined as attempting to estimate costs and benefits were the comprehensive programs. They reported on suboutcomes such as pain, quality of life, healthcare utilization, and disability claims. They concluded that this model provided the most efficacious treatment for persons with chronic pain. This model was shown to be more cost-effective than "conventional" serial medical interventions. The numbers were impressive considering that chronic pain rehabilitation programs are often the "last resort" when all other approaches have failed, or the insurance company refuses to pay for any more treatment.

They concluded that it is indeed unfortunate that these programs are not used early in an illness, before maladaptive behaviors on the part of patients, significant others, physicians, attorneys, and insurers all conspire to condemn the patient to a lifetime of misery.

Robinson et al.[63] reviewed the data of 2032 injured workers between January 1991 through May, 1993. Of these, 1226 were treated and 776 were evaluated only. They found that pain center treatment did not produce significant beneficial effects on time loss outcome. However, they identified limitations including the retrospective nature, nonrandomized assignment, nonspecific diagnostic categorization and the use of the unvalidated time loss status as the outcome measure. They justified its use on the grounds that it is an unambiguous administrative measure available on 100 percent of claimants. Return to work measures are less reliable and not necessarily related to the original injury. They subsequently confirmed their earlier finding that there was no evidence that pain center treatment affected either disability status or clinical status of injured workers.[64] The authors were aware of the opposite confounding factors to the Hooten et al. study,[49] and that this study was not likely to be generalizable either.

Hatten et al.[65] studied a different group of patients using different outcome measures. Traditional cost-utility analysis (CUA) supplemented with conversion of SF-36 data into quality-adjusted life year data. They reviewed a consecutive sample of 121 patients with a primary diagnosis of chronic spinal pain. Four groups were identified:

1. interdisciplinary management alone (I), $n = 59$;
2. interdisciplinary+anesthesia procedures (I = P), $n = 22$;
3. medications alone (M), $n = 16$;
4. medications+anesthesia procedures (M+P) $n = 24$.

They found that the groups M and M+P reported significantly higher pain intensities that the other groups. They also found that the order of increasing effectiveness (median incremental cost/QALY gained) was able to be calculated only for the groups that included interdisciplinary management, because the medication groups had decreased QALY. Patrick et al.[33] indicated that the favorable outcomes may be quite durable, at least over 13 years.

Attempts have been made by the Institute for Clinical Systems Improvement (www.icsi.org) which has published "evidence-based" clinical guidelines for both acute and chronic pain management on its web site.

CONCLUSIONS

Comprehensive interdisciplinary pain rehabilitation programs have matured beyond those originally conceived by Bonica. Evidence has accumulated that the current concept of individualized programs may be more robust from both cost–benefit and cost-effective standpoints. Unfortunately, factors such as the political climate and reimbursement priorities have a more profound impact on treatment options than outcome data and patient need.

REFERENCES

1. Melzack R, Wall PD. Pain mechanisms: a new theory. *Science.* 1965; **150**: 971–9.
2. Robinson JP. Pain rehabilitation. *Physical Medicine and Rehabilitation Clinics of North America.* 2006; **17**: xiii–xix.
3. United States Congress. The Decade of Pain Control and Research. H.R. 3244, Title IV, Sec. 1603. 2000: US Congressional Record.
4. Bonica J. *The management of pain.* Philadelphia, PA: Lea and Febiger, 1953.
* 5. Stanos S, Houle TT. Multidisciplinary and interdisciplinary management of chronic pain. *Physical Medicine and Rehabilitation Clinics of North America.* 2006; **17**: 435–50, vii.
6. Turk DC. Here we go again: outcomes, outcomes, outcomes. *Clinical Journal of Pain.* 1999; **15**: 241–3.
7. Turk D, Okifuji A. Treatment of chronic pain patients: clinical outcomes, cost-effectiveness, and cost-benefits of

multidisciplinary pain centers. *Critical Reviews in Physical and Rehabilitation Medicine.* 1998; **10**: 181–208.

8. Swanson DW, Swenson WM, Maruta T, McPhee MC. Program for managing chronic pain. I. Program description and characteristics of patients. *Mayo Clinic Proceedings.* 1976; **51**: 401–8.

9. Long D. The Development of the Comprehensive Pain Treatment Program at Johns Hopkins. In: Cohen M, Campbell J (eds). *Pain treatment centers at a crossroads: a practical and conceptual reappraisal. Progress in pain research and management.* Seattle, WA: IASP Press, 1996: 3–24.

10. Turk DC. Customizing treatment for chronic pain patients: who, what, and why. *Clinical Journal of Pain.* 1990; **6**: 255–70.

11. Sanders S. Why do most patients with chronic pain not return to work? In: Cohen M, Campbell J (eds). *Pain treatment centers at a crossroads: a practical and conceptual reappraisal. Progress in pain research and management.* Seattle, WA: IASP Press, 1996: 193–201.

12. Maruta T, Swanson DW. Problems with the use of oxycodone compound in patients with chronic pain. *Pain.* 1981; **11**: 389–96.

* 13. Turk DC. Clinical effectiveness and cost-effectiveness of treatments for patients with chronic pain. *Clinical Journal of Pain.* 2002; **18**: 355–65.

14. Swanson DW, Maruta T, Swenson WM. Results of behavior modification in the treatment of chronic pain. *Psychosomatic Medicine.* 1979; **41**: 55–61.

15. Flor H, Fydrich T, Turk DC. Efficacy of multidisciplinary pain treatment centers: a meta-analytic review. *Pain.* 1992; **49**: 221–30.

16. Keel P. Pain management strategies and team approach. Best Practice and Research. *Clinical Rheumatology.* 1999; **13**: 493–506.

17. Morley S, Eccleston C, Williams A. Systematic review and meta-analysis of randomized controlled trials of cognitive behaviour therapy and behaviour therapy for chronic pain in adults, excluding headache. *Pain.* 1999; **80**: 1–13.

18. Fishbain D, Cutler RB, Rosomoff HL, Rosomoff RS. What is the quality of the implemented meta-analytic procedures in chronic pain treatment meta-analyses? *Clinical Journal of Pain.* 2000; **16**: 73–85.

19. Kori S, Miller R, Todd D. Kinesiophobia: a new view of chronic pain behavior. *Pain Management.* 1990; **3**: 35–43.

20. Argoff CE *et al.* Consensus guidelines: treatment planning and options. Diabetic peripheral neuropathic pain [erratum appears in Mayo Clin Proc. 2006 Jun;81(6):854]. *Mayo Clinic Proceedings.* 2006; **81**: S12–25.

21. Wittink H. Physical fitness, function and physical therapy in patients with pain: clinical measures of aerobic fitness and performance in patients with chronic low back pain. *IASP refresher course on pain management.* Seattle, WA: IASP Press, 1999: 137–44.

22. Okifuji A, Turk D, Curran S. Anger in chronic pain: investigations of anger targets and intensity. *Journal of Psychosomatic Research.* 1999; **47**: 1–12.

23. Finestone HM, Stenn P, Davies F *et al.* Chronic pain and health care utilization in women with a history of childhood sexual abuse. *Child Abuse and Neglect.* 2000; **24**: 547–56.

24. Liebschutz JM, Feinman G, Sullivan L *et al.* Physical and sexual abuse in women infected with the human immunodeficiency virus: increased illness and health care utilization. *Archives of Internal Medicine.* 2000; **160**: 1659–64.

25. Coker AL, Smith PH, Bethea L *et al.* Physical health consequences of physical and psychological intimate partner violence. *Archives of Family Medicine.* 2000; **9**: 451–7.

26. Maruta T, Osborne D, Swanson DW, Halling JM. Chronic pain patients and spouses: marital and sexual adjustment. *Mayo Clinic Proceedings.* 1981; **56**: 307–10.

27. Pilowsky I. Abnormal illness behaviour: a 25th anniversary review. *Australian and New Zealand Journal of Psychiatry.* 1994; **28**: 566–73.

28. Townsend CO, Sletten CD, Bruce BK *et al.* Physical and emotional functioning of adult patients with chronic abdominal pain: comparison with patients with chronic back pain. *Journal of Pain.* 2005; **6**: 75–83.

29. Jensen MP, Nielson WR, Romano JM *et al.* Further evaluation of the pain stages of change questionnaire: is the transtheoretical model of change useful for patients with chronic pain? *Pain.* 2000; **86**: 255–64.

30. Turner J, Keefe F. Cognitive–behavioral therapy for chronic pain. *IASP refresher course on pain management.* Seattle: IASP Press, 1999: 523–33.

31. Schonstein E, Kenny DT, Keating J, Koes BW. Work conditioning, work hardening and functional restoration for workers with back and neck pain. Cochrane Back Group. *Cochrane Database of Systematic Reviews* 2003; **CD001822**.

32. Currie SR, Wilson KG, Pontefract AJ, deLaplante L. Cognitive-behavioral treatment of insomnia secondary to chronic pain. *Journal of Consulting and Clinical Psychology.* 2000; **68**: 407–16.

* 33. Patrick LE, Altmaier EM, and Found EM. Long-term outcomes in multidisciplinary treatment of chronic low back pain: results of a 13-year follow-up. *Spine.* 2004; **29**: 850–5.

34. Norrefalk JR, Linder J, Ekholm J, Borg K. A 6-year follow-up study of 122 patients attending a multiprofessional rehabilitation programme for persistent musculoskeletal-related pain. *International Journal of Rehabilitation Research.* 2007; **30**: 9–18.

35. McQuay H. Opioids in pain management. *Lancet.* 1999; **353**: 2229–32.

36. Saarto T, Wiffen. Antidepressants for neuropathic pain *Cochrane Database of Systematic Reviews* 2005; **CD005454**.

37. Coluzzi F, Mattia C. Mechanism-based treatment in chronic neuropathic pain: the role of antidepressants. *Current Pharmaceutical Design.* 2005; **11**: 2945–60.

38. Sullivan MD, Robinson JP. Antidepressant and anticonvulsant medication for chronic pain. *Physical Medicine and Rehabilitation Clinics of North America.* 2006; **17**: 381–400.

39. Savage S. Chronic pain and the disease of addiction: the interfacing roles of pain medicine and addiction medicine. *IASP refresher course on pain management.* Seattle: IASP Press, 1999: 115–23.

40. American Academy of Pain Medicine, American Pain Society. *Joint consensus statement regarding the use of opioids for the treatment of pain.* Glenview, IL: AAPM, 1996.

41. American Society for Addiction Medicine. Public policy statement: rights and responsibilities of physicians who use opioids for the treatment of pain. *Journal of Addictive Diseases.* 1998; **17**: 131–2.

42. Portenoy R. Chronic opioid therapy in nonmalignant pain. *Journal of Pain and Symptom Management.* 1990; **5**: S46–62.

43. Fishman SM, Bandman TB, Edwards A, Borsook D. The opioid contract in the management of chronic pain. *Journal of Pain and Symptom Management.* 1999; **18**: 27–37.

44. United States Federation of State Medical Boards, Inc. *Model guidelines for the use of controlled substances in the treatment of pain.* Last updated May 2004; cited February 2008. Available from: www.fsmb.org/pdf/2004_grpol_Controlled_Substances.pdf.

45. Fishbain DA, Cutler RB, Rosomoff HL, Rosomoff RS. Validity of self-reported drug use in chronic pain patients *Clinical Journal of Pain.* 1999; **15**: 184–91.

* 46. Ballantyne JC, LaForge KS. Opioid dependence and addiction during opioid treatment of chronic pain. [see comment][erratum appears in Pain. 2007; 131: 350]. *Pain.* 2007; **129**: 235–55.

47. Wesson DR, Ling W, Smith DE. Prescription of opioids for treatment of pain in patients with addictive disease. *Journal of Pain and Symptom Management.* 1993; **8**: 289–96.

48. Jamison RN, Kauffman J, Katz NP. Characteristics of methadone maintenance patients with chronic pain. *Journal of Pain and Symptom Management.* 2000; **19**: 53–62.

49. Hooten W, Townsend C, Sletten C *et al.* Treatment outcomes after multidisciplinary pain rehabilitation with analgesic education withdrawal for patients with fibromyalgia. *Pain Medicine.* 2007; **8**: 8–16.

50. Franche R.-L *et al.* Workplace-based return-to-work interventions: a systematic review of the quantitative literature. *Journal of Occupational Rehabilitation.* 2005; **15**: 607–31.

51. Franche R.-L *et al.* Workplace-based return-to-work interventions: optimizing the role of stakeholders in implementation and research. *Journal of Occupational Rehabilitation.* 2005; **15**: 525–42.

52. Maruta T, Swanson DW, McHardy MJ. Three year follow-up of patients with chronic pain who were treated in a multidisciplinary pain management center. *Pain.* 1990; **41**: 47–53.

53. Maruta T, Malinchoc M, Offord KP, Colligan RC. Status of patients with chronic pain 13 years after treatment in a pain management center. *Pain.* 1998; **74**: 199–204.

54. Fishbain DA, Cutler RB, Rosomoff HL *et al.* Prediction of "intent", "discrepancy with intent", and "discrepancy with nonintent" for the patient with chronic pain to return to work after treatment at a pain facility. *Clinical Journal of Pain.* 1999; **15**: 141–50.

55. Leonard MT, Cano A. Pain affects spouses too: personal experience with pain and catastrophizing as correlates of spouse distress. *Pain.* 2006; **126**: 139–46.

56. Gauntlett-Gilbert J, Eccleston C. Disability in adolescents with chronic pain: Patterns and predictors across different domains of functioning. *Pain.* 2007; **131**: 132–41.

57. Palermo TM, Chambers CT. Parent and family factors in pediatric chronic pain and disability: an integrative approach. *Pain.* 2005; **119**: 1–4.

58. Barrett AM, Lucero MA, Le T *et al.* Epidemiology, public health burden, and treatment of diabetic peripheral neuropathic pain: a review. *Pain Medicine.* 2007; **8**: S50–62.

59. Cross MJ, March LM, Lapsley HM *et al.* Patient self-efficacy and health locus of control: relationships with health status and arthritis-related expenditure. *Rheumatology.* 2006; **45**: 92–6.

60. Nagyova I, Stewart RE, Macejova Z *et al.* The impact of pain on psychological well-being in rheumatoid arthritis: the mediating effects of self-esteem and adjustment to disease. *Patient Education and Counseling.* 2005; **58**: 55–62.

* 61. Stewart WF, Ricci JA, Chee E *et al.* Lost productive time and cost due to common pain conditions in the US workforce. *Journal of the American Medical Association.* 2003; **290**: 2443–54.

* 62. Gatchel RJ, Okifuji A. Evidence-based scientific data documenting the treatment and cost-effectiveness of comprehensive pain programs for chronic nonmalignant pain. *Journal of Pain.* 2006; **7**: 779–93.

63. Robinson JP, Fulton-Kehoe D, Martin DC, Franklin GM. Outcomes of pain center treatment in Washington State workers' compensation. *American Journal of Industrial Medicine.* 2001; **39**: 227–36.

64. Robinson JP, Fulton-Kehoe D, Franklin GM, Wu R. Multidisciplinary pain center outcomes in Washington State Workers' Compensation. *Journal of Occupational and Environmental Medicine.* 2004; **46**: 473–8.

* 65. Hatten AL, Gatchel RJ, Polatin PB, Stowell AW. A cost-utility analysis of chronic spinal pain treatment outcomes: converting SF-36 data into quality-adjusted life years. *Clinical Journal of Pain.* 2006; **22**: 700–11.

50

Organization of pediatric pain services

GEORGE CHALKIADIS

KEY LEARNING POINTS

- Effective treatment of children's pain is a basic standard of care.
- Pain management in children is suboptimal in many hospitals.
- Biological, developmental, psychological, and parental factors distinguish children from adults, and influence organization and service delivery.
- Institutional and departmental support is vital to establish an effective pediatric pain service.
- A goal-orientated approach helps prioritize the introduction of new initiatives.

- Available resources must be considered prior to introducing new analgesic techniques to maintain patient safety.
- Barriers to effective pain management must be identified.
- Regular pain assessment and its documentation as the fifth vital sign increases the likelihood that poorly managed pain is treated.
- Education, quality improvement, and research are important roles of a pediatric pain service.
- Utilizing existing resources can save time and effort.

INTRODUCTION

There are many analgesic drugs, routes for their administration, and nonpharmacological techniques available to treat pain in children. The challenge is in organizing the safe and rational provision of effective analgesia in an individual institution.[1] This chapter will address historical aspects and describe what constitutes a comprehensive pediatric pain service. It is important to recognize that wide differences exist worldwide and that diverse local environments, economics, and culture influence organizational aspects of pediatric pain service provision.

HISTORY

The last 30 years have seen a major cultural change take place. For many years, pain was considered inevitable and of no consequence, and pain relief dangerous by medical and nursing staff. Pain assessment and analgesia were low priorities for hospitals, surgeons, anesthesiologists, and nurses.[2] More importantly, no healthcare provider was accountable for poor analgesia.

For many years we relied upon surgeons, usually their junior inexperienced residents who received little if any undergraduate education in pain management,[3] to prescribe and manage postoperative analgesia. Analgesia was safer to prescribe in small doses, and infrequently, to avoid side effects such as opioid-induced respiratory depression. We relied upon ward nurses to assess that the child was in enough discomfort to deserve its administration. Nursing education systems also provided little, if any, education in pain assessment and management.[4] Rather than focus on providing effective analgesia, staff's responsibilities were absolved by providing some, albeit insufficient, pain relief without killing the child or discharging them as an opioid addict.[5] Sadly, this is still the case in many countries.[6, 7] A recent survey of 383 German anesthesia departments of hospitals in which pediatric surgery was performed revealed that 20.9 percent never administered intravenous opioids to children and that 15.4 percent regularly prescribed intramuscular analgesia.[8]

THE BIRTH OF PAIN SERVICES

The first multidisciplinary pain clinic for adults was established by Bonica at the University of Washington, Seattle, in 1961. Concerns regarding the treatment of acute postoperative pain were voiced in an anonymous editorial[9] published in 1976. In 1983, a survey of adults undergoing general surgical procedures showed that one-third experienced moderate, severe, or unbearable, unalleviated pain. Such surveys led to the introduction of continuous intravenous opioid infusions and more frequent use of regional analgesia in adult teaching hospitals.[10, 11] Subsequently, the development of an anesthesiology-based postoperative pain management service was described in 1988.[12] National guidelines followed. In 1988, the National Health and Medical Research Council in Australia published guidelines for the management of severe pain.[13] These were followed by guidelines published by The Royal College of Surgeons of England and the College of Anaesthetists in 1990[14] and by the US Department of Health and Human Services in 1992.[15] Although national guidelines may influence the accreditation of teaching hospitals for training,[16] they do not ensure the commitment of all hospitals.[17, 18] In the USA, the Joint Commission on Accreditation of Healthcare Organizations (JCAHO) is an independent not-for-profit organization that sets healthcare standards. JCAHO standards require that hospitals assess, treat, and document patients' pain, guarantee the competence of their staff in pain assessment and management, and educate patients and families about effective pain management.[19] Adherence to these standards determines, in

part, accreditation of healthcare facilities. In contrast to the flurry of activity to conform to the JCAHO guidelines in the US,[20, 21, 22, 23, 24] 17 percent of UK National Health Service hospitals performing more than 1000 operations annually do not have an acute pain service.[17] It would seem that the most effective way to effect organizational change is therefore to institute standards that hospitals must adhere to in order to achieve and maintain accreditation. These standards strongly indicate that the assessment and treatment of acute pain is no longer optional. It is a basic standard of care.

THE BIRTH OF PEDIATRIC PAIN SERVICES

Documentation of how and when pain services for children and adolescents first began is sparse.[25, 26] In most locations where organized pain services exist, one can trace back the origins of acute pain services to individual anesthesiologists who provided more vigilant aftercare when using more effective and complex analgesic techniques such as continuous intravenous administration of opioids and epidural analgesia for adults[12, 27] and children[25, 26, 28, 29, 30, 31, 32] undergoing major surgery. Children benefited from more effective methods of analgesic administration.[33] Early audit studies that demonstrated many children often did not receive analgesia,[34, 35, 36, 37] or received less than adults undergoing similar surgery,[37, 38] overwhelmingly supported this notion. Underlying these observations were outmoded beliefs including the following.

- Newborn infants do not experience pain.[39]
- Children rarely required drugs for pain.[36]
- Pain is merely a symptom, and not necessarily harmful in itself.[40]
- Effective analgesia makes diagnosis difficult or impossible.[41, 42]
- Effective analgesia delays discharge.

In turn, that led to variability in prescribing practices.[43]

- Postoperative analgesia was frequently not prescribed.
- Prescribed doses were too small or too infrequent.
- Prescribed analgesia was not administered by nursing staff, often because children preferred to suffer pain than receive intramuscular analgesia.

CHANGING ATTITUDES AND BARRIERS TO CHANGE

Fortunately, attitudes to pain relief were changing rapidly.[44] A survey of members of the Association of Paediatric Anaesthetists in the UK and Eire, published in 1988, found that 13 percent thought that newborn infants do not feel pain and 23 percent were undecided.[39] Only 10 percent, however, prescribed opioid analgesia for major surgery in the newborn. A repeat survey in 1995[44] revealed that there was almost universal agreement that all age groups perceived pain. Although 91 percent of respondents prescribed opioid analgesia in 1995, 31 percent cited the lack of a designated pain service as a factor limiting analgesia prescribing.

Early concerns limiting analgesia prescription centered around safety – remember there were no published dosage guidelines available for children, sedation scores were not recorded, the use of pulse oximeters was not widespread, and nurses were unfamiliar with these new techniques.[31, 32] Children receiving specialized analgesic infusions were nursed in high dependency units, if available.[45] In order to safely provide effective analgesia to children, it was clear that prescription and monitoring guidelines, staff and parent education, equipment purchases and standardization within an institution, and availability to troubleshoot and guide treatment were necessary. Clearly this was beyond the scope of what the interested anesthesiologist could take on in addition to their clinical workload.[46] In order to effect these changes and establish a sustainable model of service delivery, acute pain services, comprising initially anesthesiologists and later nurses, were established in leading pediatric centers.[47] Other centers rapidly followed in providing pain management programs,[48] although most acute pain services limited their service to children receiving patient-controlled analgesia (PCA) or regional analgesia and did not obtain funding for a multidisciplinary acute and chronic pain service until some years later.

For years, anesthesiologists were consulted sporadically by pediatricians, oncologists, and surgeons to help manage children with persistent pain and cancer pain because of their ability to perform nerve blocks and their familiarity with analgesic drugs. Over time, the role of other healthcare providers from various disciplines including psychologists, physiotherapists, occupational therapists, psychiatrists, oncologists, neurologists, rheumatologists, pediatricians, and surgeons evolved. There was greater appreciation of the biopsychosocial factors that contribute to, and maintain, persistent pain in children and adolescents, leading to the establishment of integrated pediatric multidisciplinary pain services.[48]

Procedural pain management services were also provided in some centers from the mid-1980s.[48] These centers utilized nonpharmacological techniques[49] and/or provided pharmacological sedation.[50] Despite these initiatives, the management of procedural pain in neonates and older children remains problematic today.[51, 52][IV]

In 1987, the first International Symposium on Pediatric Pain was convened in Seattle. This conference is now held triennially, addressing all aspects of pediatric pain management including basic science research, acute, persistent, procedural, and cancer pain (for future meetings see: www.childpain.org).

From an organizational perspective, it is useful to separate acute, persistent, procedural, and cancer pain as the demand, skills, and resources for each differs. Furthermore, poorly resourced fledgling pain services cannot realistically encompass all successfully. Acute pain management requires the least resources and the referral base is usually finite, limited to pain secondary to surgery, trauma and, less commonly, medical conditions such as sickle cell disease or mucositis. With adequate resource and direction, integration of these services is beneficial, facilitating strategic planning, research, and consistency within an institution, with the potential for economic benefits from streamlining clinical service delivery.

ACUTE PAIN

The principle objective of a pediatric acute pain service is the safe provision of effective analgesia (often utilizing specialized techniques) in the hospital environment whilst minimizing side effects. An acute pain service must also keep abreast of new developments, deliver education and training to medical, nursing, and allied health staff, and parent and child education. Ideally, an acute pain service should also conduct research and engage in audit and quality assurance. Whilst these goals are similar for adult pain services, there are important differences that must be considered in the pediatric setting that influence service delivery.

- Biological factors
  - Size: adjusting the amount of drug in any given volume as a multiple of the child's weight results in standardized infusion rates in all children, reducing the likelihood for calculation error (**Figure 50.1a**).
  - Immaturity of physiological systems: neonates and infants have immature enzyme systems that reduce drug clearance, influencing, for example, the safe duration of the administration of local anesthetic drugs.[53]
  - Anatomy: caudal epidural catheters can be threaded cephalad in neonates and infants to the thoracic region.[54]
  - Pathology: children with cerebral palsy often undergo orthopedic surgery that results in painful muscle spasms.[55]
- Developmental factors
  - Cognition: influences the choice of pain assessment tool, pain behavior, and the age at which patient-controlled devices can be used.
  - Verbal ability: pain behavior may be difficult to distinguish from other causes of distress in nonverbal children.
  - Emotional development: nursing and medical staff must consider the child's emotional development. Play and music therapy and distraction techniques appropriate to the child's developmental stage can reduce procedure-related distress.

- Psychological factors – children with chronic illnesses often require repeated hospitalization. Previous experiences associated with poor analgesia (failure of, or delays in its administration), suboptimal and distressing routes of administration (e.g. repeated intramuscular injections or rectal suppositories) or side effects such as nausea and vomiting may cause anticipatory fear during subsequent admissions.[52]
- Parental factors – parents may have fears regarding the use of opioid or epidural analgesia. Parents' own emotional distress around their child's pain and suffering can influence the child's pain behavior.[56] [III] Parents may also draw upon past traumatic experiences of their own or of their children.[57][III]
- Regulatory constraints – many drugs are not licensed for use in children.[58]
- Segregation of child and adult health care – a recently published survey on acute pain services in all hospitals performing more than 1000 operations annually in the UK excluded those concerned solely with pediatric services[17] without any explanation why.

These considerations demonstrate that the optimal provision of effective pain relief in children requires specialized knowledge and organization.

THE IDEAL COMPREHENSIVE PEDIATRIC ACUTE PAIN SERVICE MODEL

An acute pain service has many tasks and responsibilities, including clinical service provision, education, quality improvement, and research. A significant administrative workload accompanies these. An ideal pediatric acute pain service model is described below.

Clinical service delivery organization

AVAILABILITY

The acuity, unpredictable nature, and unpleasantness of inadequate analgesia and its side effects demand immediate action. New referrals may occur at any time, as may queries related to analgesia after hospital discharge. It is therefore essential that acute pain service staff are available 24 hours per day, seven days per week.[59]

In teaching hospitals, after-hours cover for the acute pain service is often provided by anesthesiology staff who are required to be present in hospital at all times.[60] Competing demands for their attention in the operating theater may result in delays in responding to pain service calls. Some hospitals allocate separate staff to answer pain calls.[61] In private hospitals or smaller hospitals without resident medical staff, the anesthesiologist who treated the patient or the surgeon is responsible.

CONTACTABILITY

Clear guidelines must be established so that nursing and medical staff know whom to contact and how. Providing easy "one number at all times" contact, either via mobile phone or a pager that the duty physician carries, facilitates prompt notification of pain issues and response. This has the additional benefit that adequate handover from one duty physician to the next occurs. Hospitals that enter patient information into a database can print out lists of patients, their location, and the analgesia prescribed to facilitate handover and communication of pain management issues.

REGULAR PATIENT REVIEW

Twice daily ward rounds, including weekends, ensures a review of patients who most recently underwent surgery and the response to interventions instituted on earlier rounds.

It is the responsibility of the pain service to ensure that analgesia is prescribed in appropriate doses and administered by an appropriate route. If side effects of analgesia occur, they should be treated or alternative effective analgesia should be substituted.

Direct prompt communication with the surgeon responsible for a patient's care is necessary if a serious adverse event related to analgesia occurs or if unexpected increasing analgesic requirements require exclusion of a surgical complication such as compartment syndrome.

Blocks of service by pain service personnel facilitate continuity of care allowing day-to-day comparison of each patient's progress and assessment of their response to therapeutic interventions. The clinician's knowledge of what analgesia is required after certain procedures improves, whilst building rapport with the child, their parents or guardian, and the primary healthcare team caring for the child. This is advantageous in more complex patients who require acute pain service input for more than a few days.

WHICH PATIENTS ARE REVIEWED BY THE ACUTE PAIN SERVICE?

Some acute pain services routinely review only those patients receiving PCA or epidural analgesia. This approach trivializes the assessment and treatment of pain in the most vulnerable children, those that are unsuitable for PCA, the very young, and the cognitively impaired. All patients prescribed non-oral analgesia and those requiring titration or weaning of strong analgesia should be reviewed by the acute pain service.

CAPTURING REFERRALS

There must be clear communication to the acute pain service that a patient has been referred. At the Royal

Page 1

ROYAL CHILDREN'S HOSPITAL

UR NUMBER

SURNAME

GIVEN NAME(S)

Opioid infusion attachment
Fifty (50) mL dilution

DATE OF BIRTH

AFFIX PATIENT LABEL HERE ↑

Weight: _____ kg

Guidelines   50 mL dilution can be used for any age, calculate dose according to lean body weight

Morphine

- Add **0.5 mg/kg** to a total volume of **50 mL** diluent of choice (any IV maintenance solution of electrolytes and/or glucose) to make infusion.
- Infuse at **0–4 mL/hr**: equivalent to 0–40 microgram/kg/hr.
- Recommended initial bolus: **5 mL** (50 microgram/kg) of infusion.
- Recommended bolus for pain or painful procedures: **1–2 mL** (10–20 microgram/kg) of infusion at intervals of no less than **10 minutes.**

Fentanyl

- Add **15 microgram/kg** to a total volume of **50 mL** diluent of choice (any IV maintenance solution of electrolytes and/or glucose) to make infusion.
- Infuse at **0–4 mL/hr**: equivalent to 0–1.2 microgram/kg/hr.
- Recommended initial bolus: **2 mL** (0.6 microgram/kg) of infusion.
- Recommended bolus for pain or painful procedures: **1 mL** (0.3 microgram/kg) of infusion at intervals of no less than **5 minutes.**

Medical instructions

☐ **Tick if instructions differ from guidelines**

1. Add _____ **mg/microgram** of _____ to a total of **50 mL** of _____

2. Infuse from _____ **mL/hr** to _____ **mL/hr** as required for analgesia

3. Start infusion at _____ **mL/hr**

4. Administer initial bolus _____ **mL** of infusion

5. Administer _____ **mL** bolus of infusion PRN for pain or painful procedures, at intervals of no less than _____ **minutes**

6. Notify doctor if respirations less than _____ per minute or sedation score ≥ 3

Opioid toxicity   • STOP the infusion   • CALL **MET 777** if required   • Notify CPMS (pager 5773)

Dilute NALOXONE 0.4 mg to 20 mL with normal saline 0.9% (this dilution = 20 microgram per mL)

For excess sedation:

(difficult to rouse, respiratory depression, sedation score ≥ 3)

Administer **NALOXONE 2 microgram/kg IV**, repeat each **1–2 minutes** PRN (max. 5 doses)

Administer _____ **microgram** = _____ **mL** IV

Date				
Time				
Initials				

For resuscitation:

(minimal respirations or cardiorespiratory arrest, sedation score 4)

Administer **NALOXONE 10 microgram/kg IV**, repeat each **1–2 minutes** PRN (max. 5 doses)

Administer _____ **microgram** = _____ **mL** IV

Date				
Time				
Initials				

Prescriber's signature _____ Print name _____ Date _____

Record of infusion (please sign for each new syringe)

Date	Time	Initials	Initials		Date	Time	Initials	Initials

Infusion ceased: Date _____ Time _____

See overleaf for record of rate changes and bolus doses given

Pharmacy initials	

For more details please read the 'Opioid Infusion guidelines' in the Children's Pain Management Service guidelines on The Royal Children's Hospital intranet.

This attachment is a legal prescription

(a)

Opioid infusion attachment (50 mL)

This order is not valid unless securely attached to designated area on MR52

Figure 50.1   (a) RCH opioid prescription chart. Note that the range of hourly rate of infusion is standardized regardless of patient weight by diluting the opioid according to weight (continued over).

Page 2

Opioid infusion attachment (50 mL)

Record of infusion rate changes and/or bolus doses given

Date	Time	Reason for rate change / bolus	Response	Initials
Rate change	Bolus given (mL)			
Date	Time	Reason for rate change / bolus	Response	Initials
Rate change	Bolus given (mL)			
Date	Time	Reason for rate change / bolus	Response	Initials
Rate change	Bolus given (mL)			
Date	Time	Reason for rate change / bolus	Response	Initials
Rate change	Bolus given (mL)			
Date	Time	Reason for rate change / bolus	Response	Initials
Rate change	Bolus given (mL)			
Date	Time	Reason for rate change / bolus	Response	Initials
Rate change	Bolus given (mL)			
Date	Time	Reason for rate change / bolus	Response	Initials
Rate change	Bolus given (mL)			
Date	Time	Reason for rate change / bolus	Response	Initials
Rate change	Bolus given (mL)			
Date	Time	Reason for rate change / bolus	Response	Initials
Rate change	Bolus given (mL)			
Date	Time	Reason for rate change / bolus	Response	Initials
Rate change	Bolus given (mL)			
Date	Time	Reason for rate change / bolus	Response	Initials
Rate change	Bolus given (mL)			
Date	Time	Reason for rate change / bolus	Response	Initials
Rate change	Bolus given (mL)			
Date	Time	Reason for rate change / bolus	Response	Initials
Rate change	Bolus given (mL)			
Date	Time	Reason for rate change / bolus	Response	Initials
Rate change	Bolus given (mL)			
Date	Time	Reason for rate change / bolus	Response	Initials
Rate change	Bolus given (mL)			
Date	Time	Reason for rate change / bolus	Response	Initials
Rate change	Bolus given (mL)			
Date	Time	Reason for rate change / bolus	Response	Initials
Rate change	Bolus given (mL)			
Date	Time	Reason for rate change / bolus	Response	Initials
Rate change	Bolus given (mL)			

Stock No. 306516 – ERC 051464 January 2006

This attachment is a legal prescription

Opioid infusion attachment (50 mL)

This order is not valid unless securely attached to designated area on MR52

(b)

Figure 50.1 RCH opioid prescription chart (continued). (b) The reverse side of this chart were changes in infusion rate and bolus administrations, why the changes were instituted and the child's response to these measures are recorded.

Children's Hospital in Melbourne, anesthesiologists prescribe the postoperative analgesia and simultaneously complete an acute pain service referral form (**Figure 50.2a**). This form includes relevant demographic details, patient location, relevant medical history, the procedure they underwent, what analgesia and antiemetics were administered in theater, and what has been prescribed postoperatively. This form is placed in a tray in the recovery room. The forms are collected prior to each acute pain service ward round by the pain service personnel and are easily accessible if required afterhours.

WHO CAN REFER PATIENTS?

Only medical staff should refer patients to the acute pain service. Patients are admitted to hospital under one doctor who is ultimately responsible for their management. If referrals are accepted from nursing staff, allied health staff, and medical staff, the potential for conflict arises. Some problems include:

- multiple referrals for the same patient;
- surgical or medical review of the patient may not occur if the primary team have not been informed that the patient has pain;
- resident and registrar doctors become less skilled at pain management;
- primary team may not wish for pain service involvement.

Nonmedical staff should contact the primary team to review the patient's medical or surgical condition, their analgesia and, if necessary, make a referral to the acute pain service.

CHARTING AND DOCUMENTATION

Clear prescription and documentation assist acute pain services to fulfill their responsibilities to the child and their parents, as well as to the hospital and its staff. It is important to consider these when establishing and reviewing an acute pain service as they can guide direction, continuing improvement, and development.

DOCUMENTATION OF PATIENT OBSERVATIONS

Pain and sedation scores

Provision should be made on the main patient observation chart for pain and sedation scores. The regular assessment of pain at rest, with movement, and its documentation as the fifth vital sign increases the likelihood that children and adolescents receive effective and appropriate analgesia. In addition to recording respiratory rate and oxygen saturation, sedation scores should also be documented as increasing sedation usually precedes respiratory depression.[40][IV]

Treatment plan

A clear treatment plan should be written for each patient after pain service review to facilitate communication between the acute pain service, nursing, and medical teams. This records that the patient was reviewed, what was found, and the management plan.

It is important to distinguish inadequate analgesia from the development of surgical complications, as escalating analgesic requirements may herald the onset of a surgical complication hitherto unsuspected. Increasing pain is often the first and most prominent symptom of developing compartment syndrome, preceding changes in neurovascular observations. Should the latter be suspected, the surgeon should be notified and a record of this made in the treatment plan.

PRESCRIPTION CHARTS

Clear prescription charts should be designed for specialized analgesic techniques offered by the acute pain service. Liaison with chart committees and pharmacy representatives ensure pain service charts comply with hospital standards.

Printed dosage guidelines and standardization of the delivery systems and the preparation of analgesic solutions minimize the potential for errors in prescription (**Figures 50.1a**, **50.3a**, and **50.4a**). In addition to the analgesic prescription, reversal agents should also be prescribed on the same chart in the event that they are required urgently.

Safe prescribing includes ensuring that children do not have multiple orders for analgesia prescribed on separate prescription charts that could lead to side effects, overdose, or drug interactions. Computerized prescribing reduces the likelihood of this. In the absence of computerized prescribing at the Royal Children's Hospital, an adhesive strip along the left margin of an analgesic prescription chart is used to stick the analgesic attachment chart to the main prescription chart. Multiple analgesic charts can be attached (e.g. **Figures 50.1**, **50.3**, and **50.4**). The prescription and administration of all medications is clearly visible on one chart thereby reducing the potential for error.

Regular (annual) review of charts should occur with view to modification to ensure clarity and ease of prescription.

ALGORITHMS

Certain situations lend themselves to algorithms to promote safe, timely, and effective intervention that improve analgesia and management of side effects. Examples include:

- Intravenous morphine bolus administration (**Figure 50.3a**):
  - facilitates dose titration;
  - standardized volume regardless of age and size;
  - facilitates administration after acute trauma.[62]

- Management of breakthrough pain, for example the rapid optimization of analgesia should be facilitated by the prescription of bolus doses and increased infusion rate if appropriate. If pain remains unrelieved despite the prescribed interventions, the acute pain team and surgical teams should be notified to review the analgesic technique and to exclude surgical complications.
- Postoperative nausea and vomiting: its effective management may be delayed considerably if the antiemetic drug prescribed postoperatively was ineffective or not prescribed at all. Prior to the introduction of an algorithm to manage postoperative nausea and vomiting, the following illustrative example was a common scenario. A child would return from theatre and vomit. No antiemetic was prescribed. The ward nurse would call a junior doctor on-call after hours who was busy and unable to attend immediately. The doctor was not familiar with the patient and not prepared to give a phone order. On attendance, an antiemetic was prescribed and eventually administered. This was ineffective. The cycle would resume or the nurses would readminister the same antiemetic that had been ineffective when it was due again. Prescribing several antiemetics to be administered in an order decided upon by the anesthesiologist (**Figure 50.4**) facilitates more rapid control of postoperative nausea and vomiting, overcoming the delays outlined above and reducing the risk of side effects from the repeated administration of an antiemetic that has clearly been ineffective.[63, 64] In addition, if postoperative nausea and vomiting persist after trying a number of antiemetics, medical review is encouraged.
- It has been suggested that a visual analog scale (VAS) pain score above 3 be promptly treated.[65] This approach lends itself to algorithm management, although it does not take into consideration interindividual variability and patient satisfaction. An alternative and preferable approach is to ask the patient if they desire an intervention to improve analgesia.

DISCHARGE ADVICE AND FOLLOW-UP

Written discharge advice for parents is desirable to inform them what analgesia should be administered after hospital discharge, when to give it, how to obtain it, where to obtain further prescriptions if required, and what to do if pain relief is inadequate.

Specific discharge advice regarding potential complications following major regional techniques and their symptoms should be given to parents and the family general practitioner should also be notified. A discharge letter for the general practitioner should also include the postoperative analgesic plan following major procedures where children are likely to require analgesia for some time, facilitating its prescription.

Phone follow-up with the child and their family after major procedures where oral opioid titration is required after hospital discharge, for example after scoliosis surgery, is good practice.

Administrative aspects relating to clinical service delivery

CHOOSING PAIN ASSESSMENT SCALES

Age and cognition appropriate pain assessment tools must be used (see Chapter 38, Pain assessment in children). A multitude of pain assessment tools exist.[66] It is important to standardize the tools used within any institution to facilitate staff proficiency in their use.

CHOOSING ANALGESIC TECHNIQUES AND DRUGS

Nursing staff competency, the nurse:patient ratio, and the availability of equipment and monitoring will determine which analgesic techniques can be safely administered in any given hospital environment.

There are an increasing number of opioids, non steroidal anti-inflammatory drugs (NSAID), and local anesthetic agents available and suitable for systemic, regional, and oral administration in children. It is preferable to limit the number prescribed routinely. The likelihood of prescription and administration errors is less when nursing and medical staff are familiar with drugs, their dose, and route of administration. There is also the potential to reduce costs by decreasing the workload for the hospital pharmacy and negotiating discounts with pharmaceutical companies.

PROTOCOLS AND GUIDELINES

Clear dosage, prescription, administration and monitoring protocols, and guidelines must be published for available analgesic therapies. These should include which patient observations should be monitored, how these should be recorded, and their frequency for various modalities. The nurse:patient ratio, the availability of monitoring, and staff competency will also influence in which ward environment specialized analgesic techniques can be utilized safely.

Guidelines should standardize the dose prescribed, the dilution and volume of drugs, and the delivery system and its labeling. They should include reference to the co-prescription of medications with the potential for interaction, such as benzodiazepines and opioids. Protocols and guidelines should be reviewed annually.

CHILDREN'S PAIN MANAGEMENT SERVICE, RCH (REFERRAL)

```
┌─────────────────────────────────┐      Ward: _____
│                                 │      Room: _____
│                                 │      Insurance: _____
│   PATIENT IDENTIFICATION LABEL  │
│                                 │      Weight: _____ kg
│                                 │
└─────────────────────────────────┘
```

Referral date: ..../........./..........

Surgical/Medical Consultant: _____ CPMS Consultant: _____ (if applicable)

Anaesthetist: _____ Anaes Signature: _____

Procedure/Problem: _____

Relevant medical history: _____

INTRAOPERATIVE ANALGESIA:
Spinal ☐   Caudal ☐   Epidural ☐

Nerve block(s) ☐   *Details:* _____

Wound infiltration ☐   *Details:* _____

Morphine ☐   Fentanyl ☐   Ketamine ☐   Clonidine ☐   NSAID ☐   Other: _____

ANTIEMETICS GIVEN:
Metoclopramide ☐   Granisetron ☐   Dexamethasone ☐   Other: _____

POST-OPERATIVE ANALGESIA PRESCRIBED: (OR *Current analgesia if pre-surgical or medical referral*)
Oral analgesia
Paracetamol ☐   Codeine ☐   NSAID ☐   Oxycodone ☐   Tramadol ☐   Diazepam ☐   Other: _____

Intermittent IV analgesia
Morphine ☐   Tramadol ☐   Clonidine ☐   NSAID ☐   Paracetamol ☐   Other: _____

Infusion
Morphine ☐   Fentanyl ☐   Ketamine ☐   Tramadol ☐   Hydromorphone ☐   Other: _____

PCA
Morphine ☐   Fentanyl ☐   Hydromorphone ☐   Tramadol ☐   Other: _____

Regional Infusion (*please tick and complete insertion details box below*)
Epidural ☐   Intrathecal ☐   Extrapleural/Paravertebral ☐   Interpleural ☐   Femoral ☐   Wound ☐

Other nerve catheter ☐   *Details:* _____

Urinary catheter in situ ☐   *Epidural D/C Info given pre discharge* ☐

REGIONAL CATHETER INSERTION DETAILS:

Catheter (1)	Catheter (2)
Solution: _____	Solution: _____
Infusion rate (ml/hr)_____(ml/kg)_____	Infusion rate (ml/hr)_____(ml/kg): _____
Epidural kit /catheter (brand & size): _____	Epidural kit /catheter (brand & size): _____
Insertion level: _____	Insertion level: _____
Skin to space distance (cm): _____	Skin to space distance (cm): _____
Catheter mark at skin (cm): _____	Catheter mark at skin (cm): _____
Dressing material used: _____	Dressing material used: _____
Complications at insertion: _____	Complications at insertion: _____

(a)

Figure 50.2 (a) RCH acute pain service referral form. This serves to summarize the anesthetist's intervention intraoperatively, what analgesia has been prescribed postoperatively, and functions as a referral form satisfying the Health Insurance Commission's requirements (continued over).

Date/Time							
Reviewer(s)							
Plan written (✓)							
Oral analgesia	Paracetamol (oral / IV)						
	Codeine						
	NSAID						
	Oxycodone						
	Oxycontin SR						
	Diazepam						
	Tramadol (oral / IV)						
Other:							
Infusion or IV bolus	Morphine						
	Fentanyl						
	Ketamine						
Other:							
PCA Bolus dose = _____	Morphine						
	Fentanyl						
	Background mL / hr						
	Tries total / good						
Opioid total	mg/day						
Pain assessment 0 = no pain 10 = worst pain *Excellent Good Satisfactory Dissatisfactory*	At rest / on palpation						
	On moving / physio						
	Patient satisfaction						
	Parent satisfaction						
	CPMS satisfaction						
Vomit/Nausea	No. of times (V or N)						
Antiemetic(s) given	Metoclopramide						
	Granisetron						
	Droperidol						
	Promethazine						
	Dexamethasone						
Other:							
Sedation score							
Pruritis & Rx							
Resp probs & Rx							
Regional Catheter — Catheter (1)	Solution						
	Rate mL / hr						
	Catheter cm at skin						
Catheter (2)	Solution						
	Rate mL / hr						
	Catheter cm at skin						
	LEFT dermatomes						
	RIGHT dermatomes						
	Bromage score						
	Bolus given (✓)						
Regional Catheter checks / problems *NB Document problems in patient's medical record*	Temperature						
	Urinary retention / IDC						
	Bradycardia/ Low BP						
	Rx given						
	Catheter site check						
	Dressing changed						
	Pressure area check						
	Major problems						

SEDATION SCORE: 0= Awake 1= Awake, tired/sleepy 2= Sedated/Asleep easily roused 3= Sedated/Asleep hard to rouse 4 = Unrousable S= sleeping
BROMAGE SCORE: 0= none/full flexion knees feet 1= partial/just moves knees 2= almost complete/moves feet only 3= complete/unable to move legs

(b)

Figure 50.2 RCH acute pain service referral form (continued). (b) The reverse side serves as the Acute Pain Service paper record of daily visits to the patient.

Page 1

**ROYAL
CHILDREN'S
HOSPITAL**

Intermittent IV morphine bolus administration attachment

UR NUMBER

SURNAME

GIVEN NAME(S)

DATE OF BIRTH

AFFIX PATIENT LABEL HERE

Weight: _____ kg

Guidelines   Circle the box required for this patient

Child under 12 months

Add 0.2 mg/kg of morphine made up to 10 mL with normal saline 0.9%

Recommended bolus size is **1 mL** IV from the syringe

1 mL = 0.02 mg/kg (20 microgram/kg)

Child over 12 months, and under 50kg

Add 0.2 mg/kg of morphine made up to 10mL with normal saline 0.9%

Recommended bolus size is **2 mL** IV from the syringe.

2 mL = 0.04 mg/kg (40 microgram/kg)

Child weighs over 50kg

Add 10 mg of morphine made up to 10 mL with normal saline 0.9%

Recommended bolus size is **2 mL** IV from the syringe

2 mL = 2 mg

Medical instructions

1. Add _____ **mg** of **morphine** and dilute to a total volume of **10 mL** with normal saline 0.9% in a syringe

2. Bolus size is _____ **mL**. Administer intravenously from the syringe according to the numbered administration steps overleaf.

3. Specify single or multiple use:

☐ **Single use**

OR

☐ **Multiple use**
for example, in the setting of painful procedures at intervals, such as dressing changes when there is no background or continuous pain present, i.e. there is no need for PCA or opioid infusion

Opioid toxicity   • STOP opioid administration   • CALL **MET 777** if required

Dilute NALOXONE 0.4 mg to 20 mL with normal saline 0.9% (this dilution = 20 microgram per mL)

For excess sedation:
(difficult to rouse, respiratory depression, sedation score ≥ 3)
Administer **NALOXONE 2 microgram/kg IV**, repeat each **1–2 minutes** PRN *(max. 5 doses)*

Administer _____ **microgram** = _____ **mL** IV

Date					
Time					
Initials					

For resuscitation:
(minimal respirations or cardiorespiratory arrest, sedation score 4)
Administer **NALOXONE 10 microgram/kg IV**, repeat each **1–2 minutes** PRN *(max. 5 doses)*

Administer _____ **microgram** = _____ **mL** IV

Date					
Time					
Initials					

Prescriber's signature _____   Print name _____   Date _____

Pharmacy initials	

See overleaf for record of bolus doses given

For more details please read the 'Intermittent morphine bolus administration guidelines' in the Children's Pain Management Service guidelines on The Royal Children's Hospital intranet.

This attachment is a legal prescription

Intermittent IV morphine bolus administration attachment

This order is not valid unless securely attached to designated area on MR52

(a)

Figure 50.3   RCH intermittent intravenous morphine bolus administration chart. This was designed to facilitate the timely administration and titration of effective analgesia in situations such as drain tube removal or the initial management of acute trauma pain. Note the prescription for naloxone and the capacity to use the order on more than one occasion to treat intermittent procedural pain (continued over).

Page 2   **Intermittent IV morphine bolus administration attachment**

Administration steps

1   **Check patient before administering IV morphine bolus:**

- Moderate or severe pain or anticipated pain
- Sedation level: awake or easily roused to voice
- Respiratory rate: >20/min if under 12 months
                        >15/min if under 50 kg
                        >12/min if over 50 kg

Do NOT administer bolus if patient does not meet all these criteria

2   Administer bolus as prescribed

3   Wait 5 minutes

4   Is the pain resolved? Is the child comfortable?

Yes ⟶ No further boluses

No ⟶ Go back to step 1 and repeat cycle

Single use   Maximum 5 boluses – the order is valid for 24 hours after first bolus given

Date:	Time given:	Initials	Initials
Bolus 1 ☐			
Bolus 2 ☐			
Bolus 3 ☐			
Bolus 4 ☐			
Bolus 5 ☐			
Total dose given: mL			
Amount discarded:			

If pain is unresolved after 5 boluses, consider urgent referral to the Children's Pain Management Service page 5773 (24 hours).

Multiple use   The order is valid for 6 days after first bolus given

Date:	Time given:	Initials	Initials
Bolus 1 ☐			
Bolus 2 ☐			
Bolus 3 ☐			
Bolus 4 ☐			
Bolus 5 ☐			
Total dose given: mL			
Amount discarded:			

Date:	Time given:	Initials	Initials
Bolus 1 ☐			
Bolus 2 ☐			
Bolus 3 ☐			
Bolus 4 ☐			
Bolus 5 ☐			
Total dose given: ml			
Amount discarded:			

Date:	Time given:	Initials	Initials
Bolus 1 ☐			
Bolus 2 ☐			
Bolus 3 ☐			
Bolus 4 ☐			
Bolus 5 ☐			
Total dose given: mL			
Amount discarded:			

Date:	Time given:	Initials	Initials
Bolus 1 ☐			
Bolus 2 ☐			
Bolus 3 ☐			
Bolus 4 ☐			
Bolus 5 ☐			
Total dose given: mL			
Amount discarded:			

Date:	Time given:	Initials	Initials
Bolus 1 ☐			
Bolus 2 ☐			
Bolus 3 ☐			
Bolus 4 ☐			
Bolus 5 ☐			
Total dose given: mL			
Amount discarded:			

Date:	Time given:	Initials	Initials
Bolus 1 ☐			
Bolus 2 ☐			
Bolus 3 ☐			
Bolus 4 ☐			
Bolus 5 ☐			
Total dose given: mL			
Amount discarded:			

If the order is inadequate for pain management, consider referral to the Children's Pain Management Service page 5773 (24 hours).

Stock No. 306515 – ERC 060570 Updated May 2006   **This attachment is a legal prescription**

(b)

Intermittent IV morphine bolus administration attachment

This order is not valid unless securely attached to designated area on MR52

Figure 50.3   RCH intermittent intravenous morphine bolus administration chart (continued).

Figure 50.4 RCH postoperative nausea and vomiting chart. This chart was designed to overcome barriers to the timely administration of antiemetics such as the availability of an alternative prescribed antiemetic should one be ineffective, variability in prescribed doses, the unpredictable availability, willingness and knowledge of ward residents to prescribe antiemetics when required (continued over).

Page 2

Post-operative nausea and vomiting (PONV) attachment

☐ **Give Dexamethasone [0.15mg/kg]** _____ **mg IV/PO daily prn [maximum 8mg per dose per day only].**
This can be repeated once if another antiemetic fails [no more than 2 post-operative doses].

Date:_____ Time given:_____ Route:_____ Initials:_____ Initials:_____   Date:_____ Time given:_____ Route:_____ Initials:_____ Initials:_____

If ineffective i.e. PONV occurs within 1–20 hours of receiving Dexamethasone: **cease** and proceed to next numbered antiemetic.

☐ **Give Droperidol [0.01mg/kg]** _____ **mg IV 8 hourly prn [maximum 0.625mg/dose]   (NB: 2.5mg ampoule).**
Continue if effective i.e. vomiting recurs more than 7 hours after last Droperidol dose.

Date:_____ Time given:_____ Initials:_____ Initials:_____   Date:_____ Time given:_____ Initials:_____ Initials:_____

Date:_____ Time given:_____ Initials:_____ Initials:_____   Date:_____ Time given:_____ Initials:_____ Initials:_____

Date:_____ Time given:_____ Initials:_____ Initials:_____   Date:_____ Time given:_____ Initials:_____ Initials:_____

If ineffective I.e. PONV occurs within 0.5–7 hours of receiving Droperidol: **cease** and proceed to next numbered antiemetic.

☐ **Give Promethazine [0.5mg/kg]** _____ **mg IV/PO 8 hourly prn [maximum 25mg/dose].**
Continue if effective i.e. vomiting recurs more than 7 hours after last Promethazine dose.

Date:_____ Time given:_____ Route:_____ Initials:_____ Initials:_____   Date:_____ Time given:_____ Route:_____ Initials:_____ Initials:_____

Date:_____ Time given:_____ Route:_____ Initials:_____ Initials:_____   Date:_____ Time given:_____ Route:_____ Initials:_____ Initials:_____

Date:_____ Time given:_____ Route:_____ Initials:_____ Initials:_____   Date:_____ Time given:_____ Route:_____ Initials:_____ Initials:_____

If ineffective i.e. PONV occurs within 0.5–7 hours of receiving Promethazine: **cease** and proceed to next numbered antiemetic.

☐ **Give** _____ _____ **mg/kg** _____ **mg**
Route _____ / _____ _____ **hourly prn**

Date:_____ Time given:_____ Route:_____ Initials:_____ Initials:_____   Date:_____ Time given:_____ Route:_____ Initials:_____ Initials:_____

Date:_____ Time given:_____ Route:_____ Initials:_____ Initials:_____   Date:_____ Time given:_____ Route:_____ Initials:_____ Initials:_____

Date:_____ Time given:_____ Route:_____ Initials:_____ Initials:_____   Date:_____ Time given:_____ Route:_____ Initials:_____ Initials:_____

If ineffective i.e. PONV occurs within _____ – _____ hours of receiving this medication: **cease** and proceed to next numbered antiemetic.

If PONV persists or occurs after 0.5 hours of administering all numbered antiemetics,
contact Children's Pain Management Service (CPMS) Pager 5773 (24 hours).

Prescriber's   Print
signature   name   Date
_____   _____   _____

For full details of hospital guidelines concerning PONV, see the Children's Pain Management Service Guidelines
or on The Royal Children's Hospital intranet.

ERC 061503

(b)

Post-operative nausea and vomiting (PONV) attachment

Figure 50.4   RCH postoperative nausea and vomiting chart (continued).

CHOOSING AND MANAGING EQUIPMENT

Pumps for intravenous continuous or intermittent infusion should be standardized throughout the hospital to reduce the potential for programming error. Some pumps allow programming of named drugs that comply with the local hospital dilutions and administration guidelines. The decision regarding which pumps to purchase is best made together with the hospital bioengineering department.

Pumps for epidural or regional local anesthetic infusions should be distinguishable from intravenous infusion pumps with distinctly colored tubing to reduce the likelihood of inadvertent connection to an intravenous cannula.

An adequate number of pumps must be purchased. Consideration must be given to repair and maintenance of pumps that necessitate them to be taken out of service. It is important to identify whose responsibility it is, and where disused pumps must be returned to, in order to effectively manage the equipment pool. Logistics systems can be employed to keep track of equipment whereabouts and availability.

PERSONNEL

The administrative aspects, clinical workload, and the complexity of medical and surgical conditions treated necessitate adequate staffing, office space, and equipment. The principal objective is to create a capable team that can work well together and be entrusted to provide a comprehensive clinical service and fulfill its administrative, quality improvement, and research responsibilities and activities.

CORE STAFF (EMPLOYED BY THE PAIN MANAGEMENT SERVICE)

Director of pediatric pain management

A director of pediatric pain management should be appointed to provide leadership, coordinate and be responsible for service provision. As with any leadership role, consideration should be given to leadership and management training and succession planning.

Core acute pain management staff should be responsible to the director whilst the resources of others could be utilized as needed.

Anesthesiology and pain medicine

The anesthesiologist is ideally placed to lead an acute pain service because of their training and understanding of pharmacology and pain management techniques, their relationship with surgeons and ward nurses, and their technical ability to perform specialized analgesic techniques. The anesthesiologist's perspective on perioperative care is helpful, starting preoperatively when the decision to employ specialized analgesic techniques is made after

discussion of the risks and benefits, and continuing through to the intraoperative and postoperative periods, when these are implemented.

Communication with other anesthesiologists is easier, facilitating individual feedback when insufficient analgesia has been prescribed or complications from analgesia arise. Furthermore, anesthesia department morbidity and mortality meetings provide an opportunity to raise concerns amongst peers and discuss complications.

In many countries, only medical practitioners can prescribe drugs. In addition, knowledge of medical and surgical complications, withdrawal syndromes, and specialized analgesic techniques is essential. Involvement in an acute pain service provides trained anesthesiologists, and those in training, with an opportunity to follow-up patients postoperatively, assess the quality of analgesia initiated intraoperatively, and an appreciation for what analgesia is required after each surgery and its duration.

Nursing

Nursing staff can lead clinical service provision, provide education, and advocate and deliver quality patient care.[67, 68] Furthermore, there are economic advantages. Some countries have developed nurse practitioner/advanced practice nurse roles and these nurses can prescribe a limited range of drugs.

Secretarial

Adequate secretarial support is necessary.

CORE STAFF APPRAISAL

Job satisfaction is paramount to provide excellent service, encourage innovation, research, and good staff morale. Staff appraisal gives each staff member the opportunity to voice any issues, ideas, and criticisms they may have, and allows their manager an opportunity to air and resolve issues and discuss staff development and aspirations. Many hospitals have structured formats to aid conducting appraisals.

Adequate provision must be made to share the clinical workload and perform administrative duties to avoid staff burnout. Professional development must be supported and adequate provision for leave (annual, sickness, maternity, paternity, study, conference, and sabbatical leave) should be made. Adequate staffing should be planned for as the workload increases.

NONCORE STAFF WHOSE SERVICES CAN BE ACCESSED WITHOUT BEING EMPLOYED BY THE PAIN MANAGEMENT SERVICE DIRECTLY

Pharmacists

A good working relationship with the pharmacy department is helpful. Many advantages are apparent including the economical choice of drugs, ensuring drug availability in the hospital and on wards, the establishment of hospital-wide analgesia guidelines, the participation in hospital staff, child and parent education, and the standardization of available preparations when available in different concentrations, for example oral paracetamol.

Psychologists

Psychological support is often neglected in the setting of acute pain service provision. Children may have post-traumatic stress disorder following accidents, burns, and poorly managed procedural pain.[69, 70][III] Pain itself may cause anxiety, fear, and depression.

It is extremely important to address issues relating to some children perceiving pain as punishment.

Concurrent issues may benefit from counseling, for example parental separation. In adults, relaxation training, procedural information, cognitive coping methods, and behavioral instruction have been shown to improve pain intensity and reduce analgesic consumption.[71]

Child life specialists, play therapists, and music therapists

Nonpharmacological strategies can diminish the pain experience.[72][III]

IT support

This is required to establish, maintain, support, update and upgrade databases, online competencies, and websites.

Accounting

In some centers, billing for services provided is necessary to maintain the viability of the service. Some centers are required to submit business plans.

Education

NURSING

Teaching hospitals affiliated to schools of nursing or universities employ educators who, in conjunction with pain service staff, can devise a curriculum for undergraduate and postgraduate pediatric nurses. Education packages should be delivered prior to undertaking competency assessment. Attending acute pain service ward rounds and pain clinics provides valuable practical experience.

Pain resource nurse programs

The pain resource nurse program requires the more intense training of a select number of nurses from each surgical ward who then function as a resource that other nurses can call upon for pain management advice.[68] This type of program inspires confidence in nurses' ability to manage and troubleshoot pain management issues, reduces the number of calls to an acute pain service, and encourages nurses to improve specific pain management practices on their ward whilst providing practical experience otherwise unavailable.

Competencies

Existing and newly employed nursing staff should undergo annual competency assessment that reinforces the need for pain assessment, its documentation, and treatment.

At the Royal Children's Hospital in Melbourne, an online secure system has been developed that can be accessed by nursing staff from any computer terminal connected to the intranet. This system is:

- convenient – allows completion of part or whole of each nursing competency package at any time;
- time and labor saving – competency package is marked online;
- efficient – automatic feedback reports to acute pain service and area unit managers which staff have or have not completed their competency package;
- confidential – nurses are each provided with a unique access code.

Separate competency packages have been designed for intravenous opioid, epidural and regional analgesia, and nitrous oxide administration.

MEDICAL

A pediatric pharmacopoeia that details analgesic drug dosage should be distributed to junior doctors.

New junior medical staff usually commence work at predictable times of the year. Orientation for these staff should include information on pain assessment and its management within the institution. Orientation provides an opportunity to explain the hospital's commitment to pain management, what the pain service does, and how to contact them.

Anesthesiologists in particular must appreciate what postoperative analgesia is required to decide what analgesia is administered intraoperatively and prescribed postoperatively for any given surgical procedure. Attendance on the daily acute pain service rounds provides invaluable experience and opportunity to observe and document adverse outcomes that might otherwise not reach their attention.

Ideally, senior medical and surgical staff should also receive education regarding pain and its management. In large hospitals, this can be difficult to achieve due to the busy schedules of senior staff. However, new appointees could receive this information as part of an orientation package, familiarizing them with the resources available and the culture of the organization regarding pain management.

PHYSIOTHERAPISTS

Educating physiotherapists regarding the timing of and administration of analgesia prior to physiotherapy has the potential to reduce movement-related pain and facilitate rehabilitation. Communicating analgesia issues to the acute pain service should be encouraged.

PARENTS AND CHILDREN

Preoperative education regarding postoperative pain, how it will be managed, what to do if analgesia is inadequate, and what resources are available to manage pain should be communicated to parents and children. This information can be reinforced through the provision of child-friendly and age-appropriate information leaflets explaining analgesic techniques for children and information leaflets for parents that include potential risks and benefits.

QUALITY IMPROVEMENT AND RESEARCH

It is essential to periodically assess whether the acute pain service is providing a satisfactory service to identify its strengths and weaknesses and strategies for future development and improvement.[46] Opinion should be sought from hospital staff, parents, and children.

The provision of an acute pain service does not ensure that all patients are receiving optimal analgesia, that analgesia is adjusted and titrated as required, or that patients and/or their parents are satisfied with the service they receive. One must differentiate between the advantages of the analgesic techniques themselves and those conferred by the increased specialist supervision and education provided by the dedicated staff of an acute pain service.[73]

Audit

Audit is essential to monitor and maintain standards in a clinical service. A cumulative sum technique has been described to monitor the performance of an acute pain team, in particular the failure rate of epidural analgesia, in a teaching hospital environment.[74] This type of analysis can be incorporated into a database, generating regular audit cycles and systematically identifying unexpected deviations in local practice. Auditing of calls after hours may help identify the need to change staffing practices as the pain service gets busier.

The following can be used as benchmarks for quality assurance:

- documentation of pain and sedation scores;
- variability of analgesic prescription by doctors – prescription of mediocre, but not overtly dangerous analgesia may identify need for targeted education;

- audit of nurse competency assessment completion;
- parent and child satisfaction surveys which may include promptness of response to complaints of unrelieved pain.

Databases

Databases can be time-consuming and costly to design, and data entry is labor-intensive regardless of whether information is recorded prospectively at the bedside using palm-held devices or retrospectively at a desk. Establishing what information an acute pain service wishes to extract from the database will determine which fields need to be included and how the information should be entered to enable meaningful results from a query. It is easy to record too much and irrelevant information in a format that will not provide meaningful data later or that will never be used. The more labor-intensive it is to record and enter data, the less likelihood of compliance in completing each field. **Box 50.1** outlines further benefits of establishing a database.

Significant advantages exist in combining data from various centers. The French-Language Society of Pediatric Anesthesiologists published data from a one-year prospective survey that demonstrated a low complication rate following regional techniques in children; 51 percent of their membership responded.[78][IV] The UK National Paediatric Epidural Audit is an initiative whereby all pediatric hospitals prospectively record the same data for all children receiving epidural analgesia and submit these to a nominated coordinating center that collates data. Data were collected from over 10,600 patients over five

---

Box 50.1 Benefits of establishing a database for an acute pain service

An acute pain database can be used to:

- record acute pain service activity;
- audit analgesia use and its complications;[74]
- document side effects and establish their incidence;[75]
- assess changes in the incidence of side effects and complication after the introduction of new initiatives;[76]
- document outcomes;[76]
- document staff, parent, and child satisfaction;
- generate active patient lists to facilitate handover and review by afterhours staff;
- generate patient accounts;
- store information as part of computerized patient record;[77]
- facilitate time-efficient and useful data extraction.

years, that can be used to establish the incidence of rare complications and facilitate benchmarking between institutions.[79]

FREQUENT FLYER CONCEPT

Some children and adolescents undergo multiple surgical procedures. Implementing an alert system whereby patients attending frequently have recorded details of previous analgesia problems[77] encourages better pain relief by avoiding:

- medications that may not work (e.g. codeine);[80]
- techniques that have not worked (e.g. radiographically demonstrated epidural septum resulting in unilateral analgesia);
- medications associated with side effects in that patient:
  - for example pruritis with morphine but not with fentanyl;
  - opioid analgesia causing severe constipation.

Adverse events

An adverse events reporting system should be established. Adverse events including prolonged inadequate analgesia; side effects and complications should be discussed in regular morbidity and mortality meetings with a view to identifying why a problem occurred and how it may be prevented from recurring.

Complaints

Complaints and comments regarding the pain service should be acknowledged and investigated.

HOW TO ESTABLISH AND PROVIDE AN ACUTE PAIN SERVICE

Institutional support

Institutional support is less likely to be a barrier to establishing an acute pain service in some countries, for example the USA where accreditation of each hospital is based on the institution's compliance with JCAHO pain management guidelines.[19]

In other countries, national guidelines may exist but do not compel individual hospitals to provide an acute pain service. It is important to raise awareness of the importance of providing a pain service at the highest level within the hospital (Chief Executive Officer (CEO)), to ensure institutional commitment to children's pain management. Obtaining funding, resources, and establishing institutional pain management guidelines

will be very difficult without this high-level institutional support.[81]

System of governance

Clearly established systems of governance ensure that responsibility for the pain service rests with individuals appointed to manage the institution. Problems encountered can be communicated to the next level of management (**Figure 50.5**).

In establishing an acute pain service and its governance, it is important to consider whether the primary responsibility for the provision of analgesia rests with the acute pain service or with the primary team responsible for the patient's management.

A team of healthcare providers whose role within a hospital is solely the assessment and management of pain, will develop specialized knowledge and clinical acumen that is beyond the scope of pre- and postgraduate medical and nursing curriculums.

This is not always feasible. In smaller hospitals, private hospitals, and in pediatric hospitals with limited resources and where surgeons, pediatricians, and anesthesiologists visit sporadically, the clinician under whom the patient is admitted takes responsibility for prescribing analgesia.[7, 82]

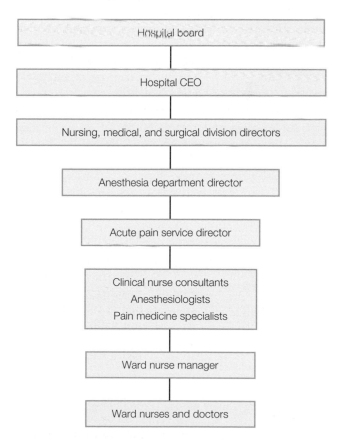

Figure 50.5 Pain service governance.

In smaller organizations

In smaller organizations, one person (e.g. the director of nursing) should be appointed to assume responsibility for appointing a multidisciplinary committee (that could comprise nursing staff, surgeons, anesthesiologists, pharmacists, and pediatricians) that delegates responsibility for:

- obtaining information from external sources (guidelines, protocols);
- regular pain assessment and its documentation utilizing appropriate pain assessment tools;
- disseminating hospital guidelines after multidisciplinary committee deliberation;
- quality improvement;
- regular review of guidelines and protocols.

STAFFING

The full-time or sufficient part-time employment of anesthesiologists or pain medicine specialists is not feasible in many hospitals due to either financial constraints[83] or the sporadic attendance of doctors that are renumerated by private insurers rather than the hospital.

Several models have been described and shown to be effective, including pain services led by surgeons in Germany,[84] nurses and clinical pharmacists in community hospitals, and large referral centers in the USA.[21, 24, 85] [IV] It is important to consider that some children, often those with pain unrelated to surgery, consume most of the pain physician's time.[86]

Goal-orientated approach

The list of tasks and responsibilities of an acute pain service outlined above can only be achieved with adequate staffing and financial support. Each hospital should identify and prioritize their objectives according to their pediatric case load and specify realistic timelines to achieve them. **Box 50.2** lists the minimum requirements that all hospitals should provide.

UTILIZATION OF EXISTING RESOURCES

Major centers are more likely to have resources to formulate guidelines and protocols that can be adapted by smaller hospitals in the same region subjected to the same laws and regulations regarding prescription, nursing care, etc. An acute pain service should be available to advise community pediatricians, anesthesiologists, general practitioners, and nurses regarding analgesia for children.

Establishing a pain service is time-consuming. Individuals asked to be involved should ensure that adequate time is allocated for this purpose if existing resources are utilized.

Box 50.2 The minimum provisions by an acute pain service applicable in any hospital that treats children

- Regular pain assessment and its documentation (fifth vital sign).
- Institutional agreement regarding which pain assessment tools to use.
- Analgesia guidelines and algorithms to ensure:
  - safe prescription of adequate analgesia;
  - assessment of pain treatment and timely revision if necessary;
  - discharge analgesic medication and parent education.
- Equipment to administer prescribed analgesia.
- Nurse education (pain assessment, preoperative education regarding unrelieved pain, and analgesia).
- Nursing competency regarding pain assessment and management.
- Education of anesthesiologists, surgeons, pediatricians, and ward doctors (analgesia prescription).

Existing guidelines, charts, and protocols from other institutions can be adapted for use. The following Internet links may be useful:

- pediatric pain assessment tools: www.medal.org (click on pediatrics);
- pediatric pain protocols, policies, and pamphlets: www.pediatric-pain.ca;
- pediatric pain protocols and charts (PCA, opioid, ketamine, and regional infusions): www.rch.org.au/anaes/pain.

PROCEDURAL PAIN MANAGEMENT

Painful medical procedures are performed every day and throughout a hospital by a wide range of staff with varied experience and knowledge regarding pharmacological and nonpharmacological pain management. Repeated attempts at intravenous cannulation on a single occasion or repeated procedures over time, such as intramuscular botulinum toxin injections for children with cerebral palsy or lumbar puncture and bone marrow aspiration in children with cancer, are distressing and traumatic for the child and their parents, and more so if physical restraint is required.[52][IV] The effective management of procedural pain is important to minimize distress at the time and to reduce the likelihood of adverse long-term psychological consequences and hospital and needle phobia.[87] Poor procedural pain management may diminish the effect of adequate analgesia in subsequent procedures.[88][IV]

In order to identify the organizational changes that need to take place, it is important to understand why procedural pain continues to be poorly managed in many hospitals.

In a review of pediatric pain management at the Royal Children's Hospital in Melbourne, 454 staff members were interviewed. Many staff commented on the "culture" of the hospital with reference to:

- an unchanging culture – whereby the tendency for beliefs and practices to prevail for long periods legitimized inadequate pain management;
- the "Nike" or "just do it" culture – whereby time constraints (often due to inadequate planning) or a perception that there was no alternative resulted in the use of forcible physical restraint to perform procedures;
- the "don't ask" culture – whereby junior medical staff perceived a culture against asking for help from senior or more experienced colleagues.

A number of barriers to improving care were identified including:

- variability in practice – both nursing and junior medical staff identified that variability of beliefs and practices amongst senior medical staff influenced procedural pain management;
- outmoded beliefs – that included notions that infants do not feel pain in the same way as adults, that children forget pain, that children are distressed and anxious rather than in pain, and that the risks associated with analgesia outweigh the benefits of effective pain management;
- inadequate knowledge and skills with regards to optimization of pharmacological and nonpharmacological options;
- inadequate time – this included insufficient time to prepare children and their parents for procedures;
- insufficient resources.

Changing the culture of an organization requires support of its leadership. The stated support of the CEO and financial support to employ a Project Officer to improve procedural pain management have led to a growing awareness amongst staff of the institution's commitment to change.

Parental empowerment can also drive organizational change. Described as a media and health system-wide campaign directed towards improving pain management for children during all phases of illness or injury, The Children's Hospital of Wisconsin developed a program called "The Comfort Zone" that resulted in a number of improvements in pain management. An important concept was the pledge by the hospital and therefore an expectation of hospital staff to provide effective pain management. Another early initiative was "The Ouchless Place," an innovative program established at the St Francis Hospital and Medical Center in Hartford, Connecticut, a community hospital with a small pediatric inpatient unit, that demonstrated effective procedural pain management is achievable in smaller hospitals.[89] Isolated islands of informed practitioners can drive reform and advocate for their patients. The challenge however, lies in isolating recalcitrant practitioners who hold on to outmoded beliefs to the detriment of children under their care. Both "The Comfort Zone" and "The Ouchless Place" empowered parents to advocate for their child's comfort.

A project officer was appointed at the Royal Children's Hospital to oversee, coordinate and implement procedural pain management initiatives after it became clear that the work required was too great to be added to existing busy clinical work schedules. Through organizational support and commitment, staff, parent and child education, establishment of hospital guidelines by multidisciplinary committees for sedation, and pharmacological and nonpharmacological procedural pain management and their implementation, a tidal wave is sweeping the organization driving improvements and cultural change.

Procedure specific guidelines outlining acceptable management for example intravenous cannulation reflect the multiple recommendations.

- Topical local anesthetic cream should be applied one hour prior to intravenous cannulation:
  - in a region where veins are clearly visible to a nurse;
  - or by the proceduralist themselves if the veins are not immediately obvious.
- Nonpharmacological techniques including positioning for comfort, distraction, and parental coaching should be employed wherever possible. Sitting the child on a parent's lap allows the child's arm to be placed behind the parent's back, so that the child can be distracted whilst intravenous cannulation is painlessly performed out of their direct line of sight.
- Thoughtfulness regarding the anxiety provoking performance ritual – preparing needles and syringes in front of the child and over-zealous skin preparation prior to intravenous cannulation heighten the child's expectation that something terrible is about to happen.
- Each proceduralist is allowed a finite number of failed attempts at cannulation before calling upon more senior staff to help out.

Recalcitrant healthcare providers will stand out; quality assurance and adverse event reporting of inadequate pain management for procedures will force a response that may require individual counseling and education.

PERSISTENT PAIN

Whereas most, if not all, hospitals that treat children should have an acute pain service, the management of children with persistent pain is:

- multidisciplinary;
- labor-intensive;
- preferably managed outside of the acute hospital environment;
- involves smaller numbers of patients;
- requires specialized skills.

Children referred for management of persistent pain fall into three broad categories:

1. persistent pain with no clear diagnosis from clinical examination and investigations, for example recurrent abdominal pain;
2. persistent pain with identifiable pathology, for example hip pain in children with cerebral palsy;
3. sympathetic maintained or neuropathic pain.

The role of persistent pain clinics includes the diagnosis and management of the presenting pain complaint and the functional disability that commonly results. Children will often have undergone assessment, multiple investigations, and treatment prior to referral;[90] those in whom pain persists are then referred. Some adolescents by this stage have "retired from life," avoiding school and social activities with their peers. The complexity of persistent pain in childhood mandates comprehensive multidisciplinary assessment and treatment (see Chapter 44, Chronic pain in children, in the *Chronic Pain* volume of this series).

An interdisciplinary model in which a team of diverse specialist healthcare providers integrate information about the child and their family, and jointly develop a comprehensive treatment plan, affords synergistic benefits over a multidisciplinary approach with serial involvement involving the same disciplines.[91]

The interdisciplinary approach acknowledges that persistent pain in childhood and adolescence may be caused, contributed to, and maintained by a diverse range of biopsychosocial factors. Elucidating their relative contribution helps formulate an integrated, individualized goal-orientated treatment plan that, delivered with intensity, constitutes a therapeutic tidal wave.

Some key differences exist between persistent pain and its management in adults and children providing opportunities for intervention.

- Parents and schools are usually motivated to be included in the treatment plan.
- The school year provides useful incentive for health care providers, children, and their families if children are to pass the school year along with their peers. Staying down a year can be detrimental to self-esteem and make the child vulnerable to teasing.

Referrals

In Australia, only medical practitioners can refer patients to medical specialists. This is advantageous because:

- the referral is made by the doctor coordinating that child's medical care;
- the child may already be under the care of one or more practitioners from disciplines that comprise the multidisciplinary pain team. There is potential:
  - to overwhelm the child and family with appointments;
  - that therapists may undermine each others work.

Who should be involved?

TEAM GOVERNANCE

A director of the multidisciplinary team must be appointed to oversee the administrative aspects that may include:

- seeking adequate funding for clinical service provision including secretarial and receptionist support;
- seeking adequate consulting and office space;
- coordination and triage of appointments;
- establishing a booking system that minimizes disruption to schooling and family commitments;
- coordinating staff leave;
- facilitating communication within the team and with medical practitioners, including general practitioners and specialists, other healthcare providers, and schools.

MEDICAL PRACTITIONERS

It is important for the therapists, the child, and their family that any hitherto undiagnosed treatable condition that may be responsible for persistent pain has been excluded. Some parents are clearly unhappy about the explanations offered so far (often a problem of communication or compounded by the accusation that the pain "is in their child's head") or harbor lingering suspicion that doctors have missed an organic problem responsible for their child's pain. Encouraging self-efficacy to manage persistent pain is contrary to, and undermined, by specialists who continue, "for the sake of completeness," to serially order further investigations they do not really believe will reveal a cause for the pain complaint.

In organizing interdisciplinary team composition, a balance must be struck between involving too many subspecialties and inefficient use of their resource and the benefits of a broad knowledge base. The pain medicine physician has comprehensive knowledge of pain assessment, diagnosis, and treatment whilst other specialists can provide complementary specific and specialized diagnostic skills.

Interdisciplinary pain assessment is a scarce and time-consuming resource. A triage system has worked well at the Royal Children's Hospital in Melbourne whereby children with recurrent headaches, for example, first consult a neurologist who then refers the child to the pain clinic if required. By the time the child is seen in the pain clinic:

- appropriate investigations will have been performed and their results available;
- parents have been reassured sinister causes such as a brain tumor are not responsible for their child's symptoms;
- multidisciplinary treatment can be started immediately.

Thus, not all children with headaches are referred to the clinic, effectively reducing the waiting times for initial assessment whilst selecting those who may benefit most from the pain program.

An alternative would be to include a neurologist or neurosurgeon as part of the interdisciplinary team. The limited availability of medical and surgical specialists to assess the child and to attend team meetings make it less likely for this to work in the Australian system.

Including a child and adolescent psychiatrist as part of the team is, on the other hand, useful. We have found their input invaluable in assessing and treating depression, anxiety, and other conditions such as Asperger syndrome. The psychiatrist works closely together with the psychologist in an advisory capacity and to provide individual and family therapy when required.

PSYCHOLOGIST

A psychologist is an essential team member. Individually they coordinate behavioral programs, conduct learning assessments, and teach children coping skills to deal with family and peer issues such as bullying at school. They can devise and implement strategies to optimize the school and family environments.

PHYSIOTHERAPISTS

A physiotherapist possesses diagnostic and treatment skills that can be effective for the primary problem that has resulted in pain as well as addressing secondary deconditioning.

OCCUPATIONAL THERAPIST

An occupational therapist assesses fine motor skills and ergonomic issues such as school desk, chairs, and lighting, establishes goal setting for individual patients and, in our institution, provides pain education for children and their families and relaxation training.

NURSES

In some pain clinics, nurses are employed to respond to calls from patients and their families regarding medication or other issues and to coordinate the clinic.

How the staff should be employed

Utilizing the services of the therapists available through the hospital may help initially establish a pain clinic. Competing demands for therapists' time, however, makes it difficult to provide coordinated care. Many pain clinics now employ the therapists ensuring their availability for pain clinic assessment, treatment, and meetings.

Staff selection

Treating children with persistent pain and their families requires therapists who are motivated to treat this population. They must be capable of being firm, compassionate, clear communicators and above all able to function within a team environment.

Practical issues

The process at the Royal Children's Hospital in Melbourne is described below to illustrate some important points.

INITIAL ASSESSMENT

Each child is accompanied by one or both parents to the initial assessment. The child and their parent(s) are seen by a:

- pain physician;
- psychologist and psychiatrist jointly;
- physiotherapist and occupational therapist jointly.

The above then meet as a team outlining the relevant history, examination findings, and investigations before jointly formulating a treatment plan. A case manager is appointed who is responsible for making future appointments. The case manager is also the person that the family contact if the need arises. The pain physician then meets with the child and their parent(s) to present the team's findings and suggestions. The pain physician then writes to the referring doctor summarizing the assessment findings and outlining the treatment plan. Copies of this letter are forwarded to the referring doctor, general practitioner, and other relevant healthcare providers.

FOLLOW-UP APPOINTMENTS

An important treatment goal is to restore normal function, including school attendance. The case manager coordinates interdisciplinary team follow-up appointments to occur on the same day and, where possible, after school.

TEAM COMMUNICATION

The team meets regularly to discuss each child's progress. Treatment goals are reset as necessary. Each team member summarizes their involvement.

DISCHARGE

Once treatment goals have been achieved, the child is discharged from the clinic and referred locally for community services if necessary. A discharge summary letter is sent to the referring doctor, the general practitioner, and other relevant healthcare providers.

CANCER PAIN

Children with cancer pain may experience acute pain, persistent pain, and procedural pain (see Chapter 25, Pediatric cancer pain in the *Cancer Pain* volume of this series). Integrating pain services into pediatric oncology seems logical.[92] On the other hand, singling out children with cancer may be seen to trivialize the pain experiences of other children with lifelong conditions necessitating frequent operative and procedural intervention such as those with cerebral palsy or cystic fibrosis. Hospital programs to identify children with a pain-sensitive temperament could help target those most in need of early intervention.[93]

LESSER DEVELOPED COUNTRIES

The large proportion of the world's children and adolescents live in lesser developed countries where analgesic drugs and basic medical care are limited or simply unavailable. Local barriers include political instability, corruption, warfare, distance and isolation, the availability and cost of medication, opioid-phobia, and cultural practices that involve the mutilation of children, often without anesthesia or analgesia. The considerations outlined earlier in this chapter are different in these populations.[94]

The relief of pain in children and adolescents in lesser developed countries should be considered important by governments and relief and aid organizations. Non-pharmacological pain strategies can be taught and implemented for little cost, whilst nonexpensive opioid analgesics such as morphine should be made available to relieve acute and cancer pain. To achieve change, local doctors who can influence policy and practice must be persuaded of the benefits of providing good analgesia.

Initiatives such as sponsoring delegates from lesser developed countries to attend conferences for pediatric pain, such as the triennial ISPP meeting, could help generate enthusiasm. The Society of Paediatric Anaesthesia of New Zealand and Australia (www.spanza.org.au) sponsors a delegate from a lesser developed country to attend its annual scientific meeting each year with good results, fostering the potential for collaboration with established centers.[95]

REFERENCES

1. Schafheutle EI, Cantrill JA, Noyce PR. Why is pain management suboptimal on surgical wards? *Journal of Advanced Nursing*. 2001; **33**: 728–37.
2. Gould TH, Crosby DL, Harmer M *et al*. Policy for controlling pain after surgery: effect of sequential changes in management. *British Medical Journal*. 1992; **305**: 1187–93.
3. Benedetti C, Dickerson ED, Nichols LL. Medical education: a barrier to pain therapy and palliative care. *Journal of Pain and Symptom Management*. 2001; **21**: 360–2.
4. Twycross A. Educating nurses about pain management: the way forward. *Journal of Clinical Nursing*. 2002; **11**: 705–14.
5. Cohen FL. Postsurgical pain relief: patients' status and nurses' medication choices. *Pain*. 1980; **9**: 265–74.
6. Wang XS, Tang JY, Zhao M *et al*. Pediatric cancer pain management practices and attitudes in China. *Journal of Pain and Symptom Management*. 2003; **26**: 748–59.
7. Karling M, Renstrom M, Ljungman G. Acute and postoperative pain in children: a Swedish nationwide survey. *Acta Paediatrica*. 2002; **91**: 660–6.
* 8. Stamer UM, Mpasios N, Maier C, Stuber F. Postoperative analgesia in children - current practice in Germany. *European Journal of Pain*. 2005; **9**: 555–60.
9. Anonymous. Editorial: Postoperative pain. *Anaesthesia and Intensive Care*. 1976; **4**: 95.
10. Donovan BD. Patient attitudes to postoperative pain relief. *Anaesthesia and Intensive Care*. 1983; **11**: 125–9.
11. Maier C, Kibbel K, Mercker S, Wulf H. [Postoperative pain therapy at general nursing stations. An analysis of eight year's experience at an anesthesiological acute pain service]. *Anaesthesist*. 1994; **43**: 385–97.
12. Ready LB, Oden R, Chadwick HS *et al*. Development of an anesthesiology-based postoperative pain management service. *Anesthesiology*. 1988; **68**: 100–6.
13. National Health and Medical Research Council (Australia). *Management of severe pain*. Canberra: NHMRC, 1988.

14. The Royal College of Surgeons of England and the College of Anaesthetists. *Report of the Working Party on Pain after Surgery.* London: HMSO, 1990.

15. US Department of Health and Human Services. *Clinical practice guideline. Acute pain management: operative or medical procedures and trauma.* Rockville, MD: Agency for Health Care and Policy and Research, 1992.

16. Windsor AM, Glynn CJ, Mason DG. National provision of acute pain services. *Anaesthesia.* 1996; **51**: 228–31.

17. Powell AE, Davies HT, Bannister J, Macrae WA. Rhetoric and reality on acute pain services in the UK: a national postal questionnaire survey. *British Journal of Anaesthesia.* 2004; **92**: 689–93.

18. Harmer M. When is a standard, not a standard? When it is a recommendation. *Anaesthesia.* 2001; **56**: 611–2.

* 19. Phillips DM. JCAHO pain management standards are unveiled. Joint Commission on Accreditation of Healthcare Organizations. *Journal of the American Medical Association.* 2000; **284**: 428–9.

20. Bell A, Wheeler R. Improving the pain management standard of care in a community hospital. *Cancer Practice.* 2002; **10**: S45–51.

21. Gordon DB, Pellino TA, Enloe MG, Foley DK. A nurse-run inpatient pain consultation service. *Pain Management Nursing.* 2000; **1**: 29–33.

22. Larson L. Treating pain: three models. *Trustee.* 2000; **53**: 25–6.

23. Ryan M, Ambrosio DA, Gebhard C, Kowalski J. Pain management: an organizational commitment. *Pain Management Nursing.* 2000; **1**: 34–9.

24. Zolnierz M, Dobbs R, Sesin P. Clinical pharmacists' pain consult service in a community hospital. *Journal of Pain and Symptom Management.* 2002; **23**: 92–3.

* 25. Lloyd-Thomas AR, Howard R. A pain service for children. *Paediatric Anaesthesia.* 1994; **4**: 3–15.

26. Lloyd-Thomas AR, Howard R. Postoperative pain control in children. *British Medical Journal.* 1992; **304**: 1174–5.

27. Brodsky JB, Brose WG, Vivenzo K. A postoperative pain management service. *Anesthesiology.* 1989; **70**: 719–20.

28. Ecoffey C, Dubousset AM, Samii K. Lumbar and thoracic epidural anesthesia for urologic and upper abdominal surgery in infants and children. *Anesthesiology.* 1986; **65**: 87–90.

29. Desparmet J, Meistelman C, Barre J, Saint-Maurice C. Continuous epidural infusion of bupivacaine for postoperative pain relief in children. *Anesthesiology.* 1987; **67**: 108–10.

30. Bray RJ. Postoperative analgesia provided by morphine infusion in children. *Anaesthesia.* 1983; **38**: 1075–8.

31. Beasley S, Tibbals J. Efficacy and safety of continuous morphine infusion in children. *Australian and New Zealand Journal of Surgery.* 1987; **57**: 233–7.

32. Murat I, Delleur MM, Esteve C *et al.* Continuous extradural anaesthesia in children. Clinical and haemodynamic implications. *British Journal of Anaesthesia.* 1987; **59**: 1441–50.

33. Gaukroger PB, Tomkins DP, van der Walt JH. Patient-controlled analgesia in children. *Anaesthesia and Intensive Care.* 1989; **17**: 264–8.

34. Campbell NN, Reynolds GJ, Perkins G. Postoperative analgesia in neonates: an Australia-wide survey. *Anaesthesia and Intensive Care.* 1989; **17**: 487–91.

35. Purcell-Jones G, Dormon F, Sumner E. The use of opioids in neonates. A retrospective study of 933 cases. *Anaesthesia.* 1987; **42**: 1316–20.

36. Swafford LI, Allan D. Pain relief in the pediatric patient. *Medical Clinics of North America.* 1968; **52**: 131–6.

37. Eland JM, Anderson JE. The experience of pain in children. In: Jacox A (ed.). *Pain: a source book for nurses and other health professionals.* Boston: Little Brown, 1977.

38. Beyer JE, DeGood DE, Ashley LC, Russell GA. Patterns of postoperative analgesic use with adults and children following cardiac surgery. *Pain.* 1983; **17**: 71–81.

39. Purcell-Jones G, Dormon F, Sumner E. Paediatric anaesthetists' perceptions of neonatal and infant pain. *Pain.* 1988; **33**: 181–7.

40. Australian and New Zealand College of Anaesthetists and Faculty of Pain Medicine. *Acute pain management: scientific evidence.* Canberra: National Health and Medical Research Council, 2005.

41. Green R, Bulloch B, Kabani A *et al.* Early analgesia for children with acute abdominal pain. *Pediatrics.* 2005; **116**: 978–83.

42. Kim MK, Strait RT, Sato TT, Hennes HM. A randomized clinical trial of analgesia in children with acute abdominal pain. *Academic Emergency Medicine.* 2002; **9**: 281–7.

* 43. Mather L, Mackie J. The incidence of postoperative pain in children. *Pain.* 1983; **15**: 271–82.

44. de Lima J, Lloyd-Thomas AR, Howard RF *et al.* Infant and neonatal pain: anaesthetists' perceptions and prescribing patterns. *British Medical Journal.* 1996; **313**: 787.

45. Lynne A, Opheim K, Tyler D. Morphine infusion after pediatric cardiac surgery. *Critical Care Medicine.* 1984; **12**: 863–6.

46. Kitowski T, McNeil H. Evaluation of an acute pain service. *Journal of Perianesthesia Nursing.* 2002; **17**: 21–9.

47. Berde C, Cahill C. Multidisciplinary programs for pain management. In: Schechter NL, Berde CB, Yaster M (eds). *Pain in infants, children and adolescents.* Baltimore: Williams & Wilkins, 1993.

48. Berde C, Sethna NF, Masek B *et al.* Pediatric pain clinics: recommendations for their development. *Pediatrician.* 1989; **16**: 94–102.

49. Zeltzer L, LeBaron S. Hypnosis and nonhypnotic techniques for reduction of pain and anxiety during painful procedures in children and adolescents with cancer. *Journal of Pediatrics.* 1982; **101**: 1032–5.

50. Marx CM, Stein J, Tyler MK *et al.* Ketamine-midazolam versus meperidine-midazolam for painful procedures in pediatric oncology patients. *Journal of Clinical Oncology.* 1997; **15**: 94–102.

* 51. Walker SM. Management of procedural pain in NICUs remains problematic. *Paediatric Anaesthesia*. 2005; **15**: 909–12.

52. Crock C, Olsson C, Phillips R *et al*. General anaesthesia or conscious sedation for painful procedures in childhood cancer: the family's perspective. *Archives of Disease in Childhood*. 2003; **88**: 253–7.

53. Chalkiadis GA, Anderson BJ. Age and size are the major covariates for prediction of levobupivacaine clearance in children. *Paediatric Anaesthesia*. 2006; **16**: 275–82.

54. Bosenberg AT, Bland BA, Schulte-Steinberg O, Downing JW. Thoracic epidural anesthesia via caudal route in infants. *Anesthesiology*. 1988; **69**: 265–9.

55. Nolan J, Chalkiadis GA, Low J *et al*. Anaesthesia and pain management in cerebral palsy. *Anaesthesia*. 2000; **55**: 32–41.

56. Goubert L, Eccleston C, Vervoort T *et al*. Parental catastrophizing about their child's pain. The parent version of the Pain Catastrophizing Scale (PCS-P): a preliminary validation. *Pain*. 2006; **123**: 254–63.

57. Ramchandani PG, Stein A, Hotopf M, Wiles NJ. Early parental and child predictors of recurrent abdominal pain at school age: results of a large population-based study. *Journal of the American Academy of Child and Adolescent Psychiatry*. 2006; **45**: 729–36.

58. Wilson JT. An update on the therapeutic orphan. *Pediatrics*. 1999; **104**: 585–90.

59. Wigfull J, Welchew EA. Acute pain service audit. *Anaesthesia*. 1999; **54**: 299.

60. Norman AT, Jackson IJ. Acute pain services: a 24-h commitment. *Anaesthesia*. 1998; **53**: 1228–9.

61. Duncan MA, Victory R. An audit of the pain management work done by anaesthetists during on-call time in a teaching hospital. *Anaesthesia*. 2001; **56**: 608.

62. Alexander J, Manno M. Underuse of analgesia in very young pediatric patients with isolated painful injuries [see comment]. *Annals of Emergency Medicine*. 2003; **41**: 617–22.

63. Yis U, Ozdemir D, Duman M, Unal N. Metoclopramide induced dystonia in children: two case reports. *European Journal of Emergency Medicine*. 2005; **12**: 117–9.

64. Mejia NI, Jankovic J. Metoclopramide-induced tardive dyskinesia in an infant. *Movement Disorders*. 2005; **20**: 86–9.

* 65. Rawal N. Organization, function, and implementation of acute pain service. *Anesthesiology Clinics of North America*. 2005; **23**: 211–25.

66. Finley GA, McGrath PA. Measurement of Pain in Infants and Children. In: Finley GA, McGrath PA (eds). *Progress in pain research and management*, Vol. 10. Seattle: IASP Press, 1998.

67. VanDenKerkhof EG, Goldstein DH, Wilson R. A survey of directors of Canadian academic acute pain management services: the nursing team members role – a brief report. *Canadian Journal of Anaesthesia*. 2002; **49**: 579–82.

68. Ferrell BR, Grant M, Ritchey KJ *et al*. The pain resource nurse training program: a unique approach to pain management. *Journal of Pain and Symptom Management* 1993; **8**: 549–56.

69. Rennick JE, Morin I, Kim D *et al*. Identifying children at high risk for psychological sequelae after pediatric intensive care unit hospitalization. *Pediatric Critical Care Medicinc*. 2004; **5**: 358–63.

70. Rennick JE, Johnston CC, Dougherty G *et al*. Children's psychological responses after critical illness and exposure to invasive technology. *Journal of Developmental and Behavioral Pediatrics*. 2002; **23**: 133–44.

71. Johnston M, Vogele C. Benefits of psychological preparation for surgery: a meta-analysis. *Annals of Behavioral Medicine*. 1993; **15**: 245–56.

72. Huth MM, Broome ME, Good M. Imagery reduces children's post-operative pain. *Pain*. 2004; **110**: 439–48.

73. Rawal N. Acute pain services revisited–good from far, far from good? *Regional Anesthesia and Pain Medicine*. 2002; **27**: 117–21.

74. Hammond EJ, Veltman MG, Turner GA, Oh TE. The development of a performance indicator to objectively monitor the quality of care provided by an acute pain team. *Anaesthesia and Intensive Care*. 2000; **28**: 293–9.

75. Tsui SL, Irwin MG, Wong CM *et al*. An audit of the safety of an acute pain service. *Anaesthesia*. 1997; **52**: 1042–7.

76. Story DA, Shelton AC, Poustie SJ *et al*. Effect of an anaesthesia department led critical care outreach and acute pain service on postoperative serious adverse events. *Anaesthesia*. 2006; **61**: 24–8.

77. Goldstein DH, VanDenKerkhof EG, Rimmer MJ. A model for real time information at the patient's side using portable computers on an acute pain service. *Canadian Journal of Anaesthesia*. 2002; **49**: 749–54.

78. Giaufre E, Dalens B, Gombert A. Epidemiology and morbidity of regional anesthesia in children: a one-year prospective survey of the French-Language Society of Pediatric Anesthesiologists. *Anesthesia and Analgesia*. 1996; **83**: 904–12.

79. Llewellyn N, Moriarty A. The national pediatric epidural audit. *Paediatric Anaesthesia*. 2007; **17**: 520–33.

80. Williams DG, Patel A, Howard RF. Pharmacogenetics of codeine metabolism in an urban population of children and its implications for analgesic reliability. *British Journal of Anaesthesia*. 2002; **89**: 839–45.

81. Jiang HJ, Lagasse RS, Ciccone K *et al*. Factors influencing hospital implementation of acute pain management practice guidelines. *Journal of Clinical Anesthesia*. 2001; **13**: 268–76.

82. Jacob E, Puntillo KA. Variability of analgesic practices for hospitalized children on different pediatric specialty units. *Journal of Pain and Symptom Management*. 2000; **20**: 59–67.

83. Mackey DC, Ebener MK, Howe BL. Patient-controlled analgesia and the acute pain service in the United States: Health-Care Financing Administration policy is impeding optimal patient-controlled analgesia management. *Anesthesiology*. 1995; **83**: 433–4.

84. Lempa M, Gerards P, Eypasch E *et al.* [Organization of pain therapy in surgery–comparison of acute pain service and alternative concepts]. *Chirurg.* 2003; **74**: 821–6.

85. Shapiro A, Zohar E, Kantor M *et al.* Establishing a nurse-based, anesthesiologist-supervised inpatient acute pain service: experience of 4,617 patients. *Journal of Clinical Anesthesia.* 2004; **16**: 415–20.

86. Shapiro BS, Cohen DE, Covelman KW *et al.* Experience of an interdisciplinary pediatric pain service. *Pediatrics.* 1991; **88**: 1226–32.

87. Chen E, Zeltzer LK, Craske MG, Katz ER. Children's memories for painful cancer treatment procedures: implications for distress. *Child Development.* 2000; **71**: 933–47.

∗ 88. Weisman SJ, Bernstein B, Schechter NL. Consequences of inadequate analgesia during painful procedures in children. *Archives of Pediatrics and Adolescent Medicine.* 1998; **152**: 147–9.

89. Schechter NL, Blankson V, Pachter LM *et al.* The ouchless place: no pain, children's gain. *Pediatrics.* 1997; **99**: 890–4.

∗ 90. Sleed M, Eccleston C, Beecham J *et al.* The economic impact of chronic pain in adolescence: methodological

considerations and a preliminary costs-of-illness study. *Pain.* 2005; **119**: 183–90.

∗ 91. Turk D, Stieg R. Chronic pain: the necessity of interdisciplinary communication. *Clinical Journal of Pain.* 1987; **3**: 163–7.

92. Meyer MJ. Integration of pain services into pediatric oncology. *International Anesthesiology Clinics.* 2006; **44**: 95–107.

93. Chen E, Craske MG, Katz ER *et al.* Pain-sensitive temperament: does it predict procedural distress and response to psychological treatment among children with cancer? *Journal of Pediatric Psychology.* 2000; **25**: 269–78.

94. Kumar A. Organization and development of pain clinics and palliative care in developing countries. *European Journal of Anaesthesiology.* 2004; **21**: 169–72.

95. Williams JE, Chandler A, Ranwala R *et al.* Establishing a cancer pain clinic in a developing country: effect of a collaborative link project with a UK cancer pain center. *Journal of Pain and Symptom Management.* 2001; **22**: 872–8.

51

Where does pain fit within healthcare delivery systems and organizations?

BRIAN R THEODORE, CHETWYN CH CHAN, AND ROBERT J GATCHEL

KEY LEARNING POINTS

- Pain should be considered the fifth vital sign, in addition to pulse, blood pressure, core temperature, and respiration.
- One of the best assessment methods of pain is the patient's self-report of pain, measured unidimensionally as pain intensity, or multidimensionally (e.g. functional status and psychosocial well-being, in addition to pain intensity).
- The biopsychosocial model of pain posits an interaction among physiological, psychological, and social factors; each of these factors play a role in exacerbating and perpetuating the experience of pain. The interactions among these factors become more complex, and harder to treat, as pain progresses from the acute to the chronic stage.
- Multidisciplinary pain management is the best evidence-based model for treating pain, and has

- demonstrated improved treatment outcomes and is significantly more cost-effective compared to single discipline treatment modalities.
- Levels of care for pain can be divided into three broad categories (primary, secondary, and tertiary care), differentiated by the patient's level of physical deconditioning and psychosocial comorbidity. Within each level of care, a psychosocial component is required, varying only in intensity of intervention that increases from primary to tertiary care.
- Increased efforts on education about the efficacy and cost-effectiveness of multidisciplinary pain management are required for personnel at all levels within healthcare organizations and delivery systems.

INTRODUCTION

Pain is the most commonly reported symptom in the primary care setting, and has been estimated to account for more than 80 percent of all visits.[1, 2] Healthcare costs related to back pain alone was estimated at upwards of $90 billion in 1998.[3] The experience of pain is now known to be associated with several other factors, including psychopathology (such as depression and anxiety), poor occupational and psychosocial functioning, and lower quality of life in general. Such factors play a major role in indirect costs, such as lost productivity, greatly increasing the total costs related to pain in an exponential manner.[1, 4]

Due to the major impact of pain on the healthcare system, as well as its related socioeconomic costs, greater attention and resources have been devoted to understanding pain and its related impact on patients as well as the healthcare system. The importance of pain treatment, research, and control is underscored by the International Association for the Study of Pain's (IASP's) declaration of the Global Year Against Pain, with the year from September 2006–October 2007 declared as IASP's Global Year Against Pain in Older Persons. In the United States, the 106th Congress passed H.R. 3244, signed into law by President Clinton, declaring the Decade of Pain Control and Research starting from January 1, 2001.[5] In addition, the Joint Commission on Accreditation of Healthcare Organizations (JCAHO) has issued guidelines requiring that pain be considered the fifth vital sign, in addition to pulse, blood pressure, core temperature, and respiration.[6] As a result, several clear guidelines have emerged on how pain fits within healthcare delivery systems and organizations.

Given the importance of the role pain plays within clinical settings, attention to pain should be a part of every level within healthcare systems. The clinical focus would be differentiated by levels of care depending on the severity of patients' pain symptoms and the extent of physical and psychosocial comorbidity. The first step would of course be a reliable, and preferably multi-dimensional, assessment of pain and its related symptoms. Following assessment, relevant treatment can be efficiently planned based upon Von Korff's[7] stepped-care framework to reflect the level of care required based on pain symptom, extent, severity, and related comorbidity. Central to both the assessment and the clinical interventions for pain is a firm understanding of the biopsychosocial perspective of pain, and the process of progression from acute to chronic pain. Thus, a review of these and their underlying characteristics is warranted.

BIOPSYCHOSOCIAL PERSPECTIVE OF PAIN

The traditional focus on pain was based on the philosophy of biomedical reductionism, which proposed a mind–body duality. A consequence of this was that medical assessments only focused on identifying a physiological basis for pain. When none could be found, as is the case with many chronic pain conditions, the pain was attributed to psychological causes with no real basis for treatment with the usual medical regimens. This duality greatly diminished the understanding of pain symptoms and their related phenomena, since pain often triggers psychosocial responses, and, more importantly, these psychosocial responses, in turn, affect how pain is perceived.

When Melzack and Wall[8] formulated their gate control theory of pain, it was the first evidence-based model that elaborated on a physiological basis for the role played by psychosocial factors in pain perception.[9] The biopsychosocial approach to medicine was first formulated by Engel,[10] and it conceptualizes physical disorders (including pain) as a complex interaction among physiological, psychological, and social factors. Each of these factors may play a role in exacerbating and perpetuating the disorder; resulting in distress, maladaptive behavior, and the adoption of a sick role. Since then, the biopsychosocial approach has been applied in the research and treatment of various disorders, including pain, and has now replaced the biomedical reductionism paradigm. This new paradigm has resulted in a greater understanding of pain and its related phenomena, but more importantly it has provided an effective treatment model for dealing with pain.

PROGRESSION OF PAIN

The progression of pain from acute to chronic is best described by Gatchel's[11, 12] three-stage model. The acute phase of pain is described in stage 1, and consists of the normal reactions to pain, and serves as a protective function that motivates the individual to reduce or remove the pain, by seeking medical attention for example. These responses of general psychological distress include:

- fear;
- anxiety;
- worry.

Stage 2 of the model describes the situation in which pain has persisted beyond the duration of what is considered the normal healing period (two to four months), and indicates the beginning of the development of a chronic pain condition. This stage is marked by the exacerbation of physiological and behavioral problems. The nature and extent of the progression in stage 2 is dependent upon preexisting factors, such as an individual's personality and psychosocial health, as well as socioeconomic and environmental conditions. Common symptoms observed during stage 2 include:

- learned helplessness;
- anger;
- somatization;
- substance abuse;
- psychophysiological disorders;
- emergence of personality disorders.

Continued exacerbation and the feedback loop between physiological and psychosocial symptoms eventually lead to Stage 3 of the progression model. At this stage, the pain is chronic in nature and is more strongly driven by psychological factors and psychosocial barriers than it is by any identifiable physiological problem. An individual at this stage will often develop the sick role, which is characterized by:

- focus on pain;
- development of secondary gains;
- avoidance of responsibility;
- poor occupational and social functioning.

Understanding the progression of pain from acute to chronic, and the underlying characteristics in each stage, allows for reliable assessment and planning of treatment. Furthermore, it highlights the importance of addressing pain during the acute stage and preventing the complications of various complex and interacting factors found in chronic pain conditions.

ASSESSMENT

Present guidelines in the United States require physicians to document pain severity using a pain scale.[6] These self-report measures can be obtained using tools such as a pain numeric rating scale or a visual analog scale.[13] Such measures provide a number, usually ranging from 0 to 10, reflecting the severity of pain according to the patient. Additionally, there are various multidimensional measures, such as the McGill Pain Questionnaire[14] and the Brief Pain Inventory,[15] that allow scaling of multiple dimensions of subjective experience of pain and its related impact on activities of daily living and functional status.[16] In addition to the measure of pain severity, the JCAHO guidelines also require the following assessments:

- pain described in patient's own words;
- duration and location of pain;
- associated aggravating and alleviating factors of pain;
- present pain management regimen and its effectiveness;
- effects of pain;
- patient's pain goal;
- physical examination.

The above guidelines constitute the assessment of pain during an initial evaluation, and are applicable to both malignant and nonmalignant pain, as well as across treatment settings and levels of care.[17] Clinicians should also be able to assess pain in populations where verbal communication or ability to provide numerical ratings may not be possible. For example, facial expressions in response to pain can be observed and scored in patients from such clinical subpopulations, such as children.[18, 19]

One crucial aspect of reliable assessment at the primary care level is the ability to determine the risk of acute pain developing into a chronic pain condition for any given patient. In addition to the unpleasantness experienced by the patient, the complicated interactions among the various factors characteristic of chronic pain would require more healthcare resources for treatment, thus increasing costs. Identifying high-risk patients allows the clinician to administer early/preventative interventions to prevent development of chronicity. Risk can be determined using predictive algorithms based upon multidimensional assessments of psychosocial functioning.[20] The benefits of early intervention for pain conditions in high-risk patients are well documented, resulting in better occupational and functional outcomes in high-risk acute low back pain patients,[21] and reduced pain levels and improved psychosocial functioning in high-risk acute temporomandibular disorder patients.[22] Additionally, early intervention for acute pain patients (regardless of risk) have also demonstrated better outcomes compared to controls who had no early intervention. These benefits include:

- improved occupational and functional outcomes;[23, 24]
- reduced risk for disability;[25]
- improved psychosocial well-being and quality of life.[26]

Once a reliable assessment has been made, the appropriate level of treatment for the patient can be determined.

LEVELS OF CARE

Levels of care are categorized into primary care, secondary care, and tertiary care. This categorization reflects a progressively increasing level of intensity in treatment approach commensurate with the severity of pain symptoms and any comorbidity. In addition to treatment intensity, this distinction among the three levels of care also reflects the different types of biopsychosocial approaches that need to be incorporated into the treatment regimen.[12]

Primary care

In general, primary care is designed to efficiently deal with pain of limited severity during the acute stage. The main goals in primary care are to control the symptoms of pain and to set the stage for adequate healing of the pathophysiology to prevent deconditioning.[27] Additionally, the clinician should address any psychosocial barriers to recovery, such as anxiety about the pain, by reassuring the patient that acute pain is temporary and will soon be alleviated. As mentioned earlier, pain is the most common symptom presented at the primary care setting. As such, this setting is a crucial step in being able to identify the extent of the problem and to provide referrals and subsequent management of specialty care services beyond the primary care level. In order to better provide pain management services within the primary care setting, there should be efficient integration and coordination between a psychosocial component and the traditional primary care setting. One way to achieve this is by having a clinical health psychologist as part of the primary care team.[17]

A useful assessment and treatment model for pain in the primary care setting is the stepped-care framework developed by Von Korff.[7] While Von Korff's original conception of this model was developed for managing low back pain in the primary care setting, it is applicable to dealing with pain symptoms in general.[17] This stepped-care framework consists of three steps of progressively increasing intervention commensurate with the severity of the presenting symptoms (including comorbidity). **Table 51.1** details the three steps in Von Korff's model. Step 1 is the lowest intensity of treatment, and is provided in complement to standard primary care treatment modalities for pain control. This level of treatment includes addressing possible psychosocial barriers, such as anxiety about the pain, while offering education and advice about self-care and resuming activities of daily living. Step 2 of this framework is targeted at patients who continue to suffer from pain six to eight weeks after the initial episode of pain, and who start demonstrating functional limitations and some psychosocial barriers to recovery. Step 3 of this framework addresses the complicated and interacting factors of physical and psychosocial deconditioning in a chronic pain patient.

It should be noted that steps 2 and 3 are analogous to the distinctions of levels of care for secondary and tertiary care interventions (to be discussed below under Secondary care and Tertiary care). Von Korff suggests a stratified approach in order to match the patients to the appropriate level of care depending on symptom severity, without necessarily requiring the patient to progressively go through each step of the model.[7] If a patient arrives at a primary care setting demonstrating advanced physical deconditioning and psychiatric comorbidity, the application of step 3 may be warranted without necessarily going through steps 1 and 2.

Secondary care

Secondary care is targeted at patients who do not recover after the timeframe of the normal healing process, are presenting with psychosocial barriers to recovery, or require additional interventions for helping with the transition from primary care (or surgical intervention) to resuming activities of daily living or return to work. The goal of secondary care is reactivation of the area of injury and to prevent the development of long-term physical and psychosocial deconditioning. Treatment modalities here usually include structured exercise programs, functional training for improving general health and work capacity, and cognitive-behavioral interventions designed to address psychosocial barriers to recovery that play a role in the development of chronicity. Previous studies found that the control of the pain level, optimization of workload, and balanced lifestyle are important factors for achieving the therapeutic goals.[13, 28]

Health care at this point should involve an interdisciplinary team consisting of clinical psychologists, physical therapists, occupational therapists, and nurses or health educators, in addition to the primary care physician. There is evidence-based support for the efficacy of an interdisciplinary approach for pain interventions at the secondary care level.[29] The benefits of such a secondary care approach have also been evaluated in several randomized controlled trials.[24, 30, 31, 32] Benefits include:

- reduction in occurrence of daily and bothersome pain;
- improved general health and self-efficacy;
- increased treatment satisfaction;
- lower healthcare costs;
- improved return-to-work outcomes.

Tertiary care

For patients who do not respond well to primary or secondary care interventions, and present with significant psychiatric comorbidity, tertiary care is required to prevent permanent disability. Treatment at this level is more complex and requires a multidisciplinary healthcare team

---

Table 51.1 Elements of intervention recommended by Von Korff's stepped-care framework.

Step 1	Step 2	Step 3
Address fear/avoidance beliefs	Structured exercise programs	Address psychiatric comorbidity
Education	Cognitive-behavioral interventions	Address secondary gain issues
Information	Extended or multiple visits	Address physical deconditioning
Advice	Interdisciplinary intervention recommended	Multidisciplinary intervention required
Initial primary care visit		

to plan and implement a tailored intervention to address physical and psychosocial deconditioning, as well as psychosocial barriers to recovery such as secondary gains that play a role in perpetuating pain-related disability and the sick role.[33] Healthcare team members should include clinical psychologists or psychiatrists, physical therapists, occupational therapists, disability case managers, and nurses or health educators in addition to the primary physician. Usually, such services may not be provided at a primary care setting and may require referral to a specialty pain management program.

Treatment modalities in tertiary care can take two broad approaches. The overlapping goals of these two approaches are in managing pain and associated disability, while the differences are in terms of treatment intensity and the focus on improving function. The ultimate goal of such an approach, besides managing pain and its associated disability, is preparing the patient for full or partial/modified resumption of occupational status and activities of daily living. One example of the more intense approach is functional restoration[34] and return-to-work programs.[35] These programs include:

- narcotic detoxification;
- cognitive-behavioral therapy;
- disability and occupational case management;
- psychotropic medication for any psychiatric comorbidity;
- structured graded exercises aimed at improving functional capacity;
- work hardening and skills training aimed at improving work capacity and employability;
- individual placement and support for returning to work.

The other approach to tertiary care is palliative pain management, the goal of which is simply to manage pain without any focus on restoring functional status.[27] Treatment modalities include pain-relieving narcotics, psychotropic medication for any psychiatric comorbidity, and psychological interventions aimed at increasing pain and stress management and coping techniques. The latter is useful in helping patients deal with a lifestyle of reduced function.[27, 36]

Cohort studies and randomized controlled trials provide evidence for the benefits of tertiary care approaches such as functional restoration.[34, 37, 38, 39, 40] Positive outcomes include:

- increased return-to-work rates;
- increased resumption of activities of daily living;
- decreased healthcare utilization;
- reduced levels of pain intensity;
- improved readiness to change;
- improved psychological well-being;
- resolution of outstanding medicolegal issues.

These findings were also consistent in a two-year post-treatment follow-up study.[41] Additionally, the efficiency of such an approach has been shown to be generalized across markedly different economic and social conditions as well as medicolegal systems.[42, 43, 44, 45] The multidisciplinary intervention for chronic pain also results in better outcomes compared to standard conservative care, pharmacological treatment, surgery, spinal cord stimulators, and implantable drug delivery systems.[4, 46] Finally, it should also be noted that intensive multidisciplinary approaches to managing chronic pain have also been demonstrated to be cost-effective compared to standard conservative treatment.[4, 47, 48]

HEALTHCARE DELIVERY SYSTEMS AND ORGANIZATION ISSUES

Education of healthcare providers and organizations

A chapter on where pain fits within healthcare systems and organizations will not be complete without addressing issues related to education in pain management and adherence to treatment guidelines and protocols. Several studies have documented the fact that medical school education in pain management and residency training has not been adequate.[49, 50] Within healthcare settings, several studies in the last decade have also found deficits in proper knowledge of pain management.[51, 52, 53, 54] Despite the increased attention and research findings on pain within the last six years, a recent study found that many of the deficits in proper pain management still hold true.[55] This study on clinical nurses' pain assessment indicated that:

- patients' self-report of pain were ignored (except for older patients);
- pain assessment influenced by patients' age;
- pain assessment influenced by patients' behavior (grimace);
- nurses were reluctant to administer appropriate doses of analgesia (fear of respiratory depression).

These deficits in knowledge, however, can be reversed with proper training and educational programs for healthcare professionals. This should also be mandated for third-party payers who have the responsibility of authorizing assessment and treatment requests in an educated manner based upon the best evidence-based data available. Education on up-to-date pain management techniques has been shown to result in significant gains in knowledge, adopting of appropriate attitudes regarding pain management, and improved self-efficacy among the targeted healthcare professionals.[56] Education and training aimed towards improving assessment of postoperative pain in surgical wards have also resulted in significantly greater adherence to protocols in assessing pain, as demonstrated during annual audits over a period of three years.[57] This study suggests the following elements within an in-house training and education program for pain management:

- mandatory training;
- regular staff meetings;
- regular audits;
- feedback to staff members based on audit.

The major problem of treatment "carve out" practices of managed care organizations

As Gatchel and Okifuji[4] and Gatchel et al.,[58] have recently highlighted, a major obstacle to the employment of effective multidisciplinary pain programs is the lack of understanding by third-party payers who often refuse to cover such programs. Efforts by third-party payers to contain costs have paradoxically steered patients away from treatments that demonstrably reduce healthcare utilization and towards more expensive therapies with poorer outcomes. As noted by Turk,[59] (page 13) "Greater collaboration is required among professional groups, consumers of healthcare services, governmental agencies and third-party payers to ensure that the more clinically effective and cost-effective treatments are provided to all likely to benefit from them".

Unfortunately, managed care organizations are currently "carving out" portions of comprehensive multidisciplinary programs (i.e. sending patients to different providers for their various needs outside of the comprehensive programs), thus diluting the proven successful outcome of such comprehensive programs, in an effort to cut costs.[60, 61, 62] In the long run, however, such "cost cutting" efforts are counterproductive because they significantly reduce the ability of patients to resume productive lives, and are actually less cost-effective from the perspective of healthcare, tax, legal, and economic factors. Indeed, in a recent study by Hatten et al.,[63] the cost-utility (expressed in cost/quality-adjusted life years (QALY)) of multidisciplinary programs for chronic spinal pain was evaluated. The calculation of QALYs involves the costs of a specific intervention, relative to the desired improvement in health (in this case, increased functioning and decreased pain). Results of the study revealed that, relative to a "carve out" unimodal medication treatment with or without anesthetic procedure, the multidisciplinary treatment was associated with a better QALY. Such cost-utility findings again indicate that such comprehensive, non-carve-out treatment programs are both less costly and more effective than the other options.

In addition to cost-utility issues, there is evidence that such "carve-out" practices result in poorer clinical outcomes among patients. For example, patients who linger within the healthcare system without adequate multidisciplinary pain management will develop very complex psychosocial disorders characteristic of stage 3 chronic pain, as described above under Progression of pain. When such patients eventually reach a medical and financial end point, and receive multidisciplinary pain management at the tertiary care level, the increased chronicity has been found to be associated with poorer rehabilitation outcomes.[64] Additionally, undertreated pain, as a result of noncomprehensive pain management programs, has been identified as a risk factor for increased abuse of prescription opioids.[65] The resulting opioid dependence has also been identified as a risk factor for poorer rehabilitation outcomes, even when chronic pain is later addressed within a multidisciplinary pain management setting.[66] Finally, comprehensive pain management approaches that address psychosocial barriers to effective pain management have been shown to increase the effectiveness of pharmacological interventions.[67]

CONCLUSION

Research on pain has made great advances over the last decade, and is still making continued immense progress. While the fruits of pain research have been successfully applied to treatment modalities and protocols to control and alleviate pain in clinical settings, research findings have also indicated that there is a need for improvement "across the board," including education of patients, healthcare providers, managed care organizations, and governmental or regulatory agencies. The key component in facilitating the appropriate position of pain within healthcare organizations and delivery systems is the recognition of pain as a multidimensional phenomenon that is moderated by biological, psychological, and social/environmental factors. Thus, there is no "one-size-fits-all" approach in dealing with pain, without taking into account the various predisposing, co-occurring, and consequent factors associated with pain. This biopsychosocial perspective of pain is the best evidence-based model to date, resulting in greater treatment satisfaction, improved patient outcomes, and greater clinical- and cost-effectiveness, compared to the traditional unimodal approaches of dealing with pain in clinical settings. Appreciation of this model and its successful implementation should be a part of every level of healthcare organizations and delivery systems, from the primary care setting to specialty pain management facilities.

ACKNOWLEDGMENTS

The writing of this chapter was supported in part from Grants No. 2R01 DE10713, 2R01 MH46452, and K05 MH071892 from the National Institutes of Health, and Grant No. DAMD17-03-0055 from the Department of Defense.

REFERENCES

1. Gatchel RJ, Turk DC. *Psychological approaches to pain management: a practitioner's handbook.* New York: Guilford Publications, 1996.

2. Kerns RD, Otis J, Rosenberg R, Reid MC. Veterans' reports of pain and associations with ratings of health, health-risk behaviors, affective distress, and use of the healthcare system. *Journal of Rehabilitation Research and Development.* 2003; **40**: 371–9.

* 3. Luo X, Pietrobon R, Sun SX *et al.* Estimates and patterns of direct health care expenditures among individuals with back pain in the United States. *Spine.* 2004; **29**: 79–86.

* 4. Gatchel RJ, Okifuji A. Evidence-based scientific data documenting the treatment and cost-effectiveness of comprehensive pain programs for chronic nonmalignant pain. *Journal of Pain.* 2006; **7**: 779–93.

5. Lippe PM. The decade of pain control and research. *Pain Medicine.* 2000; **1**: 286.

* 6. Joint Commission on Accreditation of Healthcare Organizations. *Pain assessment and management: An organization approach.* Oakbrook Terrace, IL: Author, 2000.

* 7. von Korff M. Pain management in primary care: An individualized stepped-care approach. *Psychological Factors in Pain.* 1999; **22**: 360–70.

* 8. Melzack R, Wall PD. Pain mechanisms: a new theory. *Science.* 1965; **150**: 971–9.

* 9. Turk DC, Monarch ES. Biopsychosocial perspective on chronic pain. In: Turk DC, Gatchel RJ (eds). *Psychological approaches to pain management: a practitioner's handbook*, 2nd edn. New York: Guilford, 2002.

* 10. Engel GL. The need for a new medical model: a challenge for biomedicine. *Science.* 1977; **196**: 129–36.

* 11. Gatchel RJ. Early development of physical and mental conditioning in painful spinal disorders. In: Mayer TG, Mooney V, Gatchel RJ (eds). *Contemporary conservative care for painful spinal disorder.* Philadelphia: Lea and Febiger, 1991: 278–89.

* 12. Gatchel RJ. Psychological disorders and chronic pain: Cause and effect relationships. In: Gatchel RJ, Turk DC (eds). *Psychological approaches to pain management: a practitioner's handbook.* New York: Guilford, 1996: 33–52.

13. Chan CCH, Li CWP, Hung LK, Lam PCW. A standardized clinical series for work-related lateral epicondylitis. *Journal of Occupational Rehabilitation.* 2000; **10**: 143–52.

14. Melzack R. The McGill Pain Questionnaire: major properties and scoring methods. *Pain.* 1975; **1**: 277–99.

15. Cleeland CS, Ryan KM. Pain assessment: global use of the Brief Pain Inventory. *Annals of the Academy of Medicine, Singapore.* 1994; **23**: 129–38.

16. Turk DC, Melzack R (eds). *Handbook of pain assessment*, 2nd edn. New York: Guilford Press, 2001.

17. Gatchel RJ, Oordt MS. *Clinical health psychology and primary care: practical advice and clinical guidance for successful collaboration.* Washington, DC: American Psychological Association, 2003.

* 18. Keefe FJ, Williams DA, Smith SJ. Assessment of pain behaviors. In: Turk DC, Melzack R (eds). *Handbook of pain assessment*, 2nd edn. New York: Guilford Press, 2001: 170–89.

* 19. Craig KD, Prkachin KM, Grunau RE. The facial expression of pain. In: Turk DC, Melzack R (eds). *Handbook of pain assessment*, 2nd edn. New York: Guilford Press, 2001: 153–69.

* 20. Pulliam C, Gatchel RJ, Gardea MA. Psychosocial differences in high risk versus low risk acute low back pain differences. *Journal of Occupational Rehabilitation.* 2001; **11**: 43–52.

* 21. Gatchel RJ, Polatin PB, Noe CE *et al.* Treatment- and cost-effectiveness of early intervention for acute low back pain patients: A one-year prospective study. *Journal of Occupational Rehabilitation.* 2003; **13**: 1–9.

* 22. Gatchel RJ, Stowell AW, Wildenstein L *et al.* Efficacy of an early intervention for patients with acute temporomandibular disorder-related pain: A one-year outcome study. *Journal of the American Dental Association.* 2006; **137**: 339–47.

* 23. Linton SJ, Hellsing AL, Andersson D. A controlled study of the effects of an early intervention on acute musculoskeletal pain problems. *Pain.* 1993; **54**: 353–9.

24. Hagen EM, Eriksen HR, Ursin H. Does early intervention with a light mobilization program reduce long-term sick leave for low back pain? *Spine.* 2000; **25**: 1973–6.

25. Cooper JE, Tate RB, Yassi A, Khokhar J. Effect of an early intervention program on the relationship between subjective pain and disability measures in nurses with low back injury. *Spine.* 1996; **21**: 2329–36.

26. Wand BM, Bird C, McAuley JH *et al.* Early intervention for the management of acute low back pain: a single-blind randomized controlled trial of biopsychosocial education, manual therapy, and exercise. *Spine.* 2004; **29**: 2350–6.

* 27. Mayer TG, Press JM. Musculoskeletal rehabilitation. In: Vaccaro A (ed.). *Orthopedic knowledge update.* Chicago, IL: AAOS Press, 2005: 655–61.

28. Chan HHK, Li-Tsang WPC, Chan CCH *et al.* Psychosocial aspects of injured workers' returning to work (RTW). *Hong Kong Journal of Occupational Therapy.* 2007; **17**: 279–88.

* 29. Karjalainen K, Malmivaara A, van Tulder M *et al.* Multidisciplinary biopsychosocial rehabilitation for subacute low back pain in working-age adults: a systematic review within the framework of the Cochrane Collaboration Back Review Group. *Spine.* 2001; **26**: 262–9.

30. Indahl A, Haldorsen EH, Holm S *et al.* Five-year follow-up study of a controlled clinical trial using light mobilization and an informative approach to low back pain. *Spine.* 1998; **23**: 2625–30.

* 31. Karjalainen K, Malmivaara A, Mutanen P *et al.* Mini-intervention for subacute low back pain: two-year follow-up and modifiers of effectiveness. *Spine.* 2004; **29**: 1069–76.

* 32. Lindstrom I, Ohlund C, Eek C et al. The effect of graded activity on patients with subacute low back pain: a randomized prospective clinical study with an operant-conditioning behavioral approach. *Physical Therapy*. 1992; **72**: 279–90; discussion 91–3.

* 33. Dersh J, Polatin PB, Leeman G, Gatchel RJ. The management of secondary gain and loss in medicolegal settings: strengths and weaknesses. *Journal of Occupational Rehabilitation*. 2004; **14**: 267–79.

* 34. Mayer TG, Gatchel RJ, Kishino N et al. Objective assessment of spine function following industrial injury. A prospective study with comparison group and one-year follow-up. *Spine*. 1985; **10**: 482–93.

* 35. Li EJ, Li-Tsang CW, Lam CS et al. The effect of a "training on work readiness" program for workers with musculoskeletal injuries: A randomized control trial (RCT) study. *Journal of Occupational Rehabilitation*. 2006; **16**: 529–41.

36. Lau OWY, Leung LNY, Wong LOL. Cognitive behavioral techniques for changing the coping skills of patients with chronic pain. *Hong Kong Journal of Occupational Therapy*. 2002; **12**: 13–20.

37. Hazard RG, Fenwick JW, Kalisch SM et al. Functional restoration with behavioral support. A one-year prospective study of patients with chronic low-back pain. *Spine*. 1989; **14**: 157–61.

* 38. Becker N, Sjogren P, Bech P et al. Treatment outcome of chronic non-malignant pain patients managed in a Danish multidisciplinary pain centre compared to general practice: a randomised controlled trial. *Pain*. 2000; **84**: 203–11.

* 39. Guzman J, Esmail R, Karjalainen K et al. Multi-disciplinary rehabilitation for chronic low back pain: systematic review. *British Medical Journal*. 2001; **322**: 1511–16.

40. Patrick LE, Altmaier EM, Found EM. Long-term outcomes in multidisciplinary treatment of chronic low back pain: results of a 13-year follow-up. *Spine*. 2004; **29**: 850–5.

41. Mayer TG, Gatchel RJ, Mayer H et al. A prospective two-year study of functional restoration in industrial low back injury. An objective assessment procedure. *Journal of the American Medical Association*. 1987; **258**: 1763–7.

* 42. Bendix AF, Bendix T, Vaegter K et al. Multidisciplinary intensive treatment for chronic low back pain: a randomized, prospective study. *Cleveland Clinic Journal of Medicine*. 1996; **63**: 62–9.

43. Hildebrandt J, Pfingsten M, Saur P, Jansen J. Prediction of success from a multidisciplinary treatment program for chronic low back pain. *Spine*. 1997; **22**: 990–1001.

44. Corey DT, Koepfler LE, Etlin D, Day HI. A limited functional restoration program for injured workers: A randomized trial. *Journal of Occupational Rehabilitation*. 1996; **6**: 239–49.

45. Jousset N, Fanello S, Bontoux L et al. Effects of functional restoration versus 3 hours per week physical therapy: a randomized controlled study. *Spine*. 2004; **29**: 487–93; discussion 94.

* 46. Turk DC. Clinical effectiveness and cost effectiveness of treatment for patients with chronic pain. *Clinical Journal of Pain*. 2002; **18**: 355–65.

47. Turk DC, Okifuji A. Multidisciplinary pain centers: Boons or boondoggles? *Journal of Workers' Compensation*. 1997; **6**: 9–26.

* 48. Skouen JS, Grasdal AL, Haldorsen EM, Ursin H. Relative cost-effectiveness of extensive and light multidisciplinary treatment programs versus treatment as usual for patients with chronic low back pain on long-term sick leave: randomized controlled study. *Spine*. 2002; **27**: 901–09; discussion 9–10.

49. Billings JA, Block S. Palliative care in undergraduate medical education. Status report and future directions. *Journal of the American Medical Association*. 1997; **278**: 733–8.

50. Green CR, Wheeler JR, Marchant B et al. Analysis of the physician variable in pain management. *Pain Medicine*. 2001; **2**: 317–27.

* 51. Acute Pain Management Guideline Panel. *Acute pain management: operative or medical procedures and trauma: Clinical practice guideline*. Washington, DC: Agency for Health Care Policy and Research, Public Health Service, US Dept of Health and Human Services, 1992.

52. McCaffery M, Ferrell BR. Nurses' assessment of pain intensity and choice of analgesic dose. *Contemporary Nurse*. 1994; **3**: 68–74.

53. Closs SJ. Pain and elderly patients: a survey of nurses' knowledge and experiences. *Journal of Advanced Nursing*. 1996; **23**: 237–42.

54. Drayer RA, Henderson J, Reidenberg M. Barriers to better pain control in hospitalized patients. *Journal of Pain and Symptom Management*. 1999; **17**: 434–40.

55. Horbury C, Henderson A, Bromley B. Influences of patient behavior on clinical nurses' pain assessment: implications for continuing education. *Journal of Continuing Education in Nursing*. 2005; **36**: 18–24; quiz 46–7.

56. Chiang LC, Chen HJ, Huang L. Student nurses' knowledge, attitudes, and self-efficacy of children's pain management: evaluation of an education program in Taiwan. *Journal of Pain and Symptom Management*. 2006; **32**: 82–9.

57. Karlsten R, Strom K, Gunningberg L. Improving assessment of postoperative pain in surgical wards by education and training. *Quality and Safety in Health Care*. 2005; **14**: 332–5.

* 58. Gatchel RJ, Noe C, Kishino N. "Carving-out" services from multidisciplinary chronic pain management programs: Negative impact on therapeutic efficacy. In: Schatman ME, Campbell A (eds). *Chronic pain management: a guidebook for multidisciplinary program development*. New York: Informa Healthcare, 2007: 39–48.

* 59. Turk DC. Progress and directions for the agenda for pain management. *American Pain Society Bulletin*. 2004; **14**: 3–13.

60. Gatchel RJ, Noe C, Gajraj N et al. The negative impact on an interdisciplinary pain management program of

insurance "treatment carve-out" practices. *Journal of Workers Compensation*. 2001; **10**: 50–63.

61. Keel PJ, Wittig R, Deutschmann R *et al.* Effectiveness of in-patient rehabilitation for sub-chronic and chronic low back pain by an integrative group treatment program (Swiss Multicentre Study). *Scandinavian Journal of Rehabilitation Medicine*. 1998; **30**: 211–19.

* 62. Robbins H, Gatchel RJ, Noe C *et al.* A prospective one-year outcome study of interdisciplinary chronic pain management: compromising its efficacy by managed care policies. *Anesthesia and Analgesia*. 2003; **97**: 156–62.

* 63. Hatten AL, Gatchel RJ, Polatin PB, Stowell AW. A cost-utility analysis of chronic spinal pain treatment outcomes: converting SF-36 data into quality-adjusted life years. *Clinical Journal of Pain*. 2006; **22**: 700–11.

64. Jordan KD, Mayer TG, Gatchel RJ. Should extended disability be an exclusion criterion for tertiary rehabilitation? Socioeconomic outcomes of early versus late functional restoration in compensation spinal disorders. *Spine*. 1998; **23**: 2110–16; discussion 7.

65. Katz NP, Adams EH, Benneyan JC *et al.* Foundations of opioid risk management. *Clinical Journal of Pain*. 2007; **23**: 103–18.

66. Mayer TG, Dersh J, Towns B *et al.* Opioid dependencies associated with worse socioeconomic outcomes of spinal rehabilitation. *Spine Journal*. 2006; **6**: 95.

67. Chapman E, Hughes D, Landy A *et al.* Challenging the representations of cancer pain: experiences of a multidisciplinary pain management group in a palliative care unit. *Palliative and Supportive Care*. 2005; **3**: 43–9.

PART V

OTHER ISSUES

52

The use of guidelines, standards, and quality improvement initiatives in the management of postoperative pain

TONE RUSTOEN AND CHRISTINE MIASKOWSKI

KEY LEARNING POINTS

- Evidenced-based clinical practice guidelines (CPGs) have been developed in a number of countries to improve the effectiveness and safety of acute postoperative pain management.
- Despite the development and dissemination of these CPGs, the undertreatment of acute postoperative pain remains a significant clinical problem worldwide.
- Studies need to be carried out to determine the most effective approaches to change clinicians' behaviors to be in concert with recommendations in CPGs.

- While no perfect measures of quality exist, longitudinal data support the validity of a core set of quality indicators that could be used to obtain benchmark data for quality improvement (QI) initiatives in pain management.
- Additional studies are needed to determine which indicators are most effective in determining the quality of postoperative pain management.

INTRODUCTION

While the total number of surgeries performed worldwide is not known, recent surveys from the United Kingdom, Sweden, Norway, Germany, Italy, Switzerland, the United States, Australia, Asia, and Africa demonstrate that the undertreatment of postoperative pain remains an international problem.[1, 2, 3, 4, 5, 6, 7, 8, 9] In fact, in a recent review[10] it was noted that approximately 70 percent of patients experienced moderate to severe pain following surgery. The consequences of unrelieved postoperative pain can be serious and include increased morbidity and

mortality, the development of chronic pain, increased hospital stay, and decreased quality of life.

GUIDELINES FOR POSTOPERATIVE PAIN MANAGEMENT

Over the past 15 years, attempts have been made to improve postoperative pain management through the publication and dissemination of clinical practice guidelines (CPG). This work began in the USA with the development of a CPGs Program by the Agency for

Health Care Policy and Research (AHCPR). Based on recommendations from the Institute of Medicine, evidenced-based CPGs were defined as systematically developed statements that were to be used to assist practitioners and patients in making decisions about appropriate health care for specific clinical circumstances.[11] One of the first CPGs published by the AHCPR was entitled Acute pain management: operative or medical procedures and trauma.[12]

While the federal government in the US no longer develops CPGs, this work sparked the development of a number of CPGs for postoperative pain management throughout the world. Most of these CPGs were developed by professional organizations or by professional organizations in collaboration with federal governments. Four of these CPGs for postoperative pain management that are representative of international efforts to improve postoperative pain management are:

1. *Acute pain management in the perioperative setting* – American Society of Anesthesiologists;[13, 14]
2. *Acute pain management: scientific evidence* – Australian and New Zealand College of Anesthetists and Faculty of Pain Medicine;[15]
3. *Pain management services – good practice* – The Royal College of Anesthetists and The Pain Society[16] and *Guidelines for the provision of anesthetic services* – The Royal College of Anesthetists;[17]
4. *Postoperative pain management – good clinical practice* – European Society of Regional Anesthesia and Pain Therapy.[18]

Acute pain management in the perioperative setting – American Society of Anesthesiologists

In 1995, the American Society of Anesthesiologists published evidence-based *Practice guidelines for acute pain management in the perioperative setting.*[13] This CPG was updated in 2004.[14] The purposes of this CPG are to: (1) facilitate the efficacy and safety of acute pain management in the perioperative setting; (2) reduce the risk of adverse outcomes; (3) maintain the patient's functional status; and (4) enhance the quality of life for patients with acute pain during the perioperative period.[13, 14] The 2004 update provides recommendations on a wider range of pain management techniques, including:

- institutional policies and procedures for providing perioperative pain management;
- preoperative evaluation of the patient;
- preoperative preparation of the patient;
- perioperative techniques for pain management;
- multimodal techniques for pain management;
- patient subpopulations.

Acute pain management: scientific evidence – Australian and New Zealand College of Anesthetists and Faculty of Pain Medicine

In 1994, the National Health and Medical Research Council (NHMRC) of Australia took the initiative to develop an evidence-based CPG on all aspects of acute pain management. In 2005, this CPG was revised by a multidisciplinary committee.[15] The aim of the report is to "combine the best available evidence for acute pain management with current clinical and expert practice." In addition, a substantial amount of evidence currently available on the management of acute pain is summarized in a concise and easily readable form. The specific areas addressed in the guide are:

- physiology and psychology of acute pain;
- assessment and measurement of acute pain and its treatment;
- provision of safe and effective acute pain management;
- systemically administered analgesic drugs;
- regionally and locally administered analgesic drugs;
- routes of systemic drug administration;
- techniques of drug administration;
- nonpharmacological techniques;
- management of acute pain in specific clinical situations;
- management of acute pain in specific patient groups.

The document begins with a summary of the key messages in each chapter, as well as the level of evidence that supports each message. An extensive bibliography is included at the end of the text.

The chapter on the physiology and psychology of acute pain includes information on the definition of pain, pain perception, and pain pathways, as well as various psychological aspects of acute pain. The chapter concludes with discussions of the progression from acute to chronic pain, the use of preemptive and preventive analgesia, and the adverse effects of unrelieved pain.

The chapter on the assessment and measurement of acute pain and its treatment provides a comprehensive summary of approaches that can be used to assess pain in patients who can provide a verbal report as well as those with special needs. Emphasis is placed on the multidimensional nature of pain and the need to address outcomes other than pain (e.g. physical functioning, psychological functioning, adverse events). The chapter on the provision of safe and effective acute pain management outlines the requirements for patient and staff education. In addition, the minimal requirements that must be in place at the organizational level to provide effective acute pain management are enumerated.

Four chapters are devoted to the pharmacologic management of acute postoperative pain. These chapters provide detailed information on the systemic and regional administration of analgesic medications. In addition, recommendations are made regarding all of the major routes of drug administration. The chapter on non-pharmacologic interventions for acute postoperative pain summarizes the available evidence on a variety of psychological interventions, transcutaneous nerve stimulation (TENS), acupuncture, and physical therapy. The text concludes with two chapters on the management of acute pain in special conditions or populations. The chapter on special conditions provides information on acute pain management in a variety of chronic medical conditions (e.g. spinal cord injury), acute medical conditions (e.g. abdominal pain), acute cancer pain, and acute pain management in the intensive care unit and emergency department. The final chapter addresses pain management in special populations (e.g. children, pregnant women, elderly patients, Aboriginal and Torres Strait Islander peoples).

Pain management services – good practice – The Royal College of Anesthetists and The Pain Society and *Guidelines for the provision of anesthetic services* – The Royal College of Anesthetists

In 2003, the Royal College of Anesthetists and the Pain Society (i.e. The British Chapter of the International Association for the Study of Pain) published a document entitled *Pain management services – good practice*.[16] The summary statement in this document states that relief of pain should be the fundamental objective of any health service. In addition, as listed in **Box 52.1**, 11 requirements are enumerated for the provision of effective and safe management of acute and chronic pain in hospitals. This document focuses on the structures and processes that need to be in place in hospitals to achieve effective and safe pain management.

In 2004, the Royal College of Anesthetists published *Guidelines for the provision of anesthetic services*.[17] This comprehensive document contains a chapter on acute pain management which is consistent with and supplements the publication referenced in the previous paragraph.[16] The chapter entitled "Guidance on the provision of anesthetic services for acute pain management" is divided into two main sections (i.e. the importance of acute pain management services and levels of provision of service). The first section emphasizes the undertreatment of acute pain and the deleterious effects of unrelieved pain. Explicit in this CPG is the statement that the provision of an organized, multidisciplinary acute pain team is an effective approach for providing high quality pain relief in a hospital setting. In addition, emphasis is placed on the importance of ongoing staff education and the

---

Box 52.1 Requirements for the effective and safe management of acute and chronic pain in hospitals

1. The provision of services for acute pain management in all hospitals.
2. The provision of core services for chronic pain management in all district general hospitals and most specialist hospitals.
3. The provision of specialized services for pain management on a regional basis.
4. Adequate resources to provide an appropriate number of fixed sessions for consultants (specialists in pain management), other health care professionals, secretarial and administrative staff, as well as appropriate accommodation, facilities, and equipment.
5. Recognition that anesthetists who have sessions in pain management need to have job plans that differ from those of most anesthetists who work in operating theaters, obstetric units, and critical care units.
6. Close liaison between pain management and other health care groups (including primary care and palliative care services) in order to provide an individualized, inter-disciplinary approach to pain management for each patient.
7. Specific arrangements for the treatment of vulnerable groups such as the elderly, children, nonverbal, disabled, intellectually handicapped, and those whose primary language is not English.
8. Equity of access and service provision for all patients taking into account clinical, socio-economic, and cultural factors.
9. The provision of properly constructed pain management programmes which aim to promote restoration of normal physical and psychological function, and to decrease the inappropriate use of healthcare resources by patients with chronic pain.
10. An active programme of education in the understanding of pain, its presentation, and its management, for all health professionals who care for patients with pain both the primary and secondary services.
11. Continuing education and audit of pain management services.

Reprinted with permission from *Pain management services: good practice*, The Royal College of Anaesthetists and The Pain Society, London, UK.

development of appropriate guidelines or protocol to facilitate the provision of care.

The second section provides recommendations about acute pain services. In terms of staffing requirements for acute pain services, they should include a physician with expertise in acute pain management and clinical nurse specialists. In addition, effective collaborations should occur between the acute pain service and physical therapists, pharmacists, and psychologists.

The document emphasizes the need for appropriate equipment, support services, and facilities. In addition, the need for CPGs and protocols that are focused on pain assessment, the use of various analgesic modalities, and monitoring for adverse events are specified in the chapter. Additional topics include: the management of pain in patients with special needs; the need for education and training in pain management; the need for audits of the quality of pain management; the appropriate governance structure that needs to be in place to insure effective pain management; and the need for patient education.

Postoperative pain management – good clinical practice – European Society of Regional Anesthesia and Pain Therapy

In 2004, a consensus document entitled *Postoperative pain management – good clinical practice* was published by a panel of European anesthesiologists in consultation with the European Society of Regional Anesthesia and Pain Therapy.[18] The purpose of the document was to raise awareness of recent advances in pain control and to provide advice on how to achieve effective postoperative analgesia. The recommendations are general in nature rather than specific to surgical procedures.

The guideline is not evidenced-based but provides comprehensive, up-to-date information on:

- goals of pain treatment;
- physiology of pain;
- assessment of pain;
- patient education;
- treatment options;
- structure of an acute pain management service;
- day case surgery;
- pediatric analgesia;
- patient groups with special problems in pain management;
- risk management/discharge criteria.

The specific goals of effective and appropriate pain management are to:

- improve the quality of life of the patient;
- facilitate rapid recovery and return to full function;
- reduce morbidity;
- allow early discharge from hospital.

These goals will be achieved if clinicians understand the negative consequences of unrelieved pain and initiate appropriate assessment and management procedures to provide effective postoperative pain management.

The physiology section provides information on the physiological basis of pain, the positive and negative aspects of pain, and the mechanisms for peripheral and central pain sensitization. The section on pain assessment emphasizes that the assessment of pain is a vital element of effective postoperative pain management. The specific principles of successful pain management are enumerated in **Box 52.2**.

The next section outlines specific topics for patient and family education including:

- the importance of treating postoperative pain;
- available methods of pain treatment;
- pain assessment routines;
- goals of pain management;
- the patient's participation in the treatment of pain.

In the section on treatment options, emphasis is placed on: good nursing care, the use of nonpharmacologic techniques (e.g. distraction), and the use of balanced (multimodal) analgesia. The definition of balanced or multimodal analgesia is "the use of two or more analgesic agents that act by differing mechanisms to achieve a superior analgesic effect without increasing the adverse events compared with increased doses of single agents."[18]

An entire section of the CPG is devoted to the structure of an acute pain management service. One of the principles in this section is that the treatment of postoperative pain requires good multidisciplinary and multiprofessional cooperation. In addition, every unit where surgery is performed should provide a pain management team that is structured according to local needs. All staff involved in the treatment of postoperative pain should have education and training about pain management and be updated on a regular basis. This section concludes with a model for how to organize a postoperative pain management program.

The section on day surgery notes that as more surgery is carried out on an outpatient basis, attention needs to be placed on effective pain control in this setting. Recommendations are made on the requirement for effective pain management in day surgery; the role of regional analgesia; postoperative pain management; and the assessment, documentation, and management of pain following discharge.

Separate sections of the CPG are devoted to the management of pain in children and special populations. The document concludes with a discussion of risk management and discharge criteria, namely: need for a safe discharge; need to define a maximum permissible pain score at discharge; need to give patients written information about the appropriate analgesics to take home; need to give patients a hospital phone number for any questions; and need to instruct parents to assess and treat pain in their children.

Box 52.2 Principles of successful pain management

- Assess pain both at rest and with movement to evaluate the patient's functional status.
- The effect of a given treatment is evaluated by assessing pain before and after every treatment intervention.
- In the surgical Post Anesthesia Care Unit (PACU) or other circumstances where pain is intense, evaluate, treat, and reevaluate frequently (e.g. every 15 minutes initially, then every one to two hours as pain intensity decreases).
- On the surgical ward, evaluate, treat, and reevaluate regularly (e.g. every four to eight hours) both the pain and the patient's response to treatment.
- Define the maximum pain score above which pain relief is offered (i.e. the intervention threshold). For example, verbal rating score of 3 at rest and 4 on moving, on a 10-point scale.
- Pain responses to treatment, including adverse events, are documented clearly on easily accessible forms, such as the vital sign sheet. This is useful for treatment, good communication between staff, auditing, and quality control.
- Patients who have difficulty communicating their pain require particular attention. This includes patients who are cognitively impaired, severely emotionally disturbed, children, patients who do not speak the local language, and patients whose level of education and cultural background differs significantly from that of their health care team.
- Unexpected intense pain, particularly if associated with altered vital signs (hypotension, tachycardia, fever) is immediately evaluated. New diagnoses, such as wound dehiscence, infection, or deep venous thrombosis should be considered.
- Immediate pain relief without asking for a pain rating is given to patients with obvious pain who are not sufficiently focused to use a pain rating scale.
- Family members are involved where appropriate.

Reprinted from Postoperative Pain Management – Good Clinical Practice – European Society of Regional Anesthesia and Pain Therapy, with permission.

Dissemination and implementation of CPGs for the management of postoperative pain

All of the CPGs cited above are available on the World Wide Web (see reference list). In addition, professional organizations and governmental agencies have disseminated these documents widely to their respective constituencies. Therefore, it is reasonable to ask why the undertreatment of acute postoperative pain persists in all countries of the world.[1, 2, 3, 4, 5, 6, 7, 8, 9]

In a recent review, Barosi[19] noted that interventions designed to effectively implement and disseminate CPGs fall into different categories: dissemination of educational materials (e.g. journal articles, audiovisual materials); decision-support systems and reminders (e.g. automated prompts in electronic medical records); educational meetings, educational outreach visits; and audit and feedback. To date, the major strategies that have been used to disseminate the various CPGs for postoperative pain management include the dissemination of educational materials and educational meetings. However, these strategies are the least likely to result in changes in clinicians' behaviors. In addition, many clinicians cite high staff turnover, the pressures of day-to-day practice, and limited clinician time with patients as major barriers to the implementation of CPG

recommendations in general.[20, 21] Another reason why CPGs are not implemented is that some clinicians believe that they are too prescriptive and do not allow for individualization of treatment regimens. Systematic investigations need to be carried out to determine which implementation strategies are most effective in changing clinicians' behaviors so that the management of postoperative pain improves.

STANDARDS FOR POSTOPERATIVE PAIN MANAGEMENT

On January 1, 2001, pain standards developed by JCAHO were implemented in the US. JCAHO is a private organization that accredits all patient care organizations (i.e. ambulatory care, behavioral health, healthcare networks, home care, hospitals, long-term care, and long-term care pharmacies) in the US. While this accreditation process is voluntary, it is necessary to have this "seal of approval" from JCAHO to obtain reimbursement for healthcare services from the federal government and private insurance companies. While JCAHO primarily accredits healthcare organizations in the US, it is expanding its services to the international community.

The pain standards represent a landmark initiative by JCAHO, as well as a rare and important opportunity for widespread and sustainable improvements in how pain is managed in the US.[22, 23, 24] The JCAHO pain standards were developed in recognition of the widespread undertreatment of both acute and chronic pain. While they were developed in the US, they are applicable throughout the world. The pain standards require all organizations to:

- recognize the right of patients to appropriate assessment and management of their pain;
- identify patients with pain in an initial screening assessment;
- perform a more comprehensive assessment when pain is identified;
- record the results of the assessment in a way that facilitates regular assessment and follow-up;
- educate relevant providers in pain assessment and management;
- determine and assure staff competency in pain assessment and management;
- address pain assessment and management in the orientation of all new staff;
- establish policies and procedures that support appropriate prescription or ordering of effective pain medications;
- ensure that pain does not interfere with participation in rehabilitation;
- educate patients and families about the importance of effective pain management;
- address patient needs for symptom management in the discharge planning process;
- collect data to monitor the appropriateness and effectiveness of pain management.

These standards have prompted every patient care organization to build an institutional commitment to pain management. As part of this commitment, many healthcare organizations have integrated the treatment of pain into their mission statements. In addition, throughout the organization, universal screening for pain is instituted so that every patient who comes to an inpatient or outpatient setting is asked about the presence of pain. In order to "institutionalize pain management," organizations must follow a series of steps that are outlined in **Table 52.1**.[22, 23, 25]

The majority of US healthcare organizations have adopted the use of a standardized approach to pain assessment using either 0 (no pain) to 10 (worst pain imaginable) numeric rating scales or 0 (no pain) to 5 (severe pain) descriptive ratings scales to perform routine pain assessments. In addition, the education of physicians, nurses, allied health professionals, and patients about the importance of pain treatment has become a priority in healthcare organizations. Finally, healthcare institutions have started to include pain management as one of their quality indicators.

QUALITY IMPROVEMENT INITIATIVES IN PAIN MANAGEMENT

The field of pain management has a long tradition of evaluating the quality of pain management. Initially, these surveys reported on the undertreatment of acute and chronic pain.[26, 27] These studies provided the impetus for professional organizations, as well as government and regulatory agencies, to publish CPGs for acute and cancer pain management. The majority of these CPGs recommended that the quality of pain management should be evaluated after the implementation of the CPGs' recommendations.

The process of continuous quality improvement

An integral part of any evaluation of the quality of patient care is the process of continuous quality improvement (CQI). This process, illustrated in **Figure 52.1**, provides organizations with the ability to collect benchmark data, determine the effectiveness of various treatment strategies, and evaluate whether systematic changes in patient care strategies improve the quality of care that patients receive.[26, 27, 28] In this section, the CQI process is applied to a specific pain management problem.

In many healthcare organizations, an interdisciplinary committee is established to conduct various quality improvement (QI) studies. Typically, they consist of physicians, nurses, pharmacists, physical therapists, and other clinicians who are involved in postoperative pain management. The first step in the CQI process is to determine the specific aspect of care that requires evaluation. For example, the QI committee may choose to evaluate nurses' adherence with a pain assessment policy that states that pain assessments will be documented every four hours for the first 24 hours following surgery.

The second step in the CQI process involves the evaluation study. The QI committee decides to conduct the pain assessment study on the orthopedic surgery and neurosurgery units. A total of 30 patients' charts from each unit are evaluated and data on adherence with the pain assessment policy are collected so that an analysis can be carried out to evaluate for differences in adherence rates across the different nursing shifts. The third step of the CQI process involves the actual analysis of the study data and the presentation of the study findings to the QI committee.

Once the data are gathered and the findings are presented, the QI committee needs to determine which processes of care require modification. This part of the CQI process usually involves a comparison of the study findings with some predetermined benchmark. For example, prior to the initiation of the study, the QI committee determined that their benchmark for adherence with the pain assessment policy would be 90 percent.

Table 52.1 Steps to institutionalize pain management.

Steps to institutionalize pain management

1. Develop an interdisciplinary committee to create the plan to institutionalize pain management
   a. Identify the key "stake-holders" in the institution and establish their buy-in with the plan
   b. Members of the interdisciplinary committee should include, at a minimum, physicians, nurses, pharmacists, administrators
   c. Invite participation from individuals who might be most resistant to change
   d. Include patient and family member participation when appropriate
2. Perform an analysis of pain management practices within the organization
   a. Identify areas for improvement in pain management practices
   b. Collect data to verify the need for improvement in a variety of pain management practices
   c. Evidence of deficits facilitates the buy-in of key opinion leaders
3. Develop a plan to institutionalize pain management
   a. Establish the goals of the program
   b. Establish a timeline for implementation
   c. Determine which policies and procedures need to be written and disseminated
      i. Pain assessment
      ii. Use of pharmacologic interventions for pain management
      iii. Use of nonpharmacologic interventions for pain management
      iv. Use of technology for pain management
   d. Allocate resources to implement the plan
4. Establish accountability for pain management
   a. Determine which staff will be responsible for which components of the pain management plan
   b. Develop competency based assessment tools to evaluate staff performance
   c. Integrate the principles of effective pain management and assign responsibility for pain management into policies, procedures, and job descriptions
5. Provide education to all personnel involved in pain management
   a. Provide education on pain assessment
   b. Provide education on both pharmacologic and nonpharmacologic interventions for pain management
   c. Provide education on the use of new technologies for pain management
6. Incorporate effective pain management into the mission statement of the organization
   a. Inform patients and family members on admission of their right to prompt pain treatment
   b. Explain to patients and family members why pain management is an important part of their care
   c. Teach patients and family members how to report pain using established pain assessment tools
7. Use quality improvement approaches to evaluate pain management practices
   a. Implement a variety of quality improvement approaches to evaluate various aspects of pain management
      i. Review of medical records
      ii. Review of adherence with specific policies and procedures
      iii. Patient interviews
      iv. Competency evaluations of staff
      v. Family member interviews

Findings from the study found a 95 percent adherence rate on the day shift, 80 percent on the evening shift, and 70 percent on the night shift. Based on this analysis, the QI committee determined that adherence rates with the pain assessment policy on the evening and night shifts were not acceptable.

The fifth step in the CQI process involves the development and implementation of a plan to improve care. This step requires a careful examination of all of the factors within the organization that may impede the ability of clinicians to adhere to a particular policy. In this case, the QI committee evaluated the evening and night staff's knowledge about the pain assessment policy, as well as factors that interfered with their ability to complete pain assessments in a timely manner. Based on a series of meetings with the nursing staff, the QI committee determined that the nurses were not aware of how often pain assessments were to be performed in the immediate postoperative period. A series of educational sessions on pain assessment were conducted for nurses on the two units. The final step in the CQI process involved a reevaluation of the pain assessment policy three months after the educational program. At that time, 95 percent adherence rates with the policy were achieved on both surgical units and on all three shifts.

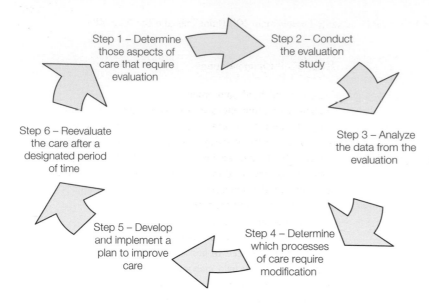

Figure 52.1 The process of continuous quality improvement.

QI indicators in pain management – the experience in the United States

To improve the quality of acute and cancer pain management, the American Pain Society (APS) and the AHCPR outlined a specific set of QI recommendations for institutions in the early 1990s.[29] These recommendations included a Patient Outcome Questionnaire (POQ) that could be used to evaluate the quality of acute and cancer pain management. Several studies were carried out with the POQ[28, 30, 31, 32, 33, 34] and consistently found that patients reported high levels of satisfaction with pain management despite significantly high levels of pain.

In 1995, the APS QI guidelines were revised based on published reports and clinical experience.[35] An interdisciplinary committee concluded that efforts to improve the quality of pain management must move beyond assessment and communication about pain to implementation and evaluation of improvements in pain treatment that are timely, safe, evidence-based, and multimodal. The key elements in this revision of the QI guidelines were to:

- assure that a report of unrelieved pain raised a "red flag" that attracted clinicians' attention;
- make information about analgesics convenient where orders are written;
- promise patients responsive analgesic care and urge them to communicate pain;
- implement policies and safeguards for the use of modern analgesic technologies;
- coordinate and assess implementation of these measures.

A revision of the POQ was included in this paper. The main revisions included the addition of five items on how pain interferes with function from the Brief Pain Inventory[36] and seven items from the Patient Barriers Questionnaire.[37] In addition, emphasis was placed on using CQI processes to improve pain management and to facilitate the recognition of institutional barriers to optimal pain treatment.

Over the next ten years, several QI studies were published that used the POQ.[2, 3, 25, 30, 38] An extensive review of these QI studies[30] identified six quality indicators for hospital-based pain management initiatives.

1. Pain intensity is documented with a numeric or descriptive rating scale.
2. Pain intensity is documented at frequent intervals.
3. Pain is treated by a route other than intramuscular.
4. Pain is treated with regularly administered analgesics, and when possible a multimodal approach is used.
5. Pain is prevented and controlled to a degree that facilitates function and quality of life.
6. Patients are adequately informed and knowledgeable about pain management.

In 2005, the APS Quality of Care Task Force published a revision of their QI recommendations.[39] Differences between the 1995 and 2005 APS recommendations are summarized in **Table 52.2**. This interdisciplinary task force concluded that efforts to improve pain management must move beyond merely improving assessment and documentation. What is required to improve the quality of acute pain management is the implementation of customized, evidenced-based treatment regimens. In addition, patients must actively participate in pain management. Finally, emphasis was placed on the routine use of quality measures that are specific to pain management.

A final outcome of the APS Quality of Care Task Force's work was the development of a new set of quality indicators and suggested measures for acute pain management. These quality indicators and measures are summarized in **Table 52.3**. The authors acknowledged

Table 52.2   Comparison of the 1995 American Pain Society (APS) Quality Improvement (QI) Guidelines and the 2005 APS Recommendations.

1995 APS QI guidelines	2005 APS recommendations

Recognize and treat pain promptly
  Routine assessment of pain intensity
  Routine documentation of pain intensity
	Recognize and treat pain promptly
	  Emphasis on comprehensive pain assessment
	  Emphasis on the importance of the prevention of pain
	  Emphasis on prompt recognition and treatment of pain

Make information about analgesics readily available in places where clinicians write medication orders	Involve patients and families in the pain management plan
	  Emphasis on the need to customize the pain management plan
	  Emphasis on the importance of having the patient participate in the pain management plan

Promise patients attentive analgesic care
  Urge patients to report pain to clinicians
	Improve treatment patterns
	  Eliminate inappropriate practices
	  Emphasis on the need to provide multimodal therapy

Develop explicit policies for analgesic technologies
  Patient-controlled analgesia
	Reassess and adjust pain management plan as needed
	  Emphasis placed on the need to respond not only to pain intensity scores but to changes in patient's functional status and side effects

Spinal administration of opioids and anesthetics Examine the processes and outcomes of pain management with the goal of continuous quality improvement	Monitor processes and outcomes of pain management Emphasis on new standardized QI indicators

Table 52.3   Quality indicators and measures for acute pain management.

Quality indicator	Measures
Intensity of pain is documented	Is there any documentation of pain in the medical record?
Numeric rating scale (i.e. 0 to 10)	In charts with documentation of pain, was a pain rating scale used?
Descriptive rating scale (i.e. none, mild, moderate, severe)	
Pain intensity is documented at frequent intervals	How many pain intensity ratings were documented in a 24-hour period?
Pain is treated by a route other than intramuscular injection	Percentage of patients who received an intramuscular injection of an analgesic in the postoperative period
Pain is treated with regularly administered analgesics	Percentage of patients who received an analgesic on a regular schedule Percentage of patients who received meperidene
Pain is treated, when possible with multimodal approaches	Percentage of patients who received only a single analgesic modality Percentage of patients who received combinations of therapeutic approaches (nonopioid, opioid, local anesthetic, regional techniques) Percentage of patients who received both pharmacologic and nonpharmacologic approaches
Pain is prevented and controlled to a degree that facilitates function and quality of life	Measurement of worst pain in past 24 hours Amount of time the patient was in moderate to severe pain in the past 24 hours Level of pain's interference with sleep, walking ability, mood (0 = does not interfere to 10 = completely interferes)
Patients are adequately informed and knowledgeable about pain management	Patient's rating of the adequacy of information received about pain and pain management while in the hospital (1 = poor to 5 = excellent)

that improvements in the quality of patient care are influenced by a wide variety of internal and external factors. In order to improve the quality of pain management, multilevel approaches are needed that involve patients, clinicians, and organizations. Therefore, a scientific and systems-oriented approach to changing pain management behaviors is crucial to the achievement of the goal of improved pain management.

QI indicators in pain management – the experience in Sweden

In a series of studies,[2, 40, 41, 42] researchers in Sweden developed and tested an instrument entitled *Strategic and clinical indicators in postoperative pain management*. The patient version of the instrument consists of 14 items about communication, action, trust, and the environment; two questions about general patient satisfaction; and three questions about pain intensity. The individual items on the scale are listed in **Table 52.4**. The initial Cronbach's alpha for the total scale was 0.84. A four-factor structure emerged from an orthogonal factor analysis that explained a cumulative variance of

61.4 percent.[42] Some of the items on this instrument evaluate similar indicators to those proposed by the APS. Additional studies are warranted with both instruments to determine which indicators are most effective in determining the quality of postoperative pain management.

RECOMMENDATIONS FOR CLINICAL PRACTICE AND RESEARCH

Recommendations contained within the various CPGs for postoperative pain management represent a synthesis of the "best practices" in the field that should result in improvements in patient care. Based on the experience in the US with the JCAHO pain standards, the implementation of systematic approaches to pain management that are coupled with clinician education about pain assessment and management are leading to some improvements in patient care.[25] However, to continue to make progress in the management of postoperative pain, healthcare organizations need to design and implement CQI programs that provide ongoing feedback

Table 52.4 Individual items on the strategic and clinical quality indicators in postoperative pain management – patient version.

	Score

Communication

1. Before my operation, I was told about the type of pain treatment that I would be offered after surgery
2. When nurses come on duty, they know "everything" about how much pain I have had and the pain treatment I have received
3. The nurses and doctors have cooperated in treating my pain

Action

1. After my operation, I talked with a nurse about how I wanted my pain to be treated
2. I received support or help in finding a comfortable position in bed to help avoid pain
3. The staff asked me about the pain I had when I breathed deeply, sat up, or moved around
4. To determine my level of pain, a member of the staff asked me to pick a number between 0 and 10 at least once every morning, afternoon, and evening

Trust

1. Even if I did not always ask for it, I was given pain medication
2. The nurses helped me with pain treatment until I was satisfied with the effects of pain relief
3. The nurses are knowledgeable about how to relieve my pain
4. The nurses believe me when I tell them that I am in pain

Environment

1. I was given the opportunity for peace and quiet so I could sleep during the night
2. I have a pleasant room
3. There have been enough nurses on duty for someone to respond quickly to my request for pain relief

Items are rated on a five-point Likert scale (1 = strongly disagree to 5 = strongly agree).
Three additional items evaluate pain intensity (i.e. worst, least, pain right now) in the past 24 hours.
Two items evaluate expectations about pain and satisfaction with pain management.
Adapted from Idvall E, Hamrin E, Sjostrom B, Unosson M. Patient and nurse assessment of quality of care in postoperative pain management. *Quality and Safety in Health Care.* 2002; **11**: 327–34, with permission from the BMJ Publishing Group.

to clinicians about how to improve the systems and professional practices that are critical for effective postoperative pain management.

REFERENCES

1. Rawal N, Langford RM. Current practices for postoperative pain management in Europe and the potential role of the fentanyl HCl iontophoretic transdermal system. *European Journal of Anaesthesiology.* 2007; **24**: 299–308.

2. Idvall E, Hamrin E, Sjostrom B, Unosson M. Patient and nurse assessment of quality of care in postoperative pain management. *Quality and Safety in Health Care.* 2002; **11**: 327–34.

3. Dihle A, Helseth S, Kongsgaard UE *et al.* Using the American Pain Society's patient outcome questionnaire to evaluate the quality of postoperative pain management in a sample of Norwegian patients. *Journal of Pain.* 2006; **7**: 272–80.

4. Wilder-Smith OH, Mohrle JJ, Martin NC. Acute pain management after surgery or in the emergency room in Switzerland: a comparative survey of Swiss anaesthesiologists and surgeons. *European Journal of Pain.* 2002; **6**: 189–201.

5. Arnold S, Delbos A. [Evaluation of 5 years of postoperative pain management in orthopaedic surgery, in a private hospital, following quality standard management]. *Annales Françaises d'Anesthésie et de Reanimation.* 2003; **22**: 170–8.

6. Dolin SJ, Cashman JN, Bland JM. Effectiveness of acute postoperative pain management: I. Evidence from published data. *British Journal of Anaesthesia.* 2002; **89**: 409–23.

7. Geissler B, Neugebauer E, Angster R, Witte Dagger J. [Quality management during postoperative pain therapy]. *Chirurg.* 2004; **75**: 687–93.

8. Myles PS, Williams DL, Hendrata M *et al.* Patient satisfaction after anaesthesia and surgery: results of a prospective survey of 10,811 patients. *British Journal of Anaesthesia.* 2000; **84**: 6–10.

9. Apfelbaum JL, Chen C, Mehta SS, Gan TJ. Postoperative pain experience: results from a national survey suggest postoperative pain continues to be undermanaged. *Anesthesia and Analgesia.* 2003; **97**: 534–40.

10. Neugebauer EA, Wilkinson RC, Kehlet H, Schug SA. PROSPECT: a practical method for formulating evidence-based expert recommendations for the management of postoperative pain. *Surgical Endoscopy.* 2007; **21**: 1047–53.

11. Field MJ, Lohr KN. *Clinical practice guidelines – directions for a new program.* Washington, DC: National Academy Press, 1990.

12. Panel APMG. *Acute pain management: operative or medical procedures and trauma. Clinical practice guideline.* Rockville, MD: Agency for Health Care Policy and Research, Public Health Service, US Department of Health and Human Services, 1992.

13. Practice guidelines for acute pain management in the perioperative setting. A report by the American Society of Anesthesiologists Task Force on Pain Management, Acute Pain Section. *Anesthesiology.* 1995; **82**: 1071–81.

* 14. Practice guidelines for acute pain management in the perioperative setting: an updated report by the American Society of Anesthesiologists Task Force on Acute Pain Management. *Anesthesiology.* 2004; **100**: 1573–81.

* 15. Medicine AaNZCoAaFoP. *Acute pain management: scientific evidence.* Melbourne: Australian and New Zealand College of Anaesthetists; 2005.

* 16. The Royal College of Anaesthetists & The Pain Society. Pain management services – good practice. Last updated: May 2003; cited December 2007. Available from: www.rcoa.ac.uk/docs/painservices.pdf.

* 17. The Royal College of Anaesthetists. Guidelines for the provision of anaesthetic services. Last updated July 2004; cited December 2007. Available from: www.rcoa.ac.uk/docs/GPAS.pdf.

* 18. European Society of Regional Anaesthesia and Pain Therapy. Postoperative pain management – good clinical practice. Last updated September 2005; cited December 2007. Available from: www.esraeurope.org/PostoperativePainManagement.pdf.

19. Barosi G. Strategies for dissemination and implementation of guidelines. *Neurological Sciences.* 2006; **27**: S231–4.

20. Brand C, Landgren F, Hutchinson A *et al.* Clinical practice guidelines: barriers to durability after effective early implementation. *Internal Medicine Journal.* 2005; **35**: 162–9.

21. Ockene JK, Zapka JG. Provider education to promote implementation of clinical practice guidelines. *Chest.* 2000; **118**: 33S–9.

22. Berry PH. Getting ready for JCAHO – just meeting the standards or really improving pain management. *Clinical Journal of Oncology Nursing.* 2001; **5**: 110–12.

23. Berry PH, Dahl JL. The new JCAHO pain standards: implications for pain management nurses. *Pain Management Nursing.* 2000; **1**: 3–12.

24. Phillips DM. JCAHO pain management standards are unveiled. Joint Commission on Accreditation of Healthcare Organizations. *Journal of the American Medical Association.* 2000; **284**: 428–9.

25. Stevenson KM, Dahl JL, Berry PH *et al.* Institutionalizing effective pain management practices: practice change programs to improve the quality of pain management in small health care organizations. *Journal of Pain and Symptom Management.* 2006; **31**: 248–61.

26. Miaskowski C. Monitoring and improving pain management practices. A quality improvement approach. *Critical Care Nursing Clinics of North America.* 2001; **13**: 311–17.

27. Miaskowski C. New approaches for evaluating the quality of cancer pain management in the outpatient setting. *Pain Management Nursing.* 2001; **2**: 7–12.

28. Bookbinder M, Coyle N, Kiss M *et al*. Implementing national standards for cancer pain management: program model and evaluation. *Journal of Pain and Symptom Management*. 1996; **12**: 334–47; discussion 331–3.

29. Acute pain management in adults: operative procedures. Agency for Health Care Policy and Research. *American Family Physician*. 1992; **46**: 128–38.

∗ 30. Gordon DB, Pellino TA, Miaskowski C *et al*. A 10-year review of quality improvement monitoring in pain management: recommendations for standardized outcome measures. *Pain Management Nursing*. 2002; **3**: 116–30.

31. Bostrom BM, Ramberg T, Davis BD, Fridlund B. Survey of post-operative patients' pain management. *Journal of Nursing Management*. 1997; **5**: 341–9.

32. Lin CC. Applying the American Pain Society's QA standards to evaluate the quality of pain management among surgical, oncology, and hospice inpatients in Taiwan. *Pain*. 2000; **87**: 43–9.

33. Miaskowski C, Nichols R, Brody R, Synold T. Assessment of patient satisfaction utilizing the American Pain Society's quality assurance standards on acute and cancer-related pain. *Journal of Pain and Symptom Management*. 1994; **9**: 5–11.

34. Ward SE, Gordon D. Application of the American Pain Society quality assurance standards. *Pain*. 1994; **56**: 299–306.

35. Quality improvement guidelines for the treatment of acute pain and cancer pain. American Pain Society Quality of Care Committee. *Journal of the American Medical Association*. 1995; **274**: 1874–80.

36. Daut RL, Cleeland CS, Flanery RC. Development of the Wisconsin Brief Pain Questionnaire to assess pain in cancer and other diseases. *Pain*. 1983; **17**: 197–210.

37. Ward SE, Goldberg N, Miller-McCauley V *et al*. Patient-related barriers to management of cancer pain. *Pain*. 1993; **52**: 319–24.

38. Mann C, Beziat C, Pouzeratte Y *et al*. [Quality assurance program for postoperative pain management: impact of the Consensus Conference of the French Society of Anesthesiology and Intensive Care]. *Annales Françaises d'Anesthésie et de Reanimation*. 2001; **20**: 246–54.

∗ 39. Gordon DB, Dahl JL, Miaskowski C *et al*. American pain society recommendations for improving the quality of acute and cancer pain management: American Pain Society Quality of Care Task Force. *Archives of Internal Medicine*. 2005; **165**: 1574–80.

40. Idvall E, Hamrin E, Rooke L, Sjostrom B. A tentative model for developing strategic and clinical nursing quality indicators: postoperative pain management. *International Journal of Nursing Practice*. 1999; **5**: 216–26.

41. Idvall E, Hamrin E, Sjostrom B, Unosson M. Quality indicators in postoperative pain management: a validation study. *Scandinavian Journal of Caring Sciences*. 2001; **15**: 331–8.

∗ 42. Idvall E, Hamrin E, Unosson M. Development of an instrument to measure strategic and clinical quality indicators in postoperative pain management. *Journal of Advanced Nursing*. 2002; **37**: 532–40.

53

The expert medicolegal report

PETER JD EVANS

KEY LEARNING POINTS

- Medical negligence and personal injury claims show an increasing trend.
- Most claims arise because there is a belief that an injustice has occurred.
- An expert needs to show impartiality, accuracy, and a depth of knowledge in the chosen field.

- Where possible, opinions need to be supported by evidence-based medicine.
- The appointment of "single" joint experts accelerate cases and reduce court attendance rates.
- Chronic pain syndromes and somatoform pain disorders are recognized conditions.

INTRODUCTION

Trends in litigation

Medical litigation is a regrettable but essential aspect of medical practice. Whilst the comments in this chapter reflect practices within the UK, the majority of the principles have wide applicability. Perfection in health care does not exist and all healthcare professionals have the capacity to err. Similarly, no intervention is without risk so the recipient of care needs to be intimately involved in the decision-making process and be fully informed of the positive and negative aspects of care. Nevertheless, providing informed consent does not absolve the clinician from the risk of being sued if it can be demonstrated that the treatment was negligently performed. However, it should help to reduce the vexatious claims from plaintiffs who for whatever reason become dissatisfied with the outcome of care. All treatments have failure rates!

The development of clinical governance within primary and secondary health care has helped to raise the awareness of best practice and provided guidance on healthcare decision-making. Similarly, the advent of Clinical Incident Reporting provides the ability to analyze adverse events in a calm and constructive manner so that lessons can be learned and changes in practice adopted (see The National Forum for Risk Management in the Public section, www.alarm-uk.org).

The Cochrane Collaboration[1] has been an important driver in the approach to best medical practice and, although not established as a result of litigation, its analyses offer a way to look more critically at issues of quality. The concept of the "evidence-based review" distilling the international experience of treatment to provide critical evaluations has helped provide a greater understanding of the efficacy of individual clinical practice. It is not the only approach and others advocate the use of graded scales to measure efficacy.[2]

In the UK, there have been a number of high profile criminal cases that have involved lapses of good medical practice. These have influenced public opinion adversely and undermined confidence in standards of medical practice. Some doctors have, publicly, been shown to have failed to maintain expected standards of care. Sadly, the many are implicated by the few and the medical profession has been put under great pressure to visibly "put its house in order."

Even more concerning is the recent trend that has left doctors unprotected from immunity from prosecution when as a result of their "expert opinion" criminal convictions have been obtained which have subsequently been reversed on appeal. The implication is that the expert, by giving erroneous or inaccurate testimony, has by default committed a criminal act.

Within the practice of pain management there are many situations that could give rise to litigation (**Table 53.1**).

Britain has enjoyed a privileged position with a relatively low level of medical litigation. This is now changing as patients are more readily going to court to settle grievances or seek financial compensation.[3] It has long been recognized that within medicine the surgical disciplines, including obstetrics, have carried greater risk.[4] Pain management is also becoming an area of concern. This reflects a greater recourse to invasive or destructive procedures (spinal cord stimulation, radiofrequency lesioning), as well as increased expectation by the patient of what should or can be achieved.

Why do people complain

In an ideal world, all treatment would be successful and no complications would occur. In general, the public accept that life is imperfect and mistakes can occur. They see imperfection in every aspect of daily life and most are happy to accept that some problems and side effects may occur as a result of normal medical treatment. However, it is when they feel that an injustice has been done that they tend to litigate. Over 57 percent of patients take an action because they just want an answer.[5] They may feel that for whatever reason "the facts" have been hidden, obscured, or suppressed. They may also feel that the clinician is not sincere in his explanation.

Too often doctors provide overoptimistic projections with regard to outcomes and may minimize the risks associated with surgical or other procedures. So it is not surprising that a significant number use the courts as a means of financial redress.

A review of 227 patients who were claiming negligence highlighted some important issues.[5] Over 70 percent of the respondents had been seriously affected by the incidents causing the litigation. The events had created long-term affects on work and social life. Often the decision that finally determined legal action was the poor communication and insensitive handling of the original injury. Where explanations had been given, less than 15 percent were considered satisfactory. Four themes emerged from the analysis:

1. Concern with standards of care – to prevent future events occurring.
2. An explanation – to know how and why the event happened.
3. Compensation for loss – pain, suffering, income, and future care.
4. Accountability – admission of fault, honesty.

What do they complain about

Motor vehicle accident and work-related injury represent the largest number of cases that involve persistent pain as a primary component (**Table 53.2**). The majority of these claims are settled "out of court" but nevertheless the process can be drawn out. Often liability is admitted early on, but agreeing the quantum can take many years. The defendants will always wish to leave a protracted period so that the maximum recovery will take place and disability will be minimized. Plaintiffs may resist attempts to recover early, as it may appear to weaken their cases.[6]

It is now recognized that prolonged litigation leads to chronicity, both for pain and disability.[7] Furthermore, the concept of "compensation neurosis" is ill founded. There

Table 53.1 Potential sources for medical litigation.

Acute pain	Chronic pain
Lack of consent	Personal injury
Complication of therapy	Inadequate preparation
Inappropriate treatment	Medical negligence
Assault	Work – compensation
Issues around competence	Lack of informed consent
	Unlicensed preparations
	Missed diagnoses

Table 53.2 Types of litigation: as presented to the author (1997–2007).

Problem	%
Work-related injury	37
Road traffic accident	18
Medical negligence	40
Acute pain	(9)
Chronic pain	(31)
Lack of consent	1
Lack of care/treatment	3

is evidence that the emotional distress caused by the compensation process can produce long-term psychological damage.[8]

WHAT SHOULD CONCERN THE EXPERT?

Standards of care

It should seem obvious that maintaining the highest standard of care would be normal. However, often lapses in care, failure to do the expected preparatory work, failure to adhere to normal care pathways, and failure to even examine the patient have led to complaints being upheld. Often the doctor concerned knew what should have been done, but failed in the implementation. The expert in a report should seek to understand how the injury or event occurred and what omissions or failures on behalf of the doctor contributed to the event. At all times, the expert has to acknowledge that reports are addressed to the courts and should be impartial.

Personal loss and suffering

In an expert report it will be necessary to assess the impact of the injury on the loss or distress experienced by the patient. The financial value of such loss is for the court to determine. Nevertheless, it is reasonable to suggest how life has altered and what limitation is imposed on daily existence because of the personal injury. This may be a big concern where the symptoms and loss of mobility are great, yet the physical findings are limited.

The subjective nature of pain may require a greater reliance on secondary characteristics to address the impact on the individual:

- the state of anxiety;
- the presence of reactive depression;
- the use of avoidance behavior;
- the appearance of elaborated responses to examination;
- the presence of post-traumatic stress (flashbacks, autonomic evoked responses);
- disturbances to sleep patterns;
- sickness records for those who still continue in employment;
- attendance rates with healthcare professionals;
- the use of allowances and benefits;
- the role of carers and in home support;
- the impact of locally provided social services for individual or family support.

Such data provide a more realistic picture of the impact and disability of chronic pain.

Probably the most difficult aspect is to assess the influence that on-going pain has on an individual's functional capacity. Most chronic pain sufferers will indicate that they do not undertake actions or tasks because these trigger or aggravate pain. There are numerous scales that can be applied, the majority assess simple tasks:

- brushing teeth, shaving;
- bathing or showering;
- combing or washing hair;
- putting on socks or stockings, dressing and undressing;
- climbing stairs;
- undertaking household tasks: cleaning, cooking, gardening etc.;
- driving or sitting in a vehicle;
- walking distance and standing times;
- ability to lift and carry objects;
- ability to enjoy pleasurable activities: eating out, attending movies or theater.

Such limitation in activity may prove difficult to explain in the absence of any recorded muscular or neurological disease. It will be necessary to explore these aspects with the claimant and record all restrictions to daily living.

The courts are well aware of the development of "illness behavior" and it is perfectly acceptable to link impaired functioning to the original injury or accident. The term "chronic pain syndrome" is widely recognized.

The competence or otherwise of the clinician

When assessing the events it will be an important consideration to investigate the skill of the doctor in relation to the treatments undertaken. Competence must be related to experience in the subject or field. It may become necessary to address the advisability of undertaking a procedure when experience is limited. Clearly the perspective is different if the case is an emergency or life threatening occasion than when the procedure is a cold elective event.

The suitability of the treatment planned or undertaken

The establishment of organizations such as National Institute for Clinical Excellence (NICE) have influenced the basis on which clinical decision-making is achieved. In the past, the "Bolam" concept[9] acknowledged that there could be differing clinical opinions. Today, much greater emphasis is placed upon what is felt to be the most appropriate course of action. The application of clinical guidelines and the involvement of multidisciplinary teams (MDTs) are important in answering such a question. It is accepted that doctors do not work in isolation.

Opinions must reflect the knowledge and understanding that was held at the time the incident or injury occurred. Over the prolonged period that a negligence claim may be pursued, opinions may change and new evidence could be published. It would be unreasonable to review competence only on the basis of current day standards.

The nature of the incident or complication

All therapy carries risk and part of the process of informed consent is to identify as far as possible the known risks. If a complication is rare but has been described, then it is less likely that claims for negligence will arise unless it can be shown that the risk was increased because of a poor technique or because the treatment itself was inappropriate.

Where the complication is quite common, claims may arise because of the way the problem was managed rather than for the event itself.

Informed consent

This is an issue that applies to both acute and chronic pain management. The difficulty for the clinician is to decide what level of detail should be provided to inform, but not frighten, patients.

For a patient to make a valued judgment, it is necessary to know not only what can go wrong and the likely incidence, but also the comparative efficacy of the treatment being offered.

To advise a patient with acute sciatica that following an epidural block with steroids there is a 1 in 5000 chance of a serious adverse event has a very different weighting to stating that one in six patients will derive improvement not achieved by other means.[10] A process of shared decision-making offers one method of improving consent.[11]

The assessment of risk, or more precisely the risk to benefit ratio, of treatment has yet to be fully evaluated. Systematic reviews and randomized controlled trials provide guidance. Many treatments for chronic pain have never been subjected to rigorous analysis. Sometimes it is difficult to establish a control group (e.g. acupuncture) and sometimes, because the control arm also involves an invasive procedure (e.g. radiofrequency lesion generation), it may not be possible to run a true double-blind study.

Robust guidelines are available for dealing with the issue of consent.[12]

Lack of consent

Most written consent forms that are signed by patients carry a caveat to "include all necessary procedures at the time of surgery." This is not an opportunity for clinicians to disregard their expected responsibilities. Issues can arise out of seemingly straightforward pain-relieving procedures.

For example, if a local anesthetic block is performed on an anesthetized patient, a laudable pain-relieving consideration, it may not be considered part of the basic anesthetic technique, particularly if this issue was not discussed at the anesthetic preassessment meeting. Should the patient suffer nerve injury or find the postoperative paralysis and anesthesia unacceptable, then potentially there are grounds for complaint. Obtaining consent, written if necessary, in advance of the event will provide the only safe form of defense against a charge of assault. Should nerve injury be the consequence, greater support will be given if the technique involved nerve stimulation and adherence to sound anatomical principles.[13]

Drugs used "off label" and outside the remit of their product licences pose another area of concern, particularly if patients are not advised of this fact. Whilst it is recognized that a large number of older drugs are routinely given in this manner for the treatment of chronic pain, newer compounds cannot enjoy this "wide exposure" privilege.

Malingering – false claims

A small percentage of patients will exaggerate claims for financial gain. This is more common in claims related to work injury and road traffic accidents. If the plaintiff feels aggrieved because a job has been lost, the injury was not their fault, the employer made unreasonable demands or provided inadequate support and protection, then one can understand how these emotional triggers will influence symptoms and behavior.

It should be noted that for some medical conditions a whole litigation industry has developed to deal with ever increasing demands and claims. A good example is "whiplash syndrome" where pain and injury is experienced by claimants for long periods of time in the absence of any truly defined clinical pathology.[6]

It is most unusual to see plaintiffs who clearly have "made the whole thing up." Insurance companies are always looking for these scenarios and invest considerable resources in investigating claimants. Video evidence is increasingly being used to observe claimants in their home environment. The findings can surprise even the most experienced medical examiner and can, on occasion, cause an expert to appear ill informed.

Sadly this type of pernicious investigation of claimants only adds to the distress of the genuine plaintiff, but is a necessary consequence of any form of compensation process. Experts will be expected to view video evidence and provide suitable commentary.

CLINICAL GOVERNANCE

Clinical governance has a broad remit and covers all aspects of current medical practice. Its introduction has changed the way medicine is delivered. In time it should help to clarify one of the key elements, "best practice." It is within this context that one should seek to look at the medicolegal basis upon which claims are based.

- Was there a duty of care?
- Upon whom lay that duty?
- Was there a failure to fulfil that duty?
- Did actual harm occur?
- If there was a breach of duty, did it cause the damage?

Improving standards is a slow process and involves both willingness and a commitment by all staff to make the change. There are some useful drivers.

A complaints procedure

The establishment of a complaint procedure is a healthy sign. It encourages openness in practice, exposes shortcomings, and highlights failure in service. Learning from errors can lead to improvements, if positive changes in practice are adopted.

Not all complaints are valid and the majority never results in litigation. Addressing issues early and expressing honest responses will defuse most situations. Such action will certainly aid in greater understanding and communication between the patient and the healthcare team even if issues cannot be resolved.

Best practice

Best practice is an attempt to discover the consensus within a discipline or speciality for a particular practice or procedure. The strength of evidence to support a view can be determined. A systematic review, for example, would have high weighting. Such studies have their limitations and sometimes when the evidence is in short supply it may be impossible to make a valued judgment on efficacy. A number of other measures need to be considered. Useful tools include clinical audit, complication rates, outcome studies, personal series, and individual case reports. All these help to generate a picture of the relevance of a particular treatment and will enable the determination of indexes such as the number needed to treat (NNT) and number needed to harm (NNH).[14]

Clinical guidelines

Finally, it is possible to approach best practice by looking at clinical guidelines and trying to develop a process and pathway by which a treatment can be introduced or maintained within given parameters. This practice must also involve disregarding therapies which no longer have a place or have been shown to have extremely limited efficacy. Whilst some guidelines may be locally based, many more are being adopted nationally and are being endorsed by learned societies and colleges (Royal College of Anaesthetists (www.rcoa.ac.uk), British Pain Society (www.britishpainsociety.org)).

LEGAL STANDING

For many years the basis on which medical negligence was assessed was based on a case, Bolam v Friern.[9] However, such an approach has been challenged and there have been recent changes in the law.

Bolam

The determination of negligence is for the courts. It is not the role of the clinician to apportion blame or culpability. The medical expert should attempt to give a balanced view of what is current best practice and what is perhaps appropriate for the level of skill and training of the doctor involved in litigation. It is acknowledged that the skill employed by a trainee doctor would, in normal circumstances, be less than that displayed by a consultant.[15]

Sometimes it may be difficult to define an absolute course of action and the expert must give an opinion as to what he or she would have done in the same circumstance. Evidence to support such opinions is normally derived from published articles although personal extensive experience with a procedure is always of additional merit.

It is easy for the expert to reflect on a particular incident and be critical of individual performance. It is always difficult for those involved in an adverse event to be analytical since crisis management may not be routinely practiced.

Where the body of medical opinions supports a particular action there is little difficulty. The problems tend to occur if less conventional approaches are adopted and something goes wrong. Then the decision might be to decide whether the issue was one of mishap or negligence.

To succeed in litigation, the plaintiff must be able to demonstrate that the defendant owed a legal duty of care. Furthermore, it must be demonstrated that such care fell below the standard required by the law and that the defendant could reasonably have foreseen that the careless behavior in question could have damaged the plaintiff. Damage must have occurred and a causal link between behavior and damage must be proved.

Nevertheless, "a doctor is not negligent, if he is acting in accordance with a practice accepted as proper by a reasonable body of medical men skilled in that particular art, merely because there is a body of such opinion that takes a contrary view."[9]

Woolf recommendations

Since April 2000 the conduct of medical litigation has changed dramatically. It has been acknowledged that the process of "going to court" has become extremely costly. In the UK the National Health Service (NHS) has to put aside some many millions of pounds to cover the cost of current cases trawling through the courts.

Lord Woolf[16] chaired a number of working parties on the subject of negligence. The groups concluded that the civil justice system had become excessively adversarial, slow, complex, and expensive. This was particularly true of medical negligence. There were five areas of great concern.

1. The relationship between the costs of the litigation and the amount involved was particularly disproportionate. The costs were particularly excessive in low value cases.
2. The delay before claims were resolved was unacceptable.
3. Unmeritorious cases were pursued and clear-cut claims defended for longer than happens in other areas of litigation.
4. The success rate was lower than in other personal injury litigation.
5. The lack of cooperation between the parties to the litigation and the mutual suspicion as to the motives of the opposing party was frequently more intense than in other classes of litigation.

As a result of the working parties a number of changes have been introduced, the effect of which has been to change and speed up the process:

- the introduction of "fast track" mechanisms for minor cases;
- restrictions in the application of legal aid;
- the development of mediation as an alternative to court;
- the imposition of strict timetables by the courts on all aspects of cases;
- the reduction in the number of expert witnesses that can be called;
- the alternative use of a single "joint medical expert" by both parties;
- conferences of medical experts to agree the medical findings to minimize the need for court attendances.

Far too few treatments for chronic pain have been subjected to rigorous analysis, hence the risk of litigation is potentially greater. The majority of claims result from personal injury and loss of income from work-related incidents (**Table 53.2**). Nevertheless, claims for medical negligence are increasing.

The clinician may also become involved in assessing pain as part of a claim for personal injury or when determining the prognosis and future management of a patient suffering pain and disability from a work-related injury.

Acute pain management is not exempt either. Litigation may result from intraoperative pain procedures such as injections or blocks. It could also result from a failure to consent and has led on occasion to charges of assault. Claims may also arise because of ongoing symptoms following an otherwise normal procedure. Examples might include post-spinal headache and low back pain following epidural anesthesia (**Table 53.1**).

PREPARATION OF THE REPORT

There are three principal elements to a report: the history, the physical and other findings, and then the comment and opinion.

Most medical reports are structured in this format. The content may well run to several thousand words so it is important that the report is annotated effectively. This can be by paragraph but it is often easier to number each individual statement or comment. Of course one should use an easy-to-read type face and font size which is appropriate. Double line spacing also adds to clarity. Another approach is to write it like a manuscript with each section titled, with an index at the front, and a summary or conclusion at the end.

Preparing a useful medical report involves time and deliberation. It is necessary to assess the injury and the circumstances around the event. Reference to general practitioner records will give insight into the patient's past behavior and previous relevant problems. The history should be extensive, details of all relevant problems, events, investigations, treatments, and responses should be recorded. Consistency of these facts across all medical reports strengthens the plaintiff's case.

The examination should be an opportunity to substantiate the patients' claims. It can be an opportunity to assess their demeanour and how tasks such as removing garments and putting on shoes are performed. It is also important to look for features, which may suggest enhancement of the patient's problem (**Box 53.1**). Invariably lawyers will want assessments on future progress so a request may be made for condition and prognosis reports. It is most difficult to estimate future disability and responses largely depend on the personal experience of the examiner.

The inclusion of recognized scale results can be useful for example:

- pain rating scales (McGill, Melzack);[17]
- depression (Beck);[18]
- disability (Roland-Morris);[19]
- health status (SF 36).[20]

When preparing the report it is important to evaluate the validity of claims and the opinions of other experts.

Box 53.1 The "litigious" patient frequently exhibit some of the following

- Previous pain problems
- Family experience
- Illness behavior
- Medication abuse
- Poor response to previous treatment
- Poor compliance with treatment
- Exaggerated responses to examination
- Inappropriate symptoms and signs
- Lack of eye contact
- Difficult communication/consultation
- Anger and resentment

Box 53.2 Source information for medical reports

- GP records
- Hospital notes
- Nursing reports
- Therapy reports (physiotherapy, occupational etc.)
- Accident and Emergency records
- Previous medical reports
- Written correspondence
- Social service reports

Reference to published studies is always extremely valuable. When drawing a conclusion it is useful to record the initial problems and level of disability and to relate that to the recovery made unto the time of the examination. Giving a prognosis is difficult and often it is more relevant to provide advice on further lines of support or treatment. However, when the prospects of further improvement are slim this should be clearly stated.

HISTORY

The history is an opportunity to explore the background to the problem. The expert should gather as much information as possible relating to the problem (**Box 53.2**). This is a time-consuming activity, but provides great understanding of the patient and the problem. Information should be recorded in chronological manner and particular reference made to relevant issues. It is not appropriate to be judgmental. However, in a patient making a claim for a work-related back injury it is essential to record past episodes of back pain, even previous claims. One will be asked to give an opinion as to the relative impact of past disease on the present complaint.

Previous behavior can provide an illuminating background on the patient. A history of psychiatric disease or affective disorder will give an insight into the ability of the patient to manage "life events." Similarly, patients who are failing to cope will tend to consult their GP's frequently, some attending 60–80 times in a single year. Records demonstrate how trivial the symptoms often are.

The sickness record is also an indicator to recovery. Patients who maintain a work ethic, even if the scale of duties is reduced, have a better prognosis. Those who remain off sick for two years or more are unlikely to return to useful employment.

The impact of previous treatment needs to be recorded.

The social and domestic framework in which the patient exists should be included. If the patient has been significantly disabled by the injury it often results in socioeconomic difficulties (**Table 53.3**). There is often major disruption to lifestyles, there may be role reversal by family members, support needed for children, and the individual may become socially isolated and depressed. All of this information should be recorded in the body of the history.

THE EXAMINATION

This is the most critical part of the whole process and generally provides "the substance" to the claim. Here there can be a factual representation of the plaintiff's problems.

A full physical examination is required, but emphasis must be placed on the musculoskeletal and neurological systems.

Neurological examination

One is looking for evidence of loss of function including obvious sensory changes, failure of coordination, and any dissociative losses. One should observe the usual parameters including reflexes, coordination, position sense, gait, and overall fitness.

Particular emphasis should be noted of the areas of distribution of the changes and are they consistent with nerve injury. The use of pain drawings can assist. Likewise the availability of electromyogram (EMG) reports will add support to any conclusions.

The presence of altered sensation (allodynia and hyperalgesia) is extremely important, particularly when one is assessing neuropathic or complex regional pain syndromes. It may be necessary to resort to qualitative sensory testing to confirm the nature of small fiber damage or sympathetic fiber impairment.

Table 53.3 Social impact of injury.

Work	Home
Loss of employment	Income reduction
	Care assistants
Benefits cycle	Driving support
	Domestic cleaning
Medical retirement	Care facilities for children
	Meals preparation
	Bathing aids
	Boredom and depression
	Social isolation
	Family conflict
	Recrimination and anger
	Inability to enjoy social pleasure
	Dining, theater, sports
	Impaired sexual relationships

A simpler approach can be to measure the impairment of the sympathetic systems by testing the responses to heat and cold.

When there are advanced changes (e.g. Sudek's atrophy), photographic evidence is invaluable.

Musculoskeletal system

One is obviously looking for physical deformity, loss of joint range, and evidence of disuse such as muscle wasting.

Simple measurement observations can be used to record the degree of restriction, such as flexion, extension, or rotation. Measuring muscle girth can assess evidence of muscle wasting. The more subjective measures of muscle power and muscle spasm should be recorded. There are a number of mechanical grip strength recorders available and these can be used. Various categorical scales are used to assess lumbar muscle spasm but they remain very subjective.

It is necessary to differentiate if the restrictions in movement are due to the onset of pain or as a consequence of a fixed deformity. One should look for inappropriate signs and these are particularly relevant in managing back-related problems.[21]

As many patients suffer from limited mobility it is important to observe their locomotion and in particular how patients manage changes in posture, for instance getting on to an examination couch or out of a chair.

Likewise, valuable information can be gleaned by the way the patient sits during the history taking. Is there evidence of rigid posture, fidgeting, position changing, or other features indicative of discomfort? In assessing illness behavior, is the plaintiff displaying evidence of elaborated responses, movements, or posture and using any support such as a splint, crutch, or corset.

THE CONCLUSION AND OPINION

The purpose of the report is to present to the court an analysis of the plaintiff's condition structured around the history and physical examination. It is then necessary to form an opinion as to how the present state arose and whether or not such a condition can be linked to any antecedent event. At all times the report should be objective and succinct. It is often worthwhile attaching explanations for common conditions, such as illness behavior and neuropathic pain by way of explanation.

If one is of the opinion that the plaintiff has suffered injury then it is imperative that one presents a suitable case by drawing out the salient facts and demonstrating a causal link. One should not only explore one's own personal experience but seek to back up any comment or view by reference to the published medical literature. It may also be relevant to include recommendations from professional bodies such as the Royal Colleges or National Societies.

Increasingly, the courts are requesting that medical experts meet after reports have been exchanged so that a joint statement can be produced identifying the areas of commonality and disagreement in the evidence.

Whilst this can help reduce the attendance of experts in court and is to be encouraged, it does sometimes diminish the possibility of a fuller explanation of the opinion in court, perhaps under cross-examination.

Cases in which the primary disability is pain are often the most difficult to present. The lack of physical signs and the subjective nature of symptoms can add to the confusion. Nevertheless, more reliance is now placed on behavioral aspects of cases and psychologists are frequently consulted to add weight to the observation of the pain clinician. Likewise, the concept of post-traumatic stress disorder and somatoform pain disorder are more readily accepted.

Frequently one is asked to give recommendations as to the prognosis and the eventual return of the plaintiff to a more normal existence. There are no hard rules and the conclusion is often based on the experience of the clinician from within their own clinical practice (**Table 53.4**).

Finally, it must be remembered that anything that one writes in a medical report may be studied very closely by lawyers for either party. Therefore one must always be certain to check all direct statements for clarity and accuracy and ensure that all opinions can be substantiated.

A typical report would be structured to the following format:

- reason for the report;
- information available: statements, records and reports provided for analysis;
- statement of impartiality;
- summary of findings and opinion;
- background medical history and relevant treatment related to incident;

- past medical history, previous injuries, vulnerability, psychological factors;
- present situation and review of principle issues:
  - overall impact of injury;
  - the effects of ongoing pain and suffering;
  - changes in physical capabilities;
  - emotional disturbances, past and present;
  - impact on home life, the family unit, and activities of daily living;
  - impact on social and sporting activities.
- review of general practitioner, hospital, and other records;
- clinical examination findings (should an attendance for examination be required);
- opinion:
  - causation;
  - condition and prognosis;
  - recommendations for future care and management.
- analysis and comments concerning defendant/plaintiff reports provided;
- conclusion.

Table 53.4 Predicted time "off sick" after acute injury (years) for those involved in litigation (author's case review).

Condition	Persistent pain	Functional recovery	Full recovery
Simple fracture	No	1	1
Neuropathic pain	Yes	2	5
Low back pain	Yes	2	3–5
Acute sciatica	No	1	1
Back pain on benefit	Yes	10	?
Neuropathy	Yes	?	?
Fibromyalgia	No	3–5	5–7
Nerve entrapment	No	1–2	1–2

Functional recovery reflects the time period in which the plaintiff should be able to return to former or equivalent employment.

REFERENCES

1. UK Cochrane Centre. The Cochrane Collaboration homepage. Available from: www.cochrane.co.uk/en/collaboration/html.
2. Bandolier. Evidence-based everything. *Bandolier Journal.* 1995; **12**. Available from: www.jr2.ox.ac.uk/bandolier/band12/b12-1.html.
3. Aikenhead AR. The pattern of litigation against anaesthetists. *British Journal of Anaesthesia.* 1994; **73**: 10–21.
4. Coleman NA. Litigation in anaesthesia. *British Journal of Hospital Medicine.* 1996; **55**: 62–4.
* 5. Vincent C, Young M, Phillips A. Why do people sue doctors? A study of patients and relatives taking legal action. *Lancet.* 1994; **343**: 1609–13.
* 6. Malleson A. *Whiplash and other useful diseases.* Montreal: McGill-Queen's University Press, 2002.
7. Mendelson G. Compensation and chronic pain. *Pain.* 1992; **48**: 121–3.
8. Guest GH, Drummond PD. Effects of compensation on emotional state and disability in chronic back pain. *Pain.* 1992; **48**: 125–30.
9. Bolam v Friern Barnet. *HMC* [1957] 2 AER 118.
* 10. McQuay HJ, Moore RA, Eccleston C *et al.* Systematic review of outpatient services for chronic pain. *Health Technology Assessment.* 1997; **1**: i-iv, 1–135.
11. Charles C, Gafni A, Whelan T. Shared decision-making in the medical encounter: what does it mean? *Social Science and Medicine.* 1997; **44**: 681–92.
12. Department of Health UK. *Reference guide to consent for examination or treatment.* London: HMSO, 2001.
13. Selander DE. Regional anaesthesia: thoughts and some honest ethics; about needle bevels and nerve lesions, and back pain after spinal anaesthesia. *Regional Anaesthesia and Pain Medicine.* 2007; **32**: 339–50.
14. Moore RA, McQuay HJ. Getting NNT's. *Bandolier.* 1997; **36**: 1–3.
15. Dawson J. *Rights and responsibilities of doctors.* London: British Medical Association, 1998. ISBN 0 7279 0236 9.
* 16. Woolf L. Medics, lawyers and the courts. *Journal of The Royal College of Physicians.* 1997; **31**: 686–93.
17. Melzack R. *Pain measurement and assessment.* New York: Raven Press, 1983. ISBN 0-89004-893-2.
18. Richter P, Werner J, Heerlein A *et al.* On the validity of the Beck Depression Inventory, a review. *Psychopathology.* 1998; **31**: 160–8.
19. Stratford PW, Binkley J, Solomon P *et al.* Defining the minimum level of detectable change for the Roland–Morris questionnaire. *Physical Therapy.* 1996; **76**: 359–65.
20. Ruta DA, Hurst NP, Kind P *et al.* Measuring health status in British patients with rheumatoid arthritis: reliability, validity and responsiveness of the short form 36-item health survey (SF-36). *British Journal of Rheumatology.* 1998; **37**: 425–36.
* 21. Waddell G, McCulloch JA, Kummel E, Venner RM. Non-organic physical signs in low back pain. *Spine.* 1980; **5**: 117–25.

Index

This index covers the chapters in this volume only. A combined index covering all four volumes in the *Clinical Pain Management* series is available as a pdf on the accompanying website: www.clinicalpainmanagement.co.uk

An *F* following a page reference indicates that the reference is to a figure; a *T* indicates that the reference is to a table.

Notes

To save space in the index, the following abbreviations have been used:

APS – Acute Pain Service(s)
NHS – National Health Service
PCA – patient-controlled analgesia
SCS – spinal cord stimulation
TENS – transcutaneous electrical nerve stimulation